CALCIUM ANTAGONISTS
Pharmacology and Clinical Research

ANNALS OF THE NEW YORK ACADEMY OF SCIENCES
Volume 522

CALCIUM ANTAGONISTS
Pharmacology and Clinical Research

Edited by P. M. Vanhoutte, R. Paoletti, and S. Govoni

The New York Academy of Sciences
New York, New York
1988

Library of Congress Cataloging in Publication Data

Calcium antagonists.

(Annals of the New York Academy of Sciences, ISSN 0077-8923; v. 522)
Proceedings of a conference held Feb. 10–13, 1987 in New York, N.Y., sponsored by Fondazione Giovanni Lorenzini and the New York Academy of Sciences.
Includes bibliographies and index.
1. Calcium—Antagonists—Congresses. 2. Calcium—Antagonists—Therapeutic use—Congresses. I. Vanhoutte, Paul M. II. Paoletti, Rodolfo. III. Govoni, Stefano, 1950– . IV. Fondazione Giovanni Lorenzini. V. New York Academy of Sciences. VI. Series. [DNLM: 1. Calcium—metabolism—congresses. 2. Calcium Channel Blockers—pharmacology—congresses. 3. Calcium Channel Blockers—therapeutic use—congresses. 4. Cardiovascular Diseases—drug therapy—congresses. 5. Central Nervous System Diseases—drug therapy—congresses. 6. Ion Channels—physiology—congresses.
W1 AN626YL v. 522/QV 150 C1437 1987]
Q11.N5 vol. 522 [RM666.C243] 500 s 88-5280
ISBN 0-89766-419-1 [615′.2393]
ISBN 0-89766-420-5 (pbk.)

SP
Printed in the United States of America
ISBN 0-89766-419-1 (Cloth)
ISBN 0-89766-420-5 (paper)
ISSN 0077-8923

ANNALS OF THE NEW YORK ACADEMY OF SCIENCES

Volume 522
March 31, 1988

CALCIUM ANTAGONISTS[a]
Pharmacology and Clinical Research

Editors and Conference Organizers
P. M. VANHOUTTE, R. PAOLETTI, and S. GOVONI

International Advisory Committee
S. EBASHI, C. FIESCHI, A. FLECKENSTEIN, T. GODFRAIND, L. H. OPIE,
H. REUTER, A. SCHWARTZ, W. N. SCOTT, and M. SPEDDING

CONTENTS

[a]This volume is the result of a conference entitled Calcium Antagonists: Pharmacology and Clinical Research held from February 10 to February 13, 1987 in New York, N.Y., sponsored by Fondazione Giovanni Lorenzini, Giovanni Lorenzini Medical Foundation, and The New York Academy of Sciences.

Part III. Biochemical Pharmacology

Poster Papers

Part IV. Physiology and Pharmacology

Poster Papers

Part V. Modulatory Influences

Poster Paper

Part VI. Pathophysiology

Poster Papers

Part VII. Cardiovascular Diseases

Poster Papers

Part VIII. Neurological Disease

Poster Papers

Part IX. Other Therapeutic Indications

Poster Papers

Major funding for this conference was provided by:

- BAYER AG (Leverkusen, FRG)
- JANSSEN PHARMACEUTICA (Beerse, Belgium and Rome, Italy)
- MARION LABORATORIES, INC. (Kansas City, USA)
- TANABE SEIYAKU CO., LTD. (Osaka, Japan)
- U.S. ARMY MEDICAL RESEARCH AND DEVELOPMENT COMMAND (Fort Detrick, USA)

Financial assistance was received from:

- AMERICAN CRITICAL CARE (McGraw Park, USA)
- AMERICAN CYANAMID (Pearl River, USA)
- BRISTOL MYERS (Wallingford, USA)
- E.I. DU PONT DE NEMOURS & CO. (Wilmington, USA)
- ELI LILLY & CO. (Indianapolis, USA)
- ITALIAN MINISTRY OF FOREIGN AFFAIRS
- KNOLL AG (Ludwigshafen, FRG)
- MCNEIL PHARMACEUTICAL (Spring House, USA)
- MERCK SHARP & DOHME (Rahway, USA)
- MERREL DOW (Cincinnati, USA and Strasbourg, France)
- PFIZER CENTRAL RESEARCH (Groton, USA)
- SCHERING CORPORATION (Bloomfield, USA)
- SEARLE LABORATORIES (Skokie, USA)
- SMITH KLINE & FRENCH (Philadelphia, USA)
- THE SQUIBB INSTITUTE FOR MEDICAL RESEARCH (Princeton, USA)
- SYNTEX LABORATORIES (Palo Alto, USA)
- THE UPJOHN COMPANY (Kalamazoo, USA)

Preface

P. M. VANHOUTTE,[a] R. PAOLETTI,[b] AND S. GOVONI[b]

[a]*Department of Physiology*
and Biophysics
Mayo Clinic and Mayo Foundation
Rochester, Minnesota 55905

[b]*Institute of Pharmacological Sciences*
University of Milan
Via Andrea del Sarto 21
I-20129 Milan, Italy

The new pharmacodynamic principle of calcium antagonism was first proposed in the sixties by A. Fleckenstein of the University of Friburg and T. Godfraind of the University of Louvain and originally applied to drugs active in the cardiovascular field. Since then, the number of active molecules has increased tremendously, forcing the reappraisal of the concept of calcium antagonism in the different tissues and of the class of drugs based on this concept.

This is the goal of this volume containing the proceedings of an international symposium on Calcium Antagonists: Pharmacology and Clinical Research, which has provided a forum in which most of the leading workers in the field have discussed the research progress on calcium and calcium channel pharmacology as well as the clinical applications of the old and the newest calcium antagonists.

We hope that as a whole these proceedings will be greater than the sum of the parts (as the meeting was); this volume is both of theoretical and practical application, it is essentially interdisciplinary and based on the most recent development of research into calcium homeostasis control. Basic research has exploited the use of these drugs and new specific toxins to define the existence of various types of calcium channels.

Both from the experimental and the clinical point of view, great attention has been paid to the possibility that calcium antagonists may exert a significant action on central nervous system functioning. The clinical reports on their use in neurology (e.g., epilepsia) are in support of this concept.

In addition this volume considers the utilization of calcium antagonists to obtain protection of the tissue from insults of various types, mostly of ischemic origin. The events triggered by exaggerated calcium influx and release are undoubtedly devastating and contribute to cell death. Along this line, new avenues to pursue the control of excessive calcium ion influx, to facilitate intracellular calcium buffering, or to counteract calcium-evoked reactions have been debated during the meeting.

Important new uses or effects of calcium antagonists in the cardiovascular field as well as in other areas of interest (renal, gynecological, endocrinological, etc.) have also been discussed.

The work pointing to the emerging application in long-term diseases, in particular atherosclerosis, is of great prospective interest. Experimental results indicate that verapamil and verapamil analogues enhance low density lipoprotein uptake through an increase of low density lipoprotein receptors. These data suggest that calcium antagonists may have so far unexplored actions at the gene level, affecting mRNA and protein synthesis, and open, from a general point of view, new avenues of research on drugs affecting calcium homeostasis.

Finally, we would like to acknowledge the advice and the aid provided by the staff of the New York Academy of Sciences and by the Fondazione Giovanni Lorenzini (Houston and Milan). We are also grateful for the financial support of the sponsors that have made this conference possible.

Historical Overview

The Calcium Channel of the Heart

ALBRECHT FLECKENSTEIN

Study Group for Calcium Antagonism
Physiological Institute
University of Freiburg
Hermann-Herder-Strasse 7
D 7800 Freiburg, Federal Republic of Germany

One of the most surprising developments in present cardiovascular pharmacology consists of the Ca^{++} antagonist boom that is actually sweeping the European countries, Japan, and particularly the United States. National and international meetings on this topic have become abundant, and naturally the question arises as to where the concept of Ca^{++} antagonism and the compounds that embody this principle in a specific form came from.

BLOCKADE OF CALCIUM-DEPENDENT MYOCARDIAL EXCITATION-CONTRACTION COUPLING WITH VERAPAMIL AND PRENYLAMINE

The story about the origin of specific Ca^{++} antagonism I have to tell began 24 years ago, i.e., in November 1963, when I was asked by two German pharmaceutical companies (Knoll and Hoechst) to have a look at two newly synthesized coronary vasodilators with unexplained cardiodepressant side effects. One of these compounds was prenylamine. The other, more powerful compound had not yet a name, but was later called Isoptin, iproveratril, or the generic name verapamil. And to our surprise, it rapidly turned out that both compounds, in particular verapamil, mimicked the cardiac effects of simple Ca^{++} withdrawal (FIGURE 1). We had studied in our laboratory the influence of Ca^{++} deprivation in previous physiological investigations over a couple of years,[1] so we could realize the striking similarity between the actions of verapamil and those of Ca^{++} withdrawal without long experimentation. As I reported in 1964, both substances, like Ca^{++} deficiency, inhibited cardiac excitation-contraction coupling in that they diminished contractile force without a major change of the single fiber action potentials.[2,3] Extra calcium restored contractility.

FIGURE 2 shows original experiments with verapamil on three isolated guinea pig papillary muscles, observations that we published in 1967. As shown from top to bottom, contractility was selectively suppressed by verapamil but recovered upon addition of epinephrine or norepinephrine or after a fourfold increase in extracellular Ca^{++} concentration.[3] Cardiac glycosides acted similarly. In FIGURE 3, published one year later, the contractile responses disappeared completely with 1×10^{-5} M verapamil, whereas, again, the single fiber action potentials persisted.[4] On the bottom, systolic force returned to normal with the help of the β-adrenergic stimulant isoproterenol. As is generally known, adrenergic β-receptor stimulation—like administration of extra calcium or cardiac glycosides—is able to improve Ca^{++} supply to the contractile system so that contractility recovers promptly, even in the presence of the Ca^{++}-antagonistic inhibitors. As shown in FIGURE 4, verapamil only suppressed

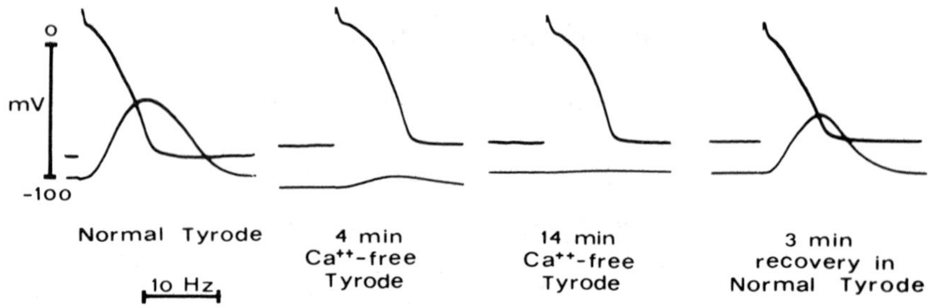

FIGURE 1. Selective loss of contractility of an isolated rabbit papillary muscle in a Ca^{++}-free Tyrode solution at 37°C. Rapid recovery in ordinary Tyrode solution containing 2 mM Ca^{++}. Rate of stimulation: 3 shocks/minute. Potentials were measured with intracellular microelectrodes of conventional type. Isometric tensions were recorded with transducer valves (RCA 5734). The solutions were vigorously gassed with 95% O_2 and 5% CO_2.[1]

Ca^{++}-dependent isometric tension, but did not reduce the Na^+-dependent maximal upstroke velocity of the action potentials.[5]

CALCIUM-DEPENDENT UTILIZATION OF HIGH-ENERGY PHOSPHATES IN ACTIVE MYOCARDIUM; MODULATION BY CALCIUM ANTAGONISTS AND CALCIUM PROMOTERS

The selective decline of contractility always occurred on a clear biochemical background since we could demonstrate in extensive parallel studies on several hundred guinea pig ventricles and rabbit atria that Ca^{++}-deprived myocardial fibers as well as those treated with verapamil or related compounds eventually lose their ability to utilize the high-energy phosphate stores for contraction. Our conclusion was that the Ca^{++}-dependent myofibrillar ATPase by which phosphate-bond energy is transformed into mechanical work no longer operated if the Ca^{++} supply had become defective. As in a motor car, the engine stops not only if the gasoline tank is empty, but also if gasoline utilization fails, due to a defect in internal combustion. And this is exactly what happens to the ATP utilization in a Ca^{++}-deficient myocardial fiber.[1–7]

In consequence, myocardial contractile failure of this type was always accompanied by abnormally high ATP and (particularly) creatine phosphate contents (FIGURE 5). Accordingly, the ratio of creatine phosphate to inorganic phosphate rose considerably above normal (that is to say up to a value of about 4) when tension development decreased upon treatment with Ca^{++} antagonists or Ca^{++} withdrawal.[3–7] Moreover, as could be expected, there was a drop in oxygen demand per heartbeat because contractile force and activity-related oxygen uptake diminished in parallel (FIGURE 6). As to the therapeutic issue, this action of Ca^{++} antagonists opened a new way of downward regulation of mechanical energy output and oxygen requirement of heart muscle, for instance in hyperkinetic disorders.

But again, all these inhibitory effects of verapamil, prenylamine, and related compounds on high-energy phosphate utilization and contractile force could be overcome in isolated myocardium and hearts *in situ* with the help of additional Ca^{++}, β-adrenergic catecholamines, or cardiac glycosides. Or more precisely, under the influence of measures that are able to restore the Ca^{++} supply to the contractile system, high-energy phosphate utilization recovered and the ratio creatine phosphate over inorganic phosphate fell to the normal range (this is a value of 1 or 2). Simultaneously, oxygen requirement per systole went up to its original level.

All these observations justified the conclusion that the principal action of verapamil and prenylamine consisted of an interference with the mediator function of Ca^{++} in excitation-contraction coupling of heart muscle. Therefore, to characterize this mechanism of action, we coined the term "calcium antagonist" in 1966 (see

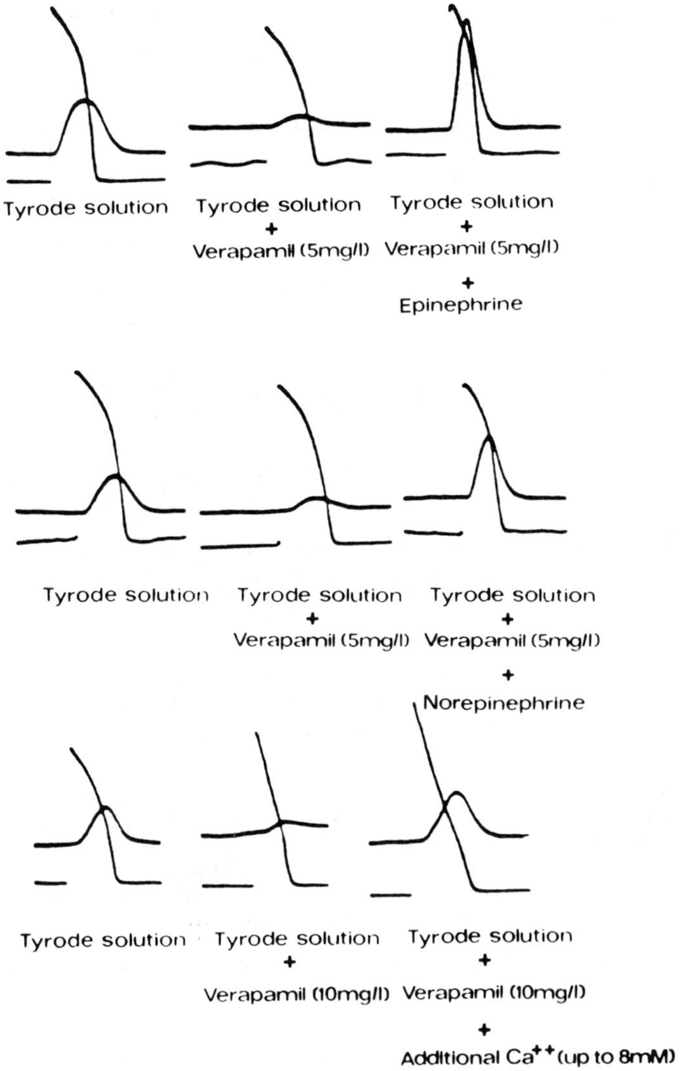

FIGURE 2. Strong inhibition by verapamil of Ca^{++}-dependent excitation-contraction coupling in three isolated guinea pig papillary muscles.[3] Overshooting restitution of contractile force with epinephrine, nonrepinephrine, or extra calcium. Methods as in FIGURE 1.

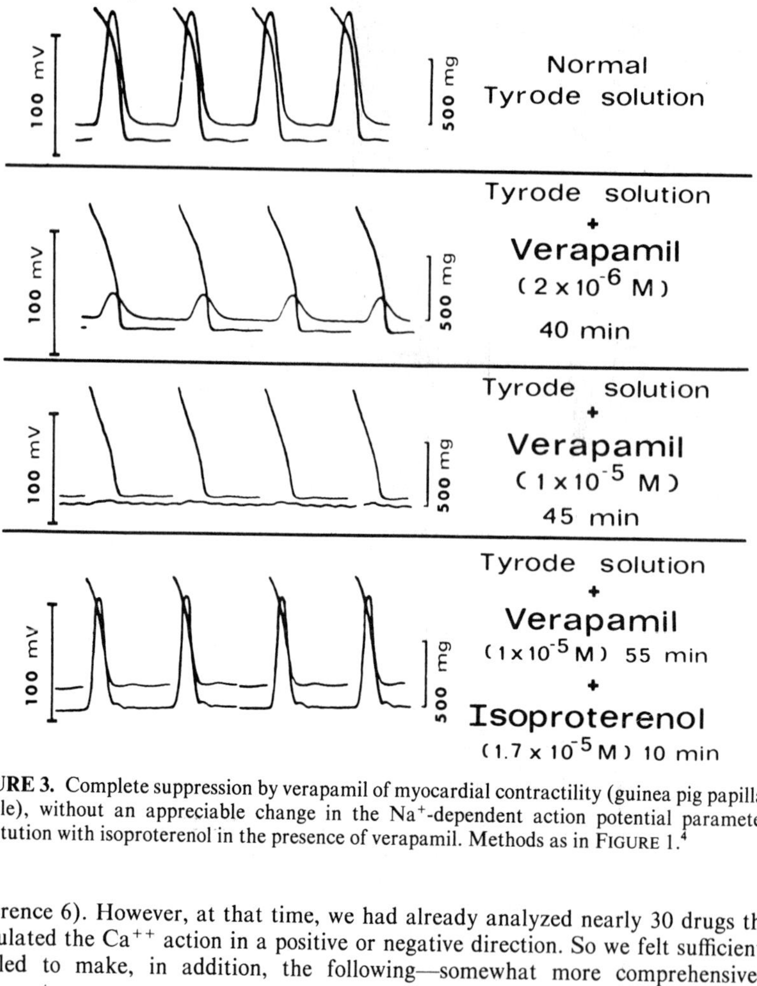

FIGURE 3. Complete suppression by verapamil of myocardial contractility (guinea pig papillary muscle), without an appreciable change in the Na^+-dependent action potential parameters. Restitution with isoproterenol in the presence of verapamil. Methods as in FIGURE 1.[4]

Reference 6). However, at that time, we had already analyzed nearly 30 drugs that modulated the Ca^{++} action in a positive or negative direction. So we felt sufficiently entitled to make, in addition, the following—somewhat more comprehensive—statement:

> The key role of Ca in activity metabolism becomes even more evident by virtue of the fact that many substances with a positive or a negative inotropic effect on heart muscle exert this influence by enhancing Ca action on utilization of high-energy phosphates or by interfering with it. As to the inhibitors of utilization, they seem either to block the movements of Ca from the excited fibre membrane to the myofibrils or to compete with Ca for the active sites in the contractile system where ATP is split.
>
> Our experiments show that there are many inhibitors and promoters of the Ca action in excitation-contraction coupling. By this basic mechanism, they can intensify or restrict the utilization of high-energy phosphates in the contractile machinery or even block it.[6]

DISCOVERY OF FURTHER OUTSTANDING CALCIUM ANTAGONISTS (GALLOPAMIL =D 600, NIFEDIPINE AND ITS DERIVATIVES)

The following years brought a further growth of the Ca^{++} antagonist family. Thus in 1968, Dr. Ferdinand Dengel (the chief chemist of the Knoll company) handed me a methoxy derivative of verapamil and asked me to test this substance also. By the way, he told me that this agent was the 600th compound he had synthesized in his carrier. Therefore, it was decided to give this drug the name D 600. The substance turned out to be much stronger than verapamil on both myocardium and smooth muscle. Myocardial contractility of guinea pig papillary muscle was totally abolished by a 1×10^{-6} M concentration without a major change in Na^+-dependent action potential (see FIGURE 7A). At a low extracellular Ca^{++} concentration the Ca^{++}-antagonistic drug effects were greatly increased, whereas they promptly disappeared in a Ca^{++}-rich medium.

The next important achievement of our laboratory consisted of the identification of the outstanding Ca^{++}-antagonistic drug nifedipine.[5,7–10] We had received this substance under the code name "Bay a 1040" in 1969 from Professor Kroneberg (Bayer/Germany) with the request to clarify the molecular mechanism of its negative-inotropic and coronary vasodilative action. FIGURE 7B shows one of our experiments on an isolated guinea pig papillary muscle with increasing concentrations of nifedipine. With 1 mg nifedipine per liter, Ca^{++}-dependent contractility was totally abolished. In the upper curve, the Na^+-dependent maximal upstroke velocity of the action potentials (dV/dt_{max}) was directly registered. This Na^+-dependent parameter is obviously not affected by nifedipine since the rate of upstroke remained at a steady

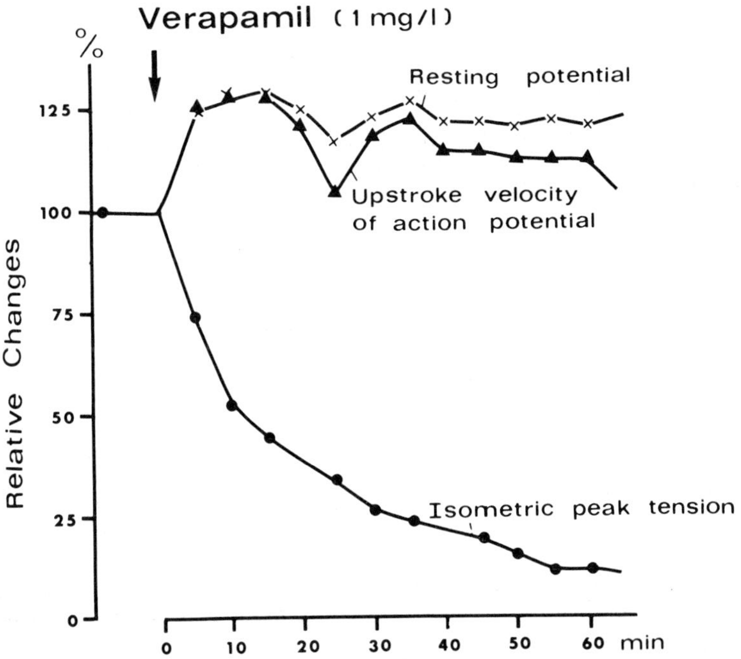

FIGURE 4. Selective reduction of Ca^{++}-dependent contractile force of guinea pig papillary muscle to one-tenth of normal by 1 mg/1 verapamil within 60 minutes. In contrast, velocity of upstroke of action potential (dV/dt_{max}) did not decrease, but followed the small spontaneous fluctuation of resting potential. Continuous microelectrode recordings from the same fiber during 90 minutes. The absolute values (=100%) at the beginning were as follows: resting potential −75 mV; upstroke velocity 130 V/second, isometric tension 700 mg; temperature 36°C; frequency of stimulation 2/second (see Reference 5).

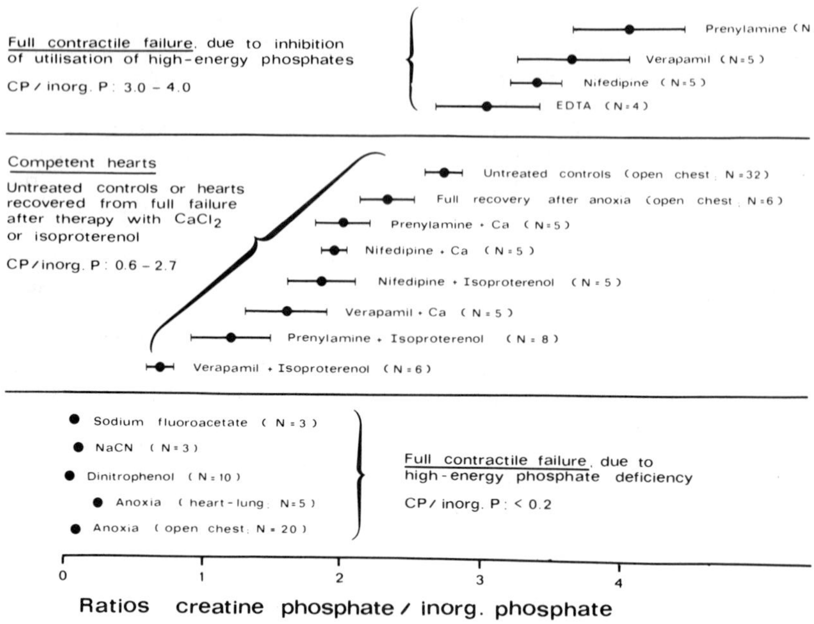

FIGURE 5. Increase of the creatine phosphate/inorganic phosphate ratio (up to a value of 3–4) in the left ventricular myocardium of guinea pig hearts *in situ* (open chest preparations) during contractile failure produced by inhibition of Ca^{++}-dependent high-energy phosphate utilization. Rapid return of this elevated ratio to the normal value of 1 or 2 as soon as high-energy phosphate utilization (and consequently contractility) is restored with the help of intravenous injections of extra calcium or isoproterenol (observations of Fleckenstein *et al.* and Fleckenstein).[3–7]

level of about 150 volts/second. No doubt, the discovery of the top Ca^{++} antagonist nifedipine marked the definite breakthrough of the concept of Ca^{++} antagonism and induced enormous efforts by the pharmaceutical industry to expand the new Ca^{++}-antagonistic drug family by further syntheses. For instance, FIGURE 8 contains a host of Ca^{++}-antagonistic derivatives of the prototypical substance nifedipine. Admittedly, this enumeration is not comprehensive.

SELECTIVE BLOCKADE OF SLOW-CHANNEL-MEDIATED CALCIUM INFLUX BY SPECIFIC CALCIUM ANTAGONISTS

Although it was clear from our studies that the Ca^{++} antagonists restricted the Ca^{++} supply to the contractile system, the exact site of action remained a matter of speculation until 1969. In this decisive year, we could establish with radioactive ^{45}Ca that the Ca^{++} antagonists inhibit the transmembrane uptake of calcium.[11] Moreover, rather simultaneously, the studies of Reuter and Beeler provided new means to measure the transsarcolemmal Na^{+} and Ca^{++} currents in heart muscle independently of each other.[12] With this technique we were enabled to approach the urgent problem of whether Ca^{++} antagonists such as verapamil, D 600, or nifedipine interfere with the slow inward Ca^{++} current specifically. The electrical device used in our experiments corresponded to Stämpfli's classical sucrose gap technique[13] in a modification by Haas, Kern, and Einwächter.[14] The separation of the transmembrane Na^+ and Ca^{++} currents was done according to the conditioning clamping technique described by Reuter and Beeler in 1969.[12] The results of our studies (FIGURE 9) supported not only our own notion, but also Reuter's two-channel concept. As shown together with Dr. Kohlhardt,[15] the slow transmembrane Ca^{++} current was indeed selectively suppressed by verapamil and D 600 (and the same was later shown by us also for nifedipine).[16] On the other hand, there was no influence of these highly specific Ca^{++} antagonists on the fast-channel-mediated transmembrane Na^+ influx that produces the action potential upstroke. With these findings, we delivered in 1970 the experimental basis for the terms "slow channel blocker" or "Ca^{++} entry blocker." Our first communication of the selective blockade of the slow transmembrane Ca^{++} channel by the Ca^{++} antagonist D 600 (at a cardiodepressant concentration of 0.5 mg/liter) was made at a meeting of the European Section of the International Study Group for Research in Cardiac Metabolism on September 6th, 1970, in London.[5]

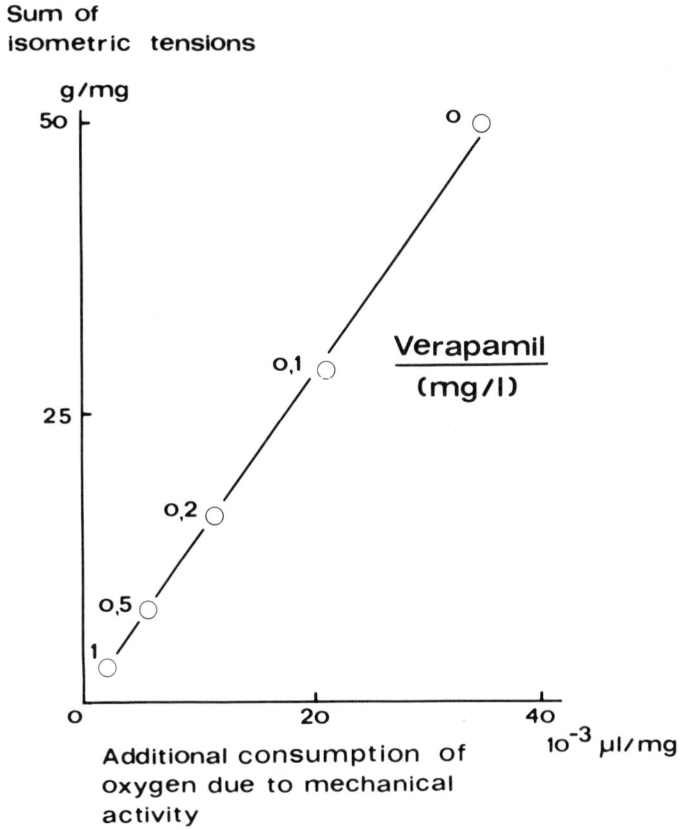

FIGURE 6. Linear reduction of isometric tension and activity-related extra consumption of oxygen (above the resting respiration) by increasing concentrations of verapamil (0.1–1.0 mg/l) [from Byon and Fleckenstein (1969), see References 3, 5, 7, and 10].

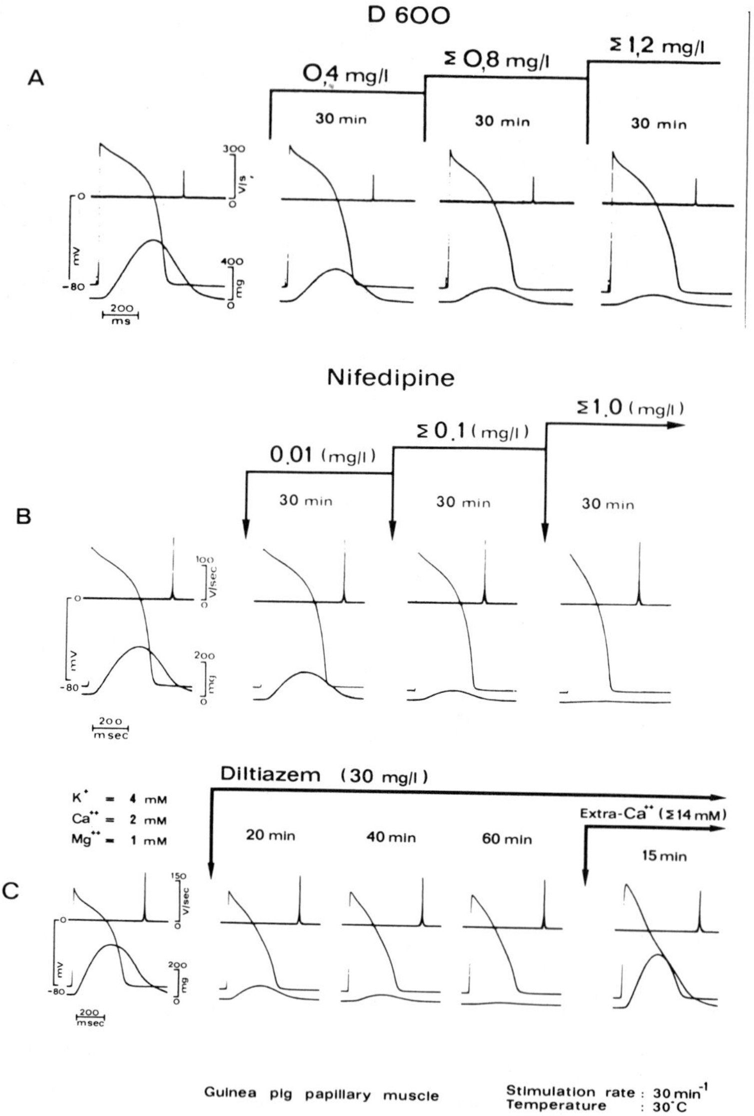

FIGURE 7. Selective suppression of myocardial contractility with D 600 (gallopamil), nifedipine, or diltiazem. No change in the Na^+-dependent action potential parameters such as height of action potential and maximal upstroke velocity (dV/dt_{max}). The latter parameter was directly registered (upper record in each experiment) and remained at an absolutely constant level of about 175 V/second in the Ca^{++}-antagonist-containing environment.[7,9,10]

The allotted time does not allow me to discuss here in detail our further electrophysiological, biochemical, and isotope studies since 1972. They were depicted by Fleckenstein in a monograph[10] and in several review articles by our group.[8,9,17] However, first of all, I must apologize for not dealing with the latest ligand binding studies on Ca^{++} transport proteins by other laboratories. No doubt, this highly qualified Ca^{++} antagonist research and the use of patch clamp techniques have enormously advanced the fundamental knowledge about the interference of Ca^{++} antagonists with transmembrane Ca^{++} influx. However, the experts in these fields will have an opportunity to depict during this conference their own important results.

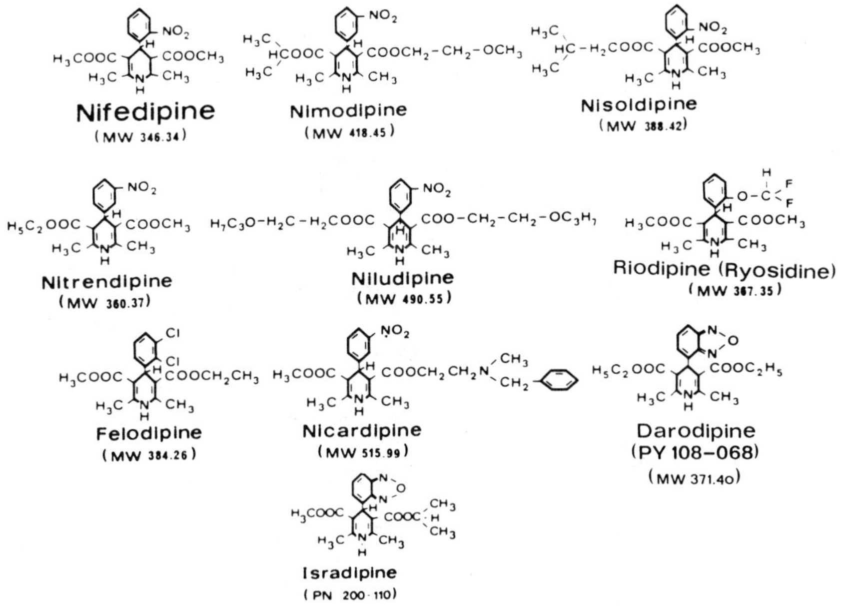

FIGURE 8. 1,4-Dihydropyridine compounds that share their fundamental Ca^{++}-antagonistic properties with the prototypical nifedipine. Nifedipine was identified as a highly potent and selective Ca^{++} antagonist by Fleckenstein in 1969 and 1970 (also see References 5, 7–10, 19, and 20). The code number of nifedipine was Bay a 1040; the trade name is Adalat.

CLASSIFICATION OF CALCIUM ANTAGONISTS BASED ON SPECIFICITY CRITERIA

In concluding this report, I should like to say a word about the problem of classification of Ca^{++} antagonists. In fact, one of the most important aims of our studies was to identify drugs that embodied the new Ca^{++}-antagonistic principle of action in a specific manner.[18] Specificity of a Ca^{++} antagonist means, according to our early definition, that the Ca^{++}-antagonistic action is so predominant that all other pharmacological effects are practically negligible, at least in a reasonable dosage range. Therefore, our main concern was a careful selection of top Ca^{++} antagonists out of a host of about 100 agents that exerted Ca^{++} antagonism less specifically or as a side effect.

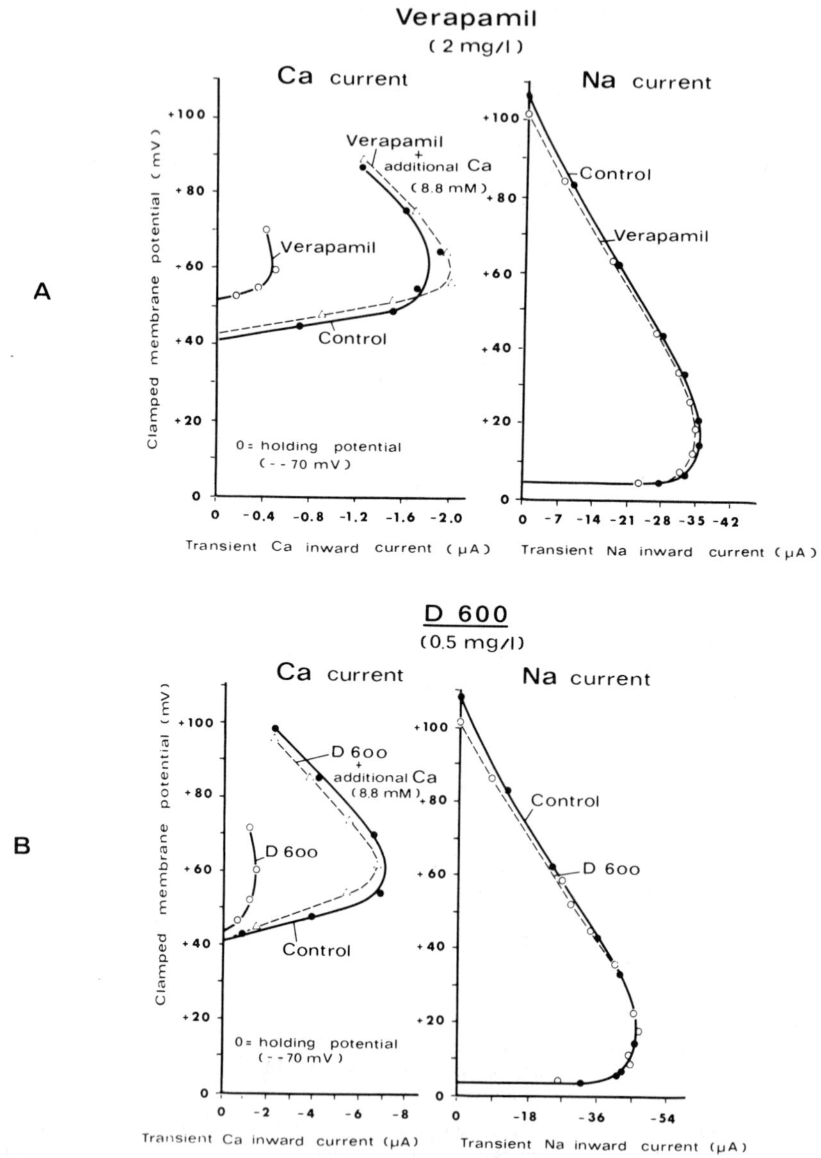

FIGURE 9. Current-voltage-relationship curves of the slow transmembrane Ca^{++} current and the fast Na^{+} current under the influence of verapamil (2 mg/l) or D 600, i.e., gallopamil (0.5 mg/l). With these strong negative-inotropic concentrations, the transmembrane Ca^{++} currents are reduced to very low values. On the other hand, there is no significant change in the fast Na^{+} currents. The voltage-clamp measurements were carried out on trabeculae from right ventricles of cats.[15]

As already emphasized above, the first decisive criterion of a highly specific Ca^{++} antagonist consists of its ability to block slow-channel-mediated transsarcolemmal Ca^{++} entry without a major inhibitory action on the fast inward Na^{+} current. However, a second specificity criterion, which has also proven in our experiments to be particularly useful, is the ability of top Ca^{++} antagonists to suppress, on partially depolarized myocardial fibers, Ca^{++}-dependent action potentials without inhibition of Mg^{++}-induced bioelectric membrane phenomena.[9,10,19,20] We consider it as a further success that, using these two tests, we were able to characterize *diltiazem* as another Ca^{++} antagonist of outstanding specificity (FIGURE 7C). Diltiazem had first been launched by Japanese researchers as a Ca^{++} antagonist.[21] However, its first-class position in the Ca^{++} antagonist family had not been realized in the introductory papers.

Our efforts, over almost a quarter of a century, have established that there are, up to now, only three prototypical Ca^{++} antagonists that fulfill the ultimate expectations of Ca^{++}-antagonistic specificity, namely, verapamil, nifedipine, and diltiazem (see FIGURE 10), with inclusion of derivatives such as gallopamil (D 600) or the nifedipine-

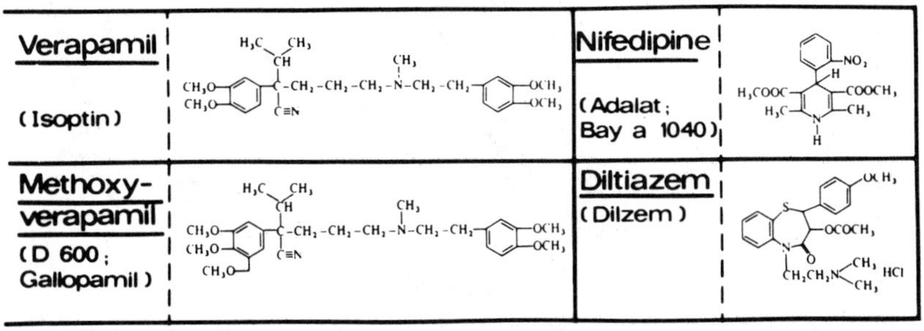

FIGURE 10. Prototypes of highly specific Ca^{++} antagonists of group A. The above-listed drugs cover about 80% of the prescriptions of calcium antagonists for therapeutic purposes. A subdivision of group A into classes I, II, and III for verapamillike, nifedipinelike, and diltiazemlike Ca^{++} antagonists has recently been suggested by a World Health Organization committee.

like 1,4-dihydropyridines listed in FIGURE 8. We have categorized these three sorts of highly specific compounds as Ca^{++} antagonists of group A.

The substances of group A are capable of inhibiting Ca^{++}-dependent excitation-contraction coupling of the mammalian ventricular myocardium by 90–100%, before the fast Na^{+} influx, during the rising phase of action potential, is also affected. Moreover, they do not interfere with electrogenic membrane effects of Mg^{++} ions.[9,10,19,20] Another proof of the outstanding Ca^{++}-antagonistic specificity of verapamil, nifedipine, and diltiazem came from recent ligand binding studies. In fact, only these three prototypical agents (and their close derivatives) can be bound stereospecifically at individual receptor sites of the Ca^{++} transport proteins that act as "slow channels."[22] Following a World Health Organization proposal, one may subdivide the group A Ca^{++} antagonists into the classes I, II, and III for verapamillike, nifedipine-like, and diltiazemlike agents.[23]

Our group B, on the other hand, includes substances like *prenylamine, fendiline, terodiline, caroverine, perhexiline,* etc. These Ca^{++} antagonists are somewhat less potent and specific than the agents of group A. Under their influence, a concomitant inhibition of the Na^+-dependent excitatory process can be seen, when Ca^{++}-dependent contractile tension development of isolated papillary muscles has been reduced by 50–70%.[10] Moreover, the substances of group B are also unable to discriminate clearly between Ca^{++}- and Mg^{++}-induced bioelectric membrane effects. There are some indications that *cinnarizine* (first identified as a Ca^{++} antagonist in 1968/69 by Godfraind and his associates)[24] as well as *flunarizine* also belong to group B, but the poor water solubility of these drugs did not allow us a satisfactory electrophysiological analysis on isolated myocardial tissue. Bepridil, on the other hand, exhibited all characteristic features of a group B Ca^{++} antagonist.

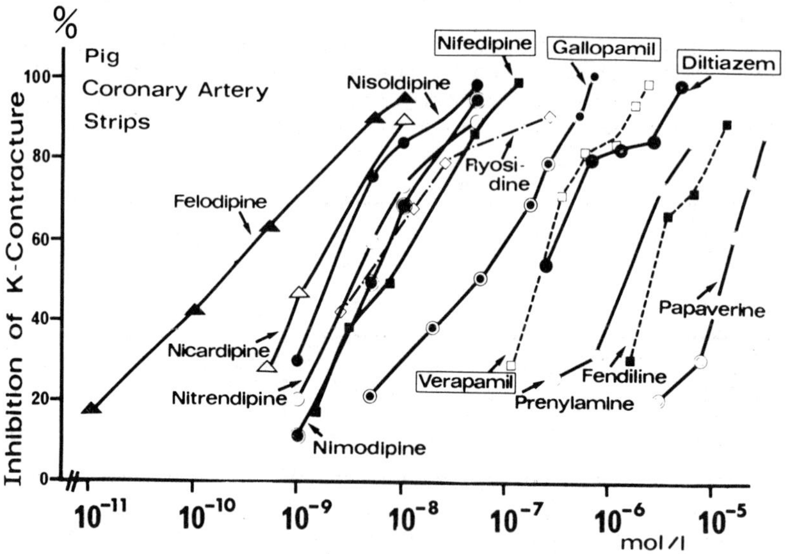

FIGURE 11. Suppression by various Ca^{++} antagonists of tonic contractures of isolated pig coronary artery strips, arising from voltage-dependent transmembrane Ca^{++} influx in a depolarizing K^+-rich (43 mM KCl) Tyrode solution. Nifedipine, ryosidine (riodipine), nitrendipine, and nimodipine were about 3000 times stronger than the reference substance papaverine. Gallopamil (D 600) surpassed papaverine by approximately 300 times, verapamil and diltiazem by about 50 to 100 times. Felodipine, nisoldipine, and nicardipine turned out to be the most potent coronary vasodilators; they produced a 50% relaxation of spasms of the vasculature of the great extramural coronary stem arteries still in a concentration range of 10^{-10} to 10^{-9} M. Needless to say, for therapeutic purposes, such differences in strength can be compensated by adaptation of dose (observations of Fleckenstein-Grün *et al.*).[26]

It is to be stressed in this context that arterial smooth muscle cells which are not provided with a special Na^+ transport system [in the form of tetrodotoxin (TTX) sensitive fast Na^+ channels] were a priori *inadequate* for such specificity tests, because they did not allow the assessment of Ca^{++}-antagonistic drug effects separately from Na^+-antagonistic potencies. Similarly, arterial smooth muscle is blind with respect to differentiation by Ca^{++} antagonists of Ca^{++}-dependent from Mg^{++}-induced bioelectric membrane responses. Nevertheless, it was an astonishing fact that the same prototypical inhibitors of slow-channel-mediated Ca^{++} influx that we had identified primarily on the myocardium also exerted equal or even stronger Ca^{++}-antagonistic effects against phasic and particularly tonic vascular smooth muscle activity[8–10,17,24,26] (see FIGURE 11). Interestingly, the sensitivity of arterial and arteriolar vasculature to some derivatives of nifedipine such as nitrendipine, nimodipine, felodipine, nicardipine, darodipine, or isradipine may be a hundredfold that of ventricular myocardium. Needless to say here, the Ca^{++} antagonists of group A represent the most important spasmolytic agents for the large extramural coronary trunk arteries, the great nutrient arteries of brain, gut, and kidneys, as well as for the small systemic resistance vessels.

Thus it is not surprising that the Ca^{++} antagonists of group A have become the drugs of choice for patients with spastic Prinzmetal's "variant angina," cerebral artery constriction after subarachnoidal hemorrhage, or peripheral circulatory troubles as in Raynaud's disease. Moreover, verapamil, diltiazem, and nifedipine (including their derivatives) are powerful relaxants of spastically narrowed resistance vessels in systemic circulation. Therefore these drugs play an increasing role, not only in the treatment of acute hypertensive crises, but also in the long-term therapy of essential or renal hypertension (for more details see References 27–29).

Lastly, one should not forget that the Ca^{++} transport systems that operate in spontaneously firing nomotopic or ectopic pacemaker cells also resemble the "slow channels" of ordinary myocardial fibers with respect to their drug sensitivity.[8–10] It is well known that the fundamental process of sinoatrial and atrioventricular node automaticity—as well as atrioventricular conduction—is obligatorily linked with a transmembrane influx of Ca^{++} ions as electric charge carriers. This applies even more to ectopic pacemaker activity arising from altered atrial or ventricular fibers which, in this state, are liable to excessive transmembrane Ca^{++} intrusion. This means that cardiac automaticity is also susceptible to the inhibitory action of Ca^{++} antagonists, particularly if it originates from ectopic centers. Here, due to a drop in membrane potential, the excitatory process turns form its regular Na^{+}-dependent form into the slow-channel-mediated Ca^{++}-dependent type, characteristic of partially depolarized myocardium.[8–10] Hence, Ca^{++} antagonists ("the fourth class" of antidysrhythmic drugs according to the nonmenclature of Vaughan Williams)[30] extinguish such preferentially Ca^{++}-dependent ectopic foci. Ca^{++} antagonists also block Ca^{++}-dependent slow-channel-mediated reentry pathways in altered myocardium, leaving normal Na^{+}-dependent atrial or ventricular excitation and conduction unaffected. According to clinical observations, verapamil is particularly useful for the suppression of reciprocating atrioventricular (AV) tachyarrhythmias. This drug slows down Ca^{++}-dependent impulse conduction through the AV node more effectively than other specific Ca^{++} antagonists do. Hence, verapamil is particularly suited to a dramatic interruption of such atrioventricular reentry loops. This was first demonstrated by Krikler and his group.[31,32]

SUMMARY

The present historical paper concentrates on the roots of the pharmacodynamic concept of Ca^{++} antagonism, and on the various therapeutic consequences of transmembrane Ca^{++} entry inhibition, i.e., normalization of hyperkinetic cardiac disorders, suppression of arterial and arteriolar spasms, relief of systemic arterial hypertension, stopping of cardiac dysrhythmias. Obviously in all these cases, medicine makes use of the different manifestations of one and the same fundamental action, that is to say, dose-dependent restriction of transmembrane inward Ca^{++} movements in active myocardium, vascular smooth muscle, or cardiac pacemaker cells. Interestingly, the origin of the principle of Ca^{++} antagonism and the discovery of drugs that possess Ca^{++}-antagonistic potencies preceded the detection of the "slow Ca^{++} channels" by some years. However, the subsequent identification of the "slow channels" (or analogous Ca^{++} transport systems) as the decisive site of action of specific Ca^{++} antagonists has to be considered a keystone of the actual concept.

The present paper does not treat tissue protection by Ca^{++} antagonists which is provided against intracellular Ca^{++} overload and its histopathological sequelae, as for instance Ca^{++}-induced myofibrillar or mitochondrial disintegration. However, the inclusion of morphological topics, such as preservation of myocardial and vascular integrity by Ca^{++} antagonists, would exceed the limits of this article.

REFERENCES

1. FLECKENSTEIN, A. 1963. Metabolic aspects of the excitation-contraction coupling. *In* The Cellular Functions of Membrane Transport. J. F. Hoffman, Ed.: 71–93. Prentice Hall Inc. Englewood Cliffs, N.J.
2. FLECKENSTEIN, A. 1964. Die Bedeutung der energiereichen Phosphate für Kontraktilität und Tonus des Myocards. Verh. d. Deutsch. Gesell. f. Innere Medizin, 70. Kongress: 81–99.
3. FLECKENSTEIN, A., H. KAMMERMEIER, H. J. DÖRING & H. J. FREUND (with the collaboration of G. GRÜN & A. KIENLE). 1967. Zum Wirkungsmechanismus neuartiger Koronardilatatoren mit gleichzeitig Sauerstoff-einsparenden Myokard-Effekten, Prenylamin und Iproveratril. Ztschr. f. Kreislaufforsch. **56:** 716–744; 839–858.
4. FLECKENSTEIN, A. 1968. Experimental heart failure due to disturbances in high-energy phosphate metabolism. *In* Proceedings of the Fifth European Congress of Cardiology, Athens, Greece, Sept. 1968: 255–269.
5. FLECKENSTEIN, A. 1970/71. Specific inhibitors and promoters of calcium action in the excitation-contraction coupling of heart muscle and their role in the prevention or production of myocardial lesions. *In* Calcium and the Heart. P. Harris & L. Opie, Eds.: 135–188. Academic Press. London & New York.
6. FLECKENSTEIN, A., H. J. DÖRING & H. KAMMERMEIER. 1966/67. Experimental heart failure due to inhibition of utilisation of high-energy phosphates. *In* Proceedings of an International Symposium on the Coronary Circulation and Energetics of the Myocardium, Milano 1966: 220–236. Karger. Basel & New York.
7. FLECKENSTEIN, A., H. TRITTHART, H. J. DÖRING & Y. K. BYON. 1972. Bay a 1040—ein hochaktiver Ca^{++}-antagonistischer Inhibitor der elektro-mechanischen Koppelungsprozesse im Warmblüter-Myokard. Arzneimittel-Forsch. (Drug Res.) **22:** 22–33.
8. FLECKENSTEIN, A. 1977. Specific pharmacology of calcium in myocardium, cardiac pacemakers, and vascular smooth muscle. Annu. Rev. Pharmacol. Toxicol. **17:** 149–166.
9. FLECKENSTEIN, A. 1983. History of calcium antagonists. *In* Calcium Channel-Blocking Drugs: a Novel Intervention for the Treatment of Cardiac Disease. Am. Heart Assoc. Monogr. No. **95:** 3–16.
10. FLECKENSTEIN, A. 1983. Calcium Antagonism in Heart and Smooth Muscle—Experimental Facts and Therapeutic Prospects. John Wiley & Sons, Inc. New York, Chichester, Brisbane, Toronto & Singapore.
11. FLECKENSTEIN, A. 1969/71. Pathophysiologische Kausalfaktoren bei Myocardnekrose und Infarkt. Ztsch. f. Inn. Med. **52:** 133–143.
12. REUTER, H. & G. W. BEELER. 1969. Calcium current and activation of contraction in ventricular myocardial fibres. Science **162:** 399–401.
13. STÄMPFLI, R. 1954. A new method for measuring membrane potential with external electrodes. Experientia (Basel) **10:** 508–509.
14. HAAS, H. G., R. KERN & H. M. EINWÄCHTER. 1970. Electrical activity and metabolism in cardiac tissues. An experimental and theoretical study. J. Membr. Biol. **3:** 180–209.
15. KOHLHARDT, M., B. BAUER, H. KRAUSE & A. FLECKENSTEIN. 1972. Differentiation of the transmembrane Na and Ca channel in mammalian cardiac fibres by the use of specific inhibitors. Pflügers Arch. ges. Physiol. **335:** 309–322.
16. KOHLHARDT, M. & A. FLECKENSTEIN. 1977. Inhibition of the slow inward current by

nifedipine in mammalian ventricular myocardium. Naunyn-Schmiedebergs Arch. Pharmacol. **298:** 267–272.

17. FLECKENSTEIN-GRÜN, G., M. FREY & A. FLECKENSTEIN. 1984. Calcium antagonists: mechanisms and therapeutic uses. Trends Pharmacol. Sci. **5:** 283–286.
18. FLECKENSTEIN, A., H. TRITTHART, B. FLECKENSTEIN, A. HERBST & G. GRÜN. 1969. Eine neue Gruppe kompetitiver Ca^{++}-Antagonisten (Iproveratril, D 600, Prenylamin) mit starken Hemmeffekten auf die elektromechanische Koppelung im Warmblüter-Myokard. 35. Pflügers Arch. ges. Physiol. **307:** R25.
19. FLECKENSTEIN, A. & F. SPÄH. 1982. Excitation-contraction uncoupling in cardiac muscle. *In* Advances in Pharmacology and Therapeutics II. Cardio-Renal and Cell Pharmacology. H. Yoshida, Y. Hagihara & S. Ebashi Eds. **3:** 97–110. Pergamon Press. Oxford & New York.
20. FLECKENSTEIN, A. 1985. Calcium antagonists and calcium agonists: fundamental criteria and classification. *In* Cardiovascular Effects of Dihydropyridine-Type Calcium Antagonists and Agonists. A. Fleckenstein, C. van Breemen, R. Gross & F. Hoffmeister, Eds.: 3–31. Springer. Berlin, Heidelberg, New York & Tokyo.
21. NAKAJIMA, H., M. HOSHIYAMA, K. YAMASHITA & A. KIYOMOTO. 1975. Effect of diltiazem on electrical and mechanical activity of isolated cardiac ventricular muscle of guinea-pig. Jpn. J. Pharmacol. **25:** 383–392.
22. GLOSSMANN, H., D. R. FERRY, A. GOLL, J. STRIESNIG & G. ZERNIG. 1985. Calcium channels and calcium channel drugs: recent biochemical and biophysical findings. Arzneimittel-Forsch. (Drug Res.) **35:** 1917–1935.
23. VANHOUTTE, P. M. & R. PAOLETTI. 1987. The WHO classification of calcium antagonists. Trends Pharmacol. Sci. **8:** 4–5.
24. GODFRAIND, T., A. KABA & P. POLSTER. 1968. Differences in sensitivity of arterial smooth muscles to inhibition of their contractile response to depolarization by potassium. Arch. Int. Pharmacodyn. **172:** 235–239.
25. GRÜN, G. & A. FLECKENSTEIN. 1972. Die elektro-mechanische Entkoppelung der glatten Gefässmuskulatur als Grundprinzip der Coronardilatation durch 4-(2′-Nitrophenyl)-2,6-dimethyl-1,4-dihydropyridin-3,5-dicarbonsäure-dimethylester (Bay a 1040, Nifedipin). Arzneimittel-Forsch. (Drug Res.) **22:** 334–344.
26. FLECKENSTEIN-GRÜN, G., Y. MAKITA, Y. K. BYON & A. FLECKENSTEIN. 1985. Effects of Ca^{++}-agonistic and Ca^{++}-antagonistic 1,4-dihydropyridine compounds on tonic and phasic activation of extramural coronary vasculature. *In* Cardiovascular Effects of Dihydropyridine-Type Calcium Antagonists and Agonists. A. Fleckenstein, C. van Breemen, R. Gross & F. Hoffmeister, Eds.: 290–305, Springer. Berlin, Heidelberg, New York & Tokyo.
27. FLECKENSTEIN, A., M. FREY & G. FLECKENSTEIN-GRÜN. 1986. Antihypertensive and arterial anticalcinotic effects of calcium antagonists. Am. J. Cardiol. **57:** 1D–10D.
28. FLECKENSTEIN, A., M. FREY, J. ZORN & G. FLECKENSTEIN-GRÜN. 1985. Experimental basis of the long-term therapy of arterial hypertension with calcium antagonists. Am. J. Cardiol. **56:** 3H–14H.
29. FLECKENSTEIN, A., G. FLECKENSTEIN-GRÜN, M. FREY & J. ZORN. 1987. Future directions in the use of calcium antagonists. Am. J. Cardiol. **59:** 177B–187B.
30. VAUGHAN WILLIAMS, E. M. 1975. Classification of antiarrhythmic drugs. J. Pharmacol. Ther. **1:** 115–138.
31. KRIKLER, D. 1974. A fresh look at cardiac arrhythmias. Lancet: 851, 913, 974, and 1034.
32. KRIKLER, D. & R. A. J. SPURRELL. 1974. Verapamil in the treatment of paroxysmal supraventricular tachycardia. Postgrad. Med. J. **50:** 447–453.

Calcium Channels in the Heart[a]

Properties and Modulation by Dihydropyridine Enantiomers

H. REUTER, H. PORZIG, S. KOKUBUN, AND B. PROD'HOM

Department of Pharmacology
University of Berne
Friedbühlstrasse 49
3010 Berne, Switzerland

INTRODUCTION

The important role of Ca ions in the regulation of many cellular functions is widely recognized. Ca channels in surface membranes of cells contribute to the regulation of the free cytosolic Ca concentration in various cell types. These channels are integral membrane proteins forming pores through which Ca ions can flow into the cell. The gating of these channels, that is, their opening and closing kinetics, can be investigated by means of the patch clamp technique.[1] Application of this method to cardiac cells has provided evidence for at least two types of Ca channels, T-type and L-type.[2,3] These channel types can be distinguished not only by their respective ion selectivities and by their distinct modes of gating, but also by their different sensitivities to 1,4-dihydropyridines.[2,3] The L-type Ca channel but not the T-type is sensitive to these drugs. Previous studies have shown that the action of dihydropyridines on these channels is strongly voltage dependent.[4–6] Moreover, two enantiomers of the dihydropyridine derivative Sandoz 202-791 (FIGURE 1) have opposite effects on Ca channels in cardiac cells.[7,8] One enantiomer [(+)-(S)-202-791] acts as a Ca channel activator by prolonging the open state of the channel, while the other enantiomer [(−)-(R)-202-791] is a Ca channel blocker, that is, it inhibits channel openings. We have studied the voltage dependencies of these changes in Ca channel gating and compared them with the voltage dependence of radioligand binding of these drugs in tissue-cultured cardiac cells. Our results show that at least two cooperatively interacting binding sites for 1,4-dihydropyridines are present in L-type Ca channels. An extensive account of these results has recently been published.[9]

PROPERTIES OF SINGLE Ca CHANNELS

Ca channels in neuronal and muscle tissues have been extensively analyzed by the patch clamp method over the last few years. With this method a very small area of membrane is electrically isolated from its surrounding.[1] Such a membrane patch may contain one or more functional Ca channels which can open and close if the potential across the membrane is changed. FIGURE 2 shows elementary currents flowing through

[a]Financial support by the Swiss National Science Foundation (grants 3.154-0.81 and 3.059-0.84) is gratefully acknowledged.

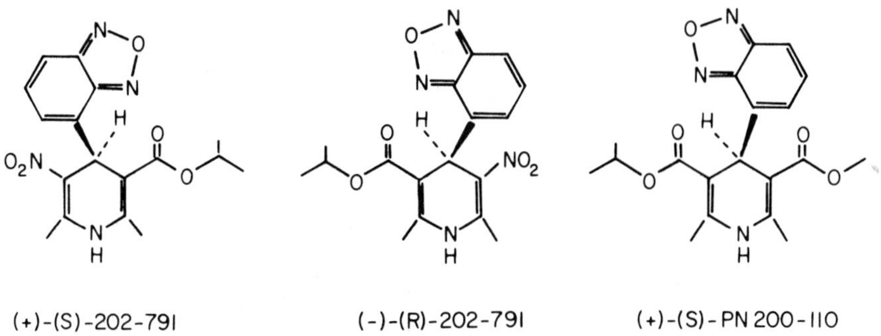

FIGURE 1. Structures of the enantiomers of Sandoz 202-791 and PN 200-110.

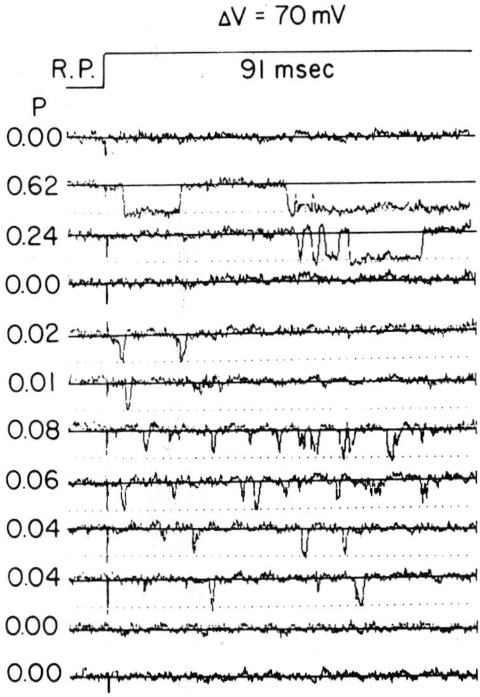

FIGURE 2. Elementary Ca channel currents recorded from a cell-attached membrane patch in a cultured cardiac cell (day 2). The pipette was filled with 96 mM/l $BaCl_2$; thus the current carrier was Ba^{2+}. Depolarizing clamp steps (ΔV) of 70 mV amplitude were applied from a holding potential identical to the resting potential (~ -70 mV). Pulse duration was 91 mseconds. Twelve consecutive single channel current records are shown. The numbers on the left-hand side of each current record indicate the open state probability, *p*, of the channel during that pulse. The heavy lines indicate the closed state of the channel; the dotted lines, the open state current.

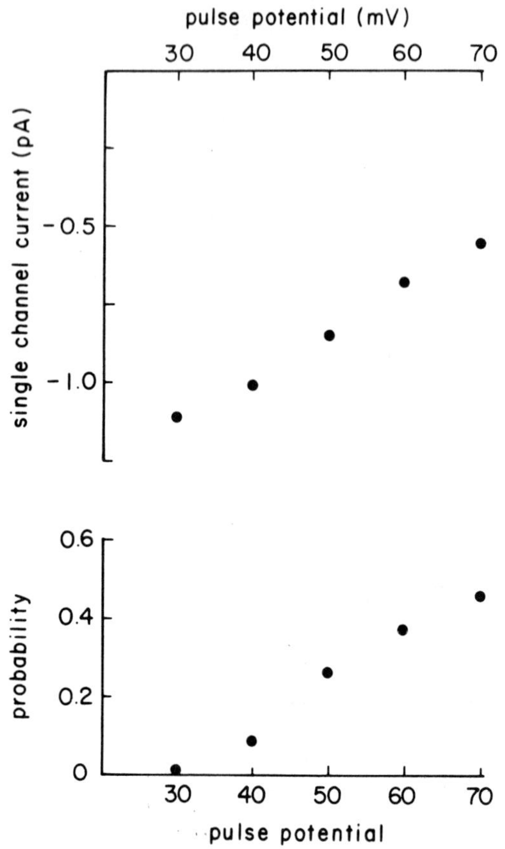

FIGURE 3. Voltage dependencies of open channel current (upper part) and of open state probabilities of the channel (lower part). Each point is the average of at least 100 single-channel current traces at each potential.

a single L-type Ca channel as recorded from a cultured neonatal rat heart cell. The charge carriers were Ba^{2+} ions. Depolarizing step pulses of 70 mV amplitude were applied from a holding potential identical to the resting potential (RP $\sim$ -70 mV). Ca channel openings often occur in bursts separated by longer intervals of closures (mode 1).[6] Quite rarely very long openings can also be observed (mode 2),[6] and sometimes the channel does not open at all during repetitive depolarizations (mode 0).[6] The open state probability, p, of the channel increases with increasing depolarization. With $p = 1$ the channel would be open all the time throughout the voltage step, while with $p = 0$ it would remain closed. The open state probability can be calculated form $I = N \times p \times i$, where I is the time-averaged mean current flowing through an open channel during depolarizing pulses, i is the magnitude of the single channel current which decreases with increasing depolarizing step sizes because the driving force for the inward moving Ba^{2+} ions decreases (FIGURE 3), and N is the number of functioning channels in the small membrane patch ($N = 1$ in FIGURES 2 and 3). Open times of Ca channels are exponentially distributed with time constants, ($\tau_0 \sim 1$ msec) that are only a little voltage dependent (FIGURE 4).[10–13] Closed time histograms of Ca channels can be fitted by double exponential curves (FIGURE 4).[11–13] The short time constant, τ_{C1}, corresponds to the brief closures during the bursts of openings, while the longer time constant, τ_{C2}, describes the distribution of closed time intervals between the bursts. While τ_{C1} does not seem to be voltage dependent, τ_{C2} decreases with increasing depolarization.

THE ACTION OF DIHYDROPYRIDINE ENANTIOMERS ON SINGLE Ca CHANNELS

1,4-Dihydropyridines are highly lipid soluble compounds which seem to have access to individual Ca channels through the lipid phase of the membrane.[14] Some chemically closely related 1,4-dihydropyridines have opposite effects on Ca channels. The main group, which also has therapeutic applications (nifedipine, nitrendipine, nimodipine, nisoldipine), reduces Ca currents (blockers), while another group (CGP 28392, BAY K 8644) increases these currents (activators).[15,16] Most interestingly two enantiomers of the same compound (Sandoz 202-791, FIGURE 1) also have opposite

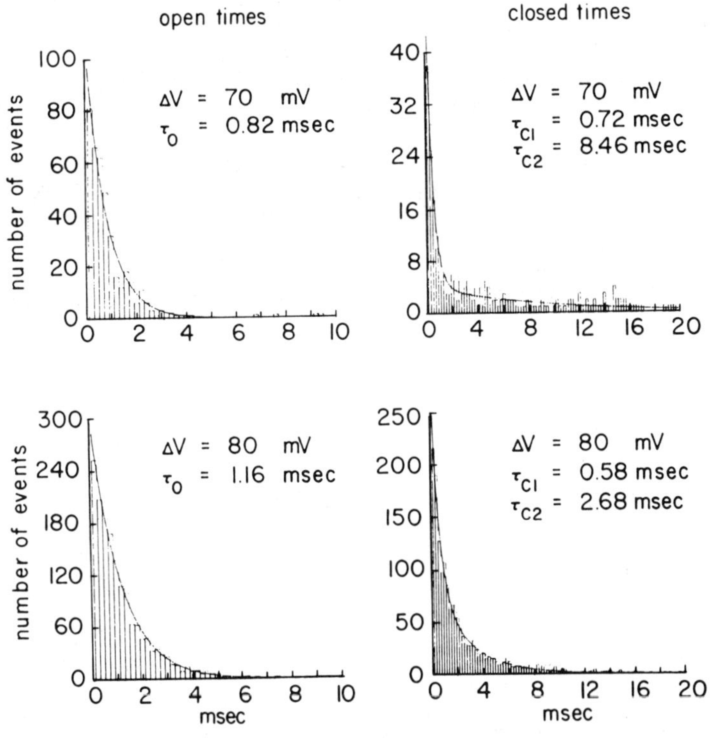

FIGURE 4. Open time histograms (left) and closed-time histograms (right) of Ca^{2+} channel openings and closings at two different membrane potentials (depolarizing clamp steps, ΔV, of 70 and 80 mV, respectively, from a holding potential around −70 mV). Histograms were fitted by nonlinear regression analysis with single exponentials (open times) or the sum of two exponentials (closed times). The respective time constants (τ) of the exponentials are indicated as insets.

effects on Ca channels.[7–9] FIGURE 5 shows current traces obtained with these two enantiomers. The membrane potential of the patch was held at the resting level (FIGURE 5, left-hand side), or 40 mV positive to the resting potential (FIGURE 5, right-hand side). The depolarizing voltage steps eliciting Ca channel activity were 60 mV and 20 mV, respectively. The Ca channel activity was greatly increased shortly after application of (+)-(S)-202-791. The increase in the averaged currents is due to a considerable prolongation of the mean open times of the channels by the drug.[9] The (+)-(S)-enantiomer acts as a Ca channel activator by promoting mode 2 behavior of the channel.[9] When the (−)-(R)-enantiomer was also added, there was a pronounced increase in the rate of decay of Ca channel activity during the pulse[9] and consequently an accelerated rate of inactivation of the averaged current, although the peak inward current was increased (FIGURE 5). The latter effect has been shown to be due to positive cooperative interaction between the enantiomers.[9] The (−)-(R)-enantiomer alone rather acts as a Ca channel blocker mainly by promoting mode 0 of Ca channel activity.[9] This blocking effect was strongly dependent on the membrane potential.[9] When the holding potential was depolarized, the blocking potency of the (−)-(R)-enantiomer was greatly increased.[9] This is shown more systematically in FIGURE 6A, where the relative peak amplitudes of averaged Ca channel currents, *I*, have been plotted as a function of the holding potential. In the absence of the drug, *I* decreases as the holding potential is made more positive. This inactivation is due to a decrease of the overall opening probability of individual Ca channels when the holding potential is depolarized. The Ca channel blocking enantiomer (−)-(R)-202-791 causes a shift of the inactivation curve towards more negative holding potentials. This shift is consistent

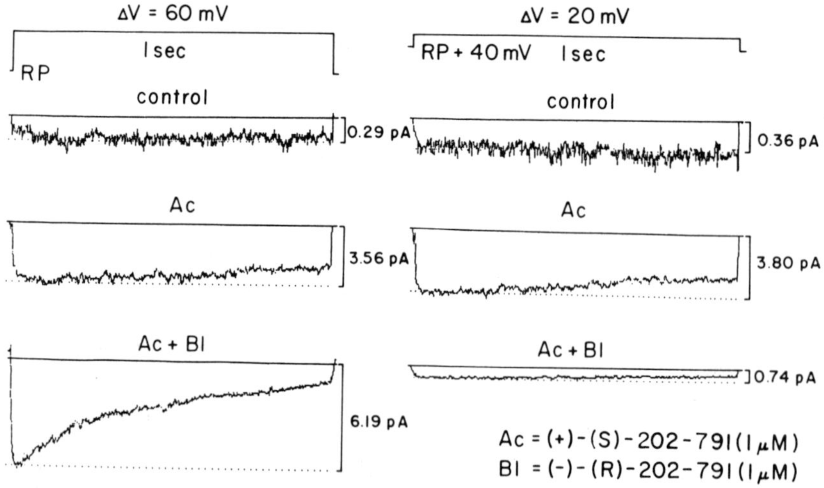

FIGURE 5. Averaged current traces recorded from an adult rat heart cell at two different holding potentials in the absence and presence of (+)-(S)-and (−)-(R)-enantiomers of the drug 202-791. Ba^{2+} ions were the charge carriers. There were at least six Ca channels in the membrane patch. Increased average current in the presence of the activator (Ac) drug is due to marked prolongation of the open times of the channel. Left: holding potential was equal to the resting potential (∼ −70 mV), and voltage clamp pulses of 60 mV amplitude lasted 1 second. Right: holding potential was adjusted 40 mV positive to the resting potential, and pulse potentials of 20 mV amplitude were applied. Note marked dependence on holding potential of averaged currents in the presence of both activating (Ac) and blocking (Bl) enantiomers.

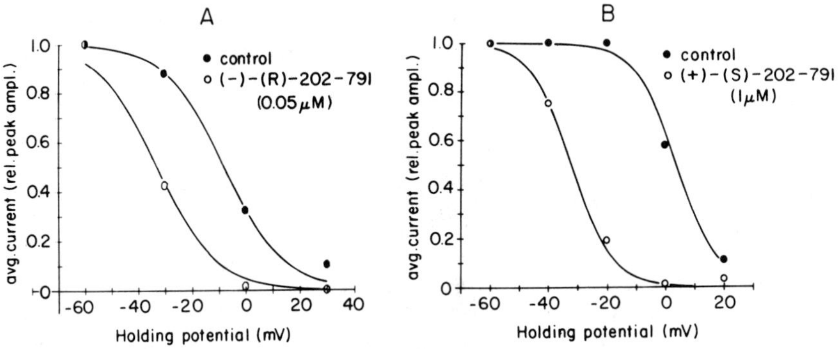

FIGURE 6. Effect of (−)-(R)-202-791 (A, channel blocker) and of (+)-(S)-202-791 (B, channel activator) on the voltage dependence of averaged Ca channel currents. Normalized current scales (ordinates). Pulse potential was always +40 mV from different holding potentials (abscissas). Lines were drawn according to $(1 + \exp[(V_m - V_{0.5})/K])^{-1}$.

with an increase in the binding affinity of the blocking drug and agrees qualitatively with similar results obtained with other dihydropyridine compounds.[4,5] The action of the (+)-(S)-enantiomer (activator) is also voltage dependent. At negative holding potentials, the average current amplitude is greatly increased (FIGURE 5), while with increasing depolarization of the holding potential the average current amplitude decreases. At potentials positive to −20 mV, the Ca current is inhibited, that is, the activating activity of the (+)-(S)-enantiomer turns over into a blocking effect.[9] A plot of the normalized peak currents in the absence and presence of (+)-(S)-202-791 illustrated a shift along the voltage axis by the drug (FIGURE 6B) similar to that obtained with the (−)-(R)-enantiomer (FIGURE 6A).

In conclusion, the electrophysiological evidence with the two enantiomers of the Sandoz compound 202-791 clearly shows an interference with Ca channel gating. The (−)-(R)-enantiomer (blocker) predominantly favors the inactivated (mode 0) state of the channel, thereby reducing the Ca current, while the (+)-(S)-enantiomer (activator) primarily stabilizes the prolonged open (mode 2) state of the channel, which causes enhancement of the current. Both enantiomers seem to have the capability of producing both effects, but one of them prevails. Combination of the enantiomers produces effects consistent with positive cooperative interaction.[9]

RADIOLIGAND BINDING OF DIHYDROPYRIDINE ENANTIOMERS

Electrophysiological studies have provided indirect evidence that the binding affinity of dihydropyridines to inactivated channels is much higher than to channels that are available to open (see above and References 7–9). Therefore, it would be expected that binding affinities of radioactively labeled 1,4-dihydropyridine ligands in intact cardiac cells depend on the membrane potential. This has first been shown to be the case with [^{3}H]-nimodipine.[16] FIGURE 7 shows an experiment where the dihydropyridine enantiomer ^{3}H-(+)-PN-200-110 has been bound to Ca channels in cultured cardiac cells at two different membrane potentials. (+)-PN-200-110 is chemically closely related to 202-791 (FIGURE 1) and acts as a Ca channel blocker. In a Ca-free Hank's solution with 137 mM NaCl and 5.4 mM KCl the K_D value of the drug is approximately 12 times higher than in depolarized cells where all the NaCl in the Hank's solution has been replaced by KCl. The membrane potentials under those conditions were -38 ± 4 mV and about 0 mV, respectively. This shows directly that binding of 1,4-dihydropyridines to Ca channels is voltage dependent and agrees, at least qualitatively, with the corresponding electrophysiological experiments. Quantitative discrepancies may be due to differences in membrane potential under the various experimental conditions, and/or in the voltage dependence of the binding constants of dihydropyridines with different structures.

We have also used ^{3}H-(+)-PN 200-110 as a radiolabel to characterize the binding properties of the two enantiomers of the compound Sandoz 202-791. In cultured cells from rat hearts ^{3}H-(+)-PN 200-110 was applied at concentrations of 0.7 nM in NaCl-containing Hank's solution or 0.06 nM in KCl Hank's solution. This corresponds to the respective K_D values of the radioligand in normal and depolarized cultured cells (see FIGURE 7). When the radioligand was added together with increasing concentrations of the (−)-(R)-enantiomer or (+)-(S)-enantiomer of the compound 202-791, there was competition in binding between the radioligand and the enantiomers in NaCl solution as well as in KCl solution. FIGURE 8 shows such competitive displacement curves under equilibrium conditions. The antagonistic (−)-(R)-enantiomer displaced the radioligand in a one-to-one fashion in both solutions. However, the respective K_D values were very different in these solutions. The calculated K_D value for the (−)-(R)-enantiomer in the NaCl solution was 1.3×10^{-7} M, while in a KCl solution it was 2.7×10^{-9} M indicating a 38-fold increase in the binding affinity of this enantiomer. The cells depolarized by approximately 40 mV in the KCl solution. The agonistic (+)-(S)-enantiomer also showed considerable voltage dependence of its binding. However, in NaCl solution the displacement curve was much steeper (Hill coefficient 2.1) than in KCl solution (Hill coefficient 1.0). This indicates allosteric interaction of binding sites for the activator enantiomer at negative membrane

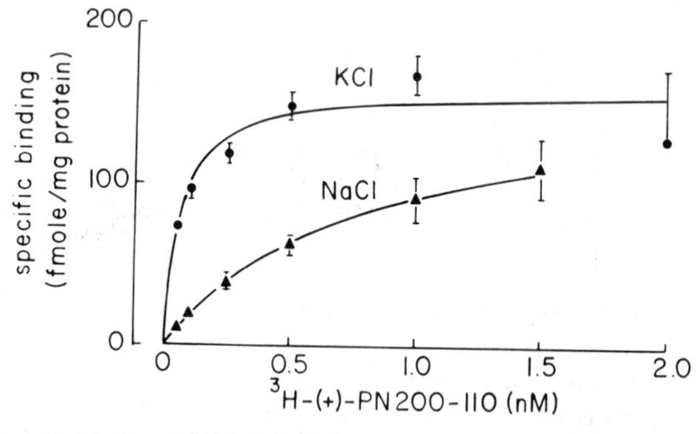

FIGURE 7. Specific binding of ^{3}H-(+)-PN 200-110 in living cardiac cells is voltage dependent. Equilibrium binding of the ligand was measured in tissue cultures of rat myocardial cells attached to glass coverslips. The apparent dissociation constant (K_D) for (+)-PN 200-110 in normal Hank medium (in mM; 137 NaCl, 5.4 KCl, a 0.8 Mg SO_4, 4.2 Na HCO_3, 0.34 Na_2HPO_4, 0.44 KH_2PO_4, 20 HEPES, 5.5 glucose) was 0.73 ± 0.13 nM (triangles); in K-rich medium (137 KCl, 5.4 NaCl, other components as above) the K_D was 0.059 ± 0.005 nM (circles). The maximal binding capacities (B_{max}) were not significantly different under both conditions (158.9 and 158.3 fmol/mg protein, respectively). The K_D values were estimated from computerized nonlinear least-square fits to the experimental data. For the fitting procedure a single homogenous population of binding sites was assumed for both conditions.

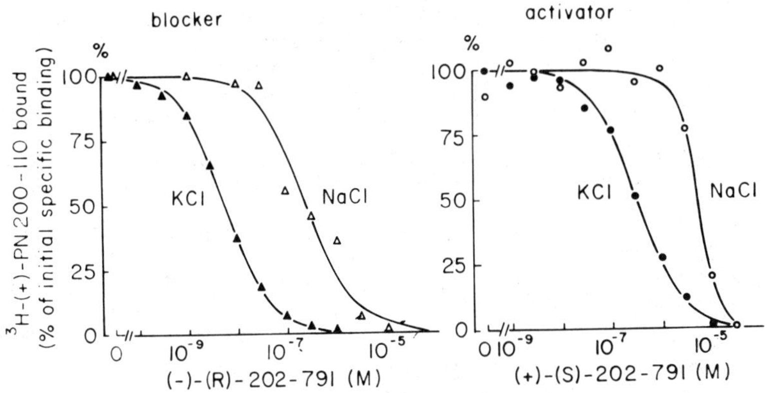

FIGURE 8. Normalized equilibrium displacement curves of the ^{3}H-labeled dihydropyridine enantiomer (+)-PN 200-110 by the enantiomers (−)-(R)-202-791 (blocker; left) and (+)-(S)-202-791 (activator; right). NaCl (open symbols) and KCl (filled symbols) indicate cultured cardiac cells kept in NaCl-containing Hank's medium or KCl-containing medium (for compositions see FIGURE 7). The average membrane potentials were −38 ± 4 mV in NaCl medium and about 0 mV in KCl medium. Depolarization shifts the displacement curves for blocker and activator to the left by factors of 38 and 12, respectively.

potentials. In the depolarized cells the affinity of the (+)-(S)-enantiomer was greater than in cells incubated in NaCl solution and, as with the blocking enantiomer, the radioligand was displaced in a one-to-one fashion (FIGURE 8). This agrees with the electrophysiological experiments which also showed that Ca channel activation by (+)-(S)-202-791 turns over into a blocking effect if the cells are depolarized (see above).[9] At low concentrations (10^{-9}–10^{-7} M) the (+)-(S)-enantiomer increased the binding of ^{3}H-(+)-PN 200-110 in polarized but not in depolarized cells.[9] This could be attributed to an increase in the binding affinity of the radioligand due to a positive cooperative effect. The blocking (−)-(R)-entiomer had no such effect, but behaved like a purely competitive ligand.[9]

The demonstration of voltage-dependent binding of the ligands together with the electrophysiological results provides strong evidence that these drugs are bound at or near the site of the channel that is responsible for its voltage-dependent gating. The binding sites are not independent from each other, but show positive cooperativity when simultaneously occupied by enantiomers with opposite effects.

ACKNOWLEDGMENTS

The authors thank Charlotte Becker for unfailing experimental help with the binding experiments. They also thank Dr. R. Hof, Sandoz AG, Basel, for providing them with the enantiomers of the compound 202-791.

REFERENCES

1. HAMILL, O. P., A. MARTY, E. NEHER, B. SAKMANN & F. J. SIGWORTH. 1981. Pflügers Arch. **391:** 85–100.
2. BEAN, B. P. 1985. J. Gen. Physiol. **86:** 1–30.

3. NILIUS, B., P. HESS, J. B. LANSMAN & R. W. TSIEN. 1985. Nature **316:** 443–446.
4. SANGUINETTI, M. C. & R. S. KASS. 1984. Circ. Res. **55:** 336–348.
5. BEAN, B. P. 1984. Proc. Nat. Acad. Sci. USA **81:** 6388–6392.
6. HESS, P., J. B. LANSMAN & R. W. TSIEN. 1984. Nature **311:** 538–544.
7. HOF, R. P., V. T. RÜEGG, A. HOF & A. VOGEL. 1985. J. Cardiovasc. Pharmacol. **7:** 689–693.
8. WILLIAMS, J. S., I. L. GRUPP, G. GRUPP, P. L. VAGHY, L. DUMONT, A. SCHWARTZ, A. YATANI, S. HAMILTON & A. M. BROWN. 1985. Biochem. Biophys. Res. Commun. **131:** 13–21.
9. KOKUBUN, S., B. PROD'HOM, C. BECKER, H. PORZIG & H. REUTER. 1986. Mol. Pharmacol. **30:** 571–584.
10. REUTER, H., C. F. STEVENS, R. W. TSIEN & G. YELLEN. 1982. Nature **297:** 501–504.
11. FENWICK, E. M., A. MARTY & E. NEHER. 1982. J. Physiol. **331:** 599–635.
12. CACHELIN, A. B., J. E. DE PEYER, S. KOKUBUN & H. REUTER. 1983. Nature **304:** 462–464.
13. HAGIWARA, S. & H. OHMORI. 1983. J. Physiol. **336:** 649–661.
14. KOKUBUN, S. & H. REUTER. 1984. Proc. Nat. Acad. Sci. USA **81:** 4824–4827.
15. JANIS, R. A. & D. J. TRIGGLE. 1984. Drug Dev. Res. **4:** 257–274.
16. REUTER, H., H. PORZIG, S. KOKUBUN & B. PROD'HOM. 1985. Trends Neurosci. **8:** 396–400.

Calcium Channel Modulation by Dihydropyridines in Vascular Smooth Muscle[a]

KENT HERMSMEYER,[b] MICHAEL STUREK,[c] AND NANCY J. RUSCH[d]

Department of Pharmacology
The Cardiovascular Center
University of Iowa
Iowa City, Iowa 52242

INTRODUCTION

Dihydropyridine calcium antagonists such as nitrendipine are effective on calcium channels in many kinds of cells. Tsien and Reuter have provided surveys of calcium channels in a number of cell types.[13,9] One of the consistent findings in various kinds of cells is the occurrence of at least two different functionally important types of calcium channels distinguished by kinetic, voltage, and permeability characteristics, as recently reported in vascular muscle,[2] cardiac muscle,[1] and secretory cells.[7]

Calcium channels in vascular muscles are of particular interest, because both functional (electrophysiological) and biochemical data are consistent with a nanomolar or higher affinity of the vascular muscle calcium channel for nitrendipine.[2,10] Because of the importance of understanding the cellular effect of nitrendipine and related compounds on calcium channels in vascular muscle, we have reviewed experiments characterizing the action of the calcium antagonist nitrendipine and the calcium agonist Bay k8644 on these cells. Our discussion focuses on which type of calcium channels the dihydropyridines act on, and what can be surmised about modulation of calcium channel function from their actions.

CONTRAST OF TWO VASCULAR MUSCLE CALCIUM CHANNEL TYPES

Publications from several laboratories have reported two kinds of calcium channels in vascular muscle cells.[2–4,6a,12,14] Our laboratory has shown that in freshly isolated single cells from mesenteric artery,[2] and in cultured single vascular muscle cells from the azygos vein of neonatal rats,[12] there is both a transient calcium channel ("T" channel) and a sustained or long duration calcium channel ("L" channel). Calcium current through the T channel inactivates rapidly (within tens of milliseconds), while the current through the L channel can be maintained for minutes (FIGURES 3 and 4).

[a]This research was supported by grants HL16328 and HL32295 from the National Institutes of Health.

[b]Present affiliation: Cardiovascular Laboratory, Chiles Research Institute, Providence Medical Center, Portland, Oregon 97213.

[c]Present affiliation: Department of Physiology, University of Missouri School of Medicine, Columbia, Missouri 65212.

[d]Present affiliation: Department of Physiology, Medical College of Wisconsin, Milwaukee, Wisconsin 53226.

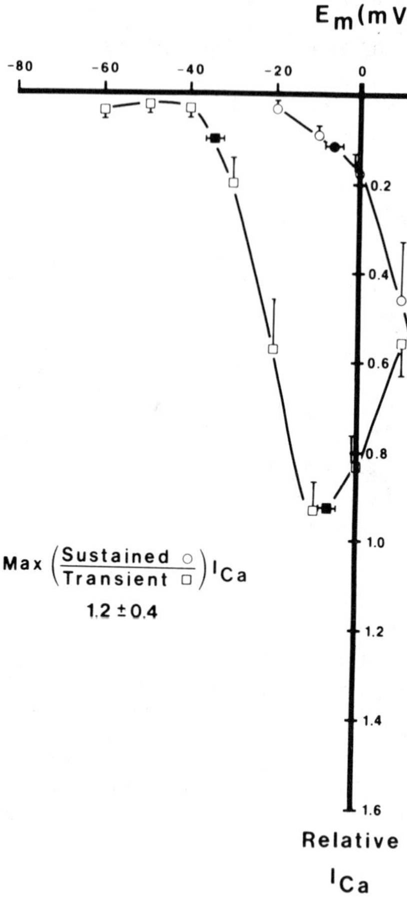

FIGURE 1. Activation current-voltage relationships for transient ("T") calcium current and sustained or long duration ("L") calcium current are shown for neonatal rat azygos venous cells. T current is plotted as squares ($n = 4$ cells) and L current is plotted as circles ($n = 15$ cells). Values plotted are means ± standard error of the mean (SEM) and represent peak calcium currents recorded during depolarization to the pulse potentials shown on the abscissa from the holding potential of −80 mV for the T current and −30 mV for the L current. L currents were 20% greater than T currents in this cell sample. Upper dark symbols show the threshold voltage (10% of maximal current), which was −38 mV for T and −6 mV for L currents. Lower dark symbols show that the voltage for peak current was −4 mV for T and +40 mV for L channels. External solution was composed of (mM): 20 CaCl, 135 TEA Cl, 1 MgCl, 10 HEPES, 10 dextrose, buffered to pH = 7.4 by TEA OH. Pipette solution was composed of (mM): 150 CsGlutamate, 10 EGTA, 1 MgCl, 10 HEPES, buffered to pH = 7.4 by CsOH.

Voltage ranges for activation (FIGURE 1) and inactivation (FIGURE 2) of the T and L currents are separate, allowing isolation and analysis of the two channel types by selection of different holding potentials in voltage clamp experiments. A more complete explanation of the methods and analysis of the two current types is available in earlier papers.[2,12] Similar observations of two kinetically distinct calcium channels in isolated vascular muscle cells have been reported recently by other investigators.[3,4,6a,14]

In addition to the voltage and kinetic differences between these two types of calcium channels, there are also differences in their permeabilities to divalent ion charge carriers. For example, during whole-cell voltage clamp of vascular muscle, replacement of 20 mM calcium with 20 mM barium as the charge carrier in the external solution enhances the L channel peak current by a factor of four, while the peak magnitude of the T channel current is unchanged (FIGURE 3). The difference in current amplitude enhancement by barium suggests the contrasting selectivity characteristics of L and T channels.

Most importantly for the present discussion, the L channel appears to be selectively affected by the dihydropyridines. Concentrations of only a few nanomolar caused significant reductions of L channel currents, and higher concentrations completely blocked them. The basic electrophysiological distinction of two types of calcium channels permits us to determine more clearly the gating behavior of the channels via actions of dihydropyridine drugs.

ACTIONS OF THE DIHYDROPYRIDINES ON L-TYPE CALCIUM CHANNELS

In the first report on the effect of the dihydropyridines on voltage-clamped vascular muscle cells, nitrendipine had no apparent effect on the T channel current in freshly

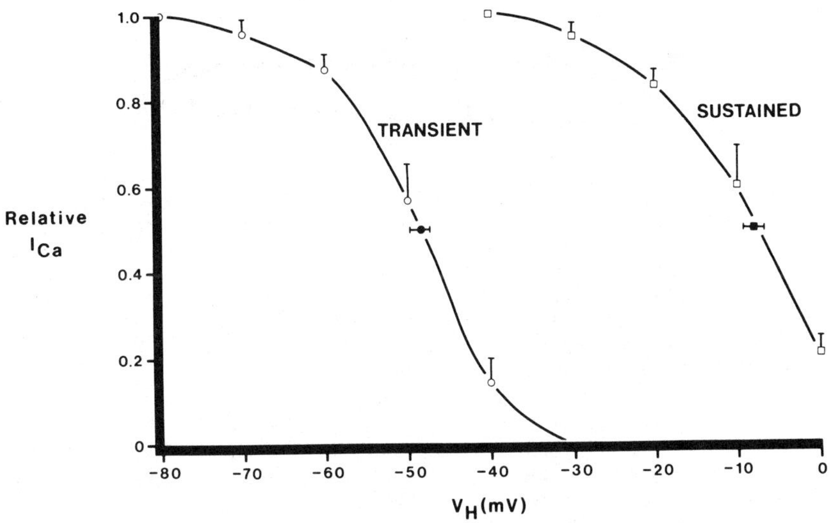

FIGURE 2. Current-voltage relationships show the steady-state inactivation of the T and L channel currents by depolarization. T current is plotted as circles and L current is plotted as squares. Values plotted are means ± SEM of the peak currents during the command potentials for 7 cells. The T current was obtained by depolarizing to a command potential of 0 mV from the holding potentials (V_H) indicated on the abscissa, while the L current was obtained by depolarizing to a command potential of +30 mV from the indicated holding potentials (V_H), which were held for 25 seconds before the command potential. The holding potential at which half-maximal inactivation occurred is shown by the solid symbols, and was −48 mV for T and −8 mV for L currents. Curves were fit by visual approximation, and solution compositions were the same as for FIGURE 1. A more detailed explanation can be found in Reference 12.

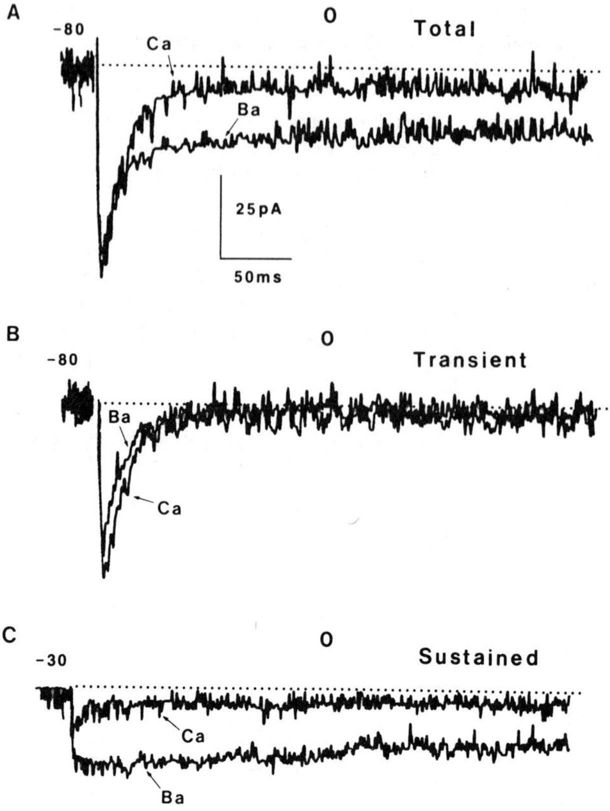

FIGURE 3. When 20 mM calcium (Ca) was replaced with 20 mM barium (Ba) in the external solution, L but not T current was enhanced. (A) Total cell current was elicited by depolarizing from −80 mV to 0 mV and shows the selective L current enhancement. (B) The transient channel current was not significantly changed, as shown more clearly in these difference (A–C) records. (C) The L channel current was clearly potentiated, in this cell fourfold, when 20 mM calcium was replaced with 20 mM barium in the external solution. Although not apparent from these records, barium replacement also prolonged the L currents, suggesting that increases in intracellular calcium contributed to inactivation of the L currents.

dissociated cells from rat mesenteric artery. However, nitrendipine selectively blocked the L channel current in the same cells.[2] Complete block of the L channel current by nitrendipine occurred at 3 micromolar (FIGURE 4).

Nitrendipine-induced block was highly dependent on the holding potential when 100 nM nitrendipine was used (FIGURE 4); the block was much stronger when calcium current was elicited by depolarizing from more positive holding potentials. More generally, plots of the current-voltage relationship in rat mesenteric artery showed that nitrendipine shifted the steady-state inactivation curve to the left, and also decreased the L channel current even at negative holding potentials[2] (FIGURE 4). While the leftward shift implies strong binding to the inactivated state of the channel, the decreased current at negative membrane potentials implies binding of nitrendipine to the resting state of the channel.[1] Using the modulated receptor hypothesis adapted to binding sites on calcium channels, equilibrium dissociation constants for nitrendipine binding to the inactivated state were calculated as below one nanomolar,[2] which concurs with the high affinity binding site reported for radiolabeled nitrendipine in vascular muscle.[10] From the same modulated receptor hypothesis, binding to resting state calcium channels in vascular muscle is 220 nanomolar[2] compared to 600 nanomolar in cardiac muscle, also reported by Bean.[1] Worley *et al.* also showed a potent block of vascular muscle calcium channels at negative holding potentials.[14]

The action of the calcium channel agonist Bay k8644 provides information on the gating of calcium channels in vascular muscle.[2] Our findings on vascular muscle are similar to those reported in cardiac Purkinje fibers,[11] in that Bay k8644 increases the calcium current through the L channel by at least severalfold and causes a hyperpolarizing (leftward) shift of both the activation and inactivation current-voltage curves. This hyperpolarizing shift of the activation curve by Bay k8644 is in marked contrast to nitrendipine, which does not affect the voltage dependency of calcium channel activation, and suggests that there is a second dihydropyridine interaction site on the calcium channel for Bay k8644.

In this characteristic, the L calcium channel in vascular muscle seems to behave similarly to the L calcium channel in cardiac muscle, where cooperative interactions

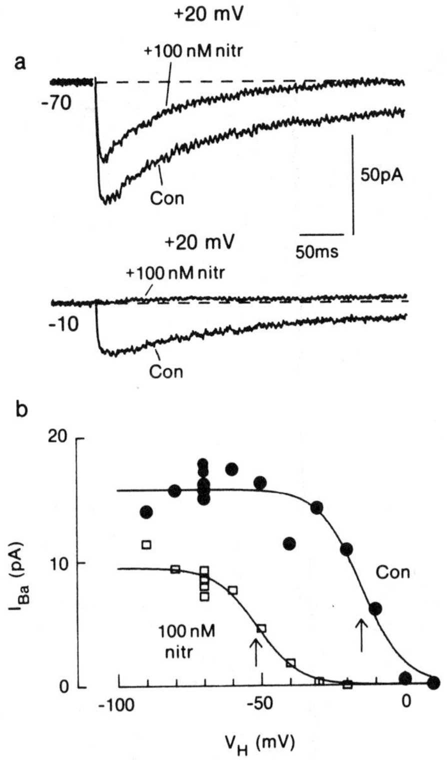

FIGURE 4. Block of L calcium channels was voltage dependent and occurred even in the resting state in adult rat mesenteric arterial muscle cells. (Reproduced from Reference 2 with permission of the American Heart Association.)

among multiple dihydropyridine binding sites have been reported recently.[6] However, we found a greater than 10-fold enhancement of current in mesenteric artery cells while investigators usually find less than a 5-fold increase in cardiac myocytes.[5] We also found, as shown in FIGURE 5, that Bay k8644 enhances the L-type calcium current in the azygos vein by nearly 10-fold without changing the transient current. The important drug interactions noted and the voltage shifts seen support the concept that interactions between membrane potential and multiple drug binding sites provide many possibilities for modulating current through L-type calcium channels in vascular muscle cells.

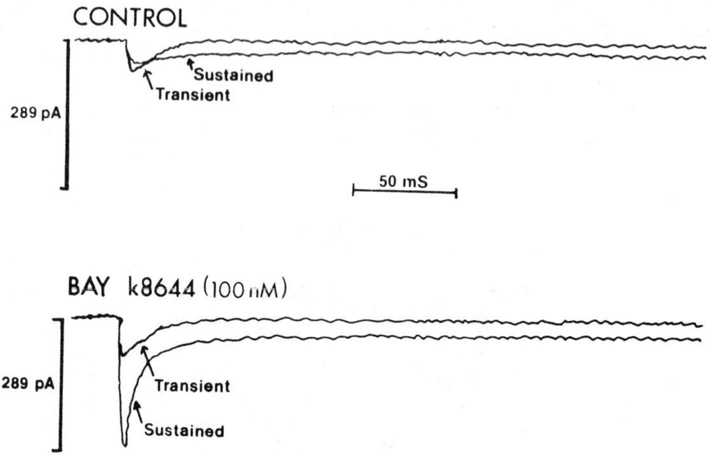

FIGURE 5. The calcium agonist Bay k8644 at 100 mM markedly increased L calcium channel currents in neonatal rat azygos vein vascular muscle. Solutions were as in FIGURE 1. Transient current was separated from sustained current by different holding potentials (T current is completely inactivated by a holding potential of −30 mV) and command potentials, as more completely explained in Reference 12.

CONCLUSION

The data reviewed in this paper show the powerful modulation by agonist and antagonist dihydropyridines of L-type calcium channels in vascular muscle. These calcium channels, which are thought to be important for the regulation of vascular muscle contraction, appear to be more potently modulated by dihydropyridines than by other drugs. Furthermore, results from our lab[2] and others[14] suggest that dihydropyridine calcium antagonists also bind to the resting state of the vascular muscle calcium channel with higher affinity than is found in cardiac muscle.[1,5] These results suggest the existence of fundamental differences among vascular, cardiac, and neuronal calcium channels, as also recently suggested by Ohya *et al.*[8] The potency of both antagonist and agonist dihydropyridines and the multiplicity of interactions provide important tools for future investigations of the physiological and pharmacological properties of voltage-dependent calcium channels in vascular muscle.

REFERENCES

1. Bean, B. P. 1984. Nitrendipine block of cardiac calcium channels: high affinity binding to the inactivated state. Proc. Nat. Acad. Sci. USA **81:** 6388–6392.
2. Bean, B. P., M. Sturek, A. Puga & K. Hermsmeyer. 1986. Calcium channels in muscle cells isolated from rat mesenteric arteries: modulation by dihydropyridine drugs. Circ. Res. **59:** 229–235.
3. Bolton, T. B., R. J. Lang, T. Takewaki & C. D. Benham. 1985. Patch and whole-cell voltage clamp of single mammalian visceral and vascular smooth muscle cells. Experientia **41:** 887–894.
4. Friedman, M., G. Kaczorowski, R. Vandlen, G. Katz & J. P. Reuben. 1985. Calcium and calcium-activated K+ currents in cultured smooth muscle cells (abstr). Fed. Proc. **44:** 452.
5. Hess, P., J. B. Lansman & R. W. Tsien. 1984. Different modes of calcium channel gating behavior favoured by dihydropyridine calcium agonists and antagonists. Nature **311**(5986): 538–544.
6. Kokubun, S., B. Prod'hum, C. Becker, H. Porzig & H. Reuter. 1986. Studies on calcium channels in intact cardiac cells: voltage-dependent effects and cooperative interactions of dihydropyridine enantiomers. Mol. Pharmacol. **30:** 571–584.

6a. Loirand, G., P. Pacaud, C. Mironneau & J. Mironneau. 1986. Evidence for two distinct calcium channels in rat vascular smooth muscle cells in short-term primary culture. Pflugers Arch **407:** 566–568.

7. Miller, R. J. 1987. Multiple calcium channels and neuronal function. Science **235:** 46–52.
8. Ohya, Y., K. Terada, K. Kitamura & H. Kumyama. 1987. D600 blocks the Ca^{2+} channel from the outer surface of smooth muscle cell membrane of the rabbit intestine and portal vein. Pflugers Arch. **408:** 80–82.
9. Reuter, H. 1983. Calcium channel modulation by neurotransmitters, enzymes, and drugs. Nature **301**(5901): 569–574.
10. Sarmiento, J. G., R. A. Janis, D. Jenkins & D. J. Triggle. 1984. Characteristics of [3H] nitrendipine binding to vascular smooth muscle membranes. *In* Nitrendipine. A. Scriabine, S. Vanov & K. Deck, Eds.: 153–160. Urban and Schwarzenberg, Inc. Baltimore, Md.
11. Sanguinetti, M. C., D. S. Krafte & R. S. Kass. 1986. Voltage-dependent modulation of calcium channel current in heart cells by Bay k8644. J. Gen. Physiol. **88:** 369–392.
12. Sturek, M. & K. Hermsmeyer. 1986. Calcium and sodium channels in spontaneously contracting vascular muscle cells. Science **233:** 475–478.
13. Tsien, R. W. 1983. Calcium channels in excitable cell membranes. Annu. Rev. Physiol. **45:** 341–358.
14. Worley, J. F., W. Jochim, W. Deitmer & M. T. Nelson. 1986. Single nisoldipine-sensitive calcium channels in smooth muscle cells isolated from rabbit mesenteric artery. Proc. Nat. Acad. Sci. USA **83:** 5746–5750.

Voltage-Dependent Calcium Channel in Intestinal and Vascular Smooth Muscle Cells[a]

T. B. BOLTON, P. I. AARONSON, AND I. MACKENZIE

Department of Pharmacology
St George's Hospital Medical School
Cranmer Terrace
London SW17 0RE, United Kingdom

The calcium channels in a variety of cell types have been studied using single channel recording methods. In neurons, three types have been identified;[1] in cardiac muscle, two.[2] There is still some uncertainty, however, as to how these channel types contribute to the transient and more sustained components of the whole-cell current. There is evidence that the shape of the inward current in rat sensory neurons can be modified by guanosine triphosphate (GTP) analogues implying that G protein binds to the channels and alters their kinetics (see Reference 3), which may indicate that calcium channel types can be interconverted under certain conditions. In vascular smooth muscle, evidence for two channel types has been obtained.[4–7] It is not certain as yet, however, that the additional component of more rapidly inactivating inward current that appears when holding at −80 mV, rather than −30 mV, is contributed solely by the activity of a T-type channel and that the more slowly inactivating component of inward current is due only to the activity of high-threshold L-type channels as has been claimed or implied.[5,8–11]

Stepping from negative (say −70 mV) holding potentials to positive potentials should activate current through both T- and L-type channels. If the L-type channel is distinctly more sensitive to dihydropyridine-type (DHP) calcium entry blocking drugs than are T channels as has been claimed[1,5] (but see References 6 and 7) in all cells where an additional inward current component appears upon holding at −70 mV rather than −30 mV, an equal component of inward current resistant to DHP drug blockade should be found. What is more generally reported is the ability to identify separate cells, some with a DHP-drug-resistant transient inward current component and others with more sustained, DHP-sensitive, current.[5,10,11] Clear biphasic concentration-effect curves for the effect of DHP drug on inward current at a test potential where both T and L channels are activated have not yet been described; the two phases would correspond to progressive effects first on the L and then on the T channels as the concentration of DHP drug was increased. Since both channels had been held at the same potential prior to stepping to the test potential, complications associated with increased voltage-dependent binding of DHP drug at more positive holding potentials would be avoided in the interpretation of such records.

The inward current has been studied in single cells of rat uterus,[12,13] urinary bladder[14,15] and longitudinal muscle of guinea pig,[16–18] and rabbit intestine.[19,20] Half activation of inward current has been reported to be −14 mV in bladder,[15] about −12 mV in uterus,[21] and −27 mV in guinea pig ileum using barium[16] with half inactivation

[a]This work is supported by the Medical Research Council (United Kingdom).

at −43 mV and −55 mV in bladder and ileum respectively. The inward current can be carried by calcium, barium, or strontium ions, or by sodium if the divalent cation concentration is low[12,19,21,22] and is blocked by manganese, cadmium, cobalt, or nickel.[15,17,19,23] Inactivation is all but complete within a few hundred milliseconds and can be described by two or more exponentials. The rate accelerates with depolarization at first but at positive membrane potentials it becomes slower again.[17] The biphasic nature has been explained by the amount of charge transferred by calcium entering the cell,[17] and it is known that, if calcium is the charge carrier, inactivation of the inward current system tested following a conditioning pulse is greater when the inward current evoked by the conditioning pulse is greater.[17,21] However, if inward current is carried by two channel types that have different thresholds for activation, the slowing of inactivation that occurs at positive potentials may have a contribution from the recruitment of a second type of channel with slower kinetics. It is not certain which of these explanations is correct, or whether both are contributory.

RESULTS

Characterization of Inward Current

Experiments were done on single cells separated from longitudinal muscle layer of rabbit jejunum by collagenase treatment. Comparisons will be made with results obtained on single cells obtained from the media of rabbit ear artery by collagenase and elastase treatment.[24] All experiments were done using standard patch-clamp technique.

Single jejunal cells when held at membrane potentials negative to −45 mV were generally quiescent but overshooting action potentials were generated if a depolarizing pulse was applied. This was in contrast to single arterial cells which, under the same conditions, showed inward rectification and did not discharge regenerative action potentials upon application of depolarizing pulses. However, if tetraethylammonium (TEA) was added to the solution bathing the cells, then weak spiking activity could generally be seen upon application of a depolarizing current pulse in arterial cells.

Activation Characteristics

In solutions of normal composition (1.5 mM calcium) inward current was triggered by depolarizations from a holding potential of −50 to −90 mV. Its form is shown in FIGURE 1. The current increased to reach a peak after stepping to the depolarized potential and then declined so that, by 500 mseconds, about 90% of the current had inactivated. This proportion is larger than in arterial cells in the same solution (1.5 mM Ca, FIGURE 1) and may be related to the higher current density in jejunal cells (about 10 times higher). This would result in a greater concentration of calcium accumulating close to the inside of the membrane during inward current flow which may contribute to the greater degree of inactivation of the current.

The rate of inactivation of inward current was slowed if 5 mM barium was substituted for 5 mM calcium in the bathing solution in both jejunal and arterial cells. The rate of inactivation was accelerated if calcium concentration was increased from 1.5 mM to 5 mM in jejunal cells, or up to 90 mM in arterial cells (FIGURES 2 and 3). In 90 mM calcium, inward current in arterial cells also increased in size. The greater degree of inactivation as calcium concentration was raised may explain its inhibitory effect on tension in high potassium solutions.[25] The results suggest that the greater rate of inactivation observed as the calcium concentration was increased may be the result of the increased calcium current density. In calcium-containing solutions the rate of inactivation was faster than when barium replaced calcium at the same concentration (FIGURE 2). The inward current in arterial cells was much larger in 110 mM barium than in 1.5 mM calcium.

If a two pulse protocol was used, the second pulse following the first after a period sufficient for deactivation but not sufficient for much recovery from inactivation, then the relationship between the size of the inward current evoked by the first and the

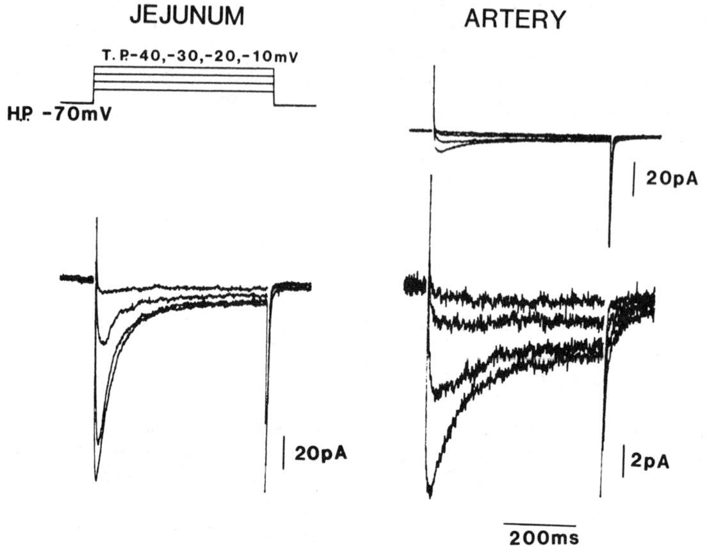

FIGURE 1. Inward current recorded in single jejunal and arterial smooth muscle cells. Cells were held at −70 mV and stepped for 500 mseconds to the indicated test potentials. Inward current is "leakage corrected" in this and subsequent figures by estimating the resting membrane conductance from small hyperpolarizing steps and subtracting the outward current through this (non-voltage-dependent) conductance at each test potential. Notice the much smaller inward current in arterial cell and its lesser degree of inactivation. Same records from artery are shown at two voltage sensitivities. The outward current in all experiments was suppressed by the use of a pipette solution containing Na 130 mM; TEA 10 mM; Mg 3.2 mM; H_2PO_4 1 mM; glucose 11.5 mM; MgATP 2 mM; SO_4 3.2 mM; Hepes 5 mM; EGTA 2.0 mM, which was at pH 7.2. The bathing solution contained Ca 1.5 mM and Na 129 mM; K 6 mM; Mg 1.2 mM; Cl 137 mM; glucose 11.5 mM; HEPES 10 mM and was at pH 7.2. All experiments at room temperature (20–25°C).

degree of inactivation of the second inward current could be studied. Inactivation of the second inward current was greatest when the inward current evoked by the first pulse was greatest in both jejunal cells in 1.5 mM calcium and in arterial cells in 90 mM calcium. Depolarization during the first pulse which exceeded that needed for maximum peak inward current (i.e., polarization to potentials approaching the reversal potential for the current) produced a lesser degree of inactivation (FIGURE 4). In calcium-free, 5 mM barium solution this latter effect was very slight; inactivation approached a plateau level with increasing size of first pulse with only a slight decline from the plateau level of inactivation with further depolarization.

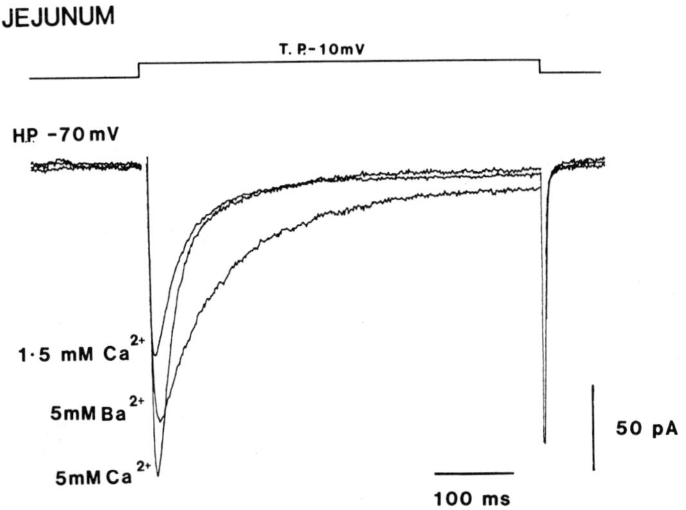

FIGURE 2. Effect of altering concentration and identity of cation carrying inward current. Single cell of jejunum holding at −70 mV and stepping to −10 mV in 1.5 mM calcium, 5 mM calcium, and calcium-free 5 mM barium-containing solution. Increasing the calcium concentration increases the peak current and its rate of inactivation. Barium substitution for calcium slightly reduces peak current and strongly delays inactivation. All records from the same cell.

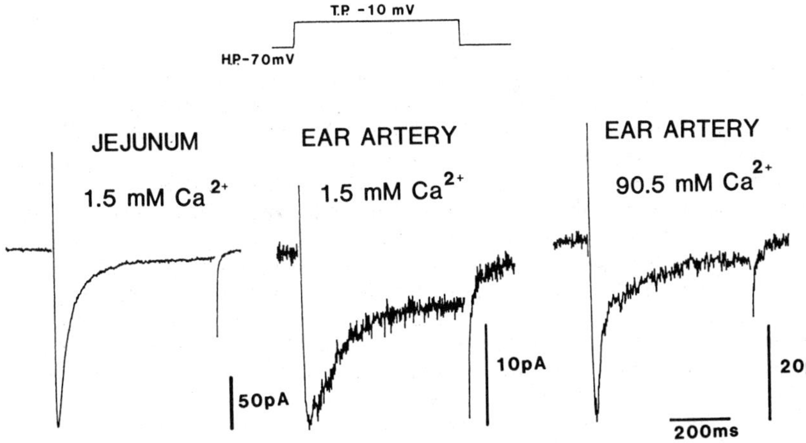

FIGURE 3. Inactivation of inward current in arterial cell is less than in jejunal and is increased if current is increased by raising the calcium concentration.

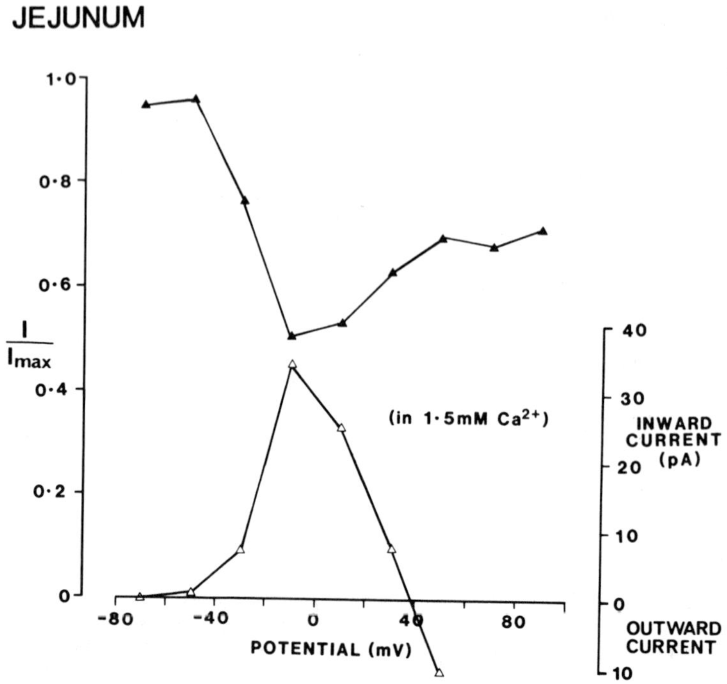

FIGURE 4. Inactivation of current evoked by a second, test, pulse following a first, conditioning, pulse. A 200 msecond pulse to various potentials in 1.5 mM calcium evoked an inward current plotted as open triangles. A second pulse of 500 mseconds, 100 mseconds after the first, and always to −10 mV evoked an inward current, *I*, which is expressed as a fraction of this current when it was maximum, I_{max} (filled triangles). Notice that the second pulse is most reduced when the first inward current is largest (at −10 mV) and depolarizations to more positive potentials evoked smaller inward currents and produced less inactivation.

The activation of current was examined in jejunal cells when stepping to various potentials from a holding potential in the range −60 to −90 mV. Inward current was activated generally at −50 mV, sometimes −40 mV, and was appreciable positive to −30 mV. The half-activation point was about −20 mV. Full activation was generally achieved by 0 mV (FIGURE 5). The results in single vascular smooth muscle cells were surprisingly similar even though inward current density was much lower (FIGURE 5).

The smaller inward current in arterial cells means that its measured size was much more affected by leakage currents through other channels. These were minimized by the use of a sodium (130 mM) and TEA (10 mM) solution inside the pipette. Sodium was used in preference to cesium as both have equally low permeability through calcium-activated K channels in smooth muscle[26] and seal formation was easier using sodium. Pipette solution of identical composition was used for arterial and jejunal cells; it contained 2 mM EGTA and was buffered to pH 7.2 with 5 mM sodium HEPES. Despite the precautions taken to minimize other currents, as the reversal potential was approached, inward current was very small and uncertainty must exist concerning its size (and direction) on account of possible contaminating current through other channel types; this was much less of a problem in jejunal cells where the current was much larger. Errors in the measurement of the reversal potential of the inward current due to contaminating currents may confound attempts to construct its activation curve and may produce artifactual differences between arterial and jejunal cells, where the reversal potential of the inward current can be more accurately measured. For this reason comparison was made between the potentials at which maximum peak inward current occurred in arterial and jejunal cells. These were within 2–3 mV. Likewise the potentials at which peak inward current achieved 25%, 50%, and 75% of its maximum value were also within a few millivolts in the two cell types. The similarity of the relationship of inward current activation to potential was confirmed in experiments on one arterial cell where inward current was particularly large so that a reasonable estimate of reversal potential, and hence the position on the voltage axis of the activation curve, could be made (FIGURE 5).

A comparison of inward current was made in arterial cells in 1.5 mM calcium and in 110 mM barium solutions. In the same cell, inward current was greatly increased in high-barium solution and the peak current occurred at +30 mV instead of at −10 mV or 0 mV in 1.5 mM calcium. The current-voltage curve was shifted to more positive potentials; the potential at which half-maximum current was observed was also some 30–40 mV more positive.

Availability

The effect of holding potential on the peak of current activated upon stepping to 0 mV was examined in jejunal cells in 1.5 mM Ca. In most cells the current measured in

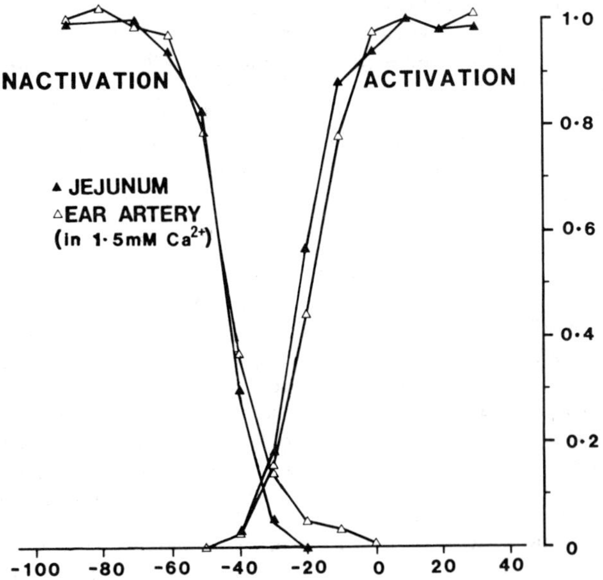

FIGURE 5. Inactivation and activation of inward current in jejunal and in arterial cells in 1.5 mM calcium. Inactivation (or availability) was measured as the fractional size of the peak current at 0 mV after holding at various potentials before the test pulse (see FIGURE 6). The activation curves were constructed from a holding potential of −70 mV (jejunum) and −60 mV (artery).

this way was almost fully available at −60 mV, although in some a small increase in availability occurred upon holding at −90 mV (in some cells this reduced the availability). Half the current was available when holding at about −45 mV and very little was available positive to −30 mV (see FIGURE 6). In artery, the half-availability point was almost the same (within 2 mV) but there was evidence that in some cells the availability curve was less steep especially positive to −30 mV so that proportionally more current could be activated from this potential than in jejunal cells (FIGURE 5). In 110 mM barium the availability of current was shifted about 30 mV in a positive direction.

Thus in normal calcium concentrations (1.5 mM) the activation and inactivation (availability) of inward current in jejunal and arterial cells were very similar, despite the greater membrane current density in the former. Small quantitative differences were detected however.

Pharmacological Properties

In jejunal cells, inward current was sensitive to DHP drugs. Nifedipine, for example, reduced inward current above about 0.01 μM; at 1 μM about 80–90% reduction was observed. Current measured at the end of a 500 msecond pulse was slightly more sensitive than peak current. These results were very similar to observations made in arterial cells, and no significant differences between the two cell types in their sensitivity to nifedipine were observed.

The sensitivity to nickel of the inward current in jejunal and arterial cells was examined. Effects were observed at 50 μM and 80–90% block was seen at 500 μM. Jejunal and arterial cells were similarly sensitive and, unlike with nifedipine, current at the end of a 500 msecond pulse was not noticeably more sensitive than peak current.

Bay K 8644 increased inward current in arterial cells in 1.5 mM calcium; it had a modest (1- to 2-fold) potentiating effect in jejunal cells at 1 μM also. A 10-fold increase in inward current was seen in arterial cells in 90 mM barium (no calcium) if 1 μM Bay K 8644 was applied. In jejunal or arterial cells in 1.5 mM calcium, the position of the inward current curve on the voltage axis was not noticeably affected but in 90 mM barium (calcium-free) solution, the current-voltage curve was shifted to more negative potentials in Bay K 8644.

DISCUSSION

In solutions of normal composition and containing 1.5 mM calcium, the activation and inactivation characteristics of inward current were surprisingly similar in jejunal and in arterial cells even though current density was about 10 times higher in the former. Regenerative action potentials are seen in jejunal cells but not generally in arterial cells (these differences hold in the whole tissues before dispersal also).[27–29] The lack of regenerative action potentials in arterial cells seems to reflect a weak inward current system, probably attributable to a lower calcium channel density, combined with a vigorous outward current system.

Inward current systems in both cell types were about equally sensitive to DHP drugs; this was also true for nickel. In the experimental protocol used in these experiments no transient, DHP-resistant, inward current component was encountered, although sustained current was slightly more sensitive than peak current. This is to be expected if DHP drug binding is voltage dependent and increased by increasing membrane positivity. Thus, upon stepping from a holding potential to a more positive

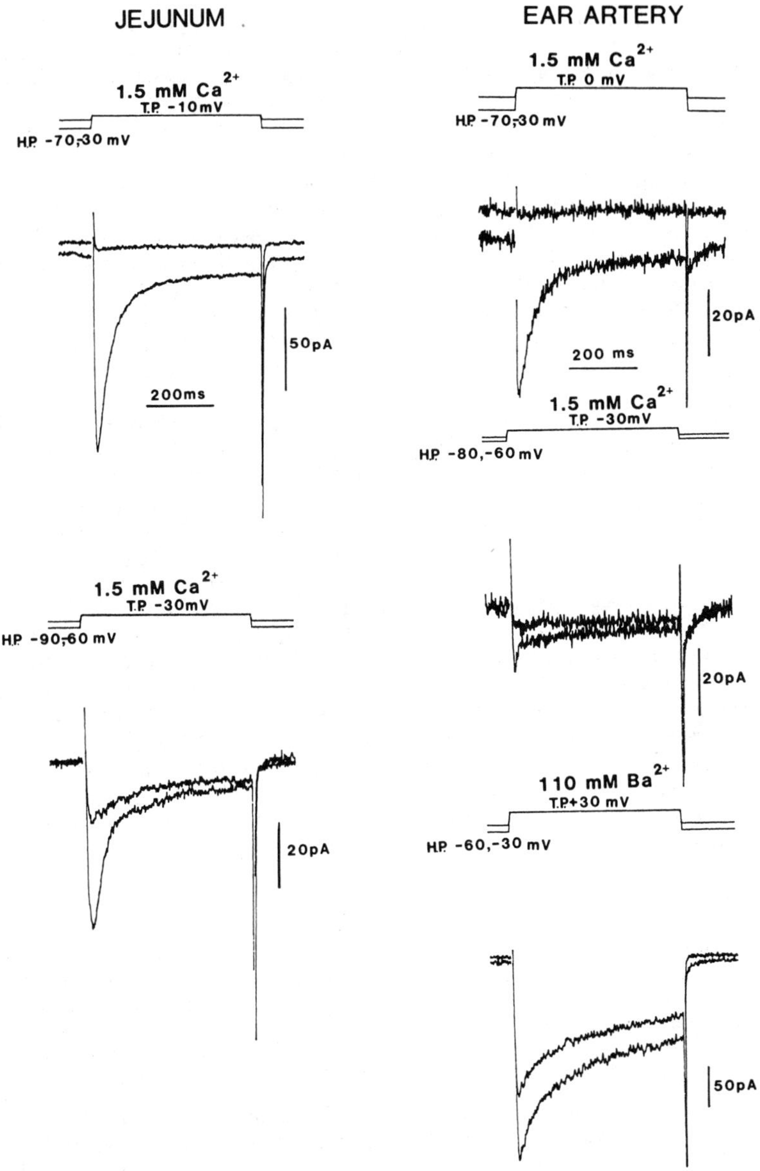

FIGURE 6. Effect of holding potential on availability of inward current in arterial and jejunal single cells in 1.5 mM calcium and in 110 mM barium. In jejunum and artery, holding at −30 mV resulted in almost complete inactivation of current (top records). Notice the difference in artery in 110 mM barium at −30 mV (lower right); in this case the more negative holding potential results in the appearance of a more rapidly inactivating component of current (difference between the traces). This phenomenon is easily demonstrated in both jejunum and artery in 1.5 mM calcium (middle records) if the holding potentials are set more negative so that they lie on the inactivation curve (see FIGURE 5).

potential which evokes inward current, peak current that occurs earlier will be less reduced than later current at DHP drug concentrations that produce incomplete block.[30] Our interpretation of these results is at variance with the interpretations given by others using different protocols.[5,10,11] In rat portal vein smooth muscle cells, sustained inward current was noticeably more sensitive to nifedipine (0.5 μM) than peak current in cells showing both components;[11] this may be explicable by the voltage-dependent block mentioned above. In some cells of portal vein, 50 nM nifedipine abolished the sustained current that was seen. This was completely abolished both at early and late times (i.e., transient current was apparently absent in these cells).[11] Similar observations were made by Bean *et al.*,[10] who also show a 35 mV negative shift in the availability of inward current by a DHP drug; this would be expected if binding of DHP drug were voltage dependent. The relative contributions of T- and L-type channels to peak and sustained inward current in an individual cell cannot be definitely identified, so quantitative arguments based on this are not convincing.[10]

Much emphasis has been placed in single cell work on protocols in which the cell is held at strongly negative potentials (e.g., −70 mV) where it is believed T channels are not inactivated, and at more positive potentials (e.g., −30 mV) where they are inactivated but L channels are still available, before stepping to a positive test potential (e.g., +20 mV).[31] This type of protocol results in a component of more rapidly inactivating current which appears when stepping from the more negative holding potential. This type of phenomenon can be observed also in jejunal cells in 1.5 mM calcium, and arterial cells in the same solution behave likewise (FIGURE 6). The interpretation advanced by others is that there are two types of channel and the extra component with more rapid kinetics is made available by holding at more negative potentials. Two types of unitary conductance of 8 and 24 pS approximately, which allow barium to pass, and with short and longer mean open times have been described.[4] However, their individual contributions to current at various potentials is by no means certain or easily established, especially in 1.5 mM calcium rather than 90 or 110 mM barium solution. It is conceivable that the kinetic behavior of a single population of channels may alter depending on the length of time they have been held at some potential; for example, it is possible that the degree of phosphorylation or association with G proteins may be affected by this. Such changes might well affect their kinetics when stepped to a test potential especially at early times; at longer times their kinetics would be expected to relax back to those characteristic of the test potential. At early times binding of DHP drugs may also be altered. Such possibilities seem not to have been explored in smooth muscle. In other cells, such as neurons, there is evidence that current kinetics can be drastically altered by G proteins if these are activated or deactivated by nonhydrolyzable analogues of GTP such as GTP-γ-S or GDP-β-S.[32] If full concentration-effect curves were constructed for the effect of DHP drugs on inward current, under conditions when voltage-dependent binding did not change, evidence for two types of calcium channel underlying inward current would be expected if both T- (DHP-insensitive) and L-type (DHP-sensitive)[2,31] channels were involved. This needs to be established. However, the unitary conductance of "calcium" channels in high-barium conditions has been described as 8 pS[5-7] and 12 pS,[6] 15 pS,[7] or 24 pS.[5] Two groups describe all channels as sensitive to DHP drugs whereas Benham *et al.* say only their 24 pS channels are sensitive.[5] The situation is confused at present.

The differences between arterial and jejunal cells were small. The potential of half-activation of inward current was almost the same in arterial and in jejunal cells as was the half-inactivation potential. However, some arterial cells had less steep inactivation (availability) curves such that proportionally more current was available positive to −30 mV. In jejunal cells virtually no inward current is available positive to this potential after a few seconds (FIGURES 5 and 6). Inactivation of the current was generally more rapid and more complete in jejunal cells; this may be related to the 10-fold (about) greater inward current density. These differences require further exploration.

REFERENCES

1. NOWYCKY, M. C., A. P. FOX & R. W. TSIEN. 1985. Three types of neuronal calcium channel with different calcium agonist sensitivity. Nature **316:** 440–443.
2. NILIUS, B., P. HESS, J. B. LANSMAN & R. W. TSIEN. 1985. A novel type of cardiac calcium channel in ventricular cells. Nature **316:** 443–446.
3. SCOTT, R. H. & A. C. DOLPHIN. 1986. Regulation of calcium currents by a GTP analogue: potentiation of (−)-baclofen-mediated inhibition. Neurosci. Lett. **69:** 59–64.
4. AARONSON, P. I., C. D. BENHAM, T. B. BOLTON, P. HESS, R. J. LANG & R. W. TSIEN. 1986. Two types of single-channel and whole-cell calcium or barium currents in single smooth muscle cells of rabbit ear artery and the effects of noradrenaline. J. Physiol. **377:** 36P.
5. BENHAM, C. D., P. HESS & R. W. TSIEN. Two types of calcium channels in single smooth muscle cells from rabbit ear artery studied with whole cells and single channel recordings. Circ. Res. (In press.)
6. CAFFREY, J. M., I. R. JOSEPHSON & A. M. BROWN. 1986. Calcium channels of amphibian stomach and mammalian aorta smooth muscle cells. Biophys. J. **49:** 1237–1242.
7. WORLEY, J. F., J. W. DEITMER & M. T. NELSON. 1986. Single nisoldipine-sensitive calcium channels in smooth muscle cells isolated from rabbit mesenteric artery. Proc. Nat. Acad. Sci. USA **83:** 5746–5750.
8. STUREK, M. & K. HERMSMEYER. 1986. Calcium and sodium channels in spontaneously contracting vascular muscle cells. Science **233:** 475–478.
9. FRIEDMAN, M. E., G. SUAREZ-KURTZ, G. J. KACZOROWSKI, G. M. KATZ & J. P. REUBEN. 1986. Two calcium currents in a smooth muscle cell line. Am J. Physiol. **250:** H699–H703.
10. BEAN, B. P., M. STUREK, A. PUGA & K. HERMSMEYER. 1986. Calcium channels in muscle cells isolated from rat mesenteric arteries: modulation by dihydropyridine drugs. Circ. Res. **59:** 229–235.
11. LOIRAND, G., P. PACAUD, C. MIRONNEAU & J. MIRONNEAU. 1986. Evidence for two distinct calcium channels in rat vascular smooth muscle cells in short-term primary culture. Pflügers Arch. **407:** 566–568.
12. JMARI, K., C. MIRONNEAU & J. MIRONNEAU. 1986. Canaux calciques des cellules musculaires lisses. J. Physiol. Paris **81:** 168–176.
13. MOLLARD, P., J. MIRONNEAU, T. AMÉDÉE & C. MIRONNEAU. 1986. Electrophysiological characterization of single pregnant rat myometrial cells in short-term primary culture. Am. J. Physiol. **250:** C47–C54.
14. KLÖCKNER, U. & G. ISENBERG. 1985. Action potentials and net membrane currents of isolated smooth muscle cells (urinary bladder of the guinea pig). Pflügers Arch. **405:** 329–339.
15. KLÖCKNER, U. & G. ISENBERG. 1985. Calcium currents of cesium loaded isolated smooth muscle cells (urinary bladder of the guinea pig). Pflügers Arch. **405:** 340–348.
16. DROOGMANS, G. & G. CALLEWAERT. 1986. Ca^{2+}-channel current and its modification by the dihydropyridine agonist BAY K 8644 in isolated smooth muscle cells. Pflügers Arch. **406:** 259–265.
17. GANITKEVICH, V. Y., M. F. SHUBA & S. V. SMIRNOV. 1986. Potential-dependent calcium inward current in a single isolated smooth muscle cell of the guinea-pig taenia caeci. J. Physiol. **380:** 1–16.
18. BURYI, V. A., A. V. ZHOLOS & M. V. SHUBA. 1986. Electrical properties and transmembrane ionic current of single smooth muscle cells. Bull. Exp. Biol. Med. **101:** 259–263.
19. OHYA, Y., K. TERADA, K. KITAMURA & H. KURIYAMA. 1986. Membrane currents recorded from a fragment of rabbit intestinal smooth muscle cell. Am. J. Physiol. **251:** C335–C346.

20. BOLTON, T. B., R. J. LANG, T. TAKEWAKI & C. D. BENHAM. 1985. Patch and whole-cell voltage clamp of single mammalian visceral and vascular smooth muscle cells. Experientia **41:** 887–894.
21. AMÉDÉE, T., C. MIRONNEAU & J. MIRONNEAU. The calcium channel current of single pregnant rat myometrial cells in short-term primary culture. J. Physiol. (In press.)
22. MIRONNEAU, J., D. EUGÈNE & C. MIRONNEAU. 1982. Sodium action potentials induced by calcium chelation in rat uterine smooth muscle. Pflügers Arch. **395:** 232–238.
23. MOLLARD, P., J. MIRONNEAU, T. AMÉDÉE & C. MIRONNEAU. 1985. Action potential and Ca^{2+} inward current in isolated pregnant rat myometrial cells. Colloques d'INSERM **124:** 43–54.
24. BENHAM, C. D. & T. B. BOLTON. 1986. Spontaneous transient outward currents in single visceral and vascular smooth muscle cells of the rabbit. J. Physiol. **381:** 385–406.
25. VAN BREEMEN, C., O. HWANG & K. D. MEISHERI. 1981. The mechanism of inhibitory action of diltiazem on vascular smooth muscle contractility. J. Pharmacol. Exp. Ther. **218:** 459–463.
26. BENHAM, C. D., T. B. BOLTON, R. J. LANG & T. TAKEWAKI. 1986. Calcium-activated potassium channels in single smooth muscle cells of rabbit jejunum and guinea-pig mesenteric artery. J. Physiol. **317:** 45–67.
27. BOLTON, T. B. 1972. The depolarizing action of acetylcholine or carbachol in intestinal smooth muscle. J. Physiol. **220:** 647–671.
28. SUZUKI, H. & K. KOU. 1983. Direct and indirect effects of histamine on the smooth muscle cells of the guinea-pig main pulmonary artery. Pflügers Arch. **399:** 46–53.
29. DROOGMANS, G., L. RAEYMAEKERS & R. CASTEELS. 1977. Electro- and pharmacomechanical coupling in the smooth muscle cells of the rabbit ear artery. J. Gen. Physiol. **70:** 129–148.
30. SANGUINETTI, M. C. & R. S. KASS. 1984. Voltage-dependent block of calcium channel current in the calf cardiac purkinje fiber by dihydropyridine calcium channel antagonists. Circ. Res. **55:** 336–348.
31. BEAN, B. P. 1985. Two kinds of calcium channels in canine atrial cells. J. Gen. Physiol. **86:** 1–30.
32. DOLPHIN, A. C. & R. H. SCOTT. 1987. Calcium channel currents and their inhibition by (−)-baclofen in rat sensory neurones: modulation by guanine nucleotides. J. Physiol. **386:** 1–17.

Monoclonal Antibody Characterization of the 1,4-Dihydropyridine Receptor of Rabbit Skeletal Muscle

ALBERT T. LEUNG,[a] TOSHIAKI IMAGAWA,[b] AND KEVIN P. CAMPBELL[c,d]

Department of Physiology and Biophysics
The University of Iowa
Iowa City, Iowa 52242

The 1,4-dihydropyridine receptor (DHPR) of the voltage-dependent Ca^{2+} channel has been purified from transverse tubular membranes of skeletal muscle.[1,2] Curtis and Catterall have shown that it consists of three polypeptides of 160,000 daltons, 50,000 Da, and 32,000 Da and that under reducing conditions the apparent molecular weight of the 160,000 Da subunit shifted to 130,000.[1] Borsotto *et al.* have identified three polypeptides of 142,000 Da, 33,000 Da, and 32,000 Da in their preparation of the dihydropyridine receptor.[2] Furthermore, they have shown by immunoblotting with polyclonal antibodies that the 142,000 Da and 32,000 Da subunits are produced by the reduction of a 170,000 Da polypeptide.[3] We report here the identification and characterization with monoclonal antibodies (MAb) of an additional high molecular weight subunit of the DHPR which is distinct from that described by Curtis and Catterall[1] and Borsotto *et al.*[3]

Monoclonal antibodies capable of specifically immunoprecipitating the [^{3}H]PN200-110-labeled DHPR of rabbit skeletal muscle were produced by immunizing BALB/c mice initially with skeletal muscle triad vesicles followed by booster immunizations with purified DHPR from skeletal muscle triads. Hybridoma supernatants were screened for the production of anti-DHPR antibodies with an immunodot assay. Supernatants that reacted positively against the partially purified DHPR were then tested for their ability to immunoprecipitate the [^{3}H]PN200-110-labeled receptor from digitonin-solubilized triads (see TABLE 1).

All three MAbs (IIC12, IIF7, IIID5) that were capable of immunoprecipitating the DHPR recognized a protein with an M_r of 170,000 on nitrocellulose transfers of skeletal muscle triads and transverse tubular membranes separated on sodium dodecyl sulfate–polyacrylamide gel electrophoresis (SDS-PAGE) under nonreducing conditions (FIGURE 1a). Wheat-germ agglutinin (WGA) peroxidase stained a 175,000 Da protein on similar nitrocellulose transfers. Neither the 170,000 Da polypeptide nor the 175,000 Da polypeptide was detected in light sarcoplasmic reticulum vesicles, a preparation devoid of DHPR. Under reducing conditions, the M_r of the 170,000 Da

[a]American Heart Association Medical Student Research Fellow (1985–86) and Iowa Graduate Fellow.

[b]Muscular Dystrophy Association Postdoctoral Fellow.

[c]Established Investigator of the American Heart Association. Recipient of a grant from the National Institutes of Health (HL-37187).

[d]To whom correspondence should be addressed.

polypeptide on SDS-PAGE remained unchanged whereas the M_r of the glycoprotein shifted from 175,000 to 150,000.

The DHPR was purified from skeletal muscle triads using a modification of the procedure according to Curtis and Catterall.[1] The purified DHPR was shown to consist of four subunits of M_r 175,000, 170,000, 50,000, and 30,000 on a 5–16% polyacrylamide gel under nonreducing conditions (FIGURE 1b). Under reducing conditions, the M_r of the 175,000 Da subunit shifted to 150,000. On nitrocellulose transfers, the 170,000 Da subunit was stained by the anti-DHPR MAbs and its M_r did not change with reduction. The 175,000 Da subunit was stained by WGA-peroxidase and the M_r of this glycoprotein shifted to 150,000 Da upon reduction. These results are consistent with the results of anti-DHPR MAb and WGA-peroxidase staining of immunoblots of skeletal muscle transverse tubular membranes and triads. Results from our laboratory have further demonstrated that the M_r 170,000 polypeptide and not the M_r 175,000 glycoprotein is a phosphoprotein[4] and binds dihydropyridines.[5]

TABLE 1. Immunoprecipitation of [^{3}H]PN200-110-Labeled Receptor Using Various Monoclonal Antibody Beads

	Amount of [^{3}H]PN200-110-Labeled Receptor (fmol)[a]
Controls	
GAM-IgG beads	2.1 ± 0.3
GAM-IgG beads preincubated with RPMI-1640	3.8 ± 0.8
MAb IIID5-GAM-IgG beads incubated with [^{3}H]PN200-110 in the absence of solubilized triads	3.4 ± 0.8
GAM-IgG beads preincubated with preimmune serum	6.7 ± 2.0
GAM-IgG beads preincubated with immunized mouse serum	17.6 ± 1.2
WGA-Sepharose	106.0 ± 6.8
Monoclonal antibody beads	
MAb IIC12-GAM-IgG beads	63.8 ± 8.8
MAb IIF7-GAM-IgG beads	52.9 ± 1.7
MAb IIID5-GAM-IgG beads	48.8 ± 1.6

[a]Monoclonal antibody beads were prepared by incubating 15 bed volumes of hybridoma supernatants with goat-anti-mouse IgG Sepharose (Cooper, diluted to an IgG binding capacity of 1 mg/ml with Sepharose CL 4B) to form MAb-GAM-IgG beads. Triad vesicles were labeled with 10 nM [^{3}H]PN200-110 and solubilized with 1% digitonin in 0.5 M NaCl and 50 mM Tris-HCl (pH 7.4). The solubilized membranes were then diluted 1:10 with 50 mM Tris-HCl (pH 7.4). Five hundred μl of this mixture were incubated with 50 μl of MAb-GAM-IgG Sepharose at 4°C for 2 hours with gentle mixing. The mixture was then centrifuged in an Eppendorf centrifuge, and the supernatants were removed and assayed for dihydropyridine receptor activity using the PEG precipitation assay. The beads were washed twice with 1 ml of buffer (100 mM NaCl, 50 mM Tris-HCl pH 7.4) containing 0.1% digitonin and then counted in a scintillation counter.

In summary, our results demonstrate that the 1,4-dihydropyridine receptor of the voltage-dependent Ca^{2+} channel from rabbit skeletal muscle contains two distinct high molecular weight subunits, a glycoprotein of M_r 175,000 and a polypeptide of M_r 170,000.

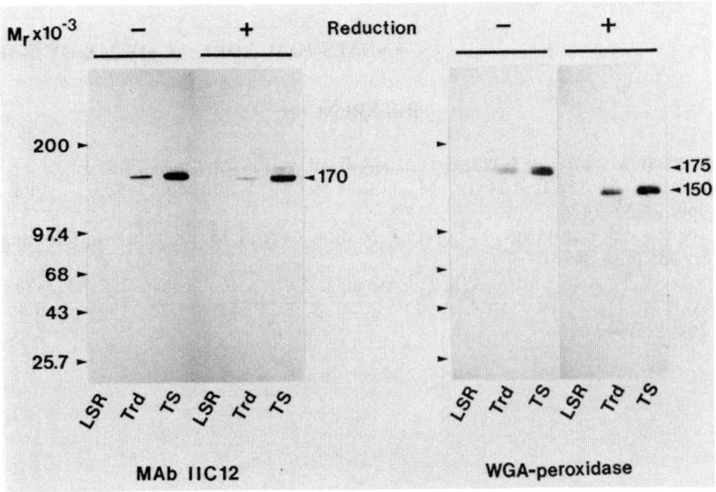

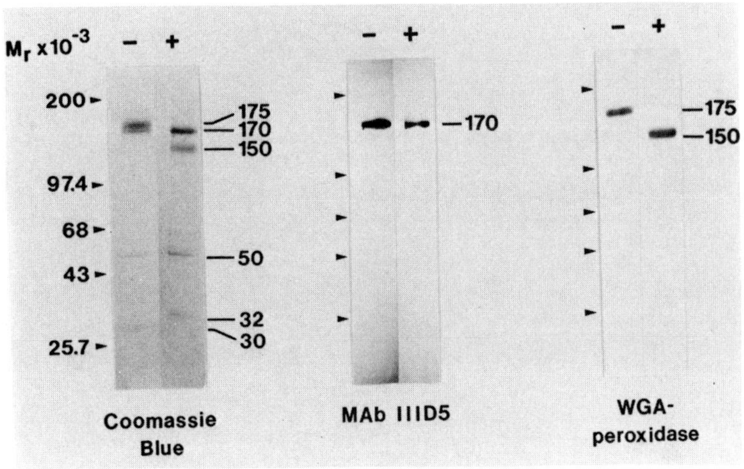

FIGURE 1. Coomassie Blue staining and immunoblot staining of rabbit skeletal muscle membrane fractions and purified dihydropyridine receptor. Light sarcoplasmic reticulum (LSR), triads (Trd), and transverse tubular (TS) membrane (30–50 μg) or the purified dihydropyridine receptor (20 μg) was subjected to SDS-PAGE on a 3–12% polyacrylamide gradient gel under nonreducing (+ 20 mN *N*-ethylmaleimide) and reducing (+ 10 mM dithiothreitol) conditions and stained with Coomassie Blue or transferred to nitrocellulose membranes. BLOTTO—Bovine Lacto Transfer Technique Optimizer (50 mM NaH_2PO_4, 0.9% NaCl, 5% nonfat dry milk, pH 7.4)—was used for blocking of the nitrocellulose transfers and dilution of the antibodies. Nitrocellulose transfers were first incubated with hybridoma supernatants (1:10 or 1:20 dilution) and then with peroxidase-conjugated goat-anti-mouse immunoglobulin G (IgG) secondary antibody (Cooper, 1:1000 dilution). WGA-peroxidase (Sigma) was used to stain WGA-positive glycoproteins on nitrocellulose transfers. The nitrocellulose transfers were blocked with 0.05% Tween-PBS (50 mM NaH_2PO_4, 0.9% NaCl, pH 7.4) and incubated with WGA-peroxidase (1:2000) in 0.05% Tween-PBS. The color was developed in both cases using 4-chloro-1-naphthol as the substrate. (a-top) The left panel shows nitrocelluose transfers of the gel stained with monoclonal antibody IIC12. The right panel shows nitrocellulose transfers of the gel stained with WGA-peroxidase. (b-bottom) The purified dihydropyridine receptor was subjected to SDS-PAGE on a 5–16% polyacrylamide gradient gel. The left panel is a photograph of a Coomassie Blue stained gel. The center panel shows a nitrocellulose transfer of the gel stained with monoclonal antibody IIID5, illustrating the insensitivity of the relative mobility of the 170,000 Da subunit to reduction. The right panel shows a nitrocellulose transfer of the gel stained with WGA-peroxidase, illustrating the shift of the relative mobility of the 175,000 Da subunit to 150,000 Da upon reduction.

REFERENCES

1. CURTIS, B. M. & W. A. CATTERALL. 1984. Biochemistry **23:** 2113–2118.
2. BORSOTTO, M., J. BARHANIN, M. FOSSET & M. LAZDUNSKI. 1985. J. Biol. Chem. **260:** 14255–14263.
3. SCHMID, A., J. BARHANIN, T. COPPOLA, M. BORSOTTO & M. LAZDUNSKI. 1986. Biochemistry **25:** 3492–3495.
4. IMAGAWA, T., A. T. LEUNG & K. P. CAMPBELL. 1987. J. Biol. Chem. **262:** 8333–8339.
5. SHARP, A. H., T. IMAGAWA, A. T. LEUNG & K. P. CAMPBELL. 1987. J. Biol. Chem. **262:** 12309–12315.

Membrane Potential Regulates Dihydropyridine Inhibition of Single Calcium Channels and Contraction of Rabbit Mesenteric Artery[a]

M. T. NELSON, I. LAHER, AND J. WORLEY

Department of Pharmacology
University of Vermont College of Medicine
Burlington, Vermont 05405

Dihydropyridine drugs (DHP) such as nisoldipine, nimodipine, and nifedipine are potent vasodilators whose effectiveness varies among vascular beds[1] and is altered by disease (e.g., hypertension).[2] Therefore, understanding the regulation of DHP action is critical for the development of appropriate drug strategies. In this study, we demonstrate that depolarization of the membrane potential increases inhibition by DHP of vascular smooth muscle contraction and single calcium channel activity.

The effects of resting (holding) potential (V_m) on DHP inhibition of high K (84 mM) evoked contraction of ring segments of rabbit mesenteric artery were determined. Changing external K levels between 5 mM and 45 mM produced corresponding changes of V_m between about -70 mV and -30 mV. In the presence of a fixed concentration of DHP, contraction evoked by the high K test pulse was a steep function of V_m, with 7.5 mV depolarization causing an *e*-fold decrease in contraction over the steepest part of the relationship (FIGURE 1). Increasing the DHP concentration shifted this curve to more negative potentials without affecting the slope factor ($k = 7.5$ mV), i.e., the degree of inhibition depends on V_m. One explanation for these results is that membrane depolarization promotes a high-affinity DHP-binding form of the calcium channel (K_d for nisoldipine = 0.07 nM), with the drug-bound form of the channel being incapable of conducting calcium.

To determine the molecular basis for the voltage dependence of DHP action on contraction, the effect of V_m on inhibition by DHP of the activity of single calcium channels was examined in excised patches from cells isolated from mesenteric arteries.[3] Single calcium channels were activated by test pulses to 0 mV. Depolarizing V_m attenuated the peak average current through single channels elicited by the test pulse; i.e., depolarization promotes an inactivated form of the channel. DHP shifted the relationship between peak average current and holding potential in the negative direction without affecting its slope (7.5 mV) (FIGURE 2B). At the single channel level, DHP (<30 nM) increased the fraction of test pulses without openings, i.e., promoted an inactivated form of the channel (FIGURE 2A) and did not affect channel open and closed times. The results from the intact artery as well as from single channel experiments indicate that the high-affinity DHP-binding form of the calcium channel is the inactivated state.[4] In addition, DHP can be used to estimate the positions (midpoint range in rabbit mesenteric artery -11 to -32.5 mV) and shapes of

[a]Supported by grants from the American Heart Association (AHA), Miles Laboratories, National Institutes of Health (BRSG), fellowships from the AHA (I.L.) and Muscular Dystrophy Association (J.W.). M.T.N. is an Established Investigator of the AHA.

1a.

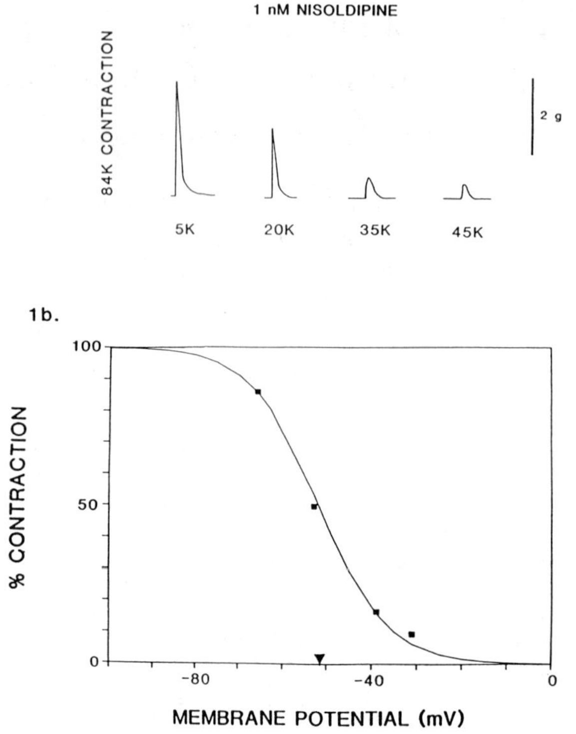

FIGURE 1. Voltage dependence of nisoldipine inhibition of contraction. (A) Original contraction records showing the effects of changing the resting level of potassium (i.e., membrane potential) on high K contractions in the presence of 1 nM nisoldipine. High potassium (84 mM) contractions were measured (upward deflections) at 37°C in a physiological salt solution that contains 1.8 mM calcium. Isometric vessel wall tension was measured by a resistance vessel myograph.[5] Prior to commencing the experiments, the vessels are exposed for one hour to phenoxybenzamine (1 μM), an irreversible multireceptor blocker. The holding potential was varied by changing the level of K from 5 mM to 40 mM. Equilibration of added nisoldipine (1 nM final concentration) was determined as the time that the high K contractions had reached a steady level (usually from 1–2 hours). The level of high K evoked contraction at each resting level of K was independent of the sequence of changes in the resting level; i.e., the sequence of resting K changes 45–35–20–5 mM gave the same results as 5–20–35–40 mM. To assure that the DHP was in equilibrium with the artery at the holding potential, the durations of the high K pulses (<1 minute) were always much shorter than the time intervals at the holding potential (>7 minutes) and much shorter than the expected equilibration times of DHP with the artery under high K conditions (>4 minutes). (B) Relationship between contraction and V_m. The reduction in high K contraction as a function of the holding potential is shown. The squares are the average of simultaneous measurements performed on four different arterial segments. Resulting K levels were translated into membrane potentials using the values from Makita *et al.*[6] Maximum contraction was the 5K to 84K contraction in the absence of drug. This relationship can be described by the equation, $1/(1 + \exp(V_m - V_{0.5})/k)$, where V_m is the membrane potential determined by the resting level of K, $V_{0.5}$ is the membrane potential where the contraction is reduced in half, k is the slope factor and is equal to 7.5 mV (determined from a least-squares fit of the ln-transformed data). $V_{0.5}$ at this drug concentration was −51 mV, indicated by the black triangle.

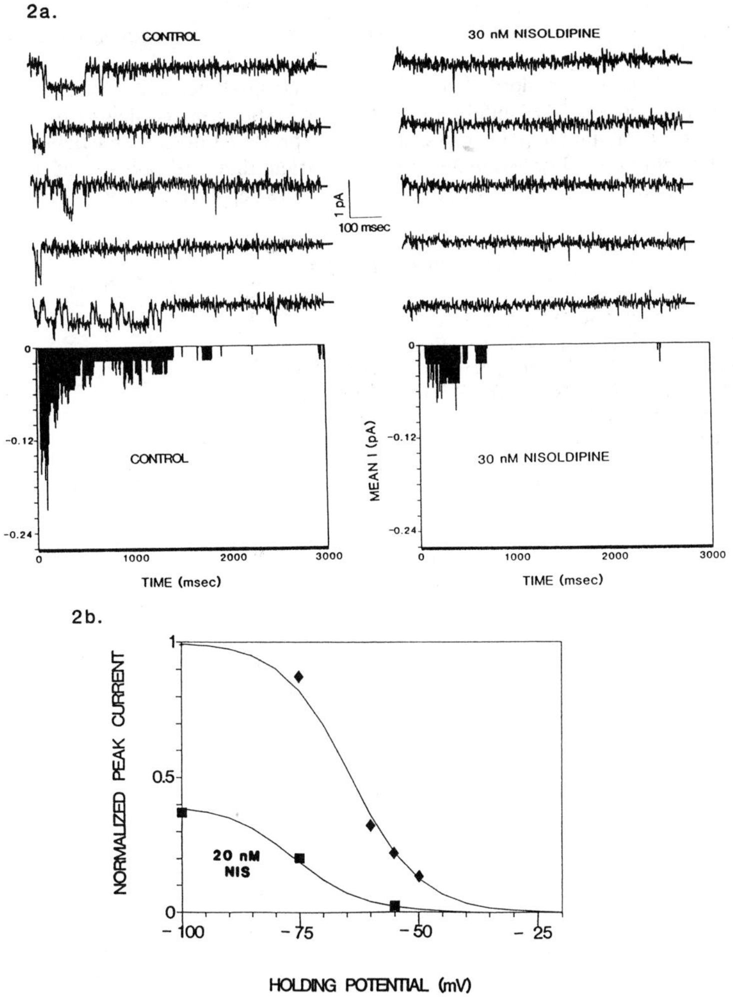

FIGURE 2. Inhibition of single calcium channels by nisoldipine. (A) Nisoldipine inhibition of single channel activity. Single channel currents were measured with barium as the charge carrier (80 mM) in excised membrane patches from single mesenteric artery cells of the rabbit (see Reference 3 for details of the experimental conditions). The holding potential was −75 mV and the test potential was 0 mV. The closed level is indicated at the right of each trace by a solid line. Channel openings are grouped toward the beginning of the pulse. The average currents (from 100–200 pulses) through the 8 pS calcium channel are shown. (B) The effect of nisoldipine on the relationship between the holding potential and the peak probability of the calcium channel being open at 0 mV. In the absence of nisoldipine, steady state inactivation was voltage dependent and can be described by the equation (solid curve), $1/(1 + \exp(V_m - V_{0.5})/k)$, with $k = 7.5$ mV and $V_{0.5} = -64$ mV. Nisoldipine (20 nM) shifted the curve in the hyperpolarized direction with the new $V_{0.5}$ being −76 mV and reduced the peak average current at −100 mV, with an apparent inhibition constant of 12.1 nM to the resting state. Filter, 300 Hz.

inactivation curves in various intact arteries. Furthermore, these findings indicate that the pharmacological characterization of vascular smooth muscle calcium channels requires, minimally, knowledge of V_m, k, and the position of the inactivation curve, as shown here.

The functional implications of our results are that small depolarizations of V_m will substantially increase DHP inhibition and that variations in the degree of channel inactivation by any factor (e.g., V_m) could have a profound impact on calcium influx and DHP inhibition. For example, the observation that the potency of DHP is increased[2] could simply be a reflection of slightly more depolarized resistance vessels.

REFERENCES

1. JANIS, R., *et al.* Adv. Drug Res. **16.** (In press.)
2. SHARMA, J. N., *et al.* 1984. Can. J. Pharmacol. **62:** 241.
3. WORLEY, J., *et al.* 1986. Proc. Nat. Acad. Sci. USA **83:** 5746.
4. BEAN, B. 1984. Proc. Nat. Acad. Sci. USA **81:** 6388.
5. BEVAN, J. A. & J. V. OSHER. 1972. Agents Actions **2:** 257.
6. MAKITA, Y., *et al.* 1983. Naunyn Schmiedeberg's Arch. Pharmacol. **324:** 302.

Historical Overview

Calcium Ion and Contractile Proteins

SETSURO EBASHI

National Institute for Physiological Sciences
Myodaiji, Okazaki 444, Japan

INTRODUCTION

The calcium ion is now widely accepted as the most fundamental regulator of intracellular processes of all living organisms. This important fact was first noticed and developed in muscle research, as listed in TABLE 1.

More than one century ago, Ringer made an epoch-making discovery, i.e., that Ca is necessary for maintaining the contractility of frog heart muscle.[1] Since a considerable part of Ca^{2+} affecting contractile proteins in the heart muscle is derived from the solution bathing the heart, Ringer's finding tacitly involved the present-day Ca concept, but it was not possible then to have such a view because of the scientific level at that time. The role of Ca was interpreted in a rather misleading way, i.e., that a subtle balance between Ca^{2+} and K^+ would be necessary for maintaining the physiological state of cardiac muscle.

Suggested by Ringer's discovery, the necessity of Ca^{2+} for smooth muscle contraction was reported at the beginning of this century.[2] The explanation of this observation naturally followed that of Ringer, and did not reach the truth about Ca.

Since then, these two kinds of muscle have never been prominent in the development of the Ca concept. Today's Ca concept has been derived entirely from studies on skeletal muscle.

HEILBRUNN'S POSITION

It is well known that the first person who clearly declared the essential role of Ca^{2+} in contractility was Heilbrunn.[3] His first experiment to show the action of Ca^{2+} was not very convincing[3]; substantial evidence for his postulation was later supplied by a Ca^{2+} injection experiment performed by Kamada and Kinosita[4] and Heilbrunn himself and Wiercinski.[5]

It must be emphasized, however, that experiments similar to those mentioned above had been carried out previously by several workers.[21,22] In spite of this, they did not claim the physiological role of Ca^{2+} in triggering muscle contraction. Perhaps these people never imagined that such a simple agent as Ca^{2+} could induce a mysterious physiological function. They might have agreed if electricity had been nominated as the direct triggering factor. In this connection, we are reminded of the historical fact that some physiologists stuck to the idea of electrical transmission at neuromuscular junctions of skeletal muscle for many years after the establishment of the chemical transmission mechanism.

DISCOVERY OF TROPONIN

Heilbrunn's proposal did not awaken the interest of muscle biochemists. They were more enthusiastically attracted by the fascinating idea of Albert Szent-Györgyi that the interaction of two distinct proteins, actin and myosin, in the presence of ATP is the mechanism underlying muscle contraction,[23,24] for which Ca^{2+} was not apparently required. No doubt the actomyosin system was one of the most remarkable events not

TABLE 1. Early Ca Research

Subjects	Date	References
Without Ca in bathing solution, no contraction of frog heart is observed	1883	1
Ca activates smooth muscle contraction	1901	2
Injured muscle fibers contract strongly in isotonic $CaCl_2$ (the first proposal of the Ca concept)	1940	3
Ca injection into myoplasm elicits local contracture or shortening of fibers	1943 1947	4 5
Muscle extract contains a factor that induces swelling of muscle homogenate in the presence of ATP (discovery of relaxing factor)	1951	6
EDTA mimics the relaxing factor	1954 1955	7 8
The relaxing factor is identical with Kielley-Meyerhof's microsomal ATPase	1955	9
Activation of myofibrillar ATPase and superprecipitation of natural actomyosin requires about 1 μM Ca^{2+}	1959 –61	10 11, 12
The relaxing factor, identified with sarcoplasmic reticulum, accumulates Ca in the presence of ATP; this activity can remove essential Ca^{2+} from the actomyosin system (the mechanism of the relaxing factor)	1960 –62	11–13
"Native tropomyosin" is essential for Ca^{2+} regulation	1963	14
Superprecipitation of cardiac natural actomyosin requires Ca^{2+} in the same manner as that of skeletal natural actomyosin	1964	15
Glycerinated muscle fibers and natural actomyosin of smooth muscle have the same Ca^{2+} sensitivity as that of skeletal and cardiac muscle contractile systems	1965	16, 17
Native tropomyosin is composed of tropomyosin and troponin, the Ca^{2+} receptive protein (discovery of troponin)	1965 1967	18, 19
Phosphorylase b kinase requires Ca^{2+} of around 1 μM for its activation (emancipation of Ca^{2+} from muscle contraction)	1967	20

only in muscle research, but also in biological sciences in general, as it was the first success in reconstructing important physiological functions on the molecular level. Overlooking the Ca^{2+} effects on the contractile proteins was due to the incredibly low concentrations of Ca^{2+} required for muscle contraction, a concentration that could not easily be achieved in those days.

As emphasized in previous review articles,[25,26] the Ca^{2+} concept was developed mainly by two groups working on "relaxing factors," i.e., Weber's group being concerned with EDTA, a chemical relaxing factor,[7,8] and Ebashi's group with a natural relaxing factor, identical with Kielley-Meyerhof's granular ATPase.[6,9] From today's point of view it might appear odd that most muscle biochemists were absorbed in the idea of a "soluble relaxing factor," an imaginary factor of small molecular weight, which was supposed to be produced from the relaxing factor in the presence of ATP and the production of which would be repressed by Ca^{2+}. This misdirection might have been partly due to the ambition of those biochemists to be the discoverer of a novel substance, but also due to the general feelings held by most biochemists at that time, i.e., that Ca^{2+} is an odd agent.

It was the discovery of troponin[18,19] that had an important biological significance in general; it introduced the concept of "Ca binding protein," or "Ca receptor protein," into biological science. From the viewpoint of muscle research, however, the discovery of "native tropomyosin"[14] prior to that of troponin had a greater impact. First of all, it challenged the contemporary idea of muscle biochemistry that two distinct proteins, viz., myosin and actin, should have represented the essential features of muscle contraction. Secondly, it revealed the function of tropomyosin, which had been discovered by Bailey as early as in 1946,[27] but the role of which had remained unknown. The fact that pure actomyosin was insensitive to Ca^{2+} appeared to those people who still believed in "soluble relaxing factor" that crude actomyosin preparations should have contained fragmented sarcoplasmic reticulum as a contaminant which could confer Ca^{2+} sensitivity on actomyosin by producing "soluble relaxing factor." Therefore, the presence of native tropomyosin in the contractile system as the third factor, in addition to myosin and actin, smashed the last hope of finding the "soluble relaxing factor."

SIGNIFICANCE OF Ca^{2+} ACTIVATION OF PHOSPHORYLASE b KINASE

The discovery of troponin had afforded a firm ground to the Ca concept, but people still believed that the Ca^{2+} action should be specific to muscle contraction: this idea was, in a sense, in accord with the belief of most people in those days that actin and myosin should be dedicated only to muscle contraction. However, Ebashi's group postulated a much wider role of Ca^{2+} and pursued the triggering role of Ca^{2+} in metabolic processes (cf. Reference 25). It was quite natural to think of glycolytic processes as the candidate, which are triggered simultaneously with the onset of contraction. Indeed, Ozawa *et al.* showed that phosphorylase b kinase was activated by Ca^{2+} in the same concentration range as that for contraction.[20] Furthermore, cyclic AMP stimulation of this enzyme was also shown to be dependent on Ca^{2+} (FIGURE 1).[28] These findings had three important meanings. First, such a common metabolic process as glycolysis was shown to be regulated by Ca^{2+}, indicating a much more universal role of Ca^{2+}, not confined to muscle contraction. Second, Ca^{2+} regulation seemed more fundamental than the cyclic AMP regulation. Third, this was the first demonstration of calmodulin-dependent reaction,[29] though at that time no one dreamed of such an important implication.

In spite of this, Ca^{2+} studies still could not get out of muscle tissue. The studies of troponin and Ca^{2+} activation of phosphorylase b kinase, however, stimulated Kakiuchi, who had been working on cyclic AMP metabolism, to find out about Ca^{2+} activation of brain phosphodiesterase[30] and isolation of Ca^{2+}-related activating factor.[31,32] Quite independently of this, Cheung, who had also been working on phosphodiesterase, reached the same factor.[33]

The factor isolated by Cheung as well as Kakiuchi was still in a preliminary stage in its chemical characterization. A little later Wang and his colleagues brought the factor to a homogeneous state, and showed that it was an acidic protein of 17K daltons with Ca^{2+} binding ability.[34,35]

Thus Ca^{2+} was completely liberated from the field of muscle and became the common property of all biological scientists. Further progress in the study of this factor, calmodulin, is well known to all and need not be described here (cf. References 36–38).

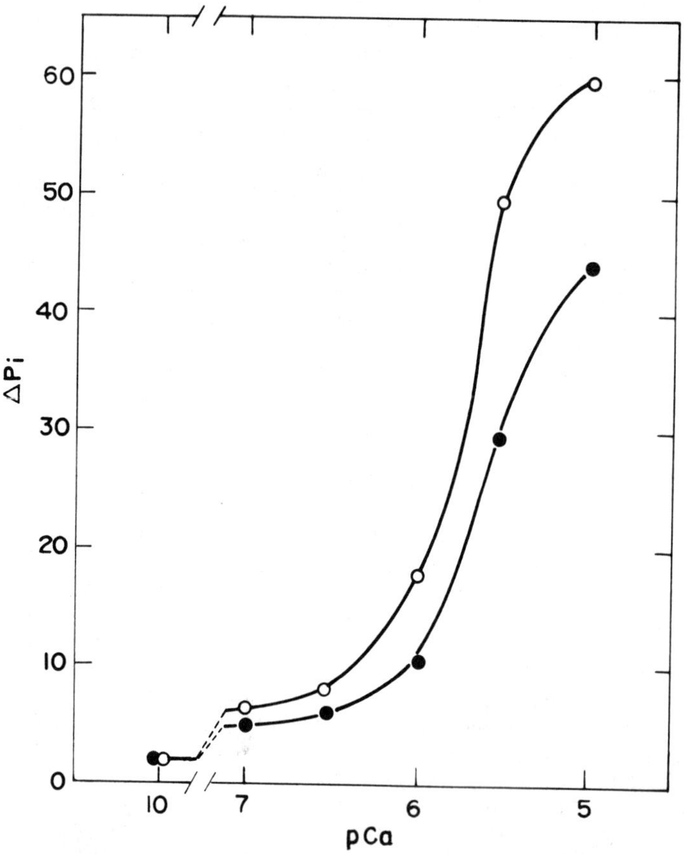

FIGURE 1. Ca^{2+} activation of phosphorylase b kinase from rabbit cardiac muscle in the presence and absence of cyclic AMP. Note that cyclic AMP–stimulated activity is also dependent on Ca^{2+}. For the experimental conditions, see Reference 28. (Reproduced from Reference 28.)

Although the discovery of calmodulin was made in nonmuscle tissue, it brought rich rewards to muscle research from which the Ca^{2+} concept emerged. One of the most important contributions was the role of Ca^{2+} regulation of smooth muscle contraction as the Ca^{2+} receptive site.

A few more words may be said about smooth muscle regulation. The majority of smooth-muscle workers believe that Ca^{2+} activation of myosin light chain kinase should be the activating mechanism (cf. Reference 39), but a small group has not yet accepted this view and believes that an actin-linked factor, leiotonin, may be a regulatory factor in collaboration with calmodulin.[40] In this connection, two things may be noted. First, myosin light chain kinase is an actin-binding protein. Secondly, caldesmon, a calmodulin-binding protein, isolated by Kakiuchi and his colleagues as an actin-binding factor in the absence of Ca^{2+},[41] is claimed to play some regulatory role in smooth muscle regulation.

MYOSIN-LINKED SYSTEMS

The troponin-tropomyosin system seemed to be a mechanism common to all kinds of muscle, at least to those concerned with body movement, but Kendrick-Jones *et al.* showed that molluscan striated muscle did not contain troponin and that the Ca-binding sites resided in the myosin molecule.[42] This regulatory system, widely called the "myosin-linked system," was later shown to be widely distributed in the animal kingdom, particularly in the protostomia.[43]

Lehman has insisted, however, that molluscan muscle also contains troponin or a troponinlike protein(s).[44] In partial agreement with his view, an actin-linked factor, without which Ca^{2+} regulation does not fully operate, has been found.[45] Furthermore, troponin, the subunits of which can be hybridized with those of rabbit skeletal troponin, has been isolated from nematodes.[46] It appears that troponin has a much wider distribution than once thought; perhaps the development of protease inhibitors contributed to the success of its isolation from protease-rich tissues.

Ca regulation of smooth muscle, which is believed to be mediated by the phosphorylation of myosin light chain, is also a myosin-linked type, but usually it is not called a "myosin-linked system." In the case of smooth muscle, too, the presence of actin-linked regulation has been asserted as mentioned above.

Ca regulation in slime mold,[47,48] described more in detail in the next section, is also a kind of myosin-linked regulation. In this case, the presence of an actin-linked regulation is also noted (see below).

Generally speaking, muscles regulated by myosin-linked systems in a wide sense seem to contain also an actin-linked regulatory system, whereas, in the case of vertebrate skeletal muscle (perhaps also in cardiac muscle), no myosin-linked regulation has been found. It is certain that vertebrate skeletal muscle (and cardiac muscle, too) contains a strong light chain kinase[49] and phosphorylation of light chain certainly takes place under physiological conditions,[50] but this phosphorylation does not play a significant physiological part.

ACTOMYOSIN IN CELL MOTILITY OTHER THAN MUSCLE CONTRACTION

Actomyosin is responsible not only for muscle contraction but also for cytoplasmic streaming of plants and ameboid movement of various kinds of cells. Slime mold is a very unique organism, i.e., it shows morphological conversion from plasmodial type, which exhibits vigorous cytoplasmic streaming like some plants, to ameboid type, which is close to ameba, a primitive animal, and *vice versa*. This might be considered as a kind of conversion from vegetable kingdom to animal kingdom.

It was controversial whether Ca^{2+} would activate or repress cytoplasmic streaming. Although not finally settled, the opinion that the streaming is repressed by Ca has gradually become dominant.[51] Then, how is this movement related to Ca regulation of the actomyosin system?

Kohama and his colleagues elaborated this problem and finally came to the conclusion that Ca^{2+} inhibits the actin-myosin-ATP interaction of both types of slime mold.[48,52–54]

The mode of Ca regulation was different from muscle to muscle, but in any case the final consequence induced by Ca^{2+} was activation and people had believed that Ca should be an activator of all contractile systems. Now we had an entirely different case—Ca^{2+} acting as a real repressor. Thus Ca^{2+} regulation is quite diverse in its modes of action.

The Ca-binding site of slime mold resides in the 14K light chain. Different from the expectation, this light chain is phylogenetically different from EDTA light chain of molluscan muscle or phosphorylatable light chains, but is akin to alkali light chain of skeletal muscle. It should also be stressed that the light chain is common for plasmodial and amebal types, whereas the heavy chain and the other light chain are quite different between two types of slime mold.[55,56]

More interestingly, 14K light chain exists also in cytoplasm (this means that it exists more abundantly than the heavy chain) and seems to exert Ca^{2+} regulation through the actin filament as briefly mentioned before.[57]

Thus Physarum seems to have all the aspects of Ca^{2+} regulation of muscle in a very primitive manner.

Recently Yanagida *et al.* have shown that under specified conditions where almost no load or resistance is present, the myosin head shifts almost 10 times faster than the maximum speed of contraction, and in this situation, one mole ATP allows the myosin head to displace a distance of more than 10 actin molecules.[58] This means that the speed of mutual dislocation of actin and myosin filaments could achieve the same level as that of cytoplasmic streaming.

Thus muscle contraction and cytoplasmic streaming, though very different in their apparent expression, seem to be based on the same process. The mechanism of Ca^{2+} regulation should be reconsidered in this new light.

CONCLUDING REMARKS

The mechanism of how Ca^{2+} regulates the actin-myosin-ATP interaction is very different from tissue to tissue. Initiated by the troponin-tropomyosin system, different types of Ca^{2+} regulation have appeared one by one. Recently, an unexpected type of regulation has been found in the actomyosin system of the slime mold, where Ca^{2+} represses the myosin-actin-ATP interaction, almost in an opposite way to conventional belief.

Since Ca^{2+} regulation is no longer confined to muscle but is in the matter of all the living organisms, it is very likely that the more we learn about Ca^{2+}, the more we will realize the diversity of the mode of Ca^{2+} action. In spite of such a diversity, there is a common feature underlying Ca^{2+} regulation, i.e., cytoplasm is virtually devoid of Ca^{2+} in the resting state.

It is, therefore, a fascinating question as to why and how the living organism created such an interior milieu, in spite of the abundant presence of Ca in the medium outside the cell, i.e., the sea when life was born. It is also an interesting problem from the evolutionary point of view as to how the living organism has developed a great variety of subtle devices to utilize Ca^{2+}. These important aspects should be more rightly appreciated in ongoing evolutionary studies.

REFERENCES

1. RINGER, S. 1883. A further contribution regarding the influence of the blood on the contraction of the heart. J. Physiol. **4:** 29–42.
2. STILES, P. G. 1903. On the rhythmic activity of the oesophagus and the influence upon it of various media. Am. J. Physiol. **5:** 338–357.
3. HEILBRUNN, L. V. 1940. The action of calcium on muscle protoplasm. Physiol. Zool. **13:** 88–94.
4. KAMADA, T. & H. KINOSITA. 1943. Disturbances initiated from naked surface of muscle protoplasm. Jpn. J. Zool. **10:** 469–493.
5. HEILBRUNN, L. V. & F. J. WIERCINSKI. 1947. The action of various cations on muscle propoplams. J. Cell. Comp. Physiol. **29:** 15–32.
6. MARSH, B. B. 1951. A factor modifying muscle fibre syneresis. Nature **167:** 1065–1066.
7. BOZLER, E. 1954. Relaxation in extracted muscle fibers. J. Gen. Physiol. **38:** 149–159.
8. WATANABE, S. 1955. Relaxing effects of EDTA on glyceroltreated muscle fibers. Arch. Biochem. Biophys. **54:** 559–562.
9. KUMAGAI, H., S. EBASHI & F. TAKEDA. 1955. Essential relaxing factor in muscle other than myokinase and creatine phosphokinase. Nature **176:** 166.
10. WEBER, A. 1959. On the role of calcium in the activity of adenosine 5′-triphosphate hydrolysis by actomyosin. J Biol. Chem. **234:** 2764–2769.
11. EBASHI, S. 1960. Calcium binding and relaxation in the actomyosin system. J. Biochem. **48:** 150–151.
12. EBASHI, S. 1961. Calcium binding activity of vesicular relaxing factor. J. Biochem. **50:** 236–244.
13. EBASHI, S. & F. LIPMANN. 1962. Adenosine triphosphate–linked concentration of calcium ions in a particulate fraction of rabbit muscle. J. Cell Biol. **14:** 389–400.
14. EBASHI, S. 1963. Third component participating in the superprecipitation of 'natural actomyosin'. Nature London **200:** 1010.
15. OTSUKA, M., F. EBASHI & S. IMAI. 1964. Cardiac myosin B and calcium ions. J. Biochem. **55:** 192–194.
16. FILO, R. S., D. F. BOHR & J. C. RUEGG. 1965. Glycerinated skeletal and smooth muscle calcium and magnesium dependence. Science **147:** 1581–1583.
17. IWAKURA, H. 1965. New contractile protein of smooth muscle. I. Native tropomyosin from smooth muscle. J. Med. Sci. Tokyo **73:** 49–57.
18. EBASHI, S. & A. KODAMA. 1965. A new protein factor promoting aggregation of tropomyosin. J. Biochem. **58:** 107–108.
19. EBASHI, S., F. EBASHI & A. KODAMA. 1967. Troponin as the Ca^{++}-receptive protein in the contractile system. J. Biochem. **62:** 137–138.
20. OZAWA, E., K. HOSOI & S. EBASHI. 1967. Reversible stimulation of muscle phosphorylase b kinase by low concentration of calcium ion. J. Biochem. **61:** 531–533.
21. CHAMBERS, R. & H. P. HALE. 1932. The formation of ice in protoplasm. Proc. R. Soc. London Ser. B **110:** 336–352.
22. KEIL, E. M. & F. J. M. SICHEL. 1936. The injection of aqueous solutions, including acetylcholine, into the isolated muscle fiber. Biol. Bull. **71:** 402.
23. SZENT-GYÖRGYI, A. 1942. *In* Studies from Szeged: Myosin and Muscular Contraction. S. Karger & R. Gergely, Eds. **1:** 1–72. Karger. Basel & New York.
24. SZENT-GYÖRGYI, A. 1947. The Chemistry of Muscular Contraction. Academic Press. New York, N.Y.
25. EBASHI, S. & M. ENDO. 1968. Calcium ion and muscle contraction. Prog. Biophys. Mol. Biol. **18:** 123–183.
26. EBASHI, S. 1980. Regulation of muscle contraction (Croonian Lecture, 1979). Proc. R. Soc. London Ser. B **207:** 259–286.
27. BAILEY, K. 1946. Tropomyosin a new asymmetric protein component of the muscle. Nature **157:** 368–369.
28. OZAWA, E. & S. EBASHI. 1967. Requirement of Ca ion for the stimulating effect of cyclic 3′,5′-AMP on muscle phospholylase b kinase. J. Biochem. **62:** 285–286.
29. COHEN, P., A. BURCHELL, J. G. FOULKES, P. T. W. COHEN, T. C. VANAMAN & A. C.

NAIRN. 1978. Identification of the Ca^{2+}-dependent modulator protein as the fourth subunit of rabbit skeletal muscle phosphorylase kinase. FEBS Lett. **92:** 287–293.
30. KAKIUCHI, S. & R. YAMAZAKI. 1970. Stimulation of the activity of cyclic 3′,5′-nucleotide phosphodiesterase by calcium ion. Proc. Jpn. Acad. **46:** 387–392.
31. KAKIUCHI, S., R. YAMAZAKI & H. NAKAJIMA. 1969. Studies on brain phosphodiesterase (2). Bull. Jpn. Neurochem. Soc. **8:** 17–20.
32. KAKIUCHI, S., R. YAMAZAKI & H. NAKAJIMA. 1970. Properties of a heat stable phosphodiesterase activating factor isolated from brain extract. Proc. Jpn. Acad. **46:** 587–592.
33. CHEUNG, W. Y. 1970. Cyclic 3′,5′-nucleotide phosphodiesterase: demonstration of an activator. Biochem. Biophys. Res. Commun. **38:** 533–538.
34. TEO, T. S., T. H. WANG & J. H. WANG. 1973. Purification and properties of the protein activator of bovine heart cycle adenosine 3′, 5′-monophosphate phosphodiesterase. J. Biol. Chem. **248:** 588–595.
35. TEO, T. S. & J. H. WANG. 1973. Mechanism of activation of a cyclic adenosine 3′:5′-monophosophate phosphodiesterase from bovine heart by calcium ions. J. Biol. Chem. **248:** 5950–5955.
36. CHEUNG, W. Y., Ed. 1980. Calcium and Cell Function. **1.** Calmodulin. Academic Press. New York, N.Y.
37. KLEE, C. B. & T. C. VANAMAN. 1982. Calmodulin. Adv. Protein Chem. **35:** 213–321.
38. EBASHI, S. & Y. OGAWA. 1987. Troponin C and calmodulin as calcium receptors: mode of action and sensitivity to drugs. *In* Handbook of Experimental Pharmacology. P. F. Baker, Ed. **83:** 31–56. Springer Verlag. Berlin, FRG.
39. HARTSHORNE, D. J. & R. F. SIEMAMKOWSKI. 1981. Regulation of smooth muscle actomyosin. Annu. Rev. Physiol. **43:** 519–530.
40. EBASHI, S., T. MIKAWA, H. KUWAYAMA, M. SUZUKI, H. IKEMOTO, Y. ISHIZAKI & R. KOGA. Ca^{2+} regulation in smooth muscle; dissociation of myosin light chain kinase activity from activation of actin-myosin interaction. *In* Smooth Muscle Contraction Symposium. N. L. Stephens *et al.*, Eds. Alan R. Liss, Inc. New York, N.Y. (In press.)
41. SOBUE, K., K. MORIMOTO, M. INUI, K. KANDA & S. KAKIUCHI. 1982. Control of actin-myosin interaction of gizzard smooth muscle by calmodulin- and caldesmonlinked flip-flop mechanism. Biomed. Res. **3**(2): 188–196.
42. KENDRICK-JONES, J., W. LEHMAN & A. G. SZENT-GYÖRGYI. 1970. Regulation in molluscan muscle. J. Mol. Biol. **54:** 313–326.
43. LEHMAN, W. & A. G. SZENT-GYÖRGYI. 1975. Regulation of muscular contraction, distribution of actin control and myosin control in the animal kingdom. J. Gen. Physiol. **66:** 1–30.
44. LEHMAN, W. 1981. Thin-filament-linked regulation in molluscan muscles. Biochim. Biophys. Acta **668:** 349–356.
45. YAZAWA, Y. 1985. Actin-linked regulation in scallop striated muscle. Proc. Jpn. Acad. **61:** 497–500.
46. KIMURA, K., T. TANAKA, H. NAKAE, & T. OBINATA. Troponin from nematode: purification and characterization of troponin from ascaris body wall muscle. Comp. Biochem. Physiol. (In press.)
47. HATANO, S. 1970. Specific effect of Ca^{2+} on movement of plasmodial fragment obtained by caffeine treatment. Exp. Cell Res. **61:** 199–203.
48. KOHAMA, K. & S. EBASHI. 1986. Inhibitory Ca^{2+}-regulation of the Physarum actomyosin system. *In* The Molecular Biology of *Physarum polycephalum.* W. F. Dove, *et al.*, Eds.: 175–190. Plenum Publishing Corp. New York, N.Y.
49. PIRES, E. M. B. & S. V. PERRY. 1977. Purification and properties of myosin light chain kinase from fast skeletal muscle. Biochem. J. **167:** 137–146.
50. BÁRÁNY, K., M. BÁRÁNY, J. M. GILLIS & M. J. KUSHMERICK. 1980. Myosin light chain phosphorylation during the contraction cycle of frog muscle. Fed. Proc. **39:** 1547–1551.
51. YOSHIMOTO, Y. & N. KAMIYA. 1984. ATP and calcium-controlled contraction in a saponin model of *Physarum polycephalum.* Cell Struct. Funct. **9:** 135–141.
52. KOHAMA, K., K. KOBAYASHI & S. MITANI. 1980. Effects of Ca ion and ADP on superprecipitation of myosin B from slime mold, *Physarum polycephalum.* Proc. Jpn. Acad. **56:** 591–596.

53. KOHAMA, K. 1981. Co-dependent inhibitory factor for the myosin-actin-ATP interaction of *Physarum polycephalum*. J. Biochem. **90:** 1829–1832.
54. KOHAMA, K. 1985. Inhibitory Ca^{2+}-control of movement of beads coated with Physarum myosin along actin-cables in chara internodal cells. Protoplasma **129:** 88–91.
55. KOHAMA, K. & H. TAKANO-OHMURO. 1984. Stage specific myosins from amoeba and plasmodium of slime mold, *Physarum polycephalum*. Proc. Jpn. Acad. **60:** 431–434.
56. KOHAMA, K., H. TAKANO-OHMURO, T. TANAKA, Y. YAMAGUCHI & T. KOHAMA. 1986. Isolation and characterization of myosin from amoebae of *Physarum polycephalum*. J. Biol. Chem. **261:** 8022–8027.
57. KOHAMA, K., T. Q. P. UYEDA, H. TAKANO-OHMURO, T. TANAKA, T. YAMAGUCHI, K. MARUYAMA & T. KOHAMA. 1985. Ca^{2+}-binding light chain of Physarum myosin confers inhibitory Ca^{2+}-sensitivity on actin-myosin-ATP interaction via actin. Proc. Jpn Acad. **61:** 501–505.
58. YANAGIDA, T., T. ARATA & F. OOSAWA. 1985. Sliding distance of actin filament induced by a myosin crossbridge during one ATP hydrolysis cycle. Nature **316:** 366–369.

Vascular Smooth Muscle Sarcoplasmic Reticulum[a]

Function and Mechanisms of Ca^{2+} Release

C. VAN BREEMEN, K. SAIDA, H. YAMAMOTO,
K. HWANG, AND C. TWORT

Department of Pharmacology
University of Miami School of Medicine
Post Office Box 016189
Miami, Florida 33101

The sarcoplasmic reticulum (SR) of smooth muscle is a membranous tubular system that has components closely underlying the surface membrane as well as deeper portions that are contiguous with the rough endoplasmic reticulum and the nuclear envelope.[1] Its functions are (1) to transport Ca^{2+} actively from the cytoplasm into its lumen via a Ca^{2+} ATPase in order to produce relaxation, (2) to release its luminal Ca^{2+} rapidly into the cytoplasm upon smooth muscle stimulation by neurotransmitters and autocoids, and (3) to buffer Ca^{2+} entry from the extracellular space into the myoplasm. In this presentation we explore the mechanisms of Ca^{2+} release from the SR and investigate the SR's function in amplifying and dampening the Ca^{2+} influx.

Ca^{2+}-INDUCED Ca^{2+} RELEASE

The development of the technique of saponin skinning of smooth muscle cells which permeabilizes the plasmalemma while preserving the integrity of the SR has made it possible to study the Ca^{2+} transport mechanisms of the *in situ* SR.[2,3] Since caffeine has been shown to induce Ca^{2+} release from isolated skeletal SR,[4] it has been used as an SR marker in skinned muscle. This appears to be valid also for smooth muscle where it has been shown to release the same intracellular Ca^{2+} fraction that is sensitive to norepinephrine (NE), but not to affect mitochondrial Ca^{2+} content.[5–7] Thus, using the caffeine contraction of skinned vascular smooth muscle, bathed in a Ca^{2+}-free medium, as a measure of SR Ca^{2+} content, it was found that a short period of elevated Ca^{2+} concentration could partially deplete the SR.[8,9] FIGURE 1 shows this decrease in SR Ca^{2+} content upon elevation of the ambient Ca^{2+} concentration, as well as the stimulation of this effect by cAMP and its inhibition by Mg^{2+} and procaine.[10] These data show that the mechanism of Ca^{2+}-induced Ca^{2+} release (CICR) that has been reported for skeletal and cardiac SR is also present in vascular smooth muscle.[11,12]

Ryanodine, another marker for the Ca^{2+}-activated SR Ca^{2+} channels,[13,14] has been postulated to inhibit Ca^{2+} release in smooth muscle.[15] FIGURE 2 presents evidence for the presence of ryanodine-sensitive sites in rabbit aortic smooth muscle; it also reveals that the mechanism of action of ryanodine is a slow release of Ca^{2+} from the SR rather than an inhibition of release.[16,17] Application of ryanodine induces a slow release of

[a]The work presented from our laboratory was supported by National Institutes of Health grant HL 29467, and Charles Twort was supported by an M.R.C. Travelling Fellowship.

labeled Ca^{2+} from these smooth muscle cells; this depletes the source from which norepinephrine releases Ca^{2+} during a subsequent application. FIGURE 2 shows that the Ca^{2+} released by ryanodine is equal in quantity to the subsequent reduction in release by norepinephrine; this accounts for the delayed inhibition of the norepinephrine contraction by ryanodine, which occurs in Ca^{2+}-free solution when only SR Ca^{2+} is available for activation.

In spite of the ample evidence for CICR in vascular smooth muscle, it has not yet been possible to demonstrate its physiological role. One critical question addressed in FIGURE 3 is whether CICR, which is observed in skinned fibers, contributes to Ca^{2+}

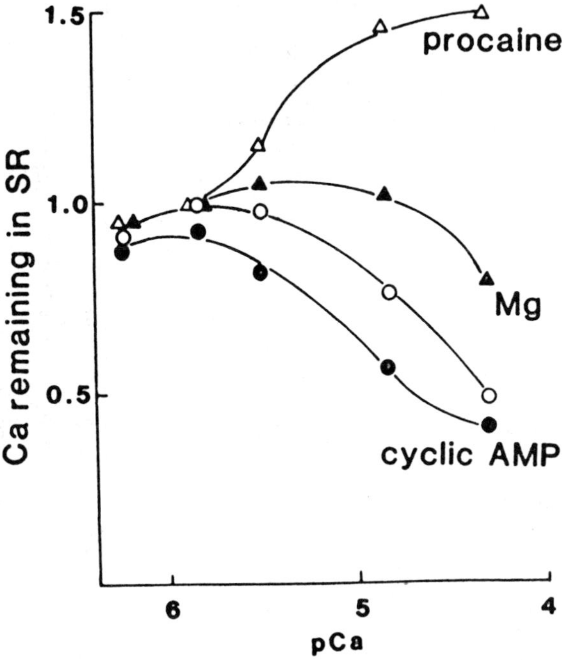

FIGURE 1. Ca^{2+}-induced Ca^{2+} release from the SR in skinned smooth muscle. The saponin-skinned smooth muscle was loaded with 10^{-6} M Ca^{2+} for 3 minutes and then exposed to various concentrations of Ca^{2+} (pCa) with or without 10 mM procaine, 10 mM Mg^{2+}, and 10^{-5} M cyclic AMP for 30 seconds. The amount of Ca^{2+} remaining in the SR was estimated by the contraction induced by 25 mM caffeine in the presence of 0.1 mM EGTA.

activation during membrane depolarization and stimulated Ca^{2+} influx in intact muscle. In order to test this, we investigated the effect of Ca^{2+} influx, stimulated by high K^+ depolarization, on the Ca^{2+} content of the SR in the small branches of rabbit mesenteric arteries. These vessels contract and relax rapidly upon applying and removing 80 mM K^+, and are therefore well suited for rapid fluctuations in tension and Ca^{2+} uptake. FIGURE 3 shows that even a few seconds of depolarization loads the SR with Ca^{2+} which sheds doubt on the assumption that in smooth muscle Ca^{2+} entry releases SR Ca^{2+}, or that depolarization could be a stimulus for physiological SR Ca^{2+} release.[3,18] Norepinephrine (NE), however, which is known to release SR Ca^{2+} even in

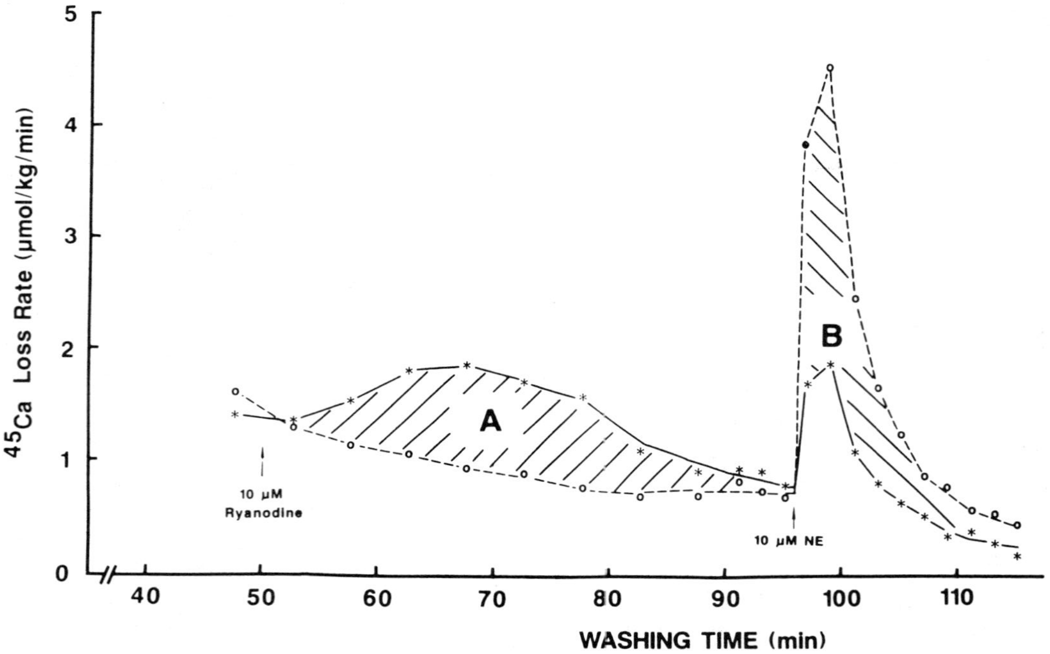

FIGURE 2. Effects of NE (10 μM), and sequential ryanodine (10 μM) and NE on ^{45}Ca efflux from the rabbit aorta. Ryanodine (asterisks) caused a small prolonged increase in ^{45}Ca efflux, whereas NE caused a large transient stimulation of ^{45}Ca efflux (circles). The 10 μM NE-induced ^{45}Ca loss rate (98–116 minutes) was suppressed by ryanodine treatment (asterisks). The cumulative ^{45}Ca loss of both groups during both treatments (50–116 minutes) was identical; 76.1 ± 2.6 μM kg in the absence of ryanodine and 77.9 ± 2.2 μM kg in its presence. The ryanodine-induced stimulation of ^{45}Ca loss (area A, 19.5 ± 1.9 μM kg) was similar to the ryanodine-induced inhibition on NE-stimulated ^{45}Ca loss (area B, 17.7 ± 2.1 μM kg). The results presented are means of six experiments. The standard errors of the mean on ^{45}Ca efflux rates are less than 5% and are not shown for clarity.

the absence of extracellular Ca^{2+}, is seen to cause a transient decrease in SR Ca^{2+} content. The fact that the SR Ca^{2+} recovers after prolonged norepinephrine exposure, is thought to be due to the presence of the second component of SR, which, intact fibers, releases Ca^{2+} upon stimulation by caffeine but not by norepinephrine.[19] This second, probably deeper, SR component is therefore thought to function mainly in relaxation, and refilling the more superficial Ca^{2+}-releasing SR component.

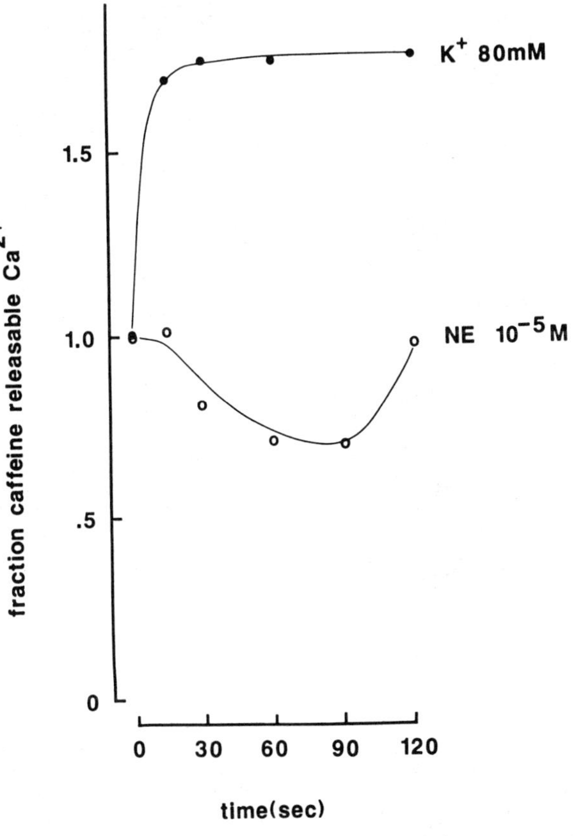

FIGURE 3. The amount of Ca^{2+} remaining in the SR of mesenteric artery smooth muscle after exposure to 80 mM K^+ (filled circles) or 10^{-5} M NE (open circles) for various time periods. After the application of agonist for various time periods the muscle was bathed in Ca^{2+}-free PSS containing 2 mM EGTA for 2 minutes; then 25 mM caffeine in the presence of 2 mM EGTA was applied in order to estimate the amount of Ca^{2+} in the SR.

INOSITOL-1,4,5-TRISPHOSPHATE (IP_3) INDUCED Ca^{2+} RELEASE

The discovery that IP_3 is generated upon receptor activation and can release Ca^{2+} from the endoplasmic reticulum in nonmuscle cells constituted a major breakthrough in the field of excitation-function coupling.[20,21] The same Ca^{2+}-release mechanism has subsequently been identified in permeabilized smooth muscle.[22-25] FIGURE 4 shows an

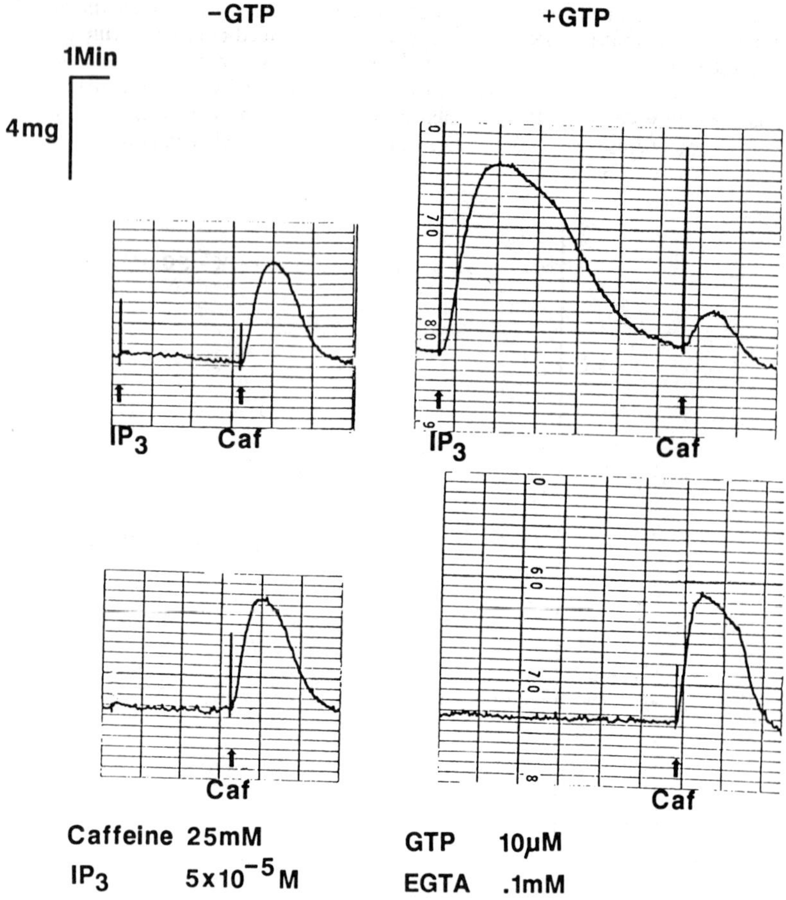

FIGURE 4. IP_3-induced Ca^{2+} release from the SR in a skinned vascular smooth muscle. After the SR was loaded with Ca^{2+} by bathing the skinned preparation in the Ca^{2+}-loading solution with 4×10^{-7} M Ca^{2+} for 3 minutes, the skinned preparation was bathed in the relaxing solution with 0.1 mM EGTA. Left: application of 5×10^{-5} M IP_3 (upper) and control experiment (lower). Right: application of 5×10^{-5} M IP_3 in the presence of 10 μM GTP (upper) and control experiment (lower). The amount of Ca^{2+} in the SR was estimated by application of 25 mM caffeine.

IP_3-induced contraction in saponin-treated skinned mesenteric artery. The contraction requires GTP or the nonhydrolyzable GTP analogue GppNHp as a cofactor, suggesting that a GTP binding protein may be involved in the transduction of receptor activation by IP_3 to the opening of Ca^{2+} release channels in the SR (Saida & van Breemen, *Biochemical and Biophysical Research Communications,* in press). However, we have not ruled out the possibility that GTP stimulates local production of IP_3 by activating phospholipase C in the saponin-skinned fibers or that a GTP-dependent kinase is involved in smooth muscle SR Ca^{2+} release.

We have found that the quantitative and kinetic aspects of SR Ca^{2+} release could be more accurately studied in saponin-skinned monolayers of primary cultured smooth muscle cells[23,26] rather than in skinned smooth muscle bundles. FIGURE 5 illustrates the dependence on ambient free Ca^{2+} concentration of the ATP-dependent and IP_3-sensitive Ca^{2+} fractions of the skinned cultured smooth muscle. In this preparation, the SR, which is sensitive to IP_3 and insensitive to Na^+-azide, is half-maximally loaded with Ca^{2+} at an ambient Ca^{2+} concentration of 300 nM; this is near the middle of the range over which Ca^{2+} fluctuates under physiological conditions.[27,28] Mitochondria take up Ca^{2+} only at 10× higher Ca^{2+} concentrations[26] than are required for SR. The relatively lower procaine sensitivity of IP_3-induced Ca^{2+} release illustrated in FIGURE 6 suggests that this mechanism is distinct from CICR since procaine is known to inhibit CICR (FIGURE 1). FIGURE 6 demonstrates that the IP_3 concentration necessary for the release of half the SR Ca^{2+} content is 1.7 μM. Addition of GTP to the assay mixture

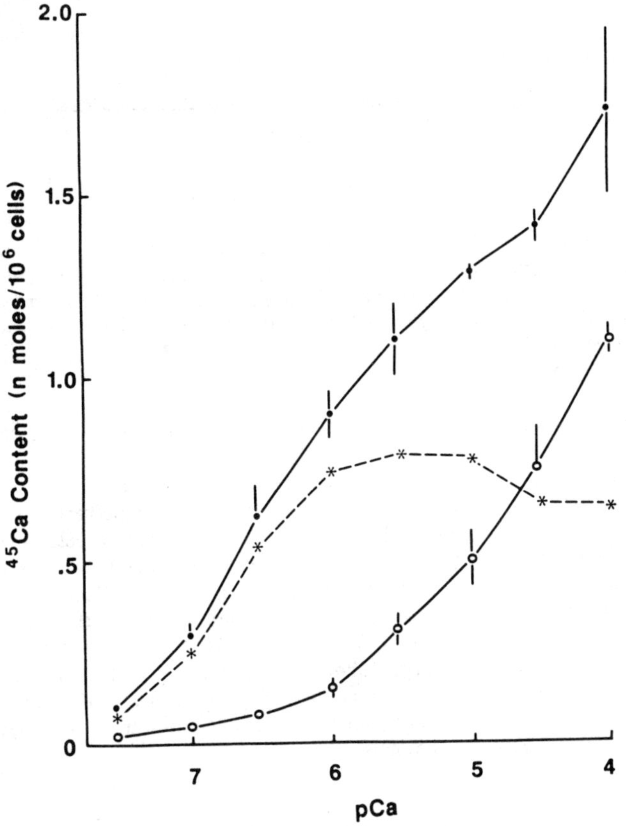

FIGURE 5. IP_3-releasable ^{45}Ca uptake at various concentrations of free Ca^{2+}. The skinned cells were loaded with ^{45}Ca at various concentrations of free Ca^{2+} (pCa, abscissa) for 20 minutes (see Reference 7) and subsequently exposed to 100 μM of IP_3 in the same solution for 1 minute. The IP_3-releasable ^{45}Ca uptake (asterisks) was determined as the difference between ^{45}Ca uptake in the control cells (filled circles) and that in the cells exposed to IP_3 (open circles). Each point and bar represent the mean and the standard deviation from three independent experiments.

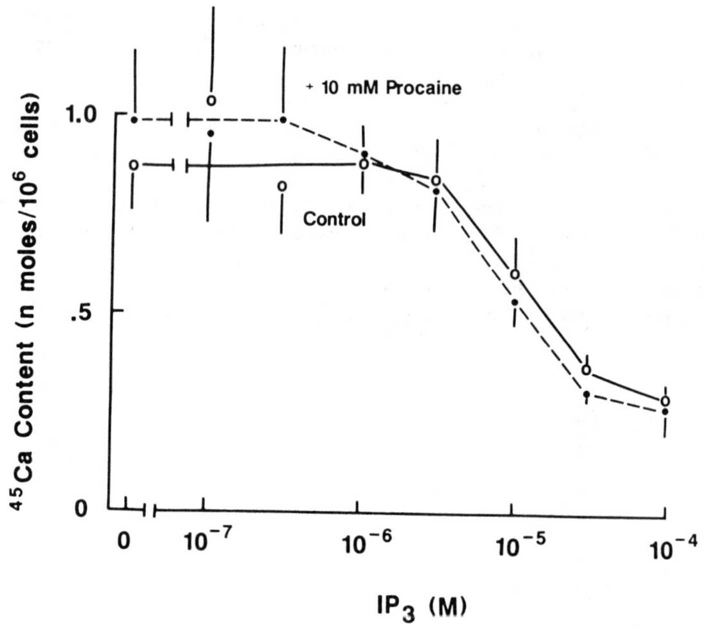

FIGURE 6. Effect of 10 mM procaine on IP_3-induced Ca^{2+} release. The skinned cells were loaded with ^{45}Ca in 1 μM of free Ca^{2+} for 20 minutes and incubated with various concentrations of IP_3 for 1 minute in the presence of 10 mM of procaine (open circles). Procaine was omitted in the control cells (filled circles). Each point and bar represent the mean and the standard deviation from three experiments.

further reduces this ED_{50} to 0.8 μM, which is well within a physiologically plausible range.

In order to examine the rates of Ca^{2+} release from the SR, uncomplicated by the activity of the plasmalemmal Ca^{2+} ATPase, we performed unidirectional ^{45}Ca efflux experiments on previously labeled skinned cultured smooth muscle cells, an example of which is illustrated in FIGURE 7. It can be seen that under nonstimulated control conditions, the efflux of ^{45}Ca from the sarcoplasmic reticulum proceeds in an exponential fashion with a rate constant of 0.05 $minute^{-1}$. IP_3 was the most effective in stimulating ^{45}Ca efflux, releasing approximately 90% of the SR at a maximal rate of 2 $minute^{-1}$. Compartmental analysis showed that caffeine and ATP released from 80–90% of the SR at slower rates. Since the ATP-induced Ca^{2+} release is sensitive to procaine, it is assumed, as has been suggested for skeletal muscle SR, that ATP and Ca^{2+} activate the same Ca^{2+} channels.

CYCLIC NUCLEOTIDES

A number of hormones modulate smooth muscle function through the intracellular messengers cAMP and cGMP. Cyclic AMP has been reported to enhance CICR in skinned fibers and Ca^{2+} release during the initial phase of norepinephrine contraction in intact vascular smooth muscle.[9] However, the main effect of cAMP on arterial tone is to cause relaxation through activation of the SR Ca^{2+} pump, presumably by a stimulation of phosphorylation of phospholamban.[29,30] In addition to its effect on cytoplasmic Ca^{2+} concentration, cAMP stimulates phosphorylation of myosin light chain kinase, resulting in a lower affinity of this enzyme for the calmodulin-Ca^{2+} complex. The significance of this latter process with respect to tension regulation of intact smooth muscle is as yet unclear.[31]

The recent discoveries of atrial natriuretic peptides (ANP) and endothelium-derived relaxing factor (EDRF), which activate particulate and soluble guanylate cyclase respectively, have focused interest in the second messenger cGMP. Since ANP has been reported to inhibit intracellular Ca^{2+} release,[32] we tested the effect of cGMP

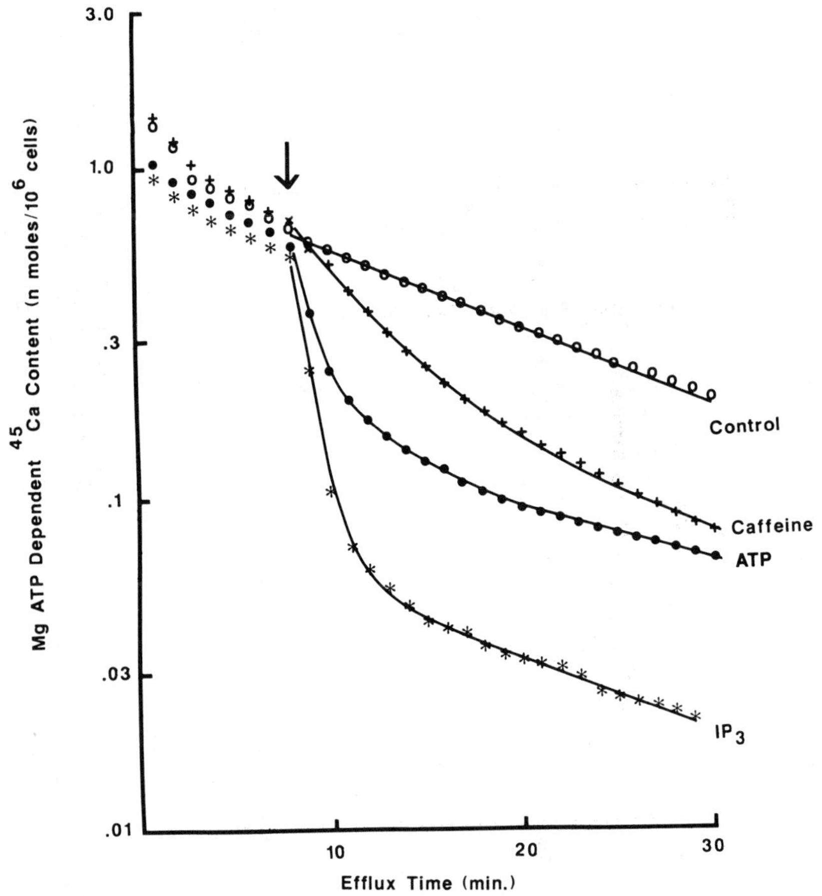

FIGURE 7. Free ATP–induced Ca^{2+} release in the absence of $MgCl_2$. The skinned cells were loaded with ^{45}Ca in 1 μM free Ca^{2+} for 20 minutes and then washed with the efflux solution containing no ATP and no $MgCl_2$. The efflux solution was changed every 1 minute. At 8 minutes the following additions were made: 25 mM caffeine (crosses), 3 mM ATP (filled circles), and 10 mM IP_3 (asterisks). No addition was made to the control (open circles). The MgATP-dependent ^{45}Ca content was plotted as a function of efflux time. Data are the means of two experiments.

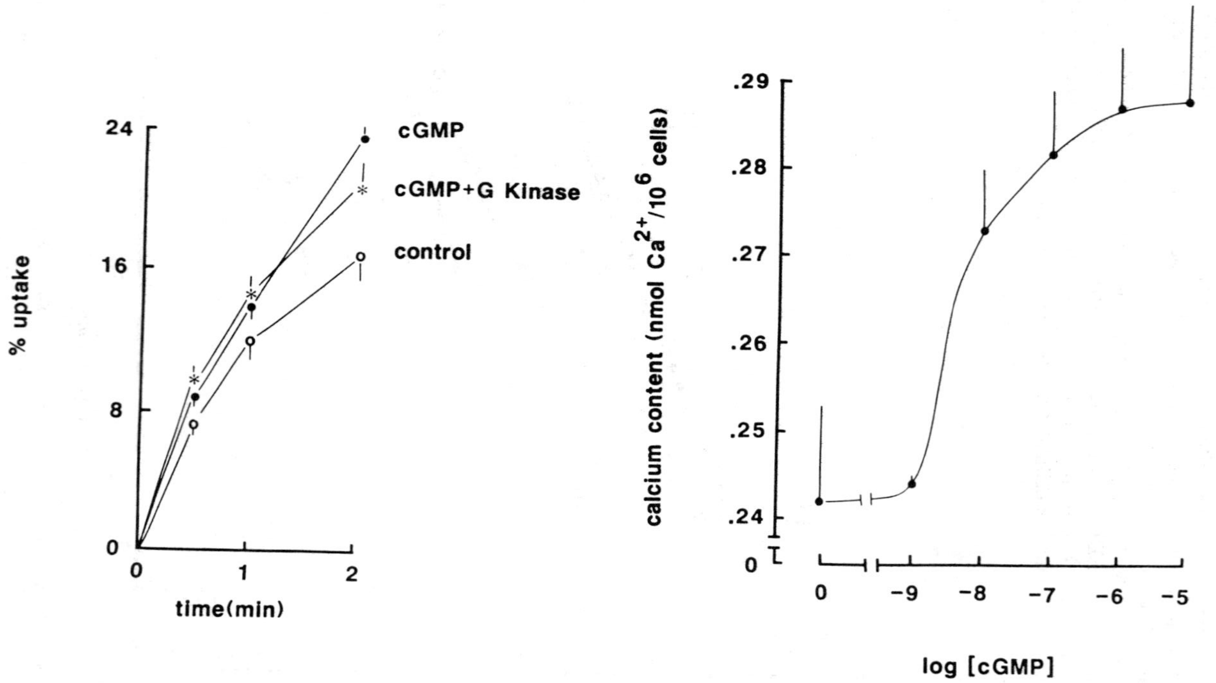

FIGURE 8. Effect of cGMP on Ca^{2+} uptake by skinned monolayers of cultured rat aortic smooth muscle cells. Left: Time course of Ca^{2+} uptake (expressed as percent of maximum uptake at 20 minutes) in the absence of cGMP (open circles) and in the presence of cGMP 1 μM (filled circles), and of cGMP 1 μM together with cGMP-dependent protein kinase 10 nM (asterisks); n = 6–9. (cGMP-dependent protein kinase was the generous gift of Dr. T. Lincoln, University of South Alabama). Right: Dose response of initial Ca^{2+} uptake to cGMP. Ca^{2+} content was measured after 2 minutes of uptake, with varying doses of cGMP (M); n = 6.

on the IP_3-induced Ca release from the SR of skinned cultured aortic smooth muscle cells. We could demonstrate no effect of cGMP on the release of Ca^{2+} from the SR, but instead we found that it did stimulate Ca^{2+} uptake into the SR (FIGURE 8). The increase in the initial rate of uptake amounted to 20% and was not further enhanced by exogenous cGMP-dependent protein kinase, which suggests that endogenous cGMP-dependent kinase is not lost during saponin skinning. (The relationship between this effect and the phosphorylation of an SR protein needs to be investigated.) The dose-response curve for the cGMP-mediated stimulation of SR Ca^{2+} accumulation yielded a K_D of $\sim 10^{-8}$ M (FIGURE 8). We thus propose that cGMP stimulation of the SR Ca^{2+} pump contributes to its physiological role in reducing smooth muscle tone. In addition there is convincing evidence that a rise in cGMP concentration signals stimulation of Ca^{2+} extrusion from vascular smooth muscle,[33,34] although other mechanisms such as inhibition of phospholipase C[35,36] and a direct inhibitory effect on the contractile apparatus[37] have also been suggested.

THE "SUPERFICIAL BUFFER BARRIER"

It was proposed in 1977 that a fraction of the Ca^{2+} entering arterial smooth cells during depolarization is accumulated by peripherally located SR before it is able to raise the cytosolic [Ca^{2+}] and so activate the myofilaments.[38] Increasing the Ca^{2+} content of this peripheral SR would potentially diminish such a buffering action. This hypothesis has subsequently been confirmed by the experiment illustrated in FIGURE 9.[39] Depletion of the SR Ca^{2+} by exposing aortic rings bathed in Ca-free (2 mM EGTA) physiological saline solution to NE, diminished the effectiveness in activating tension (FIGURE 9A) of a subsequent high K^+ depolarization–stimulated Ca^{2+} influx (FIGURE 9B). It was found that high K^+ depolarization could induce tension only if the norepinephrine- or caffeine-releasable intracellular Ca^{2+} store (the SR) was refilled to near its physiological level.[40] These results made it clear that the buffering of Ca^{2+} influx occurred before Ca^{2+} reached the deeper myoplasm, hence the SR located close to the plasmalemma was proposed to act as a "superficial buffer barrier."[40] According to this hypothesis, Ca^{2+} entering the myoplasm from the extracellular space has to cross two barriers in series before it can activate the bulk of the myofilaments: (1) the surface membrane containing its various Ca^{2+} transport mechanisms; and (2) a superficial cytoplasmic region which is rich in SR which also contains Ca^{2+} pumps and various ion channels. The superficial buffer barrier hypothesis predicts (1) that an irregular, outwardly directed Ca^{2+} gradient exists in a narrow region (in the order of tens of nanometers) just beneath the plasmalemma and (2) that the proportion of the Ca^{2+} crossing the surface membrane that is taken up into the superficial SR is crucial in determining the threshold value of Ca^{2+} influx that can initiate contraction. The first prediction has not been directly verified although some indirect support for this concept exists. For example, den Hertog has shown that α stimulation of intestinal smooth muscle simultaneously increases the Quin 2 fluorescent signal and decreases contractile tension.[41] This is interpreted as resulting from a local increase of [Ca^{2+}] near the Ca^{2+}-activated K^+ channels of the surface membrane, which causes hyperpolarization which inhibits voltage-gated Ca^{2+} channels localized in specific areas and thus simultaneously decreases myoplasmic [Ca^{2+}].[41] The second prediction is clearly verified by the data shown in FIGURE 10. Rabbit aortic contractions initiated by either norepinephrine or high K^+ are characterized by a rapid shortening phase lasting a few minutes followed by maintained tension lasting for an hour or more (tonic phase). During the tonic phase a maintained increase in Ca^{2+} influx can be measured, while the net Ca^{2+} content increases during the first 5–10 minutes after which it reaches a

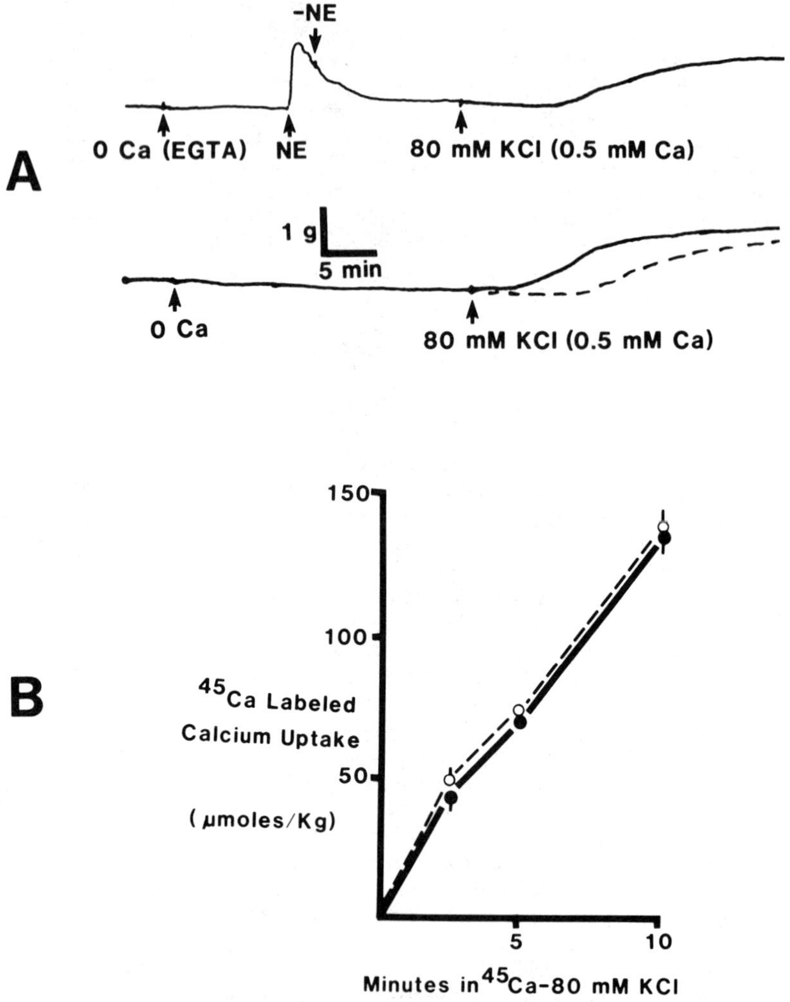

FIGURE 9. (A) Tracings of contractions produced by addition of 80 mM KCl-PSS containing 0.5 mM Ca^{2+} after incubation in 0 Ca^{2+}-PSS containing 2 mM EGTA. Depletion of the agonist-releasable calcium pool by norepinephrine increases the delay in onset of the contraction (upper tracing and dashed line). (B) ^{45}Ca uptake during the two conditions illustrated in A. The ^{45}Ca uptake of tissues in which the agonist-sensitive pool had been depleted by NE (open circles) was identical to that of controls (filled circles). Both groups of tissues were preincubated in 0 Ca^{2+}, 2 mM EGTA for 22 minutes before being placed in ^{45}Ca-labeled 0.5 mM Ca^{2+}, 80mM KCl-PSS.

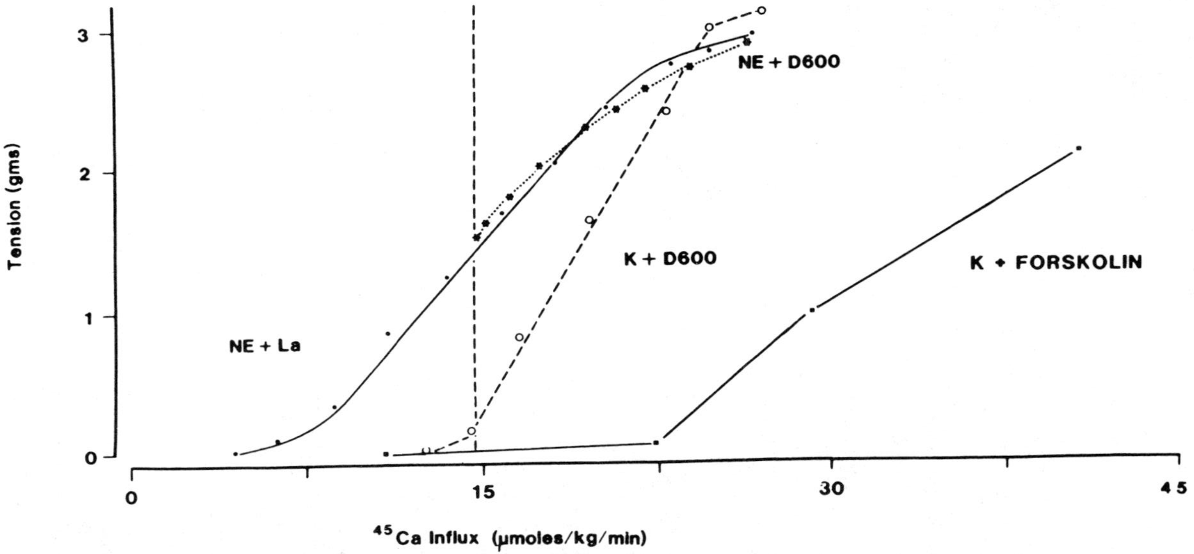

FIGURE 10. Relation between tonic tension and ^{45}Ca influx during stimulation by 6×10^{-5} M norepinephrine (NE), 80 mM KCl, and 80 mM potassium (K) with 10^{-5} M forskolin in the presence of variable concentrations of Ca^{2+} entry blockers. Rings of rabbit aorta were exposed to high K^+ or NE in the absence and presence of various concentrations of D600 or La. The maintained contractions were measured at 5 minutes. At this time point, parallel aortic rings from the same animals were exposed for 90 seconds to ^{45}Ca to measure calcium influx. Open circles = D600 (10^{-8}–10^{-6} M) + 80 mM KCl. Asterisks = D600 (10^{-8}–10^{-6} M) + NE. Filled circles = La^{3+} (3×10^{-5}–3×10^{-3} M) + NE. Squares = 80 mM KCl + M forskolin + D600 10^{-8}–10^{-6} M). Vertical dashed line represents basal ^{45}Ca influx through the intrinsic Ca^{2+} "leak."

steady state.[42] Norepinephrine transiently releases Ca^{2+} from the SR and apparently maintains the SR in a state of enhanced permeability. Since the Ca^{2+} supply from the SR decays rapidly, the tonic NE contraction must depend on Ca^{2+} influx as, of course, does the tonic phase of the depolarization-induced contraction. However the quantitative aspects of the dependencies on Ca^{2+} influx for the development of tension by these two agonists are quite different. When the high K^+–stimulated Ca^{2+} influx is inhibited by D600, tension falls in parallel with the fall in Ca^{2+} influx[43]; however, a similar degree of inhibition of the norepinephrine-stimulated Ca^{2+} influx only reduces the tonic tension by 50%. Abolition of NE-induced tonic tension also requires blockade of the leak Ca^{2+} influx by lanthanum, demonstrating a reduction in the Ca^{2+} influx threshold for contraction when the superficial SR is prevented from taking up Ca^{2+}.

Forskolin stimulates adenylate cyclase to increase cAMP, which has been shown to stimulate the SR Ca^{2+} pump. This process would enhance the effectiveness of the superficial buffer barrier by removing a greater portion of the entering Ca^{2+}, so shifting the threshold of influx for tension development to higher values; this is also shown in FIGURE 10.

Although we have presented considerable experimental data consistent with the superficial buffer barrier hypothesis, changes in the Ca^{2+} sensitivity of the contractile mechanism—such as an increase in sensitivity with norepinephrine and a decrease with cAMP—could also explain some of the observations. However, new data from our laboratory show that only 30%, at most, of the NE-induced tonic contraction can be attributed to a more Ca^{2+}-sensitive C-kinase-related mechanism (Khalil and van Breemen, unpublished results), and that in cultured aortic cells forskolin does reduce the intracellular free Ca^{2+} Fura 2 signal associated with high K^+–stimulated Ca^{2+} influx (Hwang and van Breemen, unpublished results).

CONCLUSION

Ca^{2+} can be released from vascular smooth muscle SR via two separate mechanisms, one stimulated by Ca^{2+}, which can also be activated by caffeine, free ATP, and ryanodine, and another mechanism activated by IP_3. Experiments have so far failed to demonstrate the presence of CICR in intact cells and have instead supported the hypothesis that Ca^{2+} entry is buffered by superficial SR. The result of this superficial buffering is a peripheral Ca^{2+} gradient which may complicate conclusions drawn from average intracellular free-Ca^{2+} measurements. The extent of superficial buffering and consequently the relationship between Ca^{2+} influx and tonic tension are regulated by the intracellular messengers IP_3 and the cyclic nucleotides. A model for continued Ca^{2+} buffering by the superficial SR during maintained Ca^{2+} influx is presented in Reference 44.

REFERENCES

1. SOMLYO, A. 1980. Ultrastructure of vascular smooth muscle. *In* Handbook of Physiology, Section 2. D. F. Bohr, A. P. Somlyo & H. V. Spacles, Eds. **2:** 33–69. American Physiological Society. Bethesda, Md.
2. SAIDA, K. & Y. NONOMURA. 1978. J. Gen. Physiol. **72:** 1–14.
3. SAIDA, K. 1982. J. Gen. Physiol. **80:** 191–202.
4. WEBER, A. & R. HERZ. 1968. J. Gen. Physiol. **52:** 750–759.
5. DETH, R. & R. CASTEELS. 1977. J. Gen. Physiol. **69:** 401–416.
6. LEIJTEN, P. & C. VAN BREEMEN. J. Physiol. **357:** 327–339.
7. YAMAMOTO, H. & C. VAN BREEMEN. 1986. J. Gen. Physiol. **87:** 369–389.

8. SAIDA, K. & C. VAN BREEMEN. 1984. Blood Vessels **21:** 43–52.
9. SAIDA, K. & C. VAN BREEMEN. 1984. J. Gen. Physiol. **84:** 307–318.
10. SAIDA, K. & C. VAN BREEMEN. 1984. Inserm **124:** 183–192.
11. ENDO, M. 1977. Physiol. Rev. **57:** 71–108.
12. FABIATO, A. 1985. J. Gen. Physiol. **85:** 247–289.
13. SUTKO, J. L., K. KTO, & J. L. VENYON. 1985. Fed. Proc.: 2984–2988.
14. PESSAH, I. N., A. L. WATERHOUSE & J. E. CASIDA. 1985. Biochem. Biophys. Res. Commun. **128:** 449–456.
15. STEINSLAND, O. S., R. F. FURCHGOT & S. M. KIRPELIAR. 1973. Circ. Res. **32:** 49–58.
16. HWANG, K. S. & C. VAN BREEMEN. 1987. Pfluegers Arch. **408:** 343–350.
17. HWANG, K. S., K. SAIDA & C. VAN BREEMEN. 1987. Biochem. Biophys. Res. Commun. **142** (3): 674–679.
18. KOBAYASHI, S. 1985. Biochem. Biophys. Res. Commun. **129.**
19. LEIJTEN, P. A. A. & C. VAN BREEMEN. 1986. Br. J. Pharmacol. **89:** 739–747.
20. BERRIDGE, M. J. 1984. Biochem. J. **220:** 345–360.
21. BERRIDGE, M. J. & R. F. IRVINE. 1984. Nature London **312:** 315–321.
22. SUEMATSU, E., M. HIRATA, T. SASAGURI & H. KURIYAMA. 1984. Biochem. Biophys. Res. Commun. **120:** 481–485.
23. YAMAMOTO, H. & C. VAN BREEMEN. 1985. Biochem. Biophys. Res. Commun. **130:** 270–274.
24. SOMLYO, A. V., M. BOND, A. P. SOMLYO, A. SOMLYO & A. SEARPA. 1985. Proc. Nat. Acad. Sci. USA **82:** 5231–5235.
25. HASHIMOTO, T., M. HIRATA, T. ITOH, Y. KANMURA & H. KURIYAMA. 1986. J. Physiol. London **370:** 605–618.
26. YAMAMOTO, H. & C. VAN BREEMEN. 1986. J. Gen. Physiol. **87:** 369–389.
27. MORGAN, J. P. & K. G. MORGAN. 1984. J. Physiol. London **351:** 155–167.
28. WILLIAMS, D. A., K. E. FOGARTY, R. Y. TSIEN & F. S. FAY. 1985. Nature **318:** 558–561.
29. MUELLER, E. & C. VAN BREEMEN. 1979. Nature **281:** 682–683.
30. RAEYMAEKERS, L., F. WUYTACK & R. CASTEELS. 1985. Biochim. Biophys. Acta **815:** 441–454.
31. KAMM, K. E. & J. T. STULL. 1985. Am. Rev. Pharmacol. Toxicol. **25:** 593–620.
32. MEISHERI, K. D., C. J. TAYLOR & H. SANEII. 1986. Am. J. Physiol. **250**(Jan.): C171–174.
33. SUEMATSU, E., M. HILATA & H. KURIYAMA. 1984. Biochim. Biophys. Acta **773:** 83–90.
34. POPESAU, L. M., C. PANOIU, M. HINESCU & D. NUTU. 1985. Eur. J. Pharmacol. **107:** 393–394.
35. FUJII, K., T. ISHIMATSU & H. KURIYAMA. 1985. J. Physiol. **377:** 315–332.
36. RAPAPORT, R. M. 1986. Circ. Res. **58:** 407–410.
37. PFITZER, G., F. HOFFMANN, J. DISALVO & J. C. RÜEGG. 1984. Pfluegers Arch. **401:** 277–280.
38. VAN BREEMEN, C. 1977. J. Physiol. **272:** 317–329.
39. LOUTZENHISER, R. & C. VAN BREEMEN. 1983. Circ. Res. **52**(Suppl 1): 97–103.
40. VAN BREEMEN, C., K. HWANG, R. LOUTZENHISER, S. LUKEMAN, & H. YAMAMOTO. 1985. *In* Cardiovascular Effects of Dihydropyridine-Type Calcium Antagonists and Agonists. A. Fleckenstein, C. van Breemen, C. R. Gross & F. Hoffmeister, Eds.: 58–75. Springer Verlag. Berlin, FRG.
41. DAN HERTOG, A. & S. A. NELEMANS. 1986. Proc. Smooth Muscle Funct. Symp. Banijf 3-p2:93.
42. HWANG, K. S. & C. VAN BREEMEN. 1987 Eur. J. Pharmacol. **134:** 155–162.
43. LUKEMAN, S. & C. VAN BREEMEN. 1985. *In* Recent Aspects in Calcium Antagonism. P. R. Lichtlen, Ed.: 49–65. Schattauer. Stuttgart, FRG.
44. VAN BREEMEN, C., P. LEIJTEN, H. YAMAMOTO, P. AARONSON & C. CAUVIN. 1986 Hypertension **8**(Suppl. 2): II89–II95.

Calmodulin and Its Activation by Cadmium Ion[a]

WAI YIU CHEUNG

Department of Biochemistry
St. Jude Children's Research Hospital
Memphis, Tennessee 38101

INTRODUCTION

Calmodulin was discovered as a protein activator of cyclic 3′5′-nucleotide phosphodiesterase in the late 1960s.[1,2] It is a calcium-binding protein found in all eukaryotes; the protein also modulates the intracellular concentration of calcium ion. The name calmodulin is merely abstracted from *cal*cium *modul*ated prote*in*.[3] Ca^{2+} regulates a wide spectrum of basic cellular processes: endo- and exocytosis, metabolic activities, muscle contraction, cell motility, chromosome movement, and cell division.[4,5] In fact, the cation is involved in almost all aspects of cellular activities. Many, but not all, of the Ca^{2+}-regulated processes are mediated through a homologous class of Ca^{2+}-binding portions, of which calmodulin appears to serve as a major intracellular Ca^{2+} receptor.

BIOCHEMICAL PROPERTIES OF CALMODULIN

Only a brief introduction is attempted below. For general information, the reader is referred to more comprehensive reviews and monographs.[6,7] Calmodulin is a single polypeptide with 148 amino acids and a molecular weight of 16,700.[8] Some 30% of its amino acids consist of aspartate and glutamate; the abundance of acidic amino acids accounts for its low isoelectric point (4.3). The protein contains no cysteine, hydroxyproline, or tryptophan, but does contain a trimethylated lysine at position 115. Calmodulin isolated from marine organisms contains no trimethylated lysine and appears to be as active. The lack of cysteine and hydroxyproline allows calmodulin to have a flexible tertiary structure, a desirable feature for a multifunctional protein that interacts with many different receptor proteins. One striking feature of calmodulin is its tenacity to retain biological activity after exposure to harsh experimental conditions. A second is that calmodulins from a wide variety of sources possess essentially identical physicochemical properties. In fact, calmodulins isolated from mammalian tissues have identical tryptic peptide maps and essentially identical amino acid sequences; thus, calmodulin lacks both tissue and species specificities. As depicted in FIGURE 1, calmodulin contains four Ca^{2+}-binding domains each of which comprises a 12-residue Ca^{2+}-binding loop, flanked on each side by an 8-residue α-helix. The four domains appear homologous, with affinity for Ca^{2+} in the micromolar range. The three-dimensional structure of calmodulin has been determined crystallographically at 3.0 Å resolution.[9] Calmodulin molecules crystallized at pH 5.6 display two globular

[a]The work in our laboratory was supported by National Institutes of Health grants CA21765, GM36734, and HL36314 and by American-Lebanese-Syrian Associated Charities.

lobes connected by a long exposed α-helix (FIGURE 2). Each lobe binds two Ca^{2+} through a helix-loop-helix domain similar to those of other Ca^{2+}-binding proteins. Differential kinetic labeling studies suggest that the long helix between the lobes may be involved in the interactions of calmodulin with various target proteins or drugs.[10] Studies on structure-function relationship indicate that the biological activity of

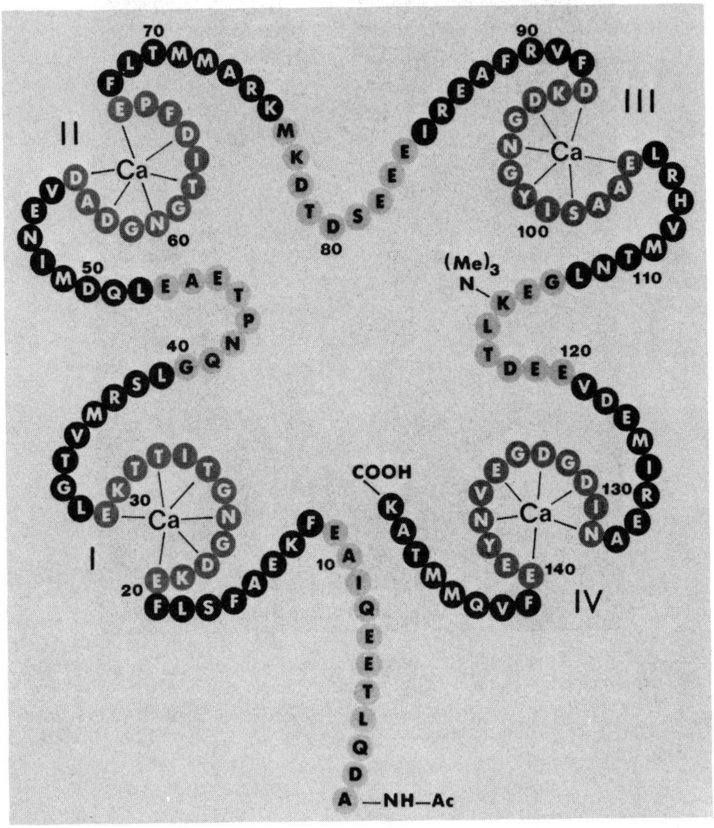

FIGURE 1. Amino acid sequence of bovine brain calmodulin. The calcium-binding loops (I–IV) indicated (gray circles, white letters), are flanked on each side by an eight amino acid α-helix (dark circles, white letters). The amino acids are designated by the one-letter code: A = alanine; R = arginine; N = asparagine; H = histidine; D = aspartic acid; Q = glutamine; E = glutamic acid; G = glycine; K = lysine; M = methionine; F = phenylalanine; P = proline; S = serine; T = threonine; Y = tyrosine; V = valine. (Reproduced from Reference 1 with permission from the publisher.)

calmodulin relies heavily on the integrity of the entire molecule. Conceivably, the role of calmodulin in cellular functions is of such fundamental importance that any mutation resulting in a gross change of the primary structure of the molecule may be lethal to the cell. Supporting this notion is the recent finding that disruption or deletion of the calmodulin gene in yeast results in a recessive-lethal mutation, indicating that

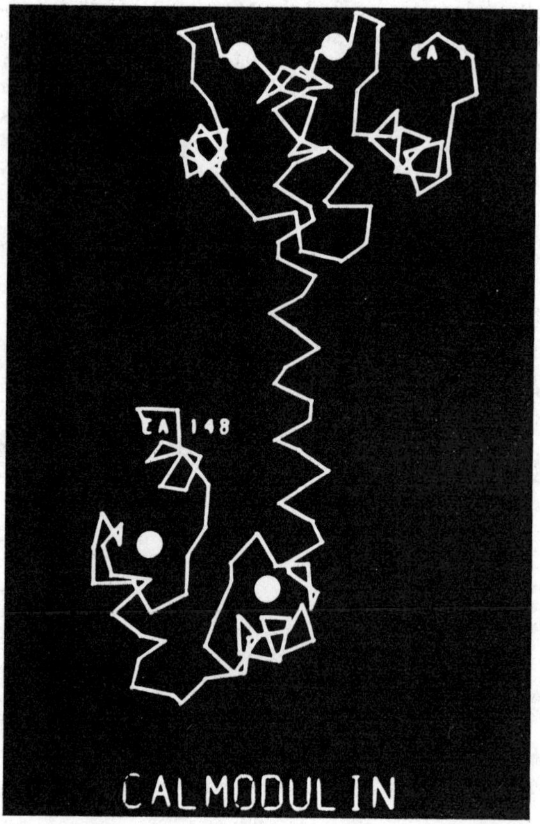

FIGURE 2. The three-dimensional structure of rat testis calmodulin. The positions of the four calcium ions are indicated (white dots). CA1 indicates the N-terminus, and CA148 indicates the C-terminus. The overall shape of the molecule is that of a dumbbell, with the two lobes connected by an eight-turn α-helix and no contacts between the two lobes. (Reproduced from Reference 9 with permission from the publisher.)

TABLE 1. Biological and Biochemical Properties of Calmodulin

1. Found in all eukaryotes
2. Lacks species specificity
3. Cellular level usually constant
4. Single polypeptide, amino acid sequence highly conserved
5. M_r 16,700, pI 4.3
6. Four Ca^{2+}-binding sites, $K_d = \mu M$
7. K_d for target enzymes = nM
8. Stoichiometry for CaM · E = 1.1
9. Increases V_{max}, no change in K_m
10. Intact molecule required for activity

calmodulin is essential for the growth of yeast.[11] Some of the salient features of calmodulin are summarized in TABLE 1.

BIOLOGICAL FUNCTIONS OF CALMODULIN

The functional status of calmodulin is unique; it has no intrinsic enzymatic activities but has the ability to regulate the activity of many enzymes. TABLE 2 lists the known calmodulin-dependent enzymes and their cellular functions. These enzymes deal with the metabolism of cyclic nucleotides, Ca^{2+}, glycogen, and NAD, the contractility and mobility of cells, cross-linking of proteins, and the phosphorylation and dephosphorylation of various proteins, which constitute a major cellular regulatory mechanism.

TABLE 2. Calmodulin-Dependent Enzymes and Their Functions[a]

Enzyme	Cellular Function
1. Adenylate cyclase	Synthesis of cAMP
2. Guanylate cyclase	Synthesis of cGMP
3. Cyclic 3′,5′-nucleotide phosphodiesterase	Hydrolysis of cAMP and cGMP
4. Ca^{2+}-ATPase	Ca^{2+} pump
5. NAD kinase	Synthesis of NADP
6. Phosphorylase kinase	Glycogen degradation
7. Glycogen synthetase kinase	Glycogen synthesis
8. Myosin light chain kinase	Contractility and motility
9. Calmodulin-dependent protein kinases	Phosphorylation of various proteins
10. Calmodulin-dependent protein phosphatase	Dephosphorylation of various proteins
11. Transglutaminase	Cross-linking of proteins

[a]Glycogen synthetase kinase appears similar to one of the calmodulin-dependent protein kinases. The evidence that enzymes 1 to 10 are calmodulin dependent is well documented (see References 6 and 7), but that for transglutaminase appears preliminary.[12]

MECHANISM OF ACTION OF CALMODULIN

The mechanism by which calmodulin activates an enzyme has been extensively characterized. In response to a stimulus, Ca^{2+} flows into the cell or is released from the cell membrane or internal organelles and binds to calmodulin. Binding of Ca^{2+} causes calmodulin to assume a more helical structure, exposing a hydrophobic patch that appears to interact with a receptor enzyme to form an activated quarternary complex. Kinetic evidence suggests that binding of Ca^{2+} proceeds sequentially, first to domains III and IV, and then to domains I and II. Direct comparison of Ca^{2+} requirements for calmodulin interaction with and activation of calmodulin-dependent phosphatase indicates that filling of the first two Ca^{2+} sites permits calmodulin to form a complex with the enzyme, but this complex is not active; full activation requires additional filling of the remaining one or two sites.[13] Complex formation is reversible, and under physiological conditions, its direction is thought to be controlled by the cellular flux of Ca^{2+} rather than the cellular concentration of calmodulin. An increase of Ca^{2+} favors the formation of the active calmodulin enzyme complex and a decrease favors its dissociation, thus terminating the Ca^{2+} signal.

STIMULATION OF CALMODULIN BY METAL CATIONS

We have mentioned that many of the biological functions of Ca^{2+} are mediated through calmodulin. We have shown previously that Tb^{3+}, which has an ionic radius (0.92 Å) comparable to that of Ca^{2+} (0.99 Å), effectively substitutes for Ca^{2+} in calmodulin stimulation of cyclic 3′,5′-nucleotide phosphodiesterase.[14] We have further shown that other cations including heavy metals such as Pb^{2+}, Hg^{2+}, and Cd^{2+} having comparable ionic radii also replace Ca^{2+} effectively in supporting calmodulin-dependent phosphodiesterase activity.[15] In this article, we will use phosphodiesterase as an assay system to illustrate the effects of Cd^{2+} on calmodulin activity.

GENERAL EXPERIMENTAL APPROACH

The sequence leading to activation of calmodulin can be arbitrarily divided into several steps. When calmodulin binds Ca^{2+}, its conformation is changed; the change can be monitored by an increase in its intrinsic tyrosine fluorescence, and by a differential mobility change in acrylamide gel electrophoresis.[15] Coupled to the conformational change is exposure of a hydrophobic region that interacts with calmodulin antagonists such as trifluoperazine, or with receptor enzymes such as phosphodiesterase.[16,17] We have examined the ability of various metal cations to substitute for Ca^{2+} in all these attributes.[15] We will summarize herein the experimental results from studies on Cd^{2+}.[18]

Cd^{2+} BINDING TO CALMODULIN

A Sephadex G-25 column was equilibrated with 50 mM Tris-HCl (pH 7.4) containing various concentrations of $^{109}CdCl_2$. A sample of calmodulin was loaded to the column and eluted with the same buffer. A peak of ^{109}Cd radioactivity appeared in the void volume, which coincided with the elution profile of calmodulin. The amount of Cd^{2+} bound to calmodulin was calculated by integrating the trough area[19] trailing the protein peak.

FIGURE 3 shows the binding of Cd^{2+} to calmodulin as a function of various concentrations of Cd^{2+}. At a concentration of 50 μM Cd^{2+}, calmodulin bound 3.5 mol Cd^{2+}, presumably to the Ca^{2+}-binding sites; in a parallel experiment with 50 μM Ca^{2+}, calmodulin bound 3.8 mol Ca^{2+}. At 100 μM Cd^{2+}, calmodulin bound about 4 mol Cd^{2+}; at higher concentrations, calmodulin bound 7–8 mol Cd^{2+} with a K_d of about 140 μM, indicating nonspecific binding probably to the methionine or histidine residues of calmodulin (which lacks cysteine). The inset shows a Scatchard plot of these data. The plot is not linear, but when a straight line is drawn after correction for nonspecific binding,[20] the data indicate that calmodulin bound at least 2 mol Cd^{2+} with a K_d of 4.5×10^{-6} M. A cautionary note should be added—a nonlinear Scatchard plot invariably does not give an accurate determination of the number or the affinity of ligand binding.[21]

CONFORMATIONAL CHANGES OF CALMODULIN BY Cd^{2+}

Of the many metal ions tested for their ability to substitute for Ca^{2+} in calmodulin, Cd^{2+} was one of the most effective, as measured by an increase of intrinsic tyrosine fluorescence or differential mobility change in acrylamide gel electrophoresis.[15] The change in tyrosine fluorescence caused by Cd^{2+} was 80% of that caused by Ca^{2+}, and the electrophoretic mobility of calmodulin in both native gel and sodium dodecyl sulfate gel was indistinguishable from that in the presence of Ca^{2+}.[15] These results suggest that Cd^{2+} induced a conformational change in calmodulin comparable to that by Ca^{2+}.

EFFECT OF Cd^{2+} ON BINDING OF CHLORPROMAZINE TO CALMODULIN

Calmodulin exhibited two classes of binding affinities for antipsychotic drugs such as chlorpromazine in the presence of Ca^{2+}, one class with two molecules of chlorproma-

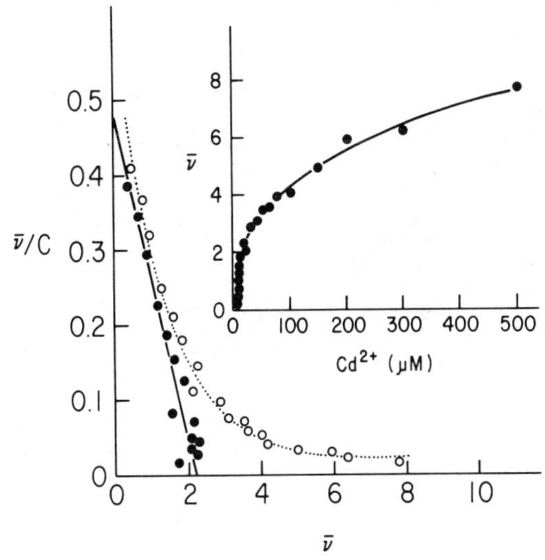

FIGURE 3. Determination of ^{109}Cd binding to calmodulin by gel filtration. A column of Sephadex G-25 (0.9 × 12 cm) was equilibrated with 50 mM Tris-HCl (pH 7.4) and various concentrations of $^{109}CdCl_2$ (0.1 μCi/ml). After equilibration, 50 μl of calmodulin (5.2 nmol) were applied to the column, which was eluted with the same buffer. Fractions (500 μl) were collected, and the radioactivity was determined. The amount of Cd^{2+} bound was calculated from the trough fractions.[19] Inset: The amount of bound Cd^{2+} (moles of Cd/mole of calmodulin) is plotted against the concentration of Cd^{2+} (μM). The Scatchard plot of these data is also presented; $\bar{\nu}$, mole of Cd^{2+} bound/mole of calmodulin; *C*, free Cd^{2+} concentration (μM) in the buffer. (Reproduced from Reference 18 with permission from the publisher.)

zine per molecule of calmodulin, with a K_d of 1 μM, and another with 24 chlorpromazines per molecule of calmodulin with a K_d of 5 mM.[22] LaPorte *et al.* and Tanaka and Hidaka demonstrated that the binding of Ca^{2+} exposed in calmodulin a hydrophobic region,[16,17] which apparently interacts with hydrophobic drugs or target proteins such as phosphodiesterase. FIGURE 4 (panel A) shows that the amount of [^{3}H]chlorpromazine bound to calmodulin was comparable whether in the presence of Cd^{2+} or Ca^{2+}.

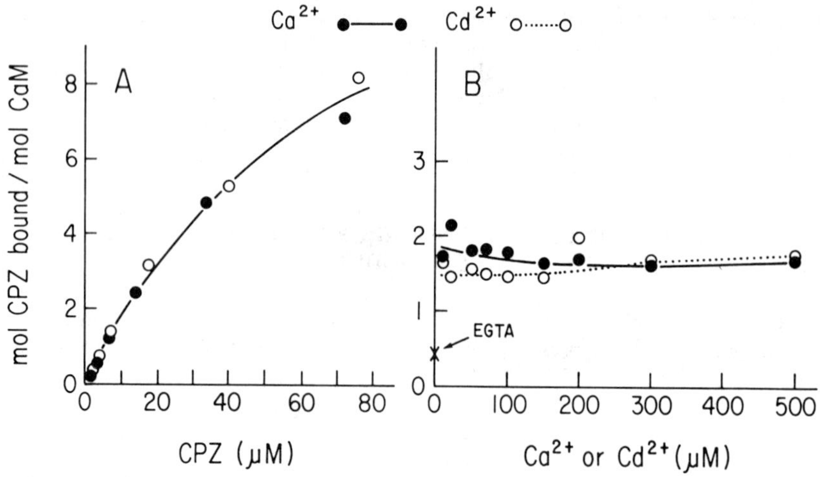

FIGURE 4. Effect of Cd^{2+} on chlorpromazine binding to calmodulin. Binding of [^{3}H]chlorpromazine to calmodulin was done by equilibrium dialysis in an acrylic plastic cell (1 ml/side, Fisher Scientific, Pittsburgh, Pa.). Both the outer and inner solutions consisted of 0.5 ml sample. The dialysis membrane was boiled for 5 minutes in 50 mM EDTA and 5% $NaCO_3$, and then washed extensively with double-distilled water. A. Calmodulin (15 μg) was added to the inner solution and was dialyzed against 50 mM Tris-HCl (pH 7.4) and various concentrations of chlorpromazine in the presence of either 200 μM Cd^{2+} or 200 μM Ca^{2+} for 20 hours at 22°C. B. Calmodulin (30 μg) was dialyzed against 50 mM Tris-HCl (pH 7.4) and 10 μM [^{3}H]chlorpromazine at various concentrations of Ca^{2+} or Cd^{2+} for 20 hours at 22°C. The arrow indicates binding in the presence of 1 mM EGTA. The amount of [^{3}H]chlorpromazine bound to calmodulin was calculated from the difference in radioactivity between the inside and outside solutions. (Reproduced from Reference 18 with permission from the publisher.)

When the concentration of [^{3}H]chlorpromazine was held constant, about 2 mol chlorpromazine were bound per mole of calmodulin at various concentrations of either Cd^{2+} or Ca^{2+} (panel B). These results suggest that the binding of chlorpromazine to calmodulin in Cd^{2+} was indistinguishable from that in Ca^{2+}.

COMPLEX FORMATION BETWEEN CALMODULIN AND PHOSPHODIESTERASE IN THE PRESENCE OF Cd^{2+}

Phosphodiesterase was passed through a calmodulin-Sepharose affinity column equilibrated with 1 mM Cd^{2+}. No phosphodiesterase activity was detected in the flow-through fractions (FIGURE 5), indicating that the enzyme bound to the affinity column. When eluted with 2 mM EGTA, essentially all the activity emerged in one fraction, indicating that the binding of the enzyme to the calmodulin-Sepharose column was dependent on Cd^{2+}. In a parallel experiment, a similar elution profile was obtained when Cd^{2+} was replaced by Ca^{2+} (data not shown). In previous experiments with a Sepharose column, we have shown that phosphodiesterase did not bind to the column,[23] suggesting that the enzyme interacted with the immobilized calmodulin and not with the Sepharose matrix.

EFFECTIVENESS OF Ca^{2+} AND Cd^{2+} IN STIMULATING PHOSPHODIESTERASE ACTIVITY IN THE PRESENCE OF EACH OTHER

FIGURE 6 shows the activity of phosphodiesterase as a function of Ca^{2+} in the presence or absence of 5 μM Cd^{2+} (panel A), or as a function of Cd^{2+} in the presence or absence of 5 μM Ca^{2+}. In the presence of 5 μM Cd^{2+} (panel A), which raised phosphodiesterase activity to some 60% of the maximum, the titration curve by Ca^{2+} gradually increased the activity to the maximum, which remained unchanged thereafter, similar to the titration curve by Ca^{2+} alone. The peak phosphodiesterase activity was obtained at 10 μM Ca^{2+} in the presence of 5 μM Cd^{2+} and at 15 μM Ca^{2+} in the absence of Cd^{2+}. The activity of phosphodiesterase was generally higher in the presence of Cd^{2+} at each of the Ca^{2+} concentrations below 10 μM, but the final maximal activities were identical, suggesting that the effects of the two cations are not strictly additive. In the presence of 5 μM Ca^{2+} (panel B), which increased phosphodiesterase activity to some 70% of the maximum, the titration curve by Cd^{2+} also gradually increased to the maximum (comparable to that in panel A). Cd^{2+} at concentrations higher than 20 μM inhibited phosphodiesterase activity in a manner qualitatively similar to that by Cd^{2+} alone. The peak phosphodiesterase activity was obtained in the presence of 10 μM Cd^{2+} in the presence of 5 μM Ca^{2+}, and 15 μM Cd^{2+} in the absence of Ca^{2+}. Although Cd^{2+} alone could not activate phosphodiesterase to the maximal level, the addition of 5 μM Ca^{2+} did. Ca^{2+} at 5 μM could only stimulate phosphodiesterase submaximally. These data suggest that the presence of Cd^{2+} does not interfere with the effectiveness of Ca^{2+} to activate calmodulin; in fact, Cd^{2+} accentuates the

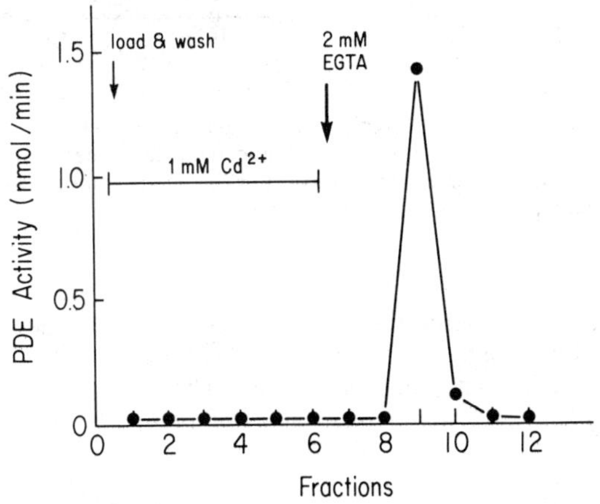

FIGURE 5. Complex formation between phosphodiesterase and calmodulin immobilized to Sepharose 4B in the presence of Cd^{2+}. Phosphodiesterase in 150 μl (4.5 μg, 3.6 units/mg) was applied to a calmodulin-Sepharose 4B affinity column (0.6 × 7 cm) equilibrated with 50 mM Tris-HCl (pH 7.4) and 1 mM $CdCl_2$. The column was washed with the same buffer. Where indicated, the column was eluted with 50 mM Tris-HCl (pH 7.4) and 2 mM EGTA. Fractions (400 μl) were collected and each fraction was dialyzed against 50 mM Tris-HCl (pH 7.4) for 12 hours at 4°C. Aliquots (40 μl) were assayed for phosphodiesterase activity in the presence of 200 μM Ca^{2+} and 1.1 μg calmodulin. The recovery of phosphodiesterase activity was 94%. (Reproduced from Reference 18 with permission from the publisher.)

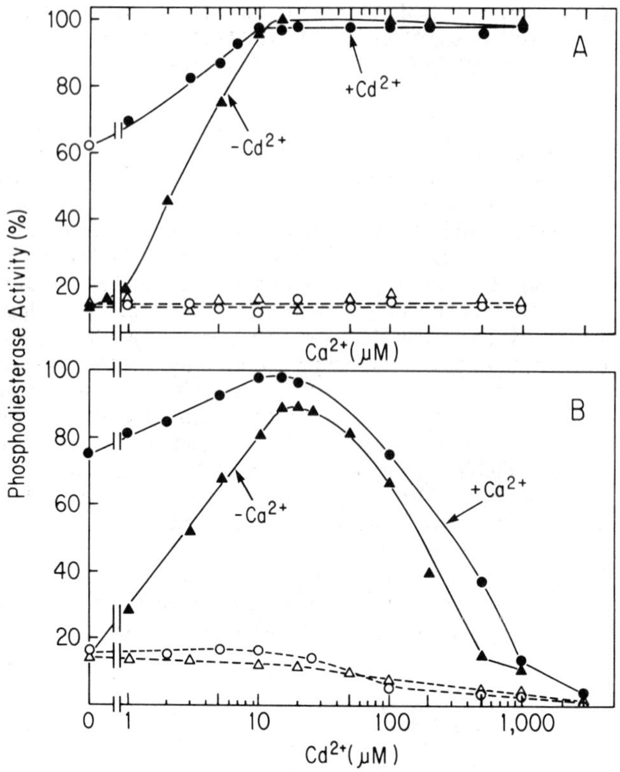

FIGURE 6. Effect of Ca^{2+}, Cd^{2+}, or both on phosphodiesterase activity. A. 5 μM Cd^{2+} and indicated concentration of Ca^{2+}; B. 5 μM Ca^{2+} and indicated concentration of Cd^{2+}. Open symbols depict phosphodiesterase activities assayed in the absence of calmodulin. (Reproduced from Reference 15 with permission from the publisher.)

effectiveness of Ca^{2+}. Similarly, Ca^{2+} accentuates the effectiveness of Cd^{2+}. These results are compatible with the notion that these cations occupy the same binding sites as Ca^{2+} on calmodulin, and that these sites, when occupied by Cd^{2+}, support calmodulin activity.

EFFECTS OF VARIOUS SULFUR-CONTAINING REAGENTS ON Cd^{2+}-ACTIVATED PHOSPHODIESTERASE ACTIVITY

Mammalian cells contain millimolar concentrations of glutathione,[24] and Cd^{2+} is known to bind to sulfhydryl groups with a high affinity.[25,26] We determined whether Cd^{2+} can activate calmodulin in the presence of various sulfur-containing reagents.

FIGURE 7 shows the effect of these reagents on calmodulin-dependent phosphodiesterase activity in the presence of Cd^{2+}. Dithiothreitol, which has two sulfhydryl groups, was the most effective in abolishing calmodulin-dependent phosphodiesterase activity. Its effectiveness was followed by cysteine and β-mercaptoethanol, each of which has one sulfhydryl group. Methionine, oxidized dithiothreitol, or oxidized cysteine was ineffective. At a concentration of 10 mM, glutathione had no significant effect on Cd^{2+} activation of calmodulin. Separate experiments showed that these reagents did not affect basal or calmodulin-supported phosphodiesterase activity in the presence of Ca^{2+} (data not shown).

EFFECTS OF CALMODULIN CONCENTRATION ON PHOSPHODIESTERASE ACTIVITY IN THE PRESENCE OF Cd^{2+} AND GLUTATHIONE

Although glutathione had no effect on Cd^{2+} activation of phosphodiesterase activity under the conditions shown in FIGURE 7, it could reverse the effect of Cd^{2+} at lower calmodulin concentrations. At 1 μM calmodulin, a concentration found in many mammalian tissues (other tissues such as brain and testis[27] have considerably higher concentrations), 5 mM glutathione did not affect Cd^{2+} stimulation of calmodulin (see FIGURE 8). At lower concentrations of calmodulin (e.g., 0.5 μM), 5 mM glutathione reversed the Cd^{2+} effect by about 50%; at 0.2 μM calmodulin, 100 μM glutathione reversed the effect by 50%. This is understandable, because the activation of

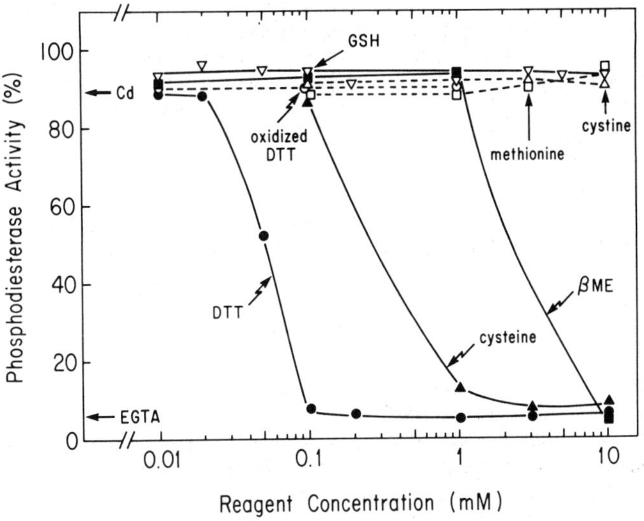

FIGURE 7. Effects of various sulfur-containing reagents on calmodulin-supported phosphodiesterase activity in the presence of Cd^{2+}. Enzyme activity was assayed in the presence of 20 μg phosphodiesterase and 1 μM calmodulin. Control activity in the presence of 100 μM Ca^{2+} and 1 μM calmodulin was 0.5 μmol/mg protein per minute, which was expressed as 100% activity. A 30 μM solution of Cd^{2+} was made with a mixture of 50 μM Cd^{2+} and 20 μM EGTA. The arrows at the left of the figure show the activities in the presence of 30 μM Cd^{2+} or 1 mM EGTA without sulfur-containing reagents. The order of addition in the reaction mixture was buffer, calmodulin, phosphodiesterase, sulfur reagents, and Cd^{2+}. After the addition of Cd^{2+}, the mixture was preincubated for 30 minutes at 30°C. The reaction was started by the addition of cAMP and incubated for an additional 10 minutes. (Reproduced from Reference 18 with permission from the publisher.)

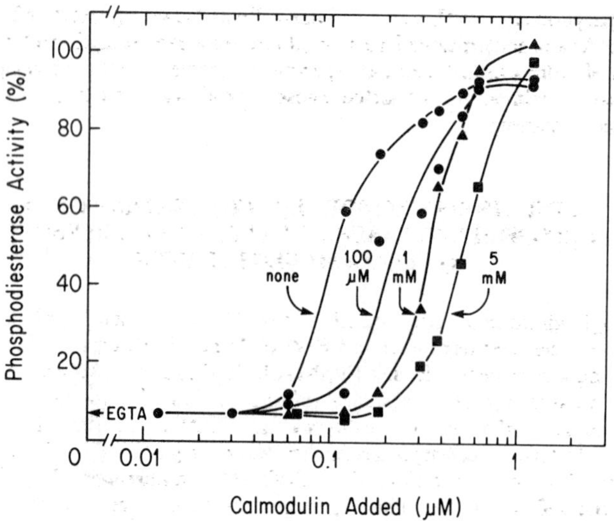

FIGURE 8. Calmodulin concentration dependence of Cd^{2+} activation of phosphodiesterase activity in the presence of glutathione (GSH). Enzyme activity was assayed in the presence of 20 μg phosphodiesterase, and 30 μM Cd^{2+} (50 μM Cd^{2+} plus 20 μM EGTA). Calmodulin concentrations were varied as indicated. Phosphodiesterase activity in the presence of 100 μM Ca^{2+} and 1 μM calmodulin (0.5 μmol/mg per minute) is taken as 100%. The arrow at the left of the figure shows the basal activity in the presence of 1 mM EGTA and 1 μM calmodulin. The order of addition was the same as that in FIGURE 7. (Reproduced from Reference 18 with permission from the publisher.)

calmodulin by Cd^{2+} depends not only on the concentration of calmodulin, but also on that of glutathione, which competes with calmodulin for Cd^{2+}.

DISCUSSION

We have examined the ability of Cd^{2+} to substitute for Ca^{2+} in calmodulin, and found that Cd^{2+} substitutes for Ca^{2+} in all the criteria examined: (1) binding to calmodulin; (2) inducing conformational change in calmodulin; (3) binding of chlorpromazine to calmodulin; (4) complex formation between calmodulin and phosphodiesterase; and (5) activating phosphodiesterase.

The binding of Cd^{2+} to calmodulin appears more complicated than that of Ca^{2+}. Using $^{109}Cd^{2+}$, we found that calmodulin exhibited two high-affinity binding sites with a K_d of 4.5 μM. This K_d value may be an underestimation because Cd^{2+} interacts with the Tris-HCl buffer in the reaction mixture.[25] Two relatively low-affinity sites were also apparent, but they were difficult to determine since the Scatchard plot (FIGURE 3) was nonlinear. In addition, there were low-affinity sites which were apparent only at a Cd^{2+} concentration over 100 μM. These sites were probably nonspecific, since Cd^{2+} interacts with methionine or histidine residues of proteins.[26] These nonspecific binding sites did not seem to interfere with the binding of Cd^{2+} to the Ca^{2+}-binding sites necessary for bringing about the active conformation of calmodulin.

Cd^{2+} is known to affect many biologic processes, presumably by interacting with the sulfhydryl groups of certain enzymes.[28] Nathanson and Bloom reported that Cd^{2+} is a potent inhibitor of phosphodiesterase,[29] and Cox and Harrison correlated Cd^{2+} toxicity with the inhibition of calmodulin-supported phosphodiesterase activity.[30] The concentration of Cd^{2+} used in their experiments was high, and it appears likely that Cd^{2+} inhibited the basal enzyme activity. As seen in FIGURE 6, the effect of Cd^{2+} on phosphodiesterase activity was biphasic: activation below 20 μM and inhibition at higher concentrations.

There are at least 10 calmodulin-dependent enzymes (see TABLE 2); none of them share a common subunit. Although it has been generally believed that calmodulin interacts with its target enzymes through a Ca^{2+}-exposed hydrophobic region, recent findings suggest that the nature of this interaction may vary with different enzymes, that multiple sites on calmodulin may be involved, and that different enzymes may display different structural requirements.[31]

In this study, we have used phosphodiesterase as a model to probe the effectiveness of $CaM \cdot Cd^{2+}$ to interact with target enzymes. Mazzei *et al.* recently reported that Cd^{2+} activated a myosin light chain kinase,[32] an enzyme involved in the control of contraction of smooth muscle and nonmuscle cells, suggesting that the effectiveness of Cd^{2+} to substitute for Ca^{2+} in calmodulin is not unique with respect to phosphodiesterase. The effectiveness of Cd^{2+} in supporting calmodulin-dependent activities of other enzymes has not been examined carefully. To address this question, it is necessary that Cd^{2+} does not inhibit the basal activity of the enzyme; for example, Cd^{2+} inhibits the basal activity of Ca^{2+}-ATPase of human erythrocytes (Chao and Cheung, unpublished experiments).

Cd^{2+} is a serious environmental pollutant in areas in which cadmium-nickel batteries are manufactured.[33] It accumulates in tissues such as kidney, liver, brain, or bone with a very slow turnover, and causes serious disorders.[34–36] With chronic exposure, Cd^{2+} accumulation in the kidney may reach 200 μM. Obviously, this does not necessarily correspond to its free concentration; Cd^{2+} may bind to methionine and cysteine of various proteins, to glutathione, and especially to metallothionein, a protein inducible by Cd^{2+} and rich in sulfhydryl groups.[26,28]

In many mammalian tissues, the intracellular concentrations of glutathione reach

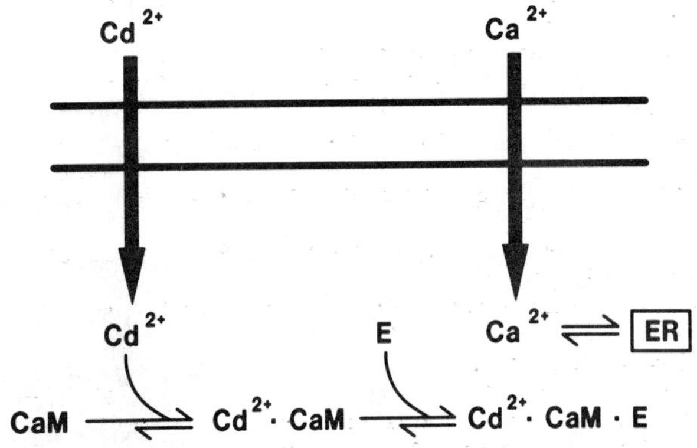

FIGURE 9. A speculative scheme depicting stimulation of calmodulin by Cd^{2+}. Cd^{2+} could effectively substitute for Ca^{2+} in calmodulin and could accentuate the effectiveness of Ca^{2+}, raising the possibility that a combination of both ions may fully activate calmodulin at a suboptimal concentration of Ca^{2+}. Such a condition could usurp the normal regulation of calmodulin by Cd^{2+} and precipitate disturbances to the many vital cellular functions.

millimolar, but such concentrations appear not to affect significantly the ability of Cd^{2+} to stimulate calmodulin-dependent phosphodiesterase *in vitro,* provided that the concentration of calmodulin is at the physiological micromolar range. Thus, it appears that glutathione is not a particularly good cellular constituent to counteract the effect of Cd^{2+}.

Most of the Cd^{2+} accumulated in mammalian tissues probably is chelated to metallothioneins and other proteins. But if some of the cation in the cellular milieu does find its way to calmodulin, it could lead to a prolonged activation of this important intracellular Ca^{2+} receptor, whose activity is normally regulated by the cellular flux of Ca^{2+} (FIGURE 9). Since calmodulin mediates many of the Ca^{2+}-regulated cellular processes, its prolonged activation could precipitate serious pathological consequences. This notion is speculative, but it offers an alternative view to other postulated mechanisms of toxicity at the molecular level, namely, the cation affects the structure of nucleic acids (DNA, tRNA) and the activities of certain enzymes by reacting with their sulfydryl groups.[25,26,28] Further experiments are necessary to establish whether there exists a link between Cd^{2+} activation of calmodulin *in vitro* and its tissue toxicity.

ACKNOWLEDGMENTS

The contributions of Drs. Sheng-Hao Chao, Yasuhiro Suzuki, and John R. Zysk to this study and of Ms. P. A. Suttle to the preparation of the manuscript are gratefully acknowledged.

REFERENCES

1. CHEUNG, W. Y. 1981. J. Cyclic Nucleotide Res. **7:** 71–84.
2. CHEUNG, W. Y. 1980. Science **207:** 19–27.
3. CHEUNG, W. Y., T. J. LYNCH & R. W. WALLACE. 1978. Adv. Cyclic Nucleotide Res. **9:** 233–251.
4. CAMPBELL, A. K. 1983. Intracellular Calcium. Its Universal Role as Regulator. Wiley Press. New York, N.Y.
5. KRETSINGER, R. H. 1980. CRC Crit. Rev. Biochem. **8:** 119–174.
6. MANALAN, A. S. & C. B. KLEE. 1984. Adv. Cyclic Nucleotide Protein Phosphorylation Res. **18:** 227–278.
7. CHEUNG, W. Y., Ed. 1980–1986. Calcium and Cell Function: **1–7.** Academic Press. Orlando, Fla.
8. WATTERSON, D. M., F. S. SHARIEF & T. C. VANAMAN. 1980. J. Biol. Chem. **255:** 962–975.
9. BABU, Y. S., J. S. SOCK, T. J. GREENHOUGH, C. E. BUGG, A. R. MEANS & W. J. COOK. 1985. Nature: 37–40.
10. JACKSON, A. E., K. L. CARRAWAY III, D. PUETT & K. BREW. 1986. J. Biol. Chem. **261:** 12226–12232.
11. DAVIS, T. N., M. S. URDEA, F. R. MASIAOZ & J. THORNER. 1986. Cell: 423–431.
12. PUSZKIN, E. G. & V. RAGHURAMAN. 1985. J. Biol. Chem. **260:** 16012–16020.
13. KINCAID, R. L. & M. VAUGHAN. 1986. Proc. Nat. Acad. Sci. USA **83:** 1193–1197.
14. WALLACE, R. W., E. A. TALLANT, M. E. DOCKTOR & W. Y. CHEUNG. 1982. J. Biol. Chem. **257:** 1845–1854.
15. CHAO, S. H., Y. SUZUKI, J. R. ZYSK & W. Y. CHEUNG. 1984. Mol. Pharmacol. **26:** 75–82.
16. LAPORTE, D. C., W. A. TOSCANO, JR. & D. R. STORM. 1979. Biochemistry **18:** 2820–2825.
17. TANAKA, T. & H. HIDAKA. 1980. J. Biol. Chem. **255:** 11078–11080.

18. SUZUKI, Y., S. H. CHAO, J. R. ZYSK & W. Y. CHEUNG. 1985. Arch. Toxicol.: 205–211.
19. HUMMEL, J. P. & W. J. DREYER. 1962. Biochim. Biophys. Acta **63:** 530–532.
20. CHAMNESS, G. C. & W. L. MCGUIRE. 1975. Steroids **26:** 538–542.
21. LIN, Y. M. & W. Y. CHEUNG. 1975. Int. J. Biochem. **6:** 271–280.
22. LEVIN, R. M. & B. WEISS. 1977. Mol. Pharmacol. **13:** 690–697.
23. LIN, Y. M., Y. P. LIU & W. Y. CHEUNG. 1975. FEBS Lett. **49:** 356–360.
24. KOSOWER, N. S. & E. M. KOSOWER. 1978. Int. Rev. Cytol. **54:** 109–160.
25. HANLON, D. P., D. S. WATT & E. W. WESTHEAD. 1966. Anal. Biochem. **16:** 225–233.
26. JACOBSON, K. B. & J. E. TURNER. 1980. Toxicology **16:** 1–37.
27. SMOAKE, J. A., S. Y. SONG & W. Y. CHEUNG. 1974. Biochim. Biophys. Acta **341:** 402–411.
28. VALLEE, B. L. & D. D. ULMER. 1972. Annu. Rev. Biochem. **41:** 91–128.
29. NATHANSON, J. A. & F. E. BLOOM. 1976. Mol. Pharmacol. **12:** 390–398.
30. COX, J. L. & S. D. HARRISON, JR. 1983. Biochem. Biophys. Res. Commun. **115:** 106–111.
31. PUTKEY, J. A., G. F. DRAETTA, G. R. SLAUGHTER, C. B. KLEE, P. COHEN, J. T. STULL & A. R. MEANS. 1986. J. Biol. Chem. **261:** 9896–9903.
32. MAZZEI, G. J., P. R. GIRALD & J. F. KUO. 1984. FEBS Lett. **173:** 124–128.
33. FRIBERG L., M. PISCATOR, G. F. NORDBERG & T. KJELLSTROM. 1974. Cadmium in the Environment. 2nd edit. CRC Press. Cleveland, Ohio.
34. SINGHAL, R. L., Z. MERALI & P. D. HRDINA. 1976. Fed. Proc. **35:** 75–80.
35. SAMARAWICKRAMA, G. P. 1979. *In* The Chemistry, Biochemistry and Biology of Cadmium. M. Webb, Ed.: 341–408. Elsevier/Holland Biomedical Press. Amsterdam & New York.
36. GILES, W., J. R. HUME & E. F. SHIBATA. 1983. Fed Proc.: 2994–2997.

Interaction of Calcium with Receptor-Stimulated Phosphoinositide Hydrolysis in Brain and Liver[a]

F. T. CREWS, R. A. GONZALES, R. RAULLI, R. McELHANEY, N. PONTZER, AND M. RAIZADA

Department of Pharmacology
University of Florida Medical School
Box J-267 J. Hillis Miller Health Center
Gainesville, Florida 32610

Receptors coupled to phosphoinositide hydrolysis have been associated with calcium flux in a variety of tissues.[1] Phosphoinositides (PI) are a class of inositol phospholipids which include phosphatidylinositol, phosphatidylinositol 4-phosphate (PIP), and phosphatidylinositol 4,5-bisphosphate (PIP2). Recently, studies by Berridge and his colleagues have shown that phosphoinositide hydrolysis leads to the formation of inositol 1,4,5-trisphosphate (IP_3) which can release calcium from the sarcoplasmic reticulum of a number of tissues.[2] These experiments clearly demonstrate that phosphoinositide hydrolysis mobilizes intracellular stores of calcium.

The mechanism of receptor activation of plasma membrane calcium flux is still not clear. PI hydrolysis initiates a bifurcating cascade. Receptor stimulation activates a phospholipase C which hydrolyzes PIP_2 to IP_3 and diacylglycerol (DAG). Both IP_3 and DAG are second messengers. IP_3 releases calcium from intracellular stores activating a variety of calcium-requiring processes including calcium-dependent protein kinases. DAG activates a phospholipid-calcium-dependent protein kinase usually referred to as protein kinase C (PKC). PKC has a high activity in a number of excitable tissues. Thus, the PI cascade bifurcates following receptor activation of PIP_2 hydrolysis.

Although receptor-stimulated PI hydrolysis releases intracellular stores of calcium, most receptors have a partial requirement for extracellular calcium.[3,4] Cholinergic muscarinic, $alpha_1$ adrenergic, and several other receptors are inhibited by chelation of extracellular calcium. In fact, different receptors have a differential requirement for extracellular calcium.[4,5] These differences suggest multiple mechanisms of agonist-receptor coupling to PI hydrolysis. Our studies on $alpha_1$ adrenergic receptor stimulation of PI hydrolysis have suggested that there are two subtypes of $alpha_1$ adrenergic receptors, both of which are coupled to PI hydrolysis. One subtype appears to couple directly to the PI phospholipase C through a guanine nucleotide protein, whereas the second subtype appears to stimulate PI hydrolysis secondary to calcium influx.

STUDIES ON $ALPHA_1$ ADRENERGIC AGONISTS

The $alpha_1$ adrenergic receptor is known to mobilize both intracellular and extracellular calcium in a variety of tissues. We have recently investigated the actions

[a]Research supported by Grant NIAAA-AA06069 from the National Institute of Alcohol Abuse and Alcoholism.

of a number of alpha$_1$ agonists on the hydrolysis of PI in different brain regions and in liver. Norepinephrine (NE) was the most efficacious agonist in all brain regions studied (TABLE 1). The largest response was found in the hippocampus and cerebral cortex, whereas the smallest response was found in the brain stem. Several alpha adrenergic drugs were found to be partial agonists. Although the efficacy of most of the partial agonists studied remained constant in different brain regions, dihydroergotamine was significantly less efficacious in the cerebral cortex compared to the brain stem (FIGURE 1). The norepinephrine response in cortex was 161% of the brain stem response, whereas the dihydroergotamine response was slightly greater in the brain stem (TABLE 1). Similar differences in efficacy and brain regional response have been found with muscarinic cholinergic stimulation of PI hydrolysis.[3,6] The differences in agonist efficacy could be due to multiple receptor subtypes coupled to PI hydrolysis and/or differences in the coupling mechanisms of receptors to PI hydrolysis.

To determine if the efficacy of alpha$_1$ adrenergic agonists was similar in excitable (e.g., brain) and nonexcitable (e.g., liver) tissues, the efficacy of alpha$_1$ agonists was

TABLE 1. Brain Region Fractional Release of Phosphoinositides[a]

	CORTEX	HIPPO	BS	OLF BLB	STRIAT.
NE	32.26 ± 1.14	38.80 ± 2.30	19.99 ± 1.08	33.15 ± 2.33	25.72 ± 3.31
PHEN	21.37 ± 0.32	25.84 ± 1.18	14.03 ± 1.09	18.18 ± 0.52	17.41 ± 2.25
METH	20.92 ± 1.37	26.43 ± 0.96	15.44 ± 1.33	20.55 ± 1.82	15.55 ± 2.21
6-FLNE	26.14 ± 0.70	31.97 ± 2.96	14.72 ± 2.30	ND	20.62 ± 2.68
ERGOT	10.20 ± 0.55	10.17 ± 1.44	11.36 ± 0.63	10.85 ± 0.94	ND

[a]Brain regional phosphoinositide hydrolysis for various alpha$_1$ agonists. Phosphoinositide hydrolysis expressed as fractional release (FR), i.e., DPM [^{3}H]inositol phosphates released × 100/total DPM [^{3}H]inositol incorporated ± standard error the mean. Values indicated are total FR × 100 minus basal FR × 100. Basal levels ranged from 4–11% for the various brain regions. Data from cortex, hippocampus (HIPPO), and brain stem (BS) consist of six separate determinations from two experiments. Data from striatum (STRIAT) and olfactory bulb (OLF BLB) as well as 6-fluoronorepinephrine (6-FLNE) and dihydroergotamine (ERGOT) consist of three determinations from one experiment. All drugs were used at a concentration of 100 μM. NE, norepinephrine; PHEN, phenylephrine; METH, methoxamine. ND, not done.

compared between brain and liver (FIGURE 2). When compared with norepinephrine a marked difference between phenylephrine and methoxamine were noted. The efficacy of phenylephrine was 0.66 and 0.92 in brain and liver respectively, whereas that of methoxamine was 0.64 and 0.48 in brain and liver, respectively. Thus variations in alpha$_1$ agonist responsiveness occur in different brain regions and between cerebral cortex and liver.

EFFECTS OF ORGANIC CALCIUM ANTAGONISTS

A variety of data indicate that there are a number of different types of calcium channels. Organic calcium channel antagonists have been shown to modulate the opening of certain voltage-dependent calcium channels. In brain, increased extracellular K^+ has been shown to stimulate PI hydrolysis. The maximum response was observed at 18 mM K^+. Organic calcium channel antagonists can reduce this response by a maximum of 60–65%, while the organic calcium agonist BAY-K-8644 produces a

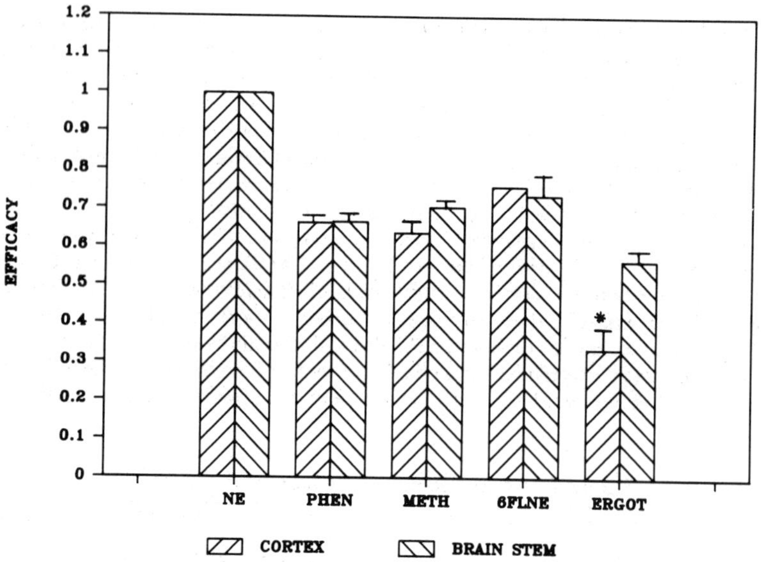

FIGURE 1. Efficacies of various alpha$_1$ agonists: cerebral cortex vs. brain stem. The fractional release (FR) for each drug is divided by the FR for NE in that region to obtain efficacy. Norepinephrine (NE), phenylephrine (PHEN), and methoxamine (METH) data consist of six determinations from two experiments. 6-Fluoronephrine (6FNE) and dihydroergotamine (ERGOT) data consist of three determinations from one experiment. All drugs were used at concentration of 100 μM. $^*p < 0.05$ as determined by Student's t-test.

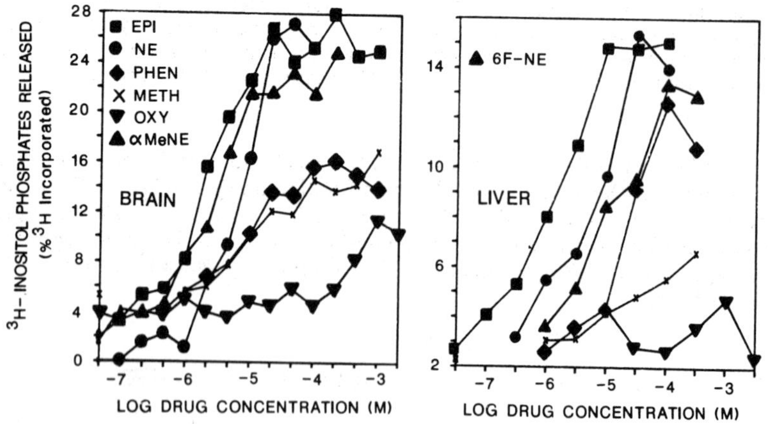

FIGURE 2. Concentration response curves for alpha$_1$ agonist–stimulated phosphoinositide hydrolysis in brain and liver slices expressed as disintegrations per minute (DPM) [^{3}H]inositol phosphates released/total [^{3}H]inositol incorporated × 100, i.e., the fractional release. Data for each drug consists of nine separate determinations from three experiments. EPI, epinephrine; NE, norepinephrine; PHEN, phenylephrine; METH, methoxamine; OXY, oxymetazoline; MeNE, alpha-methyl-norepinephrine; 6F-NE, 6-fluoronephrine.

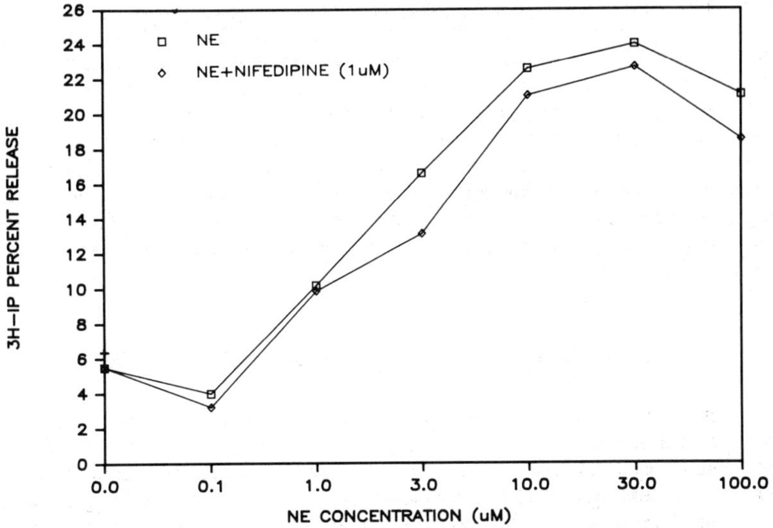

FIGURE 3. Effect of nifedipine on norepinephrine-stimulated phosphoinositide hydrolysis in rat cerebral cortical slices expressed as percent of DPM [^{3}H]inositol phosphates released/total DPM [^{3}H]inositol incorporated. Data consist of six measurements from three separate experiments.

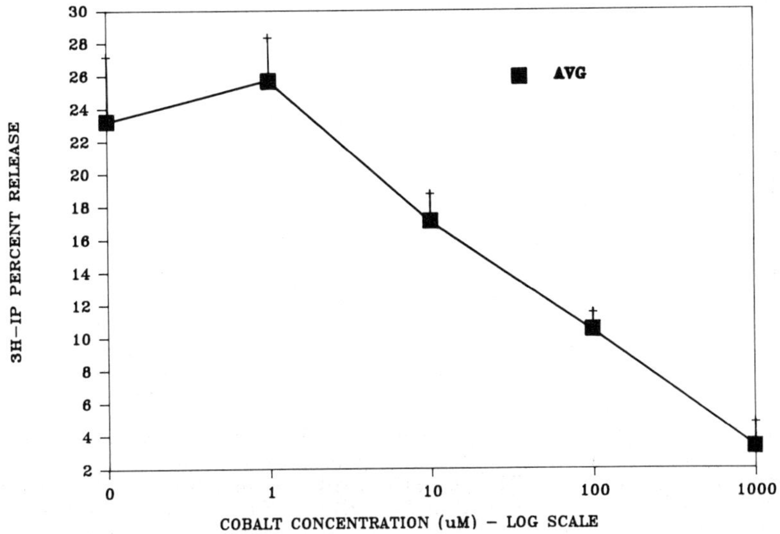

FIGURE 4. Effect of cobalt (Co) on 10 μM norepinephrine-stimulated phosphoinositide hydrolysis in rat cortical slices. Data consist of three determinations from one experiment. [^{3}H]-IP percent release represents [^{3}H]inositol phosphates released/total [^{3}H]inositol incorporated into phospholipids.

dose-related enhancement of the response. In the presence of antagonist, the dose-response curve for BAY-K-8644 is shifted to the right.[7] Thus, K^+ activation of PI hydrolysis appears to be related to the opening of voltage-dependent calcium channels and calcium influx due to depolarization may stimulate the hydrolysis of PI.

To determine if norepinephrine-stimulated PI hydrolysis in brain was altered by organic calcium antagonists, we did complete dose-response curves in the presence of nifedipine (FIGURE 3). Neither the potency nor the maximal response was altered by the presence of organic calcium antagonists. This suggests that the nifedipine-sensitive voltage-dependent calcium channels do not contribute to NE-stimulated PI hydrolysis. This is not surprising since receptor-activated channels are likely to be different from voltage-sensitive channels.

EFFECTS OF OTHER CALCIUM CHANNEL BLOCKERS

To determine if other agents that are known to alter calcium flux interfere with norepinephrine stimulation of PI hydrolysis, we investigated the effects of cobalt (Co^{2+}) and ethanol. Cobalt competes with calcium for the channel binding site and blocks calcium flux. Ethanol has been shown to inhibit Na^+/Ca^{2+} exchange,[8] increase synaptosomal membrane calcium binding,[9] and decrease fast-phase calcium influx.[10,11] We have found that Co^{2+} causes a concentration-dependent decrease in norepineph-

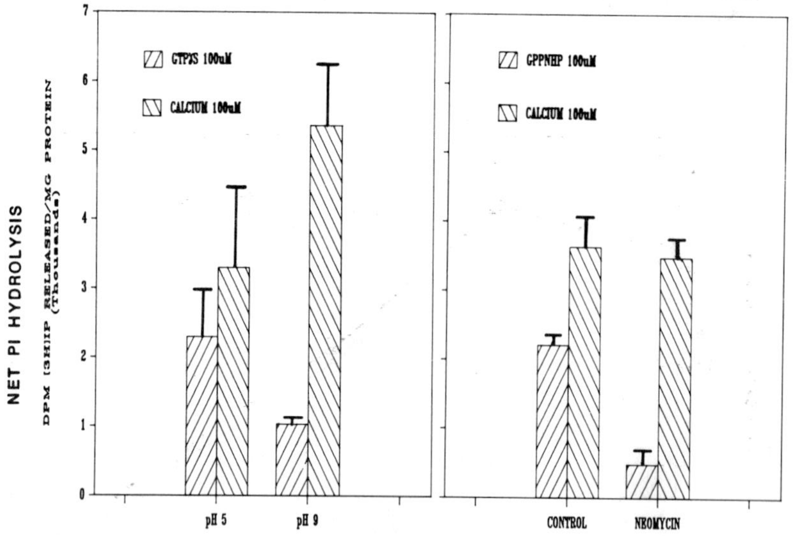

FIGURE 5. Differentiation between guanine nucleotide–stimulated and calcium-stimulated PI hydrolysis in rat cortical membranes. Cerebral cortical slices were labeled with [^{3}H]inositol, membranes were prepared, and PI hydrolysis stimulated by guanine nucleotides or calcium was determined. Assays were conducted in 20 mM Tris-HCl (pH 7.4) or in 20 mM Tris-maleate at the indicated pH for 15 minutes at 37°C. Basal values for control and neomycin-treated membranes were 1800 ± 110 and 210 ± 170 dpm/mg protein, respectively. Basal values for assays done at pH 5 and pH 9 were 4740 ± 820 and 3020 ± 510 dpm/mg protein, respectively. Data are presented as means ± standard error of the mean of three or four independent experiments.

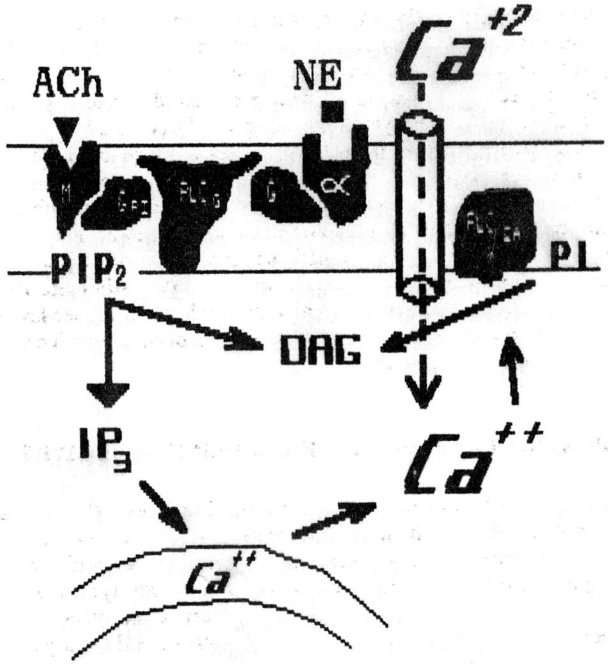

FIGURE 6. Schematic representation of mechanism by which binding of norepinephrine to the alpha adrenergic receptor may directly activate a guanine nucleotide–coupled phospholipase C (PLC_g) and also a calcium-sensitive phospholipase C (PLC_{ca}) through mobilization of both intercellular and extracellular calcium. See text for details.

rine-stimulated PI hydrolysis (FIGURE 4). Previous studies have shown that ethanol blocks both calcium influx[10] and a portion of NE-stimulated phosphoinositide hydrolysis.[13] Thus, agents that are known to block a variety of different types of calcium channels inhibit NE-stimulated PI hydrolysis. These data suggest that calcium is involved in the coupling of the alpha adrenergic receptor to PI hydrolysis.

STUDIES ON GUANINE NUCLEOTIDE-ACTIVATED AND CALCIUM-ACTIVATED PI HYDROLYSIS

To investigate the mechanisms of receptor activation of PI hydrolysis, isolated membranes labeled with [^{3}H]inositol were prepared and PI hydrolysis activated with either guanine nucleotides or calcium. We have previously shown that calcium and guanine nucleotides stimulate PI hydrolysis in membranes in an additive manner.[12] Guanine nucleotides activate phospholipase C hydrolysis of PIP_2 to form IP_3 suggesting that receptors are coupled to a PIP_2-specific phospholipase C through a guanine nucleotide binding protein.[12] Guanine nucleotide stimulation occurs in the absence of calcium. Neomycin, which is known to bind to PI, markedly inhibits guanylylimidodiphosphate (GppNHp) mediated hydrolysis while it has no effect on calcium-activated hydrolysis (FIGURE 5). Calcium stimulation of PI hydrolysis is slightly greater than GppNHp-stimulated hydrolysis at neutral pH and at pH 5. However, at pH 9 guanine nucleotide stimulation is almost completely lost whereas calcium-activated hydrolysis is markedly increased (FIGURE 5, left). These data suggest that there may be two phosphoinositide phospholipase C (PI-PLC) enzymes in brain tissue, one activated by receptors through a guanine nucleotide protein and another that is activated by calcium. These enzymes may have a differential affinity for phosphatidylinositol, PIP, and/or PIP_2. PIP_2 hydrolysis releases intracellular stores of calcium and generates DAG for activation of PKC. Hydrolysis of phosphatidylinositol would activate only the PKC side of the bifurcating PI cascade. Although the increases in cytoplasmic calcium following receptor stimulation might not be sufficient for calcium-activated PI hydrolysis, the increases that occur during pathological conditions clearly are within the range of concentrations that stimulate PI hydrolysis *in vitro*.[12] Cytoplasmic concentrations of calcium reach much higher levels in excitable tissues. Receptors in these tissues may couple PI hydrolysis through calcium flux more readily than in nonexcitable tissues.

$ALPHA_1$ RECEPTOR SUBTYPE COUPLING TO PI HYDROLYSIS

The data presented are consistent with the hypothesis that $alpha_1$ adrenergic receptors are coupled to PI hydrolysis through two separate pathways (FIGURE 6). $Alpha_1$ adrenergic receptors may interact with a guanine nucleotide protein to activate the PI phospholipase C. This activation results in the hydrolysis of PIP_2 forming IP_3 and releasing intracellular stores of calcium. Muscarinic receptors may act through a similar mechanism. $Alpha_1$ receptors may also couple directly to a plasma membrane calcium channel (FIGURE 6). The increase in cytosolic calcium due to calcium influx and the release of intracellular calcium stores may activate a second PI phospholipase C. Thus, $alpha_1$ adrenergic receptors may stimulate phosphoinositide hydrolysis directly through a guanine nucleotide protein and indirectly through the opening of calcium channels.

REFERENCES

1. MICHELL, R. H. 1975. Inositol phospholipids and cell surface receptors. Biochim. Biophys. Acta **415:** 81–147.
2. BERRIDGE, M. J. 1984. Inositol trisphosphate and diacylglycerol as second messengers. Biochem. J. **220:** 345–360.
3. GONZALES, R. A. & F. T. CREWS. 1984. Characterization of the cholinergic stimulation of phosphoinositide hydrolysis in rat brain slices. J. Neurosci. **4**(12): 3120–3127.
4. KENDALL, D. A. & S. R. NAHORSKI. 1984. Inositol phospholipid hydrolysis in rat cerebral cortical slices. II. Calcium requirement. J. Neurochem. **42**(5): 1348–1394.
5. GONZALES, R. A. & F. T. CREWS. 1985. Cholinergic- and adrenergic-stimulated inositide hydrolysis in brain: interaction, regional distribution, and coupling mechanism. J. Neurochem. **45**(4): 1076–1084.
6. FISHER, S. K. & R. T. BARTUS. 1985. Regional differences in the coupling of muscarinic receptors to inositol phospholipid hydrolysis in guinea pig brain. J. Neurochem. **45**(4): 1085–1095.
7. KENDALL, D. A. & S. R. NAHORSKI. 1985. Dihydropyridine and calcium channel activators and antagonists influence depolarization-evoked inositol phospholipid hydrolysis in brain. Eur. J. Pharmacol. **115:** 31–36.
8. MICHAELIS, M. L. & E. K. MICHAELIS. 1983. Alcohol and local anesthetic effects on Na^+ dependent Ca^{2+} fluxes in brain synaptic membrane vesicles. Biochem. Pharmacol. **32:** 963–969.

9. MICHAELIS, E. K. & S. L. MYERS. 1979. Calcium binding to brain synaptosomes: effects of chronic ethanol intake. Biochem. Pharmacol. **28:** 2081–2087.
10. LESLIE, S. W., E. BARR, J. CHANDLER & R. P. FARRAR. 1983. Inhibition of fast- and slow-phase depolarization dependent synaptosomal calcium uptake by ethanol. J. Pharmacol. Exp. Ther. **225:** 571–575.
11. DANIELL, L. C. & S. W. LESLIE. 1986. Inhibition of fast phase calcium uptake and endogenous norepinephrine release in rat brain region synaptosomes by ethanol. Brain Res. **377:** 18–28.
12. GONZALES, R. A. & F. T. CREWS. 1985. Guanine nucleotides stimulate production of inositol trisphosphate in rat cortical membranes. Biochem. J. **232:** 799–804.
13. GONZALES, R. A., C. THEISS & F. T. CREWS. 1986. Effects of ethanol on stimulated inositol phospholipid hydrolysis in rat brain. J. Pharmacol. Exp. Ther. **227:** 92–98.

Presence in Brain of an Endogenous Ligand for Nitrendipine-Binding Sites that Modulates Ca^{2+} Channel Activity

INGEBORG HANBAUER AND ENRICO SANNA[a]

Hypertension-Endocrine Branch
National Heart, Lung and Blood Institute
National Institutes of Health
Building 10, Room 7N244
Bethesda, Maryland 20892

INTRODUCTION

Ca^{2+} is considered to be an intracellular messenger because it is involved in the regulation of processes that include contractile, secretory, and neuronal activities (for review, see Reference 1). Several classes of drugs including phenylalkylamines, dihydropyridines, and benzothiazepines have been shown to inhibit Ca^{2+} flux through voltage-dependent Ca^{2+} channels.[2–6] This drug action mechanism has been established and verified by several laboratories to occur in smooth and cardiac muscle cells. In contrast, only recently was the presence of voltage-dependent Ca^{2+} channels discovered in neuronal tissues.[7–10] An important tool that facilitated the biochemical identification of Ca^{2+} channels in neuronal cells was the measurement of the specific binding of radiolabeled dihydropyridines.[11–14] In brain, recognition sites for dihydropyridines are not uniformly distributed. Autoradiographic and radioligand binding studies demonstrated that the highest densities occur in the hippocampus, the cerebral cortex, the caudate nucleus, and the granular layer of the cerebellum.[14–15] Similar results were obtained from immunofluorescence techniques using antisera raised against subunits of the dihydropyridine-binding sites.[16] In addition to the information on the distribution of dihydropyridine-recognition sites, work from this laboratory showed that ^{3}H-nitrendipine-binding sites in corpus striatum or hippocampus are mainly localized on intrinsic neurons and are only sparingly present or absent in nerve terminals emanating from other brain areas.[10] Moreover, voltage-dependent $^{45}Ca^{2+}$ uptake occurred at sites closely linked to the dihydropyridine-recognition sites, because destruction of intrinsic neurons by injecting kainic acid directly into the tissue completely impaired the veratridine-stimulated $^{45}Ca^{2+}$ uptake.[10]

Although there exists ample evidence that voltage-dependent Ca^{2+} channels can be modulated by dihydropyridines, it is still unresolved whether their recognition sites on cell membranes play a physiological role in the regulation of calcium channel activity. Recent reports in the literature demonstrated that sympathetic denervation of heart tissue caused by intravenous injections of 6-hydroxy-dopamine elicited supersensitivity of ^{3}H-nitrendipine-binding sites.[17] Similarly, an up regulation of ^{3}H-nitrendipine-binding sites in cardiac membranes was observed four weeks after bilateral adrenal demedullation (Sanna, E., to be published). Moreover, the number of ^{3}H-nitrendipine-

[a]E. Sanna was supported in part by a grant from the Scottish Rite Schizophrenia Research Program, Northern Masonic Jurisdiction, United States.

binding sites in brain synaptosomal membranes was increased in morphine-tolerant mice.[18] It is tempting to speculate that the sites to which Ca^{2+} channel antagonists bind with high affinity may be binding sites for endogenous ligands operative in Ca^{2+} channel gating.

Some information in the literature favors the concept that endogenous modulators may be operative in regulating Ca^{2+} channel activity. Recent work by Spedding showed that palmityl carnitine, a substance found in ischemic heart, directly increased Ca^{2+} channel function.[19] In contrast, recent work from this laboratory demonstrated the existence in rat brain of a substance that displaces ^{3}H-nitrendipine from its binding sites and that decreases Ca^{2+} channel activity.[20]

The present report describes an isolation procedure for the nitrendipine-displacing material, and demonstrates its modulatory effect on veratridine- and glutamic acid–stimulated Ca^{2+} uptake and cyclic GMP formation.

EXTRACTION AND ISOLATION OF AN ENDOGENOUS LIGAND FOR NITRENDIPINE-BINDING SITES FROM RAT BRAIN

Fractionation on Biogel-P10 and Silica SEP-PAK

Rat brains were homogenized in 10 v/w distilled water (Brinkman, Polytron, setting 6, 30 seconds). The homogenates were heat treated at 95°C for 5 minutes, centrifuged (35,000 × *g* for 20 minutes at 4°C) and the supernatant fraction was lyophilized. The dried residue was dissolved in 0.1 N acetic acid and loaded on Biogel-P10 (1 × 45 cm, equilibrated in 0.1 N acetic acid). The eluted fractions (1 ml) were lyophilized and then tested for ^{3}H-nitrendipine-displacing activity using a procedure for radioligand binding described by Sanna *et al.*[10] The top panel of FIGURE 1 demonstrates that ^{3}H-nitrendipine-displacing activity elutes in a single peak with a profile similar to that of a molecular weight marker of 1.2 K. Studies on the solubility showed that this endogenous ligand for nitrendipine-binding sites was insoluble in chloroform but soluble in more polar organic solvents (methanol, ethanol) and aqueous solvents with acidic or neutral pH, but precipitated in solutions with basic pH range. In order to establish a technique useful to purify the endogenous ligand, the elution profiles on various SEP-PAK cartridges were studied. The endogenous-ligand-containing material was dissolved in a small volume of ethanol and loaded on Silica SEP-PAK (Waters). The elution profile in the bottom panel of FIGURE 1 shows that endogenous ligand was retained on the cartridge if it was washed with 100% chloroform. The main activity of the endogenous ligand was eluted by increasing the polarity of the eluent such as a solvent mixture of chloroform (8 parts) and methanol (2 parts). In contrast, the endogenous ligand was not retained on a C_{18}-SEP-PAK cartridge (Waters) suggesting that the active material may contain highly charged molecular groups.

Purification of the Endogenous Ligand by High-Voltage Electrophoresis

Endogenous-ligand-containing material was loaded on a column (1.0 × 60 cm) of 0.2% agarose C equilibrated in 25 mM ammonium formate pH 4.0 or pH 5.0 at the middle height of the column and was electrophoresed at 1100 V, 4.5 mA for 6 hours. Under these conditions the nitrendipine-displacing material remained at the site of application but was separated off from other contaminating material. The lack of mobility on agarose C at the given electrophoretic conditions indicates that in acidic pH conditions the endogenous ligand may occur in a state close to its isoelectric point.

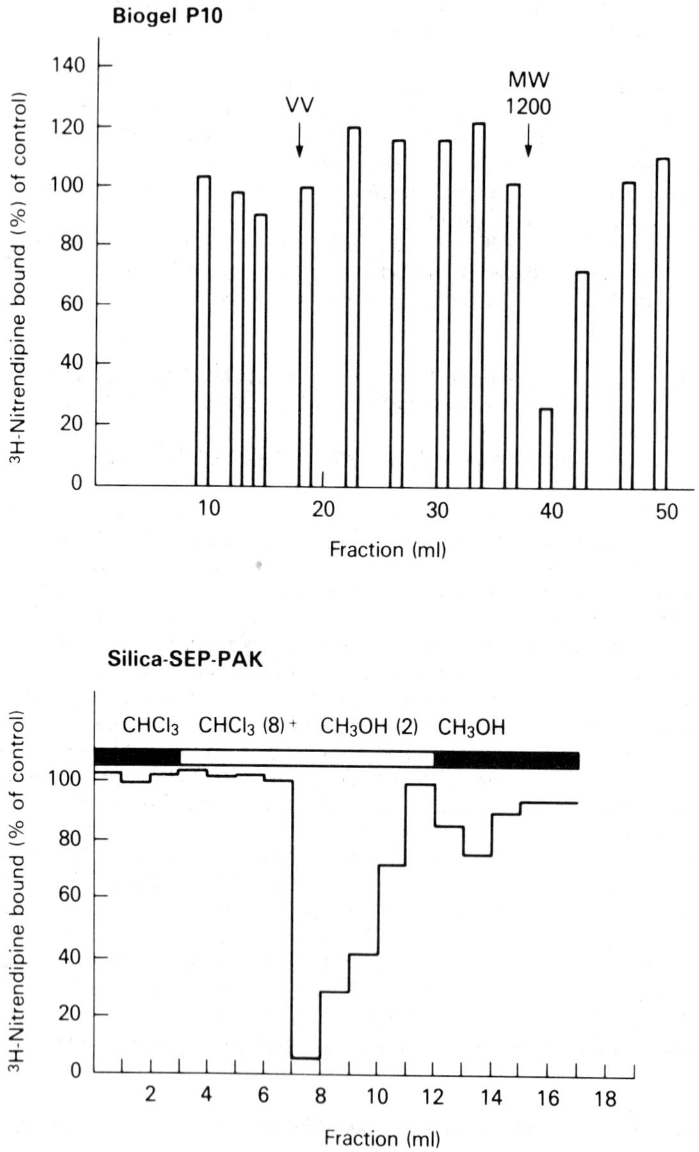

FIGURE 1. Top: Behavior of an endogenous ligand for nitrendipine-binding sites on Biogel-P10 equilibrated and eluted with 0.1 N acetic acid (1 ml/fraction). The eluates were lyophilized and then assayed for ^{3}H-nitrendipine-displacing activity. Bottom: Behavior of the endogenous ligand for nitrendipine-binding sites on Silica SEP-PAK. The cartridge was first washed with 100% chloroform, then with solvent mixture of 8 parts chloroform and 2 parts methanol that was followed by 100% methanol.

Fractionation of the Endogenous Ligand by High Performance Liquid Chromatography (HPLC) on Partisil-10SCX

The endogenous-ligand-containing fractions obtained from high-voltage electrophoresis were eluted with water, and the supernatant fractions were dried in a speed

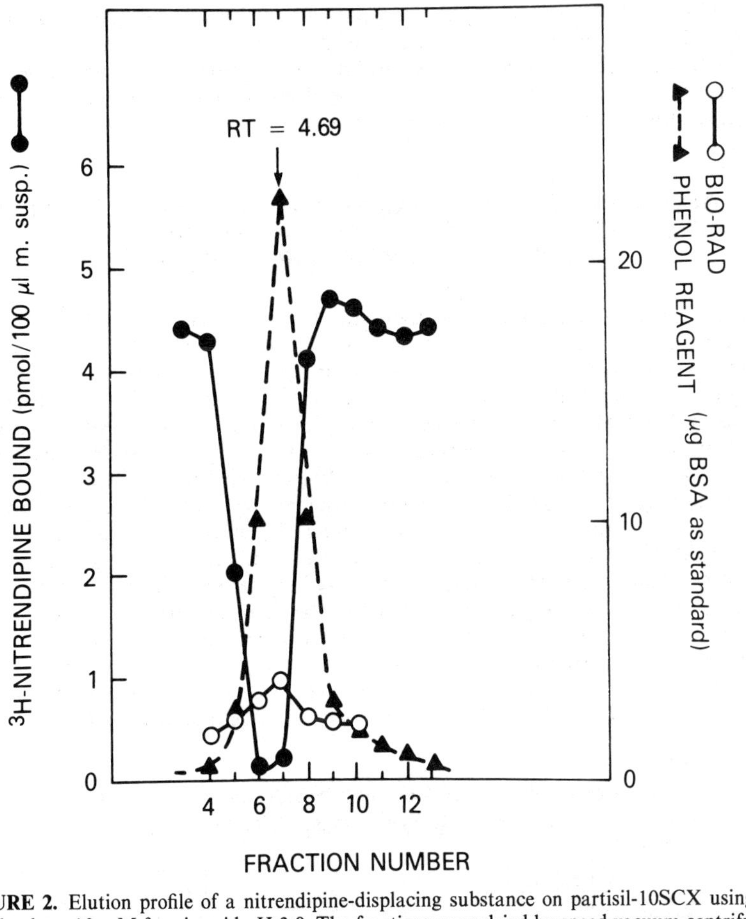

FIGURE 2. Elution profile of a nitrendipine-displacing substance on partisil-10SCX using as mobile phase 10 mM formic acid pH 3.0. The fractions were dried by speed vacuum centrifugation and redissolved in distilled water. Aliquots were tested for ^{3}H-nitrendipine-displacing activity and reactivity with Folin phenol reagent or Bio-Rad reagent using as an arbitrary standard bovine serum albumin.

vacuum concentrator at 37°C (Savant Instruments). The active material was redissolved in H_2O and injected into a HPLC system (Waters) using a partisil-10SCX column and as mobile phase 10 mM formic acid pH 3.0. The data in FIGURE 2 show that ^{3}H-nitrendipine-displacing material elutes in one single peak with a retention time of 4.7 minutes. Aliquots of the same fractions were tested with Bio-Rad protein reagent and Folin phenol reagent (Fisher). FIGURE 2 shows that the fractions that contained ^{3}H-nitrendipine-displacing activity were also reacting with the Folin phenol reagent. In comparison, the fractions containing ^{3}H-nitrendipine-displacing material showed very low reactivity with the Bio-Rad protein reagent. The discrepancy in reactivity between these two test reagents indicates that material isolated in a single peak from the partisil-10SCX column contains only a small amount of protein, but contains a large amount of phenol-residues. In order to establish whether the endogenous ligand could be characterized as a peptide, fractions containing the nitrendipine-displacing material were incubated in the absence or presence of pronase (1 mg/ml). The data shown in TABLE 1 clearly indicate that the nitrendipine-displacing activity was unaltered by the treatment with pronase and suggest that the endogenous ligand may not be a peptide but rather an organic substance possibly containing phenol groups.

MODULATION OF $^{45}Ca^{2+}$ UPTAKE INTO CULTURED CEREBELLAR GRANULE CELLS ELICITED BY AN ENDOGENOUS LIGAND FOR NITRENDIPINE-BINDING SITES

Recently, the coexistence of various types of Ca^{2+} channels in neuronal membranes has been demonstrated by patch-clamp studies.[7–8] The outcome of that work proposed that the opening of Ca^{2+} channels may occur through a voltage-dependent mechanism resembling qualitatively that of the Na^+ channel. Electrophysiological and pharmacological studies demonstrated that dihydropyridine derivatives can interact as agonists or antagonists with the voltage-dependent or long-lasting current-dependent Ca^{2+} channel. In fact, the recognition sites for dihydropyridines are considered to be a part of the supramolecular unit of the voltage-dependent Ca^{2+} channel complex. Proceeding on the assumption that ^{3}H-nitrendipine-binding sites constitute a part of the supramolecular entity of the Ca^{2+} channel, studies were carried out in this laboratory aimed to clarify whether the endogenous ligand that was shown to displace ^{3}H-nitrendipine from its specific binding sites would affect other processes associated with the Ca^{2+} channel function including Ca^{2+} influx. In cerebellar granule cells Ca^{2+} entry is mediated by channels that were shown to be regulated by specific receptors or by changes in membrane potential. The increase in Ca^{2+} influx elicited by increasing K^+ concentrations or by veratridine was shown to be attenuated by Ca^{2+} channel

TABLE 1. Decreased Specific Binding of ^{3}H-Nitrendipine to Hippocampal Membranes by a Pronase-Resistent Endogeneous Ligand Isolated from Rat Brain[a]

Endogenous Ligand		^{3}H-Nitrendipine Bound
Addition	Pretreatment	(pmol/mg protein)
no	None	85
yes	None	8.5
yes	Pronase (1 mg/ml) 1 hour at 37°C	10

[a]The values represent the mean of two different assays in triplicate. Fractions from SCX HPLC containing ^{3}H-nitrendipine-displacing activity were pooled and dried by speed vacuum centrifugation. Aliquots of the active material were incubated in the absence and presence of pronase. The pronase-treated samples were exposed to 95°C for 5 minutes, centrifuged, and the nitrendipine-displacing activity was measured as described by Sanna *et al.*[10]

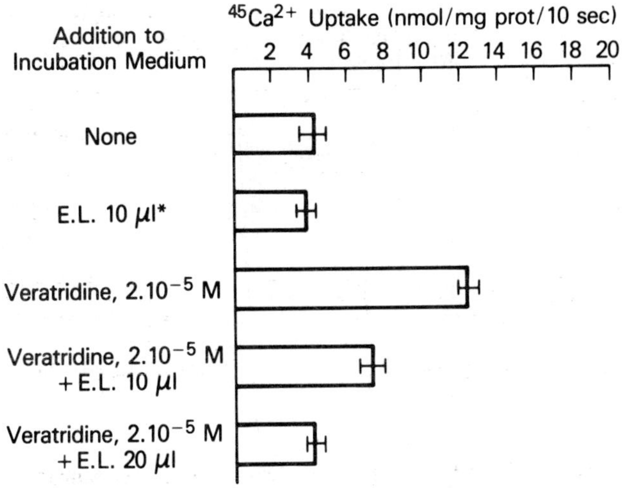

Values are means ± SE of 3 to 6 determinations

*10 μl E.L. extract decreased ^{3}H-Nitrendipine binding by 20%

FIGURE 3. Effect of an endogenous ligand for nitrendipine-binding sites purified by HPLC technique on the veratridine-stimulated increase of $^{45}Ca^{2+}$ uptake in primary cultures of cerebellar granule cells. The cells were preincubated for 20 minutes. Various amounts of endogenous ligand were added 1 minute before addition of 1.3 mM $^{45}Ca^{2+}$ and 2.10^{-5} M veratridine.

antagonists.[20–21] Primary cultures of cerebellar neurons prepared from seven-day-old rats were used for studying the effect of the endogenous ligand on $^{45}Ca^{2+}$ uptake. After about eight days in culture under conditions described by Gallo *et al.*[22] approximately 90% of the cells are granule cells and express voltage-dependent as well as glutamate-receptor-dependent Ca^{2+} channels.[21–23] Measurements of $^{45}Ca^{2+}$ uptake in cultured cerebellar cells were carried out at 37°C after replacing the culture medium with balanced salt solution[21] and after a preincubation period of about 20 minutes. The cells were incubated in the absence or presence of various amounts of endogenous ligand for 1 minute. Thereafter incubation buffer containing 1.3 mM $^{45}Ca^{2+}$ and 2×10^{-5} M veratridine (final concentration) was added and the incubation was continued for 10 seconds. The cells were then washed three times with 1 ml of incubation buffer, the proteins were precipitated with 5% trichloroacetic acid, and the amount of $^{45}Ca^{2+}$ in the supernatant fraction was measured by scintillation spectroscopy. FIGURE 3 shows that the presence in the incubation medium of 2×10^{-5} M veratridine elicts a two- to threefold increase of $^{45}Ca^{2+}$ uptake into cerebellar granule cells which was attenuated by the addition of 10^{-6} M tetrodotoxin (final concentration; data not shown). When endogenous ligand purified by HPLC technique was added to the incubation medium 15 seconds before the addition of veratridine, the $^{45}Ca^{2+}$ uptake was inhibited in a dose-dependent manner and was completely blocked by an equivalent amount of endogenous ligand that caused about 50% inhibition of ^{3}H-nitrendipine binding. Recently, it has been demonstrated that an increase of intracellular Ca^{2+} concentration initiated several biochemical processes. In cerebellar granule cells, for example, the increase in Ca^{2+} influx elicited by excitatory amino acids was associated with the

TABLE 2. Modulation of the $^{45}Ca^{2+}$ Uptake and cGMP Accumulation Elicited by Veratridine in Cerebellar Granule Cells by an Endogenous Ligand Eluted from Silica-SEP-PAK[a]

Addition of Endogenous Ligand from Silica-SEP-PAK	Incubation in Presence of Veratridine[b]	$^{45}Ca^{2+}$ Uptake (nmol/mg protein per 20 seconds)	cGMP Accumulation (pmol/mg protein per 2 minutes)
None	No	4.3	0.11
None	Yes	11.2	17.25
30 μl	Yes	8.1	11.04
60 μl[c]	Yes	5.3	5.12

[a] Values were obtained by two different measurements in triplicate.

[b] For $^{45}Ca^{2+}$ uptake and cGMP accumulation studies, 2×10^{-5} M and 5×10^{-5} M veratridine, respectively, was used.

[c] 60 μl of the endogenous-ligand-containing solution inhibited ^{3}H-nitrendipine binding by 90%.

activation of guanylate cyclase, specific protein kinases, and enhanced inositol phospholipid hydrolysis.[24-26] The data in TABLE 2 show that in cerebellar granule cells the veratridine-elicited increase of $^{45}Ca^{2+}$ uptake was also associated with an increase in cyclic GMP formation. Furthermore, addition of various amounts of endogenous ligand reduced the $^{45}Ca^{2+}$ influx and decreased cyclic GMP formation in a concentration-dependent manner. These findings show that the nitrendipine-displacing material isolated from rat brain modulates voltage-dependent Ca^{2+} uptake in a manner comparable to Ca^{2+} channel antagonists. The question arises as to whether the endogenous ligand of nitrendipine-recognition sites is specifically acting on membrane sites associated with the voltage-dependent Ca^{2+} channel. It has been shown previously that glutamic acid can stimulate Ca^{2+} influx into brain cortical slices,[27] striatal synaptosomes,[28] and cerebellar granule cells in primary culture.[23] Moreover, it has been pointed out that in neurons of various brain areas, functional subtypes of this receptor exist which can be differentiated by their sensitivity to *N*-methyl-D-aspartate, phencyclidine, and Mg^{2+}. Electrophysiological studies showed that the glutamate receptor stimulated by *N*-methyl-D-aspartate was also strongly dependent on the voltage applied to the postsynaptic cell.[29] At negative voltages this channel was immediately blocked by physiological concentrations of Mg^{2+}, while at more positive voltages Mg^{2+} was driven out and Na^{+} and Ca^{2+} were permitted to flow in resulting in

TABLE 3. Effect of an Endogenous Ligand for Nitrendipine-Binding Sites on $^{45}Ca^{2+}$ Uptake Elicited by Kainic Acid or Glutamic Acid in Cerebellar Granule Cells[a]

Number of Fraction Eluted from SCX Column	$^{45}Ca^{2+}$ Uptake (nmol/mg protein per 5 minutes)	
	Kainic Acid (10^{-4} M)	Glutamic Acid (10^{-4} M)
4	28	18
6	36	16
7	23	12
8	27	13
9	34	23
10	34	18

[a] The values are the mean of two different measurements in triplicate. The uptake of $^{45}Ca^{2+}$ in absence of kainic acid or glutamic acid was 9.8 nmol/mg protein per 5 minutes.

an excitation of the neuron. In order to assess the mechanism whereby the endogenous ligand may act on voltage-dependent Ca^{2+} uptake, studies on various types of receptor-dependent Ca^{2+} channels were carried out. In primary cultures of cerebellar granule cells, addition to the culture medium of 10^{-4} M glutamic acid or 10^{-4} M kainic acid caused a two- or threefold increase in $^{45}Ca^{2+}$ uptake (TABLE 3). The accumulation of $^{45}Ca^{2+}$ elicited by glutamic acid was effectively reduced by the nitrendipine-displacing material that eluted in fractions 7 and 8 from the partisil-10SCX column. In contrast, the same fractions failed to alter the kainic acid–stimulated $^{45}Ca^{2+}$ uptake (TABLE 3). The outcome of these experiments is compatible with the information obtained from electrophysiological studies which indicated that the glutamate-activated Ca^{2+} channel may induce a voltage-dependent conductance increase, while kainic acid and quisqualic acid were ineffective.[29]

CONCLUSION

The present report brings evidence for the existence in brain of an organic substance that appears to bind to recognition sites for dihydropyridine derivatives. By binding to these sites this substance modifies the kinetics of the dihydropyridine-

TABLE 4. Interaction of an Endogenous Ligand for Nitrendipine-Binding Sites with Various Types of Ca^{2+} Channels in Cerebellar Granule Cells

Depolarizing Agent	Ca^{2+} Flux	Cyclic GMP Formation	Inhibition by	
			Dihydropyridines	Endogenous Ligand
K^+	↑	↑	Yes	Yes
Veratridine	↑	↑	Yes	Yes
Glutamic acid	↑	↑	ND[a]	Yes
Kainic acid	↑	↑	No	No

[a]ND = not determined.

inhibited Ca^{2+} channel. Several lines of evidence indicate that dihydropyridine-recognition sites are a molecular component of the Ca^{2+} channel complex. In fact, the activity of this substance isolated from brain has been demonstrated by measuring the displacement of ^{3}H-nitrendipine from its binding sites on hippocampal membrane preparations. Moreover, some of the effects of this endogenous ligand on Ca^{2+} channel activity resemble strikingly that displayed by Ca^{2+} channel antagonists themselves. The endogenous ligand attenuates the veratridine-elicited increase in Ca^{2+} influx and reduces cyclic GMP formation in a concentration-dependent fashion. In addition, it also blocks the glutamate-receptor-stimulated $^{45}Ca^{2+}$ uptake in cerebellar granule cells, while it fails to alter Ca^{2+} accumulation elicited by kainic acid, an agonist for a specific subtype of glutamate receptors. These results clearly demonstrate that this endogenous ligand isolated from brain interacts with a specific class of Ca^{2+} channels, in that the opening of the channel appears to require an intramembrane voltage-dependent gate. It has been pointed out that at least two subtypes of glutamate-activated channels exist, one of which is allegedly voltage sensitive. The present data are not sufficient to understand whether there are differences in the molecular mechanisms operative in membrane depolarization triggered by veratridine or glutamic acid. The scheme shown in TABLE 4 depicts a working model that involves the action of the putative endogenous ligand in the regulation of certain types of Ca^{2+}

channels present in neurons. Before closing, it is tempting to suggest that the term "voltage-dependent channel" is a provisional term to indicate that it is understood that the channel can open by changing the energy levels with voltage. The energy shift that triggers channel opening may well be mediated by a specific transmitter or modulator. Certainly, this inference is in order for the Ca^{2+} channel because specific substances such as dihydropyridines were shown to be able to open or close this channel. The data on an endogenous ligand described in this report indirectly support the view that the so-called dihydropyridine-sensitive, voltage-dependent Ca^{2+} channel could turn out to be a receptor-modulated Ca^{2+} channel having as an endogenous modulator the substance that we have isolated from brain and which we are in the process of chemically characterizing.

ACKNOWLEDGMENT

The authors thank L. Elliott and A. G. Wright, Jr., for their excellent technical assistance.

REFERENCES

1. RUBIN, R. P. 1970. Pharmacol. Rev. **22:** 389–428.
2. FLECKENSTEIN, A. & G. GRUN. 1969. Pfluegers Arch. **307:** R26.
3. FLECKENSTEIN, A. 1977. Annu. Rev. Pharmacol. Toxicol. **17:** 149–166.
4. JANIS, R. A. & A. SCRIABINE. 1983. Biochem. Pharmacol. **32:** 3499–3507.
5. REUTER, H. 1984. Electrophysiology and calcium channels in the heart. *In* Calcium Antagonists and Cardiovascular Disease. L. H. Opie, Ed.: 43–51. Raven Press. New York, N.Y.
6. TSIEN, R. W. 1983. Annu. Rev. Physiol. **45:** 341–358.
7. NOWYCKY, M. C., A. P. FOX & R. W. TSIEN. 1985. Proc. Nat. Acad. Sci. USA **82:** 2178–2182.
8. NOWYCKY, M. C., A. P. FOX & R. W. TSIEN. 1985. Nature London **316:** 440–443.
9. TURNER, T. J. & S. M. GOLDIN. 1985. J. Neurosci. **5:** 841–849.
10. SANNA, E., G. A. HEAD & I. HANBAUER. 1986. J. Neurochem. **47:** 1552–1557.
11. GOULD, R. J., K. M. MURPHY & S. H. SNYDER. 1982. Proc. Nat. Acad. Sci. USA **80:** 860–864.
12. JANIS, R. A., S. C. MAURER, J. G. SARMIENTO, G. T. BOLGER & D. J. TRIGGLE. 1982. Eur. J. Pharmacol. **82:** 191–194.
13. GLOSSMANN, H. & D. R. FERRY. 1983. Naunyn Schmiedeberg's Arch. Pharmacol. **323:** 279–291.
14. CORTES, R., P. SUPAVILAI, M. KAROBATH & J. M. PALACIOS. 1983. Neurosci. Lett. **42:** 249–254.
15. QUIRION, R. 1985. Eur. J. Pharmacol. **117:** 139–142.
16. SCHMID, A., J. BARHANIN, C. MOURRE, T. COPPOLA, M. BORSOTTO & M. LAZDUNSKI. 1986. Biochem. Biophys. Res. Commun. **139:** 996–1002.
17. SKATTEBOL, A. & D. J. TRIGGLE. 1986. Eur. J. Pharmacol. **127:** 287–289.
18. RAMKUMAR, V. & E. E. EL-FAKAHANY. 1984. Eur. J. Pharmacol. **102:** 371–372.
19. SPEDDING, M. 1985. Naunyn Schmiedeberg's Arch. Pharmacol. **328:** 464–466.
20. HANBAUER, I. & E. SANNA. 1986. Clin. Neuropharmacol. 3(Suppl. 4): 220–222.
21. CARBONI, E., W. J. WOJCIK & E. COSTA. 1985. Neuropharmacology **24:** 1123–1126.
22. GALLO, V., M. T. VIOTTI, A. COLETTI, F. ALOISI & G. LEVI. 1982. Proc. Nat. Acad. Sci. USA **79:** 7919–7923.
23. WROBLEWSKI, J. E., F. NICOLETTI & E. COSTA. 1985. Neuropharmacology **24:** 919–921.
24. NOVELLI, A., F. NICOLETTI, J. T. WROBLEWSKI, H. ALHO, E. COSTA & A. GUIDOTTI. 1987. J. Neurosci. **7:** 40–47.

25. SAITOH, T. & J. H. SCHWARTZ. 1985. J. Cell Biol. **100:** 835.
26. NICOLETTI, F., J. T. WROBLEWSKI, A. NOVELLI, H. ALHO, A. GUIDOTTI & E. COSTA. 1986. J. Neurosci. **6:** 1905–1911.
27. RETZ, K. C. & J. T. COYLE. 1984. Neuropharmacology **23:** 89–94.
28. RETZ, K. C., A. C. YOUNG & J. T. COYLE. 1982. Eur. J. Pharmacol. **79:** 319–322.
29. NOWAK, L., P. BREGESTOVSKI, P. ASCHER, A. HERBET & A. PROCHIANTZ. 1984. Nature **307:** 462–465.

Cyclic Nucleotides and Calcium Regulation in Heart and Smooth Muscle Cells

JEAN-CLAUDE STOCLET, CHANTAL BOULANGER-SAUNIER, BERNARD LASSEGUE, AND CLAIRE LUGNIER

Cellular and Molecular Pharmacology Unit
UA CNRS 600
Faculty of Pharmacy
Louis Pasteur University
BP 10, F 67048 Strasbourg Cedex, France

INTRODUCTION

It is generally accepted that contractile responses of cardiac and vascular smooth muscle cells to stimulation are triggered by an increase in intracellular concentration of free Ca^{2+} ions.[1,2] There is also strong evidence that adenosine 3′,5′-monophosphate (cAMP) can control calcium movements in and out of these cells,[3,4] and a participation of guanosine 3′,5′-monophosphate (cGMP) in the regulation of contractile activity of heart and smooth muscles has also been proposed.[5,6] However, the physiological role of the two cyclic nucleotides and the biochemical mechanisms accounting for their intracellular effects are still not completely determined. For example, it is well established that cAMP is able to modulate the intracellular free calcium concentration in cardiac[3,7] and smooth muscle[8,9] cells stimulated by depolarization or by various agonists, but the reason why cAMP increases the force of contraction and augments the rate of relaxation of the heart whereas it only decreases contraction of smooth muscles is not entirely elucidated. Extensive investigations on the respective roles of cyclic nucleotides and calcium have led to the concept of a concerted regulation of cell functions by these "second messengers"—not only calcium and cyclic nucleotides appear able to modulate the intracellular level of each other in a complex fashion, but they also exert some of their effects on the same metabolic pathways. The concept that second messengers act in a concerted manner can now be extended to other molecules like inositol phosphates and diacylglycerol, which are released upon stimulation of plasma membrane receptors, and are able to trigger a calcium signal[11] and to play a role in cell responses in which calcium and cyclic nucleotides are implicated.[1,12,13]

Cyclic nucleotides are believed to produce their intracellular effects through the activation of protein kinases,[14,15] but the identities and functions of the relevant endogenous substrates are still partially unknown. Recently, protein kinases activated by Ca^{2+} ions rather than by cyclic nucleotides have been identified. One is the calcium-activated phospholipid-dependent protein kinase, or protein kinase C, which has been found to be ubiquitous in mammalian tissues.[16] Others are protein kinases activated by the calcium-calmodulin complex, such as myosin kinase, phophorylase kinase, and other kinases of which the properties and functions are still to a large extent unknown.[13,17] Interestingly, some endogenous proteins are substrates for several protein kinases. FIGURE 1 schematically illustrates the different but intricate pathways through which stimulation of receptors located on the plasma membrane may regulate intracellular functions mediated by second messenger systems. Complete understanding of the mechanisms of cell responses to stimulation would require an entire knowledge of the intracellular regulatory networks constituted by the second messengers and their target proteins. The aim of the present review is not to give a general overview of these networks, which may vary from one cell type to another and are still very partially known. It is rather to focus on some recent findings regarding cyclic nucleotide phosphodiesterases and endogenous membrane protein substrates of cAMP-dependent protein kinase and protein kinase C, in cardiac and vascular smooth muscle cells. These findings may help us to understand the regulation of cyclic

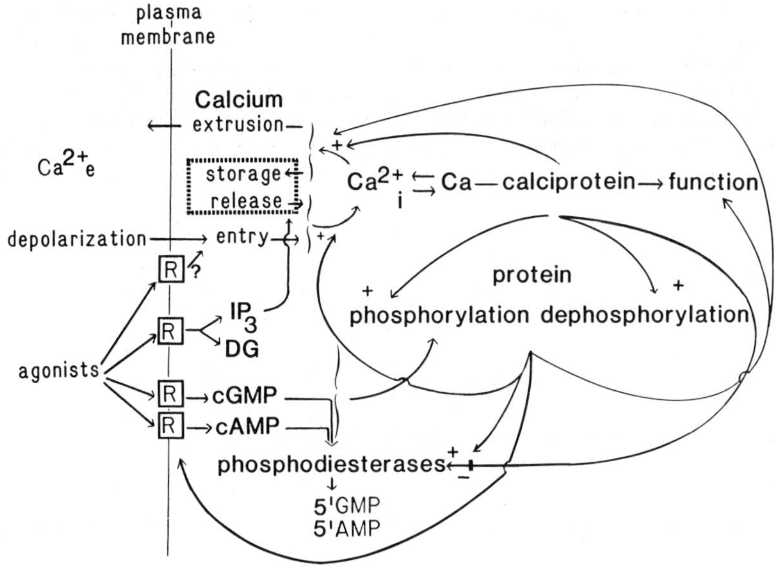

FIGURE 1. Tentative representation of concerted regulation of cell activity by calcium ions, cyclic nucleotides, and phosphoinositide hydrolysis products. IP_3 stands for inositol 1,4,5-trisphosphate, DG for diacylglycerol, and R represents different receptors. Intracellular calcium stores are indicated by a square enclosed by a dashed line.

nucleotide levels and some aspects of their role in these cells, in association with calcium and protein kinase C.

CYCLIC NUCLEOTIDE PHOSPHODIESTERASES

There has been much controversy regarding the physical and catalytic properties of the different forms of phosphodiesterase (PDE) isolated from tissues. It is now well established that several isoenzymes participate in the hydrolysis of cyclic nucleotides in cells,[18] but their repartition in different tissues and their respective role are still to a large extent unknown.

Three major isoenzymes have been purified to homogeneity or near homogeneity from bovine heart by Beavo's group.[19,21] One of these enzymes catalyzes the hydrolysis of both cAMP and cGMP and is activated by calmodulin.[15] According to a recently proposed classification,[22] this enzyme is a type I PDE. According to the same classification, a type II PDE catalyzes the hydrolysis of both cAMP and cGMP and is activated by cGMP, which acts on a site different from the catalytic site.[20] A third enzyme is a type IV PDE: it specifically catalyzes the hydrolysis of cAMP with a low K_m and is competitively inhibited by cGMP.[21]

As illustrated in FIGURES 2 and 3, the presence of the three PDEs affords the possibility of a fine regulation of cyclic nucleotide levels in heart cells. The relative participation of PDE I in this regulation may vary with intracellular calcium concentration and the degree of enzyme activation by calmodulin. Recently, it has been reported that brain PDE I contains two subunits of 60 and 63 kDa, respectively phosphorylated by cAMP-dependent[23] or calcium-calmodulin-dependent[24] protein kinases, leading to a decrease in affinity for the calcium-calmodulin complex. In both cases, dephosphorylation was catalyzed by calcineurin, a calmodulin-dependent phosphatase, but not by other phosphoprotein phosphatases. In addition, phosphorylation is completely inhibited when two calcium-calmodulin complexes are bound per PDE molecule. Sharma and Wang have suggested that these properties can contribute to the regulation of cyclic nucleotide concentrations in cells.[23,24] Whether these mechanisms

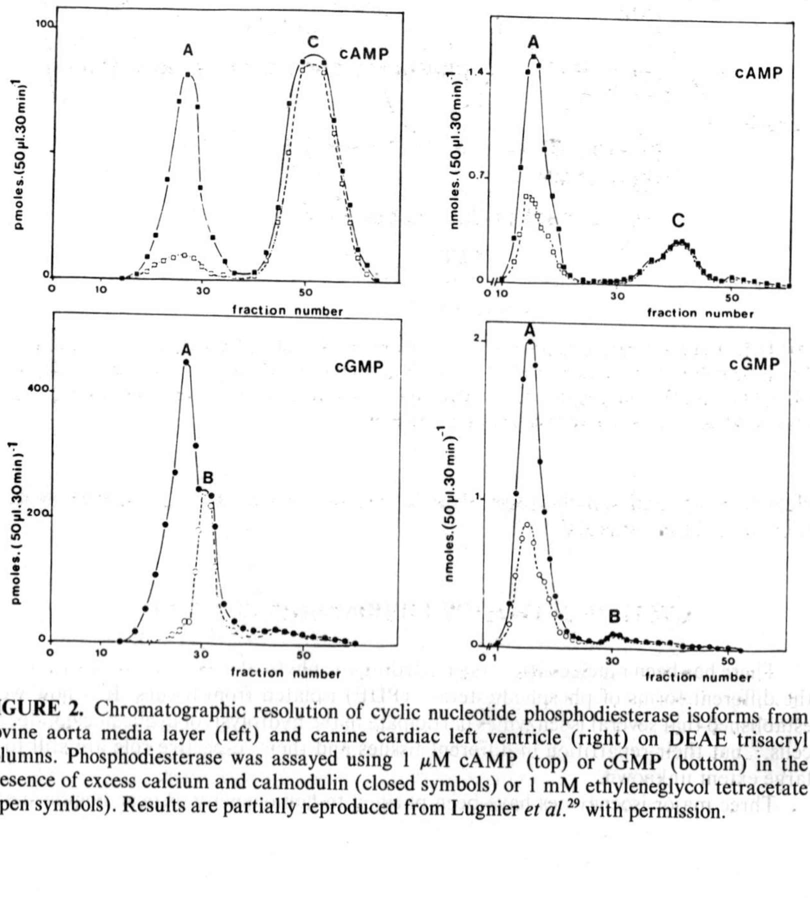

FIGURE 2. Chromatographic resolution of cyclic nucleotide phosphodiesterase isoforms from bovine aorta media layer (left) and canine cardiac left ventricle (right) on DEAE trisacryl columns. Phosphodiesterase was assayed using 1 μM cAMP (top) or cGMP (bottom) in the presence of excess calcium and calmodulin (closed symbols) or 1 mM ethyleneglycol tetracetate (open symbols). Results are partially reproduced from Lugnier *et al.*[29] with permission.

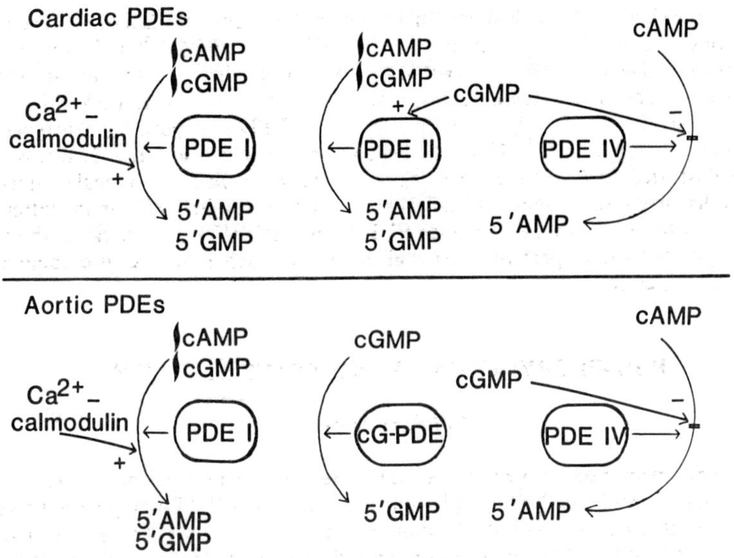

FIGURE 3. Schematic representation of cAMP and cGMP hydrolysis catalyzed by cardiac and aortic cyclic nucleotide phosphodiesterase (PDE) isoforms. PDEs I, II, and IV are classified according to Appleman *et al.*,[22] and cG-PDE designates a form that is specific for cGMP.[29]

operate under physiological conditions remains to be demonstrated. In addition, it is not known whether the properties and regulation of the heart and brain PDE I are identical. The isoenzymes purified from heart and brain are both dimeric, but they appear to have slightly different molecular weights.[25,26]

The properties of PDE II and PDE IV purified from bovine heart suggest that cGMP may modulate cAMP levels in a rather complex fashion. On the one hand, cGMP can increase cAMP breakdown by PDE II, and evidence has been reported suggesting that this mechanism could account for inhibition by cGMP of the cAMP-induced increase in the slow inward calcium current in heart cells.[27] cGMP could also play a part in the inhibition of β-adrenergic myocardial stimulation by muscarinic agents, in addition to the inhibitory effect of muscarinic receptors on adenylate cyclase.[28] On the other hand, cGMP competitively inhibits cAMP hydrolysis by PDE IV, an enzyme that is probably the receptor for cardiotonic drugs such as milrinone.[21] The K_i of cGMP for this enzyme (0.06 μM) is low enough to be consistent with a role for the latter mechanism in heart cells, but this remains to be demonstrated.

As illustrated in FIGURE 2, the existence of three PDE isoforms has also been reported in aortic smooth muscle from different species, including man.[29] Two of these isoenzymes respectively have the properties of PDE I (calmodulin activated, catalyzing cAMP and preferentially cGMP hydrolysis) and PDE IV (cAMP specific, cGMP-inhibited). The third PDE form, which has been isolated from the aorta, specifically hydrolyzes cGMP (cG-PDE). Its properties are different from those of PDE II isolated from heart, since it does not catalyze the hydrolysis of cAMP and is not allosterically stimulated by cGMP. It is also selectively inhibited by zaprinast (M&B 22,948), which is more than 100 times less active on cardiac PDE II than on aortic cG-PDE isolated as described in FIGURE 2. This cG-PDE has not been found in some other vascular smooth muscles, such as coronary arteries.[30] However, the isolation procedure used in this case did not favor separation of cG-PDE from PDE I,[31] and zaprinast is much more active in inhibiting cG-PDE than PDE I when the two enzymes are separated.[30,32] The fact that zaprinast is able to elevate the aortic cGMP level at concentrations that selectively inhibit the isolated cG-PDE supports the existence of this enzyme in aortic cells.[29] Thus, the regulation of cyclic nucleotide levels by the PDEs (illustrated in FIGURE 3) may be different in cardiac and vascular smooth muscle cells, due to the absence of PDE II and the presence of cG-PDE in the latter. It still remains to be determined whether PDE I and PDE IV are identical in the two tissues and what the respective physiological roles of each PDE are in cardiac and smooth muscle cells.

PHOSPHORYLATION OF MEMBRANE PROTEINS

Calcium Pumps

The first membrane protein to be implicated in the regulation of a calcium-transporting system by cAMP was phospholamban,[33] a 22–27 kDa polymeric protein localized in cardiac sarcoplasmic reticulum. Phospholamban can be phosphorylated at different sites by cAMP- and calmodulin-dependent protein kinases,[10] and by protein kinase C.[34,35] The three separate phosphorylations produce additive increases in calcium-pumping activity in cardiac sarcoplasmic reticulum vesicles. Recently, it has been reported that phospholamban binds the calcium-calmodulin complex and that bound calmodulin prevents phosphorylation of phospholamban.[36] It has been suggested that this mechanism operates during systole, allowing an increase in the concentration of free cytosolic Ca^{2+} ions to produce contraction without stimulating the calcium pump,[36,37] whereas cAMP-dependent phosphorylation is likely to occur only when the concentration of cytosolic Ca^{2+} ions is low, i.e., during diastole. At the present time, there is no evidence to support a role of protein kinase C in controlling calcium transport in sarcoplasmic reticulum in intact myocardium. In contrast to β-adrenergic stimulation, α-adrenergic stimulation, which may activate protein kinase C as a consequence of enhanced formation of diacylglycerol, does not produce phospholamban phosphorylation in intact myocardium.[38] In addition, its positive inotropic effect is not associated with a shorter duration of contraction. Thus, only cAMP-induced phosphorylation of phospholamban is likely to play a physiological role in cardiac cells where it increases calcium pumping by sarcoplasmic reticulum and is believed to play a part in the increased relaxation rate of the heart upon β-adrenergic stimulation.

The question of whether cAMP-dependent phosphorylation of phospholamban and subsequent activation of a calcium-pumping ATPase operate in smooth muscle cells, where they could account for, or contribute to, relaxation, has been much debated. Recently, it has been shown that the Ca^{2+}-ATPase of smooth muscle endoplasmic reticulum resembles the calcium transport ATPase of skeletal and cardiac muscle sarcoplasmic reticulum and is different from the Ca^{2+}-ATPase of the plasma membrane.[39,40] Moreover phospholamban has been identified in endoplasmic reticulum of several types of smooth muscles,[41] suggesting that it might regulate calcium transport there.

A calcium-pumping ATPase has been purified from heart sarcolemma[42] and smooth muscle plasma membrane.[43] The activity of the cardiac enzyme is enhanced by cAMP-dependent phosphorylation and deactivated by dephosphorylation.[44] This may contribute to an increased cardiac relaxation rate and to smooth muscle relaxation under the influence of cAMP, together with calcium transport in sarcoplasmic reticulum. Recently, evidence has been reported that phosphorylation by cGMP-dependent protein kinase activates the calcium-pumping ATPase in sarcolemmal vesicles from porcine coronary artery.[45] Whether and to what extent these mechanisms operate within intact cardiac and smooth muscle cells remain to be determined.

Finally, it has been proposed that cAMP-dependent phosphorylation may activate the ouabain-sensitive Na^+, K^+ ATPase in smooth muscle cells. This mechanism could indirectly decrease the intracellular concentration of free Ca^{2+} ions, which is linked to the intracellular concentration of Na^+ ions through the Na^+-Ca^{2+} exchange. In effect, exposure of *Bufo marinus* stomach cells to β-adrenergic stimulation or to dibutyryl-cAMP induces stimulation of ^{42}K influx and ^{45}Ca efflux, and these effects can be abolished by blockade of the Na^+, K^+ pump.[46,47]

Voltage-Dependent Calcium Channels

The cardiac slow calcium channel is modulated by cAMP, which increases the probability of its opening.[3,7,48,49] Recently, the channel has been purified from skeletal muscle transverse tubules, and its subunit composition has been analyzed.[50] Its major component could be phosphorylated by both cAMP-dependent and calcium-calmodulin-dependent protein kinases, and dephosphorylated by calcineurin.[51] Evidence that this mechanism may account for cAMP-dependent activation of the calcium channel is provided by the observation that injection of cAMP-dependent protein kinase into myocytes causes the activation of calcium channels.[48] Once incorporated into reconstituted membranes, the channel presents the principal electrophysiological and pharmacological properties of the cardiac slow channel, including activation by cAMP in the presence of cAMP-dependent protein kinase.[52] These findings strongly suggest that phosphorylation of the channel protein by cAMP-dependent protein kinase may account for activation of the channel by cAMP and perhaps for its positive inotropic effect. However, it remains to be determined whether cAMP-dependent phosphorylation of slow calcium channels occurs in intact cardiac and other cells. It would be important to know if there is a difference between cardiac and vascular smooth muscle cells with respect to cAMP-dependent and calcium-dependent phosphorylation of voltage-dependent calcium channels. It has been reported that cAMP decreases depolarization-induced calcium entry in vascular smooth muscle,[8] but the mechanism of this effect is unknown.

As mentioned above, there is a functional antagonism between cAMP and cGMP on calcium current in heart cells[53] which could be explained by cGMP-dependent activation of a phosphodiesterase.[27] In some tissues cGMP is implicated in the regulation of ionic channels. In the retina, for example, cGMP directly interacts with a cation channel,[54] and in snail neurones, cGMP-dependent protein kinase enhances calcium current.[55] It has been suggested that cGMP may influence the electromechanical activity of some smooth muscles[56] in which it depresses the slow inward calcium current.[57] To our knowledge, however, there is no direct evidence that cGMP itself or cGMP-dependent phosphorylation modulates a calcium channel in cardiac or vascular smooth muscle cells.

Other Plasmalemmal Proteins

A number of proteins, including sarcolemmal proteins, are phosphorylated in cardiac and smooth muscle cells under the influence of agents that elevate cAMP or cGMP levels, but the physiological relevance of the phosphorylation of these proteins often remains unclear. In intact cells, phosphorylation-dephosphorylation reactions may be secondary to variations in the intracellular concentration of free Ca^{2+} ions produced by cyclic nucleotides. Protein substrates for cyclic-nucleotide- and calcium-dependent kinases have also been found in plasmalemmal membrane preparations in various states of purity, but phosphorylation of these proteins in intact cells and its functional consequences have not always been established. For example, a phospholambanlike protein is phosphorylated in plasma-membrane-enriched preparations from cardiac cells,[58] and β-adrenergic-mediated phosphorylation of such a protein has been reported in perfused heart preparations.[59] However, whether or not this protein is a true sarcolemmal protein has been much debated. It seems that the observed phosphorylation could be due to a contamination with fragments of endoplasmic reticulum.[60]

Another cardiac sarcolemmal protein of relatively low molecular weight (15 kDa), which is distinct from phospholamban, is a substrate of cAMP-dependent protein kinase and protein kinase C, which have additive effects.[59,61] A protein of similar molecular weight (16 kDa) and identical properties with respect to phosphorylation by the two kinases has also been found in a plasmalemmal preparation from cultured rat aortic myocytes.[62,63] In both intact cardiac and smooth muscle cells, the 15 or 16 kDa protein is the principal plasmalemmal substrate phosphorylated in response to β-adrenergic stimulation.[59,62] In cardiac cells, a similar protein is also phosphorylated upon α-adrenergic stimulation (which may induce protein kinase C activation), and its phosphorylation correlates with the positive inotropic effects of either α- or β-adrenergic agonists.

Indirect evidence suggests that phosphorylation of the 15 kDa protein in heart sarcolemma is associated with an increase in slow inward calcium current.[37] In aortic smooth muscle cells, the 16 kDa protein is also phosphorylated under the influence of vasopressin and of protein kinase C activating phorbol esters.[63] In these cells, vasopressin stimulates V_1 receptors and produces the hydrolysis of plasma membrane phosphatidyl inositol 4,5-bisphosphate. The phosphoinositide hydrolysis yields two second messengers, inositol 1,4,5-trisphosphate, which releases Ca^{2+} ions from an intracellular store, and diacylglycerol, which activates protein kinase C.[1,11,16] As illustrated in FIGURE 4 calcium release[64] is transient and precedes phosphorylation of the 16 kDa protein, which reaches a maximum in about 1 minute and then returns to control values after about 7 minutes. Phosphorylation itself precedes the evolution of the contractile response, which reaches a maximum in about 5 minutes and is sustained for the next 20 minutes (not shown), as observed using an optical method described by Travo *et al.*[65] The three effects (calcium release, phosphorylation, and contraction) are quantitatively correlated.[64,65] These findings are consistent with a role for the phosphorylation of the 16 kDa protein in the sequence of events underlying contraction of aortic myocytes in response to vasopressin V_1 receptor stimulation.

Thus, there is evidence that in cardiac and vascular smooth muscle cells, stimulation of receptors activating either adenylate cyclase or phospholipase C induce phosphorylation of a 15 or 16 kDa plasmalemmal protein, via cAMP-dependent or protein kinase C activation. Whether the cardiac 15 kDa protein and the smooth muscle protein are the same and whether they are identical to a 16 kDa protein found in hepatocytes[66] are possibilities suggested by their practically identical molecular weights and properties as endogenous substrates of protein kinases. The physiological role of this or these proteins is unknown. The presence of a 15 or 16 kDa peptide associated with a calcium channel or a calcium-transporting system has not been reported. It is possible, however, that phosphorylation of a 15 or 16 kDa protein may modulate calcium fluxes through the plasma membrane in cardiac and vascular smooth muscle cells.

CONCLUSION

The mechanisms through which cyclic nucleotides and calcium modulate each other's levels and regulate heart and vascular smooth muscle contraction are still not completely understood. Recent studies of cyclic nucleotide phosphodiesterases suggest that these isoenzymes play a central role in this regulation, since the activity of some phosphodiesterase isoforms is regulated by cyclic nucleotides themselves and by the calcium-calmodulin complex. There seem to be some differences between cardiac and vascular phosphodiesterase isoforms with respect to the effect of cGMP on cAMP hydrolysis and with respect to their sensitivity to some inhibitors. However, the participation of each phosphodiesterase isoform in the hydrolysis of cyclic nucleotides in intact cells remains to be clarified.

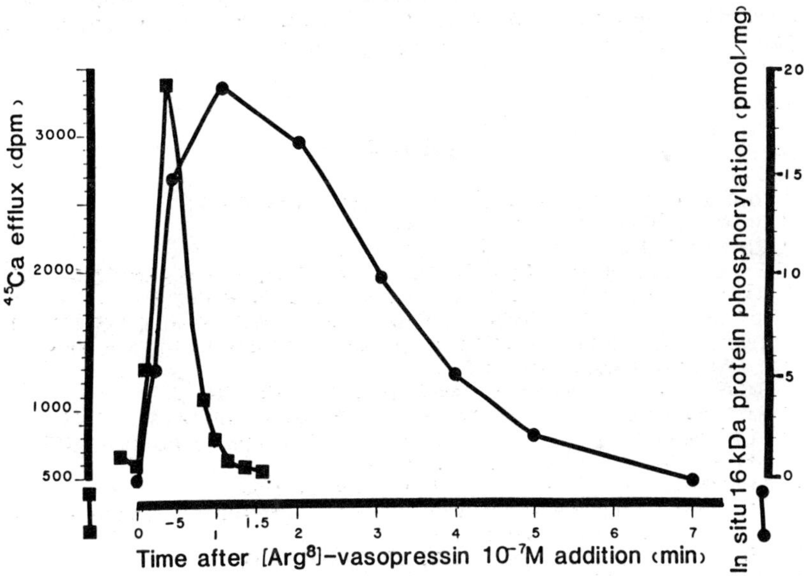

FIGURE 4. Time courses of ^{45}Ca release from intracellular stores and phosphorylation of a 16 kDa plasma membrane protein elicited by vasopressin (Arg^8 vasopressin, 10^{-7} M) in cultured rat aortic myocytes. Results based on Lassegue and Stoclet[64] and Boulanger-Saunier and Stoclet.[63]

Phosphorylation of endogenous proteins very likely represents the mechanism through which cyclic nucleotides exert their intracellular effects. Cells also contain protein kinases which are activated by calcium through an interaction with the calcium-calmodulin complex or through direct activation by Ca^{2+} ions, as in the case of protein kinase C. It has been discovered that some endogenous proteins are substrates for two or three different kinases, although the substrates are phosphorylated at different sites by the kinases. In that case, the different kinases may, or may not, phosphorylate a particular protein in intact cells, depending on the respective localization of the enzyme and of the substrate protein within the cells. Of particular interest is the finding that membrane proteins involved in calcium-transporting systems, including a protein associated with the slow calcium channel, are substrates for cAMP-dependent protein kinase, protein kinase C, or both. In most cases, the physiological role of these proteins is not entirely elucidated in intact cells. Nevertheless, it seems likely that phosphorylation of these proteins, including a 15–16 kDa sarcolemmal protein, regulates intracellular calcium concentration in cardiac and vascular smooth muscle cells. Together with phosphorylation of contractile proteins, which has not been reviewed here, these mechanisms control contractile responses of cardiac and vascular tissues to neuromediators and hormones.

Many questions regarding the role of cyclic nucleotides in the concerted regulation of the activity of cardiac and smooth muscle cells remain unsolved. For example, the reason why cAMP has a positive inotropic effect and increases the relaxation rate in cardiac myocytes but only relaxes smooth muscle cells is still not clearly determined. Also, the mechanisms of action of cGMP are still to a large extent unknown, especially in smooth muscle cells. Different cyclic-nucleotide- and calcium-dependent processes activate a variety of protein kinases and phosphatases, resulting in complex intricate phosphorylation-dephosphorylation reactions. These mechanisms may constitute regulatory networks which may be different in each cell type.

REFERENCES

1. Rasmusen, H. & P. Q. Barrett. 1984. Physiol. Rev. **64:** 938–984.
2. Bolton, T. B. 1979. Physiol. Rev. **59:** 606–718.
3. Reuter, H. 1983. Nature London **301:** 569–574.
4. Carafoli, E. 1984. Adv. Cyclic Nucleotide Protein Phosphorylation Res. **17:** 543–549.
5. Rapoport, R. M. & F. Murad. 1983. J. Cyclic Nucleotide Res. **9:** 281–296.
6. Ignarro, L. J. & P. J. Kadowitz. 1985. Annu. Rev. Pharmacol. Toxicol. **25:** 171–191.
7. Tsien, R. W., R. P. Bean, P. Hess, J. B. Lansman, B. Nillius & M. C. Nowycky. 1986. J. Mol. Cell. Cardiol. **18:** 691–710.
8. Saida, K. & C. van Breemen. 1984. J. Gen. Physiol. **84:** 307–318.
9. Saitoh, Y., J. G. Hardman & J. N. Wells. 1985. Biochemistry **24:** 1613–1618.
10. Le Peuch, C. J., J. Haiech & J. G. Demaille. 1979. Biochemistry **18:** 5150–5157.
11. Berridge, J. M. 1984. Biochem. J. **2:** 345–360.
12. Berridge, J. M. 1975. Adv. Cyclic Nucleotide Res. **6:** 1–98.
13. Stoclet, J.-C., D. Gerard, M. C. Kilhoffer, C. Lugnier, R. Miller & P. Schaeffer. 1987. Prog. Neurobiol. **29:** 321–364.
14. La Raia, P. J. & E. Morkin. 1974. Circ. Res. **35:** 298–306.
15. England, P. J. 1980. Protein phosphorylation in the regulation of muscle contraction. *In* Recently Discovered Systems of Enzyme Regulation by Reversible Phosphorylation. P. Cohen, Ed.: 153–173. Elsevier/North Holland. Amsterdam, Holland
16. Nishizuka, Y. 1984. Nature London **308:** 693–698.
17. Manalan, A. S. & C. B. Klee. 1984. Adv. Cyclic Nucleotide Protein Phosphorylation Res. **18:** 227–278.
18. Beavo, J. A., R. S. Hansen, S. A. Harrison, R. L. Hurwitz, T. J. Martins & M. C. Mumby. 1982. Mol. Cell. Endocrinol. **23:** 387–410.
19. Martins, T. J., M. C. Mumby & J. A. Beavo. 1982. J. Biol. Chem. **257:** 1973–1979.
20. Macphee, C. H., S. A. Harrison & J. A. Beavo. 1986. Proc. Nat. Acad. Sci. USA **83:** 6660–6663.
21. Harrison, S. A., D. H. Reifsnyde, B. Gallis, G. G. Cadd & J. A. Beavo. 1986. Mol. Pharmacol. **29:** 506–514.
22. Appleman, M. M., J. Beavo, Jr., J. G. Hardman, C. B. Klee & W. J. Thompson. 1984. Adv. Cyclic Nucleotide Protein Phosphorylation Res. **16:** vi.
23. Sharma, R. K., & J. H. Wang. 1985. Proc. Nat. Acad. Sci. USA **82:** 2603–2607.
24. Sharma, R. K. & J. H. Wang. 1986. J. Biol. Chem. **261:** 1322–1328.
25. Hansen, R. S. & J. A. Beavo. 1982. Proc. Nat. Acad. Sci. USA **79:** 2788–2792.
26. Sharma, R. K., A.-M. Adachi, K. Adachi & J. H. Wang. 1984. J. Biol. Chem. **259:** 9248–9254.

27. HARTZELL, H. C. & R. FISCHMEISTER. 1986. Nature London **323:** 273–275.
28. FISCHMEISTER, R. & C. HARTZELL. 1986. J. Physiol. London **376:** 183–202.
29. LUGNIER, C., P. SCHOEFFTER, A. LE BEC, E. STROUTHOU & J.-C. STOCLET. 1986. Biochem. Pharmacol. **35:** 1743–1751.
30. WELLS, J. N., C. E. BAIRD, Y. J. WU & J. G. HARDMAN. 1975. Biochim. Biophys. Acta **384:** 430–442.
31. LUGNIER, C., M. BRUCH, J.-C. STOCLET, M. P. STRUB, M. MARIVET & C. G. WERMUTH. 1985. Eur. J. Med. Chem—Chim. Ther. **20:** 121–125.
32. LUGNIER, C., A. STIERLE, A. BERETZ, P. SCHOEFFTER, A. LE BEC, C. G. WERMUTH, J. P. CAZENAVE & J.-C. STOCLET. 1983. Biochem. Biophys. Res. Commun. **113:** 954–959.
33. KATZ, A. M. 1979. Adv. Cyclic Nucleotide Res. **11:** 304–343.
34. IWASA, Y. & M. M. HOSEY. 1984. J. Biol. Chem. **259:** 534–540.
35. MOVESIAN, M. A., M. NISHIKAWA & R. S. ADELSTEIN. 1984. J. Biol. Chem. **259:** 8029–8032.
36. MOLLA, A., J. P. CAPONY & J. G. DEMAILLE. 1985. Biochem. J. **226:** 859–865.
37. LINDEMANN, J. P. & A. M. WANATABE. 1985. J. Biol. Chem. **260:** 4516–4525.
38. LINDEMANN, J. P. 1985. J. Biol. Chem. **261:** 4860–4867.
39. WIBO, M., N. MOREL & T. GODFRAIND. 1981. Biochim. Biophys. Acta **649:** 651–660.
40. WUYTACK, F., L. RAEYMAEKERS, G. DE SCHUTTER & R. CASTEELS. 1985. Biochim. Biophys. Acta **693:** 42–52.
41. RAEYMAEKERS, L. & L. R. JONES. 1986. Biochim. Biophys. Acta **882:** 258–265.
42. CARONI, P. & E. CARAFOLI. 1981. J. Biol. Chem. **256:** 3263–3270.
43. DE SCHUTTER. G., F. WUYTAK. J. VERBIST & R. CASTEELS. 1984. Biochim. Biophys. Acta **773:** 1–10.
44. NEYSES, L., L. REINLIB & E. CARAFOLI. 1985. J. Biol. Chem. **260:** 1083–1087.
45. POPESCU, L. M., C. PANOU, M. HINESCU & O. NUTA. 1985. Eur. J. Pharmacol. **107:** 393–394.
46. SCHEID, C. R. & F. S. FAY. 1984. Am J. Physiol. **246:** c415–c421.
47. SCHEID, C. R. & F. S. FAY. 1984. Am. J. Physiol. **246:** c431–c438.
48. OSTERRIEDER, W., G. BRUM, J. HESCHELER, W. TRAUTWEIN, V. FLOCKERZI & F. HOFMANN. 1982. Nature London **298:** 576–578.
49. NARGEOT, J., J. M. NERBONNE, J. ENGELS & H. A. LESTER. 1983. Proc. Nat. Acad. Sci. USA **80:** 2395–2399.
50. BORSOTTO, M., J. BARHANIN, M. FOSSET & M. LAZDUNSKI. 1985. J. Biol. Chem. **260:** 14255–14263.
51. HOSEY, M. M., M. BORSOTTO & M. LAZDUNSKI. 1986. Proc. Nat. Acad. Sci. USA **83:** 3733–3737.
52. FLOCKERZI, V., H.-J. OEKEN, F. HOFMANN, D. PELZER, A. CAVALIE & W. TRAUTWEIN. 1986. Nature London **323:** 66–68.
53. BKAILY, G. & N. SPERELAKIS. 1985. Am. J. Physiol. **248:** H745–H749.
54. FESENKO, E. E., S. S. KOLESNIKOV & A. L. LYUBARSKY. 1986. Biochim. Biophys. Acta **856:** 661–671.
55. PAUPARDIN-TRITSCH, D., C. HAMMOND, H. M. GERSCHENFELD, A. C. NAIRN & P. GREENGARD. 1986. Nature London **323:** 812–814.
56. RICHARDS, I. S, C. MURLAS, J. M. OUSTERHOUT & N. SPERELAKIS. 1986. Eur. J. Pharmacol. **128:** 299–302.
57. OUSTERHOUT, J. M. & N. SPERELAKIS. 1985. Biophys. J. (Abstr): 266.
58. RINALDI, M. L., J. P. CAPONY & J. G. DEMAILLE. 1982. J. Mol. Cell. Cardiol. **14:** 279–289.
59. HUGGINS, J. P. & P. J. ENGLAND. 1983. FEBS Lett. **163:** 297–302.
60. PRESTI, C. F., L. R. JONES & J. P. LINDEMANN. 1985. J. Biol. Chem. **260:** 3860–3867.
61. PRESTI, C. F., B. T. SCOTT & L. R. JONES. 1985. J. Biol. Chem. **260:** 13879–13889.
62. BOULANGER-SAUNIER, C., D. M. KATTENBURG & J.-C. STOCLET. 1985. FEBS Lett. **193:** 283–288.
63. BOULANGER-SAUNIER, C. & J.-C. STOCLET. 1987. Biochem. Biophys. Res. Commun. **143:** 517–524.
64. LASSEGUE, B. & J.-C. STOCLET. 1986. FEBS Lett. **205:** 251–254.
65. TRAVO, P., P. BODIN, G. BURNSTOCK & J.-C. STOCLET. 1987. Lab. Invest. **56:** 335–343.
66. COOPER, R. H., K. KOBAYASHI & J. R. WILLIAMSON. 1984. FEBS Lett. **166:** 125–130.

Calcium Antagonist Receptors[a]

Clinical and Physiological Relevance

JOHN A. WAGNER,[b] SANDY E. GUGGINO,[e]
IAN J. REYNOLDS,[f] ADELE M. SNOWMAN,[b]
AMITAVA BISWAS,[b] BALDOMERO M. OLIVERA,[g]
AND SOLOMON H. SNYDER[b,c,d,h]

[b]*Department of Neuroscience*
[c]*Department of Pharmacology and Molecular Sciences*
[d]*Department of Psychiatry and Behavioral Sciences*
Johns Hopkins University School of Medicine
725 North Wolfe Street
Baltimore, Maryland 21205

[e]*Gerontology Research Center*
National Institute on Aging
Baltimore, Maryland 21224

[f]*Department of Pharmacology and Physiological Sciences*
University of Chicago
847 East 58th Street
Chicago, Illinois 60637

[g]*Department of Biology*
University of Utah
Salt Lake City, Utah 84112

The unique pharmacologic actions of calcium antagonist drugs were simultaneously identified through their effects on cardiac and arterial smooth muscle.[1-4] The application of receptor binding techniques to the study of these drugs has considerably enhanced our insight into their mechanism of action (see reviews in References 5 and 6). In this paper, we will review some of the properties of calcium antagonist drug receptors and discuss novel calcium antagonist receptors. We will also review evidence showing that a variety of drugs not classically identified as calcium antagonists may exert their clinical effects through voltage-sensitive calcium channels (VSCC); and describe recent findings descriminating drug and ion effects on calcium flux through VSCC and the Na^+/Ca^{2+} exchange.

CALCIUM ANTAGONIST BINDING SITES

The first identification of receptor binding sites utilized the dihydropyridine (DHP) [^{3}H]nitrendipine.[7-10] The relative potencies of numerous DHP at these binding

[a]This work was supported by Public Health Service Grants MH 18501 and U.S. Public Health Service Grant DA-00074 to S.H.S. J.A.W. was supported by a National Science Foundation Predoctoral Fellowship.

[h]To whom all correspondence should be addressed.

sites closely parallel their potencies in influencing calcium-dependent contractions of smooth muscle.[11–14] Additional evidence for a link of DHP receptors to VSCC comes from the demonstration that thorough removal of calcium from membranes with chelating agents abolishes receptor binding which is restored by physiological concentrations of calcium in brain membranes.[15–18] Moreover, the ability of calcium to stimulate binding is mimicked by cations that physiologically are calcium agonists and

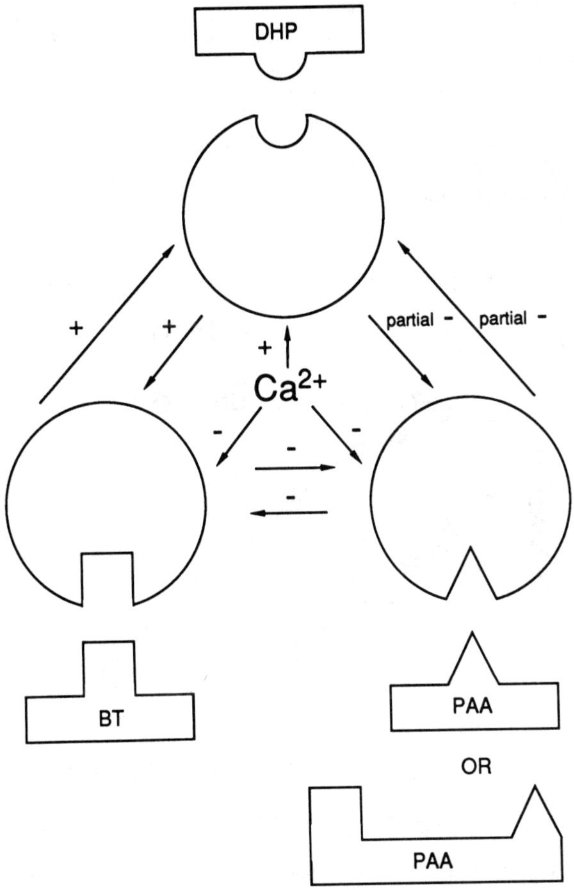

FIGURE 1. Model of the interactions of calcium antagonist binding sites. Dihydropyridine, DHP; phenylalkylamine, PAA; benzothiazepine, BT.

blocked by cations that are calcium antagonists.[15,16,19–22] Receptor binding sites are similar in brain, heart, and smooth muscle[7–10,17,23–34] but differ in some of their properties in skeletal muscle, where binding is inhibited by calcium and stimulated by chelating agents. Moreover, most DHP drugs are substantially weaker in skeletal muscle than in the other tissues.[8,9,16,35–39]

Evidence for multiplicity of calcium antagonist receptors has come from the shallow competition curve of verapamil at DHP-binding sites and the ability of diltiazem and other benzothiazepines (BT) to stimulate DHP binding.[8,16,40–45] The variable ability of verapamil and other phenylalkylamines (PAA) to maximally reduce the binding DHP and to compete with each other in this effect indicated variations in the "efficacy" of coupling of apparent verapamil receptors to DHP receptors.[8] Subsequent ligand binding studies with (−)-[^{3}H]-desmethoxyverapamil[46–49] and *d-cis*-[^{3}H]-diltiazem[48,50–52] have provided direct evidence for differences in binding sites indicating the presence of three separate subtypes of receptors selective respectively for DHP, PAA, and BT. Interactions between binding sites are summarized in FIGURE 1. Evidence that all three subtypes occur on the same macromolecular receptor protein complex derives from recent successes in purifying receptors to homogeneity with the isolated proteins recognizing all three classes of drugs.[53–58]

Recently, we discovered a novel class of (−)-[^{3}H]desmethoxyverapamil-binding sites in rat osteoblastlike osteosarcoma cells (UMR and ROS) and dissociated human osteoblasts.[59] This binding site differs substantially from binding sites observed in brain, heart, and skeletal and smooth muscle. Binding is linear with protein concentra-

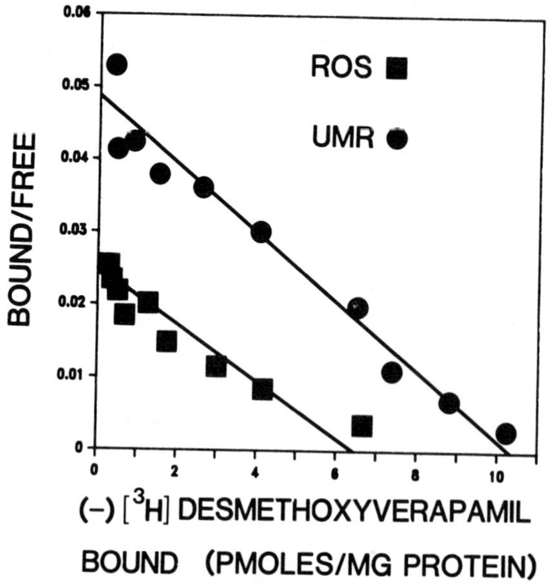

FIGURE 2. Scatchard plots of (−)-[^{3}H]desmethoxyverapamil binding to membranes prepared from the osteoblastlike osteosarcoma cell lines ROS (squares) and UMR (circles). Membranes were prepared by homogenizing cells in 50 mM HEPES, pH 7.4 using a Brinkmann polytron on half-maximal setting for 30 seconds. Homogenates were centrifuged at 40,000 ×*g* for 10 minutes. The pellet was resuspended in 50 mM HEPES, pH 7.4. The pellet was washed and resuspended in chelex-treated 50 mM HEPES, pH 7.4, 10 mM EDTA. The homogenate was incubated at 4°C for 30 minutes and then centrifuged for 40,000 ×*g* for 10 minutes. The pellet was resuspended in chelex-treated 50 mM HEPES, pH 7.4 to a concentration of 6 mg protein/ml. Membranes (0.2 mg protein/ml) were incubated for 90 minutes with 2 nM (−)-[^{3}H]desmethoxyverapamil with and without varying concentrations of cold (−)-desmethoxyverapamil in 50 mM chelex-treated HEPES, pH 7.4 with 0.4% bovine serum albumin (BSA). Assays were stopped by filtration over glass fiber filters pretreated with 0.5% polyethylenimine (PEI) and washed with two 4 ml aliquots of 4°C 50 mM NaCl. Radioactivity was assessed by liquid scintillation spectrophotometry.

TABLE 1. Pharmacology of the (−)-[^{3}H]Desmethoxyverapamil-Binding Site in ROS and UMR Osteoblastlike Osteosarcoma Cell Membranes

Drug	K_i ± Standard Error of the Mean (SEM) (nM)[a]	
	ROS	UMR
(−)Desmethoxyverapamil	53 ± 8.9	54 ± 10.3
(+)Desmethoxyverapamil	362 ± 100	523 ± 62
Verapamil	352 ± 165	426 ± 210
Methoxyverapamil	475 ± 121	610 ± 143
Bepredil	1633 ± 846	953 ± 36
Loperamide	187 ± 23	220 ± 54
Lidoflazine	5730 ± 500	5400 ± 495
Thioridazine	ND	1513 ± 231
Terfenadine	4560 ± 1070	3550 ± 690
Amiodarone	1570 ± 921	1800 ± 742
Dihydropyridine[b]	>10,000[b]	>10,000[b]

[a](−)-[^{3}H]Desmethoxyverapamil binding was performed as in the legend to FIGURE 2. K_i values were computed by an iterative curve-fitting program. K_i values for ROS cell membranes are the mean of three independent experiments performed in duplicate. K_i values for UMR cell membranes are the mean of four independent experiments performed in duplicate. ND means not determined.

[b]Dihydropyridines tested include nitrendipine, nifendipine, nisoldipine, bay K 8644, (+)PN200-110, (−)PN200-110, (+)202-791, (−)202-791, and nicardipine.

tion in the range between 0.05 and 1.0 mg/ml. FIGURE 2 depicts a typical Scatchard plot of (−)-[^{3}H]desmethoxyverapamil binding to ROS and UMR osteosarcoma cell membranes. Scatchard analysis suggests the presence of a single binding site in UMR and ROS with K_D values of 47 ± 5 and 68 ± 12 nM, respectively. The densities of binding sites (B_{max}) are 12.6 ± 4.2 and 7.5 ± 2.1 pmol/mg protein, respectively.

The pharmacology is similar to that seen in skeletal muscle, except that PAA are approximately 10-fold less potent (TABLE 1). In contrast to the pharmacology of skeletal muscle (−)-[^{3}H]desmethoxyverapamil-binding sites, DHP have no inhibitory effects up to 10 μM concentrations. We have not detected binding sites for [^{3}H]nitrendipine on these cells. Group IIa divalent cations noncompetitively inhibit binding with IC_{50}s between 1 and 5 mM. Several transition elements also noncompetitively inhibit binding. Surprisingly, several divalent cations stimulate binding (TABLES 2 and 3).

Is this (−)-[^{3}H]desmethoxyverapamil-binding site related to osteoblast calcium channels? We have recently obtained cell-attached and excised patch clamp evidence suggesting the presence of calcium conductances in ROS cells. This conductance is potently inhibited by desmethoxyverapamil (FIGURE 3). This PAA-sensitive channel may be involved in the transduction of the cellular response to parathyroid hormone (PTH). This hypothesis is supported by *in vitro* bone resorption experiments (FIGURE 4) in which (−)-desmethoxyverapamil potently inhibits PTH-induced release of $^{45}Ca^{2+}$ preloaded into fetal bone, an index of bone resorptive activity.[60] (+)-Desmethoxyverapamil also inhibits the PTH-induced release of $^{45}Ca^{2+}$, but less potently than its stereoisomer. The Ca^{2+} entering through an osteoblast calcium channel may be Ca^{2+} absorbed from the bone matrix in response to PTH, or it may cause the release of factors secreted by osteoblasts which then interact with osteoclasts.

Another new class of calcium antagonist receptors has been defined by [^{125}I]ω-conotoxin GVIA, a peptide toxin purified from the venom of the fish-hunting sea snail *Conus geographus*.[61] DHP and other calcium antagonist drugs act at the L calcium

TABLE 2. Inhibition and Enhancement of (−)-[^{3}H]Desmethoxyverapamil Binding to ROS and UMR Osteoblastlike Osteosarcoma Cell Membranes by Selected Ions

Ion	EC_{50} ± SEM (mM)[a]	
	ROS[b]	UMR[c]
Group IIa, inhibitor		
$MgCl_2$	5.2 ± 3.1	6.7 ± 2.0
$CaCl_2$	3.0 ± 1.5	2.4 ± 0.40
$SrCl_2$	1.7 ± 0.51	1.6 ± 0.29
$BaCl_2$	2.1 ± 1.7	1.4 ± 0.39
Transition, inhibitor		
$CoCl_2$	1.1 ± 1.3	3.6 ± 0.87
$MnCl_2$	4.1 ± 2.0	3.1 ± 1.2
$LnCl_3$	0.55 ± 0.47	0.41 ± 0.11
$PbNO_3$	0.60 ± 0.33	0.44 ± 0.037
Transition, enhancer		
$NiCl_2$	0.055 ± 0.041	0.043 ± 0.046
$CdCl_2$	ND	0.057 ± 0.011
$HgCl_2$	0.037 ± 0.025	0.023 ± 0.011
$ZnCl_2$	0.051 ± 0.051	0.10 ± 0.031
$CaCl_2$	0.045 ± 0.040	0.090 ± 0.007

[a] EC_{50} for inhibitor ions is IC_{50}, or the concentration for 50% inhibition of binding. EC_{50} for enhancing ions is the concentration for 50% of maximal stimulation of binding. Values are means ± SEM. (−)-[^{3}H]Desmethoxyverapamil binding was performed as in the legend to FIGURE 2.

[b] Values are derived from experiments performed in duplicate and repeated on 2–3 occasions.

[c] Values are derived from experiments performed in duplicate and repeated on 3–4 occasions.

TABLE 3. Effects of Selected Ions on (−)-[^{3}H]Desmethoxyverapamil Saturations to UMR Osteoblastlike Osteosarcoma Cell Membranes[a]

Ion	Ion Concentration (mM)	K_D (nM)	B_{max} (pmol/mg protein)
Control	0	47	12.6
Group IIa, inhibitor			
$BaCl_2$	10	32	2.6
$SrCl_2$	10	54	5.1
$CaCl_2$	10	38	4.9
$MgCl_2$	10	38	6.4
Transition, inhibitor			
$CoCl_2$	1	34	6.1
$LnCl_3$	1	35	5.1
Transition, enhancer			
$NiCl_2$	0.1	51	18.2
$CdCl_2$	0.1	44	16.6
$HgCl_2$	0.1	39	17.3

[a] (−)-[^{3}H]Desmethoxyverapamil binding was performed as in the legend to FIGURE 2.

channel, while N and T channels are resistant to DHP drug effects.[62] ω-Conotoxin GVIA potently blocks both L and N but not T channels.[63] Quantitatively, [^{125}I]ω-conotoxin GVIA binding in rat brain is much greater than that of [^{3}H]DHP.[64,65] Therefore, [^{125}I]ω-conotoxin GVIA appears to bind predominantly to N channels or to an abundant protein that interacts with both N and L channels.

We have recently further characterized [^{125}I]ω-conotoxin GVIA binding in rat brain homogenates.[66] Binding is saturable, reversible, of extreme high affinity, and linear with protein between 0.1 and 10 mg/ml. Scatchard analysis (FIGURE 5) indicates the presence of one [^{125}I]ω-conotoxin GVIA–binding site with a K_D value of 60 pM and B_{max} of 3 pmol/mg protein. Association kinetics are extremely rapid, but dissociation is very slow, although binding is completely reversible by 24 hours of dissociation. We have observed higher specific binding in fresh than in frozen brain tissue. [^{125}I]ω-Conotoxin GVIA binding is inhibited by divalent cations such as calcium with an IC_{50} of 100 μM, although binding is unaffected by pH variations between 7.0 and 8.9. [^{125}I]ω-Conotoxin GVIA binding levels vary more than 10-fold

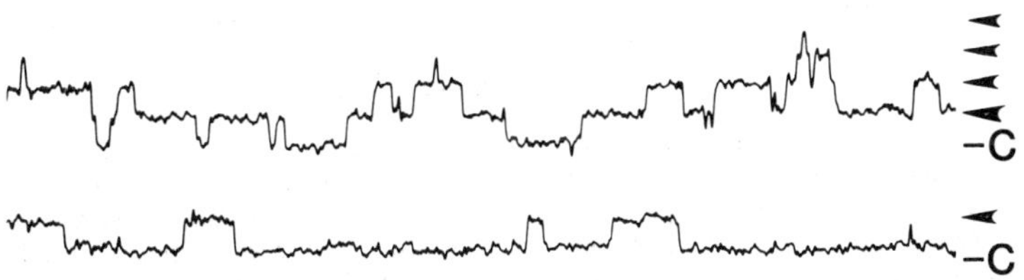

FIGURE 3. The effect of (+)-desmethoxyverapamil on the open state probability is to inhibit channel opening. This channel recording is from an excised, inside-out patch from the apical membrane of confluent cultured osteoblastlike ROS 17/2.8 osteosarcoma cells at −20 mV pipette voltage. The top trace shows control activity of four channels opening with a probability of 0.3 for each channel. The bottom trace, recorded in the presence of 1 μMRD888 on the inside of the patch, shows a decrease in opening probability to 0.05. In the absence of Ca^{2+}, an Na^{+} but not a K^{+} current flows through this channel. The single channel conductance is 13 pS with (in mM) 140 KCl, 5 NaCl, 1 $MgCl_2$, 16 KHEPES, pH 7.4 with 10^{-7} M $CaCl_2$ buffered with 5 EGTA in the pipette and 140 NaCl, 1 $MgCl_2$, 16 NaHEPES, pH 7.4 with 10^{-8} M $CaCl_2$ buffered with 5 EGTA in the bath. The channel amplitude is 0.5 pA. The recording time is 1.6 seconds for each trace. C indicates a closed state, and the arrows indicate an open state.

throughout the brain, with highest values in the cerebral cortex and lowest binding in the brain stem (TABLE 4). Similar regional variations are apparent in our autoradiographic studies (data not shown).

DRUG ACTIONS AND PATHOPHYSIOLOGICAL EFFECTS ON CALCIUM ANTAGONIST RECEPTORS OF POTENTIAL CLINICAL RELEVANCE

It is now well established that the ability of drugs such as DHP, verapamil, and diltiazem to relieve the symptoms of angina, supraventricular tachycardia, and hypertension reflects their influences upon receptor sites labeled with the ligands discussed above. The chemical structures of PAA calcium antagonists resemble many other clinically useful drugs. In a screen of a large number of drugs, we obtained evidence that drugs of other classes may exert some of their effects via calcium antagonist receptors (TABLE 5).

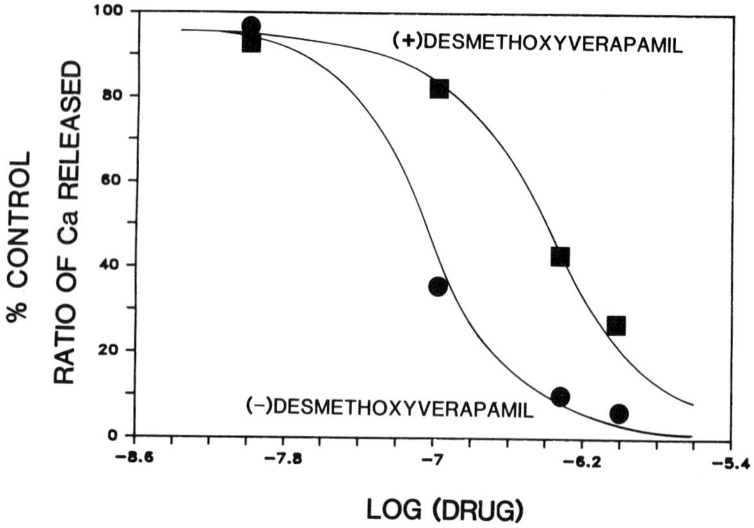

FIGURE 4. Effects of (+)- and (−)-desmethoxyverapamil (squares and circles, respectively) on PTH-stimulated *in vitro* fetal rat bone resorption. Rats, 17-days pregnant, were injected with 500 μCi $^{45}CaCl_2$. On the 19th day of gestation, pregnant rats were sacrificed and fetuses were removed. Radii and ulni were dissected away from surrounding tissues and placed in individual wells of a 24 well plate. Culture medium was 250 μl of Dulbecco's modified Eagles medium supplemented with 10% heat-inactivated fetal calf serum. Half the wells were treated with 2.5 U/ml bovine parathyroid hormone (PTH). Both PTH-treated and untreated wells were exposed to different concentrations of (+)- and (−)-desmethoxyverapamil. PTH-treated and untreated controls were run with each plate. Fetal bones were incubated for 72 hours at 37–37.5°C in 5% CO_2. At the end of the incubation, two 50 μl aliquots were removed and counted by liquid scintillation spectrophotometry. Bone resorptive activity is expressed as PTH-treated-to-untreated ratio of $^{45}Ca^{2+}$ release. Drug effects are expressed as percent remaining compared to control ratio. PTH-treated and untreated values are means of triplicates, each point determined in duplicate. Release of previously $^{45}Ca^{2+}$ labeled fetal long bones is well known as a measure for bone resorptive activity.[60]

The antipsychotic neuroleptic drugs comprise several chemical groups including the phenothiazines, butyrophenones, and diphenylbutylpiperidines (DPBP). All of these drugs share the ability to block dopamine D_2 receptors at low nanomolar concentrations, and the relative antipsychotic potencies of these drugs closely parallel their dopamine-blocking activity.[67,68] Thus it has been generally accepted that the major antipsychotic effects of these drugs derive from dopamine receptor blockade. However, conventional neuroleptics, especially of the phenothiazine and butyrophenone class, are much less effective in relieving the "negative" symptoms of schizophrenia, which involve affective withdrawal, than in treating the "positive" symptoms comprising florid hallucinations and delusions. The DPBPs are unique in their ability to relieve negative symptoms of schizophrenia, enhancing social interaction and diminishing withdrawal as has been demonstrated in numerous controlled studies comparing these agents with other neuroleptics.[67–76]

Strikingly, DPBPs are extremely potent calcium antagonists of the verapamil type both at receptor binding sites and in blocking calcium-dependent contractions of smooth muscle.[77] They are approximately as potent as calcium antagonists as they are as dopamine antagonists so that at therapeutic doses they will be influencing calcium antagonist receptors as well as dopamine receptors in the brain. By contrast, the phenothiazine and butyrophenone neuroleptics, which do not markedly influence negative symptoms of schizophrenia, are orders of magnitude weaker as calcium antagonists. Thus, we[77] and, recently, others[78] have suggested that the ability of DPBP to relieve negative symptoms of schizophrenia derives from their calcium antagonist actions.

Calcium antagonist effects may account for some side effects of neuroleptics. Phenothiazines cause cardiac arrhythmias with thoridazine being a major offender.[79–82] The electrocardiographic changes elicited by thoridazine closely resemble those produced by verapamil. Additionally, thoridazine uniquely causes inhibition of ejaculation, presumably reflecting impaired contraction of the vas deferens.[83] At therapeutic blood levels of thioridazine, the drug is highly active at calcium antagonist receptors of the verapamil type and blocks calcium-dependent contractions of the vas deferens. Thus, thioridazine's inhibition of ejaculation and possibly cardiac side effects reflect calcium antagonist influences.[84]

Loperamide is one of the major antidiarrheal drugs clinically employed. Though

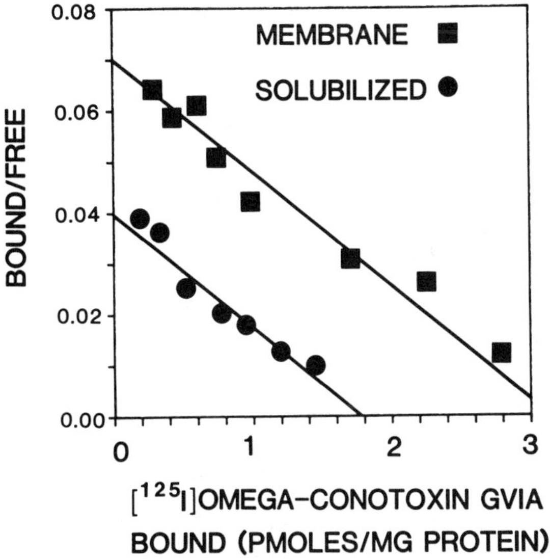

FIGURE 5. Scatchard plot of [^{125}I] ω-conotoxin GVIA binding to rat forebrain membranes (squares) and 0.75% 3-[(3-cholamidopropyl)dimethylammonio]-l-propanesulfonate (CHAPS) solubilized extract (circles). Crude brain membranes were prepared as described.[8] CHAPS detergent 0.75% was added to fresh crude membranes and homogenized by 8 strokes using a Teflon glass homogenizer. After 30 minutes at 4°C, membrane homogenates were centrifuged at 100,000 ×*g* for 90 minutes. The supernatant was aspirated and concentrated using an ultrafiltration apparatus (Amicon Corporation, Cambridge, Mass.) at 50 psi. One μg membrane protein or 10 μg solubilized extract protein was incubated with 20 pM [^{125}I]ω-conotoxin GVIA in 1 ml of buffer containing 50 mM HEPES, pH 7.4 and 0.4% BSA. Cold saturation analysis was performed with varying concentrations of cold ω-conotoxin GVIA from 1 pM to 20 nM. After 30 minutes at 22°C, assays were filtered and washed with two 4 ml aliquots of 4°C 160 mM choline chloride, 10 mM Tris pH 7.7, and 0.2% BSA. Radioactivity was assessed by liquid scintillation spectrophotometry.

TABLE 4. [^{125}I]ω-Conotoxin GVIA Binding to Different Brain Regions[a]

Brain Region	K_D (pM)	B_{max} (pmol/mg protein)
Cortex	67	8.3
Cerebellum	54	3.7
Hypothalamus	82	3.6
Striatum	71	2.0
Pituitary	313	2.2
Hippocampus	46	6.4
Midbrain	113	3.5
Brain stem	40	0.55

[a] [^{125}I]ω-Conotoxin GVIA binding was performed as in the legend to FIGURE 5.

loperamide is a potent opiate, its antidiarrheal effects are not blocked consistently by the opiate antagonist naloxone.[85,86] When administered orally in antidiarrheal doses, loperamide is an effective calcium antagonist acting as receptors in a verapamillike fashion and blocks calcium-induced smooth muscle contractions.[87] Thus, loperamide may owe all or part of its antidiarrheal therapeutic effects to calcium antagonism. Interestingly, constipation is a major side effect of verapamil therapy.[88]

Amiodarone is an effective antianginal drug whose mechanism of therapeutic action is unclear. Recently we and others have shown that therapeutic blood levels of amiodarone inhibit dihydropyridine and phenylalkylamine receptor binding.[89,90] Taken together with the fact that the general spectrum of clinical actions of amiodarone resembles that of verapamil, we suggest that amiodarone acts as a calcium antagonist.

Hypertrophic cardiomyopathy is a genetically determined clinical condition in which the hypertrophy results in an outflow tract obstruction. A genetically determined cardiomyopathy in Syrian hamsters appears to be a valid animal model of this condition.[91,92] The ability of verapamil to relieve selectively the symptoms of both human patients and the cardiomyopathic hamsters suggested that VSCC play a part in the pathophysiology. We and others have demonstrated a 50% increase in numbers of calcium antagonist receptors both of the DHP and PAA type in brain, heart, and skeletal muscle.[92–94] Since the potassium-stimulated contractions of aortic and tracheal rings, both mediated by calcium, are enhanced in these hamsters, the increased numbers of binding sites appear to have direct influence on muscle contractility.[95] The increases in receptors in very young hamsters, prior to the onset of the cardiomyopathy, and in the brain, indicate that the alterations in cardiac receptors are not secondary to the hypertrophy. Very recently, we demonstrated similar increases in these receptors in cardiac tissue of patients with hypertrophic cardiomyopathy, closely paralleling the results in hamsters and suggesting that the human clinical condition is closely related to a genetically determined abnormality in voltage-dependent calcium channels.[96]

The ability of verapamil to alleviate the symptoms of hypertrophic cardiomyopathy may simply reflect a direct blockade of calcium influx. Alternatively, chronic treatment with verapamil may influence the nature of the receptor sites. Quite recently we have demonstrated that chronic treatment of rats with verapamil produces a 50% decrease in the numbers of [^{3}H]nitrendipine-binding sites in the heart,[97] suggesting that down regulation of receptors may be responsible for therapeutic effects, such as in the treatment of hypertrophic cardiomyopathy, migraine, myocardial ischemia, and prospective use in other noncardiovascular disease.

Two other pathophysiological states are associated with alterations in [^{3}H]DHP binding. [^{3}H]Nitrendipine B_{max} alterations are observed in hypertension. Spontaneously hypertensive rats exhibit a 60% increase in the B_{max} for [^{3}H]nitrendipine in brain, but not heart, with no change in K_D.[98] Deoxycorticosterone NaCl hypertensive rats exhibit a 50% decrease in the B_{max} for [^{3}H]nitrendipine in brain stem, but not in heart or other brain regions.[99] Twenty-four month old rats exhibit an increase in K_D for [^{3}H]nitrendipine in brain with no change in B_{max} when compared to younger animals.[100]

We have also found drug interactions with the [^{125}I]ω-conotoxin GVIA–binding site. Because N channels are responsible for neurotransmitter release,[101] which is blocked by aminoglycoside antibiotics,[102] we examined the effects of aminoglycosides on [^{125}I]ω-conotoxin GVIA binding to neuronal membranes (TABLE 6).[103]

Neomycin is most potent, inhibiting binding 50% at 3 μM. Gentamycin and tobramycin are only 30% and 15% as potent, respectively, as neomycin. Streptomycin is 40% as potent as tobramycin; and kanamycin, the weakest agent, is only about 1% as potent as neomycin. Both the absolute and relative potencies of these drugs are essentially the same in inhibiting $^{45}Ca^{2+}$ uptake into synaptosomes conducted under

TABLE 5. Drug and Pathophysiologic Effects on Calcium Receptors of Potential Clinical Relevance

Drug or Condition	Receptor Effect			Reference
	DHP	PAA	Clinical	
Diphenylbutyl piperidines	K_i (nM)	K_i (nM)	Relieves negative schizophrenia symptoms	67–78
Pimozide	13	2		
Clopimozide	17	0.9		
Fluspirilene	21	0.4		
Penfluridol	30	0.9		
Phenothiazines Thoridazine	K_i (nM) 1–2	ND	Cardiac and sexual side effects in antipsychotic therapy	79–84
Antidiarrheal opiates	K_i (nM)		Antidiarrheal actions	85–87
Loperamide	10,000	ND		
Fluperamide	2,500	ND		
Diphenoxylate	1,000	ND		
Fetoxylate	500	ND		
Amiodarone	K_i (nM) 61	K_i (nM) 65	Antianginal Antiarrhythmic	89,90
Verapamil	10 mg/kg 60 days decreases cardiac [^{3}H]nitrendipine binding by 50%		Antianginal Antiarrhythmic	97
Cardiomyopathy	50% increase in DHP and PAA B_{max}		—	92–96
Hypertension	[^{3}H]nitrendipine B_{max} alterations in brain not heart		—	98, 99
Aging	Increase in K_D for [^{3}H]nitrendipine in 24-month-old rat brains		—	100

TABLE 6. Comparison of Dihydropyridines, Phenylalkylamines, and Aminoglycosides in Inhibition of [^{3}H]Nitrendipine, (−)-[^{3}H]Desmethoxyverapamil, [^{125}I]ω-Conotoxin GVIA Binding, and Synaptosomal N Channel $^{45}Ca^{2+}$ Influx

Drug	[^{3}H]Nitrendipine[a] IC_{50} or K_i (nM)	(−)-[^{3}H]Desmethoxyverapamil[b] IC_{50} or K_i (nM)	[^{128}I]ωCgTx[c] IC_{50} (μM)	Snyaptosomal[d] N Channel $^{45}Ca^{2+}$ Influx IC_{50} (μM)
Dihydropyridines				
Nifedipine	0.2–0.3	2.1	>30	>30
Nitrendipine	0.1–0.5	1.8	>30	>30
(−)-PN202-791	0.9	ND	>30	>30
(+)-PN202-791	90	ND	>30	>30
(±)-Bay K 8644	ND	9.4	>30	>30
Phenylalkylamines				
(−)-Desmethoxyverapamil	ND	2.4	>10	18
(+)-Desmethoxyverapamil	ND	45.5	>10	14
Methoxyverapamil	42	21.4	>10	16
Verapamil	180–400	40.3	<10	10
Aminoglycosides				
Amikacin	$>10^6$	ND		
Gentamycin	$>10^6$	ND	10	20
Kanamycin	$>10^6$	ND	200	500
Neomycin	$>10^6$	ND	3	5
Streptomycin	330,000	ND	50	150
Tobramycin	$>10^6$	ND	20	50

[a] [^{3}H]Nitrendipine binding values for DHP and PAA were derived from the literature.[8] Values for aminoglycosides were derived experimentally. IC_{50} values were derived from single experiments performed in duplicate and repeated twice.

[b] (−)-[^{3}H]Desmethoxyverapamil binding data were derived from the literature.[49]

[c] [^{125}I]ω-Conotoxin GVIA ([^{125}I]CgTx) binding was assayed in whole rat brain homogenates as described.[64–66] IC_{50} values were derived from single experiments performed in duplicate and repeated on two occasions.

[d] Synaptosomal $^{45}Ca^{2+}$ flux was assayed as described.[101] IC_{50} values were derived from individual experiments performed in triplicate and repeated three times. IC_{50} values represent the concentration of drug inhibiting ligand binding or $^{45}Ca^{2+}$ flux by 50%.

conditions in which calcium accumulation selectively involves N channels.[101] The relative potencies of these drugs in blocking N channels correlates closely with their relative presynaptic neuromuscular toxic actions.[103] Despite the aminoglycoside effects on [^{125}I]ω-conotoxin GVIA binding, only streptomycin inhibited [^{3}H]nitrendipine binding below 1 mM.

CALCIUM FLUX THROUGH VOLTAGE-SENSITIVE CALCIUM CHANNELS AND SODIUM/CALCIUM EXCHANGE

While calcium antagonist drugs markedly influence calcium-mediated effects in smooth and cardiac muscle, influences on nervous tissue, such as neurotransmitter

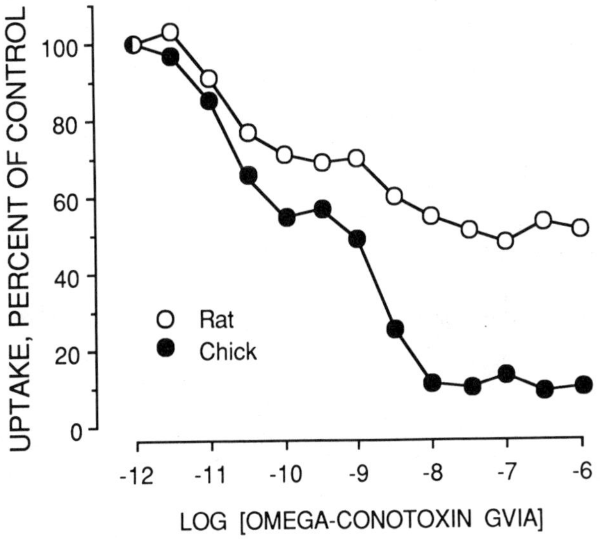

FIGURE 6. $^{45}Ca^{2+}$ uptake in chick (filled circles) and rat (open circles) synaptosomes is inhibited by ω-conotoxin GVIA. Methods are as described.[101]

release and calcium flux in synaptosomal preparations of the brain, have been difficult to demonstrate.[104–108] Recently, utilizing nervous tissue preparations such as the dorsal root ganglion, primarily cultures of brain tissue, and neuroblastoma cultures, reproducible influences on calcium flux have been shown with DHP agonists facilitating calcium entry and antagonists blocking these effects.

Some insight into the failure of calcium antagonist drugs to influence calcium flux in brain synaptosomes has come from the discrimination of subtypes of voltage-sensitive calcium channels by Tsien and co-workers.[62] Calcium antagonist drugs act primarily at the L channel, while the N and T channels are resistant to DHP drug effects.[62] ω-Conotoxin GVIA very potently blocks both L and N but not T channels.[63] We have demonstrated that the rapid influx of $^{45}Ca^{2+}$ into synaptosomes, measured at 1 second, is stimulated by depolarization indicating a voltage dependency, inhibited by predepolarization, and blocked by low concentrations of cadmium.[101] This influx is not affected by DHP and PAA calcium antagonist drugs, but is potently blocked by ω-conotoxin GVIA in both rat and chick synaptosomes (FIGURE 6).[101] The potent effects of ω-conotoxin GVIA indicate that L or N channels are involved, while the ineffectiveness of calcium antagonist drugs rules out L channels. Accordingly, the N channels predominantly account for rapid calcium influx into synaptosomes. Interestingly, in rat brain synaptosomes, the maximal effect of ω-conotoxin GVIA is to reduce calcium influx by 50%, while in chick synaptosomes almost 100% blockade of flux can be obtained (FIGURE 6).[101,110] These observations fit with findings that ω-conotoxin GVIA injected intracerebrally is substantially more toxic in chicks than in rats.[61]

The availability of calcium antagonist drugs has greatly facilitated the study of L channels. We have screened large numbers of chemicals to seek selective antagonists of N channels. Whereas DHP and PAA are quite weak at these sites, we detect influences of several aminoglycoside antibiotics on these sites at concentrations corresponding to therapeutic blood levels (TABLE 6).

TABLE 7. EC_{50} of Cations and Anions on Na^+/Ca^{2+} Exchange

Ion	Microsome	Synaptosome
	$EC_{50}(\mu M)^a$	
Group Ia, enhancer		
$RbCl$	1300	1200
$CsCl$	2700	3000
Group IIa, inhibitor		
$MgCl_2$	600	900
$SrCl_2$	43	40
$BaCl_2$	100	120
Transition, inhibitor		
$MnCl_2$	20	23
$FeCl_3$	500	700
$FeCl_2$	500	600
$CoCl_2$	18	20
$NICl_2$	20	15
$CuCl_2$	20	22
$ZnCl_2$	7	9
$PbNO_3$	3	5
$CdCl_2$	15	14
Lanthanide Series, inhibitor		
$LaCl_3$	5	30
	$IC_{50}(\mu M)$	
Anions		
Bromide	>10	>10
Iodide	10	10
Acetate	>10	>10
Citrate	0.2	0.5
Nitrate	>10	>10
Nitrate	>10	>10
Sulfite	>10	>10
Sulfate	5	5

[a] $Na^+/^{45}Ca^{2+}$ exchange experiments were performed as previously described.[111] EC_{50} for inhibitor ions is IC_{50}, the concentration for 50% inhibition of binding. EC_{50} for enhancing ions is the concentration for 50% of the maximal stimulation. Values are derived from a single experiment performed in triplicate and repeated twice.

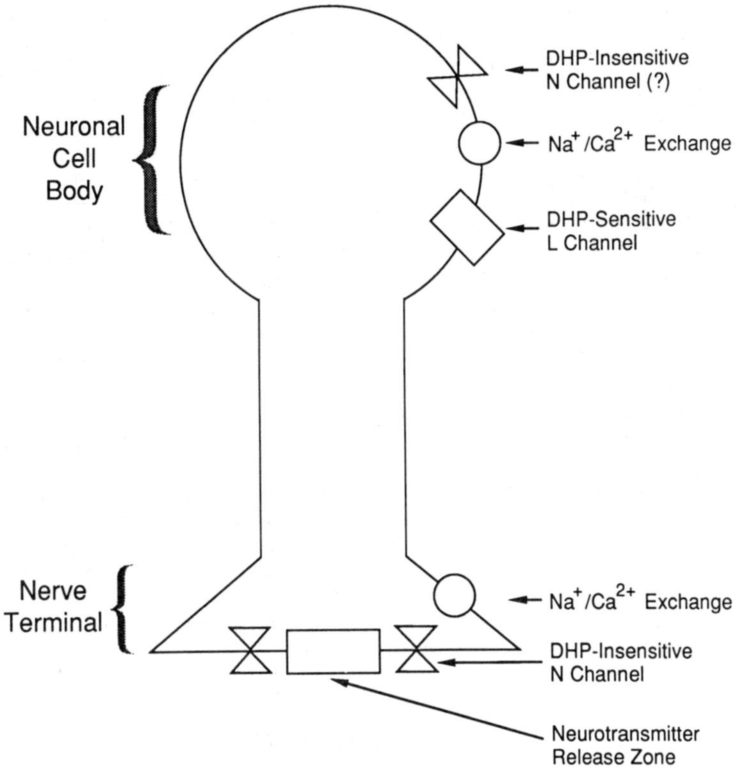

FIGURE 7. Model of typical neuron indicating hypothesized locations of different Ca^{2+} transport processes.

Many earlier studies of calcium flux into synaptosomes, first thought to involve VSCC, appear largely to reflect Na^+/Ca^{2+} exchange. To understand the physiological relevance of Na^+/Ca^{2+} exchange, we have tried to identify agents that selectively influence this exchange.

Numerous ions affect Na^+/Ca^{2+} exchange. The inhibitory actions of group IIa cations such as calcium, barium, strontium, and magnesium and the effects of transition elements such as cadmium and lanthanum in brain synaptosomes resemble the effects previously reported in the heart (TABLE 7). We have made the novel finding that group Ia monovalent cations such as rubidium and cesium also exert potent effects but in a different direction. Whereas the divalent and trivalent cations inhibit Na^+/Ca^{2+} exchange, these monovalent cations provide 50–100% increase in Na^+/Ca^{2+} exchange (TABLE 7).

CONCLUSIONS

In summary, a major advance in understanding calcium transport mechanisms has been the identification of calcium antagonist drug receptors and their association with specific subtypes of voltage-dependent calcium channels. A wide range of evidence both for biophysical and biochemical studies now supports the existence of at least three subtypes of VSCC. They can be differentiated in terms of their ion selectivity and sensitivity to inhibition by cadmium, dihydropyridines, and ω-conotoxin GVIA. The N and L channels appear to be localized, respectively, to nerve terminals and cell bodies. Thus, isolated nerve terminals display N channel calcium transport but no DHP-sensitive L channel accumulation of calcium. By contrast, neuronal cell bodies such as those in the hippocampus, dorsal root ganglion, and cell cultures[109] display DHP-sensitive and ω-conotoxin GVIA–sensitive calcium uptake. The localization of N-type channels to nerve channels suggests that they are the VSCC that mediate calcium-linked neurotransmitter release. Na^+/Ca^{2+} exchange normally functions to extrude calcium from the cell, but, in a depolarized state, might mediate calcium accumulation and may account for many reports of synaptosomal calcium uptake. Quantitatively, the Na^+/Ca^{2+} exchange mechanism can transport substantially more calcium than the VSCC in synaptosomes. Accordingly, when nerve terminals are depolarized and Na^+/Ca^{2+} exchange presumably mediates an inward movement of calcium, it might be responsible for neurotransmitter release. This may be especially important during prolonged depolarization related to pathological states. Na^+/Ca^{2+} exchange also exists in cell bodies and is readily demonstrable in cells in culture.

FIGURE 7 depicts our model of calcium transport in neurons. Clarification of subtypes of calcium channels may have even more clinical relevance than is evident today. Drugs inhibiting Na^+/Ca^{2+} exchange might display cardiac ionotropic actions. Drugs that selectively block N-type VSCC might influence neurotransmitter release in a therapeutic fashion. Moreover, it is conceivable that numerous side effects of presently employed drugs, such as neuromuscular blockade of aminoglycoside antibiotics, might stem from actions at calcium channels.

ACKNOWLEDGMENTS

A very special thank you to N. Bruce for manuscript preparation.

REFERENCES

1. FLECKENSTEIN, A. 1971. *In* Calcium and the Heart. P. Harris & L. Opie, Eds.: 135–188. Academic Press. London, England.
2. FLECKENSTEIN, A. 1977. Annu. Rev. Pharmacol. Toxicol. **17:** 149–166.
3. GODFRAIND, T. & A. KABA. 1969. Br. J. Pharmcol. **35:** 354P–355P.
4. GODFRAIND, T., A. KABA & P. POLSTER. 1968. Arch. Int. Pharmacodyn. Ther. **172:** 235–239.
5. GODFRAIND, T., R. MILLER & M. WIBO. 1986. Pharmacol. Rev. **38:** 321–416.
6. SNYDER, S. H. & I. J. REYNOLDS. 1985. N. Engl. J. Med. **313:** 995–1002.
7. BELLEMANN, P., D. FERRY, F. LUBBECKE & H. GLOSSMANN. Arzneim.-Forsch. **31:** 2064–2067.
8. MURPHY, K. M. M., R. J. GOULD, B. L. LARGENT & S. H. SNYDER. 1983. Proc. Nat. Acad. Sci. USA **80:** 860–864.
9. EHLERT, F. J., W. R. ROESKE, E. ITOGA & H. I. YAMAMURA. 1982. Life Sci **30:** 2191–2202.
10. BOLGE, G. T., P. GENGO, R. KLOCKOWSKI, *et al.* 1983. J. Pharmacol. Exp. Ther. **225:** 291–309.
11. TRIGGLE, P. J. 1981. *In* New Perspectives on Calcium Antagonists, G. B. Weiss, Ed.: 1–18. American Physiological Society. Bethesda, Md.
12. CHENG, J. B. & R. G. TOWNLEY. 1983. Arch. Int. Pharmacodyn. **263:** 228–244.

13. GRANGER, S. E., M. HOLLINGSWORTH & A. H. WESTON. 1986. Br. J. Pharmacol. **87:** 147–156.
14. HOT, R. P. & H. J. VUORELA. 1983. J. Pharmacol. Methods. **9:** 41–52.
15. GOULD, R. J., K. M. M. MURPHY & S. H. SNYDER. 1982. Proc. Nat. Acad. Sci. USA **79:** 3656–3660.
16. GOULD, R. J., K. M. M. MURPHY & S. H. SNYDER. 1984. Mol. Pharmacol. **25:** 235–241.
17. LUCHOWSKI, E. M., F. YOUSIF, D. J. TRIGGLE, S. C. MAURER, J. G. SARMIENTO & R. A. JANIS. 1984. J. Pharmacol. Exp. Ther. **230:** 607–613.
18. PTASIENSKI, J., K. K. MCMAHON & M. M. HOSEY. 1985. Biochem. Biophys. Res. Commun. **129:** 910–917.
19. BELLEMANN, P. 1984. FEBS Lett. **167:** 88–92.
20. BELLEMANN, P. 1984. J. Receptor Res. **4:** 571–585.
21. FAWZI, A. B. & J. H. MCNEILL. 1984. Eur. J. Pharmacol. **104:** 357–362.
22. GLOSSMANN, H., D. R. FERRY, F. LUBBECKE, R. MEWES & F. HOFMANN. 1982. Trends Pharmacol. Sci. **3:** 431–437.
23. BRISTOW, M. R., R. GINSBURG, J. A. LASER, B. J. MCAULEY & W. MINOBE. 1984. Br. J. Pharmacol. **82;** 309–320.
24. CHENG, J. B., A. BEWTRA & R. G. TOWNLEY. 1984. Experientia Basel **40:** 267–269.
25. GROVER, A. K., C.-Y. KWAN, E. LUCHOWSKI, E. E. DANIEL & D. J. TRIGGLE. 1984. J. Biol. Chem. **259:** 2223–2226.
26. JANIS, R. A., J. G. SARMIENTO, S. C. MAURER, G. T. BOLGER & D. J. TRIGGLE. 1984. J Pharamcol. Exp Ther. **231:** 8–15.
27. MARANGOS, P. J., J. PATEL, C. MILLER & A. M. MARINO. 1982. Life Sci. **31:** 1575–1585.
28. MILLER, W. C. & J. B. MOORE. 1984. Life Sci. **34:** 1717–1721.
29. MURAMATSU, M., A. FUJITA, M. TANAKA & H. AIHARA. 1985. Jpn. J. Pharmacol. **39:** 217–223.
30. POWERS, R. E. & W. S. COLUCCI. 1985. Biochem. Biophys. Res. Commun. **132:** 844–849.
31. RAMKUMAR, V. & E. E. EL-FAKAHANY. 1984. Eur. J. Pharmacol. **102:** 371–372.
32. RENAUD, J.-F., T. KAZAZOGLOU, A. SCHMID, G. ROMEY & M. LAZDUNSKI. 1984. Eur. J. Biochem. **139:** 673–681.
33. SARMIENTO, J. G., R. A. JANIS, A. M. KATZ & D. J. TRIGGLE. 1984. Biochem. Pharmacol. **33:** 3119–3123.
34. WILLIAMS, L. T. & L. R. JONES. 1983. J. Biol. Chem. **258:** 5344–5347.
35. FERRY, D. R. & H. GLOSSMANN. 1982. Circ. Res. **321:** 80–83.
36. FERRY, D. R. & H. GLOSSMANN. 1982. FEBS Lett. **148:** 331–337.
37. FOSSET, M., E. JAIMOVICH, E. DELPONT & M. LAZDUNSKI. 1983. Eur. J. Pharmacol. **86:** 141–142.
38. FOSSET, M., E. JAIMOVICH, E. DELPONT & M. LAZDUNSKI. 1983. J. Biol. Chem. **258:** 6086–6092.
39. GLOSSMANN, H., D. R. FERRY & C. B. BOSCHEK. 1983. Naunyn Schmiedebergs Arch. Pharmacol. **323:** 1–11.
40. BOLES, R. G., H. I. YAMAMURA, H. SCHOEMAKER & W. R. ROESKE. 1984. J. Pharmacol. Exp. Ther. **229:** 333–339.
41. DEPOVER, A., M. A. MATLIB, S. W. LEE, G. P. DUBE, I. L. GRUPP, G. GRUPP & A. SCHWARTZ. 1982. Biochem. Biophys. Res. Commun. **108:** 110–117.
42. GLOSSMANN, H., D. R. FERRY, A. GOLL & M. ROMBUSCH. 1984. J. Cardiovasc. Pharmacol. **6:** S608–S621.
43. HOLCK, M., W. FISCHLI & U. HENGARTNER. 1984. J. Receptor Res. **4:** 557–569.
44. LEE, H. R., J. A. JAROS, W. R. ROESKE, N. L. WEICH, R. URSILLO & H. I. YAMAMURA. 1985. J. Pharmacol. Exp. Ther. **233:** 611–616.
45. YAMAMURA, H. I., H. SCHOEMAKER, R. G. BOLES & W. R. ROESKE. 1982. Biochem. Biophys. Res. Commun. **108:** 640–646.
46. FERRY, D. R., A. GOLL & H. GLOSSMANN. 1984. Naunyn-Schmiedeberg's Arch. Pharmacol. **323:** 183–187.
47. GALIZZI, J.-P., M. FOSSET & M. LAZDUNSKI. 1984. Eur. J. Biochem **144:** 211–215.

48. GALIZZI, J.-P., M. FOSSET & M. LAZDUNSKI. 1985. Biochem. Biophys. Res. Commun. **132:** 49–55.
49. REYNOLDS, I. J., A. M. SNOWMAN & S. H. SNYDER. 1986. J. Pharmacol. Exp. Ther. **237:** 731–738.
50. BALWIERCZAK, J. L. & A. SCHWARTZ. 1985. Eur. J. Pharamcol. **116:** 193–144.
51. GLOSSMANN, H., T. LINN, M. ROMBUSCH & D. R. FERRY. 1983. FEBS Lett. **160:** 226–232.
52. SCHOEMAKER, H. & S. Z. LANGER. 1985. Eur. J. Pharmacol. **111:** 273–277.
53. BORSOTTO, M., J. BARHANIN, M. FOSSET & M. LAZDUNSKI. 1985. J. Biol. Chem. **260:** 14255–14263.
54. BORSOTTO, M., J. BARHANIN, R. I. NORMAN & M. LAZDUNSKI. 1984. Biochem. Biophys. Res. Commun. **122:** 1357–1366.
55. BORSOTTO, M. R. I. NORMAN, M. FOSSET & M. LAZDUNSKI. 1984. Eur. J. Biochem. **142:** 447–455.
56. CURTIS, B. M. & W. A. CATTERALL. 1984. Biochemistry **23:** 2113–2118.
57. TAKAHASHI, M. & W. A. CATTERALL. 1987. Science **236:** 88–91.
58. GLOSSMANN, H. D. R. FERRY & C. B. BOSCHEK. 1983. Naunyn-Schmiedelberg's Arch. Pharmacol. **323:** 1–11.
59. GUGGINO, S. E., J. A. WAGNER & S. H. SNYDER. In preparation.
60. RAISZ, L. G. 1965. J. Clin. Invest. **44:** 103–116.
61. OLIVERA, B. M., W. R. GRAY, R. ZEIKUB, M. MCINTOSH, J. VARGA, J. RIVIER, V. DESANTES & L. J. CRUZ. 1985. Science **230:** 1338–1343.
62. NOWYCKY, M. C., A. P. FOX & R. W. TSIEN. 1985. Nature London **316:** 440–443.
63. MCCLESKEY, E. W., A. P. FOX, D. H. FELDMAN, L. J. CRUZ, B. M. OLIVERA, R. W. TSIEN & D. YOSHIKAMI. 1987. Proc. Nat. Acad. Sci. USA **84:** 4327–4331.
64. RIVIER, J. & B. M. OLIVERA. 1986. J. Biol. Chem. **261:** 6230–6233.
65. CRUZ, L. J., P. S. JOHNSON & B. M. OLIVERA. 1987. Biochemistry **26:** 820–824.
66. WAGNER, J. A., A. S. SNOWMAN, B. M. OLIVERA & S. H. SNYDER. In preparation.
67. PEROUTKA, S. J. & S. H. SNYDER. 1980. Am. J. Psychiatry **137:** 1518–1522.
68. SEEMAN, P. 1981. Pharamcol Rev. **32:** 229–313.
69. PINDER, R. M., R. N. BROGDEN, P. R. SAWYER, T. M. SPEIGHT, R. SPENCER & G. S. AVERY. 1976. Drugs **12:** 1–40.
70. HAAS, S. & H. BECKMANN. 1982. Pharmacopsychiatry **15:** 70–74.
71. KUDO, Y. 1972. Acta Psychiatr. Belg. **72:** 685–697.
72. LAPIERRE, Y. D. & J. LAVALLEE. 1975. Curr. Ther. Res. Clin. Exp. **18:** 181–188.
73. LAPIERRE, Y. D. 1978. Am. J. Psychiatry **135:** 956–959.
74. SHOPSIN, B., H. KLEIN, L. GERBINO & G. SELZER. 1977. Psychopharmacology **55:** 157–164.
75. FRANGOS, H., N. P. ZISSIS, I. LEONTOPOULOS, N. DIAMANTAS, S. TSITOURIDIS, I. GAVRIIL & K. TSOLIS. 1978. Acta Psychiatr. Scand. **57:** 436–446.
76. SINGH, A. N. 1982. *In* Calcium Blockers, Mechanisms of Action and Clinical Applications, S. F. Flaim & R. Zelis, Eds.: 121–134. Urban and Schwarzenberg. Baltimore, Md.
77. GOULD, R. J., K. M. M. MURPHY, I. J. REYNOLDS & S. H. SNYDER. 1983. Proc. Nat. Acad. Sci. USA **80:** 5122–5125.
78. GALIZZI, J.-P., M. FOSSET, G. ROMEY, P. LADURON & M. LAZDUNSKI. 1986. Proc. Nat. Acad Sci USA **83:** 7513–7517.
79. APPLETON, W. S. 1982. J. Clin. Psychiatry. **43:** 12–27.
80. RISCH, S. C., E. P. GROOM & D. S. JANOWSKY. 1981. J. Clin. Psychiatry. **42:** 23–34.
81. RISCH, S. C., G. P. GROOM & D. S. JANOWSKY. 1981. J. Clin. Psychiatry. **42:** 47–59.
82. STIMMEL, B. 1979. Cardiovascular Effects of Mood Altering Drugs. Raven Press. New York, N.Y.
83. SHADER, R. I. & A. DIMASCIO. 1970. *In* Clinical and Theoretical Perspectives. Williams and Wilkins. Baltimore, MD.
84. GOULD, R. J., K. M. M. MURPHY, I. J. REYNOLDS & S. H. SNYDER. 1984. Am. J. Psychiatry **141:** 352–357.
85. SANDHU, B. K., J. H. TRIPP, D. C. A. CANDY & J. T. HARRIES. 1981. Gut **22:** 658–662.

86. Wuster, M. & A. Herz. 1978. Naunyn-Schmiedeberg's Arch. Pharmacol **301:** 187–194.
87. Reynolds, I. J., R. J. Gould & S. H. Snyder. 1984. J. Pharmacol. Exp. Ther. **231:** 628–632.
88. Guerrero, J. R. & S. S. Martin. 1984. Med. Res. Rev. **4:** 87–109.
89. Wagner, J. A., H. F. Weisman, A. M. Snowman, F. Sax & S. H. Snyder. In preparation.
90. Nokin, P., M. Clinet, S. Swillens, C. Pelisee, L. Meysmans & P. Chatelain. 1986. J. Cardiovasc. Pharmacol. **8:** 1051–1057.
91. Gertz, E. W. 1972. Prog. Exp. Tumor Res. **16:** 242–260.
92. Wagner, J. A., I. J. Reynolds, H. F. Weisman, P. Dudeck, M. L. Weisfeldt & S. H. Snyder. 1986. Science **232:** 515–518.
93. Finkel, M. S., E. S. Marks, R. E. Patterson, E. H. Speir, K. A. Steadman & H. R. Keiser. 1986. Am. J. Cardiology **57:** 1205–1206.
94. Finkel, M. S., E. S. Marks, R. E. Patterson, E. H. Speir, K. A. Steadman & H. R. Keiser. 1987. Life Sci. **41:** 153–159.
95. Monakata, M., L. K. Huang, J. A. Wagner & H. Menkes. Am. J. Physiol. (Submitted.)
96. Wagner, J. A., F. L. Sax, H. F. Weisman, J. Porterfield, C. McIntosh, M. L. Weisfeldt, S. H. Snyder & S. E. Epstein. In preparation.
97. Wagner, J. A., H. F. Weisman, A. M. Snowman & S. H. Snyder. In preparation.
98. Ishii, K., T. Kano & Y. Kurobe. 1983. Eur. J. Pharmacol. **88:** 277–278.
99. Lee, H. R., M. Watson, H. I. Yamamura & W. R. Roeske. 1985. Life Sci. **37:** 971–977.
100. Lee, H. R., M. Watson, H. I. Yamamura & W. R. Roeske. 1985. Life Sci. **37:** 971–974.
101. Reynolds, I. J., J. A. Wagner, S. H. Snyder, S. A. Thayer, B. M. Olivera & R. J. Miller. 1986. Proc Nat. Acad. Sci. USA **83:** 8804–8807.
102. Wright, J. & B. Collier. 1977. J. Pharmacol. Exp. Ther. **200:** 576–587.
103. Wagner, J. A., A. M. Snowman, B. M. Olivera & S. H. Snyder. In preparation.
104. Nachshen, D. A. & M. P. Blaustein. 1979. Mol. Pharmacol. **16:** 579–586.
105. Nachshen, D. A. 1985. J. Physiol. London **361:** 251–268.
106. Creha, J. A. & M. Karobath. 1986. Biochem. Biophys. Res. Commun. **134:** 1038–1042.
107. Suszkiw, J. B., M. E. O'Leary, M. M. Morawsky & T. Wang. 1986. J. Neurosci. **6:** 1349–1357.
108. Rampe, D., R. A. Janis & D. J. Triggle. 1984. J. Neurochem. **43:** 1688–1691.
109. Miller, R. J. 1987. Science **235:** 46–52.
110. Rivier, J., R. Galyeon, W. R. Gray, A. Azimi Zonouz, J. M. McIntosh, L. J. Gruz & B. M. Olivera. 1986. J. Biol. Chem. **262:** 1194–1198.
111. Wagner, J. A., I. J. Reynolds & S. H. Snyder. 1987. J. Cardiovasc. Pharmacol. (In press.)

Molecular Properties of Structure and Regulation of the Calcium Channel[a]

MICHEL LAZDUNSKI,[b] JACQUES BARHANIN,[b]
MARC BORSOTTO,[b] CHRISTIAN COGNARD,[c]
CHRISTIE COOPER,[d] THIERRY COPPOLA,[b]
MICHEL FOSSET,[b] JEAN-PIERRE GALIZZI,[b]
MARLENE M. HOSEY,[d] CHRISTIANE MOURRE,[b],
JEAN-FRANÇOIS RENAUD,[b] GEORGES ROMEY,[b]
ANNIE SCHMID,[b] AND SYLVIE VANDAELE[b]

[b]*Biochemistry Center*
National Center for Scientific Research (CNRS)
Parc Valrose
06034 Nice Cedex, France

[c]*General Physiology Laboratory*
40 Avenue du Recteur Pineau
86021 Poitiers Cedex, France

[d]*University of Health Sciences*
The Chicago Medical School
3333 Green Bay Road
North Chicago, Illinois 60064

Voltage-dependent calcium channels are known to play important roles in excitation-contraction coupling in cardiac and smooth muscles and also in a number of neurosecretory processes. They have recently become accessible to biochemical study as a result of the availability of a number of tritiated calcium channel inhibitors belonging to the dihydropyridine and the phenylalkylamine series.[1] Dihydropyridine derivatives such as nitrendipine and other calcium inhibitors such as verapamil, bepridil, and diltiazem are very important therapeutic agents in the treatment of cardiovascular disorders.[2]

One of the difficulties associated with the biochemical characterization of macromolecules that confer electrical excitability to biological membranes, such as the voltage-sensitive calcium channel, is that they are almost always present in very low amounts in membranes. For most membrane preparations in which the voltage-sensitive calcium channel has been characterized, the dihydropyridine receptor is only present at a density in the range of 0.1 to 1 pmol/mg protein.[1] Therefore, the transverse tubule (T-tubule) membrane preparation isolated from rabbit skeletal muscle appears to be exceptional in that it contains more than 50 pmol [^{3}H]dihydropyridine-binding sites/mg protein.[3] Voltage-clamp analyses of skeletal muscle have shown that essentially all specific Ca^{2+} conductances are localized in the transverse tubular system and that the channel responsible for these conductances is inhibited by low concentrations

[a]This work was supported by the Association des Myopathes, the Centre National de la Recherche Scientifique, the Fondation sur les Maladies Vasculaires, the Fondation pour la Recherche Médicale, and the Ministère de l'Industrie et de la Recherche (grant no. 83.C.0696).

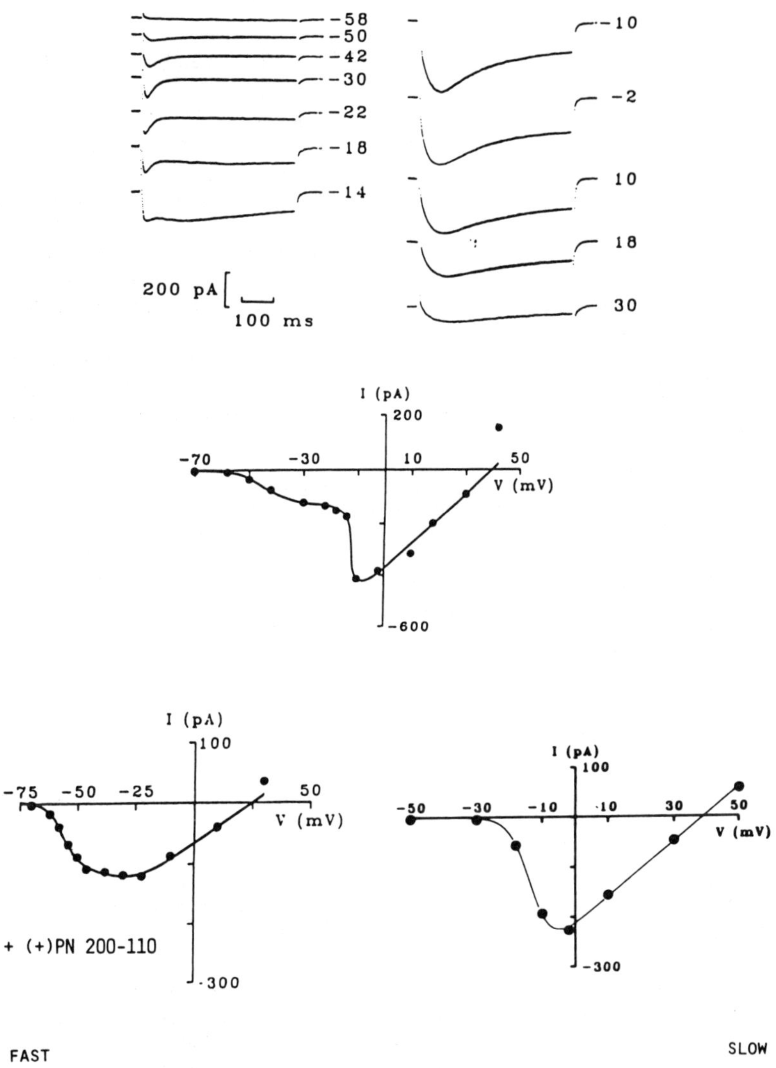

FIGURE 1. Different types of Ca^{2+} channels in rat muscle cells in culture. Top left: fast (T-type) Ca^{2+} channels. Top right: slow (L-type) Ca^{2+} channels. I–V characteristic of the fast (bottom left) and slow (bottom right) Ca^{2+} channels. The voltage-dependence of these two types of Ca^{2+} channels is different. Center: I–V characteristic of a skeletal muscle cell having both T- and L-type Ca^{2+} channels.

of dihydropyridines.[4–7]. T-tubule membranes were used to analyze the molecular pharmacology of the Ca^{2+} channel as starting material for the solubilization and purification of this channel.

DIFFERENT TYPES OF Ca^{2+} CHANNELS IN SKELETAL MUSCLE

There are at least two different types of Ca^{2+} channels in skeletal muscle (FIGURE 1).[6,7] One class of these Ca^{2+} channels activates at very low membrane potentials and opens and closes rapidly; another type of Ca^{2+} channels is much slower and only activates near −40 mV. This latter type of Ca^{2+} channel (L-type) is the only one that is sensitive to 1,4-dihydropyridines.[7]

The L-type Ca^{2+} channel is blocked by compounds such as (+)PN 200-110 and activated by Ca^{2+} channel activators such as Bay K 8644.[7] Blockade by (+)PN 200-110 is voltage dependent and is more potent when the channel is in the inactivated state (in a situation where the drug interacts with the depolarized membrane). There is an excellent correlation between binding constants determined with tritiated ligands on isolated membranes and binding constants measured by electrophysiology (voltage clamp) on depolarized cells in which the L-type Ca^{2+} channel is inactivated.[7] L-type

TABLE 1. Affinities of Different 1,4-Dihydropyridines for Binding to Rabbit Microsome Membranes from Different Tissues

Microsome Membranes	(+)[^{3}H]PN 200-110 K_D(nM)[a]	[^{3}H]Nitrendipine K_D(nM)[a]
Skeletal muscle	0.2	1.8
Heart muscle	0.06	0.3
Smooth muscle	0.4	0.4
Brain	0.04	0.1

[a] K_D is the equilibrium dissociation constant.

Ca^{2+} channels in skeletal muscle are slower than in cardiac cells and have a different voltage dependence of inactivation.

PHARMACOLOGICAL PROPERTIES FOR CALCIUM CHANNEL BLOCKER RECEPTORS

TABLE 1 indicates some of the affinities found for the binding of different 1,4-dihydropyridines to the Ca^{2+} channel protein in skeletal muscle as compared to other tissues. The most active 1,4-dihydropyridine is (+)PN 200-110. The binding of 1,4-dihydropyridines to the voltage-dependent Ca^{2+} channel in cardiac and skeletal muscle cells[7,8] is voltage-dependent, the highest affinity being found when the membrane is depolarized. The affinity of (+)PN 200-110 found from binding experiments to purified membranes is the same as that found by electrophysiology on cells having a membrane potential near 0 mV.

Verapamil, bepridil, and diltiazem are known to allosterically regulate 1,4-dihydropyridine binding sites in brain, smooth, skeletal, and cardiac muscles.[9] T-tubule membranes also have high-affinity binding sites for (−)[^{3}H]desmethoxyverapamil [(−)D888], *d-cis*-[^{3}]diltiazem, and (±)[^{3}H]bepridil. Binding at these sites is reversible and saturable with the following equilibrium dissociation constants (K_D) and maximum binding capacities (B_{max}): (−)[^{3}H]desmethoxyverapamil (K_D = 1.5 nM, B_{max} = 70 ± 10 pmol/mg protein), *d-cis*-[^{3}H]diltiazem (K_D = 50 nM, B_{max} = 50 ± 8 pmol/mg protein), and (±)[^{3}H]bepridil (K_D = 20 nM, B_{max} = 80 ± 15 pmol/mg protein). Desmethoxyverapamil, diltiazem, and bepridil are competitive for binding to skeletal muscle T-tubule membranes.[10] A high-affinity Ca^{2+}-binding site ($K_{Ca^{2+}}$ = 5 μM) modulates the affinity of binding of desmethoxyverapamil, diltiazem, and bepridil at their presumably common binding site.[11]

AFFINITY LABELING EXPERIMENTS OF BEPRIDIL, OF DILTIAZEM, AND OF 1,4-DIHYDROPYRIDINE RECEPTORS IN SKELETAL MUSCLE

Affinity labeling experiments with (±)[^{3}H]bepridil, *d-cis*-[^{3}H]diltiazem, and (+)[^{3}H]PN 200-110 have shown that a polypeptide of 170 ± 10 kDa is specifically labeled.[10] Affinity labeling results suggest that the Ca^{2+} channel structure is a large protein of 170 kDa carrying receptors for 1,4-dihydropyridines and for verapamil, D888, diltiazem, and bepridil.

PURIFICATION OF THE 1,4-DIHYDROPYRIDINE RECEPTOR COMPONENT OF THE Ca^{2+} CHANNEL

Among 14 detergents of varied chemical natures, only one, the 3-[(3-cholamido-propyl)-dimethyl-ammonio]-1 propane sulfonate (CHAPS), presented the required qualities for solubilization of the dihydropyridine receptor from T-tubule membranes.[12] Different unlabeled calcium inhibitors have been tested for their ability to interfere with the [^{3}H]nitrendipine binding on the solubilized receptor.[12] These molecules not only include dihydropyridine derivatives [(+)PN 200-110, nitrendipine, and nifedipine] but also benzothiazepine (l-*cis* and *d-cis* diltiazem), phenylalkylamine [(+) and (−)verapamil], and bepridil compounds. Rank order of potencies to inhibit 50% of binding ($K_{0.5}$) are: (+)PN 200-110 ($K_{0.5}$ = 0.7 nM) > nifedipine ($K_{0.5}$ = 7 nM) > nitrendipine ($K_{0.5}$ = 9 nM) for 1,4-dihydropyridine and (+)verapamil ($K_{0.5}$ = 500 nM) > (±)bepridil ($K_{0.5}$ = 4000 nM) > (−)verapamil ($K_{0.5}$ = 50 000 nM) ≫ l-*cis*-diltiazem for the other class of drugs. *d-cis*-Diltiazem has a potentiating effect on (+)[^{3}H]PN 200-110 binding to T-tubule membranes with a $K_{0.5}$ = 500 nM. Evidence that the solubilization procedure used in this work is useful to purify the voltage-sensitive calcium channel arises from the observations that ligand specificity and stereoselectivity are very close to those known for the membrane-bound receptor.

The CHAPS-solubilized extract from rabbit skeletal muscle microsomes was used for purification studies. The dihydropyridine receptor was substantially purified by a combination of ion exchange chromatography (DEAE), lectin affinity chromatography on wheat germ agglutinin (WGA), and gel filtration on Sephacryl S_{400}. After solubilization, a trace amount of (+)[^{3}H]PN 200-110 was added to the solubilized receptor. In this way a small part of the solubilized receptor was specifically labeled (less than 5% of the total receptor complex). This small proportion of the [^{3}H]dihydropyridine receptor complex was used to monitor the purification steps by counting aliquots of each fraction, while the total active binding site capacity can still be measured by equilibrium binding experiments.[13] Sodium dodecyl sulfate (SDS) gel electrophoresis analysis was carried out after each purification step. The protein pattern revealed that the probable subunit composition of the dihydropyridine receptor from skeletal muscle membranes under disulfide reducing conditions consisted of a protein of 142 kDa and a doublet of 32 kDa–33 kDa. These three proteins were strongly enriched by the purification procedure. This subunit composition is in good agreement with different polypeptide components determined by photoaffinity labeling: 145 kDa with [^{3}H]azidopine on guinea-pig skeletal muscle,[14] 170 kDa with

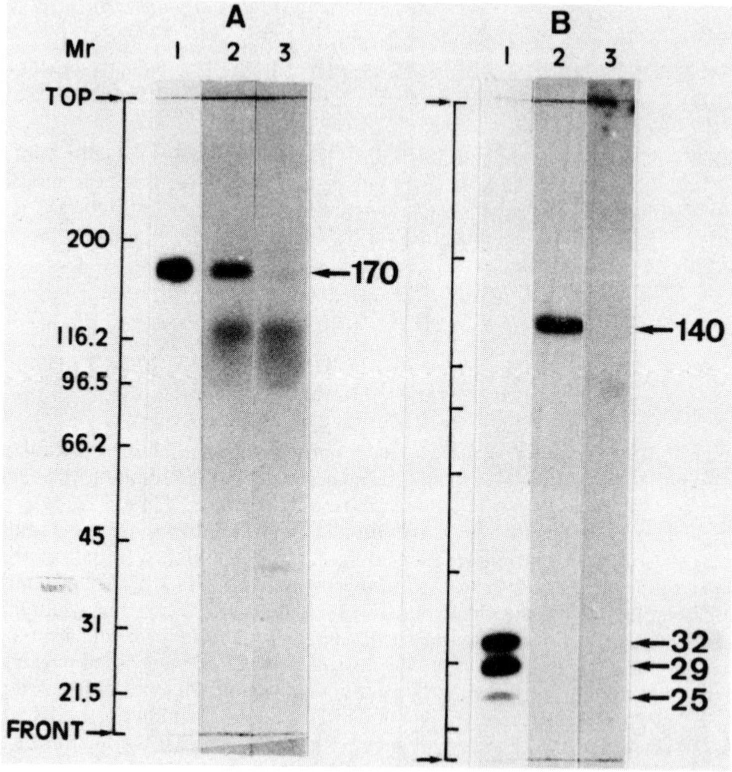

FIGURE 2. Immunoblots on rabbit skeletal muscle microsomes under nonreducing conditions (A) and under reducing conditions (B). Lane 1 with anti-32 serum (exposure time = 2 hours), lane 2 with anti-140 serum (exposure time = 7 hours), and lane 3 with control serum (exposure time = 7 hours). All the antisera are used at a 10^3 dilution. Molecular weight markers are from Biorad: myosin (200,000), β-galactosidase (116,500), phosphorylase B (96,500), bovine serum albumin (66,200), ovalbumin (45,000), carbonic anhydrase (31,000), soybean trypsin inhibitor (21,500).

(+)[^{3}H]-PN 200-110 on rabbit skeletal muscle, and 33 kDa with [^{3}H]nitrendipine on canine cardiac membrane.[15] The purified protein contains receptor for (+)PN 200-110, (−)D888, and *d-cis*-diltiazem in a 1:1:1 stoichiometry. Both the large and the small subunit are glycosylated.[16] Under nonreducing conditions both subunits are covalently linked within a 170 kDa protein unit.[16,17]

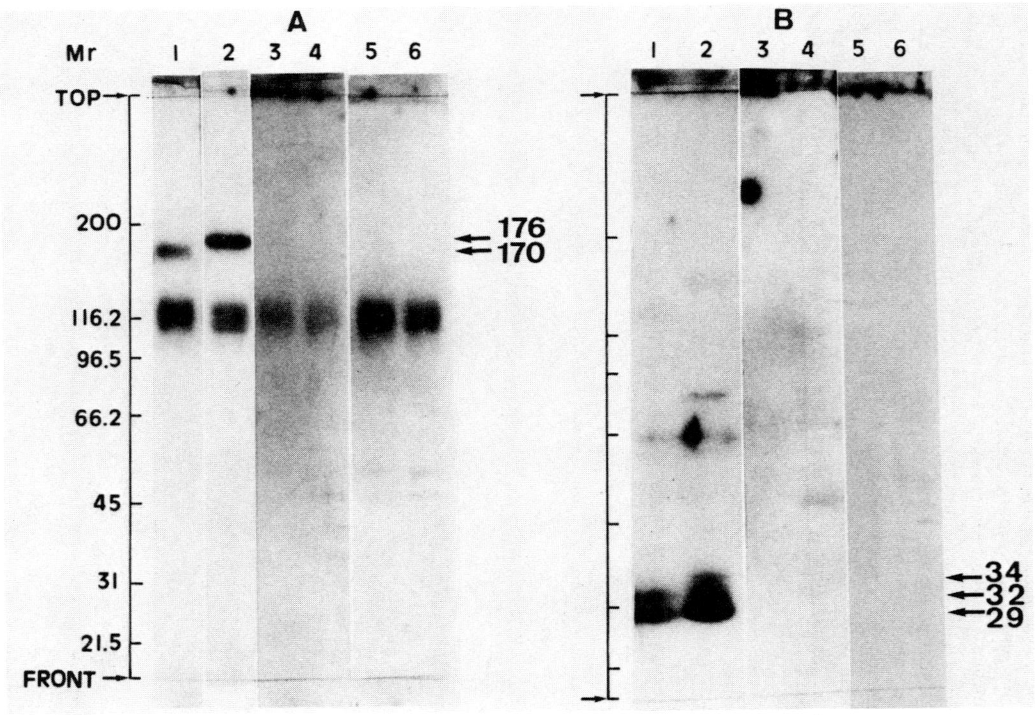

FIGURE 3. Immunoblots on rabbit cardiac and smooth muscle microsomes under nonreducing conditions (A) and under reducing conditions (B). Lanes 1, 3, and 5: smooth muscle with anti-32, anti-140, and control sera respectively. Lanes 2, 4, and 6: cardiac muscle with anti-32, anti-140, and control sera respectively. All sera are used at 10^3 dilution. Nonspecific labeling of a diffuse band of M_r 120,000 in nonreducing conditions was probably due to the presence in control and preimmune sera of immunoglobulin (IgG) against this peptide. Exposure time was 10 hours for all lanes. Molecular weight markers are the same as in FIGURE 2.

IMMUNOCHEMICAL ANALYSIS OF SUBUNIT STRUCTURES OF 1,4-DIHYDROPYRIDINE RECEPTORS ASSOCIATED WITH VOLTAGE-DEPENDENT Ca^{2+} CHANNELS IN SKELETAL, CARDIAC, AND SMOOTH MUSCLES

The skeletal muscle dihydropyridine (DHP) receptor has previously been shown to be made of two polypeptide chains of 140 kDa and 32–33 kDa.[13,17] Immunoblotting experiments performed on rabbit skeletal muscle membranes using the antiserum against the purified 140 kDa protein (anti-140 serum) showed that, under disulfide reducing conditions (2.5% of 2-mercaptoethanol), this antiserum specifically labeled the large component of the Ca^{2+} channel protein of 140 kDa as expected (FIGURE 2B, lane 2). Under nonreducing conditions (FIGURE 2A, lane 2) the anti-140 serum specifically recognized a protein with a larger structure of 170 kDa, suggesting that the small component of 32–33 kDa, identified in purification studies,[17] was probably covalently linked by disulfide bridges to the protein of 140 kDa. In order to test this

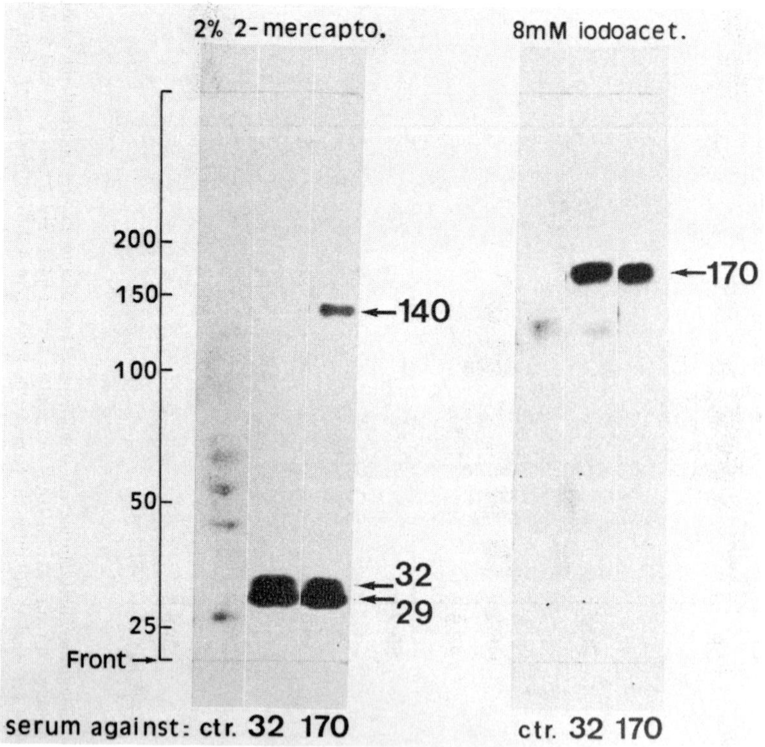

FIGURE 4. Immunoblots on rabbit brain synaptosomes. Experiments were carried out under nonreducing conditions (8 mM iodoacetamide) and under reducing conditions (2% of 2-mercaptoethanol). Lane 1: control serum (ctr.). Lane 2: anti-32 serum. Lane 3: anti-170 serum (serum directed against the large component of M_r = 170,000 of the skeletal muscle DHP receptor). All the antisera were used at 1/1000 dilution and the exposure times were 12 hours for all lanes. Molecular weight markers are the same as in FIGURE 2.

TABLE 2. Binding of (+)[^{3}H]PN 200-110 and Anti-32 Serum as Respectively Determined by Autoradiographic and Indirect Immunofluorescence Methods[a]

	Specific Binding of (+)[^{3}H]PN 200-110	Anti-32 Serum
Hippocampus		
Ammon's horn	+	+
Dentate gyrus	+++	+++
Cerebral cortex	++	++
Striatum	+	+
Thalamus	+	+
Hypothalamus	+	+
Substantia nigra	+	±
Colliculi	+	+
Cerebellum cortex		
Granular layer	+++	+++
Molecular layer	++	+

[a] +++, very high label; ++, high label; +, moderate label; ±, low label.

hypothesis, an antiserum directed against the purified 32–33 kDa component (anti-32 serum) was prepared and its ability to react with the DHP receptor of skeletal muscle was studied in immunoblots. FIGURE 2B, lane 1, shows that one band revealed by anti-32 serum under disulfide reducing conditions corresponded effectively to a low component of 32 kDa, but it also shows the presence of bands at 29 kDa and 25 kDa. Under nonreducing conditions the only peptide revealed by anti-32 serum had a structure of 170 kDa (FIGURE 2A, lane 1). Nonreducing conditions caused not only the complete disappearance of the band of 32 kDa but also the disappearance of the bands at 29 kDa and 25 kDa. This observation suggests that the two smaller polypeptides of 25 kDa and 29 kDa are degradation products of the 32 kDa component. Other structural studies carried out in this laboratory which did not involve the use of antibodies confirmed this view.[16] All these data taken together obtained both with the anti-140 serum and the anti-32 serum indicate that the DHP receptor is indeed a protein of about 170 kDa made of two chains of 140 kDa and 32 kDa covalently linked by disulfide bridge(s).

One important question was to know to what extent the molecular structure of the DHP receptor Ca^{2+} channel protein in nerve cells and in cardiac and smooth rabbit muscles was similar to that found in skeletal muscle. In order to answer this question, immunoblotting experiments were carried out using microsomal fractions from cardiac and smooth muscles and brain synaptosomes. FIGURE 3A (lanes 1 and 2) shows that proteins of 170 kDa (smooth muscle) and 176 kDa (heart) were specifically labeled by the anti-32 serum under nonreducing conditions. Under disulfide reducing conditions, after 2-mercaptoethanol treatment, the anti-32 serum revealed smaller components of 32 kDa and 29 kDa in the case of smooth muscle (FIGURE 3B, lane 1) and of 34, 32, and 29 kDa in the case of cardiac muscle (FIGURE 3B, lane 2). It is probable that the 29 kDa component in smooth muscle membranes is a degradation product of the 32 kDa peptide and that peptides at 32 kDa and 29 kDa are degradation products of the 34 kDa peptide in cardiac muscle membranes. No specific labeling of peptide bands was observed with the anti-140 serum either in the presence or in the absence of the reducing agent (FIGURE 3A and B, lanes 3 and 4). The presence in cardiac and smooth muscle membranes of the 170–176 kDa protein under nonreducing conditions and of the 32–34 kDa protein under reducing conditions clearly indicates, however, that a component of about 140 kDa exists in these tissues as in skeletal muscle. The lack of

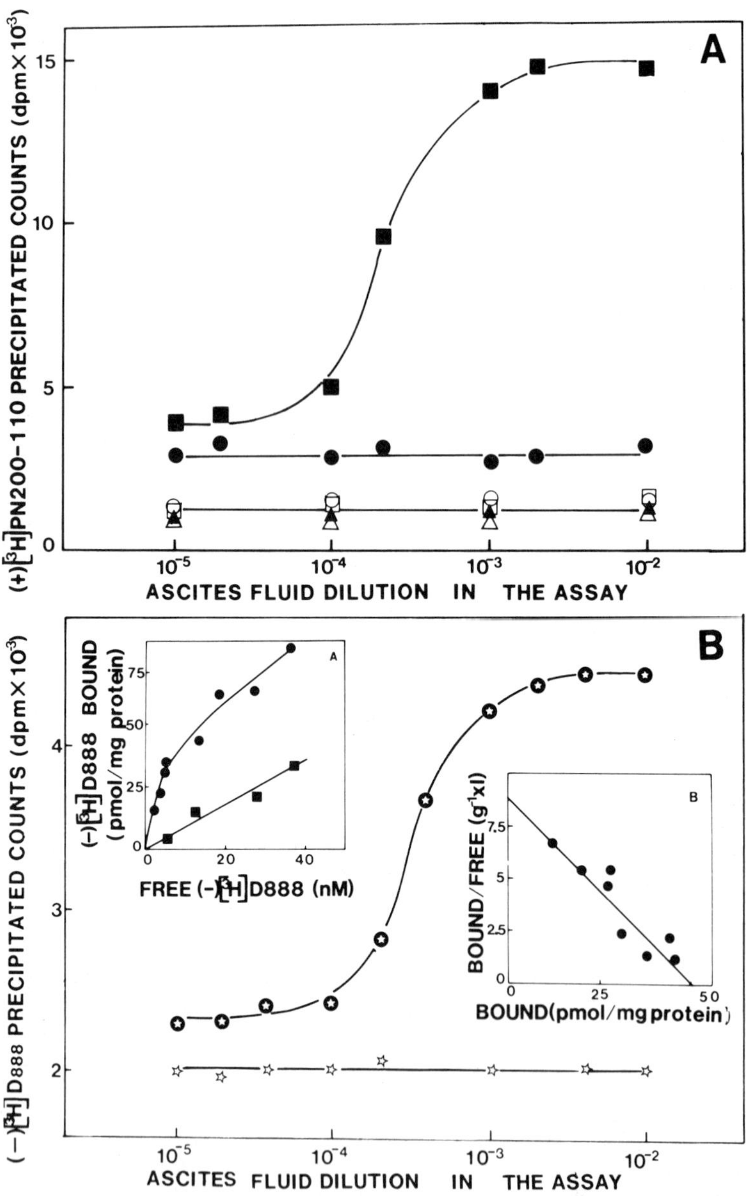

FIGURE 5. Immunoprecipitation of the (+)[^{3}H]PN 200-110 and (−)[^{3}H]D888 binding components by monoclonal antibody 3007 and equilibrium binding assay of (−)[^{3}H]D888 to T-tubule membranes in CHAPS solubilized form. Experiments were performed in duplicate. (**A**) The CHAPS-solubilized T-tubule membranes from rabbit skeletal muscle were incubated with (+)[^{3}H]PN 200-110 at increasing concentrations of ascites fluid. In this experiment, rabbit anti–mouse IgG antibodies were omitted. Immunoprecipitation with 3007 in the absence (filled squares) or in the presence (open squares) of 1 μM unlabeled (+)PN 200-110. Nonrelevant

labeling of such a polypeptide component by the anti-140 serum could be due to the fact that antigenic determinants are different in skeletal muscle and in cardiac and smooth muscle DHP receptors. It could also be due to an insufficient titer of the anti-140 serum used. This second explanation seems more likely since the titer of the anti-140 serum was lower than the titer of the anti-32 serum and since the amount of DHP receptors measured with (+)[^{3}H]-PN 200-110 in heart and in smooth muscle was considerably lower than in skeletal muscle, making these receptors more difficult to detect in these tissues. Attempts to obtain more potent anti-140 sera were unsuccessful.

FIGURE 4 shows that the same type of subunit structure exists for neuronal Ca^{2+} channels.[18] In conclusion, this work provides evidence that the DHP receptor, which presumably corresponds to the Ca^{2+} channel protein of skeletal, cardiac, and smooth muscle as well as of nerve cells, has a very similar subunit composition in all these tissues comprising a large polypeptide of about 140 kDa associated with a smaller polypeptide of 32–34 kDa by disulfide bridge(s). The small subunit could be the same polypeptide that was previously photolabeled with [^{3}H]nitrendipine in canine cardiac membranes.[15]

The series of antibodies described in this report can of course be very useful tools for future purifications of the nerve and smooth muscle Ca^{2+} channel proteins, for the analysis of the distribution of these channels, as previously done for Na^+ channels.[19] Immunofluorescence studies of brain sections have already indicated a distribution of the Ca^{2+} channel protein similar to that of 1,4-dihydropyridine-binding sites with (+)[^{3}H]PN 200-110 by autoradiographic techniques (TABLE 2).[18]

MONOCLONAL ANTIBODIES AGAINST THE DIHYDROPYRIDINE RECEPTOR

Monoclonal hybridoma cell lines secreting antibodies against the (+)PN 200-110 and the (−)desmethoxyverapamil-binding components of the voltage-dependent calcium channel from rabbit T-tubule membranes have been isolated.[20,21] The specificity of these monoclonal antibodies was established by their ability to coimmunoprecipitate (+)[^{3}H]PN 200-110 and (−)[^{3}H]desmethoxyverapamil receptors (FIGURE 5). Monoclonal antibodies described in this work cross-reacted with rat, mouse, chicken, and frog skeletal muscle Ca^{2+} channels, but not with crayfish muscle Ca^{2+} channels. Cross-reactivity was also detected with membranes prepared from rabbit heart, brain, and intestinal smooth muscle.

These antibodies were used in immunoprecipitation experiments with ^{125}I-labeled detergent (CHAPS and digitonin) solubilized membranes. They revealed a unique

ascites fluid in the absence (filled circles) or in the presence (open circles) of 1 μM (+)PN 200-110. Antibody 3007 without CHAPS-solubilized membranes in the absence (filled triangles) or in the presence (open triangles) of 1 μM (+)PN 200-110. (**B**) Inset A: T-tubule membranes at 20 μg/ml in 20 mM Hepes/NaOH buffer (pH 7.5 and 0°C) were incubated for 60 minutes (time sufficient to attain equilibrium) with increasing concentrations of (−)[^{3}H]D888 in the absence (circles) or in the presence (squares) of 1 μM (−)D888. Each sample was then CHAPS solubilized.[21] Bound (−)[^{3}H]D888 was separated from the free ligand by filtration (200 μl aliquots) through 2.8 ml Sephadex G-50 columns. Inset B: Scatchard plot for the specific (−)[^{3}H]D888 binding component. Main panel: T-tubule membranes from rabbit skeletal muscle labeled with (−)[^{3}H]D888 and CHAPS solubilized were incubated with increasing concentrations of ascites fluid.[21] Immunoprecipitation with 3007 in the absence (circled stars) or in the presence (stars) of 1 μM (−)D888.

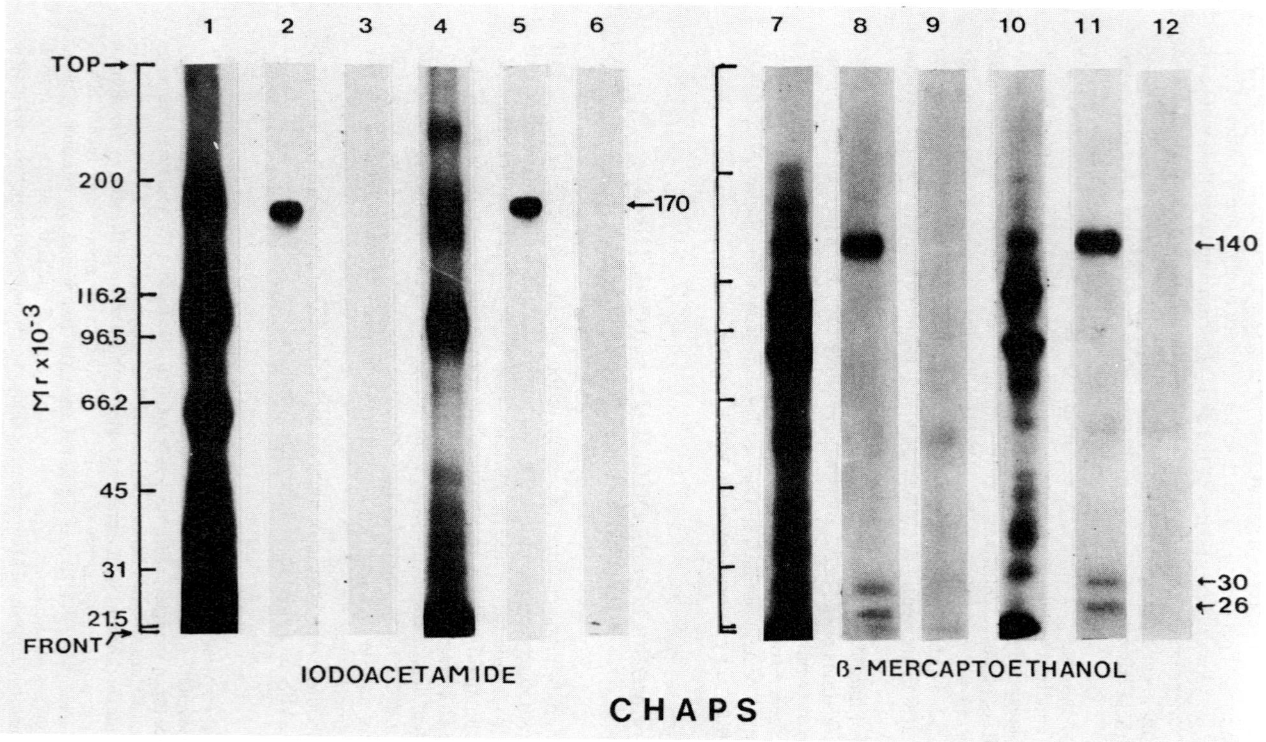

FIGURE 6. Immunoprecipitation by monoclonal antibody 3007 from the radioiodinated CHAPS-solubilized membranes and from the CHAPS-WGA extract of rabbit T-tubule membranes. These detergent extracts were iodinated and subjected to immunoprecipitation. Autoradiogram: SDS–polyacrylamide gel electrophoreses were performed in the presence of iodoacetamide (lanes 1–6) or 2-mercaptoethanol (lanes 7–12). Iodinated proteins from detergent-solubilized membranes (lanes 1 and 7; 10 μl aliquots from starting volume of 100 μl) or after immunoprecipitation by monoclonal antibody 3007 (lanes 2 and 8) and control mouse IgG (lanes 3 and 9). Iodinated proteins from WGA extract before (lanes 4 and 10) or after immunoprecipitation by monoclonal antibody 3007 (lanes 5 and 11) and control mouse IgG (lanes 6 and 12). Lanes 1, 4, 7, and 10 were exposed to the film for 5 hours; the other lanes were exposed for 24 hours. Molecular weight markers are presented at the left side of the figure.

immunoprecipitating component of 170 kDa under nonreducing conditions. After disulfide bridge reduction the CHAPS-solubilized (+)PN 200-110/(−)desmethoxy-verapamil binding component gave rise to a large peptide of 140 kDa and to smaller polypeptides of 30 kDa and 26 kDa (FIGURE 6) whereas the digitonin-solubilized receptor appeared with subunits of 170 kDa, 140 kDa, 30 kDa, and 26 kDa.

All these results taken together are interpreted as showing that both the 1,4-dihydropyridine and the phenylalkylamine receptors are part of a single polypeptide chain of 170 kDa.

PURIFICATION OF THE CARDIAC Ca^{2+} CHANNEL PROTEIN

The dihydropyridine-sensitive voltage-dependent Ca^{2+} channel from chick heart has now been purified.[20] It appears as a major component of 170 kDa linked by disulfide bridges to smaller polypeptides of 32–29 kDa. Both peptide maps of the 140 kDa peptide in cardiac and skeletal muscle preparations and studies with monoclonal antibodies suggest a high degree of homology for Ca^{2+} channels in the two tissues.

REGULATION OF Ca^{2+} CHANNEL ACTIVITY AND Ca^{2+} CHANNEL LEVEL BY ISOPROTERENOL AND cAMP

The effects of short-term stimulation of β-adrenergic receptors and elevations in intracellular cyclic adenosine monophosphate (cAMP) on nitrendipine-sensitive voltage-dependent Ca^{2+} channels of skeletal muscle cells *in vitro* have been studied using both the $^{45}Ca^{2+}$ flux technique and [^{3}H]nitrendipine binding experiments.[22] Isoproterenol increased the nitrendipine-sensitive $^{45}Ca^{2+}$ influx under depolarizing conditions. The effects of isoproterenol were additive to those of depolarization and were antagonized by alprenolol. Half-maximal inhibition of $^{45}Ca^{2+}$ influx induced both by depolarization and by isoproterenol occurred at a nitrendipine concentration of 1 nM. Treatments that resulted in an increased level of intracellular cAMP, such as treatment with 1-methyl 3-isobutylxanthine, theophylline, dibutyryl cAMP or 8-bromo cAMP also resulted in an activation of the nitrendipine-sensitive Ca^{2+} channel.

As for cardiac cells,[23] phosphorylation of the Ca^{2+} channel in skeletal muscle via a cAMP-dependent kinase increases the probability of finding the Ca^{2+} channel in the open form.

In contrast, long-term treatment of myotubes in culture with isoproterenol and other compounds that increased intracellular cAMP led to a very large increase in the number of nitrendipine receptors. This increase was accompanied by a 4- to 10-fold decrease in the affinity of the receptors for nitrendipine.[22] A similar increase has been observed in neuronal cells.[24]

Recent work from this laboratory[25] has shown that the major subunit of the Ca^{2+} channel (140–145 kDa) is phosphorylated both by cAMP and Ca^{2+}-calmodulin-dependent processes and that dephosphorylation occurs via calcineurin, a Ca^{2+}-calmodulin-dependent phosphatase.[25]

A NEW EMERGING PHARMACOLOGY FOR Ca^{2+} CHANNELS

[^{3}H]Fluspirilene, a neuroleptic molecule of the diphenylbutylpiperidine series with anxiolytic properties, binds to skeletal muscle transverse tubule membranes with a

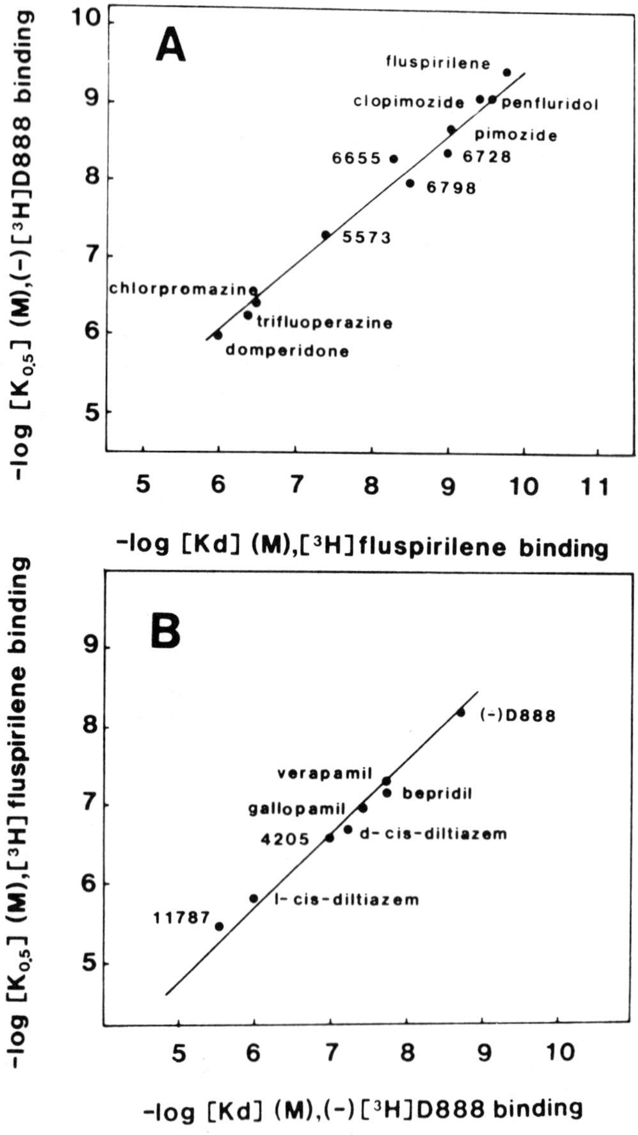

FIGURE 7. Correlation between $(-)[^3H]D888$ and $[^3H]$fluspirilene binding inhibition by neuroleptic or calcium antagonist drugs ($K_{0.5}$ is half-maximum inhibition concentrations, and K_D is equilibrium dissociation constant), $-\log[K_{0.5}]$ (for inhibition of $(-)[^3H]D888$ binding by neuroleptic drugs) was plotted versus $-\log[K_d]$ (inhibition of $[^3H]$fluspirilene binding). The plot has a slope of 0.87 and a correlation coefficient $r = 0.99$. (B) $-\log[K_{0.5}]$ for the inhibition of $[^3H]$fluspirilene binding by calcium channel inhibitors was plotted versus $-\log[K_d]$ (inhibition of $(-)[^3H]D888$ binding). The plot has a slope of 0.93 and a correlation coefficient $r = 1.0$.

high affinity corresponding to a dissociation constant $K_d = 0.11 \pm 0.04$ nM.[26] A 1:1 stoichiometry was found between [^{3}H]fluspirilene binding and the binding of (−)[^{3}H]desmethoxyverapamil, one of the most potent Ca^{2+} channel inhibitors. Ca^{2+} channel inhibitors such as desmethoxyverapamil, verapamil, gallopamil, bepridil, or diltiazem antagonize [^{3}H]fluspirilene binding besides antagonizing [^{3}H]desmethoxyverapamil binding. Neuroleptics, especially those of the diphenylbutylpiperidine family, antagonize (−)[^{3}H]desmethoxyverapamil binding besides antagonizing [^{3}H]fluspirilene binding. There is an excellent correlation between affinities found from [^{3}H]fluspirilene and from (−)[^{3}H]desmethoxyverapamil binding experiments (FIGURE 7).

Analysis of the properties of these cross-inhibitions indicates that [^{3}H]fluspirilene binds to a site that is not the same as the site for phenylalkylamine derivatives (gallopamil, verapamil, diltiazem, bepridil).

Voltage-clamp experiments have shown that fluspirilene is a very efficient inhibitor of the voltage-dependent Ca^{2+} channel with a half-maximum effect near 0.1–0.2 nM and a nearly complete blocking effect at a concentration of 1 nM. Fluspirilene blockade has very little voltage dependence.[26]

A PATHOLOGY INVOLVING THE Ca^{2+} CHANNEL

Binding experiments using tritiated dihydropyridines have shown that receptors for this drug were lacking in a mouse skeletal muscle disease.[27] The mdg/mdg mouse has muscles that are unable to contract. This lack of contraction of course prevents birth. Muscles of mdg/mdg embryos present a lack of functional Ca^{2+} channels.[28,29] This absence of Ca^{2+} channels is only observed in muscle. Ca^{2+} channels are present on both nerve and cardiac cells. The absence of Ca^{2+} channels in muscle may be linked to the fact that well-formed triads are not observed in mdg/mdg muscle.

ACKNOWLEDGMENTS

We wish to thank Dr. Busch for the gift of (+)bepridil, Dr. Schramm from Bayer AG (FRG) for CGP 28932, and Dr. Hoffmeister and Dr. Garthoff from Bayer AG (FRG) for Bay K8644 and dihydropyridines. We also thank Bayer Pharma (France) for nitrendipine, Dr. Hollmann and Dr. Traut from Knoll AG (FRG) for (−)[^{3}H]desmethoxyverapamil, and CERM (Riom, France) and CEA (France) for [^{3}H]bepridil. Thanks are due to M. T. Ravier, M. Valetti, and C. Roulinat-Bettelheim for expert technical assistance.

REFERENCES

1. JANIS, R. A. & D. J. TRIGGLE. 1984. 1,4-Dihydropyridine Ca^{2+} channel antagonists and activators: a comparison of binding characteristics with pharmacology. Drug Dev. Res. **4:** 257–274.
2. FLECKENSTEIN, R. 1977. Specific pharmacology of calcium in myocardium, cardiac pace-maker and vascular smooth muscle. Annu. Rev. Pharmacol. Toxicol. **17:** 149–166.
3. FOSSET, M., E. JAIMOVICH, E. DELPONT & M. LAZDUNSKI. 1983. [^{3}H]nitrendipine receptors in skeletal muscles. Properties and preferential localization in transverse tubules. J. Biol. Chem. **258:** 6086–6092.
4. POTREAU, D. & G. RAYMOND. 1980. Calcium-dependent electrical activity and contraction of voltage-clamped frog single muscle fibers. J. Physiol. **307:** 9–22.

5. ALMERS, W., R. FINK & P. T. PALADE. 1981. Calcium depletion in frog muscle tubules: the decline of calcium current under maintained depolarization. J. Physiol. **312:** 177–207.
6. COGNARD C., M. LAZDUNSKI & G. ROMEY. 1986. Different types of Ca^{2+} channels in mammalian skeletal muscle cells in culture. Proc. Nat. Acad. Sci. USA **83:** 517–521.
7. COGNARD C., G. ROMEY, J. P. GALIZZI, M. FOSSET & M. LAZDUNSKI. 1986. Dihydropyridine-sensitive Ca^{2+} channels in mammalian skeletal muscle cells in culture: electrophysiological properties and interactions with Ca^{2+}-channels activator (Bay K8644) and inhibitor (PN 200-110). Proc. Nat. Acad. Sci. USA **83:** 1518–1522.
8. BEAN, B. P. 1984. Nitrendipine block of cardiac channels: high affinity binding to the inactivated state. Proc. Nat. Acad. Sci. USA **81:** 6388–6392.
9. TRIGGLE, D. J. & R. A. JANIS. 1984. Calcium channel antagonists: New perspectives from the radioligand binding assay. *In* Modern Methods in Pharmacology **2:** 1–28. Alan R. Liss, Inc. New York, NY
10. GALIZZI, J. P., M. BORSOTTO, J. BARHANIN, M. FOSSET & M. LAZDUNSKI. 1986. Characterization and photoaffinity labelling of receptor sites for the Ca^{2+} channel inhibitors *d-cis*-diltiazem, (±)bepridil, desmethoxyverapamil and (+)PN 200-110 in skeletal muscle transverse tubule membranes. J. Biol. Chem. **261:** 1393–1397.
11. GALIZZI, J. P., M. FOSSET & M. LAZDUNSKI. 1985. Characterization of the Ca^{2+} coordination site regulating binding of Ca^{2+} channel inhibitors *d-cis*-diltiazem (±)bepridil and (−)desmethoxyverapamil to their receptor site in skeletal muscle transverse tubule membranes. Biochem. Biophys. Res. Commun. **132:** 49–55.
12. BORSOTTO, M., R. I. NORMAN, M. FOSSET & M. LAZDUNSKI. 1984. Solubilization of the nitrendipine receptor from skeletal muscle transverse tubule membranes. Interactions with specific inhibitors of the voltage-dependent Ca^{2+} channel. Eur. J. Biochem. **142:** 449–455.
13. BORSOTTO, M., J. BARHANIN, R. I. NORMAN & M. LAZDUNSKI. 1984. Purification of the dihydropyridine receptor of the voltage-dependent Ca^{2+} channel from skeletal muscle transverse tubules using (+)[^{3}H]PN 200-110. Biochem. Biophys. Res. Commun. **122:** 1357–1366.
14. FERRY, D. R., M. ROMBUSCH, A. GOLL & H. GLOSSMANN. 1984. Photoaffinity labelling of Ca^{2+} channels with [^{3}H]azidopine. FEBS Lett. **169:** 112–118.
15. CAMPBELL, K. P., G. M. LIPSHUTZ & G. M. DENNEY. 1984. Direct photoaffinity labelling of the high affinity nitrendipine-binding site in subcellular membrane fractions isolated from canine myocardium. J. Biol. Chem. **259:** 5384–5387.
16. BARHANIN, J., T. COPPOLA, A. SCHMID, M. BORSOTTO & M. LAZDUNSKI. 1987. The calcium channel antagonists receptor from rabbit skeletal muscle. Reconstitution after purification and subunit characterization. Eur. J. Biochem. **164:** 525–531.
17. BORSOTTO, M., J. BARHANIN, M. FOSSET & M. LAZDUNSKI. 1985. The 1,4-dihydropyridine receptor associated with the skeletal muscle voltage-dependent Ca^{2+} channel: purification and subunit composition. J. Biol. Chem. **260:** 14255–14263.
18. SCHMID, A., J. BARHANIN, C. MOURRE, T. COPPOLA, M. BORSOTTO & M. LAZDUNSKI. 1987. Antibodies reveal the cytolocalization and subunit structure of the 1,4 dihydropyridine component of the neuronal Ca^{2+} channel. Biochem. Biophys. Res. Commun. **139:** 996–1002.
19. ELLISMAN, M. H. & S. R. LEVINSON. 1982. Immunocytochemical localization of sodium channel distributions in the excitable membranes of *Electrophorus electricus*. Proc. Nat. Acad. Sci. USA **79:** 6707–6711.
20. COOPER, C. L., S. VANDAELE, J. BARHANIN, M. FOSSET, M. LAZDUNSKI & M. M. HOSEY. 1987. Purification and characterization of the dihydropyridine-sensitive voltage-dependent Ca^{2+} channel from cardiac tissue. J. Biol. Chem. **262:** 509–512.
21. VANDAELE, S., M. FOSSET, J. P. GALIZZI & M. LAZDUNSKI. 1987. Monoclonal antibodies that co-immunoprecipitate the 1,4-dihydropyridine and phenylalkylamine binding components associated with the voltage-dependent Ca^{2+} channel from skeletal muscle. Biochemistry **26:** 5–9.
22. SCHMID, A., J. F. RENAUD & M. LAZDUNSKI. 1985. Short-term and long-term effects of β-adrenergic effectors and cyclic AMP of nitrendipine-sensitive voltage-dependent Ca^{2+} channels of skeletal muscle. J. Biol. Chem. **260:** 13041–13046.

23. REUTER, H. 1983. Calcium channel modulation by neurotransmitters, enzymes and drugs. Nature **301:** 569–574.
24. NIRENBERG, M., S. WILSON, H. HIGASHIDA, A. ROTTER, K. KRUEGER, N. BASIS, R. RAY, S. KENINER & M. ADLER. 1983. Modulation of synapse formation by cyclic adenosine monophosphate. Science **222:** 794–799.
25. HOSEY, M., M. BORSOTTO & M. LAZDUNSKI. 1986. Phosphorylation and dephosphorylation of the major component of the voltage-dependent Ca^{2+} channel in skeletal muscle membranes by cyclic AMP and Ca^{2+}-dependent processes. Proc. Nat. Acad. Sci. USA **83:** 3733–3737.
26. GALIZZI, J. P., M. FOSSET, G. ROMEY, P. LADURON & M. LAZDUNSKI. 1986. Neuroleptics of the diphenylbutylpiperidine series are potent calcium channel inhibitors. Proc. Nat. Acad. Sci. USA **83:** 7513–7517.
27. PINCON-RAYMOND, M., F. RIEGER, M. FOSSET & M. LAZDUNSKI. 1985. Abnormal transverse tubule system and abnormal amount of receptors for Ca^{2+} channel inhibitors of the dihydropyridine family in skeletal muscle from mice with embryonic muscular dysgenesis. Dev. Biol. **112:** 458–466.
28. ROMEY, G., F. RIEGER, J. F. RENAUD, M. PINCON-RAYMOND & M. LAZDUNSKI. 1986. The electrophysiology expression of Ca^{2+} channels and of apamin sensitive Ca^{2+} activated K^+ channels is abolished in skeletal muscle cells from mice with muscular dysgenesis. Biochem. Biophys. Res. Commun. **136:** 935–940.
29. BEAM, K. G., C. M. KNUDSON & J. A. POWELL. 1986. A lethal mutation in mice eliminates the slow calcium current in skeletal muscle cells. Nature **320:** 168–170.

Purification and Reconstitution of Calcium Channel Drug-Receptor Sites[a]

HARTMUT GLOSSMANN,[b] JÖRG STRIESSNIG,[b] LIN HYMEL,[c] AND HANSGEORG SCHINDLER[c]

[b]*Institute of Biochemical Pharmacology*
University of Innsbruck
Peter Mayr-Strasse 1
A-6020 Innsbruck, Austria

[c]*Institute of Biophysics*
University of Linz
Altenbergerstrasse 69
A-4040 Linz, Austria

INTRODUCTION

The voltage-dependent L-type calcium channel (CC) is a transmembrane structure controlling inflow of calcium into excitable cells. The channel is involved in the regulation of numerous cell functions. CCs also exist in vertebrate skeletal muscle transverse-tubule (T-tubule) membranes.[1] The functional role in this tissue is yet unclear,[2] although the channel is believed to be important for excitation-contraction coupling.[3] Because of the high density of receptor sites[4] for the different chemical classes of CC active drugs, skeletal muscle became the prime target for the biochemical characterization and purification of CCs in the past few years.[5–9]

Three major criteria help to identify purified polypeptides as L-type CC components. First, conditions have to be established that allow reversible ligand binding with the appropriate CC-typical pharmacological profile throughout the entire purification procedure. Second, to unequivocally identify which of the isolated polypeptides carries the drug receptor(s) (i.e., must be by definition an L-type channel component), highly specific irreversible labels (e.g., photoaffinity labels) are required. Third, functional reconstitution of the purified fractions must demonstrate that not only silent receptor sites but functional channel proteins are isolated.

Earlier experiments established the basic conditions for effective solubilization, purification, and reversible labeling of skeletal muscle L-type CCs.[5] Here we report the use of potent radioligands for the 1,4 dihydropyridine (DHP) {(+)-[^{3}H]PN200-100} and phenylalkylamine (PA) drug receptor {(−)-[^{3}H]desmethoxyverapamil} together with novel arylazido photoaffinity ligands (−)-[^{3}H]azidopine and [*N*-methyl-^{3}H]LU49888 {(−)-5-[(3-azidophenethyl)[*N*-methyl-^{3}H]methylamino]-2-(3,4,5-trimethoxyphenyl)-2-isopropylvaleronitrile} to purify the CC and characterize the receptor-carrying subunit. Reconstitution experiments with the purified preparation suggest that a channel with most of the properties of a L-type CC has been purified.

[a]This work was supported by Österreichische Nationalbank, Fonds zur Förderung der wissenschaftlichen Forschung und Deutsche Forschungsgemeinschaft.

MATERIALS AND METHODS

Purification and Binding Assays

Sources of chemicals are given in References 9 and 10. Routine binding experiments for membrane-bound, solubilized, and purified receptors were carried out as described.[10] Digitonin (0.02–0.4%) was present in assays with the purified fractions. Purification of the CC (135-fold, measured by reversible 1,4 DHP binding) from T-tubulus membranes from guinea pig skeletal muscle was carried out as described.[9]

Photoaffinity Labeling Experiments

For photoaffinity labeling experiments with the enantiomers of [^{3}H]azidopine, 6.5–8 nM ligand was incubated in the absence or presence (to define nonspecific binding or incorporation, respectively) of 1 (or 3) μM (+)-PN200-110 with 3–4 pmol of solubilized, wheat germ agglutinin (WGA) sepharose eluted or purified CC for 45 minutes in the dark. Aliquots (50 μl) of the incubation mixture were removed to determine reversible binding. The incubation mixture was irradiated for 3 minutes with UV light (Philips 38W/TL UV lamp). Samples were lyophilized, resuspended in electrophoresis sample buffer containing 10 mM *N*-ethylmaleimide (alkylating conditions) or 10 mM dithiothreitol (reducing conditions), and separated on 5–15% gradient sodium dodecyl sulfate (SDS) gels. Gels were either silver stained, cut into 2 mm slices, and counted for radioactivity or processed for autoradiography as described.[9]

Photoaffinity labeling of the PA receptor with [*N*-methyl-^{3}H]LU49888 was carried out as described for [^{3}H]azidopine, but 3 μM (−)-desmethoxyverapamil was used to define nonspecific binding or incorporation, respectively.

Binding data were fitted by nonlinear methods.[9] Results are given as mean ± standard deviation (SD) from at least three experiments.

Reconstitution

Purified channel preparations were reconstituted using the fast dilution procedure.[11] Briefly, 10–50 μl were rapidly injected into 20 ml of a suspension of crude, nonvesicular soybean phospholipids (approximately 10 μg/ml in a buffer usually containing 110 mM NaCl and 10 mM HEPES-Tris, pH 7.4), which was immediately added to a 1 liter round-bottomed flask containing lipids dried to a thin film from hexane. The lipid in the flask consisted of 18 mg acetone-washed soybean phospholipids plus 3 mg cholesterol. Vesicles containing the reconstituted channels were formed by gentle mixing using several small (2 mm) glass beads. These vesicles, containing less than one 1,4 DHP receptor binding site per 10 vesicles, were freed from remaining detergent by passing them through a 0.25 ml column of Extracti-Gel D (Pierce). Vesicle-derived planar bilayers were formed by allowing these vesicles to form monolayers at the surface of the solution, which were then combined to bilayers in a 100 or 160 μm hole in a teflon septum.[12] Protein-containing vesicles were diluted with protein-free vesicles to adjust the number of channels incorporated into the planar bilayer. Typically, about 25 1,4 DHP binding sites (assumed to be functional channel molecules) were present, only on the *cis* side of the bilayer. The voltage source was connected to the *cis* side via an Ag/AgCl electrode and a current-voltage converter to the *trans* side. The output signal was filtered at 3 kHz and recorded on a PCM video cassette recorder modified to accept DC signals. Results were further filtered upon playback into a B-Scope computer system (Med-Natic, München, BRD) where they were analyzed and plotted.

RESULTS

Reversible Labeling of the Purified CC-Linked Drug Receptors

To purify the 1,4 DHP and PA receptor a rapid two-step procedure was employed.[9] Four major polypeptides comigrated with both 1,4 DHP and PA drug receptor activities on sucrose gradients with apparent molecular masses (M_r) of 165 kDa, 155 kDa, 65 kDa, and 32 kDa as revealed by nonreducing SDS–polyacrylamide gel electrophoresis (PAGE). The 165 kDa band migrated with an apparent M_r of 135 kDa under reducing conditions of SDS-PAGE (see FIGURE 2c). The potent 1,4 DHP (+)-[^{3}H]PN200-110 was routinely used to follow purification by postlabeling.[9,10] Dissociation constants (K_d) and maximal binding capacities (B_{max}) were determined after each purification step and used to calculate the purification factors. Thus, indirect calculation of purification factors and receptor recoveries as was described for prelabeled receptors[6,13] was thereby avoided.

The affinity for (+)-[^{3}H]PN200-110 was unaffected upon solubilization (K_d = 0.7 ± 0.02 nM). However, after a 15-fold purification of the CC on WGA-sepharose, the dissociation constant decreased about 3- to 4-fold (K_d = 2.7 ± 1.0 nM). D-CIS Diltiazem, which is a positive heterotropic allosteric regulator of 1,4 DHP binding in several tissues,[14] had only small effects on (+)-[^{3}H]PN200-110 binding to membrane-bound or solubilized channels but dramatically potentiated (+)-[^{3}H]PN200-110 binding to the WGA-sepharose purified material mainly by increasing the B_{max} (from 45 ± 11 to 137 ± 25 pmol per mg of protein. The K_d was almost unaffected (2.3 ± 0.2 nM). Further purification leads to a final specific activity of 1311 ± 194 pmol per mg of protein (K_d = 4.1 ± 1.7 nM) in the presence of *d-cis*-diltiazem, indicating at least 135-fold purification from the solubilized starting material. Similar results were obtained when (−)-[^{3}H]azidopine was used to follow purification. In the final preparation this ligand reversibly labeled 970 ± 181 pmol per mg of protein (K_d = 2.1 ± 1.6 nM) in the presence of *d-cis*-diltiazem.

PAs bind with lower affinity to membrane-bound CCs than do 1,4 DHPs.[14]

TABLE 1. Properties of (−)-[^{3}H]Azidopine and [N-Methyl-^{3}H]LU49888

	(−)-[^{3}H]Azidopine	[*N*-Methyl-^{3}H]LU49888
Specific activity (Ci/mmol)	>45	>75
Stability in aqueous buffers	good	good
Bindable radioactivity (%)	>90	>65
Dissociation constants (nM) (guinea pig membranes)		
Skeletal muscle	0.70 ± 1.4	2.0 ± 0.4
Hippocampus	0.11 ± 0.02	1.3 ± 0.1
Heart	0.03 ± 0.01	ND[a]
Irreversible labeling (%)		
Skeletal muscle membranes	>0.8	>0.2
Purified channel	>10	>0.8

[a]ND is not determined.

TABLE 2. Interaction of (−)-[^{3}H]Azidopine and [*N*-Methyl-^{3}H]LU49888 Reversibly Labeled Drug Receptors with Calcium Channel Active Drugs[a]

	Membrane-Bound Channel		Purified Channel	
Label/Drug	K_i(*) or IC_{50} (nM)	Maximum Inhibition or Stimulation (%)	K_i(*) or IC_{50} (nM)	Maximum Inhibition or Stimulation (%)
(−)-[^{3}H]Azidopine				
(−)-Azidopine	0.99 ± 0.1*	100	3.6 ± 0.6*	100
(+)-Azidopine	9.35 ± 1.9*	100	59.6 ± 14.8*	100
(+)-PN200-110	0.80 ± 0.2*	100	7.5 ± 4.4*	100
(−)-PN200-100	164.80 ± 33.3*	100	812 ± 261*	100
(−)-D888	ND		126 ± 65	163+
(+)-D888	ND		6600 ± 2200	94
d-cis-Diltiazem	NE at 25°C		3470 ± 940	214+
l-cis-Diltiazem	NE at 25°C		>10000	98
[*N*-Methyl-^{3}H]LU49888				
(±)-LU47781	8.18 ± 2.6*	100	113.3 ± 48.1	100
(−)-D888	5.7 ± 1.0*	100	40.1 ± 12.5	100
(+)-D888	24.4 ± 3.2*	100	ND	—
(±)-D619	5600.2 ± 610*	100	44000 ± 10780	100
d-cis-Diltiazem	163.6 ± 27.5	100	>3000	—
l-cis-Diltiazem	9140 ± 120	100	>3000	—
(+)-PN200-110	1.4 ± 0.2	46	21 ± 5	238+
(−)-PN200-110	489 ± 105	100	>10000	—

[a]Results are means ± SD from at least three experiments. Binding inhibition is defined as 100 × (1–B/B_0), and binding stimulation (+) as 100 × (B/B_0). B and B_0 are specific binding in the presence and absence of added drug, respectively. K_i values are given in case of competitive inhibition as indicated (*); ND, not determined; NE, no effect; D888, desmethoxyverapamil. LU 47781 is the racemic compound, LU 4988 the (−)- (S)-enantiomer. See also References 9 and 16 for experimental details.

[*N*-methyl-^{3}H]LU49888 is a new arylazido PA with reversible binding properties very similar to (−)-[^{3}H]desmethoxyverapamil in skeletal muscle T-tubule membranes (K_d = 2.0 ± 0.5 nM; B_{max} = 17.0 ± 0.9 pmol per mg of protein). Upon purification the decrease of affinity for both PA ligands is more pronounced than for 1,4 DHPs. Even in the presence of (+)-PN200-110, which is a positive heterotropic allosteric regulator of (−)-[^{3}H]desmethoxyverapamil binding to the purified CC [(+)-PN200-110 and other antagonistic DHPs decrease the K_d and increase the B_{max}, see Reference 10], a 20-fold lower affinity is measured for this ligand in the purified channel preparation (K_d = 48 ± 11 nM). In accordance, the K_d for [*N*-methyl-^{3}H]LU49888 increases to 62 ± 11 nM (B_{max} = 694 ± 235 pmol per mg of protein) measured in the absence of allosteric effectors. In contrast to 1,4 DHP binding, this decrease in affinity occurs upon solubilization (not shown) and is maintained throughout purification.

Photoaffinity Labeling of the Calcium-Channel-Linked Drug-Receptor Sites

(−)-[^{3}H]Azidopine and [*N*-methyl-^{3}H]LU49888 are two arylazido compounds, highly suitable for photoaffinity labeling of membrane-bound as well as purified 1,4 DHP and PA receptors, respectively.[15,16] Their properties are outlined in TABLE 1. The reversible interaction of both ligands with the particulate and purified channel is stereospecifically modulated by the three main chemical classes of CC active drugs (summarized in TABLE 2) with a CC typical profile. FIGURE 1 shows the autoradiographs of photolabeling experiments with (−)-[^{3}H]azidopine carried out for each step of the purification procedure. Control experiments were performed with the 10- to 15-fold less potent (see TABLE 1) tritiated (+)-enantiomer. Three polypeptides were labeled in the solubilized starting material with apparent molecular masses of 155 kDa, 100 kDa, and 45 kDa. Only the 155 kDa band was specifically labeled by both enantiomers, the (−)-enantiomer being more potent according to its reversible binding activity (see also legend to FIGURE 1). Nonspecific incorporation (which was identical for both enantiomers) occurred into the 100 and 45 kDa band. In 1 out of 10

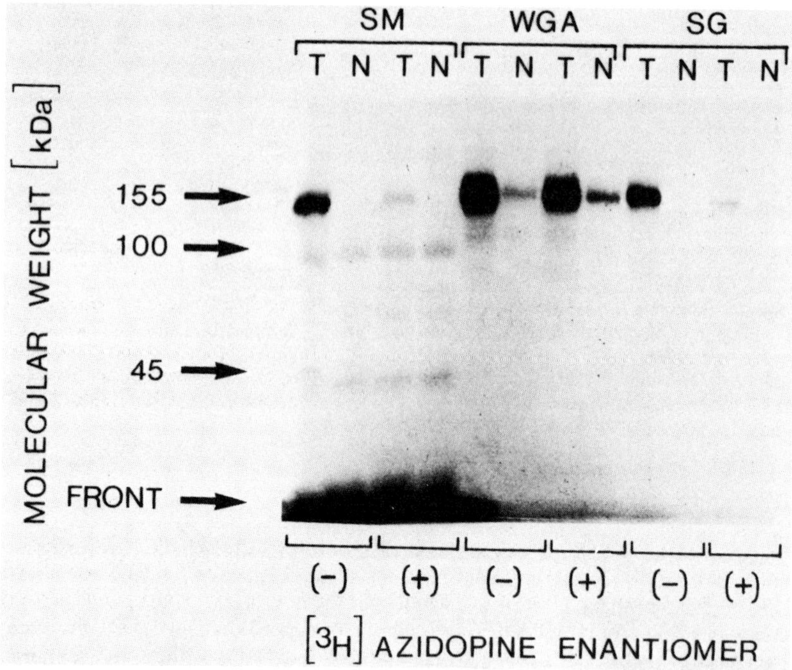

FIGURE 1. Photoaffinity labeling of the 1,4 DHP receptor with the tritiated enantiomers of [^{3}H]azidopine throughout channel purification: 7.2 nM of (+)- and (−)-[^{3}H]azidopine were incubated in parallel with solubilized starting material (SM, 131 μg of protein), WGA-purified receptor (WGA, 23.8 μg), or sucrose-gradient-purified receptor (SG, 1.5 μg) in the absence (total incorporation, T) or presence (nonspecific incorporation, N) of 3 μM (+)-PN200-110. Photoaffinity labeling and autoradiography were as described in Materials and Methods. The amount of label recovered in the 155 kDa region (determined from sliced gels run in parallel) was (−)-[^{3}H]azidopine: 94 fmol (SM), 282 fmol (WGA), 129 fmol (SG); (+)-[^{3}H]azidopine: 20 fmol (SM), 134 fmol (WGA), 8 fmol (SG).

experiments a component with an M_r slightly higher than the 45 kDa band was labeled in a specific manner which contained less than 10% of the total radioactivity in the 155 kDa band (see FIGURE 1). In WGA-sepharose-purified and the highly purified fractions, only a 155 kDa polypeptide was preferentially labeled by (−)-[^{3}H]azidopine. The increase in specific activity could also be determined by calculating the pmoles of incorporated (−)-[^{3}H]azidopine for each purification step and was 120-fold

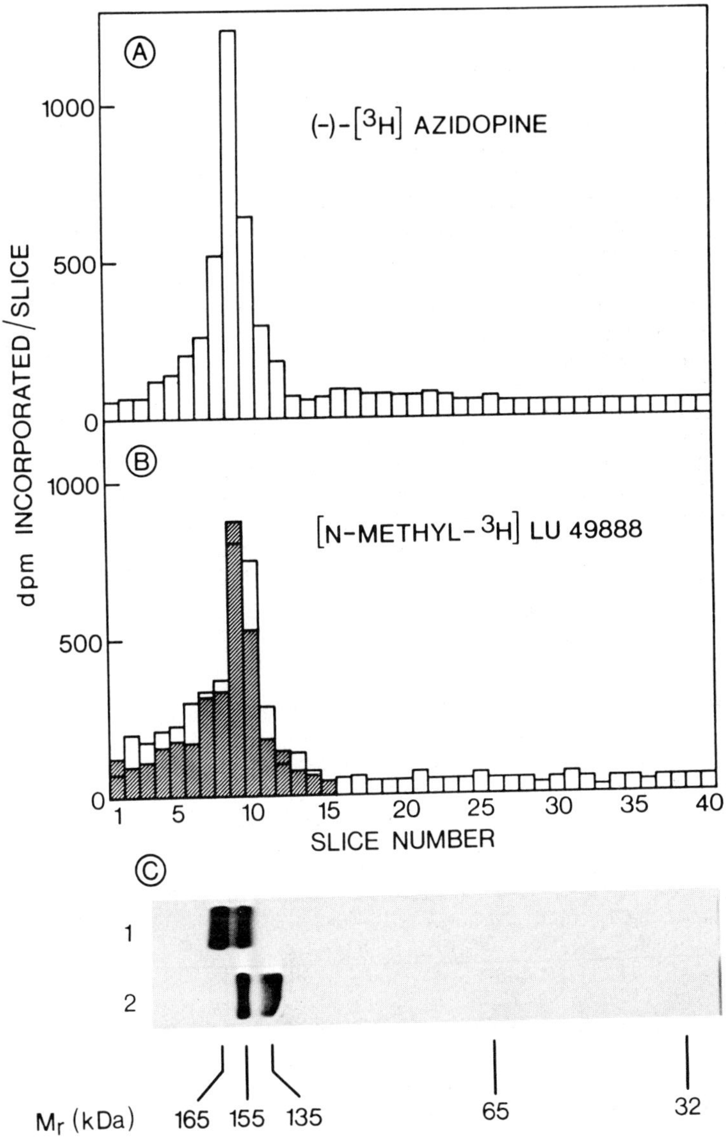

FIGURE 2. Colocalization of the 1,4 DHP and PA receptor on the 155 kDa polypeptide (alpha$_1$-subunit). A and B: 0.9 or 2.9 μg of protein from purified fractions were incubated with 4.7 nM of (−)-[^{3}H]azidopine or 15.1 nM [*N*-methyl-^{3}H]LU49888, respectively, and photoaffinity labeled as described. Gels were cut and slices counted for radioactivity. As nonspecific labeling was less than 100 dpm in all slices for both ligands, only total labeling is shown. Open columns: separation under nonreducing conditions (10 mM *N*-ethylmaleimide) of SDS-PAGE. Hatched columns: reducing conditions (10 mM dithiothreitol). C. Silver stain of the same gels as in B prior to gel slicing. Lane 1, nonreducing conditions; lane 2, reducing conditions. The 65 kDa and 32 kDa band comprise less than 15% of the total silver-stain intensity and are only weakly stained in the gels shown.

(solubilized starting material, 0.7; WGA purified, 12; sucrose gradient purified, 86 pmol per mg of protein): 11 ± 1.5% of the reversibly bound (−)-[^{3}H]azidopine was recovered in the 155 kDa band.

To prove or disprove the existence of the PA receptor on the same polypeptide, photoaffinity labeling experiments were carried out with [*N*-methyl-^{3}H]LU49888 in the purified fractions: 0.8% of the reversibly bound ligand were specifically incorporated into a 155 kDa polypeptide. No other band was labeled irreversibly. In FIGURE 2 the specific labeling profile with (−)-[^{3}H]azidopine or [*N*-methyl-^{3}H]LU49888 and the silver-staining pattern are presented side by side. After staining the lanes were photographed, cut into 2 mm slices, and counted for radioactivity. The maximum of specific (−)-[^{3}H]azidopine and [*N*-methyl-^{3}H]LU49888 incorporation migrates with the 155 kDa band under nonreducing conditions. The 155 kDa band can thus be directly identified as carrying the 1,4 DHP and the PA receptor. Recent immunological studies suggested that localization of the 1,4 DHP receptor on a 140 kDa polypeptide covalently linked to a 30 kDa polypeptide via disulfide bonds. The receptor-carrying subunit was claimed to decrease its molecular weight upon reduction by 30,000 mass units.[17,18] The molecular mass of our 165 kDa band also decreases by about 30 kDa. We next investigated the effects of reduction on the mobility of the photoaffinity labeled 155 kDa polypeptide. As shown in FIGURE 2B reduction neither shifts the peak of maximal labeling associated with the 155 kDa band nor alters the shape of the radioactivity peak. Thus, we have no evidence that the PA-receptor-carrying subunit is linked by disulfide bonds to a 30 kDa polypeptide.

Functional Reconstitution

L-Type CC Activity of Purified, Reconstituted Channels

After reconstitution by the fast dilution method and incorporation into solvent-free bilayers, the purified channels demonstrated activity consistent with the well-known properties of muscle L-type CCs.[19] Cation-selective single-channel events were observed in NaCl, $BaCl_2$, and $CaCl_2$ solutions, while no anion-selective events were detected using gradients of these salts across the membrane. Higher values were typically observed for the Na^+ conductance, which could be completely inhibited by addition of $BaCl_2$ (500 μM) or $CaCl_2$ (100 μM). The channels showed a high selectivity of Ba^{2+} over Na^+ ($P_{Ba}/P_{Na} = 294$) as revealed in FIGURE 3a by a reversal potential of −88 mV for a mixed Ba^{2+}-Na^+ solution (*cis*, 100 mM $BaCl_2$, 100 mM NaCl: *trans*, 110 mM NaCl). In addition, all observed conductances could be potently inhibited by micromolar concentrations of $CdCl_2$ (cf. FIGURE 3b).

Conductance Levels of Reconstituted CCs

The most remarkable characteristic of "single-channel" events of our reconstituted CCs is their heterogeneity of conductance levels. The various conductance states can be assigned to a mixture of differently sized channel associates. Since the fast dilution method enabled us to trap single proteins in separate vesicles, we were able to follow the association of channel proteins in the planar bilayer. This association was manifested as an increase in mean channel conductance with time. When only a small number of proteins were incorporated into the bilayer (25 binding sites/100 μm aperture), only channels of small conductance (3.7 pS in 110 mM NaCl) were seen for the first 5–10 minutes (FIGURE 3c). These channels were distinguishable from larger

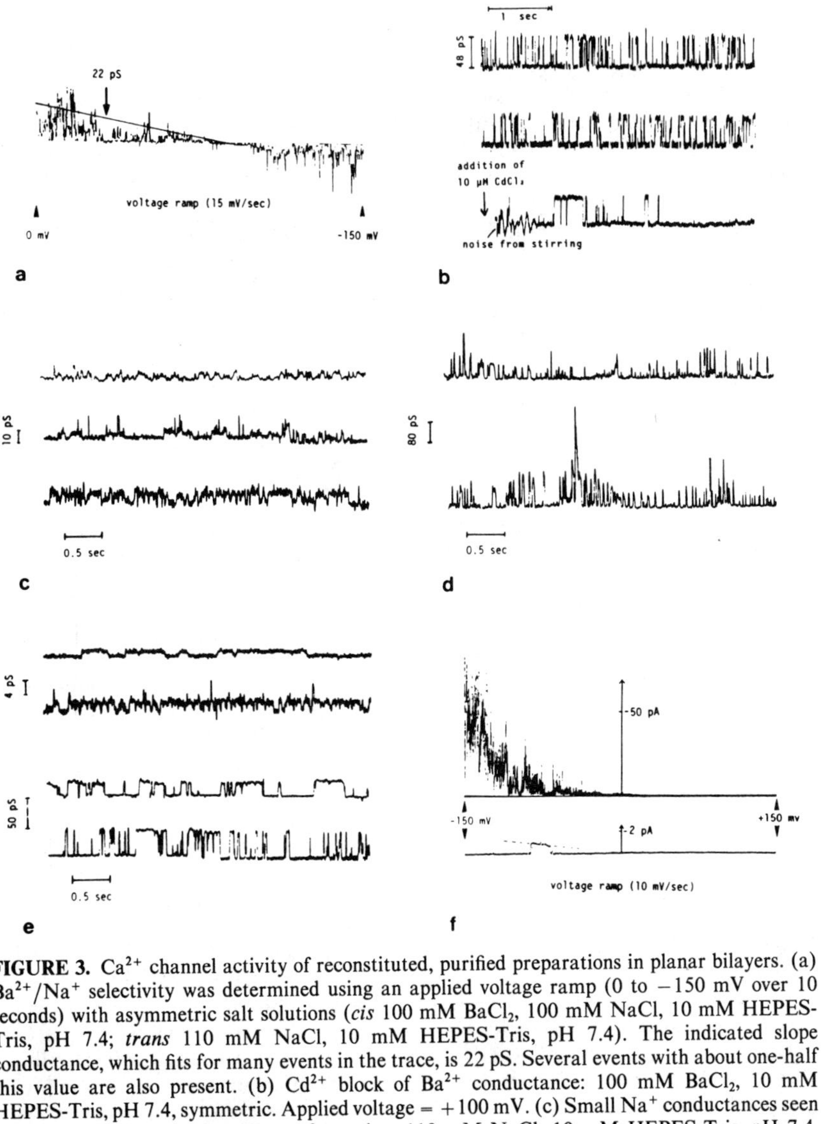

FIGURE 3. Ca^{2+} channel activity of reconstituted, purified preparations in planar bilayers. (a) Ba^{2+}/Na^{+} selectivity was determined using an applied voltage ramp (0 to −150 mV over 10 seconds) with asymmetric salt solutions (*cis* 100 mM $BaCl_2$, 100 mM NaCl, 10 mM HEPES-Tris, pH 7.4; *trans* 110 mM NaCl, 10 mM HEPES-Tris, pH 7.4). The indicated slope conductance, which fits for many events in the trace, is 22 pS. Several events with about one-half this value are also present. (b) Cd^{2+} block of Ba^{2+} conductance: 100 mM $BaCl_2$, 10 mM HEPES-Tris, pH 7.4, symmetric. Applied voltage = +100 mV. (c) Small Na^{+} conductances seen in the first 5 minutes after bilayer formation: 110 mM NaCl, 10 mM HEPES-Tris, pH 7.4, symmetric. Applied voltage = +50 mV: 25 channels per bilayer (*cis* side only). (d) Larger Na^{+} conductance levels seen after 10 minutes (same conductions as c). (e) Ba^{2+} conductance levels. Solutions as in b, +100 mV. (f) Voltage dependence of macroscopic currents (top, up to 500 pS) and small associates (bottom, 17 pS) in 110 mM NaCl, 10 mM HEPES, pH 7.4.

channels seen later by virtue of their nearly continuous burst activity (high open state probability) and their completely symmetrical and linear voltage dependence. After some 10 minutes, larger conductances were inevitably observed, often mixed with smaller ones (FIGURE 3d). Single openings of channels as large as 70 pS and more were observed in 110 mM NaCl. When much higher amounts of protein were incorporated into the planar bilayer (e.g., more than 100 binding sites/100 μm aperture), large heterogeneous "macroscopic" conductances were obtained almost immediately. It is noteworthy that under these conditions, opening events in excess of, for example, 100 pS were resolved as single events without smaller steps (time resolution 200 μseconds). Thus the channel association time and maximum observable conductance were observed to be a function of the channel protein concentration.

Similar results were obtained using $BaCl_2$, although the conductance values were somewhat smaller, the smallest values being 0.9–1.0 pS. Typical channel conductances for symmetrical 100 mM $BaCl_2$ ranged from 1–4 to 24–48 pS (FIGURE 3e).

Although small conductance events typically revealed a linear current-voltage curve, larger "macroscopic" aggregates usually demonstrated a nonlinear and, sometimes, asymmetric voltage dependence. This behavior was revealed by applying voltage ramps, as indicated in FIGURE 3f.

DISCUSSION

In this paper we describe the purification and successful reconstitution of the guinea pig skeletal muscle L-type CC. The polypeptide pattern of the fractions containing the highest specific activity of reversible and irreversible 1,4 DHP and PA binding (1300 pmol and 700 pmol per mg of protein, respectively) is almost identical to that obtained with rabbit skeletal muscle.[6–8] Curtis and Catterall identified 165 kDa, 53 kDa, and 32 kDa polypeptides ("alpha," "beta," and "gamma" subunit) under nonreducing conditions of SDS-PAGE.[6] FIGURE 2C shows that distinct polypeptides can be separated within the alpha subunit region with apparent molecular masses of 155 kDa (termed $alpha_1$-subunit) and 165 kDa (termed $alpha_2$-subunit) in 5–15% gradient gels (nonreducing conditions). As both polypeptides are diffuse bands in SDS gels (probably due to their glycoprotein nature, see Reference 9), optimal resolution (as shown in FIGURE 2C) is not always obtained in gradient gels under nonreducing conditions. However, after reduction always two distinct bands with apparent M_r of 155 kDa and 135 kDa can be clearly separated (see FIGURE 2C). Similar microheterogeneity was seen by Curtis and Catterall,[6] their alpha subunit migrating as a doublet with molecular masses 165 kDa and 135 kDa after reduction. Their interpretation was incomplete reduction of interchain disulfide bonds of one polypeptide. In earlier photoaffinity labeling experiments with (±)-[^{3}H]azidopine, the 1,4 DHP receptor was localized on a 140–158 kDa polypeptide in T-tubule membranes from different species. This polypeptide did not alter its mobility upon reduction.[15] Identical results were obtained employing [*N*-methyl-^{3}H]LU49888 to label the PA receptor irreversibly.[16] These results strongly suggest that both receptor domains are on the 155 kDa polypeptide ($alpha_1$-subunit) of the purified channel. Interestingly, Curtis and Catterall reported that the phosphorylated alpha-subunit migrated slightly more rapidly than did the nonphosphorylated portion under nonreducing conditions of SDS-PAGE (see Figure 1 in Reference 20). This was interpreted in terms of altered binding of SDS to the phosphorylated protein. However, the more plausible explanation is the selective phosphorylation of the $alpha_1$-polypeptide in the poorly resolved high M_r region, migrating with a slightly lower M_r than the $alpha_2$-component (compare FIGURE 2C) under nonreducing conditions. Presumably the $alpha_1$-polypeptide is both carrier of the

CC-linked drug receptors and substrate for cAMP-dependent phosphorylation. The silver-stain and phosphorylation pattern of the purified channel from rabbit skeletal muscle (see Figure 1, Reference 21) is in complete agreement with this interpretation. The functional importance of the other polypeptides ($alpha_2$, beta, and gamma) has not yet been elucidated, but the $alpha_1$-polypeptide is clearly an L-type channel subunit. Immunochemical studies with polyclonal antibodies claim that the $alpha_2$-polypeptide, which is covalently linked to a 30 kDa protein via disulfide bonds,[17] is the carrier of the 1,4 DHP receptor in skeletal muscle, heart muscle, smooth muscle, and brain.[17,18] However, no direct evidence was presented to demonstrate that the antibody recognizes a polypeptide carrying a CC-linked drug receptor.[17,18]

We have observed CC-activity in reconstitution experiments of purified preparations. Proof of the identity of the channel with the L-type lies in its 1,4 DHP or PA binding ability, Cd^{2+} inhibition, and strong selectivity for divalent over monovalent cations. Also typical for this channel is the approximately 4:1 ratio of Na^+:Ba^{2+} conductance values (for the monomeric channel, cf. FIGURE 3c and 3f), a property also seen in patch clamp experiments with cardiac L-type CCs,[22] reflecting the lower binding affinity of the channel pore for Na^+ than for divalents. This behavior is mirrored in the complete blockade of Na^+ currents by Ba^{2+} and more potently by Ca^{2+} in concentrations high enough to replace bound Na^+ but insufficient to produce measurable currents themselves.[22] Another characteristic of native L-type CCs, a sole unitary conductance of 20–25 pS in 90–100 mM $BaCl_2$,[19,22,23] was absent in our reconstituted preparations. Instead, we observed a variety of discrete conductance levels from 1 to 24 (and more) pS in 100 mM $BaCl_2$, and approximately 3.5 times higher levels in 110 mM NaCl. In addition, we found the conductance levels to be highly dependent on protein concentration in the planar bilayer and time after bilayer formation (FIGURE 3c–e). Since we begin with singly distributed channel proteins just after incorporation, we interprete these findings as evidence for a monomeric channel conductance on the order of 1 pS (100 mM $BaCl_2$). This would imply a native channel associate consisting of about 20–25 channel molecules, functioning under usual conditions as a synchronously switching unit (all-or-none cooperativity). Similar evidence for strong positive cooperativity between ion channels has previously been provided for bacterial porin[24] and the nicotinic acetylcholine receptor.[11]

Cooperative interactions within channel associates may prove to be the rule rather than the exception, since practically all ion channels observed up to now in planar bilayers using initial distribution assays have shown the tendency to associate and form synchronously switching larger units. In addition to inducing synchronous gating of several channel molecules, channel interactions may be a crucial factor in determining voltage-dependent gating. The strongly nonlinear current-voltage curves (FIGURE 3f) of large channel associates imply that the interaction energy required to open a highly cooperative channel complex might be the source of a nonlinear voltage dependence.

It is interesting to compare these results with those obtained by others for skeletal muscle CCs in planar bilayers. Although the native channel is usually reported to give 20 pS in 100 mM $BaCl_2$,[23] one report also showed 10 pS channels.[25] In the only other report of reconstituted CCs,[21] the main conductance discussed was also 20 pS, although both smaller and larger ones were mentioned as being observed, but not inhibitable by methoxyverapamil like the 20 pS conductance level. Unfortunately, we have been unable to reproduce these results due to poorly described methodology.

A surprising aspect of our reconstituted CCs has been their apparent insensitivity to 1,4 DHP-channel blockers, although these compounds are clearly able to inhibit physiological Ca^{2+} currents in skeletal muscle.[26] This trait, together with the lack of all-or-none cooperativity, would indicate that some component or property of the CC is not retained through the isolation and reconstitution procedures. Further work on these aspects will hopefully lead to a better understanding of the molecular functioning of the isolated polypeptides as Ca^{2+}-selective ion channels.

{**Note added in proof:** Data presented here and in References 15 and 16, namely, that the skeletal muscle 1,4 dihydropyridine and phenylalkylamine receptors are co-localized on a polypeptide (termed $alpha_1$) which does not change its molecular mass upon reduction and is distinct from the alpha subunit ($alpha_2$) described in all previous publications, have been confirmed by (1) immunochemical analysis [Morton, M. E. & S. Froehner. 1987. J. Biol. Chem. **262** (in press); Leung, A. T., *et al.* 1987. J. Biol. Chem. **262:** 7943–7946], (2) primary structure amino acid analysis of $alpha_1$ (Tanabe, T., *et al.* 1987. Nature **328:** 313–318) and N-terminal amino acid sequence analysis of $alpha_2$ (Nakayama, N., *et al.* 1987. J. Biol. Chem. **262:** 6572–6576), (3) photoaffinity labeling of $alpha_1$ [Takahashi, M., *et al.* 1987. Proc. Nat. Acad. Sci. USA **84:** 5478–5482; Vaghy, P. L., *et al.* 1987. J. Biol. Chem. **262** (in press)].}

ACKNOWLEDGMENTS

S. Daubenmerkl, H. Fluch, H.-G. Knaus, M. Grabner, and K. Moosburger were of great help in the laboratory. K. Hofer is thanked for competent secretarial assistance, and C. Trawöger for the illustrations.

REFERENCES

1. ALMERS, W., E. W. MCCLESKEY & P. T. PALADE. 1986. Prog. Zool. **33:** 61–74.
2. SCHWARTZ, L. M., E. W. MCCLESKY & W. ALMERS. 1985. Nature **314:** 747–750.
3. BEAN, B. P. 1986. Trends Neurosci. **9:** 535–536.
4. FERRY, D. R. & H. GLOSSMANN. 1982. FEBS. Lett. **148:** 331–337.
5. GLOSSMANN, H. & D. R. FERRY. 1983. Naunyn Schmiedeberg's Arch. Pharmacol. **323:** 279–291.
6. CURTIS, B. M. & W. A. CATTERALL. 1984. Biochemistry **23:** 2113–2118.
7. BORSOTTO, M., J. BARHANIN, M. FOSSET & M. LAZDUNSKI. 1985. J. Biol. Chem. **260:** 14255–14263.
8. FLOCKERZI, V., H.-J. OEKEN & F. HOFMANN. 1986. Eur. J. Biochem. **161:** 217–224.
9. STRIESSNIG, J., K. MOOSBURGER, A. GOLL, D. R. FERRY & H. GLOSSMANN. 1986. Eur. J. Biochem. **161:** 603–609.
10. STRIESSNIG, J., A. GOLL, K. MOOSBURGER & H. GLOSSMANN. 1986. FEBS. Lett. **197:** 204–210.
11. SCHINDLER, H., F. SPILLECKE & E. NEUMANN. 1984. Proc. Nat. Acad. Sci. USA **81:** 6222–6226.
12. SCHINDLER, H. 1980. FEBS Lett. **122:** 77–79.
13. BORSOTTO, M., J. BARHANIN, R. I. NORMAN & M. LAZDUNSKI. 1984. Biochem. Biophys. Res. Commun. **122:** 1357–1366.
14. GLOSSMANN, H. & D. R. FERRY. 1985. Methods Enzymol. **109:** 513–550.
15. FERRY, D. R., K. KÄMPF, A. GOLL & H. GLOSSMANN. 1985. EMBO J. **4:** 1933–1940.
16. STRIESSNIG, J., H.-G. KNAUS, M. GRABNER, K. MOOSBURGER, W. SEITZ, H. LIETZ & H. GLOSSMANN. 1987. FEBS Lett. **212:** 247–253.
17. SCHMID, A., J. BARHANIN, C. MOURRE, T. COPPOLA, M. BORSOTTO & M. LAZDUNSKI. 1986. Biochem. Biophys. Res. Commun. **139:** 996–1002.
18. SCHMID, A., J. BARHANIN, T. COPPOLA, M. BORSOTTO & M. LAZDUNSKI. 1986. Biochemistry **25:** 3492–3495.
19. NILIUS, B., P. HESS, J. B. LANSMAN & R. W. TSIEN. 1985. Nature **316:** 443–446.
20. CURTIS, B. M. & W. A. CATTERALL. 1985. Proc. Nat. Acad. Sci. USA **82:** 2528–2532.

21. FLOCKERZI, V., H.-J. OEKEN, F. HOFMANN, D. PELZER, A. CAVALIE & W. TRAUTWEIN. 1986. Nature **323:** 66–68.
22. HESS, P., J. B. LANSMAN & R. W. TSIEN. 1986. J. Gen. Physiol. **88:** 293–319.
23. AFFOLTER, H. & R. CORONADO. 1985. Biophys. J. **48:** 341–347.
24. SCHINDLER, H. & J. P. ROSENBUSCH. 1981. Proc. Nat. Acad. Sci. USA **78:** 2302–2306.
25. ROSENBERG, R. L., P. HESS, J. P. REEVES, H. SMILOWITZ & R. W. TSIEN. 1986. Science **231:** 1564–1566.
26. ALMERS, W., R. FINK & P. T. PALADE. 1981. J. Physiol. London **312:** 177–207.

Molecular Properties of Dihydropyridine-Sensitive Calcium Channels

MICHAEL J. SEAGAR,[a] MASAMI TAKAHASHI,[b] AND WILLIAM A. CATTERALL[c]

Department of Pharmacology, SJ-30
University of Washington
Seattle, Washington 98195

INTRODUCTION

Voltage-sensitive calcium channels constitute an essential link between transient changes in membrane potential and a variety of cellular responses. In nerve terminals, calcium influx couples membrane depolarization to transmitter release,[1] whereas in the soma it may activate calcium-dependent potassium channels and thus modulate repetitive firing patterns.[2,3] In cardiac and smooth muscle tissue calcium channels mediate excitation-contraction coupling, although in skeletal muscle their physiological role is still a matter for debate.[4,5]

Electrophysiological measurements have established the existence of multiple classes of calcium channels.[6–9] The most prominent type, revealed by single channel recording, has been termed the "L-channel" by Tsien and colleagues.[8] L channels, when activated by depolarization, show different modes of gating behavior. Spontaneous transitions occur between the commonest mode characterized by brief opening bursts and two other modes in which channels either show longer sustained openings or remain completely closed. Transitions between these states may be pharmacologically modulated by drugs of the 1,4-dihydropyridine family. Calcium channel "agonists" such as Bay K 8644 favor long openings whereas "antagonists" such as nimodipine stabilize periods of no channel activity, resulting in enhanced or reduced peak calcium current respectively in a whole cell recording configuration.[8]

The availability of radiolabeled dihydropyridine derivatives, which may be used as high-affinity probes, has recently allowed biochemical analysis of the components of this type of calcium channel.

ORGANIC CALCIUM ANTAGONISTS AS CALCIUM CHANNEL PROBES

[^{3}H]-labeled derivatives of nitrendipine, nimodipine, and PN200-110 have been widely used to titrate binding sites in homogenates and membrane fractions from a variety of tissues with K_D values in the 0.1 to 1 nM range.[10] In smooth muscle, the structure-activity relationships for binding site occupancy correlate well with the

[a]Permanent affiliation: CNRS-INSERM, Laboratoire de Biochimie, Fac. Med. Nord, Marseille, France.
[b]Mitsubishi-Kasei Institute of Life Sciences, Machida-Shi, Tokyo, Japan.
[c]To whom correspondence should be addressed.

concentrations of various dihydropyridines required to inhibit contraction.[11] In other tissues, although similar structure-activity relationships are observed, the concentration required to block calcium currents is often substantially higher than that required to occupy high-affinity nitrendipine-binding sites.[12]

This apparent discrepancy has now been resolved by the finding that dihydropyridine binding and the subsequent block of calcium channels is dependent on membrane potential.[13–15] In cardiac cells, half-maximal block of calcium current requires 700 nM nitrendipine at resting membrane potential; however, when cells are depolarized to −20 mV, inactivating 70% of the calcium current, half-maximal block is achieved at 0.8 nM. This value is in good agreement with the K_D for [^{3}H]-nitrendipine binding to cardiac homogenates in which most channels are presumably in an inactivated state following depolarization induced by cell disruption.[10]

Dihydropyridine-sensitive calcium currents are also blocked by chemically unrelated organic compounds such as the phenylalkylamine verapamil and the benzothiazepine diltiazem. In keeping with these observations, the binding of [^{3}H]-nitrendipine to its receptor site is modulated via an allosteric mechanism by both verapamil and diltiazem, each interacting with a distinct binding site.[16,17] Verapamil inhibits nitrendipine binding and accelerates dissociation of the nitrendipine/receptor complex, whereas diltiazem enhances binding and stabilizes nitrendipine/receptor interaction.

[^{3}H]-Nitrendipine binding to rat brain membranes is inhibited by treatment with EGTA, and this effect can be reversed by the addition of micromolar concentrations of calcium. The cations La^{+++} and Co^{++}, which are widely used as inorganic blockers of calcium currents, also inhibit [^{3}H]-nitrendipine binding and block the stimulatory effects of Ca^{++}.[18]

Considered as a whole these results provide strong support for the view that measurements of specific binding of nitrendipine or other dihydropyridines represent drug interaction with calcium channels, and suggest that channel components carry three allosterically coupled drug receptor sites associated with one or more divalent cation binding sites.

IDENTIFICATION OF CALCIUM CHANNEL COMPONENTS BY TARGET SIZE ANALYSIS AND PHOTOAFFINITY LABELING

The first estimates of the molecular size of the calcium channel were obtained by measuring the decrease in specific [^{3}H]-nitrendipine binding resulting from exposure of membranes to increasing amounts of ionizing radiation and applying target size theory. Molecular sizes of 180–210 kDa for skeletal muscle,[19,20] 210 kDa for brain, and 280 kDa for smooth muscle[21] have been reported. Results, however, appeared to depend not only on which tissue was used as a receptor source but also on the [^{3}H]-dihydropyridine that was used to assay receptors and the irradiation conditions, suggesting that the dihydropyridine-sensitive calcium channel is a complex oligomeric structure.[22]

Certain calcium antagonists are photoreactive and may be expected to form covalent complexes with receptor polypeptides when exposed to ultraviolet light. However, the generally low efficiency of this type of reaction has led one group to synthesize an arylazide radiolabeled dihydropyridine derivative [^{3}H]-azidopine which binds with high affinity to skeletal muscle membranes and on photolysis covalently labels a 145–158 kDa polypeptide.[23,24] More recent use of the intrinsic photoreactivity of [^{3}H]-PN200-110 to probe the dihydropyridine-binding site identified a similarly sized component (170 kDa), which was also labeled by [^{3}H]-bepridil and [^{3}H]-diltiazem, ligands specific for the phenylalkylamine- and benzothiazepine-binding sites, respectively.[25] This last observation suggested that all three allosterically coupled calcium antagonist receptor sites may be carried by a single high molecular weight polypeptide.

CHARACTERIZATION OF THE DETERGENT-SOLUBILIZED CALCIUM ANTAGONIST RECEPTOR

Since it is likely to be an intrinsic membrane protein, the first essential step in purification and biochemical characterization of the calcium antagonist receptor is solubilization from an appropriate membrane source and characterization of the solubilized protein. After a survey of several detergents, we concluded that digitonin is the most effective detergent for solubilization of a specific [^{3}H]-nitrendipine-receptor complex from brain and skeletal muscle transverse tubule membranes.[26,27] Up to 40% of the receptor-ligand complex is solubilized. The dissociation of bound [^{3}H]-nitrendipine from the complex is accelerated by verapamil and slowed by diltiazem through allosteric interactions between the nitrendipine-binding site and the binding sites for those ligands as previously observed in intact membranes. These results show that the three different binding sites for calcium antagonist drugs remain associated as a complex after detergent solubilization of the calcium antagonist receptor and provide further support for the conclusion that a specific receptor complex has been solubilized under conditions that allow retention of the functional allosteric regulation of dihydropyridine binding.

Sedimentation of the solubilized [^{3}H]-nitrendipine-receptor–digitonin complex through sucrose gradients gives a single peak of specifically bound nitrendipine with a sedimentation coefficient of 19 to 20S.[26] Comparison of the sedimentation behavior of the solubilized complex of brain, heart, and skeletal and smooth muscle indicates that they have identical size. These results provide support for the view that the calcium antagonist receptor in different tissues is quite similar.

Many plasma membrane proteins are glycosylated during their synthesis and transport to the cell surface. The solubilized calcium antagonist receptor from brain or skeletal muscle is specifically adsorbed to and eluted from affinity columns with immunobilized wheat germ agglutinin or other lectins.[26–29] Evidently, one or more of the subunits of the calcium antagonist receptor are glycoproteins.

SKELETAL MUSCLE TRANSVERSE TUBULES AS A MODEL SYSTEM FOR EXAMINATION OF THE BIOCHEMICAL PROPERTIES OF CALCIUM CHANNELS

Skeletal muscle fibers have substantial voltage-activated calcium currents which have been measured under voltage clamp.[30] These currents originate almost entirely in the transverse tubular system and are blocked by dihydropyridine calcium antagonists.[12] They have been presumed to play a role in excitation-contraction coupling although direct evidence for such a role has not been obtained. Transverse tubule membranes can be extensively purified from skeletal muscle by a combination of differential and density gradient centrifugation.[31] Antibodies prepared against the most highly purified fractions of T-tubule membranes stain only T-tubules and not sarcolemma or sarcoplasmic reticulum of intact muscle, indicating a high degree of purity of this preparation.[31] Analysis of [^{3}H]-nitrendipine binding to membrane fractions from skeletal muscle reveals a specific localization of the calcium antagonist receptor in the T-tubule fraction.[32,33] These membranes contain a 10-fold greater concentration of calcium antagonist receptor than any other membrane preparation described to date. Since T-tubule membranes are the most enriched source of calcium antagonist receptors and they display a substantial voltage-activated calcium current that is blocked by dihydropyridines, they provide a favorable experimental preparation for examination of the molecular properties of the calcium antagonist receptor and its relationship to voltage-sensitive calcium channels. It is anticipated that the T-tubule calcium channel will resemble those of other tissues which are blocked by dihydropyridines and therefore that information on the molecular properties of this calcium channel will give insight into others.

MOLECULAR PROPERTIES OF CALCIUM CHANNELS FROM SKELETAL MUSCLE TRANSVERSE TUBULES

Purification and Subunit Composition

We have purified the calcium antagonist receptor, solubilized from T-tubule membranes by digitonin, 330-fold by affinity chromatography on wheat germ agglutinin (WGA) Sepharose, ion exchange chromatography on DEAE-Sephadex, and velocity sedimentation through sucrose gradients.[27] Analysis of the purified protein by sodium dodecyl sulfate–polyacrylamide gel electrophoresis (SDS-PAGE) under alkylating conditions and silver staining (FIGURE 1, lane 1) revealed three classes of polypeptide which we have designated α (167 kDa), β (54 kDa), and γ (30 kDa).[27] When disulfide bonds were cleaved with dithiothreitol, the α band split into two clearly resolved protein populations with molecular weights of 175 and 143 kDa. In the initial studies from this laboratory, the anomalous behavior of the α polypeptide was ascribed to partial cleavage and/or reformation of intrachain disulfide bonds resulting in a variable fraction of the protein with smaller apparent size.[27] The more recent use of a battery of specific labeling methods has now shown that that 175 and 143 kDa polypeptides are two distinct calcium channel subunits, α_1 and α_2, which have similar size but clearly different properties.[34]

A polyclonal antibody (PAC-10), obtained from the ascites fluids of a SJL/J mouse immunized with purified calcium channel, selectively labeled the 167 kDa polypeptide before reduction of disulfide bonds (FIGURE 1, lane 3), but only the 175 kDa polypeptide after reduction (FIGURE 1, lane 4). No immunolabeling was observed with preimmune serum (FIGURE 1, lane 5) or with PAC-10 which had been preadsorbed with purified calcium channel (FIGURE 1, lane 6). These observations indicate that the 175 kDa and 143 kDa components are distinct polypeptides.

Subunit Glycosylation

Solubilized [^{3}H]-dihydropyridine receptors specifically bind to various immobilized lectins and affinity chromatography on WGA-Sepharose is the most efficient purification step.[27–29] These results imply that at least one subunit is glycosylated. The oligosaccharide chains of the purified calcium channel were detected by separating subunits by SDS-PAGE and probing the resolved polypeptides with [^{125}I]-ConA or [^{125}I]-WGA. Under alkylating conditions [^{125}I]-ConA labeled the α polypeptide (FIGURE 1, lane 7); after disulfide reduction [^{125}I]-ConA labeled only the α_2 subunit (FIGURE 1, lane 8). [^{125}I]-WGA bound to both the α and γ protein bands in gels run under alkylating conditions (FIGURE 1, lane 9), and to the α_2 and γ subunits after

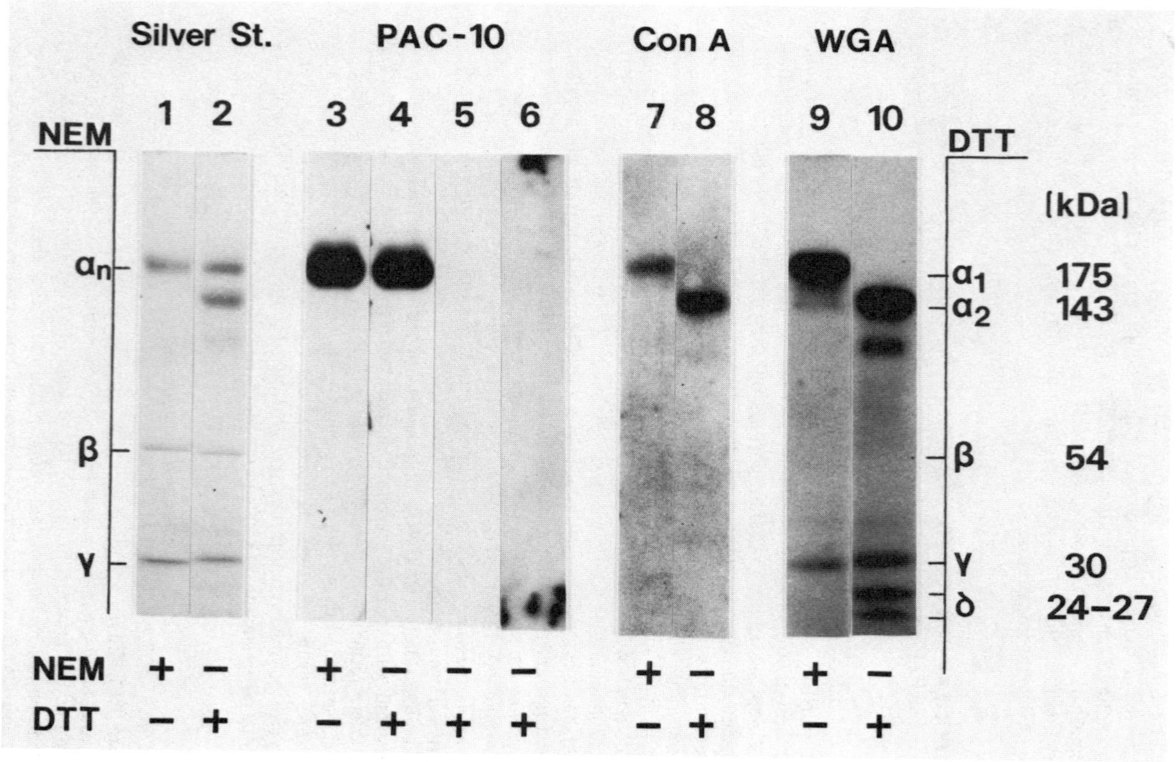

FIGURE 1. Polypeptide composition of the dihydropyridine-sensitive calcium channel. Lanes 1 and 2: purified calcium channels were analyzed by SDS-PAGE and silver staining with or without reduction of disulfide bonds as indicated beneath each lane. Lanes 3 through 6: polypeptides separated by SDS-PAGE, with or without reduction of disulfide bonds as indicated below each lane, were electrophoretically transferred to nitrocellulose strips and immunolabeled by incubation with PAC-10 (lanes 3 and 4), preimmune serum (lane 5), or PAC-10 which had been preadsorbed with purified calcium channel (lane 6), followed by incubation with ^{125}I-protein A, washing, and autoradiography. Lanes 7 and 8: calcium channel subunits were transferred to a nitrocellulose sheet and labeled with [^{125}I]-ConA. Lanes 9 and 10: calcium channel subunits were labeled directly in the gel with [^{125}I]-WGA.

dithiothreitol treatment. Disulfide reduction led to the appearance of two new [^{125}I]-WGA-labeled components at 24–27 kDa which are clearly distinct from the γ subunit. These polypeptides were also detected, but much less distinctly, by silver staining (FIGURE 1, lane 2). They appear to be disulfide linked to the α_2 subunit under nonreducing conditions; previous immunochemical evidence[35] suggests that the smaller polypeptide may be proteolytically derived from the larger so we refer to them collectively as the δ subunit. No labeling of α_1 or β was detected with either lectin. [^{125}I]-ConA and [^{125}I]-WGA binding to calcium channel subunits was blocked in the presence of 100 mM α methylmannoside or *N* acetylglucosamine, respectively (not shown).

To determine the extent of glycosylation and the core polypeptide size of the calcium channel subunits, purified channel preparations were labeled with ^{125}I, incubated with glycosidases to remove oligosaccharide chains, and analyzed by SDS-PAGE and autoradiography. Sequential deglycosylation with neuraminadase and endoglycosidase F caused a reduction in the apparent sizes of the α_2 and γ subunits reaching core polypeptide sizes of 105 kDa and 20 kDa, respectively. Poor iodination of the δ subunit prevented estimation of its carbohydrate content by this method. No shift in the mobility of the α_1 and β subunits was noted, confirming the absence of *N*-linked carbohydrate in these two subunits.

Covalent Labeling of Calcium Channel Subunits

[^{3}H]-PN200-110 and [^{3}H]-azidopine have been shown to label covalently a 145–170 kDa polypeptide in T-tubule membranes[23–25] and purified calcium channels[36] which presumably corresponds to one of the two α subunits. In our preparations, [^{3}H]-azidopine was incorporated by UV photolysis into a polypeptide which migrated as a band of 167 kDa before reduction of disulfide bonds (FIGURE 2, lane 1) and 175 kDa after dithiothreitol treatment (FIGURE 2, lane 2). The electrophoretic behavior of this polypeptide identifies it as the α_1 subunit. No labeling was observed in the presence of 2 μM PN200-110 (FIGURE 2, lane 3).

Ion channel forming polypeptides should contain transmembrane segments which may be detected using the hydrophobic probe [^{125}I]-3-(trifluoromethyl)-3-(*m*-iodophenyl)diazirine (TID). This photoreactive compound partitions into free detergent micelles and detergent associated with the major hydrophobic domains of integral membrane proteins and is specifically incorporated into these regions by photolysis. The α_1 and γ subunits were prominently labeled by TID, with a much lower level of incorporation into α_2 and δ (FIGURE 2, lanes 6 and 7). The β subunit was not detectably labeled. Quantitation of [^{125}I]TID in excised protein bands showed that the α_1 and γ subunits incorporated 10-fold more TID per unit mass than the α_2 or δ subunits did, even though, as shown below, nearly all α_1 and γ subunits are associated with an α_2 subunit. These results indicate that the α_1 and γ subunits are the principal transmembrane components of the purified calcium channel complex.

The regulation of calcium channels via a pathway involving cAMP and protein phosphorylation is now well established,[37–41] although it is not known whether the site of phosphorylation is the calcium channel itself or another intracellular protein which in turn regulates channel function. As a step toward resolving this question we have investigated whether subunits of the purified calcium antagonist receptor can serve as substrates for the catalytic subunit of cyclic adenosine monophosphate (cAMP)-dependent protein kinase. Incubation with 33 μM [γ-^{32}P]ATP and 3 μM catalytic subunit led to stoichiometric ^{32}P incorporation into the α protein band and the β

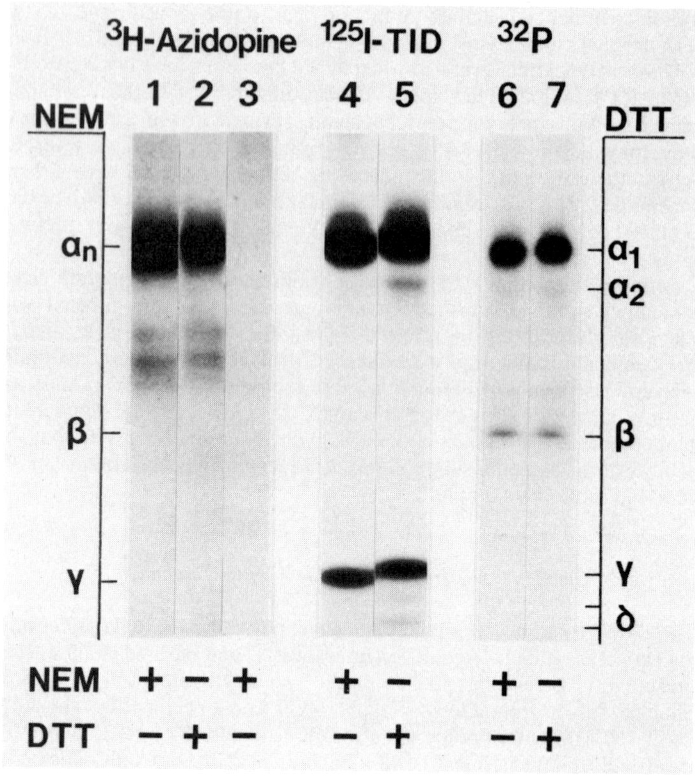

FIGURE 2. Differential labeling of calcium channel subunits. Photoaffinity labeling: T-tubule membrane (0.4 mg/ml) in 25 mM Hepes, 1 mM $CaCl_2$ adjusted to pH 7.5 with Tris base was incubated with 6 nM [^{3}H]-azidopine in the absence (lanes 1 and 2) or presence (lane 3) of 2 μM PN200-110 and was irradiated for 15 minutes at 4°C with a 30 watt UV source (λmax 356 nm). The membranes were solubilized in 1% digitonin, 10 mM Hepes, 185 mM NaCl, 0.5 mM $CaCl_2$, 0.1 mM phenylmethane sulfonyl fluoride (PMSF), 1 μM pepstatin A adjusted to pH 7.5 with Tris base, and calcium channels were partially purified by chromatography on WGA-Sepharose and analyzed by SDS-PAGE and fluorography. Hydrophobic labeling: [^{125}I]-TID (15 Ci/mmol) was prepared and purified calcium channel was labeled[46] with 100 μCi/ml [^{125}I]-TID in a buffer containing 0.1% digitonin (lanes 4 and 5). Phosphorylation: purified calcium channel was incubated with 0.3 μM cAMP-dependent kinase catalytic subunit and 0.12 μM carrier-free [γ-^{32}P]-ATP for 15 minutes at 37°C as previously described[42] (lanes 6 and 7).

subunit at rates that are consistent with a physiologically significant phosphorylation reaction.[42] Comparison of the electrophoretic mobility of the phosphorylated bands before and after reduction of disulfide bonds (FIGURE 2, lanes 6 and 7) showed that the α_1 subunit is a good substrate for this enzyme while the α_2 and δ polypeptides are not labeled. The β subunit was more weakly labeled at the low ATP concentration used in this experiment (see legend). These results identify the α_1 and β subunits of the calcium channel as potential sites of regulation of the voltage-sensitive calcium channel by cAMP-dependent phosphorylation.

Analysis of Noncovalent Subunit Interactions

By the use of several labeling techniques, we have established that α_1 has the properties expected of the calcium channel including a binding site for dihydropyridine calcium antagonists, at least one cAMP-dependent phosphorylation site, and extensive hydrophobic domains. It is important to determine whether other polypeptides present in the purified preparation are persistent impurities or specifically associated components of the oligomeric calcium channel complex.

The data presented in FIGURE 1, lane 4 demonstrate that PAC-10 antibodies recognize only the α_1 subunit of SDS-denatured calcium channel. However, this polyclonal serum produced by immunization with native calcium channel may contain antibodies that bind only to native conformations of the $\alpha_2\delta$, β, or γ subunits. To eliminate any antibodies with this specificity, a nitrocellulose strip containing α_1 subunit was used as an affinity matrix to purify anti-α_1 antibodies. Purified anti-α_1 antibodies specifically precipitated [^{3}H]-PN200-110-labeled calcium channel, while proteins from PAC-10 that were nonspecifically adsorbed to a bare nitrocellulose strip did not.

Immunoprecipitation of ^{125}I-labeled calcium channel (FIGURE 3) showed that only

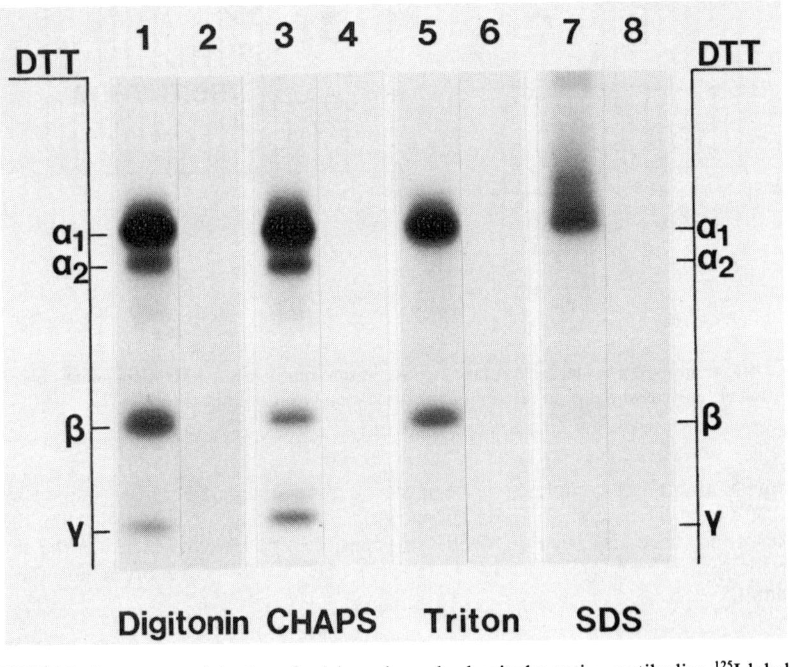

FIGURE 3. Immunoprecipitation of calcium channel subunits by anti-α_1 antibodies. ^{125}I-labeled calcium channel was immunoprecipitated as described previously[50] using affinity purified anti-α_1 antibodies (lanes 1, 3, 5, and 7) or a control preparation (lanes 2, 4, 6, and 8) in an immunoassay buffer containing the indicated detergents: 0.5% digitonin, 0.1% CHAPS, and 1% Triton X-100, or 1% SDS for 2 minutes at 100°C followed by immunoassay in 0.5% digitonin detergent after exchange by gel filtration on a 2 ml Sephadex G-50 column.

α_1 was precipitated after SDS denaturation (lane 7). In contrast, α_1, α_2, β, and γ were precipitated as a complex in 0.5% digitonin (lane 1) or 0.1% 3-[(3-cholamidopropyl)dimethylammonio]-1-propane sulfonate (CHAPS) (lane 3), detergent conditions that are known to stabilize dihydropyridine binding, allosteric coupling of the three calcium antagonist receptor sites, and ion conductance activity. A higher concentration of CHAPS (1%) caused dissociation of α_2 from the complex (data not shown). In addition, experiments in 1% Triton X-100 (lane 5) showed complete dissociation of the α_2 subunit. The β subunit and a small fraction of the γ subunit (not easily seen in FIGURE 3) were coimmunoprecipitated with α_1 in Triton X-100. The results of these immunoprecipitation experiments have been confirmed by selective elution of α_2 subunits from immune complexes. Purified calcium channels were immunoprecipitated in 0.5% digitonin as in FIGURE 3, lane 1. Resuspension in a buffer containing 1%

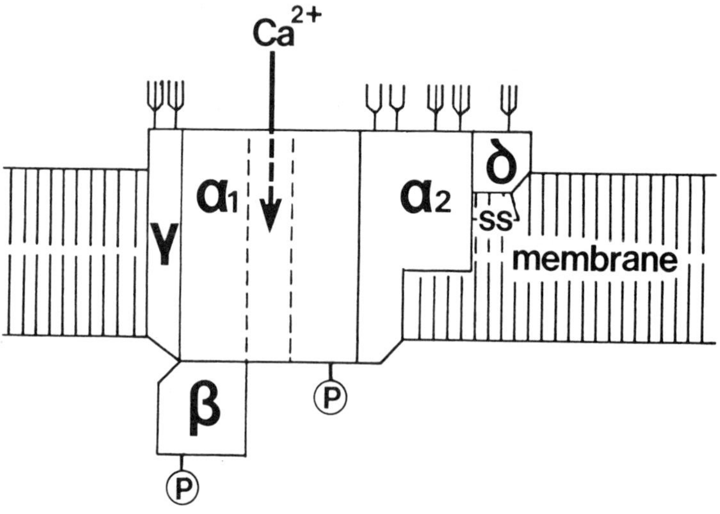

FIGURE 4. Proposed model for calcium channel structure. Sites of cAMP-dependent phosphorylation (P), glycosylation, and interaction with the membrane are illustrated.

Triton X-100 caused complete release of the $\alpha_2\delta$ dimer and partial release of γ without loss of β from the precipitate (data not shown). Complementary data supporting these observations have also been obtained using lentil lectin agarose which has the same specificity as ConA (see FIGURE 1, lane 8) and is a selective probe for the α_2 subunit.[34]

AN OLIGOMERIC MODEL FOR THE DIHYDROPYRIDINE-SENSITIVE CALCIUM CHANNEL

On the basis of present knowledge of the structure of the dihydropyridine-sensitive calcium channel, and in analogy with current models of the structure of voltage-sensitive sodium channels,[43] we propose a model (FIGURE 4) based on a central ion channel-forming element interacting with three other noncovalently associated subunits. The α_1 subunit, which contains the calcium antagonist binding sites, cAMP-dependent phosphorylation sites, and the largest hydrophobic domains, is proposed to be the central ion channel-forming component of the complex. Its apparent molecular weight of 175 kDa from SDS-PAGE is likely to be a reasonable approximation of the true polypeptide molecular weight since no *N*-glycosylation was detected. This calcium channel subunit is therefore large enough to contain four homologous transmembrane domains analogous to those of the rat brain sodium channel α subunit, whose mRNA alone encodes a functional ion channel.[44,45] Like α_1, the sodium channel α subunit also contains cAMP-dependent phosphorylation sites[43] and extensive hydrophobic domains which are efficiently labeled by TID.[46]

The β subunit is also a substrate for cAMP-dependent kinase,[42] but hydrophobic labeling indicates that it does not interact with the membrane phase and it is not a glycoprotein. It is probably therefore tightly associated with an intracellular domain of α_1.

The γ subunit of 30 kDa interacts independently with α_1, contains at least one transmembrane segment, and consists of approximately 30% carbohydrate. All these properties are similar to those of the β_1 subunit of the rat brain and skeletal muscle Na^+ channels.[43] A polypeptide of similar size appears to be associated with the apamin-sensitive calcium-activated potassium channel,[47] and it is interesting to speculate that this subunit may be a conserved constituent of voltage- or calcium-dependent ion channels.

The $\alpha_2\delta$ dimer appears to interact with α_1, although the conditions necessary to achieve dissociation result in a loss of dihydropyridine (DHP) binding activity. The 105 kDa core polypeptide of α_2 contains a heavily glycosylated extracellular domain but displays weak hydrophobic labeling, indicating a limited intramembrane domain. For this reason it seems unlikely that the ion channel is formed jointly by α_1 and α_2 at their zone of interaction.

The proposed model assumes a complex containing one of each subunit type. Our present results and previous data showing quantitative binding of solubilized calcium channels to ConA[28] suggest that each complex contains at least one α_1 and one α_2 subunit, but do not specify the stoichiometry of any subunits. α_1 and α_2 appear to be present in approximately equal amounts on silver-stained gels, and the α_1 and β subunits incorporate approximately one mole of ^{32}P per mole of complex. A complete hydrodynamic analysis of the skeletal muscle calcium channel has not been reported. However, a size of 370 kDa determined for the rat ventricular muscle dihydropyridine receptor[48] is within reasonable range of the predicted size of the complex represented in FIGURE 4 (416 kDa). Thus, an assumption of one mole of each subunit in the complex is plausible, but requires direct experimental verification.

FUNCTIONAL PROPERTIES OF THE PURIFIED CALCIUM ANTAGONIST RECEPTOR IN PHOSPHOLIPID VESICLES

We purify the calcium antagonist receptor as a preformed complex with the calcium antagonists [^{3}H]-nitrendipine or [^{3}H]-PN200-110. After solubilization, it retains allosteric interactions among the separate binding sites for verapamil, diltiazem, and dihydropyridines. However, other aspects of calcium channel function cannot be assessed in detergent solution. It is important, therefore, to return the purified calcium antagonist receptor to a membrane environment and to determine whether the purified protein is capable of mediating voltage-dependent calcium flux.

In order to maximize the probability of purification of the calcium channel in an active state, the calcium antagonist receptors in T-tubule membranes were incubated with sufficient [^{3}H]-PN200-110 to label approximately 1% of the binding sites. This label was used to identify the calcium antagonist receptor during purification as in previous studies.[27] The T-tubule membranes were then incubated in an excess of the specific calcium channel activator Bay K 8644 so that the remaining 99% of dihydropyridine sites would be occupied by this agent. The calcium antagonist receptors were then solubilized in digitonin and purified in the continued presence of Bay K 8644 using previously described procedures. Phosphatidylcholine for reconstitution was solubilized in the zwitterionic detergent CHAPS because it is poorly soluble in digitonin. Purified calcium antagonist receptor dispersed in digitonin was then mixed with phosphatidylcholine dispersed in CHAPS and single-walled phospholipid vesicles were formed by removal of the detergents by molecular sieve chromatography. Analysis of the resulting vesicle preparations by sucrose density gradient sedimentation shows that the purified calcium antagonist receptors are quantitatively incorporated into phosphatidylcholine vesicles and 15 to 25% of vesicles contain at least one calcium antagonist receptor.[49] These preparations therefore provide a suitable system for analysis of the ion transport properties of this purified protein.

Initial rates of influx of $^{45}Ca^{2+}$ or $^{133}Ba^{2+}$ into reconstituted phosphatidylcholine vesicles were measured under countertransport conditions in which the intravesicular compartment contains a high concentration of unlabeled Ca^{2+} or Ba^{2+}. These conditions greatly increase the amount of $^{45}Ca^{2+}$ or $^{133}Ba^{2+}$ uptake required to achieve isotopic equilibrium and greatly slow the approach to isotopic equilibrium as described previously for reconstituted sodium channels. They therefore maximize any ion flux mediated by reconstituted channels. Under these conditions, calcium influx into phosphatidylcholine vesicles containing reconstituted calcium antagonist receptors was two- to threefold greater than influx into protein-free phosphatidylcholine vesicles. This increase is completely blocked by verapamil at a concentration of 100 μM. If the calcium channel activator Bay K 8644 is removed from the vesicle preparation by molecular sieve chromatography, $^{45}Ca^{2+}$ influx is markedly reduced. These results show that at least a fraction of the purified calcium antagonist receptors can function as calcium channels when incorporated into phosphatidylcholine vesicles.[49]

The inhibition of the reconstituted calcium channels by different concentrations of organic calcium channel blockers from 10^{-9} M to 10^{-4} M was examined. Half-maximal inhibition was observed with approximately 1.5 μM verapamil, 1.0 μM D600, or 0.2 μM PN200-110.[49] These concentrations are similar to those that give half-maximal inhibition of voltage-activated calcium currents in intact skeletal muscle fibers, consistent with the conclusion that the calcium influx in reconstituted vesicles is mediated by functional purified calcium channels.

To determine whether the calcium influx stimulated by Bay K 8644 and blocked by PN200-110 and verapamil required the presence of the subunits of the calcium antagonist receptor and not other detectable proteins, purified preparations were sedimented through sucrose gradients and each fraction was examined for bound [^{3}H]PN200-110, polypeptide composition, and ability to mediate $^{133}Ba^{2+}$ influx when incorporated into phosphatidylcholine vesicles. A close quantitative correlation was observed between the presence of the α, β, and γ subunits of the calcium antagonist receptor and the ability to mediate barium influx.[49] Thus, these results are also consistent with the conclusion that the purified calcium antagonist receptor is capable of mediating ion flux with the pharmacologic characteristics expected of voltage-sensitive calcium channels.

IMMUNOSPECIFIC IDENTIFICATION OF CALCIUM CHANNEL COMPONENTS IN OTHER TISSUES

In order to identify the molecular components of calcium channels in tissues other than skeletal muscle, the purified calcium channel from rabbit transverse tubules was injected into mice and polyclonal antisera were obtained after multiple injections. To determine the immunological cross-reactivity of this antiserum with calcium channels from heart and brain, radioimmune assays were performed. In each tissue, calcium channels were labeled with [^{3}H]-PN200-110, solubilized with digitonin, and purified by chromatography on WGA-Sepharose. PAC-10 antiserum which we have used to characterize the α_1 subunit of the calcium channel (see FIGURES 1 and 3) showed poor cross-reactivity with other tissues. However, another antiserum, PAC-2, recognized [^{3}H]-PN200-110-labeled calcium channel in skeletal muscle, heart, and brain and the concentration dependence of immunoprecipitation was then determined. Each channel was precipitated to a similar extent by maximum concentrations of antiserum, and the ratios of antiserum for half-maximal immunoprecipitation were 1.0:1.8:7.9 for skeletal muscle, heart, and brain. These results indicate that antigenic determinants present on the skeletal muscle calcium channel are also present on calcium channels in heart and brain.

Since these antibodies recognize calcium channels in heart and brain, it is possible to use them to identify and characterize the related proteins in these tissues. For this purpose, membrane preparations from heart and brain were solubilized with digitonin and glycoproteins were purified by chromatography on WGA-Sepharose. These purified glycoproteins were labeled with ^{125}I, and the components recognized by antibodies against the skeletal muscle calcium channel were isolated by immunoprecipitation with specific antiserum and a protein A–Sepharose immunoadsorbent. In each tissue, a polypeptide with the characteristics of the calcium channel α_2 subunit was identified.[50,51] The immunoprecipitated component had a molecular weight 170 kDa in heart and 169 kDa in brain in nonreducing conditions and 141 kD and 140 kD, respectively, after reduction. In each case, immunoprecipitation was blocked by prior incubation of the antiserum with purified calcium channel. Thus, we conclude that dihydropyridine-sensitive calcium channels in skeletal muscle, heart, and brain are all associated with an α_2 subunit that is homologous, but not identical, in the three tissues. Polypeptides homologous to other subunits of the skeletal muscle calcium channel have not yet been detected using these techniques.

CONCLUSION

The molecular properties of dihydropyridine-sensitive calcium channels are now being elucidated by following a general strategy that was used previously in studies of voltage-sensitive sodium channels in this laboratory: identification by specific ligand binding and covalent labeling, solubilization and isolation by conventional protein purification methods, and reconstitution of channel function *in vitro*. The work reviewed here illustrates the substantial progress achieved with this approach to date. Future directions include further definition of the functional properties of the purified calcium channel complex in reconstituted phospholipid vesicles, analysis of the mechanism of regulation of the channel by protein phosphorylation, determination of the primary structure of the channel subunits, extension of these molecular studies to calcium channels in heart, brain, and smooth muscle, and comparison of the structural features of calcium channels with those of voltage-sensitive sodium channels in order to define common structural themes underlying the function of voltage-sensitive ion channels in general.

REFERENCES

1. KATZ, B. & R. MILEDI. 1969. J. Physiol. London **203:** 459–487.
2. ADAMS, D. J., S. J. SMITH & S. J. THOMPSON. 1980. Annu. Rev. Neurosci. **3:** 141–167.
3. GORMAN, A. L. F., A. HERMANN & M. Y. THOMAS. 1981. Fed. Proc. **40:** 2233–2239.
4. HAGIWARA, S. & L. BYERLY. 1981. Annu. Rev. Neurosci. **4:** 69–125.
5. REUTER, H. 1979. Annu. Rev. Physiol. **41:** 413–424.
6. ARMSTRONG, C. M. & D. R. MATTESON. 1985. Science **227:** 65–67.
7. CARBONE, E. & H. D. LUX. 1984. Nature **310:** 501–502.
8. NOWYCKY, M. C., A. P. FOX & R. W. TSIEN. 1985. Nature **316:** 440–443.
9. NILIUS, M. C., A. P. FOX & R. W. TSIEN. 1985. Nature **316:** 443–446.
10. JANIS, R. A. & A. SCRIABINE. 1983. Biochem. Pharmacol. **32:** 3499–3507.
11. BOLGER, G. T., P. J. GENGO, E. M. LUCHOWSKI, H. SEIGEL, D. J. TRIGGLE & R. A. JANIS. 1982. Biochem. Biophys. Res. Commun. **104:** 1604–1609.
12. ALMERS, W., R. FUNK & P. T. PALADE. 1981. J. Physiol. London **312:** 177–207.
13. BEAN, B. P. 1984. Proc. Nat. Acad. Sci. USA **81:** 6388–6392.
14. SCHWARTZ, L., E. W. MCCLESKEY & W. ALMERS. 1985. Nature **314:** 747–751.
15. UEHARA, A. & J. R. HUME. 1985. J. Gen. Physiol. **85:** 621–647.
16. MURPHY, K. M. M., R. J. GOULD, B. L. LARGENT & S. H. SNYDER. 1983. Proc. Nat. Acad. Sci. USA **80:** 860–864.
17. GARCIA, M. L., V. F. KING, P. K. S. SEIGEL, J. P. REUBEN & G. J. KACZOROWSKI. 1986. J. Biol. Chem. **261:** 8146–8157.
18. GOULD, R. J., K. M. M. MURPHY & S. H. SNYDER. 1982. Proc. Nat. Acad. Sci. USA **79:** 3656–3660.
19. FERRY, D. R., A. GOLL & H. GLOSSMANN. 1983. Naunyn-Schmiedebergs Arch. Pharmacol. **323:** 292–297.
20. NORMAN, R. I., M. BORSOTTO, M. FOSSET, M. LAZDUNSKI & J. C. ELLORY. 1983. Biochem. Biophys. Res. Commun. **111:** 878–883.
21. VENTER, J. C., C. M. FRASER, J. S. SCHABER, C. Y. JUNG, G. BOLGER & D. J. TRIGGLE. 1983. J. Biol. Chem. **258:** 9344–9348.
22. FERRY, D. R., A. GOLL & H. GLOSSMANN. 1983. EMBO J. **2:** 1729–1732.
23. FERRY, D. R., A. GOLL & H. GLOSSMANN. 1984. FEBS Lett. **169:** 112–167.
24. FERRY, D. R., K. KAMPF, A. GOLL & H. GLOSSMANN. 1985. EMBO J. **4:** 1933–1940.
25. GALIZZI, J. P., M. BORSOTTO, J. BARHANIN, M. FOSSET & M. LAZDUNSKI. 1986. J. Biol. Chem. **261:** 1393–1397.
26. CURTIS, B. M. & W. A. CATTERALL. 1983. J. Biol. Chem. **258:** 7280–7283.
27. CURTIS, B. M. & W. A. CATTERALL. 1984. Biochemistry **23:** 2113–2118.
28. GLOSSMANN, H. & D. R. FERRY. 1983. Naunyn-Schmiedebergs Arch. Pharmacol. **323:** 279–291.
29. BORSOTTO, M., J. BARHANIN, R. I. NORMAN & M. LAZDUNSKI. 1984. Biochem. Biophys. Res. Commun. **122:** 1357–1366.
30. SANCHEZ, J. A. & E. STEFANI. 1978. J. Physiol. London **283:** 197–209.
31. ROSEMBLATT, M., C. HIDALGO, C. VERGARA & N. IKEMOTO. 1981. J. Biol. Chem. **256:** 8140–8148.
32. FOSSET, M., E. JAIMOVICH, E. DELPONT & M. LAZDUNSKI. 1983. J. Biol. Chem. **258:** 6086–6092.
33. GLOSSMANN, H., D. R. FERRY & C. B. BOSCHEK. 1983. Naunyn-Schmiedebergs Arch. Pharmacol. **323:** 1–11.
34. TAKAHASHI, M., M. J. SEAGAR, J. F. JONES, B. F. X. REBER & W. A. CATTERALL. 1987. Proc. Nat. Acad. Sci. USA. **84:** 5478–5482.
35. SCHMID, A., J. BARHANIN, T. COPPOLA, M. BORSOTTO & M. LAZDUNSKI. 1986. Biochemistry **25:** 3492–3495.

36. STRIESSNIG, J., K. MOOSBURGER, A. GOLL, D. R. FERRY & H. GLOSSMANN. 1986. Eur. J. Biochem. **161:** 603–609.
37. REUTER, H. 1974. J. Physiol. London **242:** 429–451.
38. REUTER, H. 1983. Nature **301:** 569–574.
39. TSIEN, R. W., W. GILES & P. GREENGARD. 1972. Nature New Biol. **240:** 181–183.
40. BRUM, G., V. FLOCKERZI, W. OSTERRIEDER & W. TRAUTWEIN. 1983. Pfluger's Arch. **398:** 147–154.
41. SCHMID, A., J. RENAUD & M. LAZDUNSKI. 1985. J. Biol. Chem. **260:** 13041–13046.
42. CURTIS, B. M. & W. A. CATTERALL. 1985. Proc. Nat. Acad. Sci. USA **82:** 2528–2532.
43. CATTERALL, W. A. 1986. Annu. Rev. Biochem. **55:** 953–985.
44. NODA, M., T. IKEDA, H. SUZUKI, H. TAKESHIMA, T. TAKAHASHI, M. KUNO & S. NUMA. 1986. Nature **322:** 826–828.
45. GOLDIN, A. L., T. SNUTCH, H. LUBBERT, A. DOWSETT, J. MARSHALL, V. AULD, W. DOWNEY, L. C. FRITZ, H. A. LESTER, R. DUNN, W. A. CATTERALL & N. DAVIDSON. 1986. Proc. Nat. Acad. Sci. USA **83:** 7503–7509.
46. REBER, B. F. X. & W. A. CATTERALL. 1987. J. Biol. Chem. **262:** 11369–11374.
47. SEAGAR, M. J., C. LABBE-JULLE, C. GRANIER, A. GOLL, H. GLOSSMANN, J. VAN REITSCHOTEN & F. COURAUD. 1986. Biochemistry **25:** 4051–4057.
48. HORNE, W. A., G. A. WEILAND & R. E. OSWALD. 1986. J. Biol. Chem. **261:** 3588–3594.
49. CURTIS, B. M. & W. A. CATTERALL. 1986. Biochemistry **25:** 3077–3083.
50. TAKAHASHI, M. & W. A. CATTERALL. 1987. Science **236:** 88–92.
51. TAKAHASHI, M. & W. A. CATTERALL. 1987. Biochemistry **26:** 5518–5526.

Mechanism of Action of Calcium Channel Modulator Drugs[a]

Identification of a Unique, Labile, Drug-Binding Polypeptide in a Purified Calcium Channel Preparation

PAL L. VAGHY, KIYOSHI ITAGAKI, KUNIHISA MIWA, EDWARD McKENNA, AND ARNOLD SCHWARTZ[b]

Department of Pharmacology and Cell Biophysics
University of Cincinnati
College of Medicine
231 Bethesda Avenue
Cincinnati, Ohio 45267-0575

Voltage-dependent calcium channels (VDCC) are complex membrane-spanning macromolecules that form a pore and promote a rapid influx of Ca^{2+} into the cell. VDCC play a key role in excitation-contraction and excitation-secretion coupling because they are regulated by a change in the membrane potential (i.e., "voltage"). In addition to the membrane potential, VDCC can also be modulated by several endogenous and exogenous modulators such as hormones, inorganic cations, drugs, and toxins (TABLE 1). The focus of this paper is on the mechanism of action of calcium channel modulator drugs. As such, identification of the drug-binding subunit in a purified skeletal muscle calcium channel preparation is essential.

PHARMACOLOGICAL AND STRUCTURAL CLASSIFICATION

Calcium channel modulator drugs are a pharmacologically and chemically heterogeneous group of compounds which selectively interact with the VDCC. Pharmacologically, they are divided into two groups: (1) calcium channel activators or "agonists," and (2) calcium channel inhibitors or "antagonists" (TABLE 2). Such a classification is, however, artificial since their effects are membrane potential dependent. Chemically, the selective calcium channel modulator drugs belong to three distinct groups: (1) 1,4-dihydropyridines, (2) phenylalkylamines, and (3) benzothiazepines. All of the known calcium channel activators to date such as (−)Bay k 8644,[1] (+)202-791,[2] CGP 28392,[3] YC-170,[4] and (−)H 160/51[5] belong to the 1,4-dihydropyridine family.

Several peptide toxins have also been identified. These toxins can produce activation or inhibition of the VDCC. Atrotoxin[6] and β-leptinotarsin-h[7] are clacium channel activators. In contrast, ω-conotoxin is an inhibitor peptide of the neuronal calcium channels.[8-11] Maitotoxin, the most potent marine toxin isolated from toxic dinoflagellates and poisonous fish inhabiting tropical seas, is a calcium channel activator of unknown chemical structure.[12-18]

[a]This work was supported in part by United States Public Health Service Grant PO1 HL-22619-06 (1C).

[b]To whom correspondence should be addressed.

PHARMACOLOGICAL EFFECTS AND MECHANISM OF ACTION

Calcium Channel Activator Drugs

Calcium channel activator drugs induce contraction of vascular smooth muscle by acting primarily on potential-operated calcium channels.[19] When the effect of an activator is studied over a broad concentration range, a biphasic contraction-relaxation response is observed in rat tail artery,[20–21] rabbit aortic,[4,22] and pig coronary artery rings.[23,24] A concentration-dependent biphasic positive-negative inotropic effect of calcium channel activators demonstrated in isolated cardiac muscle preparations[4,25–27] is consistent with the biphasic effects observed in vascular and nonvascular smooth muscle preparations. These data suggest that the activator and inhibitor properties reside in the same 1,4-dihydropyridine molecule.

TABLE 1. Overview of Voltage-Dependent Calcium Channel Modulators

- I. Membrane potential
  - 1. Voltage-dependent activation
  - 2. Voltage-dependent inactivation
- II. Endogenous modulators
  - A. Hormones
    - 1. Activation (phosphorylation)
    - 2. Inhibition (dephosphorylation)
  - B. Inorganic cations
    - 1. Permeable cations (Ba^{2+}, Ca^{2+}, Sr^{2+}, Mn^{2+})
    - 2. Inhibitors
      - a. Occupation of Ca-binding sites (Cd^{2+}, Ni^{2+}, Co^{2+})
      - b. Stimulation of dephosphorylation (Ca^{2+})
- III. Exogenous modulators
  - A. Drugs
    - 1. Activators: (−)Bay k 8644, (+)202-791, CGP 28392, YC-170, (−)H 160/51
    - 2. Inhibitors: 1,4-dihydropyridines, such as nifedipine; phenylalkylamines, such as verapamil; and benzothiazepines, such as diltiazem
  - B. Toxins
    - 1. Activators: maitotoxin, atrotoxin, β-leptinotarsin-h
    - 2. Inhibitors: ω-conotoxin

The effect of calcium channel activators is not only concentration dependent but membrane potential dependent as well. This is indicated by studies showing that the presence of a threshold concentration of KCl (~15 mM) is needed for an optimal contractile effect of Bay k 8644 in many isolated blood vessel preparations.[4,20–22] The positive and negative inotropic effects of Bay k 8644, YC-170, and (+)202-791 are also membrane potential dependent. Calcium channel activation and positive inotropy occur under polarized conditions, and calcium channel inhibition and negative inotropy result under depolarized conditions.[4,28–30] Activators prolong the action potential duration in isolated cardiac muscle preparations[3,31] and promote long-lasting openings in single calcium channel recordings.[32–36] Calcium channel activators, both 1,4-dihydropyridine derivatives and toxins, are useful tools for studying structure and function of VDCC in different tissues.

Calcium Channel Inhibitor Drugs

Calcium channel inhibitor drugs, also called "calcium antagonists" or "calcium entry blocking agents," have great experimental and clinical significance. The term "calcium antagonism" derives from the pioneer studies carried out in the mid-1960s in Germany by Albrecht Fleckenstein and his associates who demonstrated that prenylamine and verapamil treatment mimicked the cardiac effects of Ca^{2+} withdrawal. These drug effects could be overcome by elevation of extracellular Ca^{2+} concentration.[43] The initial studies were soon followed by very extensive pharmacological, electrophysiological, and biochemical investigations[32–39] which opened up new avenues not only for studies on the mechanism of excitation-contraction and excitation-secretion coupling processes but also for the treatment of angina pectoris and hypertension.[34,40–42] Voltage-clamp experiments have revealed that the action of calcium channel inhibitors is membrane potential (i.e., "voltage") dependent; the channel inhibition is much more pronounced at depolarized conditions than at

TABLE 2. Pharmacological and Structural Classification of Calcium Channel Modulator Drugs

I. Activators		II. Inhibitors
	1. 1,4-Dihydropyridines	
(−)Bay k 8644		(+)Bay k 8644
(+)202-791		(−)202-791
CGP 28392		Nifedipine
YC-170		Nitrendipine
(−)H 160/51		(+)H 160/51
		PN200-110
	2. Phenylalkylamines	
Not known		Verapamil
		Desmethoxyverapamil
		D-600
	3. Benzothiazepines	
Not known		Diltiazem
		TA 3090

hyperpolarized conditions.[44–47] The modulated receptor hypothesis,[48,49] which assumes that the affinity of drugs for the channel is "state" dependent, is consistent with the experimental observations. This allosteric model predicts that the drugs have a high affinity for the inactivated (I) and a low affinity for the resting (R) state.[45–47] Some recent direct binding data seem to support this assumption.[50]

All the calcium channel inhibitors have a common effect which is prolongation of the recovery of VDCC from inactivation ($I \rightarrow R$ transition). This explains why the effect is frequency (use) dependent.[44,51] When depolarization pulses follow each other with a low frequency, the effect of drugs may seem to be missing. The reason for this is that there is enough time even for the prolonged $I \rightarrow R$ transition to be completed between two depolarization pulses. When the time required for the recovery from inactivation is longer than the time between two depolarization pulses (which can be the case at high-frequency pulsing), the drug effect becomes apparent.

Stereoselective and high-affinity binding sites mediating the effect of calcium channel modulator drugs have been identified in all excitable tissue containing VDCC. The basic features of these receptor binding sites have recently been reviewed.[34] A complex allosteric model, which is termed "modulated gate model," has also been advanced to explain pharmacological, electrophysiological, and radioligand binding data obtained with VDCC modulator drugs.[52] This model assumes that not only the change in the membrane potential, as the modulated receptor hypothesis predicted, but all channel modulators listed in TABLE 1 are also able to produce a conformational change in the channel macromolecule. The modulator-induced conformational changes alter affinity of gate(s) for putative "gate binding site(s)" and, therefore, alter gating, i.e., activation, inactivation, and/or recovery from inactivation. These conformational changes may or may not alter the interaction between the channel macromolecule and other channel modulator(s). Analyzing the available experimental data, a number of predictions have been made that explain the effects of individual channel modulators in the framework of a modulated gate model.[52]

VOLTAGE-DEPENDENT CALCIUM CHANNEL AS A RECEPTOR FOR DRUGS

Direct evidence demonstrating that the receptors for calcium channel modulator drugs is in fact the VDCC may come from successful purification and reconstitution of functionally intact VDCC. Previous attempts to purify skeletal and cardiac muscle VDCC have yielded important results. These studies uniformly have revealed one large (160–190 kDa) "alpha" subunit which changes its electrophoretic mobility upon reduction with either dithiothreitol or β-mercaptoethanol.[36,37,53,54] Lazdunski and his associates maintain that VDCC consists of only this single large molecular weight (~170 kDa) polypeptide which dissociates to a 140 kDa and a 30 kDa polypeptide upon reduction.[53,54,64] In contrast, beta and gamma subunits have also been identified by others.[36,55,56] In the initial purification studies, prelabeling of membrane-bound VDCC by a radiolabeled 1,4-dihydropyridine derivative guided the purification. The degree of purification was assessed by measuring the radioactivity after each purification step. The measured radioactivity was corrected by the dissociation of the drug that occurred during the purification process.[36,54]

Rabbit skeletal muscle kept frozen at −70°C for several weeks is appropriate for obtaining a T-tubular membrane fraction highly enriched in dihydropyridine (DHP) binding sites.[57,58] The yield of T-tubules was significantly increased when French press treatment was also employed.[39] In these membranes, the B_{max} for (+)[^{3}H]PN200-110 binding varied between 10 and 20 pmol/mg protein and was allosterically regulated by both (−)D888 and *d-cis*-diltiazem.[34] When prelabeling with either [^{3}H]nitrendipine or (+)[^{3}H]PN200-110 and a four step purification as described by Curtis and Catterall[36] were employed, the major component of the purified preparation was a 190 kDa polypeptide that decreased its apparent molecular mass to 150 kDa upon reduction with 10 mM dithiothreitol.[39] This polypeptide appears to be identical with the α subunit originally described by Curtis and Catterall[36] and with the single polypeptide isolated by the Lazdunski group from skeletal and cardiac muscle.[53,54,64] We have purified and determined the N-terminal sequence of this polypeptide.[39]

The above-described purification procedure can be simplified by replacing prelabeling with postlabeling and by decreasing the purification steps from four to two, maintaining only the first WGA-Sepharose column chromatography and the sucrose density gradient centrifugation. Elimination of prelabeling is necessary for carrying out direct binding studies to the purified proteins. The B_{max} for (+)PN200-110 binding was approximately 1 nmol/mg protein and was increased up to 2 nmol/mg protein with *d-cis*-diltiazem.[34] The effect of (−)D888 on (+)[^{3}H]PN200-110 binding was identical to that in T-tubular membranes, i.e., an increase in K_D.[34] In fact, the only difference between binding to the purified protein and T-tubular membranes was the B_{max} which was 75–80 times higher in the purified protein. The presence of VDCC in this preparation was demonstrated by reconstitution of purified protein into bilayers and by measurement of an ion current through the reconstituted channel(s).[59] Although the reconstitution studies clearly show the presence of VDCC in the purified protein, they do not show that percentage of the purified protein consists of functionally intact VDCC. For that, reconstitution into phospholipid vesicles and flux studies will be required, as was done in Curtis and Catterall.[60]

To show which polypeptide is responsible for the drug binding, photoaffinity

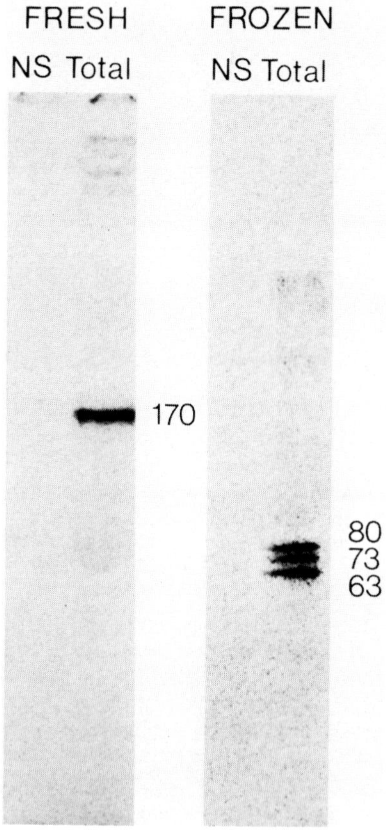

FIGURE 1. Photoaffinity labeling of the rabbit skeletal muscle 1,4-dihydropyridine receptor with [^{3}H]azidopine. T-tubular membranes isolated from rabbit skeletal muscle were photoaffinity labeled with (−)[^{3}H]azidopine as described in Reference 55. The polypeptide components were separated by sodium dodecyl sulfate polyacrylamide gel electrophoresis; the gels were impregnated with Enlightening^{TM}, a photoaffinity enhancer; and after drying, the fluorograms were exposed for three weeks at −70°C. The photoaffinity labeled polypeptides present in the membranes of frozen and fresh muscle are demonstrated.

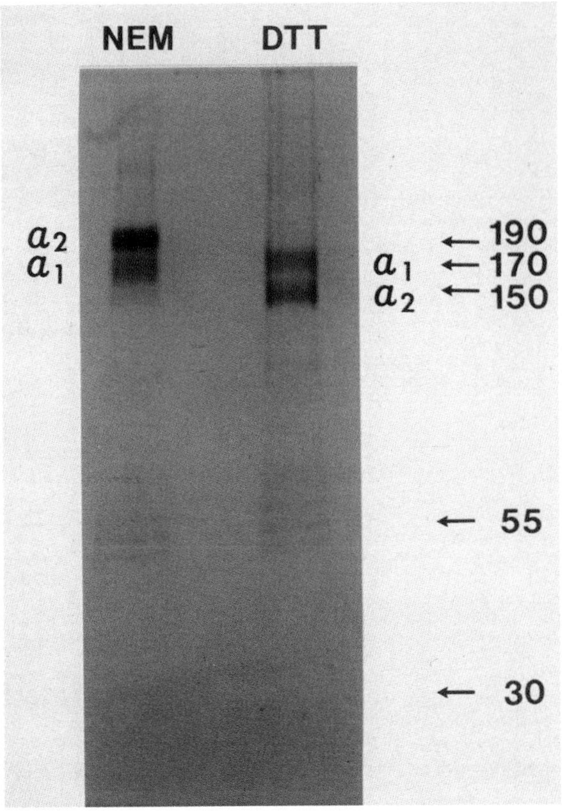

FIGURE 2. Subunit compositions of the purified rabbit skeletal muscle voltage-dependent calcium channel. One microgram purified protein was incubated at 60°C for 10 minutes with either 10 mM *N*-ethylmaleimide (NEM) or 10 mM dithiothreitol (DTT) in 100 μl sample buffer containing 2% sodium dodecyl sulfate, 10% (v/v) glycerol, and 125 mM Tris-HCl pH 6.8. The subunits of the purified calcium channel were separated on a 5–15% SDS polyacrylamide gel by electrophoresis. The polypeptides were visualized with silver staining.[63].

labeling of the purified preparation is required. We have used both a 1,4-dihydropyridine ([^{3}H]azidopine) and one phenylalkylamine derivative ([^{3}H]LU 49888) for these studies.

We found that not the 190 kDa polypeptide, which shifts its electrophoretic mobility to 150 upon reduction, but two to three polypeptides, ranging from 60 to 90 kDa, were photoaffinity labeled with (−)[^{3}H]azidopine and racemic [^{3}H]aziodopine.[61] The photoaffinity labeling experiments clearly showed that the large polypeptide, which changes its electrophoretic mobility upon reduction, is *not* the DHP-binding polypeptide. Since more than one polypeptide was labeled and the molecular weights varied in different preparations, we assumed that these photoaffinity labeled polypeptides were degradation products of a larger polypeptide. We determined that the degradation of the DHP-binding polypeptide occurred before or during isolation of

T-tubules (FIGURE 1). Elimination of French press treatment did not prevent degradation. Elimination of Ca^{2+} and inclusion of 5 mM EGTA in the incubation buffers were also ineffective in preventing degradation. It was found, however, that *the use of fresh muscle and a rapid processing of skeletal muscle from young rabbits* (body weight 1 kg or less) were essential for isolating a membrane fraction that contains only one approximately 155–170 kDa polypeptide which is specifically photoaffinity labeled with [^{3}H]azidopine (FIGURE 1). When purification from skeletal muscle membranes containing the 155–170 kDa [^{3}H]azidopine-binding protein was performed, a high-molecular-weight polypeptide 'doublet" was visualized in sodium dodecyl sulfate (SDS)–polyacrylamide gels under both alkylating and reducing conditions (FIGURE 2). The components of the "doublet," which we and Glossmann *et al.* (this volume) call here α_1 and α_2, can be identified by the criteria shown in TABLE 3. The simplest way to identify α_1 and α_2 subunits after electrophoresis is by inspection of a silver-stained gel. While the α_2 subunit, which was described in all previous studies,[36,37,53–56] is heavily stained by silver (dark gray band), the α_1 subunit is much less sensitive for this type of

TABLE 3. Criteria for Identification of Two Large-Molecular-Weight Putative Subunits of the Skeletal Muscle Voltage-Dependent Calcium Channel

Criteria	α_1	α_2
Silver/Staining	Weak (light brown)	Strong (dark gray)
Apparent M_r (SDS-PAGE)[a]		
10 mM NEM[b]	155–170 kDa	160–190 kDa
10 mM DTT[c] or βME[d]	155–170 kDa	130–150 kDa
Photoaffinity labeling		
With [^{3}H]azidopine	Yes	No
With [^{3}H]LU 49888	Yes	No
Phosphorylation (cAMP-dependent protein kinase)	Yes	No
Glycosylation	Weak	Strong

[a]Sodium dodecyl sulfate-polyacrylamide gel electrophoresis.
[b]*N*-Ethylmaleimide.
[c]Dithiothreitol.
[d]β-Mercaptoethanol.

staining (light brown band). This might be a reason for overlooking this important α_1 component of the VDCC in previous studies where less than 1 μg purified protein was used for electrophoresis. The α_1 subunit is unaltered by reduction with either dithiothreitol or β-mercaptoethanol. It is not only the DHP-binding subunit of the VDCC but it is also the phenylalkylamine binding subunit because it can be photoaffinity labeled with the phenylalkylamine [^{3}H]LU 49888.[62] The α_1 subunit can also be phosphorylated with the catalytic subunit of the cyclic adenosine monophosphate (cAMP)-dependent protein kinase (unpublished data), and it is less glycosylated than the α_2 subunit (TABLE 3). Further studies are needed to determine the exact role of α_1, α_2, β, and γ subunits of the skeletal muscle VDCC. A monoclonal antibody, 2F7, reactive with the α_1 subunit (Leung *et al.*, this volume) was used to probe a rabbit back skeletal muscle λgt11 cDNA expression library. Three clones were isolated and are presently being characterized (S. Ellis, A. T. Leung, K. Campbell, J. Robbins, M. Harpold, and A. Schwartz, unpublished data).

CONCLUSION

The voltage-dependent calcium channel in skeletal muscle T-tubules consists of at least two large-molecular-weight closely associated polypeptides. The designation "α_1" refers to a 150–170 kDa polypeptide that is characteristically labile, contains the receptors for the calcium channel modulator drugs, is phosphorylated by cAMP-dependent protein kinase, and does not change its electrophoretic mobility upon reduction with dithiothreitol or β-mercaptoethanol. The other protein "α_2" originally described by Curtis and Catterall[36] and Lazdunski *et al.*[53,54,64] is stable, does not contain the drug receptors, is not phosphorylated, and is characteristically reduced by dithiothreitol or β-mercaptoethanol to a 130–150 kDa and a 25–35 kDa polypeptide.

ACKNOWLEDGMENTS

We should like to thank Ms. Susan Koelliker and Mr. Ross Agnor for their skillful technical assistance, Ms. Kathleen Smidebush for typing the manuscript, and Ms. Gwen Kraft for preparing the figures.

REFERENCES

1. FRANCKOWIAK, G., M. BECHEN, M. SCHRAMM & G. THOMAS. 1985. The optical isomers of the 1,4-dihydropyridine Bay k 8644 show opposite effects on calcium channels. Eur. J. Pharmacol. **114:** 223–226.
2. HOF, R. P., U. T. REUGG, A. HOF & A. VOGEL. 1985. Stereoselectivity at the calcium channel: opposite action of the enantiomers of a 1,4-dihydropyridine. J. Cardiovasc. Pharmacol. **7:** 689–693.
3. PREUSS, K. C., N. L. CHEUNG, H. L. BROOKS & D. C. WARLTIER. 1984. Cardiovascular effects of the nifedipine analog, CGP 28392, in the conscious dog. J. Cardiovasc. Pharmacol. **6:** 949–953.
4. NAKAYA, H., Y. HATTORI, N. TOHSE & M. KANNO. 1986. Voltage-dependent effects of YC-170, a dihydropyridine calcium channel modulator, in cardiovascular tissues. Naunyn-Schmiedeberg's Arch. Pharmacol. **333:** 421–430.
5. GJORSTRUP, P., H. HARDING, R. ISAKSSON & C. WESTERLUND. 1986. The enantiomers of the dihydropyridine derivative H 160/51 show opposite effects of stimulation and inhibition. Eur. J. Pharmacol. **122:** 357–361.
6. HAMILTON, S., A. YATANI, M. J. HAWKES, K. REDDING & A. M. BROWN. 1985. Atrotoxin: a specific agonist for calcium currents in heart. Science **229:** 182–184.
7. CROSLAND, R. D., T. H. HSIAO & W. O. MCCLURE. 1984. Purification and characterization of β-leptinotarsin-h, an activator of presynaptic calcium channels. Biochemistry **23:** 734–741.
8. OLIVERA, B. M., W. R. GRAY, R. ZEIKUS, J. M. MCINTOSH, J. VARGA, J. RIVIER, V. DESANTOS & L. J. CRUZ. 1985. Peptide neurotoxins from fish-hunting cone snails. Science **230:** 1338–1343.
9. CRUZ, L. J., W. R. GRAY, D. YOSHIKAMI & B. M. OLIVERA. 1985. *Conus* venoms: a rich source of neuroactive peptides. J. Toxicol. Toxin Rev. **4**(2): 107–132.
10. CRUZ, L. J. & B. M. OLIVERA. 1986. Calcium channel antagonists. ω-Conotoxin defines a new high affinity site. J. Biol. Chem. **261**(14): 6230–6233.
11. REYNOLDS, I. J., J. A. WAGNER, S. H. SNYDER, S. A. THAYER, B. M. OLIVERA & R. J. MILLER. 1986. Brain voltage-sensitive calcium channel subtypes differentiated by ω-conotoxin fraction GVIA. Proc. Nat. Acad. Sci. USA **83:** 8804–8807.
12. TAKAHASHI, M., Y. OHIZUMI & T. YASUMOTO. 1982. Maitotoxin, a Ca^{2+} channel activator candidate. J. Biol. Chem. **257**(13): 7287–7289.

13. TAKAHASHI, M., M. TATSUMI, Y. OHIZUMI & T. YASUMOTO. 1983. Ca^{2+} channel activating function of maitotoxin, the most potent marine toxin known, in clonal rat pheochromocytoma cells. J. Biol. Chem. **258**(18): 10944–10949.
14. OHIZUMI, Y. & T. YASUMOTO. 1983. Contractile response of the rabbit aorta to maitotoxin, the most potent marine toxin. J. Physiol. **337:** 711–721.
15. OHIZUMI, Y., A. KAJIWARA & T. YASUMOTO. 1983. Excitatory effect of the most potent marine toxin, maitotoxin, on the guinea-pig vas deferens. J. Pharmacol. Exp. Ther. **227**(1): 199–204.
16. FREEDMAN, S. B., R. J. MILLER, D. M. MILLER & D. R. TINDALL. 1984. Interactions of maitotoxin with voltage-sensitive calcium channels in cultured neuronal cells. Proc. Nat. Acad. Sci. USA **81:** 4582–4585.
17. MIYAMOTO, T., Y. OHIZUMI, H. WASHIO & YASUMOTO. 1984. Potent excitatory effect of maitotoxin on Ca channels in the insect skeletal muscle. Pflugers Arch. Eur. J. Physiol. **400:** 439–441.
18. LOGIN, I. S., A. M. JUDD, M. J. CRONIN, K. KOIKE, G. SCHETTINI, T. YASUMOTO & R. M. MACLEOD. 1985. The effects of maitotoxin on $^{45}Ca^{2+}$ flux and hormone release in GH_3 rat pituitary cells. Endocrinology **116**(1): 622–627.
19. YAMAMOTO, H., O. HWANG & C. VAN BREEMEN. 1984. Bay k 8644 differentiates between potential and receptor operated Ca^{2+} channels. Eur. J. Pharmacol. **102:** 555–557.
20. SU, C. M., V. C. SWAMY & D. J. TRIGGLE. 1984. Calcium channel activation in vascular smooth muscle by Bay k 8644. Can. J. Physiol. Pharmacol. **62:** 1401–1410.
21. WEI, X. Y., E. M. LUCHOWSKI, A. RUTLEDGE, C. M. SU & D. J. TRIGGLE. 1986. Pharmacologic and radioligand binding analysis of the actions of 1,4-dihydropyridine activator-antagonist pairs in smooth muscle. J. Pharmacol. Exp. Ther. **239**(1): 144–153.
22. SCHRAMM, M., R. TOWART, B. LAMP & G. THOMAS. 1985. Modulation of calcium ion influx by the 1,4-dihydropyridines nifedipine and Bay k 8644. J. Cardiovasc. Pharmacol. **7:** 493–496.
23. DUBE, G. P., Y. H. BAIK & A. SCHWARTZ. 1985. Effects of a novel calcium channel agonist dihydropyridine analogue, Bay k 8644, on pig coronary artery: biphasic mechanical response and paradoxical potentiation of contraction by diltiazem and nimodipine. J. Cardiovasc. Pharmacol. **7:** 377–389.
24. DUBE, G. P., Y. H. BAIK, P. L. VAGHY & A. SCHWARTZ. 1985. Nitrendipine potentiates Bay k 8644-induced contraction of isolated porcine coronary artery: evidence for functionally distinct dihydropyridine receptor subtypes. Biochem. Biophys. Res. Commun. **128:**(3): 1295–1302.
25. SCHWARTZ, A., I. L. GRUPP, G. GRUPP, J. S. WILLIAMS & P. L. VAGHY. 1984. Effects of dihydropyridine calcium channel modulators in the heart: pharmacological and radioligand binding correlations. Biochem. Biophys. Res. Commun. **125**(1): 387–394.
26. WILLIAMS, J. S., I. L. GRUPP, G. GRUPP, P. L. VAGHY, L. DUMONT, A. SCHWARTZ, A. YATANI, S. HAMILTON & A. M. BROWN. 1985. Profile of the oppositely acting enantiomers of the dihydropyridine 202-791 in cardiac preparations: receptor binding, electrophysiological, and pharmacological studies. Biochem. Biophys. Res. Commun. **131**(1): 13–21.
27. THOMAS, G., R. GROB & M. SCHRAMM. 1984. Calcium channel modulation: ability to inhibit or promote calcium influx resides in the same dihydropyridine molecule. J. Cardiovasc. Pharmacol. **6:** 1170–1176.
28. SANGUINETTI, M. C. & R. S. KASS. 1984. Regulation of cardiac calcium channel current and contractile activity by the dihydropyridine Bay k 8644 is voltage-dependent. J. Mol. Cell. Cardiol. **16:** 667–670.
29. SANGUINETTI, M. C., D. S. KRAFTE & R. S. KASS. 1986. Voltage-dependent modulation of Ca channel current in heart cells by Bay k 8644. J. Gen. Physiol. **88:** 369–392.
30. KAMP, T. J., R. J. MILLER & M. C. SANGUINETTI. 1987. The "agonist" enantiomer of the dihydropyridine (DHP) 202-791 blocks I_{Ca} at depolarized potentials. Biophys. J. **51:** 429a.
31. THOMAS, G., M. CHUNG & C. J. COHEN. 1985. A dihydropyridine (Bay k 8644) that enhances calcium currents in guinea pig and calf myocardial cells. A new type of positive inotropic agent. Circ. Res. **56:** 87–96.

32. GLOSSMANN, H., D. R. FERRY, A. GOLL, J. STRIESSNIG & G. ZERNIG. 1985. Calcium channels and calcium channel drugs: recent biochemical and biophysical findings. Arzneim-Forsch./Drug Res. **35**(11): 1917–1935.
33. GARCIA, M. L., V. F. KING, P. K. S. SIEGL, J. P. REUBEN & G. J. KACZOROWSKI. 1986. Binding of Ca^{2+} entry blockers to cardiac sarcolemmal membrane vesicles. J. Biol. Chem. **261**(18): 8146–8157.
34. VAGHY, P. L., J. S. WILLIAMS & A. SCHWARTZ. 1987. Receptor pharmacology of calcium entry blocking agents. Am. J. Cardiol. **59:** 9A–17A.
35. GLOSSMANN, H. & D. R. FERRY. 1983. Solubilization and partial purification of putative calcium channels labelled with [^{3}H]-Nimodipine. Naunyn-Schmiedeberg's Arch. Pharmacol. **323:** 279–291.
36. CURTIS, B. M. & W. A. CATTERALL. 1984. Purification of the calcium antagonist receptor of the voltage-sensitive calcium channel from skeletal muscle transverse tubules. Biochemistry **23**(10): 2113–2118.
37. BORSOTTO, M., J. BARHANIN, M. FOSSET & M. LAZDUNSKI. 1985. The 1,4-dihydropyridine receptor associated with the skeletal muscle voltage-dependent Ca^{2+} channel. J. Biol. Chem. **260**(26): 14255–14263.
38. HORNE, W. A., G. A. WEILAND & R. E. OSWALD. 1986. Solubilization and hydrodynamic characterization of the dihydropyridine receptor from rat ventricular muscle. J. Biol. Chem. **261**(8): 3588–3594.
39. NAKAYAMA, N., T. L. KIRLEY, P. L. VAGHY, E. MCKENNA & A. SCHWARTZ. 1987. Purification of a putative Ca^{2+} channel protein from rabbit skeletal muscle: determination of the amino-terminal sequence. J. Biol. Chem. **262:** 6572–6576.
40. ELLRODT, A. G. & B. N. SINGH. 1983. Clinical applications of slow channel blocking compounds. Pharmacol. Ther. **23:** 1–43.
41. SNYDER S. H. & I. J. REYNOLDS. 1985. Calcium-antagonist drugs. Receptor interactions that clarify therapeutic effects. N England J. Med. **313:**(16): 995–1002.
42. NAYLER, W. G. & J. D. HOROWITZ. 1983. Calcium antagonists: a new class of drugs. Pharmacol. Ther. **20:** 203–262.
43. FLECKENSTEIN, A. 1983. History of calcium antagonists. Circ. Res. **52**(2 suppl I): I-3–I-16.
44. LEE, K. S. & R. W. TSIEN. 1983. Mechanism of calcium channel blockade by verapamil, D600, diltiazem and nitrendipine in single dialysed heart cells. Nature **302:** 790–794.
45. KANAYA, S., P. ARLOCK, B. G. KATZUNG & L. M. HONDEGHEM. 1983. Diltiazem and verapamil preferentially block inactivated cardiac calcium channels. J. Mol. Cell. Cardiol. **15:** 145–148.
46. BEAN, B. P. 1984. Nitrendipine block of cardiac calcium channels: high-affinity binding to the inactivated state. Proc. Nat. Acad. Sci. USA **81:** 6388–6392.
47. SANGUINETTI, M. C. & R. S. KASS. 1984. Voltage-dependent block of calcium channel current in the calf purkinje fiber by dihydropyridine calcium channel antagonists. Circ. Res. **55**(3): 336–348.
48. HILLE, B. 1977. Local anesthetics: hydrophilic and hydrophobic pathways for the drug-receptor reaction. J. Gen. Physiol. **69:** 497–515.
49. HONDEGHEM, L. M. & B. G. KATZUNG. 1977. Time- and voltage-dependent interactions of antiarrhythmic drugs with cardiac sodium channels. Biochim. Biophys. Acta **472:** 373–398.
50. KOKUBUN, S., B. PROD'HOM, C. BECKER, H. PORZIG & H. REUTER. 1986. Studies on Ca channels in intact cardiac cells: voltage-dependent effects and cooperative interactions of dihydropyridine enantiomers. Mol. Pharmacol. **30:** 571–584.
51. PELZER, D., W. TRAUTWEIN & T. F. MCDONALD. 1982. Calcium channel block and recovery from block in mammalian ventricular muscle treated with organic channel inhibitors. Pflugers Arch. **394:** 97–105.
52. VAGHY, P. L. 1987. Modulated gate model for ion permeation and drug action in voltage-dependent Ca channels. Biophys. J. **51:** 432a.
53. LAZDUNSKI, M., J. BARHANIN, M. BORSOTTO, M. FOSSET, J.-P. GALIZZI, J. F. RENAUD, G. ROMEY & A. SCHMID. 1986. Dihydropyridine-sensitive Ca^{2+} channels: molecular properties of interaction with Ca^{2+} channel blockers, purification, subunit structure, and differentiation. J. Cardiovasc. Pharmacol. **8**(suppl. 8): S13–S19.

54. Cooper, C. L., S. Vandaele, J. Barhanin, M. Fosset, M. Lazdunski & M. M. Hosey. 1987. Purification and characterization of the dihydropyridine-sensitive voltage-dependent calcium channel from cardiac tissue. J. Biol. Chem. **262**(2): 509–512.
55. Striessnig, J., K. Moosburger, A. Goll, D. R. Ferry & H. Glossmann. 1986. Stereoselective photoaffinity labelling of the purified 1,4-dihydropyridine receptor of the voltage-dependent calcium channel. Eur. J. Biochem. **161:** 603–609.
56. Flockerzi, V., H.-J. Oeken, F. Hofmann, D. Pelzer, A. Cavalie & W. Trautwein. 1986. Purified dihydropyridine-binding site from skeletal muscle t-tubules is a functional calcium channel. Nature **323:** 66–68.
57. Fosset, M., E. Jaimovich, E. Delpont & M. Lazdunski. 1983. [^{3}H]Nitrendipine receptors in skeletal muscle. Properties and preferential localization in transverse tubules. J. Biol. Chem. **258**(10): 6086–6092.
58. Galizzi, J.-P., M. Fosset & M. Lazdunski. 1984. Properties of receptors for the Ca^{2+}-channel blocker verapamil in transverse-tubule membranes of skeletal muscle. Stereospecificity, effect of Ca^{2+} and other inorganic cations, evidence for two categories of sites and effect of nucleoside triphosphates. Eur. J. Biochem. **144:** 211–215.
59. Smith, J. S., E. J. McKenna, J. Ma, J. Vilven, P. L. Vaghy, A. Schwartz & R. Coronado. Calcium channel activity in a purified dihydropyridine receptor preparation of skeletal muscle. Biochemistry. (In press.)
60. Curtis, B. M. & W. A. Catterall. 1986. Reconstitution of the voltage-sensitive calcium channel purified from skeletal muscle transverse tubules. Biochemistry **25:** 3077–3083.
61. Miwa, K., P. L. Vaghy, E. McKenna, J. L. Balwierczak, J. Striessnig, H. Glossmann & A. Schwartz. 1987. Photoaffinity labelling of the rabbit skeletal muscle 1,4-dihydropyridine receptor with (−)[^{3}H]azidopine. Fed. Proc. **46:** 395.
62. Striessnig, J., H.-G. Knaus, M. Grabner, K. Moosburger, W. Seitz, H. Lietz & H. Glossmann. 1987. Photoaffinity labelling of the phenylalkylamine receptor of the skeletal muscle transverse-tubule calcium channel. FEBS Lett. **212**(2): 247–253.
63. Ansorge, W. 1985. Fast and sensitive detection of protein and DNA bands by treatment with potassium permanganate. J. Biochem. Biophys. Methods **11:** 13–20.
64. Vandaele, S., M. Fosset, J.-P. Galizzi & M. Lazdunski. 1987. Monoclonal antibodies that coimmunoprecipitate the 1,4-dihydropyridine and phenylalkylamine receptors and reveal the Ca^{2+} channel structure. Biochemistry **26:** 5–9.

Plasticity of Neuronal L-Type Calcium Channels

S. GOVONI, F. BATTAINI,[a] S. M. MAGNONI, L. LUCCHI, R. A. RIUS, AND M. TRABUCCHI[a]

Institute of Pharmacological Sciences
University of Milan
Via Andrea Del Sarto, 21
20129 Milan, Italy

The neuron strictly controls the concentration of free intracellular calcium by means of several mechanisms including channels, pumps, and exchangers. The voltage-dependent channels are the main route of entry of calcium from the extracellular space. Nowycky *et al.* have provided evidence of the existence in peripheral neurons of three types of voltage-dependent calcium channels (VDCC) called T, L, and N.[1]

The three types of channels are activated by different levels of depolarization, have different times of inactivation, and have a specific pharmacology. The L-type is sensitive to organic calcium antagonists, in particular to dihydropyridines (DHP), whereas the T-type and the N-type are not.[1] The dihydropyridine calcium antagonists reduce the probability of channel opening while dihydropyridine agonists increase the number of long openings.[2] A peptide neurotoxin isolated from the venom of the cone snail *Conus geographus,*[3] omega-conotoxin (omega-CgTx), blocks both the L-type and the N-type channels in peripheral neurons. T-type channels are insensitive to this substance. The characteristics of VDCC in the brain are less clear.

VDCC have been investigated both by means of binding studies using labeled antagonist and functional tests examining calcium uptake and transmitter release. In synaptosomal preparations both DHP and omega-CgTx binding sites are found; the density of toxin sites is 10- to 20-fold higher than DHP receptors.[4] Studies on the anatomical distribution of the channels indicate that N channels are distributed prevalently on nerve terminals while L channels are mainly present on neuronal cell bodies.[3,4]

A recent study examining the sensitivity of voltage-dependent calcium fluxes in brain synaptosomes suggests that Ca^{2+} influx and evoked neurotransmitter release are mediated by N-type (DHP insensitive; omega-CgTx sensitive) VDCC.[4] The insensitivity of Ca^{2+} influx and neurotransmitter release to calcium antagonists found by several authors in synaptosomal preparations[5–7] might be explained by the relatively small number of DHP-sensitive channels and by their anatomical location.

On the other hand, Turner and Goldin have reported an effect of DHP at concentrations less than micromolar on calcium uptake and neurotransmitter release in synaptosomes.[8] In addition, using different experimental models, other authors have also shown an effect of calcium antagonists on neurotransmitter release. For example dihydropyridines can inhibit the calcium-agonist-stimulated release of serotonin from rat cortex slices,[9] and the K^+-stimulated release of substance P from dorsal root ganglia[10] and flunarizine (a calcium antagonist belonging to another chemical class) can inhibit the K^+-stimulated release of dopamine from striatal slices.[11,12] Moreover

[a]Chair of Toxicology, 2nd University of Rome, Via Orazio Raimondo, 00173 Rome, Italy.

the release of norepinephrine, which is insensitive to low concentrations of DHP in brain synaptosomes or in sympathetic ganglia preparations, is inhibited by nanomolar concentrations of nitrendipine (NTP) when using PC12 cells.[13] It appears therefore that the N-type channels are strategically located and mainly involved in the release of neurotransmitters while the role of L channels is less clear, although in some experimental conditions their blockade may indeed cause inhibition of transmitter release.

The interest in the role of central nervous system (CNS) DHP-binding sites is increased by several observations in the literature indicating that their density or affinity can be modified by various conditions which include treatments *in vivo* and *in vitro* with drugs or neurotoxic substances,[14–19] genetic hypertension,[20] and physiological aging[21,22] (see TABLE 1).

TABLE 1. Regulation of Calcium Antagonist Binding and Calcium Fluxes at Brain Level[a]

Condition	Brain Area	Ca^{2+} Flux	3H-NTP Binding	Reference
In vivo				
Chronic morphine	Various	i	i	16
Acute ethanol	Various	i	i	15
Chronic ethanol (low doses)	Striatum	d	d	14
Chronic ethanol (inhalation)	Cortex	—	i	27
Chronic nifendipine and verapamil	Cortex	d	d	19
Chronic chloropromazine	Whole	—	i	40
Chronic lead	Striatum Cortex	—	i	17, 41
Aging	Cortex	d	d	21
SHR	Whole	—	i	20
Cardiomyopathic hamster	Whole	i	i	31
DOCA hypertension	Brain stem	—	d	42
In vitro				
Phencyclidine	Whole	i	i	32
Lead	Striatum	—	i	43
Phenytoin	Whole	—	d	44
Substance P	Hippocampus	i	i	45

[a] i = increase; d = decrease; SHR = spontaneously hypertensive rat; DOCA = dihydroxycorticosterone acetate.

The purpose of the present paper is to review in detail some of our experience in this particular field and to present new experiments providing evidence for the plasticity of CNS DHP-binding sites after *in vivo* and *in vitro* treatments stressing that the changes present regional selectivity and may be coupled to changes in calcium uptake.

Our first experiments in this area investigated the effect of lead poisoning on ^{3}H-NTP binding in rat brain. Lead intoxication modifies various neurochemical parameters and in particular the functional state of several neurotransmitters. The effect of lead on neurotransmitters may be due to an interaction with calcium. Preliminary *in vitro* experiments showed indeed that in synaptic membranes prepared

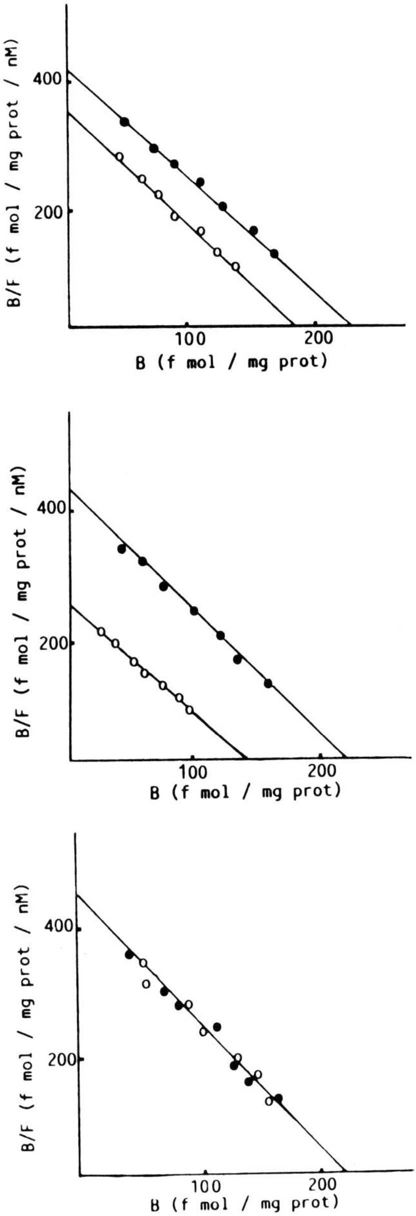

FIGURE 1. Scatchard analysis of ^{3}H-nitrendipine binding to Tris-washed membranes from cortex (upper panel), striatum (middle panel), and hippocampus (lower panel) of control (open circles) and lead-exposed rats (filled circles). Lead exposure and nitrendipine binding were performed as indicated in Reference 41.

from rat cortex, lead substituted for calcium in restoring ^{3}H-DHP binding after treatment of the membranes with chelating agents. Therefore the chronic treatment with lead had the potential of modifying DHP binding. This was indeed the case as shown in FIGURE 1.

After *in vivo* lead exposure (for over two months since the neonatal life by means of lead acetate in the drinking water) ^{3}H-NTP binding to crude synaptosomal membranes shows an increase in B_{max} in cortex (+25%) and striatum (+54%). Interestingly, studying in the same animals another brain area, the hippocampus, we found no differences in binding in the treated animals. This was the first observation in the literature indicating that CNS DHP-binding sites may display regional differences in response to a treatment.

We wanted to investigate further the *in vitro* effect of various ions on ^{3}H-NTP binding. The *in vitro* studies (TABLE 2) indicate that hippocampal nitrendipine binding has a different sensitivity to certain ions in comparison with cortex and basal ganglia. In fact, zinc stimulates the binding in all areas but the extent of stimulation is less in hippocampus (213% versus 403% in cortex and 333% in striatum); La^{3+} is always inhibitory; Pb^{2+} and Mn^{2+} stimulate the binding in striatum and cortex but not in hippocampus, where Pb^{2+} even inhibits the calcium-stimulated binding. These data shed some light on the possible mechanism of the area-selective neurotoxicity of lead and in addition strongly support the concept that DHP-sensitive voltage-dependent calcium channels may present regional differences in their characteristics.

Another substance that has the potential of modifying DHP binding when administered *in vivo* is ethanol. In fact changes of neuronal calcium metabolism have been implicated in the acute and chronic CNS effects of ethanol. In particular, the *in vivo* administration causes depletion of brain calcium content[23] and alters calcium movements.[14,24] The mechanism involved in the effect of ethanol on calcium metabolism still remain unknown, although altered calcium conductance and sensitivity have been reported.[25] Moreover in cultures of clonal neural cells the presence of ethanol (200 mM) in the medium for six days increases the number of DHP-binding sites and the K^+-stimulated $^{45}Ca^{2+}$ uptake.[26]

TABLE 2. Effect of Various Ions on ^{3}H-Nitrendipine Binding to Synaptic Membranes Prepared from Rat Cortex, Hippocampus, and Striatum[a]

Ion	Concentration (mM)	Brain Area		
		Cortex	Striatum	Hippocampus
Zn^{2+}	0.15	247	220	160
	0.30	403	333	213
	0.60	353	287	180
Pb^{2+}	0.15	280	227	90
	0.30	327	300	100
	0.60	280	327	126
Mn^{2+}	0.15	135	149	84
	0.30	141	155	110
	0.60	140	155	115
La^{3+}	0.15	40	52	55
	0.30	2	2	20
	0.60	2	2	2

[a] Values are expressed as percent of binding in absence of added ions. Each point is the mean of 5 experiments with standard error within 2–12% of the mean.

TABLE 3. Effect of the *In Vivo* Treatment with Ethanol and Acetaldehyde on ^{3}H-Nitrendipine Binding in Various Rat Brain Areas[a]

	Cortex		Hippocampus		Striatum	
	B_{max}	K_d	B_{max}	K_d	B_{max}	K_d
Control	160 ± 15	0.45 ± .04	201 ± 19	0.42 ± .04	157 ± 15	0.39 ± .04
Ethanol						
40 minutes	217 ± 17[b]	0.50 ± .05	268 ± 24[b]	0.48 ± .04	239 ± 21[b]	0.45 ± .04
8 hours	139 ± 12	0.24 ± .02[b]	170 ± 18	0.17 ± .02[b]	143 ± 14	0.19 ± .02[b]
16 hours	142 ± 14	0.28 ± .03[b]	169 ± 18	0.23 ± .03	143 ± 14	0.21 ± .02[b]
24 hours	141 ± 15	0.36 ± .04	172 ± 18	0.38 ± .04	151 ± 14	0.35 ± .04
Acetaldehyde						
5 minutes	189 ± 13	0.44 ± .05	229 ± 21	0.44 ± .03	185 ± 18	0.37 ± .04
15 minutes	225 ± 21[b]	0.37 ± .04	275 ± 26[b]	0.35 ± .04	235 ± 23[b]	0.30 ± .03
2 hours	155 ± 16	0.43 ± .04	205 ± 20	0.44 ± .05	158 ± 14	0.40 ± .04

[a] B_{max} is expressed as fmol/mg protein; K_d as nM. Values are means ± standard deviation of 4 independent experiments with triplicate samples.
[b] $p < 0.05$ two-tailed Dunnet's t test.

Along this line, we found that DHP binding can also be acutely modified. In fact, the single injection of a high dose of ethanol (3 g/kg) produces in 40 minutes an increase in DHP-binding sites in the cortex which returns to control levels within 4 hours (but at this time the affinity increases and remains high for 16 hours). Acetaldehyde administration has similar effects but its action is even quicker: the increase of DHP sites is already present (although not yet significant) 5 minutes after the administration and maximal within 15 minutes (TABLE 3).

In our hands, during chronic treatment with low doses of ethanol (6% in the drinking water for 4 weeks) the changes are opposite. In particular, we showed in a previous study that the calcium-dependent binding of nitrendipine is reduced in striatum and in the same tissue the K^+-evoked calcium uptake is also decreased.[14] These results are at variance with those of Little *et al.* who observe an increased binding after both acute and chronic treatment.[27] However, the two conditions of chronic exposure are very different, since we use low doses in the drinking water for 4 weeks (with this protocol the animals do not show withdrawal signs upon interruption of the treatment), while Little exposed the animals to a high dose of ethanol giving origin to a more drastic intoxication (with very heavy signs of withdrawal).

The molecular mechanisms by which acute ethanol first alters the number of sites and then the binding affinity are not understood. The observation that the acute ethanol modification of the calcium channel site labeled by ^{3}H-NTP is widely distributed in the CNS suggests a mechanism such as ethanol-induced changes in the structure and function of neuronal membranes. However, the observation that ethanol does not modify ^{3}H-NTP binding *in vitro* (except at very high concentrations) indicates that the interaction is either mediated by a metabolite or needs neuronal integrity to be expressed.[15]

Another condition that modifies within a brief time the binding of ^{3}H-NTP is experimental brain ischemia. Increasing evidence has pointed to the pathophysiological role of Ca^{2+} in ischemic brain.[28,29] Interruption of cerebral blood flow leads within a few seconds to the disruption of calcium homeostasis: the result is a rapid accumulation of Ca^{2+} within the cells. Further sources are mitochondria and the endoplasmic reticulum, which in the condition of ischemia releases the ion in the cytoplasm. In this

TABLE 4. Maximum Number of Binding Sites (B_{max} = fmol/mg Protein) for ^{3}H-Nitrendipine Binding to Neuronal Membranes of Various Cerebral Areas following Ischemia Induced by 1 Hour Right Carotid Occlusion[a]

	Hippocampus		Cortex		Striatum	
	Right	Left	Right	Left	Right	Left
Control	220 ± 10	220 ± 20	190 ± 20	195 ± 19	180 ± 19	183 ± 18
Right carotid occlusion	292 ± 23[b]	220 ± 21	192 ± 11	190 ± 20	180 ± 19	182 ± 19

[a]Values are means ± standard deviation of 4 independent experiments.
[b]$p < 0.05$.

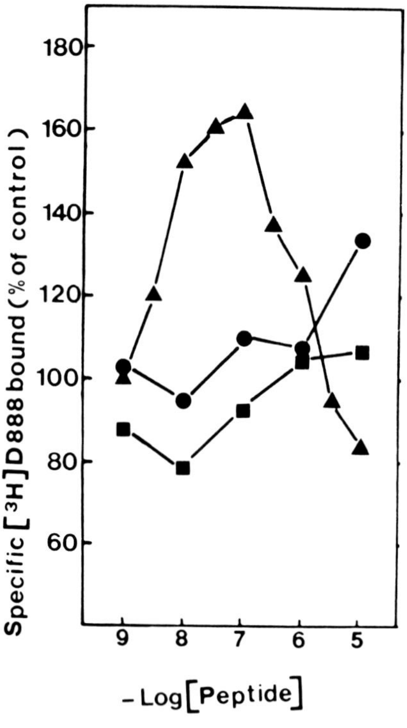

FIGURE 2. Effect of substance P (triangles), neurotensin (circles), and met-enkephalin (squares) on the binding of ^{3}H-D888 to synaptic membranes prepared from rat hippocampus. Tissues were homogenized with a motor-driven pestle (teflon in glass, 10 strokes at 700 rpm in 20 vol of 0.32 M sucrose. After centrifugation at 1000 × *g* for 10 minutes the supernatant was centrifuged at 48,000 × *g* for 15 minutes, the resulting pellet was treated with 10 mM EDTA, and then 10 mM EGTA (30 minutes at 4°C each), and washed twice in Hepes buffer. [^{3}H]D888 binding was performed in a final volume of 0.25 ml Hepes buffer with 30 μg of membrane proteins and incubated for 60 minutes at 22°C; nonspecific binding was defined by 0.1 mM (−)D600. Bound radioactivity was separated on Whatman GF/C filters presoaked in buffer containing 0.5% polyethyleneimine for 20 minutes and washed twice with 5 ml ice cold buffer.

view, we have explored the possibility that the kinetic characteristics of DHP-binding sites may be affected by ischemia. The results (TABLE 4) show that short-term mild ischemia, induced in the rat by 60 minutes of right carotid occlusion, causes in the ipsilateral hippocampus a significant increase in the number of DHP-binding sites, which may be related to an increase of Ca^{2+} influx into the cells. It is important to note that this effect is selective, at least in the beginning, for the hippocampus, a cerebral area particularly susceptible to ischemia. Presumably, the basis of this vulnerability is related to the ischemia-induced release of excitatory amino acids like glutamate, the terminals of which are particularly dense in some regions of the hippocampus.

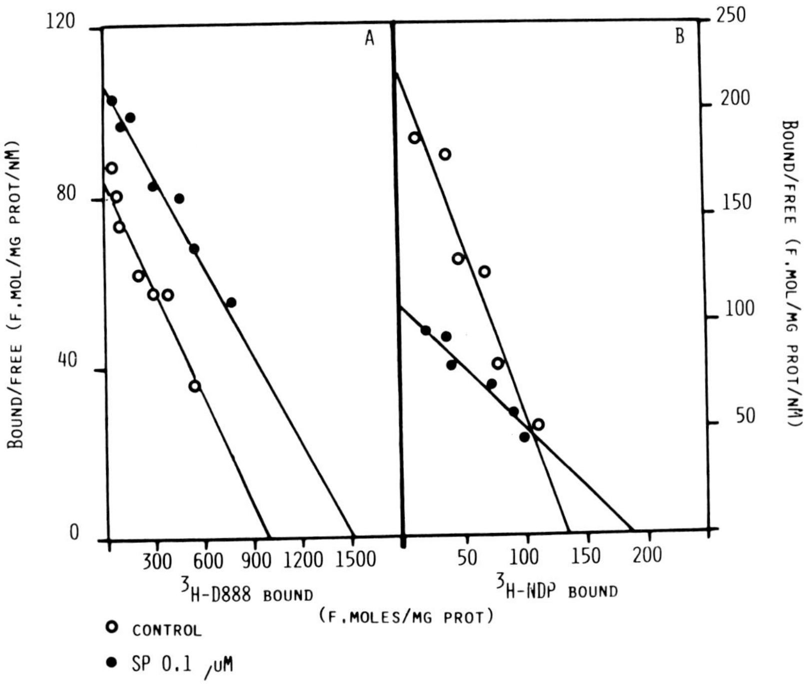

FIGURE 3. Effect of substance P on ^{3}H-D888 (panel A) and ^{3}H-nitrendipine (panel B) binding to hippocampal membranes. The figure reports the Scatchard analysis of saturation experiments performed in the presence (filled circles) or absence (open circles) of 0.1 micromolar substance P.

Excitatory amino acids are thought to cause depolarization by increasing Na^+ conductance, followed by a massive influx of Ca^{2+} into the cells. The high density of Ca^{2+} channels in the hippocampus seems to favor this view.

The increasing evidence of the plasticity of CNS DHP-binding sites prompted us to investigate whether this site may be modified by endogenous transmitters affecting calcium movements. Along this line the action of selected neuropeptides on calcium antagonist binding to synaptic membranes of various rat brain areas was investigated.

FIGURE 2 shows the effect of substance P, neurotensin and metenkephalin on ^{3}H-D888 binding to membranes prepared from rat hippocampus; this ligand labels with high affinity the phenylalkylamine subunit of calcium channel.[30] Substance P specifically increases the binding; the concentration-response curve is bell shaped and presents a peak at 10^{-7} M, while beyond 10^{-6} M binding is no longer stimulated. Substance P does not interfere with the binding of ^{3}H-D888 in a wide concentration range (10^{-9} M to 10^{-5} M) in striatal, cortical, and hypothalamic membranes (data not shown). Neurotensin and met-enkephalin have no effect on ^{3}H-D888 binding in any of the brain areas tested.

The interaction of substance P with the binding of ^{3}H-D888 to hippocampal membranes was characterized by performing saturation curves in the presence of the peptide, which revealed an increased number of binding sites for the ligand (FIGURE 3A). Substance P at 10^{-7} M also modified ^{3}H-nitrendipine binding leading to an increase in both B_{max} and K_d values (FIGURE 3B).

The effect of the substance P antagonist [(D-Pro^2, D-Trp^{7,9})-substance P] on the stimulatory action of substance P at 10^{-7} M on ^{3}H-D888 binding is shown in FIGURE 4). Preincubation of the membranes with the antagonist inhibited in a concentration-dependent manner the effect of substance P; the antagonism was complete using 10^{-5} M (D-Pro^2, D-Trp^{7,9})-substance P.

Functional studies were performed on tissue slices measuring the effect of substance P on calcium fluxes (FIGURE 5). The peptide exposure in hippocampus did not modify ^{45}Ca uptake under basal conditions (5 mM KCl), while after 50 mM KCl depolarization, substance P further increased the stimulated uptake. The concentration response curve is bell shaped reaching a maximum increase of 60% at 10^{-7} M with

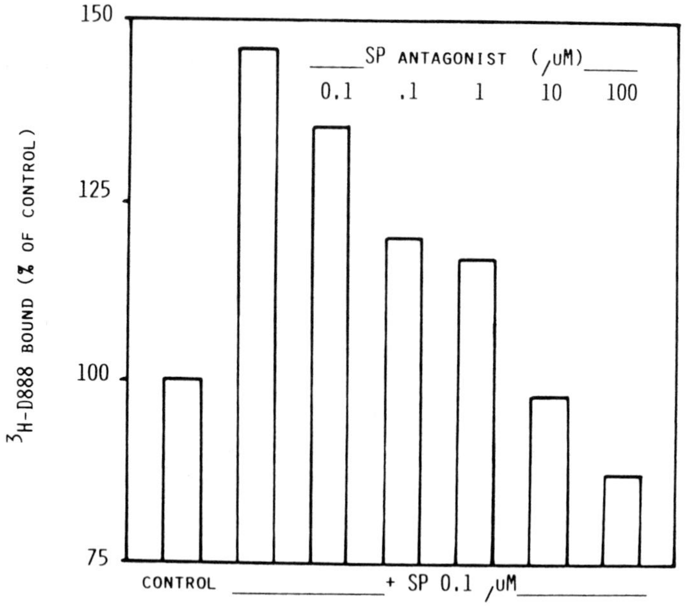

FIGURE 4. Effect of (D-Pro^2, D-Trp^{7,9}) substance P on ^{3}H-D888 binding stimulated by substance P into hippocampal membranes. Membranes were preincubated for 15 minutes in the presence of the indicated substance P antagonist concentration, then substance P and ^{3}H-D888 (5 nM) were added and samples further incubated as detailed in the legend to FIGURE 2.

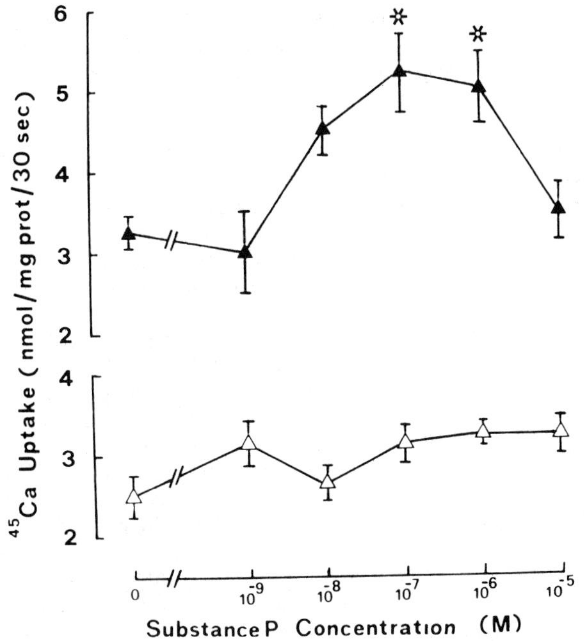

FIGURE 5. Effect of substance P on ^{45}Ca uptake into hippocampal slices under basal (open triangles) and depolarized (filled triangles) conditions. Calcium uptake assay. Uptake was performed as previously described with minor modifications.[12] Hippocampus was dissected and placed into Petri dishes with oxygenated Krebs Ringer medium (KRM) containing glucose 5.9 mM, $NaHCO_3$ 27.5 mM, NaCl 120 mM, KCl 5 mM, $MgSO_4$ 0.67 mM, KH_2PO_4 1.2 mM, $CaCl_2$ 1.0 mM, bacitracine 4 μg/ml, saturated with 5% CO_2 in O_2, pH 7.4 with NaOH. Cross-chopped slices (300 × 300 μm) were prepared with a McIlwain tissue chopper and resuspended in KRM. Aliquots of the slice suspension corresponding to 10 mg original wet weight tissue were exposed to substance P for 20 minutes. $^{45}Ca^{++}$ and ^{3}H-sucrose (0.5 and 1.0 μCi every μmol $CaCl_2$ respectively) were then added together with NaCl and KCl (final concentration 50 mM each) to basal and KCl-stimulated samples. After 30 seconds incubation, the samples were filtered under vacuum over Whatman GF/C filters, washed with 3 ml stop solution (NaCl 120 mM, KCl 5 mM, Tris 50 mM, EGTA 30 mM, pH 7.6) and 2 × 3 ml KRM without $CaCl_2$. Disintegrations per minute for ^{3}H and ^{45}Ca were determined after liquid scintillation spectrometry, using a computer-assisted program. Voltage-stimulated ^{45}Ca uptake was expressed as difference between the uptake in the presence of 50 and of 5 mM KCl.

TABLE 5. Some Characteristics of Calcium Antagonist Binding Sites in Brain

Developmental and aging modifications
Area specific modulation:
By ions
By peptides
Rapidity and reversibility of the plastic response
Parallelism with calcium fluxes

an EC_{50} of 7.2 ± 0.9 nM. Calcium fluxes were not modified by substance P under basal and depolarized conditions in striatal and cortical slices (data not shown). The increase in ^{3}H-D888 and ^{3}H-nitrendipine binding elicited by substance P in hippocampus seems therefore functionally correlated with a concomitant increase in voltage-dependent ^{45}Ca uptake in tissue slices.

Increased calcium antagonist binding, paralleled by increased K^+-dependent ^{45}Ca uptake, has been observed at brain level in other conditions such as after chronic morphine treatment,[16] in the case of cardiomyopathic hamsters[31] and after *in vitro* exposure to phencyclidine.[32] Although the action of substance P on other mechanisms controlling calcium uptake[33-35] cannot be excluded, the data suggest that the direct action on VSCC as identified with calcium antagonist binding may participate in the excitatory action of substance P in CNS.[36]

In addition to this, the effect of substance P on calcium antagonist receptors may be related to the neurotrophic action of this peptide.[37] In fact, calcium uptake into neurons is essential for synapse formation and neurite extension,[38] and these processes may be inhibited by removal of calcium ions from the extracellular space and by calcium antagonists.[39] Therefore the previously observed action of substance P in promoting neurite extension[37] could also involve a possible mediation of calcium uptake through an action on VSCC as suggested by our results. The specific action of substance P in hippocampus may suggest that a unique reinforcement process, dependent on the possibility of unmasking new VSCC may be relevant in the expression of long- and short-term events mediated by calcium in this area.

Although the function of L channels in brain is still largely unknown it may be speculated that changes in their function may contribute to modifications of neuronal activity and excitability in various conditions. The studies of their characteristics and plasticity (TABLE 5) as indicated by the binding data of tritiated calcium antagonists and the observation of an area-selective modulation will probably shed some light on their functional role and physiological regulation as well as opening new perspectives on DHP applications in the neurological and neuropsychiatric field.

REFERENCES

1. NOWYCKY, M. C., A. P. FOX & R. W. TSIEN. 1985. Three types of neuronal calcium channels with different calcium agonist sensitivity. Nature **316:** 443–446.
2. HESS, P., J. B. LANSMAN, & R. W. TSIEN. 1984. Different modes of Ca channel gating behaviour favoured by dihydropyridine Ca agonists and antagonists. Nature **311:** 538–544.
3. MILLER, R. J. 1987. Multiple calcium channels and neuronal function. Science **235:** 46–52.
4. REYNOLDS, I. J., J. A. WAGNER, S. H. SNYDER, S. A. THAYER, B. M. OLIVERA & R. J. MILLER. 1986. Brain voltage-sensitive calcium channel subtypes differentiations by a ω-conotoxin fractions GVIA. Proc. Nat. Acad. Sci. USA **83:** 8804–8807.
5. NACHSEN, D. A., M. P. BLAUSTEIN. 1979. The effect of some organic calcium antagonists on calcium influx in presynaptic nerve terminals. Mol. Pharmacol. **16:** 579–586.
6. DANIELL L. C., E. M. BART & S. W. LESLIE. 1983. $^{45}Ca^{++}$ uptake into rat whole brain synaptosomal unaltered by dihydropyridine calcium antagonists. J. Neurochem. **41:** 1455–1459.
7. RAMPE, D., R. A. JANIS & D. J. TRIGGLE. 1984. Bay K 8644: a 1,4-dihydropyridine Ca^{2+} channel activator. Dissociation of binding and functional effects in brain synaptosomes. J. Neurochem. **43:** 1688–1691.
8. TURNER, T. J. & S. M. GOLDIN. 1985. Calcium channels in rat brain synaptosomes: identification and pharmacological characterization. J. Neurosci. **5:** 841–849.

9. MIDDLEMISS, D. N. & A. SPEDDING. 1985. A functional correlate for the dihydropyridine binding site in rat brain. Nature **314:** 94–96.
10. PERNEY, T. M., L. D. HIRNING, S. E. LEEMAN & R. J. MILLER. 1986. Multiple calcium channels mediate neurotransmitter release from peripheral neurons. Proc. Nat. Acad. Sci. USA **83:** 6656–6659.
11. GOVONI, S., M. TRABUCCHI, M. S. MAGNONI, F. BATTAINI & R. PAOLETTI. 1985. Abnormal neurotransmitter release and calcium entry blockers. *In* Calcium Entry Blockers and Tissue Protection. T. Godfraind, P. M. Vanhoutte, S. Govoni & R. Paoletti, Eds.: 151–162. Raven Press. New York, NY.
12. BATTAINI, F., S. GOVONI, S. DI GIOVINE & M. TRABUCCHI. 1986. Neurotensin effect on dopamine release and calcium transport in rat striatum: interactions with diphenylalkylamine calcium antagonists. Naunyn Schmiedeberg's Arch. Pharmacol. **332:** 267–270.
13. KONGSAMUT, S. & R. J. MILLER. 1986. Nerve growth factor modulates the drug sensitivity of neurotransmitter release from PC12 cells. Proc. Nat. Acad. Sci. USA **83:** 2243–2247.
14. LUCCHI, L., S. GOVONI, F. BATTAINI, G. PASINETTI & M. TRABUCCHI. 1985. Ethanol administration in vivo alters calcium ion control in rat striatum. Brain Res. **332:** 376–380.
15. RIUS, R. A., S. BERGAMASCHI, F. DI FONSO, S. GOVONI & M. TRABUCCHI. 1987. Acute ethanol effect on calcium antagonist binding in the rat. Brain Res. **402:** 359–361.
16. RAMKUMAR, V. & E. E. EL-FAKAHANY. 1984. Increase in ^{3}H-nitrendipine binding sites in the brain in morphine tolerant mice. Eur. J. Pharmacol. **102:** 371–372.
17. RIUS, R. A., L. LUCCHI, S. GOVONI & M. TRABUCCHI. 1984. In vivo chronic lead exposure alters ^{3}H-nitrendipine binding in rat striatum. Brain Res **322:** 180–184.
18. POWERS, R. E. & N. S. COLUCCI. 1985. An increase in putative voltage-dependent calcium channel number following reserpine treatment. Biochem. Biophys. Res. Commun. **132:** 844–849.
19. PANZA, G., J. A. GREBB, E. SANNA, A. G. WRIGHT & I. HANBAUER. 1985. Evidence for down regulation of ^{3}H nitrendipine recognition sites in mouse brain after long term treatment with nifedipine or verapamil. Neuropharmacology **24:** 1113–1117.
20. ISHII, K., T. KANO, Y. KUROBE & J. ANDO. 1983. Binding of ^{3}H-nitrendipine to heart and brain membranes from normotensive and spontaneous hypertensive rats. Eur. J. Pharmacol. **88:** 277–278.
21. GOVONI, S., R. A. RIUS, F. BATTAINI, A. BIANCHI & M. TRABUCCHI. 1985. Age-related reduced affinity in ^{3}H-nitrendipine labelling of brain voltage dependent calcium channels. Brain Res. **333:** 374–377.
22. BATTAINI, F., S. GOVONI, R. A. RIUS & M. TRABUCCHI. 1985. Age-dependent increase in ^{3}H-verapamil binding to rat cortical membranes. Neurosci. Lett. **61:** 67–71.
23. ROSS, D. H., M. A. MEDINA & H. L. CARDENAS. 1974. Morphine and ethanol: selective depletion of regional brain calcium. Science **186:** 63–65.
24. FRIEDMAN, M. B., C. K. ERICKSON & S. W. LESLIE. 1980. Effects of acute and chronic ethanol administration on whole mouse brain synaptosomal calcium influx. Biochem. Pharmacol. **29:** 1903–1908.
25. LYNCH, M. A. & J. M. LITTLETON. 1983. Possible association of alcohol tolerance with increased synaptic Ca^{++} sensitivity. Nature **303:** 175–176.
26. MESSING, R. O., C. L. CARPENTER, I. DIAMOND & D. A. GREENBERG. 1986. Ethanol regulates calcium channels in clonal neural cells. Proc. Nat. Acad. Sci. USA **83:** 6213–6215.
27. J. M. LITTLETON & H. J. LITTLE. Dihydropyridine-sensitive Ca^{2+} channels in brain are involved in the central nervous system hyperexcitability associated with alcohol withdrawal states. Ann. NY Acad. Sci. (This volume.)
28. RAICHLE, M. E. 1983. The pathophysiology of brain ischemia. Ann. Neurol. **13:** 2–10.
29. SIESJO, B. K. & T. WIELOCH. 1985. Brain ischemia and cellular calcium homeostasis. *In* Calcium Entry Blockers and Tissue Protection. T. Godfraind, P. M. Vanhoutte, S. Govoni & R. Paoletti, Eds.: 135–150. Raven Press. New York, N.Y.
30. FERRY, D. R., A. GOLL, C. GADOW & H. GLOSSMAN. 1984. (–)-^{3}H-Desmethoxyverapamil labelling of putative calcium channels in brain: autoradiographic distribution and

allosteric coupling to 1-4-dihydropyridine and diltiazem binding sites. Naunyn-Schmiedebergs Arch. Pharmacol. **327:** 183–187.
31. WAGNER, J. A., I. J. REYNOLDS, H. F. WEISMAN, P. DUDEK, M. L. WEISFELDT & S. H. SNYDER. 1986. Calcium antagonist receptor in cardiomyopathic hamster: selective increases in heart, muscle and brain. Science **232:** 515–518.
32. BOLGER, G. T., M. F. RAFFERTY & P. SKOLNICK. 1985. Phencyclidine increases the affinity of dihydropyridine calcium channel antagonist binding in rat brain. Naunyn-Schmiedebergs Arch. Pharmacol. **330:** 227–234.
33. DE RIEMER, S. A., J. A. STRONG, K. A. ALBERT, P. GREENGARD & L. K. KACZMAREK. 1985. Enhancement of calcium current in Aplysia neurones by phorbol ester and protein kinase C. Nature **313:** 313–316.
34. MANTYH, P., R. D. PINNOCK, C. P. DOWNES, M. GOEDERT & S. P. HUNT. 1984. Correlation between inositol phospholipid hydrolysis and substance P receptors in rat CNS. Nature **309:** 795–797.
35. CREBA, J. A. & M. KAROBATH. 1986. The effect of dihydropyridine calcium agonists and antagonists on neuronal voltage sensitive calcium channels. Biochem. Biophys. Res. Commun. **134:** 1038–1047.
36. NICOLL, R. A., C. SCHENKER & S. E. LEEMAN. 1980. Substance P as a transmitter candidate. Annu. Rev. Neurosci. **3:** 227–268.
37. NARUMI, S. & Y. MAKI. 1978. Stimulatory effects of substance P on neurite extension and cyclic AMP levels in cultured neuroblastoma cells. J. Neurochem. **30:** 1321–1326.
38. NIRENBERG, M., S. WILSON, H. HIGASHIDA, A. ROTTER, K. KRUEGER, N. BUSIS, R. RAY, J. G. KENIMER & M. ADLER. 1983. Modulation of synapse formation by cyclic adenosine monophosphate. Science **222:** 794–799.
39. SUAREZ-ISLA, B. A., D. J. PELTO, J. F. THOMPSON & S. I. RAPOPORT. 1984. Blockers of calcium permeability inhibit neurite extension and formation of neuromuscular synapses in cell culture. Dev. Brain Res. **14:** 263–270.
40. RAMKUMAR, V. & E. E. EL-FAKAHANY. 1985. Changes in the affinity of ^{3}H-nitrendipine binding sites in the brain upon chloropromazine treatment and subsequent withdrawal. Res. Commun. Chem. Pathol. Pharmacol. **48:** 463–466
41. RIUS, R. A., S. GOVONI & M. TRABUCCHI. 1986. Regional modification of brain calcium antagonist binding after in vivo chronic lead exposure. Toxicology **40:** 191–197.
42. LEE, M. R., M. WATSON, H. I. YAMAMURA & W. R. ROESKE. 1985. Decreased ^{3}H-nitrendipine binding in the brainstem of DOCA NaCl hypertensive rats. Life Sci. **37:** 971–977.
43. RIUS, R. A., S. GOVONI, F. BATTAINI & M. TRABUCCHI. 1985. Differential sensitivity of ^{3}H-nitrendipine binding to cations of toxicological interest in various rat brain areas. Toxicol. Lett. **27:** 103–108.
44. GREENBERG, D. A., E. C. COOPER & C. L. CARPENTER. 1984. Phenytoin interacts with calcium channels in brain membranes. Ann. Neurol. **16:** 616–620.
45. BATTAINI, F., S. GOVONI, R. DEL VESCO, M. S. C. MAGNONI & M. TRABUCCHI. 1987. Interaction between substance P and calcium ion homeostasis in rat hippocampus. Biochem. Biophys. Res. Commun. **144:** 1135–1142.

Dihydropyridine-Sensitive Ca^{2+} Channels in Brain Are Involved in the Central Nervous System Hyperexcitability Associated with Alcohol Withdrawal States[a]

J. M. LITTLETON[b] AND H. J. LITTLE[c]

[b]Department of Pharmacology
King's College London
Strand
London WC2R 2LS England

[c]Department of Pharmacology
University of Bristol
Bristol BS8 1TD, England

The development of physical dependence on ethanol in the rat is associated with an increase in the number and function of dihydropyridine-sensitive Ca^{2+} channels in brain.[1] This increase might provide the basis for the increased central nervous system (CNS) excitability that underlies the ethanol physical withdrawal syndrome. This hypothesis is strengthened by our previous observation that Ca^{2+} antagonists of the dihydropyridine type are effective inhibitors of ethanol withdrawal in the rat.[2] This may, of course, not be a consequence of Ca^{2+} channel inhibition but may be due to some other property of the drugs. In these experiments we have examined the ability of the Ca^{2+} channel activator BAY K 8644 to mimic the ethanol withdrawal syndrome and to prevent the inhibitory effect of the Ca^{2+} antagonist nimodipine on this syndrome. We have also compared the effects of the stereoisomers of PN 200-110 of which the (+) isomer is an effective Ca^{2+} antagonist whereas the (−) isomer is ineffective in this respect.[3]

METHODS

Male TO Swiss mice (25–30 g) were maintained in an ethanol inhalation chamber for 10 days to induce ethanol physical dependence.[4] On removal from ethanol mice of this strain develop a characteristic pattern of seizures on suspension by the tail. Mice show tonic contractions of extended forelimbs, clonic seizures of splayed hindlimbs, an arched back, and facial grimace. These seizures can be assessed quantitatively by a scoring method that gives an estimation of the severity of the withdrawal syndrome.[5] Fifteen minutes after withdrawal from ethanol mice were injected intraperitoneally (IP) with vehicle (20% dimethylsulfoxide in saline) or with dihydropyridine drugs and were then scored blind by a trained observer. Results were analyzed statistically using the Mann-Whitney test.

[a]This work was supported by the Wellcome Trust and the Brewers' Society.

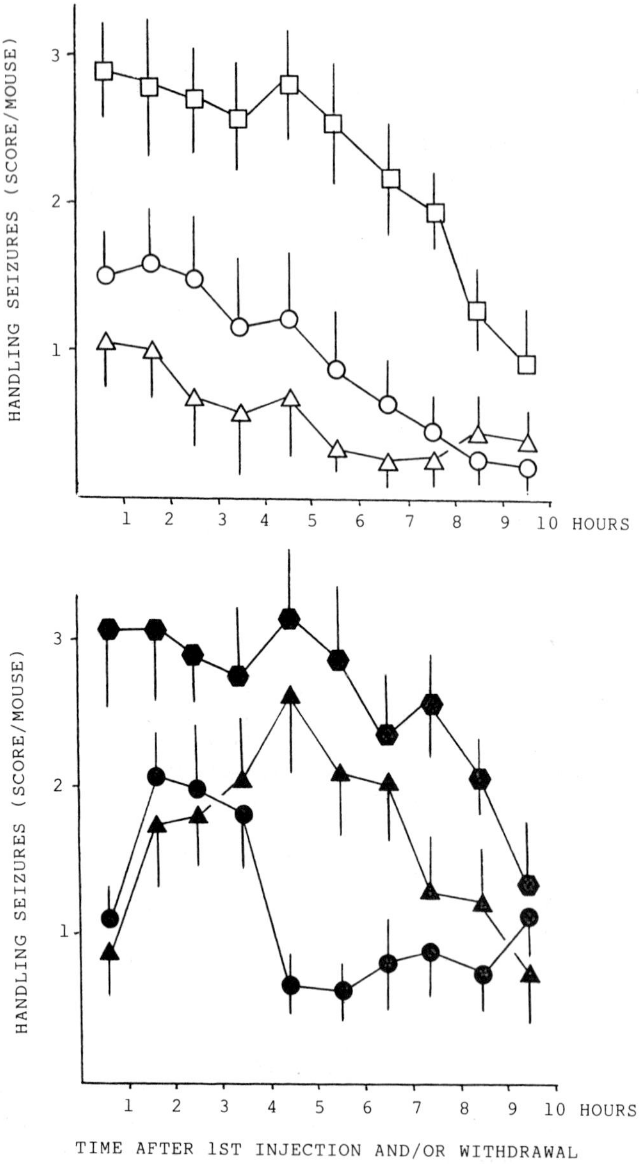

FIGURE 1. Effect of dihydropyridines on incidence of handling seizures in mice. The upper section shows the effect of 2 mg × kg^{-1} IP BAY K 8644 (squares) and 50 mg × kg^{-1} IP nimodipine (circles) on the incidence of handling seizures as compared to control mice (triangles) injected with vehicle alone. Injections were made at 0 hour and 4 hours. Results are means and standard errors of the mean (SEM) of at least 5 determinations. BAY K 8644 significantly increased the incidence of seizures. The lower section shows the effect of the same drugs on ethanol withdrawal seizures. Nimodipine 50 mg × kg^{-1} IP (circles) significantly inhibits ethanol withdrawal seizures after the second injection at 4 hours as compared to vehicle-injected animals undergoing withdrawal (triangles). Concomitant injection of BAY K 8644, 2 mg × kg^{-1} IP (hexagons), prevented the protective effect of nimodipine. Values are means ± SEM of at least 7 determinations.

RESULTS

The effect of BAY K 8644 and nimodipine on otherwise untreated mice is shown in the upper section of FIGURE 1. The Ca^{2+} channel activator produced a seizure syndrome identical in appearance to that observed in ethanol withdrawal. Control mice show a low but detectable incidence of seizures until they become used to being handled in this way. The Ca^{2+} antagonist nimodipine had no significant effect on these seizures in control animals.

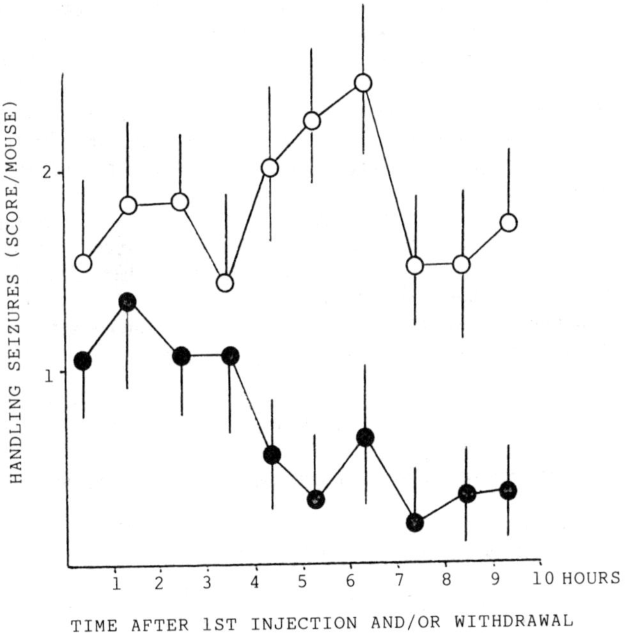

FIGURE 2. Stereoselectivity of the dihydropyridine PN 200-110 in ethanol withdrawal seizures. Results show the effects of the two isomers of PN 200-110 on handling seizures of mice undergoing the ethanol withdrawal syndrome. Mice injected at 0, 4 and 7 hours after withdrawal with 10 mg $\times$ kg^{-1} IP PN(−)200-110 (open circles) showed a typical incidence of handling seizures whereas a similar dose of the active isomer PN(+)200-110 (filled circles) markedly inhibited withdrawal seizures. Values are means ± SEM of at least 7 determinations.

The effect of these dihydropyridines on the seizure pattern of ethanol withdrawn mice is shown in the lower section of FIGURE 1. Nimodipine significantly inhibits the withdrawal seizures and this effect is reversed by the Ca^{2+} channel activator BAY K 8644. The administration of BAY K 8644 alone during ethanol withdrawal rather surprisingly did not increase seizures (data not shown).

The effects of the two isomers of PN 200-110 on ethanol withdrawal seizures are shown in FIGURE 2. PN(+)200-110, which is an effective Ca^{2+} antagonist, also proved very effective as an inhibitor of the ethanol withdrawal seizure syndrome. In contrast PN(−)200-110 did not prevent ethanol withdrawal seizures.

DISCUSSION

The results are almost exactly those predicted by our original hypothesis that ethanol withdrawal hyperexcitability is a consequence of an increased number and functional activity of dihydropyridine-sensitive Ca^{2+} channels in brain.[1] If this is so, then pharmacological activation of these channels in control animals should mimic the withdrawal hyperexcitability. We found this to be so: BAY K 8644 produced a seizure syndrome very similar to that characteristic of ethanol withdrawal. Similarly the inhibitory effects of the Ca^{2+} antagonist nimodipine on the ethanol withdrawal syndrome should be reversed by concurrent administration of BAY K 8644. This too was found to be so. Interestingly, BAY K 8644 did not potentiate ethanol withdrawal seizures, implying that these Ca^{2+} channels may already be maximally activated in this situation; this may in turn suggest the release of some endogenous activator in the withdrawn state, but this is speculative.

The ability of PN 200-110 to prevent the ethanol withdrawal seizures was shown to be dependent on its activity as a Ca^{2+} antagonist, reinforcing our belief that it is this property of the dihydropyridine drugs that is responsible for their activity in the ethanol withdrawal syndrome.

These findings are of considerable interest in relation to our understanding of the biochemical basis of ethanol dependence. At a practical level they suggest that dihydropyridine Ca^{2+} antagonists offer a method of treating the withdrawal syndrome with drugs that have little sedative effect and no known abuse potential. The Ca^{2+}-agonist-induced seizures might offer a useful model system with which to study drugs of potential value against ethanol withdrawal.

REFERENCES

1. Dolin, S., M. Hudspith, C. Pagonis, H. Little & J. M. Littleton. 1987. Neuropharmacology **26:** 275–279.
2. Little, H. J., S. Dolin & M. J. Halsey. 1986. Life Sci. **39:** 2059–2065.
3. Hof, A., U. Hof, T. Roeg, N. S. Cooke & A. Vogel. 1986. J. Cardiovasc. Pharmacol. **8:** 221–226.
4. Griffiths, P. J., J. M. Littleton & A. Ortiz. 1974. Br. J. Pharmacol. **50:** 489–498.
5. Goldstein, D. B. & N. Pal. 1971. Science **172:** 288–290.

Calcium Channel Binding Sites in Human Brain[a]

RÉMI QUIRION,[b,c] SAMARTHJI LAL,[b,c,d]
ANDRÉ OLIVIER,[e] YVES ROBITAILLE,[b,e]
N. P. VASSAVAN NAIR,[b,c]
ROBERT M. FORD,[d] AND JOSEPH G. STRATFORD[d]

[b]Douglas Hospital Research Center
[c]Department of Psychiatry
McGill University
6875 Boulevard Lasalle
Verdun, Québec, Canada H4H 1R3

[d]Montreal General Hospital
1650 Cedar Avenue
Montreal, Québec, Canada H3G 1A4

[e]Montreal Neurological Institute
3801 University Street
Montreal, Québec, Canada H3A 2B4

INTRODUCTION

The existence of highly specific binding sites for various classes of calcium channel blockers has been demonstrated in various tissues including brain.[1-3] It now appears that different classes of calcium antagonists such as the 1,4-dihydropyridines, the phenylalkylamines, and diltiazem interact with different binding sites that are allosterically coupled to induce their effects.[1-3]

In the mammalian nervous system, calcium antagonist binding sites are heterogeneously distributed being mostly concentrated in areas enriched with synaptic contacts such as the hippocampus and the cortex.[3-9] However, these sites have not been characterized in much detail in human brain. Only a few reports have described their existence and autoradiographic distribution in postmortem tissues.[6,7,10] We report here on the presence of calcium channel binding sites in human brain using postmortem as well as fresh cortical biopsied tissues.

METHODS

Comparative binding characteristics of two 1,4-dihydropyridine radioligands, [^{3}H]nimodipine (108.4 Ci/mmol, New England Nuclear, Boston, Mass.) and [^{3}H]PN200-110 (84 Ci/mmol, New England Nuclear, Boston, Mass.) were determined in fresh cortical biopsied samples as well as in postmortem tissues under incubation conditions described in detail elsewhere.[6,7] Cortical biopsied tissues were

[a]This research project has been supported by grants from Miles Institute for Preclinical Research, the Medical Research Council of Canada, and the Canadian Parkinson Society.

obtained from patients undergoing surgery for removal of brain tumors or epileptic foci. In all cases, only apparently normal tissues were used and dissected after excision, immediately brought to the laboratory, and processed rapidly for 1,4-dihydropyridine binding assays. The mean delays between removal from skull and homogenization averaged less than 60 minutes. During this period, all samples were kept at 4°C (on ice). For postmortem studies, membranes were prepared from normal control human brains (without evident neurological and psychiatric diseases) obtained at autopsy (mean delay of 18 ± 6 hours, $n = 6$), and rapidly frozen on dry ice and kept at −80°C until used. In a few experiments, the binding characteristics of the phenylalkylamine derivative [^{3}H](−)D-888 (83 Ci/mmol; gift from Knoll AG, West Germany) were also investigated for comparison.[6]

TABLE 1. Comparative Binding Characteristics of 1,4-Dihydropyridine and Phenylalkylamine Calcium Channel Antagonist Ligands in Human Biopsied and Postmortem Brain Tissues[a]

		1,4-Dihydropyridines				Phenylalkylamine	
		[^{3}H]PN200-110		[^{3}H]Nimodipine		[^{3}H](−)D-888	
Tissue		K_d	B_{max}	K_d	B_{max}	K_d	B_{max}
Biopsies—epileptic patients							
Temporal		0.15	182.3	0.82	198.1		—
Frontotemporal		0.34	180.0	0.91	196.9		—
Frontal		0.57	180.0	0.61	180.7	3.5	169.3
Frontoparietal		0.29	177.0	1.01	152.1		—
Temporoparietal		0.51	110.0	0.43	106.4		—
Parietal		0.42	87.0	0.67	74.0		—
Biopsies—brain tumors							
Temporal		0.29	191.0	0.64	182.0		—
Parietal		0.37	74.0	0.73	77.0		—
Postmortem							
Temporal	high affinity	0.8	169.0	0.9	174.0	4.1	159.0
	low affinity	25	647.0	29	691.0	ND	ND
Frontal	high affinity	1.2	142.4	1.2	129.6	3.6	141.3
	low affinity	37	651.0	32	636.0	ND	ND
Parietal	high affinity	1.3	64.0	1.2	61.3	2.9	67.4
	low affinity	39	524.0	36	542.0	ND	ND

[a] In each case, the data represent the means of at least 3–6 determinations each in triplicate and using computerized linear regression analysis to analyze the binding data (Bio-Soft, Elsevier, England). The affinity (K_d) is expressed in nanomolar while the maximal number of sites (B_{max}) is expressed in fmol/mg protein. ND = not determined.

In a second series of experiments, the autoradiographic distribution of 0.5 nM [^{3}H]PN200-110, 0.5 nM [^{3}H] nimodipine, and 0.5 nM [^{3}H](−)D-888 binding sites were studied using postmortem whole human brain hemisphere sections under incubation conditions described before.[6,7]

RESULTS AND DISCUSSION

As shown in TABLE 1, two 1-4-diydropyridine radioligands, namely [^{3}H]PN200-110 and [^{3}H]nimodipine, bind with high affinity (K_d) to an apparent single class of sites in fresh human cortical biopsies. Both ligands demonstrate similar affinities and maximal capacities (B_{max}) in the various cortical areas investigated suggesting that they are interacting with the same population of sites. Similar results have been obtained in animal brain tissues.[1-3]

The highest density of sites was found in the temporal cortex followed by frontotemporal, frontal, frontoparietal, temporoparietal and parietal cortices (TABLE 1). Very similar binding characteristics were found in biopsied tissues obtained from patients undergoing surgery for the removal of epileptic foci or brain tumors (TABLE 1), suggesting that they most likely reflect physiological conditions.

In a preliminary series of experiments, the binding characteristics of [^{3}H](−)D-888, a phenylalkylamine derivative, were also determined. This ligand apparently bound to a single class of sites in frontal cortical biopsies (TABLE 1). However, the affinity of those sites was lower than that of the 1,4-dihydropyridines (TABLE 1).

In contrast to fresh cortical biopsies, the 1,4-dihydropyridines apparently bound to two classes of specific sites in postmortem tissues (TABLE 1). The high affinity sites demonstrated characteristics that were very similar to binding sites characterized in fresh biopsied tissues and most likely represent an identical population of sites (TABLE 1). However, the lower affinity sites were only found in postmortem tissues with affinities 25- to 30-fold lower than those of high affinity sites. The absence of low affinity sites in fresh biopsied tissues suggests that this population of saturable binding sites represents an artifact of the long postmortem delays (means of 18 hours). This could also be related to a lower affinity state of calcium channel antagonist binding sites.

Unfortunately, it has not been possible to determine accurately the existence of lower affinity sites for the phenylalkylamine [^{3}H](−)D-888 in postmortem tissues since full saturation was not obtained at concentrations up to 75 nM. However, the presence of at least one population of high affinity sites was determined and its characteristics estimated by computerized analysis (TABLE 1). All these data clearly indicate that long postmortem delays alter the binding characteristics of two classes of calcium channel blockers, the 1,4-dihydropyridines and the phenylalkylamines. Thus, extrapolations from postmortem results to physiological conditions must be attempted with great care.

Finally, the autoradiographic distribution of these two classes of calcium blockers reveals that high densities of sites are located in areas enriched in synaptic contacts such as the hippocampus and the cortex. Similar results have been recently reported in animal and human brain tissues.[4-9] It should be pointed out that at the concentration of ligands (0.5 nM) used for autoradiographic experiments, it is most likely that only the population of high affinity sites was labeled. Twenty- to 30-fold higher concentrations of ligand would be necessary to bind a significant proportion of "postmortem" lower affinity sites.

In summary, 1,4-dihydropyridines and phenylalkylamines bind with high affinity to saturable populations of sites in human brain. This may be relevant for the beneficial effects of these drugs in the treatment of certain neurological and psychiatric diseases.[3,11,12]

REFERENCES

1. JANIS, R. A. & D. G. TRIGGLE. 1984. Drug Dev. Res. **4:** 257–274.
2. GLOSSMANN, H., D. R. FERRY, F. LUBBECKE, R. MEWES & F. HOFMANN. 1982. Trends Pharmacol. Sci. **3:** 431–437.
3. SNYDER, S. H. & I. J. REYNOLDS. 1985. N. Engl. J. Med. **313:** 995–1002.
4. MURPHY, K. M. M., R. J. GOULD & S. H. SNYDER. 1982. Eur. J. Pharmacol. **81:** 517–519.

5. QUIRION, R. 1983. Neurosci. Lett. **36:** 267–271.
6. QUIRION, R. 1985. Eur. J. Pharmacol. **117:** 139–142.
7. QUIRION, R., S. LAL, N. P. V. NAIR, J. G. STRATFORD, R. M. FORD & A. OLIVIER. 1985. Prog. Neuro-Psychopharmacol. Biol. Psychiatry **9:** 643–649.
8. FERRY, D. R., A. GOLL, C. GADOW & H. GLOSSMANN. 1984. Naunyn-Schmiedebergs Arch. Pharmacol. **327:** 183–187.
9. CORTES, R., P. SUPAVILAI, M. KAROBATH & J. M. PALACIOS. 1984. J. Neurol. Transm. **60:** 169–197.
10. PEROUTKA, S. J. & G. S. ALLEN. 1983. J. Neurosurg. **59:** 933–937.
11. WALSH, T. L., B. LAVENSTEIN, W. L. LICAMELE, S. BRONHEIM & J. O'LEARY. 1986. Am. J. Psychiatry **143:** 1467–1468.
12. DOSE, M., H. M. EMRICH, C. CORDING-TOMMEL & D. VON ZERSSEN. 1986. Psychoneuroendocrinology **11:** 241–243.

Morphine Treatment Increases [^{3}H]Nimodipine Binding Sites in Rat Brain

Attenuation by Nimodipine and Other Ca^{2+} Channel Antagonists of Naloxone-Precipitated Withdrawal in Morphine-Dependent Animals

VICKRAM RAMKUMAR[a] AND ESAM E. EL-FAKAHANY

Department of Pharmacology and Toxicology
School of Pharmacy
University of Maryland
Baltimore, Maryland 21201

Opiates inhibit voltage-sensitive Ca^{2+} current in neurons either directly or secondary to the activation of hyperpolarizing K^+ conductance.[1] Such inhibition might explain previous observations that acute morphine treatment in rats leads to decreased Ca^{2+} content in the brain[2] and attenuation of depolarization-induced Ca^{2+} uptake into synaptosomal preparations.[3] Inhibition of Ca^{2+} entry by opiates into the nerve terminals might account for their analgesic properties. This conclusion is supported by evidence that EGTA,[4] a Ca^{2+} chelator, and trivalent cations[5] known to block Ca^{2+} channels mediate antinociception when administered by intracerebroventricular and intrathecal routes, respectively.

Various pieces of evidence suggest that compensatory changes occur at the nerve terminals following prolonged inhibition of Ca^{2+} channel activity by opiates. For example, chronic administration of morphine[3] and levorphanol[6] in rats enhances brain synaptosomal Ca^{2+} uptake. This is presumably due to an increase in the number of Ca^{2+} channels.[7] The present study was undertaken to examine possible regulation of these channels in rat brains by morphine and to test its implication in the development of physical dependence.

The dihydropyridine (DHP) Ca^{2+} channel blocker [^{3}H]nimodipine was used to label putative Ca^{2+} channels in rat brain. For such studies, rats were made dependent by subcutaneous implantation of three morphine pellets for three days. Radioligand binding experiments were performed in 50 mM Tris-HCl buffer (pH 7.4) using several concentrations of [^{3}H]nimodipine (0.05–1.0 nM) and 1μM nifedipine to define nonspecific binding. Behavioral studies were performed on morphine-dependent rats and mice. Morphine withdrawal was initiated by administering naloxone injections [1–2 mg/kg, intraperitoneally (ip)].

Our results indicate that morphine treatment significantly increased the density of DHP Ca^{2+} channel antagonist binding sites in the brain, optimal increases being realized following treatment of rats with three morhpine pellets for three days. No change in the equilibrium dissociation constants (K_d) was observed under similar treatment conditions. Increases in [^{3}H]nimodipine binding were localized to the cortex, hippocampus, hypothalamus, and brain stem, with no change in density observed in the

[a]Present affiliation: Department of Medicine, Duke University Medical Center, Box 3444, Durham, NC 27710.

TABLE 1. Effect of Morphine Treatment on [^{3}H]Nimodipine Binding Sites in Different Brain Regions and Heart of the Rat[a]

Brain Region	B_{max} (fmol/mg protein) Placebo	B_{max} (fmol/mg protein) Morphine	K_d (nM) Placebo	K_d (nM) Morphine
Cortex	140.7 ± 11.6 (7)[b]	169.1 ± 7.3[c] (8)	0.18 ± 0.02	0.13 ± 0.01[c]
Striatum	167.1 ± 9.8 (7)	177.4 ± 8.8 (7)	0.18 ± 0.01	0.13 ± 0.01[c]
Hippocampus	174.0 ± 12.9 (6)	214.7 ± 8.7[c] (7)	0.17 ± 0.01	0.12 ± 0.01[c]
Brain stem	47.1 ± 5.4 (5)	62.7 ± 5.1[c] (5)	0.15 ± 0.05	0.13 ± 0.13
Hypothalamus	83.9 ± 9.4 (5)	105.2 ± 5.7[c] (5)	0.14 ± 0.02	0.14 ± 0.02
Cerebellum	47.1 ± 7.9 (3)	51.2 ± 2.7 (3)	0.17 ± 0.03	0.14 ± 0.08
Heart	240.2 ± 4.1 (4)	214.7 ± 13.5 (4)	0.12 ± 0.01	0.12 ± 0.01

[a]Values are expressed as the mean ± standard error of the mean (SEM).
[b]Number of brain regions used.
[c]Statistically different from control ($p < 0.05$).

striatum, cerebellum, and heart (TABLE 1). Removal of morphine pellets after three days resulted in a return to control levels by day 10. Morphine produced no changes in other receptors in the brain, such as muscarinic and phencyclidine receptors.

In order to determine the significance of the increase in DHP sites to physical dependence on morphine, we tested the effects of several Ca^{2+} channel antagonists on naloxone-precipitated withdrawal in mice and rats. In morphine-dependent mice, nisoldipine (16.6 mg/kg, ip) and nimodipine (5 and 10 mg/kg, ip) significantly attenuated the incidence of naloxone-precipitated jumping to 35% and 56% and 35% of morphine-dependent control, respectively. Similarly, nimodipine was effective in reducing the severity of naloxone-precipitated withdrawal signs in dependent rats (TABLE 2). Its effects were comparable to clonidine, a drug used clinically in the treatment of opioid withdrawal.

These studies suggest that the density of DHP Ca^{2+} channel antagonist binding sites, like several neurotransmitter receptors, can be regulated by drugs. Furthermore, a morphine-mediated increase in DHP sites might contribute to the development of physical dependence on this drug.

TABLE 2. Inhibition of Naloxone-Precipitated Withdrawal Signs in the Rat following Pretreatment with Ca^{2+} Antagonists and Clonidine[a,b]

Withdrawal Signs	Vehicle	Nimodipine (10 mg/kg; ip)	Clonidine (100 μg/kg; ip)
"Wet dog" shakes	3.4 (9)	1.3[c] (9)[d]	1.0[c] (6)
Ptosis	100	55[c]	0[c]
Teeth chattering	7.0	3.0[c]	3.8[c]
Abdominal stretching	0.9	0.5[c]	0[c]
Diarrhea	2.7	0.1[c]	0[c]

[a]All withdrawal signs were measured over a 30 minute period. "Wet dog" shakes, teeth chattering, and abdominal stretching are presented as the average number of occurrences. The percentage of animals showing ptosis and the mean severity score for diarrhea (0 = no diarrhea, 3 = severe diarrhea) are also presented.
[b]Statistical comparisons between vehicle and drug-treated groups were made using the Mann-Whitney U test for all signs except ptosis, which was analyzed by the chi-square test.
[c]Statistically different from vehicle pretreated rats administered naloxone ($p < 0.05$).
[d]Number of rats tested.

REFERENCES

1. Cherubini, E. & R. A. North. 1985. Proc. Nat. Acad. Sci. USA **82:** 1860.
2. Ross, D. H., M. A. Medina & H. L. Cardenas. 1974. Science **186:** 63.
3. Guerrero-Munoz, F., K. V. Cerreta, M. L. Guerrero & E. L. Way. 1979. J. Pharmacol. Exp. Ther. **209:** 132.
4. Kakunaga, T., H. Kaneto & K. Hano. 1966. J. Pharmacol. Exp. Ther. **153:** 134.
5. Reddy, S. V. R. & T. L. Yaksh. 1980. Neuropharmacology **19:** 181.
6. Ross, D. H., S. C. Lynn & H. L. Cardenas. 1977. *In* Neurochemical and Behavioral Mechanisms. K. Blume, Ed.: 265. Academic Press. New York, N.Y.
7. Ramkumar, V. & E. E. El-Fakahany. 1984. Eur. J. Pharmacol. **102:** 371.

Actions of Calcium on Smooth Muscle[a]

Historical Overview

DAVID F. BOHR

Department of Physiology
7710 Medical Science II
University of Michigan
Ann Arbor, Michigan 48109-0622

In 1883, Ringer alerted the biological world to the fact that calcium played an important role in muscle contraction.[1] In 1911, Cow described the extensive studies that he had carried out on isolated vascular smooth muscle.[2] He recorded the responses of this muscle to many pharmacological and physiological agents and studied the influence of calcium on these responses.

In the current review I will try to sum up what we have learned about the actions of calcium on smooth muscle since this early beginning. These actions of calcium will be reviewed from three aspects: (1) how calcium activates the contractile protein, (2) how the concentration of activator calcium is regulated, and (3) how calcium affects the plasma membrane.

CALCIUM AND THE CONTRACTILE PROTEINS

The central consideration given to the role played by calcium in muscle contraction is its activation of the chemomechanical transducing system that converts energy from the physiological fuel, ATP, to developed force. Calcium is the "spark plug" that puts the contractile proteins "in motion."

It is now well established that the role played by this activator calcium as the spark plug for contraction of vertebrate skeletal muscle is indirect. Ebashi *et al.* observed that when they combined purified actin (from which the troponin-tropomyosin system had been removed) with myosin, calcium was not necessary for super precipitation of the resultant, purified actomyosin.[3] In the intact, resting muscle and in extracted, native actomyosin, the ATPase activity of actomyosin is inhibited by a complex cooperative influence of troponin and tropomyosin. This inhibitory action of the troponin-tropomyosin system is eliminated when calcium combines with one of the troponins, TN-C. The binding of calcium to TN-C has the same calcium concentration dependence as does the activation of native actomyosin ATPase. The action of calcium is not a direct activation, but instead it is a disinhibition of the troponin-tropomyosin system. Because in the native state these inhibitory proteins are bound to actin in the thin filaments, this regulatory system is referred to as the actin or thin-filament regulatory system.

In 1965, we demonstrated that the calcium requirement for contraction of smooth muscle of the pig carotid artery was identical to that of the skeletal muscle of the rabbit psoas.[4] From these observations we concluded that the molecular mechanism by which calcium regulated the contraction of vascular smooth muscle was the same as that

[a]This work was supported by grant HL-18575 from the National Institutes of Health.

which Ebashi has characterized for striated muscle. Because of this conclusion, we credit ourselves with having delayed by a decade the correct understanding of the mechanism by which calcium activates the contractile process of smooth muscle.

It is now known that the calcium regulatory system of vertebrate smooth muscle is myosin linked as it is in molluscan muscle.[5] Bremel *et al.* observed that purified myosin from vertebrate smooth muscle could not be activated by pure actin from vertebrate skeletal muscle in the absence of calcium.[6] Calcium activated this hybrid actomyosin which had no TN-C.

In the smooth muscle cell, calcium activates a kinase that causes the phosphorylation of myosin light chain. Once phosphorylated, the actomyosin becomes an active ATPase and the myosin bridges cycle to generate active force.[7] The sensitivity of the activation of the myosin light chain kinase by calcium is increased tenfold by calmodulin.[8] In a recent study using aequorin to monitor intracellular calcium concentration in swine carotid media, Rembold and Murphy demonstrated convincingly the correlations between intracellular calcium concentration, myosin light chain phosphorylation, and cross bridge cycling rate.[9] They also observed that although these three variables were transient following stimulation of the muscle, the developed stress persisted in what they have called the "latch state." Based on these and other observations Hai and Murphy have described a kinetic model that hypothesized two types of cross bridge interactions: (1) cycling phosphorylated cross bridges and (2) noncycling dephosphorylated cross bridges ("latch bridges").[10] The only calcium-dependent regulatory mechanism in this model is myosin light chain kinase activation. They conclude that myosin phosphorylation is both necessary and sufficient for the development of the latch state.

REGULATION AND ACTIVATOR CALCIUM

These investigations have provided a comfortable understanding of the mechanism of contraction of vascular smooth muscle and have made it clear that this contraction is regulated by the concentration of calcium in the myoplasm. Parallel research has developed insight into the processes that regulate this calcium concentration. Broadly considered, these processes are involved either in the movement of calcium across the plasma membrane or in the sequestration and release of calcium from the sarcoplasmic reticulum.

In 1963 we found it possible to differentiate contractile responses to calcium from these two sources[11] when we observed that the response of the rabbit aorta was comprised of a fast and a slow component. We and others[12] established that calcium for the fast component had its origin from intracellular sequestered sites whereas that for the slow component had its origin from the extracellular calcium pool.

Calcium for the fast component of the contraction is released from the sarcoplasmic reticulum when a constrictor agonist activates its specific receptors in the plasma membrane. Somlyo and Somlyo have named this process pharmacomechanical coupling.[13] It can occur without a change in membrane potential. The role of an intracellular source of calcium in response to physiological agonist is demonstrated by the observation that vascular smooth muscle contracts phasically when stimulated with norepinephrine (NE) in a calcium-free medium.[12] Further evidence of this intracellular release of sequestered calcium in response to a receptor-agonist complex is found in the observation that ^{45}Ca efflux increases when ^{45}Ca-loaded vascular smooth muscle is stimulated with NE.[14] The signal for calcium release is transmitted to the sacroplasmic reticulum either by calcium-induced calcium release[15] or by inositol trisphosphate.[16]

In the absence of these signals the sarcoplasmic reticulum activity sequesters calcium, and it has been established that in vascular smooth muscle these microsomes hold sufficient calcium "to be both sink and source for the activator calcium in excitation-contraction coupling."[17] Van Breemen *et al.* have called our attention to the important role that the sarcoplasmic reticulum must play in buffering increments in intracellular calcium concentration.[18] They have presented evidence that NE blocks this buffering action and thereby causes a further increase in intracellular calcium concentration.

Extensive insight has also been developed into the roles played by the plasma membrane in the regulation of intracellular calcium concentration. Fundamental to this regulation is the fact that extracellular calcium concentration is approximately 10,000 times greater than that inside of the resting smooth muscle cell. For this reason the regulatory role of the plasma membrane is largely dependent on its permeability to calcium. This permeability is governed by the status of specific protein channels in the lipid bilayer of the membrane. Some channels open when the membrane is depolarized (potential-sensitive channels); others open when agonists react with their membrane receptors (receptor-operated channels).[19] Extensive evidence has established that these two classes of channels are different. For instance, they respond differently to calcium entry blockers[19] and to calcium agonists.[20]

The role of the membrane in regulating intracellular calcium concentration is influenced by the concentrations of potassium and sodium in its environment. Indirectly this influence reflects the roles that these monovalent cations have as determinants of membrane potential and hence on the opening of the potential-sensitive calcium channel. The concentration of these ions regulates membrane potential directly by their diffusion potentials and indirectly by their regulation of the activity of the electrogenic sodium pump. An increase in the activity of this pump causes membrane hyperpolarization, hence closure of the potential-sensitive channels and vascular smooth muscle relaxation.[21]

There is now being considered a more direct role for the sodium ion in regulating the transmembrane calcium movement in vascular smooth muscle. A specific sodium-calcium exchange mechanism was first critically characterized in the squid axon.[22] With the normal high transmembrane concentration gradient of sodium, the flow of this ion down its concentration gradient into the cell through this exchange system energizes the extrusion of calcium from the cell. When the sodium concentration gradient is reduced either by decreasing extracellular sodium or by increasing intracellular sodium, calcium concentration inside the cell increases. Briggs and Melvin observed that when rabbit aortic strips were exposed to a low sodium concentration, calcium influx increased by 225% and contracture developed.[23] Several investigators have attributed the contracture that develops when the sodium pump of vascular smooth muscle is inhibited, to the increase in intracellular sodium that dissipates the sodium gradient that is normally responsible for calcium extrusion via this sodium-calcium exchange system.[24-26] Although extensive arguments have been advanced supporting the physiological significance of this exchange system,[27] its importance is not universally accepted.[28]

Another substantive membrane system involved in the regulation of intracellular calcium concentration is the energy-requiring calcium-extrusion pump. When the smooth muscle cell is metabolically inhibited calcium accumulates intracellularly at the rate of its leak into the resting cell, demonstrating the essential homeostatic role of the calcium-extrusion pump.[29] The functional significance of this pump is suggested by the vasodilation by nitroglycerine that stimulates the pump,[30] and the vascular smooth muscle contraction that results from its inhibition with vanadate.[31]

CALCIUM AND THE PLASMA MEMBRANE

Not only is the plasma membrane equipped with many mechanisms that are important regulators of intracellular calcium concentration, but the function of the membrane is itself regulated by calcium. Intracellular functions are protected from excessive calcium concentration, since an increase in extracellular calcium concentration causes a decrease in cell membrane permeability to calcium. Increases in extracellular calcium concentration cause a decrease in ^{45}Ca influx in vascular smooth muscle.[32,33] This inactivation of calcium channels by increasing concentations of calcium can be demonstrated by the relaxation of vascular smooth muscle that occurs when extracellular calcium concentration is increased above physiological levels.[34] Increases in calcium concentration also cause a cessation of action potentials in the taenia coli.[35] The decrease in membrane permeability caused by the increase in calcium concentration is referred to as membrane stabilization. It is a generalized effect, as evidenced by the observations that it results in a decrease in potassium flux through the vascular smooth muscle membrane[36] and it produces identical permeability changes in the membrane of the lymphocyte.[37] The converse is also true in that a decrease in extracellular calcium concentration results in an increase in membrane excitability. Clinically this is recognized in hypocalcemic tetany, and we have observed that it causes an increase in membrane excitability in vascular smooth muscle.[11]

More recently we have used an alternate technique to evaluate the influence of membrane-bound calcium on its permeability.[38] In this technique the vascular smooth muscle is placed in a calcium-free solution for 5 minutes with the sodium pump shut down by a potassium-free solution. Calcium is then added back to the muscle bath causing a contraction, the time course of which is determined by the rate of calcium entry into the cell through the plasma membrane which, in turn, is regulated by the amount of calcium that had remained bound to the membrane during the 5 minutes exposure to the calcium-free solution. This regulatory role of calcium bound to the membrane is demonstrated by exposing the muscle to 1 mM EGTA in a calcium-free solution for 1 minute before the 5 minute period in a calcium-free solution without EGTA. The 1 minute exposure to EGTA removes calcium from the membrane. Now when the calcium is added back 5 minutes later it enters the cell easily giving rise to a much faster contractile response. Using this technique we have confirmed results of other studies[39,40] indicating that in experimental hypertension there is a deficiency of membrane binding sites on which calcium has this stabilizing action.

As characterized by Johnson *et al.* all aspects of the relationships of calcium to vascular smooth muscle functions are mediated through calcium-binding proteins.[26] The future of this field will depend on a further understanding of the role played by these proteins.

REFERENCES

1. RINGER, S. 1883. A further contribution regarding the influence of the different constituents of blood on the contraction of the heart. J. Physiol. **4:** 29–42.
2. COW, D. 1911. Some reactions of surviving arteries. J. Physiol. **42:** 125–143.
3. EBASHI, S., I. OHTSUKI, R. TSUJUI & T. FUJII. 1973. The role of regulatory protein in contractile mechanism. Excerpta Med. Int. Congr. Ser. No. 333: 419–430.
4. FILO, R. S., D. F. BOHR & J. C. RUEGG. 1965. Glycerinated skeletal and smooth muscle: calcium and magnesium dependence. Science **147:** 1581–1583.
5. KENDRICK-JONES, J., W. LEHMAN & A. G. SZENT-GYORGYI. 1973. Regulation of molluscan muscle. J. Mol. Biol. **54:** 313–326.

6. BREMEL, R. D., A. SOBIESZEK & J. V. SMALL. 1976. Regulation of actin-myosin interaction in vertebrate smooth muscle. *In* Biochemistry of Smooth Muscle. N. L. Stephans, Ed.: 533–549. University Park Press. Baltimore, Md.
7. DISALVO, J., E. GRUENSTEIN & P. SILVER. 1978. Calcium dependent phosphorylation of bovine aortic actomyosin. Proc. Soc. Exp. Biol. Med. **158:** 410–414.
8. RUEGG, J. C. & R. J. PAUL. 1982. Vascular smooth muscle. Calmodulin and cyclic AMP–dependent protein kinase alter calcium sensitivity in porcine carotid skinned fibers. Cir. Res. **50:** 394–399.
9. REMBOLD, C. M. & R. A. MURPHY. 1986. Myoplasmic calcium, myosin phosphorylation, and regulation of the cross bridge cycle in swine arterial smooth muscle. Circ. Res. **58:** 803–815.
10. HAI, C-M. & R. A. MURPHY. 1987. Crossbridge phosphorylation may be necessary and sufficient to regulate contraction in smooth muscle: a model of crossbridge kinetics. Biophys. J. **51:**338a.
11. BOHR, D. F. 1963. Vascular smooth muscle: dual effects of calcium. Science **139:** 597–599.
12. STEINSLAND, O. S., R. F. FURCHGOTT & S. M. KIRPEKAR. 1973. Biphasic vasoconstriction of the rabbit ear artery. Circ. Res. **32:** 49–58.
13. SOMLYO, A. V. & A. P. SOMLYO. 1968. Electromechanical and pharmacomechanical coupling in vascular smooth muscle. J Pharmacol. Exp. Ther. **159:** 129–145.
14. VAN BREEMEN, C., C. CAUVIN, A. JOHNS, P. LEIJTEN & H. YAMOMOTO. 1986. Ca^{2+} regulation of vascular smooth muscle. Fed. Proc. **45:**2746–2751.
15. SAIDA, K. & C. VAN BREEMEN. 1984. Cyclic AMP modulation of adrenoreceptor mediated arterial smooth muscle contraction. J. Gen. Physiol. **84:** 307–318.
16. HASHIMOTO, T., M. HIRATA, T. ITOH, Y. KANMURA & H. KURIYAMA. 1986. Inositol 1,4,5-trisphosphate activates pharmacological coupling in smooth muscle of the rabbit mesenteric artery. J. Physiol. 370:605–618.
17. FORD, G. D. & M. L. HESS. 1975. Calcium accumulating properties of subcellular fractions of bovine vascular smooth muscle. Circ. Res. **37:** 580–587.
18. VAN BREEMEN, C., P. AARONSON, R. LOUTZENHISER & K. MEISHERI. 1982. Calcium fluxes in isolated rabbit aorta and guinea pig tenia coli. Fed. Proc. **41:** 2891–2897.
19. CAUVIN, C., R. LOUTZENHISER & C. VAN BREEMEN. 1983. Mechanisms of calcium antagonist–induced vasodilation. Annu. Rev. Pharmacol. Toxicol. **23:** 373–396.
20. YAMAMOTO, H., O. HWANG & C. VAN BREEMEN. 1984. The Ca^{2+} agonist Bay K 8644 differentiates between potential- and receptor-operated Ca^{2+} channels. Eur. J. Pharmacol. **102:**555–557.
21. BONACCORSI, A., K. HERMSMEYER, O. APRIGLIANO, C. B. SMITH & D. F. BOHR. 1977. Mechanism of potassium relaxation of arterial muscle. Blood Vessels **14:**261–276.
22. BAKER, P. F., M. P. BLAUSTEIN, A. L. HODGKIN & R. A. STEINHARDT. 1969. The influence of calcium on sodium efflux in squid axons. J. Physiol. **200:** 431–458.
23. BRIGGS, A. H. & S. MELVIN. 1961. Ion movement in isolated rabbit aortic strips. Am. J. Physiol. **201:** 365–368.
24. BOHR, D. F., C. SEIDEL & J. SOBIESKI. 1969. Possible role of sodium-calcium pumps in tension development in vascular smooth muscle. Microvasc. Res. **1:** 335–343.
25. LEONARD, E. 1957. Alterations of contractile response of artery strip by a potassium-free solution, cardiac glycosides and changes in stimulation frequency. Am. J. Physiol. **189:** 185–190.
26. JOHNSON, J. D., E. J. KHABBAZA, B. L. BAILEY & T. J. GRIESHOP. 1986. Calcium-binding proteins in the regulation of muscle contraction. *In* Cardiac Muscle: the Regulation of Excitation and Contraction. R. D. Nathan, Ed.: 297–313. Academic Press. Orlando, Fla.
27. BLAUSTEIN, M. P. 1977. Sodium ions, calcium ions, blood pressure regulation, and hypertension: a reassessment and a hypothesis. Am. J. Physiol. **232:** C165–C173.
28. VAN BREEMEN, C., P. AARONSON & R. LOUTZENHIZER. 1979. Sodium-calcium interactions in mammalian smooth muscle. Pharmacol. Rev. **30:**167–208.
29. CASTEELS, R. & C. VAN BREEMEN. 1975. Active and passive Ca^{2+} fluxes across cell membranes of the guinea-pig taenia coli. Pflugers Arch. **359:** 197–207.
30. KOBAYSASHI, S., H. KANAIDE & M. NAKAMURA. 1985. Cytosolic-free calcium transients in

cultured vascular smooth muscle cells: microfluorometric measurements. Science **229:** 553–556.
31. RAPP, J. P. 1981. Aortic response to vanadate: independence of (Na, K)-ATPase and comparison of Dahl salt-sensitive and salt-resistant rats. Hypertension **3**(Suppl. I): I-168–I-172.
32. GODFRAIND, T. 1983. Action of nifedipine on calcium fluxes and contraction in isolated rat arteries. J. Pharmacol. Exp. Ther. **224:**443–450.
33. VAN BREEMEN, C., O. HWANG & K. D. MEISHERI. 1981. The mechanism of inhibitor action of diltiazem on vascular smooth muscle contractility. J. Pharmacol. Exp. Ther. **218:**559–463.
34. WEBB, R. C. & D. F. BOHR. 1978. Mechanism of membrane stabilization by calcium in vascular smooth muscle. Am. J. Physiol. **235:** C227–C232.
35. HOLMAN, M. E. 1958. Membrane potentials recorded with high-resistance micro-electrodes; and the effects of changes in ionic environment on the electrical and mechanical activity of the smooth muscle of the taenia coli of the guinea-pig. J. Physiol. **141:**464–488.
36. JONES, A. W. & R. G. HART. 1975. Altered ion transport in aortic smooth muscle during desoxycorticosterone acetate hypertension in the rat. Circ. Res. **37:** 333–341.
37. FURSPAN, P. B. & D. F. BOHR. 1986. Calcium-related abnormalities in lymphocytes from genetically hypertensive rats. Hypertension 8(Suppl. II): II-123–II-126.
38. BOHR, D. F. & R. C. WEBB. 1984. Vascular smooth muscle function and its changes in hypertension. Am. J. Med. **77:** 3–16.
39. HANSEN, T. R. & D. F. BOHR. 1975. Hypertension, transmural pressure and vascular smooth muscle response in rats. Circ. Res. **36:** 590–598.
40. POSTNOV, Y. V. & S. N. ORLOV. 1984. Cell membrane alteration as a source of primary hypertension. J. Hypertension **2:**1–12.

Calcium and Vascular Myogenic Tone[a]

ISMAIL LAHER, JOYCE HWA, AND JOHN A. BEVAN

Department of Pharmacology
University of Vermont
Given Building
Burlington, Vermont 05405

Calcium-entry inhibitors (CEIs) are used routinely in the laboratory and clinical setting. This is hardly surprising in light of the pivotal role of calcium (Ca^{2+}) in both normal and aberrant cellular function.[1] They are used because at appropriate concentrations, they would be expected to inhibit any cellular responses requiring the influx of extracellular Ca^{2+} through channels. This would provide cursory evidence for the dependence of the measured effect on Ca^{2+} influx and the involvement of Ca^{2+} channels.[2] More direct support for the involvement of channels are direct measurements of the movement of radioactive Ca^{2+} (e.g., $^{45}Ca^{2+}$) across the cell membrane,[3] unitary currents through single Ca^{2+} channels,[4] and electrophysiological recordings of macroscopic Ca^{2+} currents.[5] Direct independent evidence for the action of CEIs is essential since (a) not all responses that are inhibited in a Ca^{2+}-free solution or by inorganic CEIs such as La^{3+} or Mn^{2+} are antagonized by organic CEIs,[6] and (b) attenuation of cellular responses by CEIs may not always be due to a specific inhibition of Ca^{2+} influx through Ca^{2+} channels.[7–9]

In this presentation we will provide evidence to support our proposal that in some vascular smooth muscle preparations, Ca^{2+} influx can occur via pathways activated by stretch or distension of the blood vessel wall.[6] Such pathways would be expected to have properties that distinguish them from those activated by agonist-receptor interaction or by alterations in membrane potential. These latter [receptor (ROC) and potential operated (POC) activated] channels have been proposed independently and simultaneously by van Breemen[10] and by Bolton.[11]

The focus of this presentation is a description of studies performed in our laboratory designed to differentiate the Ca^{2+} dependency of vascular tone due to constrictor agonists, membrane depolarization, or cell membrane distension or perturbation. Since stretch-dependent tone is an important element in the response of some blood vessels to an increased transmural pressure,[12] aspects of this cardiovascular control mechanism will be described. Several excellent reviews relating to this aspect of cardiovascular function are available.[13–16]

AUTOREGULATION AND MYOGENIC TONE

Distribution of cardiac output to various organs depends primarily on the variation in local resistance to flow, which is a function of the lumen diameter particularly of middle sized arteries. From a mechanical standpoint, local blood vessel caliber is a dynamic variable determined to a great extent by the balance between two forces, the transmural pressure and the tangential wall tension.[15,16] It is well established that blood flow to a number of organs remains relatively constant despite varying perfusion pressure. This constancy of blood flow, termed autoregulation,[16] involves the interac-

[a]Supported by U.S. Public Health Service Grants HL 32985 and 32383 and by the American Heart Association (Vermont Affiliate).

tion of myogenic, neurogenic, and metabolic influences.[13,16] The capacity to autoregulate is at least in part due to the ability of smooth muscle cells in the smaller arteries to change their state of contraction—their tone—in response to stretch or distension.[12] Investigations by a number of groups have confirmed the contribution of the myogenic response to autoregulation, since alterations of blood vessel diameter still occurred in response to changes in blood pressure in vascular beds free of neurogenic regulation or after metabolic factors were virtually eliminated. The consensus is that with the possible exception of the circulation to the skin, a considerable level of vascular tone remains after most other vasoconstrictor influences have been removed. The data support the proposal that basal or intrinsic tone provides a background against which other vasoconstrictor or vasodilator influences may act.[13–16]

Using an *in vitro* method in which cannulated small cerebral arteries are pressurized,[17] Osol and Halpern observed myogenic tone and active diameter responses to rapid changes in transmural pressures.[18] Theoretical analysis of the data indicated that purely myogenic mechanisms were able to account for only a portion of the diameter adjustment required to maintain autoregulation of flow.

Considerable myogenic basal vascular tone has been observed in blood vessels supplying the brain, retina, kidney, skeletal muscle, liver, myocardium, and intestine. Such tone has been studied in vascular beds of a number of species—dogs, cats, rats, bats, calves, and rabbits.[16] It appears that basal vascular tone is a widespread phenomenon in the intact circulatory systems of mammals. Folkow revived interest in the field with his elegant studies of the perfused hindquarters of rats.[19] From such pressure-flow measurements, Folkow proposed that myogenic regulation of blood vessel diameter was essentially confined to the smaller arteries and larger arterioles. Supporting this proposal are observations that at least in the cerebral circulation, pressure-induced changes in arterial diameter are size dependent, with vessels with diameters of 200–400 μ playing a dominant role in the myogenic response.[20]

STRETCH-INDUCED MYOGENIC TONE IN ISOLATED TISSUE SEGMENTS

The earliest work on myogenic tone in isolated vessel segments was by Bayliss,[21] who reported that upon an increased intravascular pressure, dog carotid artery segments contracted. Later attempts to repeat this were largely unsuccessful and were probably a reflection of the labile nature of this cellular property. One example of myogenic tone is the rhythmic activity of portal-vein segments of a number of species.[16] Such phasic mechanical responses are accompanied by bursts of action potentials, and both measurements are influenced by the magnitude and rate of applied stretch (distension).[22] Several authors have advocated the use of the spontaneously active portal vein as a vessel representative of precapillary arterioles, which also are rhythmically active. Since vascular tone due to increased transmural pressure is also found in nonrhythmic (tonically active) small arteries and arterioles, and only smaller arteries exhibit rhythmic tone associated with spontaneous bursts of action potentials,[23,24] the intrinsic tone in the portal vein may be of a specialized form.

STRETCH-INDUCED MYOGENIC TONE IN RABBIT EAR RESISTANCE ARTERY

Myogenic tone is thought to occur predominantly in the smaller arteries, where resistance to blood flow is regulated. We have made detailed studies on the intrinsic tone that develops in branches of the rabbit ear artery.[25–27] Such vessels, which normally have unstretched lumen diameters of 75–150 μ outside diameter (O.D.) are studied *in vitro* using specially designed resistance vessel myographs.[28] The myogenic tone that develops in response to an applied stretch of resistance arteries of the rabbit ear is not influenced by the endothelium or an adrenergic nerve supply.[25] When placed in a normal physiological salt solution (PSS) and then stretched, a level of tone is attained that represents total tension due to active, intrinsic tone and passive tone due to vessel structural components. The magnitude of the active component is related to both the concentration of Ca^{2+} present in the PSS and the applied tension (FIGURE 1). Optimal levels of myogenic tone in such vessels were obtained when stretched to 2.5 times their unstretched lumen diameters. To extrapolate to *in vivo* parameters, the equivalent arterial pressure corresponding to such applied forces was calculated from the modified Laplace equation. Myogenic tone first appeared when segments were stretched to values equivalent to pressures of 10–20 mmHg, and it contributed significantly to total wall stress at 60–80 mmHg. The maximal myogenic tone when the degree of stretch and concentration of Ca^{2+} are optimized represents about 20% of the maximal contraction of such vessels (e.g., to 10 μM histamine), and is equivalent to the neurogenic tone recorded in response to sympathetic nerve activity at 2–4 Hz.

We next examined the sensitivity of both extrinsic [potassium (K^+) depolarization] and intrinsic tone (myogenic) to inhibition by agents known to inhibit influx of Ca^{2+}. Any tone changes that might be initiated by stimulation of membrane receptors were inhibited by preincubation with phenoxybenzamine (10 μM). Responses to K^+ (50 mM) were studied by isosmotic substitution of K^+ for Na^+. Such contractions presumably represent entry of Ca^{2+} via pathways activated by changes in membrane potential. Both K^+ and stretch-induced tone were dependent on extracellular Ca^{2+}, having ED_{50} values of 2.4×10^4 M ($-\log ED_{50}$ 3.6 ± 0.07 M) and 8.3×10^{-4}M ($-\log ED_{50}$ 3.1 ± 0.03M) respectively. Sensitivity to Ca^{2+} was significantly greater ($p < 0.005$) in K^+-depolarized than in stretch-activated tissues.[26]

A critical observation reported in the study by Hwa and Bevan is that Ca^{2+} influx via membrane-potential-activated pathways is not required for either initiation or maintenance of stretch-induced myogenic tone.[26] The basis for this conclusion is

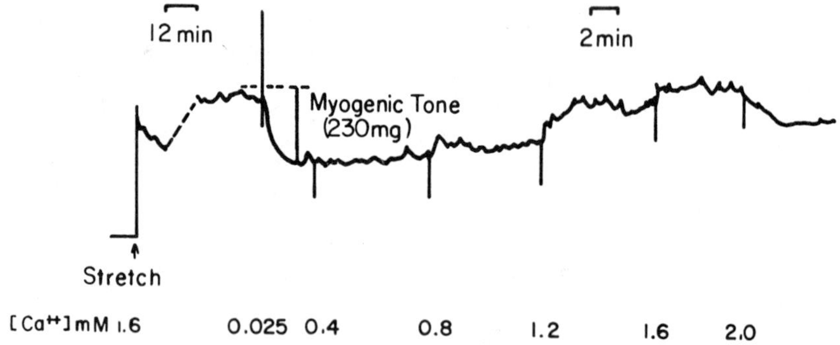

FIGURE 1. Recording of tension changes of rabbit ear arteries (75–150 μ O.D.). Vessel segments were initially stretched in physiological salt solution (PSS) containing 1.6 mM Ca^{2+}. When the developed tone was stable, the PSS was changed to one containing 25 μM Ca^{2+}, which is subthreshold for contraction. The ensuing loss of tone represents that due to stretch-activated myogenic mechanisms, while the new baseline represents passive tone. With the vessel segment still active, myogenic tone develops only when Ca^{2+} is readmitted to the PSS. (Reproduced from Reference 25 by permission of the *American Journal of Physiology*.)

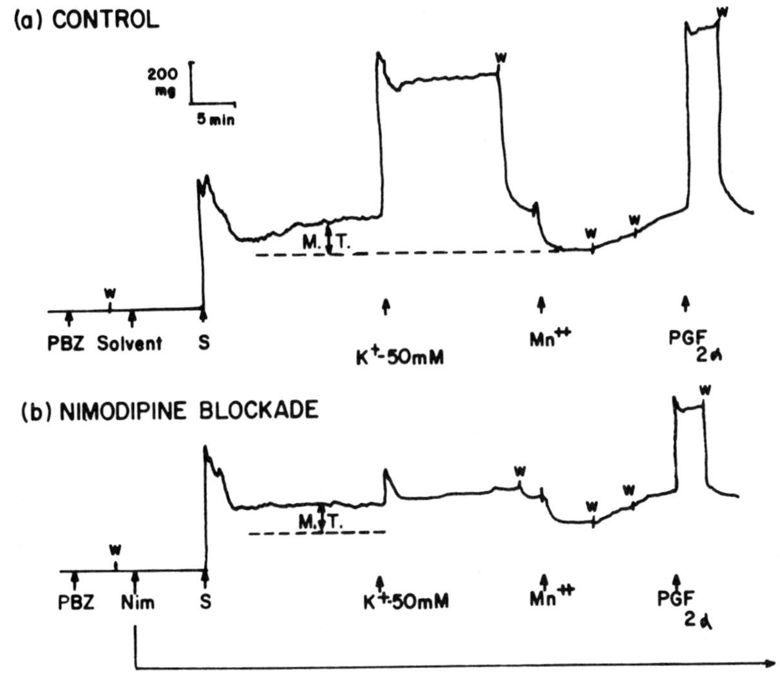

FIGURE 2. Recordings of tension changes of phenoxybenzamine (PBZ, 1 μM for 1 hour) pretreated rabbit ear arteries (75–150 μ O.D.) made in the absence (A) or presence (B) of nimodipine (0.1 μM). Vessel segments were stretched and the developed tone allowed to reach a maintained value, at which point potassium (K^+, 50 mM) was added. K^+-induced tone was not maintained in nimodipine-treated tissues. The magnitude of stretch-induced myogenic tone, as assessed by the loss of tone with manganese (Mn^{2+}, 1 mM), was similar in control and nimodipine-treated tissue segments. Subsequent addition of prostaglandin ($PGF_{2\alpha}$, 10 μM) caused a contraction in both control and nimodipine-treated segments. (Reproduced from Reference 26 by permission of the *American Journal of Physiology*.)

fourfold. First, myogenic tone is three times less sensitive than K^+-induced tone (of similar magnitude) to the reintroduction of extracellular Ca^{2+} (see above); second, whereas CEIs such as nimodipine ($-\log ID_{50}$ 8.2 ± 0.1 M), nifedipine ($-\log ID_{50}$ 8.2 ± 0.1 M) and the (−) enantiomer of PN 200-110 ($-\log ID_{50}$ 7.5 ± 0.2 M) all inhibit or abolish K^+-induced tone, they have no effect on intrinsic tone (FIGURE 2). In fact, varying the concentration of K^+ in nimodipine-treated vessels does not influence the magnitude of stretch-induced tone obtained subsequently. Since only the (−) antipode of PN 200-110 inhibited K^+-induced tone, this indicates a stereospecific effect of this dihydropyridine. Thirdly, Mn^{2+} inhibited K^+-induced tone with a lower potency ($-\log ID_{50}$ 3.1 ± 0.2 M) than it did stretch-induced tone ($-\log ID_{50}$ 3.9 ± 0.1 M) ($p < 0.002$). Finally, when nimodipine (1 μM) treated segments of rabbit ear resistance arteries were stretched in the presence of varying K^+ concentrations, it was found that the level of myogenic tone was unresponsive to changes in K^+ from 5 to 50 mM. In the central ear artery such a change in K^+ corresponds to more than 50 mV depolarization. The separation of Ca^{2+} influx via POCs and stretch-induced Ca^{2+} influx pathways represents clear evidence that membrane potential changes are not obligatory for myogenic tone and that stretch or distension of vascular smooth muscle is able to cause vascular contraction directly. Others have noted that stretch of both nonvascular[29] and vascular smooth muscle cells[30] caused a direct depolarization and a consequent activation of POC mediated Ca^{2+} influx. Such observations are not incompatible with suggestions of a stretch-activated pathway independent of depolarization.

In a subsequent study of stretch-induced myogenic tone in resistance arteries of the

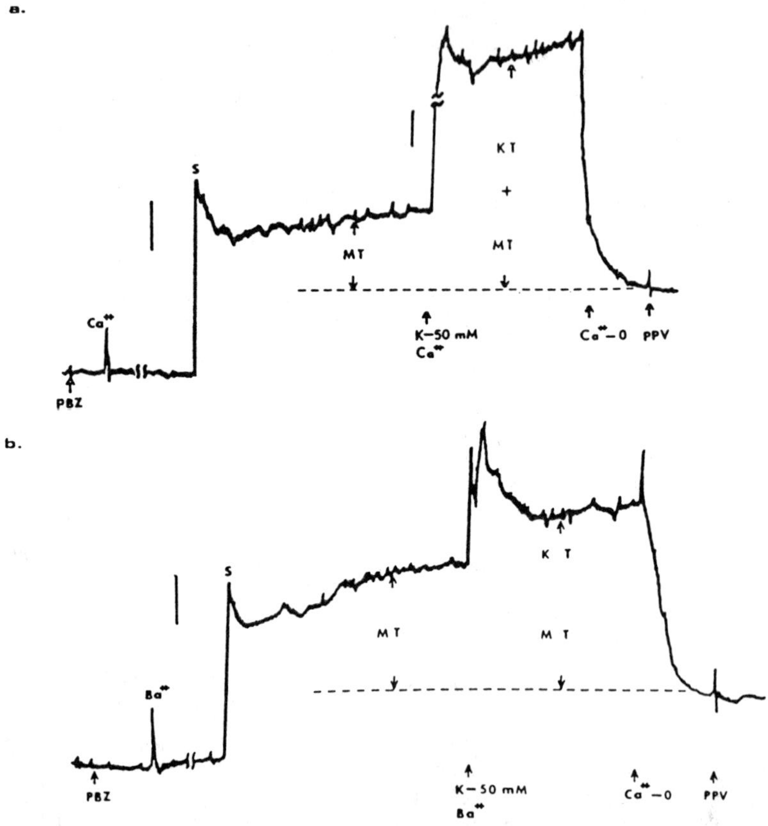

FIGURE 3. Recordings illustrating the development of myogenic tone when rabbit ear arteries (75–150 μM O.D.) are stretched in a physiological salt solution containing (a) Ca^{2+} (1.6 mM) or (b) Ba^{2+} (1.6 mM). Vessel segments were pretreated with phenoxybenzamine (PBZ, 1 μM). Ba^{2+} was less efficient than Ca^{2+} in maintaining K^+ (50 mM) induced tone, whereas it almost doubled stretch-induced tone.

rabbit ear, Hwa and Bevan provided further support for a unique Ca^{2+} entry pathway distinct from POCs and ROCs.[31] Using Ca^{2+} channel agonists (Bay K 8644, CGP 28392), they demonstrated an enhancement of stretch-induced tone at concentrations of these compounds that had no effect on high-K^+-induced tone. Additional evidence for an absence of depolarization-induced mechanisms in stretch-induced tone was obtained in ion-substitution experiments. In the rabbit ear resistance artery, myogenic tone was unaffected by changes in extracellular concentrations of K^+, Na^+, and Cl^- or by the presence of tetrodotoxin, tetraethylammonium, or ouabain. Additionally, equimolar substitution of extracellular Ca^{2+} in the PSS by Ba^{2+}, another divalent ion known to traverse Ca^{2+} entry pathways, has differential effects on stretch- and high-K^+-induced vascular tone (FIGURE 3). Whereas stretch-induced tone is augmented about twofold by this ionic substitution, the K^+-induced tone is significantly reduced.[32]

In the rat portal vein, ion substitution experiments have provided additional clues for a Ca^{2+} entry pathway unrelated to membrane potential changes. When Na^+ was substituted for by equimolar concentrations of hydrazine, mechanical responses were observed in the absence of electrical activity, whereas in choline or lithium substitution solutions electrical activity was present but contractions were abolished.[33] Since Ca^{2+} is essential for both electrical and mechanical activity in the rat portal vein, it is reasonable to suggest that at least two pathways are present—only one of which is linked to membrane potential changes.[31]

In summary, studies on the main-side branch of the rabbit ear artery have established the presence of active tone superimposed on the passive response of isolated arterial preparations to stretch. The active response is related to the concentration of extracellular Ca,$^{2+}$ is dependent on the magnitude of stretch, and is an intrinsic property of vascular smooth muscle cells (i.e., is myogenic) since it is not influenced by the removal of endothelial or neurogenic factors. There is a differential pharmacology of inhibition of tone by CEIs when responses to potassium and stretch are compared; for example, stretch-activated tone is resistant to concentrations of nimodipine that severely inhibit responses due to potassium depolarization. Such observations provide evidence for a unique Ca^{2+} entry pathway that is activated by stretch of vascular smooth muscle cells.

STRETCH-INDUCED TONE IN MYOGENIC CEREBRAL ARTERIES

Another important vascular bed that autoregulates is the cerebral circulation. Here again we have evidence based upon the differential sensitivity to CEIs for the independence of stretch-induced as compared with receptor agonist or K^+-induced tone.[34] In the rabbit basilar artery, diltiazem has a preferential action on responses to norepinephrine (ID_{50} 1×10^{-8} M), serotonin (ID_{50} 8×10^{-8} M), and K^+ contractions (ID_{50} 1×10^{-7} M). On the other hand, maintained intrinsic tone in this vessel is resistant to diltiazem.[34]

STRETCH-INDUCED MYOGENIC TONE IN THE FACIAL VEIN

The maintained myogenic tone that develops in the rabbit facial vein is dependent not only on the level of applied stretch and concentration of Ca^{2+} in the PSS, but also on the ambient temperature.[35–37] The buccal segment of this vein from a number of species is thought to function as a temperature-sensitive sphincter in cerebral thermoregulation.[38] When segments of the rabbit or feline facial vein are studied *in vitro,* maintained active responses are recorded when vessels are stretched at temperatures greater than 33°C. The magnitude of this response is related to the concentration of Ca^{2+} in the PSS, and is inhibited by inorganic ions such as Mn^{2+}.[37] However, this tone is resistant to organic CEIs; in fact compounds such as verapamil, diltiazem, and nifedipine paradoxically augment stretch-induced tone.[34,39] Several lines of evidence obtained in the rabbit facial vein promote our earlier suggestions that distension-induced tone involves Ca^{2+} influx through unique pathways. These can be summarized as follows: (1) While both agonist (histamine) and stretch (myogenic) tone are resistant to organic CEIs,[39] only the stretch-induced Ca^{2+}-dependent tone is temperature dependent.[37] (2) Whereas surgical denervation of the facial vein by superior cervical ganglionectomy causes a two- to eightfold increase in the sensitivity of the constrictor response to norepinephrine, no alteration was noted in either the magnitude or rate of development of myogenic tone under similar treatment.[40] (3) Incubation of facial veins in a moderately elevated (10 mM) K^+ containing PSS caused a significant (one- to eightfold) shift in the constrictor response to norepinephrine, while no changes were noted in the characteristics of myogenic tone under depolarizing conditions.[40] In support of a role for a Ca^{2+}-dependent myogenic tone in the rabbit facial veins are observations that the Ca^{2+} channel agonist Bay K 8644 augments myogenic tone induced by stretch activation.[41]

STRETCH-INDUCED CALCIUM INFLUX IN THE RABBIT FACIAL VEIN

Direct evidence for a stretch-activated influx of $^{45}Ca^{2+}$ in myogenically active vessels was obtained in the rabbit facial vein in collaboration with van Breemen.[41] This

TABLE 1. Measurements of $^{45}Ca^{2+}$ Influx in Rabbit Facial Veins[a]

	$^{45}Ca^{2+}$ Influx (moles/kg per minute)		
	Unstretched Control	Stretched Control	Stretched Bay K 8644
30°C	19.8 ± 3.8	19.2 ± 1.7	18.1 ± 1.4
42°C	32.8 ± 2.5	71.1 ± 5.6[b]	89.8 ± 15.7[b]

[a]One-minute unidirectional influx measurements were made in tissues without myogenic tone (unstretched, or low-temperature studies at 27°C and 30°C) or in tissues with myogenic tone [stretched at 42°C, in the absence or presence of Bay K 8644 (1 M)]. Values are the mean ± standard error of the mean of 10–25 experiments.

[b]Significantly different from unstretched control by analysis of variance ($p < 0.05$).

vessel was used since it represents a sizable myogenically active vessel that consistently develops tone with characteristics that facilitate its analysis. Unidirectional $^{45}Ca^{2+}$ influx was measured according to methods pioneered by van Breemen[42] in which tissues were exposed to PSS containing $^{45}Ca^{2+}$. Any uptake occurring over brief periods (e.g., 1 minute) represents predominantly an influx of the ion (see References 43 and 44 for details). Rabbit facial veins were prepared for iosmetric tension recordings in a Hepes-containing PSS and equilibrated at 30°C (no intrinsic tone) or at 42°C (maximal intrinsic force). Unidirectional influx of $^{45}Ca^{2+}$ was measured at these temperatures with the tissues unstretched or stretched to 0.5 *g*, both in the absence and presence of Bay K 8644 (1 μM). A large increase in unidirectional influx was measured under conditions shown to be necessary for myogenic activity (i.e., stretch and an elevated temperature), but not its association with K^+ or agonist-induced tone (see TABLE 1). The additional increase in myogenic activity caused by Bay K 8644 (1 μM) was associated with an additional increase in influx of $^{45}Ca^{2+}$. Increased $^{45}Ca^{2+}$ entry did not follow stretch at 30°C. Incubation with the calcium channel agonist for periods up to one hour failed to promote influx or contractile activity. We have also determined that CEIs that do not inhibit stretch-induced myogenic activity, such as nifedipine and nicardipine (see above), also fail to prevent the stretch-induced increase in unidirectional influx of $^{45}Ca^{2+}$ in this vessel. By comparison, when similar measurements were made in segments of facial vein lacking stretch-induced myogenic tone, we could not determine any increased influx of $^{45}Ca^{2+}$. These observations indicate that conditions that agument myogenic activity—such as stretch, increased temperature or Bay K 8644—also facilitate entry of $^{45}Ca^{2+}$ into vascular smooth muscle cells. Conversely, conditions that to do not promote stretch-dependent tone in the facial vein—such as CEIs—or that abolish it —a reduced temperature—have corresponding effects on the unidirectional influx of $^{45}Ca^{2+}$. Our results represent the first direct evidence for an increased influx of Ca^{2+} due to distension of a blood vessel.

ALTERNATE MECHANISMS FOR STRETCH-INDUCED TONE

There may be alternate explanations for the mechanism of stretch-induced myogenic tone in isolated blood vessels. The recent observations by Nakayama[45,46] suggest that stretch-induced myogenic tone in cerebral arteries is maintained by intracellular Ca^{2+} release, at least during the initial short-term active response. The observations by Hwa and Bevan,[25,26] Bevan,[34] and Winquist and Bevan[35] that stretch-induced myogenic tone in vascular segments from three vascular beds are sensitive to alterations in extracellular Ca^{2+} concentrations indicate that stretch-induced tone is independent of a Ca^{2+}-induced release of Ca^{2+} stores. Since diltiazem inhibited equally intrinsic ($-\log ID_{50}$ 6.1 ± 0.4) and K^+-induced tone ($-\log ID_{50}$ 6.3 ± 0.2) in the rabbit ear resistance artery, it is reasonable to exclude the participation of a "leak" pathway for Ca^{2+} during stretch-activated tone in that vessel. The leak pathway represents membrane permeability to Ca^{2+} when the muscle is in a resting state. Such Ca^{2+} entry characteristically is resistant to CEIs but sensitive to inhibition by La^{3+} and Mn^{2+}.[47] Another possibility is that stretch causes the direct phosphorylation of contractile proteins of vascular smooth muscle; such a mechanism is adequately explained by intracellular release of Ca^{2+}.[48] This is not the case in the initiation or maintenance of intrinsic tone in our studies.[25,26,31,34,35]

CONCLUSION

Stretch-dependent myogenic tone makes an important contribution to the autoregulation of local blood flow. Several vascular preparations develop myogenic tone when stretched *in vitro*, and can be used to study this phenomenon. Myogenic tone has been found to be dependent on the initial stretch and on the concentration of extracellular Ca^{2+}. Tone activated by stretch in rabbit arteries (ear and basilar) and in a vein (facial) appears to be dependent on a pathway for Ca^{2+} entry distinct from that associated with agonist or depolarization activation. In support of a unique stretch-activated Ca^{2+} entry pathway is evidence that (1) concentrations of dihydropyridine-type Ca^{2+} entry inhibitors such as nimodipine, which abolish contractile responses to K^+ depolarization, have no effect on stretch-activated myogenic tone; (2) contractile responses of the rabbit basilar artery to K^+, serotonin, and norepinephrine are eliminated by concentrations of diltiazem that do not affect stretch-induced myogenic tone; and (3) in the rabbit facial vein, conditions that initiate and increase myogenic tone but not other tone moieties have a parallel effect on net unidirectional influx of $^{45}Ca^{2+}$.

Our experiments support the existence of a stretch-activated Ca^{2+} influx pathway, distinct from Ca^{2+} influx pathways activated by agonists or membrane depolarization.

These findings raise the possibility of selective pharmacological manipulation of vascular tone dependent on those different factors.

REFERENCES

1. FLECKENSTEIN, A. 1977. Specific pharmacology of calcium in myocardium, cardiac pacemakers and vascular smooth muscle. Annu. Rev. Pharmacol. Toxicol. **17:** 149–166.
2. TRIGGLE, D. J. & V. C. SWAMY. 1983. Calcium antagonists. Some chemical-pharmacologic aspects. Circ. Res. **52:** 17–28.
3. CAUVIN, C., S. LUKEMAN, J. CAMERON, O. HWANG, K. MEISHERI, H. YAMAMOTO & C. VAN BREEMEN. 1984. Theoretical basis for vascular selectivity of Ca^{2+} antagonists. J. Cardiovasc. Pharmacol. **6:** S630–S638.
4. WORLEY, J. F., J. W. DEITMER & M. T. NELSON. 1986. Single nisoldipine-sensitive calcium channels in smooth muscle cells isolated from rabbit mesenteric artery. Proc. Nat. Acad. Sci. USA **83:** 5746–5750.
5. KURIYAMA, W., Y. ITO, H. SUZUKI, K. KITAMURA & T. ITOH. 1982. Factors modifying contraction-relaxation cycle in vascular smooth muscles. Am. J. Physiol. **243:** H641–H662.
6. BEVAN, J. A., R. D. BEVAN, J. J. HWA, M. P. OWEN, F. M. TAYO & R. J. WINQUIST. 1982. Calcium, extrinsic and intrinsic (myogenic) vascular tone. *In* Calcium Modulators. T. Godfraind, A. Albertini & R. Pauletti, Eds.: 125–132. Elsevier Biomedical Press. Amsterdam, Holland.
7. CAUVIN, C., R. LOUTZENHISER & C. VAN BREEMEN. 1983. Mechanisms of calcium antagonist–induced vasodilation. Annu. Rev. Pharmacol. Toxicol. **23:** 373–396.
8. LOUTZENHISER, R., P. LEIJTEN, K. SAIDA & C. VAN BREEMEN. 1985. Calcium compartments and mobilization during contraction of smooth muscle. *In* Calcium and Contractility. A. K. Grover & E. E. Daniel, Eds.: 61–92. The Humana Press. Clifton, N.J.
9. KARAKI, H. & G. B. WEISS. 1984. Calcium channels in smooth muscle. Gastroenterology **87:** 960–970.
10. VAN BREEMEN, C., P. AARONSON & R. LOUTZENHISER. 1979. Na-Ca interactions in mammalian smooth muscle. Pharmacol. Rev. **30:** 167–208.
11. BOLTON, T. B. 1979. Mechanisms of action of transmitters and other substances on smooth muscle. Physiol. Rev. **59:** 607–718.
12. BEVAN, J. A. 1985. Vascular myogenic or stetch-dependent tone. J. Cardiovasc. Pharmacol. **7:** S129–S136.
13. FOLKOW, B. 1964. Description of the myogenic hypothesis. Circ. Res. **15:** 279–287.
14. MELLANDER, S. & B. JOHANSSON. 1968. Control of resistance, exchange and capacitance functions in the peripheral circulation. Pharmacol. Rev. **20:** 117–196.
15. JOHNSON, P. C. 1977. The myogenic response and the microcirculation. Microvasc. Res. **13:** 1–18.
16. JOHNSON, P. C. 1980. The myogenic response. *In* The Handbook of Physiology. The Cardiovascular System. Vascular Smooth Muscle, Section 2. D. F. Bohr, A. P. Somlyo & H. V. Sparks. Eds. **2:** 409–442. Waverly Press. Baltimore, Md.
17. HALPERN, W. & G. OSOL. 1985. Blood vessel diameter measurement. Prog. Appl. Microcir. **8:** 32–39.
18. OSOL, G. & W. HALPERN. 1986. Myogenic properties of cerebral blood vessels from normotensive and hypertensive rats. Am. J. Physiol. **249:** H914–H921.
19. FOLKOW, B. 1949. Intravascular pressure as a factor regulating the tone of small vessels. Acta Physiol. Scand. **17:** 289–310.
20. KONTOS, H. A., E. P. WEI, R. M. NAVARI, J. E. LEVASSEUR, W. I. ROSENBLUM & J. L. PATTERSON. 1978. Responses of cerebral arteries and arterioles to acute hypotension and hypertension. Am. J. Phyiol. **234:** H371–H383.
21. BAYLISS, W. M. 1902. On the local reactions of the arterial wall to changes of internal pressure. J. Physiol. London **28:** 220–231.
22. JOHANSSON, B. & S. MELLANDER. 1975. Static and dynamic changes in the vascular myogenic response to passive changes in length as revealed by electrical and mechanical recordings from the rat portal vein. Cir. Res. **76:** 76–83.

23. KEATINGE, W. R. 1979. Blood-vessels. Br. Med. Bull. **35:** 249–254.
24. ARJAMAA, O. 1984. The effects of stretch on smooth muscle. Gen. Pharmacol. **15:** 75–77.
25. HWA, J. J. & J. A. BEVAN. 1986. Stretch-dependent (myogenic) tone in rabbit ear resistance arteries. Am. J. Physiol. **250:** H87–H95.
26. HWA, J. J. & J. A. BEVAN. 1986. A nimodipine-resistant Ca^{2+} pathway is involved in myogenic tone in a resistance artery. Am. J. Physiol. **251:** H182–H189.
27. OWEN, M. P., J. G. WALMSLEY, M. F. MASON, R. D. BEVAN & J. A. BEVAN. 1983. Adrenergic control in three segments of diminishing diameter in rabbit ear. Am. J. Physiol. **245:** H320–H326.
28. MULVANY, M. J. & W. HALPERN. 1976. Mechanical properties of vascular smooth muscle cells *in situ*. Nature London **260:** 617–619.
29. BULBRING, E. 1955. Correlation between membrane potential, spike discharge and tension in smooth muscle. J. Physiol. London **128:** 200–221.
30. HARDER, D. R. 1984. Pressure-dependent membrane depolarization in cat middle cerebral artery. Circ. Res. **55:** 197–202.
31. HWA, J. J. & J. A. BEVAN. 1986. Dihydropyridine calcium channel agonstis selectively enhance resistance artery myogenic tone. Eur. J. Pharmacol. **126:** 231–238.
32. BEVAN, J. A., J. J. HWA, I. LAHER & M. P. OWEN. 1985. Calcium, dihydropyridines and resistance vessel tone. *In* Bayer Symposium IX, Cardiovascular Effects of Dihydropyridine-Type Calcium Antagonists and Agonists. A. Fleckenstein & C. van Breemen, Eds.: 362–367. Springer-Verlag. Berlin, FRG.
33. AXELSSON, J. 1961. Dissociation of electrical and mechanical activity in smooth muscle. J. Physiol. London **158:** 381–398.
34. BEVAN, J. A. 1982. Selective action of diltiazem on cerebral vascular smooth muscle in the rabbit: antagonism of extrinsic but not intrinsic maintained tone. Am. J. Cardiol. **49:** 519–524.
35. WINQUIST, R. J. & J. A. BEVAN. 1981. In vitro model of maintained myogenic vascular tone. Blood Vessels **18:** 134–138.
36. WINQUIST, R. J. & J. A. BEVAN. 1977. Development of intrinsic muscle tone in the rabbit facial vein. Proc. West. Pharmacol. Soc. **20:** 149–152.
37. WINQUIST, R. J. & J. A. BEVAN. 1980. Temperature sensitivity of tone in the rabbit facial vein; myogenic mechanism for cranial thermoregulation? Science **207:** 1001–1002.
38. CABANAC, M. 1986. Keeping a cool head. News Physiol. Sci. **1:** 41–44.
39. WINQUIST, R. J. & E. P. BASKIN. 1983. Calcium channels resistant to organic calcium entry blockers in a rabbit vein. Am. J. Physiol. **245:** H1024–H1030.
40. WINQUIST, R. J. & J. A. BEVAN. 1979. The effect of surgical sympathetic denervation upon the development of intrinsic myogenic tone and the alpha and beta adrenergic rceptor–mediated responses of the rabbit facial vein. J. Pharmacol. Exp. Ther. **211:** 1–6.
41. LAHER, I., C. VAN BREEMEN & J. A. BEVAN. Evidence for a stretch-activated Ca^{2+}-influx pathway in a myogenically active blood vessel. (Submitted.)
42. VAN BREEMEN, C., B. R. FARINAS, R. CASTEELS, P. GERBA, F. WUYTACK & R. DETH. 1973. Factors controlling cytoplasmic Ca^{2+} concentration. Phil. Trans. R. Soc. London Ser. B **265:** 57–71.
43. VAN BREEMEN, C., K. HWANG, R. LOUTZENHISER, S. LUKEMAN & H. YAMAMOTO. 1985. Ca entry into vascular smooth muscle. *In* Bayer Symposium IX, Cardiovascular Effects of Dihydropyridine-Type Calcium Antagonists and Agonists. A. Fleckenstein & C. van Breemen, Eds.: 58–71. Springer-Verlag. Berlin, FRG.
44. MEISHERI, K. D., O. HWANG & C. VAN BREEMEN. 1981. Evidence for two separate Ca^{2+} pathways in smooth muscle plasmalemma. J. Membr. Biol. **59:** 19–25.
45. NAKAYAMA, K. 1982. Calcium-dependent contractile activation of cerebral artery produced by quick stretch. Am. J. Physiol. **242:** H760–H768.
46. NAKAYAMA, K., S. SUZUKI & H. SUGI. 1986. Physiological and ultrastructural studies on the mechanism of stretch-induced contractile activation in rabbit cerebral artery smooth muscle. Jpn. J. Physiol. **36:** 745–760.
47. VAN BREEMEN, C., S. LUKEMAN & C. CAUVIN. 1984. A theoretical consideration on the use of calcium antagonists in the treatment of hypertension. Am. J. Med. **77:** 26–30.
48. LEDVORA, R. F., K. BARANY, D. L. VANDERMEULEN, J. T. BARRON & M. BARANY. 1983. Stretch-induced phosphorylation of the 20,000-dalton light chain of myosin in arterial smooth muscle. J. Biol. Chem. **258:** 14080–14083.

Calcium and Activation of the Release of Endothelium-Derived Relaxing Factor

GABOR M. RUBANYI[a] AND PAUL M. VANHOUTTE

Department of Physiology
and Biophysics
Mayo Clinic
Rochester, Minnesota 55905

INTRODUCTION

The endothelium plays an obligatory role in mediating the relaxation of underlying vascular smooth muscle cells in response to various pharmacological agents[1,2] and increases in flow[3] by releasing a labile relaxing substance (endothelium-derived relaxing factor, or EDRF). Similar to excitation-contraction coupling in vascular smooth muscle cells, calcium ions (Ca^{2+}) must play an important role in the activation of the synthesis and/or release of EDRF from endothelial cells as evidenced by endothelium-dependent relaxation evoked by the calcium ionophore A23187.[1] Thus, facilitation of Ca^{2+} entry may have opposite effects on blood vessel tone: contraction by activation of vascular smooth muscle and relaxation by activation of the release of endothelial relaxant substances. Similarly, the vascular action of Ca^{2+} entry blockers may be the sum of such opposing effects. Therefore better understanding of Ca^{2+} activation mechanisms in endothelial cells is essential for the effective use of Ca^{2+} antagonists in various cardiovascular diseases, and also to reveal potentially selective ways of modulation of Ca^{2+} activation in these two cell types.

The purpose of this paper is to give a summary of the available data about the possible sources and mechanisms of translocation of activator Ca^{2+} in endothelial cells associated with the synthesis/release of EDRF.

SOURCES OF ACTIVATOR CALCIUM IN ENDOTHELIAL CELLS

Influx of Extracellular Calcium

Evidence that the presence of extracellular Ca^{2+} is essential for the sustained synthesis/release of EDRF was provided by experiments where endothelium-dependent vascular relaxations or increases in tissue cyclic GMP content were studied after removal of extracellular Ca^{2+}.

Exposure of the aorta of the rabbit[4] or rat[5] to Ca^{2+}-free medium depressed or abolished endothelium-dependent relaxations in response to muscarinic receptor agonists (acetylcholine and metacholine) and to the calcium ionophore A23187. Endothelium-dependent basal or acetylcholine-induced increases in tissue cyclic GMP levels in different blood vessel preparations were abolished in Ca^{2+}-free medium, while

[a]Present affiliation: Pharmacology, Berlex Laboratories, Inc., 110 East Hanover Avenue, Cedar Knolls, New Jersey 07927.

increases due to sodium nitroprusside were not affected.[6-8] However these studies did not allow a determination of whether removal of extracellular Ca^{2+} prevents the synthesis/release of EDRF or whether it blocks the action of EDRF on vascular smooth muscle. In order to distinguish between these two equally possible mechanisms, the effects of Ca^{2+} removal were studied under bioassy conditions. Perfusing aortic segments of the rat[9] or rabbit[10] with Ca^{2+}-free perfusate, while restoring a normal Ca^{2+} concentration in the perfusate before it reached the bioassay tissue, abolished basal and acetylcholine-induced release of EDRF from the endothelium of the perfused segments within seconds. These bioassay studies indicated that removal of extracellular Ca^{2+} prevented the release of EDRF, rather than its action on vascular smooth muscle.

That influx of extracellular Ca^{2+} into endothelial cells plays an important role in the activation of the release of EDRF was postulated upon the finding that the calcium ionophore A23187 (which facilitates the entry of extracellular Ca^{2+}) evokes endothelium-dependent relaxations in a variety of blood vessels isolated from different species[1] and stimulates the release of EDRF from the endothelium of perfused aorta of the rabbit[11] and cultured bovine aortic endothelial cells.[12]

More direct evidence for the occurrence of Ca^{2+} influx was presented in studies on cultured endothelial cells from bovine[13,14] and porcine[15] aorta. Stimulation of endothelial cells by bradykinin and adenosine tri- (ATP) or diphosphate (ADP) (all of which evoke endothelium-dependent relaxation in a variety of blood vessel)[1,2] triggered Ca^{2+} influx and an increase in free cytoplasmic calcium concentration as assessed by measurement of ^{45}Ca flux,[13] Ca^{2+}-dependent K^+ efflux,[15] and quin 2 fluorescence.[13,14]

Release of Calcium from Intracellular Stores

Several lines of experimental evidence suggest that Ca^{2+} can be liberated from intracellular stores in endothelial cells which may contribute to endothelium-dependent vascular relaxation. Although removal of extracellular Ca^{2+} depressed endothelium-dependent responses in the rabbit aorta, metacholine was able to evoke transient endothelium-dependent relaxations several minutes after exposure to Ca^{2+}-free solution.[4] Endothelium-dependent relaxations of the rabbit aorta in response to the bee venom polypeptide melittin were not affected by 10 minutes preincubation in Ca^{2+}-free buffer solution.[16] Indirect assessment of changes in intracellular Ca^{2+} concentration by measuring Ca^{2+}-activated potassium transport (using ^{86}Rb -efflux) in cultured porcine aortic endothelial cells revealed that after prevention of transmembrane calcium movements with lanthanum, bradykinin and ATP were able to induce one ^{86}Rb -efflux response before a complete block was established.[15] This observation suggested that the endothelium has an intracellular calcium store (or stores) from which bradykinin and ATP can liberate Ca^{2+}. Direct assessment of changes in free cytoplasmic calcium concentration in monolayers of bovine aortic endothelial cells by measuring changes in fluorescence of the calcium chelator quin 2 demonstrated that activation of purinergic receptors by ADP and ATP increased free intracellular calcium in endothelial cells, which may be essential for synthesis of prostacyclin and endothelium-derived relaxing factor.[14] In the absence of extracellular Ca^{2+}, the ability of ATP to stimulate increases in intracellular Ca^{2+} concentration was preserved. However, repetitive challenges were followed by decreasing responses. These findings confirm the postulation that ATP is able to mobilize calcium from intracellular stores in endothelial cells.

MECHANISMS OF CALCIUM TRANSLOCATION IN ENDOTHELIAL CELLS

Calcium Channels

The potential involvement of calcium channels in the entry of Ca^{2+} during activation of endothelial cells was studied by the use of Ca^{2+} channel agonists and antagonists, and also by high K^+ depolarization.

Calcium Channel Agonists

The 1,4-dihydropyridine derivative compound Bay K 8644, which is a calcium channel agonist presumably at voltage-operated Ca^{2+} channels,[17] did not evoke relaxations or increases in tissue cyclic GMP levels in rat aortic strips with endothelium.[18] Similarly, Bay K 8644 did not evoke endothelium-dependent relaxations in canine femoral or coronary artery rings.[19] In contrast to Bay K 8644, which is a racemic mixture of (+) and (−) enantiomers and can be considered as a partial agonist,[20] a more selective Ca^{2+} channel agonist—the 1,4-dihydropyridine derivative compound (+) 202,791[20]—evoked endothelium-dependent relaxations in canine femoral arteries[19] in a concentration range (10^{-11} to 10^{-9} M) that is significantly lower than the concentrations (10^{-8} to 10^{-6} M) required to induce contraction of vascular smooth muscle cells.[18,21] In coronary arterial rings of the dog (+) 202,791 did not evoke endothelium-dependent relaxations.[19] Concentration-dependent contractions of rat aorta evoked by Bay K 8644 in the presence of 12–15 mM K^+ were shifted to the right by a factor of 2, and the maximum response was inhibited by 50% in the presence of endothelium.[18] Since Bay K 8644 did not evoke endothelium-dependent relaxation or an increase in tissue cyclic GMP content, these studies suggested that the depression of Bay K 8644–induced contraction in the presence of endothelium was due to the inhibitory effect of EDRF, released continuously under basal conditions, rather than the consequence of EDRF release triggered by Bay K 8644.[18] Recent studies in the porcine coronary artery demonstrated that the Ca^{2+} channel antagonist, (−)202,791[20] augmented the contractions in response to Bay K 8644 only in the presence of endothelium.[22] These findings favor the hypothesis that, as in the canine femoral artery, the Ca^{2+} channel agonist stimulates the release of EDRF in porcine coronary artery. These observations on intact vascular rings were confirmed in bioassay studies, which demonstrated that Ca^{2+} channel agonists trigger the release of EDRF from perfused canine femoral artery segments[23] [Bay K 8644 and (+)202,791] and from bovine aortic endothelial cells[24] (Bay K 8644). The release of EDRF triggered by (+)202,791 could be prevented by nitrendipine (5×10^{-9} M).[23] Thus, endothelial cells must possess voltage-sensitive calcium channels and selective calcium agonists can trigger the release of EDRF by acting on these channels. However, voltage-operated Ca^{2+} channels in endothelial cells may not be identical with the Ca^{2+} channels of the underlying vascular smooth muscle, since much lower concentrations of the Ca^{2+} agonists seem to activate them.

High K^+ Depolarization

If voltage-operated Ca^{2+} channels exist in endothelial cells, membrane depolarization should facilitate Ca^{2+} entry and stimulate the release of EDRF. Although increases in extracellular potassium ion (K^+) concentration evoke membrane depolarization in endothelial cells,[25] so far no study demonstrated that high K^+ indeed stimulates the release of EDRF. To determine whether the negative results were due to a real absence of EDRF release, or because simultaneous exposure of vascular smooth muscle cells to high K^+ depressed the responsiveness of these cells to the released EDRF, the effect of high K^+ was tested in the bioassay system.[26] Selective stimulation of the donor blood vessel with 40 mM KCl (administering K^+ extraluminally into the organ bath where the perfused canine femoral artery segment was mounted), caused relaxation in the coronary artery bioassay ring (not exposed to high K^+). Indomethacin had no effect, but removal of the endothelium from the perfused artery segment prevented the relaxations. These observations indicated that similar to other endothelium-dependent vasodilators, the relaxations evoked by high K^+ were mediated by the release of a nonprostanoid relaxing factor from endothelial cells. Exposure of the perfused segment to other contractile agonists (e.g., prostaglandin $F_{2\alpha}$ or phenylephrine) did not stimulate the release of EDRF, indicating that the release of EDRF by high K^+ was not the nonspecific consequence of arterial contraction. Removal of extracellular Ca^{2+} abolished the response suggesting that Ca^{2+} entry is essential for high K^+–induced release of EDRF.

Although inhibitors of receptors of various known endogenous vasoactive substances (e.g., muscarinic, α- and β-adrenergic, histaminergic, serotoninergic, and purinergic) did not affect the high K^+–induced release of EDRF (Rubanyi, unpublished observations), these studies do not rule out the possibility that high K^+ triggers the release of a still unidentified mediator from the vascular wall that is responsible for the release of EDRF.

Calcium Channel Antagonists

In rabbit aortic preparations nifedipine (5×10^{-7} M) and verapamil (10^{-5} M) inhibited the maximal endothelium-dependent responses to metacholine and the calcium ionophore A23187 by about 40% without changing the EC_{50} values to these agonists or the direct smooth muscle relaxant responses to sodium nitroprusside.[4] Although these studies suggested that Ca^{2+} channels may be involved in translocation of extracellular Ca^{2+} in response to metacholine, the relative higher concentration of the antagonists needed and the inhibition of A23187-induced responses indicated nonspecific actions rather than a specific blockade of Ca^{2+} channels. Verapamil (10^{-6} to 10^{-5} M) and nifedipine (10^{-8} to 5×10^{-7} M) had no or only minor effects on EC_{50} values and maximal responses elicited by acetylcholine and A23187 in the aorta of the rat.[5] Similar negative results were obtained with verapamil in canine femoral arteries[27] and with flunarizine in rat aorta.[8] Endothelium-mediated increases in tissue cyclic GMP levels in rat aorta evoked by acetylcholine were not affected by Ca^{2+}-channel antagonists.[8] Verapamil had no effect on stimulation of ^{86}Rb efflux[15] or increase in quin 2 fluorescence[14] evoked by ATP in cultured endothelial cells. In contrast, nitrendipine (5×10^{-9} M)[23] prevented the release of EDRF from perfused canine femoral arteries triggered by Ca^{2+} channel agonists. These studies indicated that voltage-operated Ca^{2+} channels are not involved in transmembrane Ca^{2+} translocation in endothelial cells during stimulation by bradykinin and muscarinic or purinergic receptor agonists. Thus, calcium-translocation pathways, other than those sensitive to organic calcium entry blockers, must be involved in receptor-stimulation-induced release of EDRF. It is possible that, similar to other tissues,[28–30] several subclasses of Ca^{2+} channels exist in endothelial cells and receptor stimulation activates those (e.g., receptor operated) that are insensitive to organic Ca^{2+} channel antagonists.

Na^+/Ca^{2+} Exchange

Increases in intracellular sodium ion (Na^+) concentration can lead to a rise in free cytoplasmic Ca^{2+} concentration in various biological preparations either by facilitation of Ca^{2+} influx via an Na^+/Ca^{2+} exchange mechanism at the plasma membrane[3] or via Na^+-induced Ca^{2+} release from intracellular binding sites.[32] It was proposed that Na^+/Ca^{2+} exchange may play an important role in the synthesis/release of EDRF

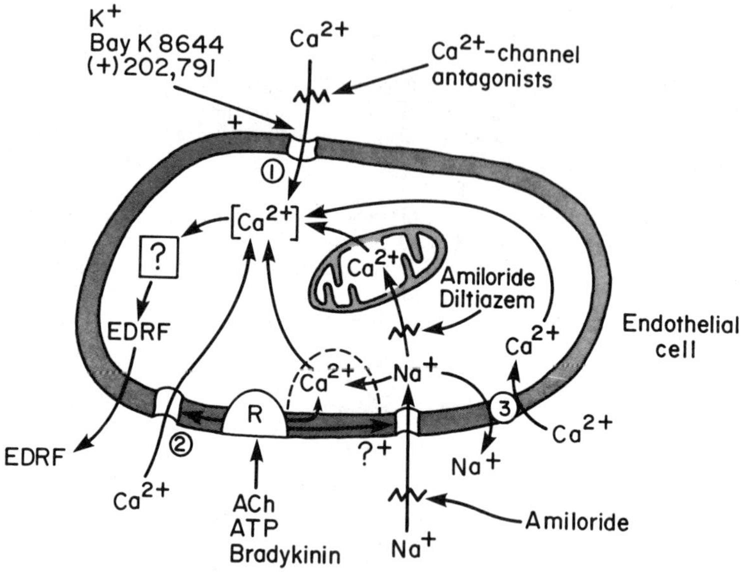

FIGURE 1. Ca^{2+} transport mechanisms that were proposed to be involved in the regulation of cytoplasmic calcium [Ca^{2+}] in endothelial cells, and could play a role in the activation of the synthesis and/or release of endothelium-derived relaxing factor (EDRF). Translocation of extracellular Ca^{2+} may occur at voltage-operated (1; VOC) and receptor-operated (2; ROC) Ca^{2+} channels, or via an Na^+/Ca^{2+} exchange mechanism at the plasma membrane (3). VOC can be activated by high K^+ and by Ca^{2+} channel agonists [Bay K 8644 and (+) 202,791] and inhibited by Ca^{2+} channel antagonists. Stimulation of endothelial receptors (R) by acetylcholine (ACh), bradykinin, or adenine nucleotides can lead to Ca^{2+} influx via ROC or by enhancing Na^+ influx and thereby stimulating Na^+/Ca^{2+} exchange; it is insensitive to Ca^{2+} channel antagonists. Receptor stimulation can lead to liberation of Ca^{2+} from intracellular stores or binding sites. It is still uncertain how an increase in [Ca^{2+}] stimulates the synthesis or the release of EDRF (?).

from endothelial cells. Replacement of sodium by lithium or sucrose in the Krebs-Ringer solution inhibited acetylcholine-induced relaxations of canine femoral artery preparations.[27] Endothelium-mediated relaxations of rat and rabbit aortic preparations in response to acetylcholine and A23187 were inhibited by dichlorobenzamil (DCB),[5] an amiloride analogue and potent inhibitor of Na^+/Ca^{2+} exchange.[31] Dichlorobenzamil did not block direct smooth muscle relaxation by atrial natriuretic factor and sodium nitroprusside.[5] Similar observations were made in the aorta of the rat[33] and canine coronary arteries.[34] In bioassay experiments, selective treatment by DCB (5×10^{-5} M) of the perfused femoral arteries, but not the superfused bioassay tissue, significantly depressed the acetylcholine-induced release of EDRF (Rubanyi, unpublished observations). This study indicated that DCB inhibited endothelium-dependent relaxations by preventing the release of EDRF, rather than its action on vascular smooth muscle. Interaction with Na^+/Ca^{2+} exchange mechanisms may also explain the stereo-selective inhibitory effect of *d-cis*-diltiazem on acetylcholine-induced release of EDRF[35] since, in contrast to other Ca^{2+} channel antagonists, low concentrations of *d-cis*-diltiazem inhibited the Na^+/Ca^{2+} exchange processes in isolated heart and brain mitochondria.[36]

It is known that amiloride and analogues, including DCB, have additional pharmacological activities.[5,31,37] That pharmacological actions of DCB other than inhibition of Na^+/Ca^{2+} exchange mechanisms may also explain the stereo-selective inhibitory effect of *d-cis*-diltiazem on acetylcholine-induced release of EDRF is indicated by the findings that the amiloride analogue was equally effective against acetylcholine- and A23187-induced relaxations.[5] The calcium ionophore A23187 promotes calcium influx into the endothelial cells most probably independent of membrane calcium channels or ion-exchange systems and therefore should be insensitive to selective blockade of Na^+/Ca^{2+} exchange. Although a series of amiloride analogues exhibited a similar rank order of potency for inhibition of endothelium-dependent relaxation in the aorta of the rat[5] and of Na^+/Ca^{2+} exchange in guinea pig cardiac sarcolemma vesicles,[31] verification of the involvement of Na^+/Ca^{2+} exchange in activation of the release of EDRF must await the discovery of more specific antagonists.

SUMMARY AND CONCLUSIONS

Indirect and direct experimental evidence demonstrates that both the entry of extracellular calcium and the liberation of calcium from intracellular stores can contribute to an increase in free cytoplasmic calcium concentration in endothelial cells, which seems to be an essential step in the synthesis and/or release of endothelium-derived relaxing factors(s). A variety of Ca^{2+} transport mechanisms may be involved in the regulation of cytoplasmic calcium in endothelial cells (FIGURE 1). Ca^{2+} entry may occur via voltage-operated Ca^{2+} channels. If they do exist, these channels may have characteristics different from those in underlying vascular smooth muscle cells. Sustained activation of the release of EDRF by various receptor agonists (e.g., acetylcholine, adenine nucleotides, and bradykinin) is also dependent on Ca^{2+} entry, but it is insensitive to organic Ca^{2+} channel antagonists. These findings indicate that, when used clinically in various cardiovascular diseases, organic calcium channel antagonists are not expected to interfere with endothelium-dependent relaxation evoked by endogenous vasoactive substances (e.g., ADP, serotonin). Since amiloride and its analogues blocked endothelium-dependent relaxations in different arterial preparations, Na^+ transport and Na^+/Ca^{2+} exchange were suggested to play a role in calcium-dependent release of EDRF. The exact nature of Ca^{2+} transport mechanisms and also the calcium-sensitive cellular processes that lead to the synthesis/release of endothelium derived relaxing factor(s) remain to be determined. However, the available data suggest that calcium handling by the vascular smooth muscle and endothelial cells may be different, allowing potentially selective modulation of Ca^{2+} activation in these two cell types.

REFERENCES

1. FURCHGOTT, R. F. 1983. Role of the endothelium in responses of vascular smooth muscle. Circ. Res. **53:** 557–573.
2. VANHOUTTE, P. M., G. M. RUBANYI, V. M. MILLER & D. S. HOUSTON. 1986. Modulation of vascular smooth muscle contraction by the endothelium. Annu. Rev. Physiol. **48:** 307–320.
3. RUBANYI, G. M., J. C. ROMERO & P. M. VANHOUTTE. 1986. Flow-induced release of endothelium-derived relaxing factor. Am. J. Physiol. **250:** H1145–H1149.
4. SINGER H. A. & M. J. PEACH. 1982. Calcium- and endothelial-mediated vascular smooth muscle relaxation in rabbit aorta. Hypertension **4**(Suppl. 2): 19–25.
5. WINQUIST, R. J., P. B. BUNTING & T. L. SCHOFIELD. 1985. Blockade of endothelium-dependent relaxation by the amiloride analog diichlorobenzamil: possible roe of Na^+/Ca^{++} exchange in the release of endothelium-derived relaxing factor. J. Pharmacol. Exp. Ther. **235:** 644–650.
6. HOLZMANN, S. 1982. Endothelium-induced relaxation by acetylcholine associated with larger rises in cylclic GMP in coronary arterial strips. J Cyclic Nucleotide Res. **8:** 409–419.
7. RAPPAPORT, R. M., M. B. DRAZNIN & F. MURAD. 1984. Mechanisms of adenosine triphosphate-, thrombin-, and trypsin-induced relaxation of rat thoracic aorta. Circ. Res. **55:** 468–479.
8. MILLER, R. C., P. SCHOEFFTER & J. C. STOCLET. 1985. Insensitivity of calcium-dependent endothelium stimulation in rat isolated aorta to the calcium entry blocker, flunarizine. Br. J. Pharmacol. **85:** 481–487.
9. LONG, C. J. & T. W. STONE. 1985. The release of endothelium-derived relaxing factor is calcium dependent. Blood Vessels **22:** 205–208.
10. GRIFFITH, T. M., D. H. EDWARDS, A. C. NEWBY, M. J. LEWIS & A. H. HENDERSON. 1986. Production of endothelium-derived relaxing factor is dependent on oxidative phosphorylation and extracellular calcium. Cardiovasc. Res. **20:** 7–12.
11. GRIFFITH, T., D. EDWARDS, M. LEWIS, A. NEWBY & A. HENDERSON. 1984. The nature of endothelium-derived relaxing factor. Nature **308:** 645–647.
12. COCKS, T. M., J. A. ANGUS, J. H. CAMPBELL & G. R. CAMPBELL. 1985. Release and properties of endothelium-derived relaxing factor (EDRF) from endothelial cells in culture. J. Cell. Physiol. **123:** 310–320.
13. BROCK, T., R. ALEXANDER & M. GIMBRONE. 1984. Bradykinin and platelet activating factor stimulate calcium flux in cultured vascular endothelial cells. *In* Program and Abstracts of Papers Presented at the 3rd International Symposium on the Biology of the Vascular Endothelial Cell: 51A. Massachusetts Institute of Technology. Cambridge, Mass.
14. LUCKHOFF, A. & R. BUSSE. 1986. Increased free calcium in endothelial cells under stimulation with adenine nucleotides. J. Cell. Physiol. **126:** 414–420.
15. GORDON, J. L. & W. MARTIN. 1983. Endothelial-dependent relaxation of the pig aorta: relationship to stimulation to ^{86}Rb-efflux from isolated endothelial cells. Br. J. Pharmacol. **79:** 531–541.
16. LOEB, A. L., R. A. JOHNS & M. J. PEACH. 1986. Phospholipase activation by melittin releases prostacyclin and an endothelium-derived relaxing factor from rabbit aorta. Blood Vessels **23:** 86.
17. SCHRAMM, M., G. THOMAS, R. TOWART & G. FRANCKOWIAK. 1983. Novel dihydropyridine with positive inotropic action through activation of Ca^{++} channels. Nature **303:** 535–537.
18. SPEDDING, M., V. SCHINI, P. SCHOEFFTER & R. C. MILLER. 1986. Calcium channel activation does not increase release of endothelial-derived relaxing factors (EDRF) in rat aorta although tonic release of EDRF may modulate calcium channel activity in the smooth muscle. J. Cardiovasc. Pharmacol. **8:** 1130–1137.
19. RUBANYI, G. M., A. SCHWARTZ & P. M. VANHOUTTE. 1986. Calcium-channel agonists stimulate the release of endothelial relaxing factor from perfused canine femoral arteries. Fed. Proc. **45:** 426.

20. HOF, R. P., U. T. RUEGG, A. HOF & A. VOGEL. 1985. Stereoselectivity at the calcium channel; opposite action of the enantiomers of a 1,4-dihydropyridine. J. Cardiovasc. Pharmacol. **7:** 689–693.
21. DUBE, G. P., Y. H. BAIK, P. L. VAGHY & A. SCHWARTZ. 1985. Nitrendipine potentiates Bay K 8644–induced contraction of isolated porcine coronary artery: evidence for functionally distinct dihydropyridine receptor subtypes. Biochem. Biophys. Res. Commun. **128:** 1295–1302.
22. WILLIAMS, J. S., Y. H. BAIK & A. SCHWARTZ. 1986. Interactions between calcium agonists and antagonists in coronary smooth muscle: role of the endothelium. Blood Vessels **23:** 55.
23. RUBANYI, G. M., A. SCHWARTZ & P. M. VANHOUTTE. 1985. The calcium agonists Bay K 8644 and (+)202,791 stimulate the release of endothelial relaxing factor from canine femoral arteries. Eur. J. Pharmacol. **117:** 143–144.
24. BUSSE, R. Personal communication.
25. NORTHOVER, B. J. 1980. The membrane potential of vascular endothelial cells. Adv. Microcirc. **9:** 135–160.
26. RUBANYI, G. M. 1986. Potassium-induced release of endothelium-derived relaxing factor. Circulation. **74:** II414.
27. DE MEY, J. G. & P. M. VANHOUTTE. 1980. Interaction between NA^+, K^+ exchanges and the direct inhibitory effect of acetylcholine on canine fermoral arteries. Circ. Res. **46:** 826–836.
28. BOLTON, T. B. 1979. Mechanisms of action of transmitters and other substances on smooth muscle. Physiol. Rev. **59:** 606–718.
29. NILIUS, B., P. HESS, J. B. LANSMAN & R. W. TSIEN. 1985. A novel type of calcium channel in ventricular cells. Nature **316:** 443–446.
30. NOWYCKY, M. C., A. P. FOX & R. W. TSIEN. 1985. Three types of neuronal calcium channel with different calcium agonist sensitivity. Nature **316:** 440–443.
31. SIEGEL, P. K. S., E. J. CRAGOE, JR., M. J. TRUMBLE & G. J. KACZOROWSKI. 1984. Inhibition of Na^+/Ca^{2+} exchange in membrane vesicle and papillary muscle preparations from guinea pig heart by analogs of amiloride. Proc. Nat. Acad. Sci. USA **81:** 3238–3242.
32. VAN BREEMEN, C., P. AARONSON & R. LOUTZENHISER. 1979. Sodium-calcium interactions in mammalian smooth muscle. Pharmacol. Rev. **30:** 167–208.
33. SCHOEFFTER, P. & R. C. MILLER. 1986. Role of sodium-calcium exchange and effects of calcium entry blockers on endothelial-mediated responses in rat isolated aorta. Mol. Pharmacol. **30:** 53–57.
34. ANN, H. S. & D. D. KU. 1986. Magnesium inhibits basal release of endothelium-derived relaxing factor in canine coronary arteries. Eur. J. Pharmacol. **130:** 353–355.
35. RUBANYI, G. M., A. SCHWARTZ & P. M. VANHOUTTE. 1985. The effect of diltiazem and verapamil on endothelium-dependent responses in canine blood vessels. ASPET-ACS-DMC. Boston, Mass.
36. MATLIB, M. A., S. W. LEE, A. DEPOVER & A. SCHWARTZ. 1983. A specific inhibitory action of certain bensothiazepines and bensodiazepines on the sodium-calcium exchange process of heart and brain mitochondria. Eur. J. Pharmacol. **89:** 327–328.
37. BESTERMAN, T. M., W. S. MAY, JR., H. LEVINE III, E. J. CRAGOE, JR. & P. CUATRECASAS. 1985. Amiloride inhibits phorbol ester–stimulated Na^+/H^+ exchange and protein kinase C. J. Biol. Chem. **280:** 1155–1159.

Calcium Antagonism and Vascular Smooth Muscle[a]

J. M. VAN NUETEN, W. J. JANSSENS, AND P. M. VANHOUTTE[b]

Department of Pharmacodynamics
Janssen Pharmaceutica
Turnhoutseweg, 30
B-2340 Beerse, Belgium

INTRODUCTION

To allow normal cellular life, the cardiovascular system ensures a continuous stream of nutrients to the extracellular space and a continuous washout of waste products from the cells. Insufficient vascular perfusion means that the amount of oxygen delivered to a tissue does not meet its actual demands. This will lead to ischemia, loss of cellular function, structural damage, and eventually symptoms of vascular insufficiency. Such impaired tissue perfusion will occur whenever the diameter of a large nutrient artery is reduced without concomitant development of collaterals. The reduction in blood flow may be caused by mechanical obstruction (e.g., due to formation of an atherosclerotic plaque), by a spastic constriction of the blood vessel wall, or moreover by a vasospasm superimposed on a partial obstruction[1,2]

These vascular constrictions ultimately are due to an increase in cytoplasmic Ca^{2+} concentration in the smooth muscle cells of the blood vessel wall. Indeed, the contractile activity of the smooth muscle is regulated by the free intracellular Ca^{2+} levels, which may rise from 0.1 μM in the resting state of 10 μM upon stimulation.[3] Disturbances in the mechanisms regulating transmembrane Ca^{2+} movements in these cells may be due to sustained membrane depolarization, to abnormally high levels of endogenous vasoactive substances, and to a number of pathological conditons.[2,4,5]

This overview discusses the protective action of calcium entry blockers (calcium antagonists) at vascular (in particular cerebral) sites, with special emphasis on the heterogeneity of some of their effects. See also recent reviews.[3,6,7]

MEMBRANE DEPOLARIZATION

When the vascular smooth muscle cell membrane is depolarized by exposure to increased levels of potassium in the presence of calcium, membrane calcium channels will open. The consecutive acceleration of Ca^{2+} entry in the cells triggers vascular contraction.[6,8–10] In blood vessels with a dense adrenergic innervation, high levels of K^+ will also induce the release of endogenous norepinephrine producing further activation of the contractile machinery.[11] In the cerebral blood vessels tested so far, contractions

[a]This work was supported in part by a grant from the Instituut voor Wetenschappelijk Onderzoek in Nijverheid en Landbouw.

[b]Department of Physiology and Biophysics, Mayo Clinic and Mayo Foundation, Rochester, Minnesota 55905.

evoked by calcium in depolarized smooth muscle are inhibited in a concentration-dependent way by all available calcium antagonists. These effects can be explained by the potential of these drugs to inhibit stimulated Ca^{2+} influx through the cell membrane of smooth muscle. However, marked differences exist among the individual compounds regarding the time course of the effect. The inhibitory action of some calcium antagonists (e.g., diltiazem, nifedipine, verapamil) is characterized by a rapid onset and short duration. In contrast, the inhibitory actions of cinnarizine, lidoflazine, nicardipine, and in particular flunarizine are progressive and sustained over a prolonged period (FIGURE 1). These individual pharmacodynamic properties and differences in the duration of action may help to explain the individual clinical application for each of these agents.[12–16]

Marked differences exist between vascular tissues of different anatomical origin from the same species in terms of their sensitivity to the individual calcium antagonists.

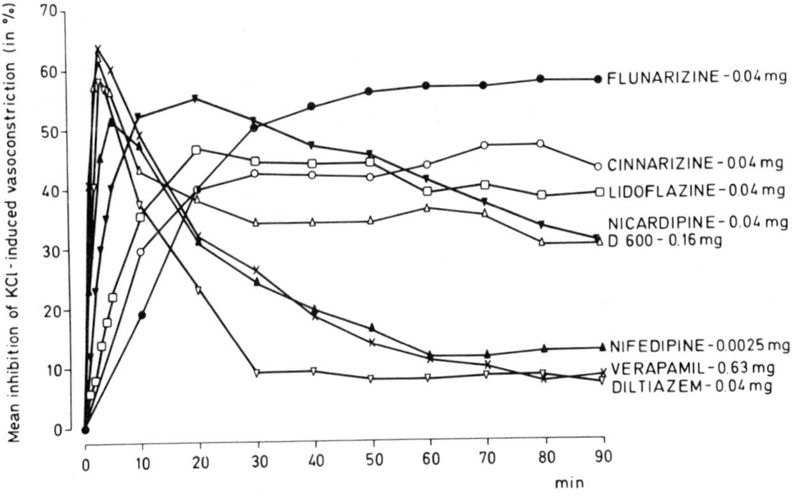

FIGURE 1. Comparison of the time-response characteristics for eight calcium antagonists that inhibit depolarization-induced vasoconstriction in the perfused ear artery of the rabbit. The compounds were added to the perfusate for 30 seconds and washed out within 10 minutes. (Reproduced from Reference 12 with permission from the publisher.)

This may indicate a different access to the calcium channels or a different configuration of these channels. For example, flunarizine and nimodipine are particularly potent in antagonizing Ca^{2+}-induced vasoconstrictor effects of cerebral blood vessels (FIGURE 2).[12,17–19] This effect is independent of the time of administration of the antagonist to the tissue (before or during a calcium-evoked contraction). This contrasts with the findings that some diphenylalkylamines, but not dihydropyridines, are less potent in reversing contractions of the smooth muscles of the taenia from the guinea pig cecum[20] or of canine coronary arteries than in preventing them. Extrapolation to pathological conditions of the similarity of the cerebrovascular effects of drugs such as flunarizine regardless of the experimental conditions implies that the compound may be effective in both preventing and interrupting cerebral vasospasms. In fact, recent experimental and clinical trials show that the calcium antagonists nimodipine and flunarizine exert

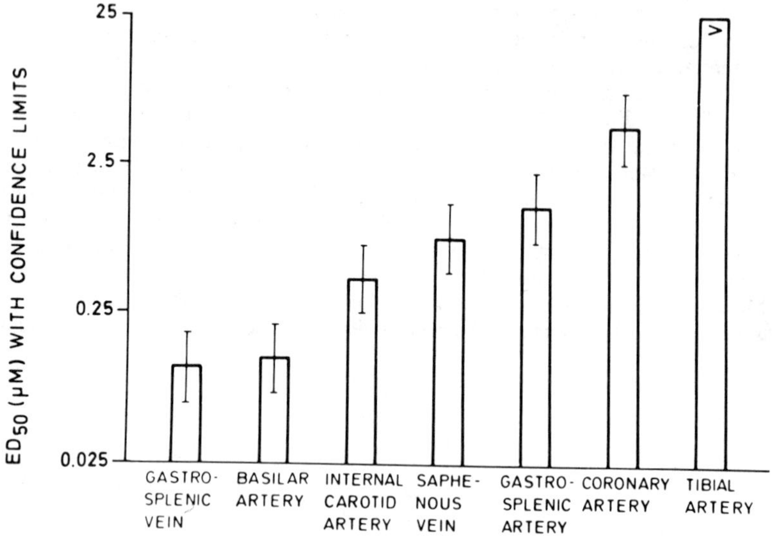

FIGURE 2. Inhibitory effects of flunarizine on calcium-induced contractions of depolarized canine arteries and veins. Data are shown as ED_{50}-molar values with confidence limits. (Reproduced from Reference 12 with permission from the publisher.)

protection against ischemic brain damage[19,21,22] (and Kornhuber, unpublished observations).

VASOCONSTRICTOR SUBSTANCES

Vasoconstrictor responses can be evoked by naturally occurring vasoactive substances, present in the blood, released from aggregating platelets, from tissue cells, from nerve endings, or from the vascular wall.[23] Interaction of these substances with receptors located at the cell membrane will result in an increase in Ca^{2+} influx leading to activation of the contractile proteins in the smooth muscle.

Alpha-Adrenergic Activation

The sympathetic nervous system plays an important role in controlling vascular function.[1] The norepinephrine released from activated adrenergic nerve endings interacts with postjunctional α-adrenoceptors of the vascular smooth muscle cells, which leads to contraction. In most vascular preparations calcium antagonists depress the contractile response to exogenous norepinephrine, but the degree of inhibition may vary among different blood vessels. In some vessels (e.g., canine saphenous vein, guinea pig aorta, ear artery of the rabbit, rat caudal artery), concentrations of calcium antagonists that inhibit Ca^{2+}-induced contractions of depolarized tissue only moderately depress the contractile response to norepinephrine.[24] In other large blood vessels (e.g., isolated splanchnic veins and coronary arteries), norepinephrine-induced contractions are inhibited at concentrations also depressing Ca^{2+}-evoked contractile responses.[10,24–27] These findings indicate that in some vascular smooth muscle part of the activation of the contractile process in response to catecholamines is due not only to an increased Ca^{2+} influx, but also to enhanced mobilization of intracellular Ca^{2+} or to differences in the properties of the vascular smooth muscle cell membrane.[24,28] The varying degrees of dependency of α-adrenergic activation upon Ca^{2+} entry probably are determined by the functional differentiation of the vascular smooth muscle cells.[24] In addition, calcium antagonists have a more pronounced inhibitory action during activation with partial than during activation with full α-adrenergic agonists.[29]

In rats and dogs, the vascular responsiveness to sympathetic stimulation and to catecholamines is decreased by the systemic administration of calcium antagonists.[30–32] In dogs, norepinephrine-induced increases in peripheral vascular resistance are prevented by flunarizine (FIGURE 3) and cinnarizine without change in systemic arterial pressure, heart rate, or basal peripheral vascular tone.[32]

Nonadrenergic Activation

In most isolated blood vessels from animals and man, vasoconstriction can be evoked by nonadrenergic vasoactive substances such as 5-hydroxytryptamine (seroto-

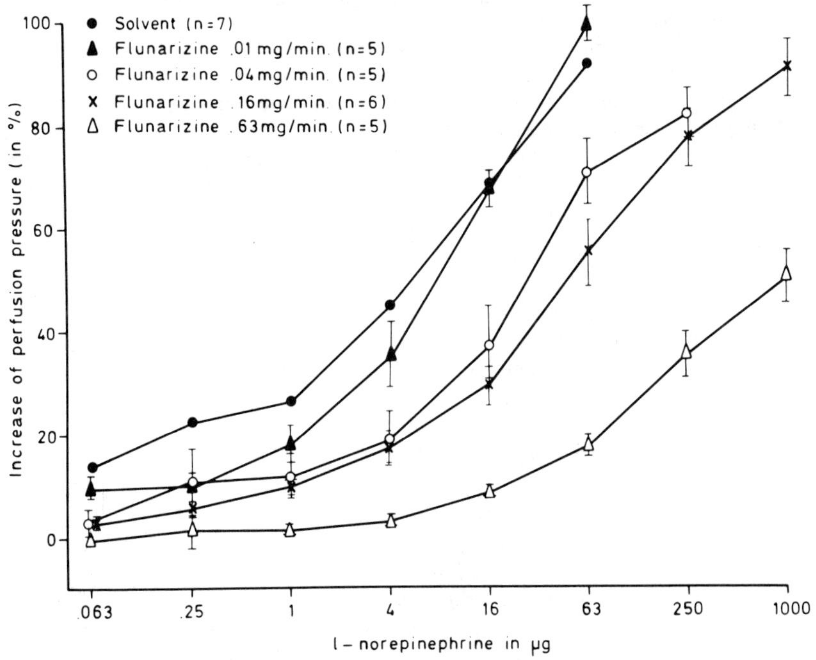

FIGURE 3. L-Norepinephrine-induced vasoconstriction in the perfused hindleg of the anesthetized dog after infusion for 1 hour of solvent or flunarizine 0.01, 0.04, 0.16, and 0.63 mg/minute. Each point represents the mean value ± standard error of the mean (SEM) of the vasoconstriction expressed in percent of the maximum obtained before infusion. (Reproduced from Reference 32 with permission from the publisher.)

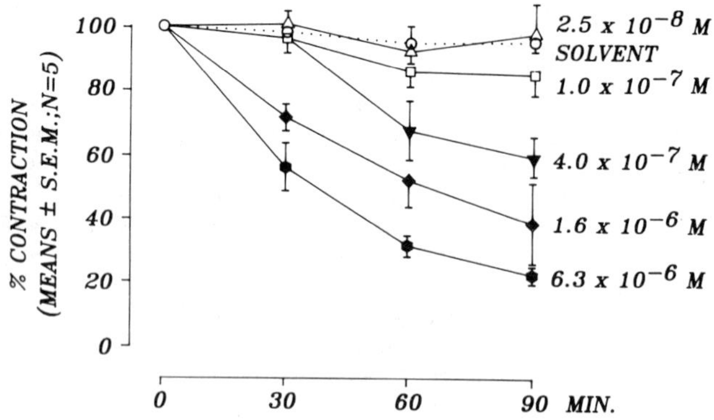

FIGURE 4. Inhibition by flunarizine of contractions of canine basilar artery in response to thrombin-activated human platelets [platelets 1.5×10^{10}/l, thrombin 0.5 National Institutes of Health (NIH) U/ml]. Filled symbols indicate that the values are significantly different from those obtained with solvent ($p < 0.05$; unpaired Student's t-test). (Reproduced from Reference 42 with permission from the publisher.)

nin), ergonovine maleate, prostaglandin $F_{2\alpha}$, thromboxane A_2, and some peptides and by exposure to blood.[24,33–39]

The calcium antagonists inhibit the vasoconstrictions induced by these nonadrenergic vasoconstrictor substances in most blood vessels, demonstrating that the activation of the contractile process depends upon the entry of extracellular Ca^{2+}.[4,17,24,40]

Exposure of vascular tissue, in particular cerebral arteries, to activated platelets from rats or humans results in contractions, which can be prevented and inhibited in a concentration-dependent way by flunarizine (FIGURE 4).[41,42] The inhibition increases gradually as a function of the incubation time with the antagonist. Aggregating blood platelets release serotonin and synthetize prostanoids, mainly thromboxane A_2, and to a lesser extent prostaglandin endoperoxides.[43,44] Pharmacological analysis demonstrates that serotonin and thromboxane A_2 are the main mediators involved in these platelet-induced contractions.[41,43] This explains the involvement of a transmembrane influx of Ca^{2+} in the initiation of the contraction of vascular smooth muscles by aggregating platelets and its inhibition by calcium antagonists.

MODULATION OF VASCULAR REACTIVITY

Pathological Conditions

The responsiveness of the blood vessel wall to vasoconstrictor substances can be modulated by acute and chronic conditions to which the vascular smooth muscle cells are exposed.[45] As an example of an acute change of the environment, a marked further increase in tension can be caused by hypoxia in coronary and cerebral arteries when these vessels first are depolarized or exposed to vasoconstrictor substances or to aggregating platelets. Such hypoxic vasoconstrictions are inhibited by calcium antagonists (e.g., bepridil, diltiazem, flunarizine, lidoflazine, nimodipine, verapamil).[24,46–48]

These findings suggest that in hypoxic conditions an exaggerated entry of Ca^{2+} may occur in vascular smooth muscle. The observation that flunarizine inhibits hypoxic vasoconstriction most potently in cerebral blood vessels (FIGURE 5) correlates with the findings that drugs such as flunarizine (and nimodipine) possess brain-protective properties both in animals with experimental cerebral damage and hypoxia and in patients with cerebrovascular pathology[18,49–54] (and Kornhuber, unpublished observations). The data available on isolated coronary arteries suggest that conditions mimicking tissue ischemia cause profound contractions of coronary vascular smooth muscle, which can be inhibited by calcium antagonists.[2]

Under certain chronic pathological conditions the vascular responsiveness to vasoconstrictor agents and to Ca^{2+} increases. For instance, segments of saphenous veins from patients with varicose veins contract to a greater extent when exposed to serotonin or to increasing amounts of Ca^{2+}. This augmented vasoconstriction is inhibited by calcium antagonists such as flunarizine (FIGURE 6).

The endothelium protects the vascular smooth muscle cells against blood-borne vasoconstrictor agents because it may constitute a physical barrier, may degrade some of the vasoconstrictors and release relaxing factors.[55] Endothelial damage experimentally induced in rats was prevented by calcium antagonists.[56] Since the formation of coronary atherosclerosis is believed to be preceded by endothelial damage and a subsequent decreased release of the endothelium-derived relaxing factor,[57] vascular smooth muscle cells will be more exposed to platelet-derived vasoconstrictor substances under these conditions.[58,59] Clinical trials are ongoing to assess if the protection against atherosclerosis as observed with some calcium antagonists in animal models[60–64] can be demonstrated in patients with this condition.[65]

Cerebral vasospasms induced by experimental subarachnoid haemorrhage in animals are reversed by some calcium antagonists (e.g., nimodipine, flunarizine). This suggests that these substances may be of value in the treatment of postischemic brain damage.[39,66–68] Actually, it appears to be the case for nimodipine[22,69,70] and flunarizine (Kornhuber, unpublished observations).

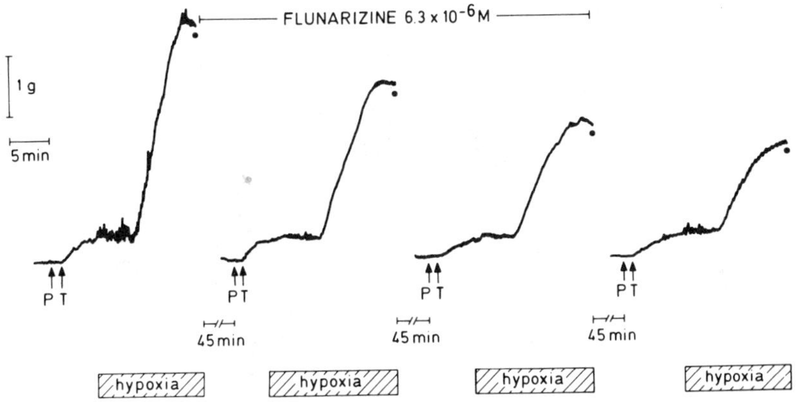

FIGURE 5. Typical experiment showing isometric tension recordings in a canine internal carotid artery segment. The preparations were first exposed to rat platelets (P, 5×10^8/l) activated with thrombin (T, 0.5 NIH U/ml). The aggregating platelets release vasoactive substances (e.g., serotonin, thromboxane A_2) causing contraction of the vascular segment. Switching the gas mixture bubbling the organ bath from 95% O_2–5% CO_2 to 95% N_2–5% O_2 results in a marked increase of the contraction. This hypoxic increase of contractile force is inhibited by the administration of flunarizine.

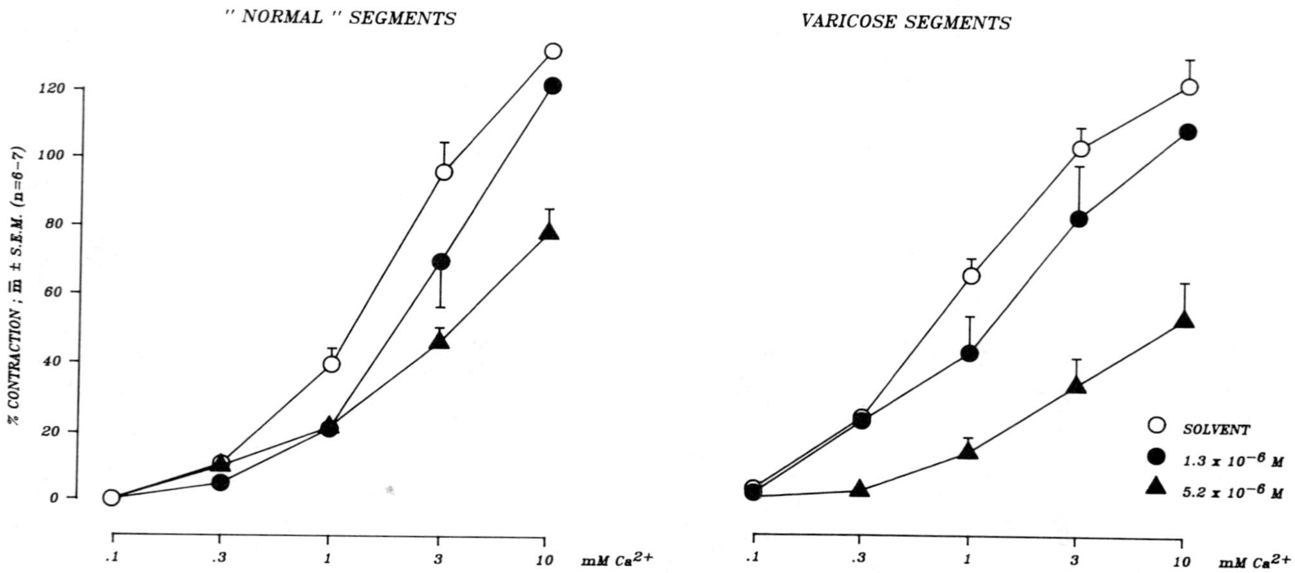

FIGURE 6. Mean increases of isometric tension (as percentage of the response to a previous exposure to 3 mM of Ca^{2+} ions) in depolarized human saphenous veins caused by increasing Ca^{2+} ion concentrations in the presence of flunarizine or its solvent. "Normal" and varicose segments were obtained from the same vessels, removed because of varicosities. Varicose segments macroscopically appeared to be affected by the disease, whereas "normal" segments had a macroscopically normal outlook. The varicose segments were more sensitive to Ca^{2+} ions as well as to the inhibitory effect of flunarizine.

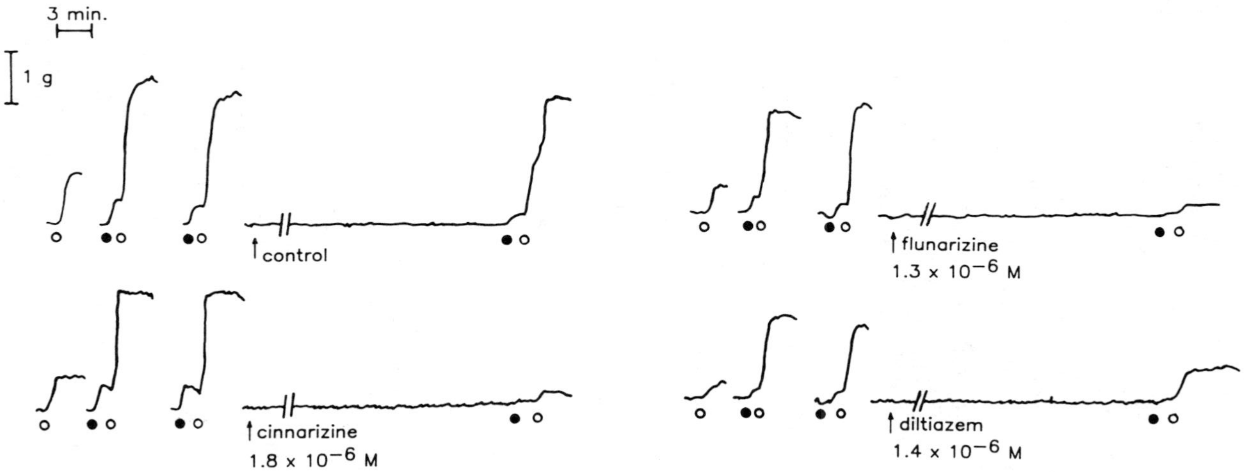

FIGURE 7. Typical experiments showing isometric tension recordings of rabbit femoral artery in response to norepinephrine (6.0×10^{-9} M) (open circles). These responses are augmented in the presence of threshold amounts of serotonin (5.8×10^{-8} M) (filled circles). These amplified contractions are inhibited by the calcium antagonists (incubation time: 90 minutes) flunarizine, cinnarizine, and diltiazem.

Interaction between Vasoactive Substances

Both in isolated blood vessels and in the intact animal or in man, serotonin augments (amplifies) the contractile response to a variety of vasoconstrictor agonists and to sympathetic stimulation.[12,71–73] Amplification has also been observed on isolated human arteries exposed to neuropeptide Y in the presence of exogenous or endogenously released noradrenaline.[74,75] Such amplifying effects, by exaggerating the constrictor effects of other neurohumoral mediators, may contribute to the etiology of vasospasms. Amplified vascular contractions are mediated by an increased influx of

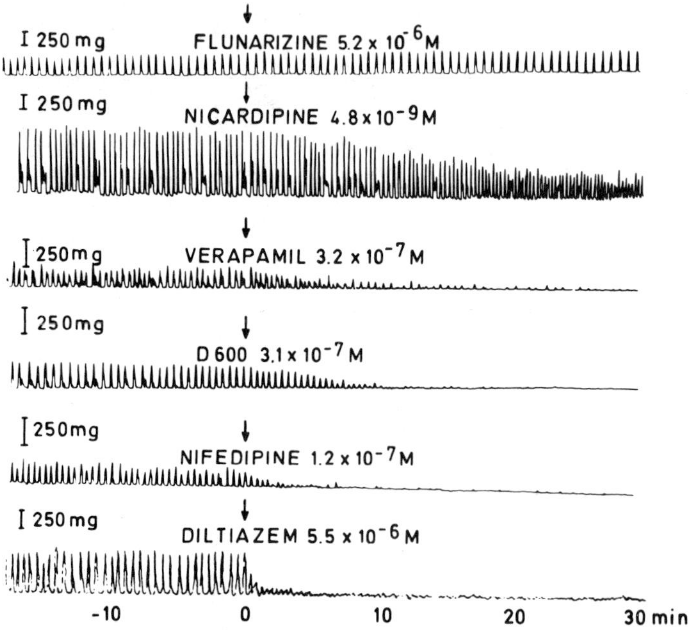

FIGURE 8. Isometric tension recordings in isolated portal-mesenteric veins of the rat. The influence of calcium antagonists on myogenic activity was studied at concentrations producing 80–100% inhibition of the response to Ca^{2+} in the same depolarized preparation. (Modified from Reference 15.)

extracellular calcium, since they are inhibited by cinnarizine, flunarizine, and diltiazem (FIGURE 7)[12] and by withdrawal of Ca^{2+} from the extracellular medium.[75]

HETEROGENEITY OF CALCIUM ANTAGONISTS

The heterogeneity of the several subgroups of calcium antagonists has been well documented.[12,15,24,76–78]

Antagonists selective for the slow Ca^{2+} channels of the myocardial cells produce a cardiac negative inotropic effect. In contrast, calcium antagonists devoid of inhibitory effects on these channels (e.g., flunarizine and cinnarizine) have no effect on contractile force of heart tissues.[14,15,79] The latter group of calcium antagonists are also devoid of inhibitory effect on myogenic activity in vascular smooth muscle, which is observed with calcium antagonists selective for slow Ca^{2+} channels (e.g., verapamil-, nifedipine-, and diltiazemlike substances) (FIGURE 8).[14,15,24,78,80]

Since myogenic tone of the arterioles depends upon the entry of extracellular Ca^{2+} via slow Ca^{2+} channels, it is not surprising that drugs such as verapamil, but not flunarizinelike compounds, inhibit the vasomotor activity of the arterioles *in vivo* (De Clerck, unpublished observations). Flunarizine therefore will interfere little with the myogenic regulation of blood flow at the precapillary level and with blood pressure.[17,24]

The observation that flunarizine does not affect myogenic tone is in agreement with the findings that it does not modify the resting blood flow to lower limbs (dogs, humans), as is the case with nifedipine in humans.[32,81]

SUMMARY AND CONCLUSIONS

Vasoconstriction results from an exaggerated increase of intracellular Ca^{2+} concentration which initiates the contractile process within the vascular smooth muscle. The dependency of these cells on extracellular Ca^{2+} to trigger the contractile process when exposed to naturally occurring vasoactive substances such as those released from aggregating blood platelets varies in different vascular areas. This is one of the factors that determine the different sensitivity to the inhibitory effect of various calcium antagonists. A blood vessel can be more reactive to some calcium antagonists than to others, depending on the vascular area.

Experiments on isolated cerebral arteries suggest that inhibition of cerebral vasoconstriction is observed with substances such as flunarizine under conditions of vascular hyperresponsiveness generated by acute or chronic pathological conditions or triggered by interaction between vasoactive substances. In this regard marked differences exist between the individual calcium antagonists. Those that are selective for slow Ca^{2+} channels will inhibit myocardial contractile force and decrease vascular myogenic activity (e.g., at the arteriolar level). Such inhibitory activity is not observed with flunarizine, which affects Ca^{2+} entry rather selectively, when calcium overload is imposed upon the vasculature, in particular at cerebrovascular sites. This suggests a potential use of this compound in a number of neurological disorders related to cerebral ischemia.

ACKNOWLEDGMENT

We wish to thank Dr. J. A. Van de Heyning-Meier for providing us with segments of human saphenous veins.

REFERENCES

1. SHEPHERD, J. T. & P. M. VANHOUTTE. 1979. The Human Cardiovascular System. Facts and Concepts. Raven Press. New York, N.Y.
2. VANHOUTTE, P. M. & R. A. COHEN. 1983. Calcium-entry blockers and cardiovascular disease. Am. J. Cardiol. **52:** 99A–103A.
3. GODFRAIND, T., R. MILLER & M. WIBO. 1986. Calcium antagonism and calcium entry blockade. Pharmacol. Rev. **38:** 321–416.

4. BOHR, D. F. 1973. Vascular smooth muscle updated. Circ. Res. **32:** 665–672.
5. SOMLYO, A. P. & A. V. SOMLYO. 1968. Electromechanical and pharmacomechanical coupling in vascular smooth muscle. J. Pharmacol. Exp. Ther. **159:** 129–145.
6. FLECKENSTEIN, A., Ed. 1983. Calcium Antagonism in Heart and Smooth Muscle. Experimental Facts and Therapeutic Prospects. John Wiley and Sons. New York, N.Y.
7. GODFRAIND, T., P. M. VANHOUTTE, S. GOVONI & R. PAOLETTI, Eds. 1985. Calcium Entry Blockers and Tissue Protection. Raven Press. New York, N.Y.
8. BOLTON, T. B. 1979. Mechanisms of action of transmitters and other substances on smooth muscle. Physiol. Rev. **59:** 606–718.
9. VAN BREEMEN, C., P. AARONSON & R. LOUTZENHISER. 1979. Sodium-calcium interactions in mammalian smooth muscle. Pharmacol. Rev. **30:** 167–208.
10. HÖGESTÄTT, E. D. & K. E ANDERSSON. 1984. Mechanisms behind the biphasic contractile response to potassium depolarization in isolated rat cerebral arteries. J. Pharmacol. Exp. Ther. **228:** 187–195.
11. VANHOUTTE, P. M., T. J. VERBEUREN & R. C. WEBB. 1981. Local modulation of the adrenergic neuroeffector interaction in the blood vessel wall. Physiol. Rev. **61:** 151–247.
12. VAN NUETEN, J. M. 1985. Calcium entry blockers and vascular smooth muscle reactivity. *In* Calcium Entry Blockers and Tissue Protection. T. Godfraind, P. M. Vanhoutte, S. Govoni & R. Paoletti, Eds.: 69–79. Raven Press. New York, N.Y.
13. GODFRAIND, T. 1981. Mechanisms of action of calcium entry blockers. Fed. Proc. **40:** 2866–2871.
14. VAN NUETEN, J. M., J. VAN BEEK & P. A. J. JANSSEN. 1978. Effect of flunarizine on calcium-induced responses of peripheral vascular smooth muscle. Arch. Int. Pharmacodyn. Ther. **232:** 42–52.
15. VAN NUETEN, J. M. 1982. Selectivity of calcium entry blockers. *In* Calcium Modulators. T. Godfraind, A. Albertini & R. Paoletti, Eds.: 199–208. Elsevier Biomedical Press. Amsterdam, Holland.
16. WADSWORTH, R. M. & J. P. MOSS. 1982. Time course of the effect of flunarizine on rabbit isolated vascular muscle. Eur. J. Pharmacol. **85:** 207–209.
17. VAN NUETEN, J. M. & P. M. VANHOUTTE. 1981. Calcium entry blockers and vascular smooth muscle heterogeneity. Fed. Proc. **40:** 2862–2865.
18. KAZDA, S. & R. TOWART. 1982. Nimodipine: a new calcium antagonistic drug with a preferential cerebrovascular action. Acta Neurochir. **63:** 259–265.
19. TOWART, R. 1981. The selective inhibition of serotonin-induced contractions of rabbit cerebral vascular smooth muscle by calcium-antagonistic dihydropyridines. An investigation of the mechanism of action of nimodipine. Circ. Res. **48:** 650–657.
20. SPEDDING, M. 1982. Assessment of "Ca^{2+} -antagonists." Effects of drugs in K^+-depolarized smooth muscle. Differentiation of antagonist subgroups. Naunyn-Schmiedeberg's Arch. Pharmacol. **318:** 234–240.
21. KAZDA, S. & D. MAYER. 1985. Postischemic impaired reperfusion and tissue damage: consequences of a calcium-dependent vasospasm? *In* Calcium Entry Blockers and Tissues Protection. T. Godfraind, P. M. Vanhoutte, S. Govoni & R. Paoletti, Eds.: 129–138. Raven Press. New York, N.Y.
22. ALLEN, G. S., H. S. AHN, T. J. PREZIOSI, R. BATTYE, S. C. BOONE, S. N. CHOU, D. L. KELLY, B. K. WEIR, R. A. CRABBE, P. J. LAVIK, S. B. ROSENBLOOM, F. C. DORSEY, C. R. INGRAM, D. E. MELLITS, L. A. BERTSCH, D. P. J. BOISVERT, M. B. HUNDLEY, M. S. RAYETTA, K. JOHNSON, J. A. STROM & R. TRANSOU. 1983. Cerebral arterial spasm—a controlled trial of nimodipine in patients with subarachnoid hemorrhage. N. Engl. J. Med. **308:** 619–624.
23. VANHOUTTE, P. M. 1981. Calcium entry blockers and cardiovascular failure. Fed. Proc. **40:** 2882–2887.
24. VANHOUTTE, P. M., T. J. RIMELE & J. M. VAN NUETEN. 1983. Calcium entry blockers and contractile responses of vascular smooth muscle. *In* Calcium Antagonists: the State of the Art and Role in Cardiovascular Disease. Symp. Frontiers Pharmacol. **2:** 65–75.
25. VANHOUTTE, P. M. 1978. Heterogeneity of vascular smooth muscle. *In* Microcirculation. G. Kaley & B. M. Altura, Eds. **2:** 181–309. University Park Press. Baltimore, Md.
26. VAN BREEMEN, C., O. HWANG & K. D. MEISHERI. 1981. The mechanism of inhibitory

action of diltiazem on vascular smooth muscle contractility. J. Pharmacol. Exp. Ther. **218:** 459–463.

27. GODFRAIND, T. & D. DIEU. 1981. The inhibition by flunarizine of the norepinephrine-evoked contraction and calcium influx in rat aorta and mesenteric arteries. J. Pharmacol. Exp. Ther. **217:** 510–515.
28. CASTEELS, R. & G. DROOGMANS. 1981. Exchange characteristics of the noradrenaline-sensitive calcium store in vascular smooth muscle cells of rabbit ear artery. J. Physiol. London **317:** 263–279.
29. COOKE, J. P., T. J. RIMELE, N. A. FLAVAHAN & P. M. VANHOUTTE. 1985. Nimodipine and inhibition of alpha adrenergic activation of the isolated canine saphenous vein. J. Pharmacol. Exp. Ther. **234:** 598–602.
30. GULATI, N., H. HUGGEL & O. P. GULATI. 1983. Pharmacological and hemodynamic studies of flunarizine. Gen. Pharmacol. **14:** 203–206.
31. HOLCK, M. & M. GEROLD. 1985. Calcium entry blockers inhibit vasoconstrictor responses to sympathetic nerve stimulation mediated by α_1-adrenoceptors. Naunyn-Schmiedeberg's Arch. Pharmacol. **330:** 22–32.
32. VAN NUETEN, J. M. & P. A. J. JANSSEN. 1973. Comparative study of the effects of flunarizine and cinnarizine on smooth muscles and cardiac tissues. Arch. Int. Pharmacodyn. Ther. **204:** 37–55.
33. FLECKENSTEIN, A. & G. FLECKENSTEIN-GRUN. 1980. Cardiovascular protection by Ca antagonists. Eur. Heart J. Suppl. B **1:** 15–21.
34. BRANDT, L., K. E. ANDERSSON, L. EDVINSSON & B. LJUNGGREN. 1981. Effects of extracellular calcium and of calcium antagonists on the contractile responses of isolated human pial and mesenteric arteries. J. Cereb. Blood Flow Metab. **1:** 339–347.
35. GODFRAIND, T. & R. C. MILLER. 1982. Actions of prostaglandin F_{2alpha} and noradrenaline on calcium exchange and contraction in rat mesenteric arteries and their sensitivity to calcium entry blockers. Br. J. Pharmacol. **75:** 229–236.
36. WHITE, R. P., M. P. CUNNINGHAM & J. T. ROBERTSON. 1982. Effect of the calcium antagonist nimodipine on contractile responses of isolated canine basilar arteries induced by serotonin, prostaglandin $F_{2\alpha}$, thrombin, and whole blood. Neurosurgery **10:** 344–348.
37. LEVY, J. V. 1975. Verapamil and diazoxide antagonism of agonist-induced contractions of aortic strips from normal and spontaneously hypertensive rats (SHR). Res. Commun. Chem. Pathol. Pharmacol. **11:** 387–404.
38. VAN NUETEN, J. M., J. VAN BEEK & P. M. VANHOUTTE. 1980. Inhibitory effect of lidoflazine on contractions of isolated canine coronary arteries caused by norepinephrine, 5-hydroxytryptamine, high potassium, anoxia and ergonovine maleate. J. Pharmacol. Exp. Ther. **213:** 179–187.
39. EDVINSSON, L., L. BRANDT, K. E. ANDERSSON & B. BENGTSSON. 1979. Effect of a calcium antagonist on experimental constriction of human brain vessels. Surg. Neurol. **11:** 327–330.
40. BOHR, D. F., S. GREENBERG & A. BONACCORSI. 1978. Mechanisms of action of vasoactive agents. *In* Microcirculation. G. Kaley & B. M. Altura, Eds. **2:** 311–348. University Park Press. Baltimore, Md.
41. DE CLERCK, F. & J. M. VAN NUETEN. 1983. Platelet-mediated vascular contractions. Inhibition by flunarizine, a Ca^{2+}-entry blocker. Biochem. Pharmacol. **32:** 765–771.
42. VAN NUETEN, J. M., W. DE RIDDER, L. VAN GORP & F. DE CLERCK. 1987. Vasoconstrictor expression of human platelet–vessel wall interactions: inhibition by the Ca^{2+} entry blocker flunarizine. Eur. J. Pharmacol. **133:** 301–308.
43. DE CLERCK, F. & J. M. VAN NUETEN. 1982. Platelet-mediated vascular contractions. Inhibition of the serotonergic component by ketanserin. Thromb. Res. **27:** 713–727.
44. ELLIS, E. F., O. OELZ, L. JACSON ROBERTS II, N. A. PAYNE, B. J. SWEETMAN, A. S. NIES & J. A. OATES. 1976. Coronary arterial smooth muscle contraction by a substance released from platelets. Evidence that it is thromboxane A_2. Science **193:** 1135–1137.
45. VANHOUTTE, P. M. 1982. Calcium entry blockers and vascular smooth muscle. Circulation **65** (Suppl. I): I-11–I-19.
46. VANHOUTTE, P. M. 1976. Effects of anoxia and glucose depletion on isolated veins of the dog. Am. J. Physiol. **230:** 1261–1268.

47. Mikkelsen, E., L. T. Jespersen & O. L. Pedersen. 1984. Effects of the two new Ca-entry blockers bepridil and nitrendipine on isolated vessels. Acta Pharmacol. Toxicol. **54:** 258–264.
48. Van Nueten, J. M., W. De Ridder & J. Van Beek. 1982. Hypoxia and spasms in the cerebral vasculature. J. Cereb. Blood Flow Metab. **2:** S29–S31.
49. Van Reempts, J. & M. Borgers. 1985. Ischemic brain injury and cell calcium: morphologic and therapeutic aspects. Ann. Emerg. Med. **14:** 736–742.
50. Wauquier, A., J. Fransen, G. Clincke, D. Ashton & H. L. Edmonds. 1985. Calcium entry blockers as cerebral protecting agents. *In* Calcium Entry Blockers and Tissue Protection. T. Godfraind, P. M. Vanhoutte, S. Govoni & R. Paoletti, Eds.: 163–172. Raven Press. New York, N.Y.
51. Deshpande, J. K. & T. Wieloch. 1985. Amelioration of ischaemic brain damage by postischaemic treatment with flunarizine. Neurol. Res. **7:** 27–29.
52. Karasaw, A., Y. Kumada, K. Yamada, K. Shuto & N. Nakamizo. 1982. Protective effect of flunarizine against cerebral hypoxia-anoxia in mice and rats. J. Pharm. Dyn. **5:** 295–300.
53. Tanaka, K., F. Gotoh, F. Muramatsu, Y. Fukuuchi, H. Okayasu & M. Kobari. 1982. Effect of nimodipine, a calcium antagonist, on cerebral vasospasm after subarachnoid hemorrhage in cats. Arzneim.-Forsch./Drug Res. **32:** 1529–1534.
54. White, B. C., D. S. Gadzinski, P. J. Hoehner, C. Krome & J. D. White. 1982. Correction of canine cerebral cortical blood flow and vascular resistance after cardiac arrest using flunarizine, a calcium antagonist. Ann. Emerg. Med. **22:** 118–127.
55. Shepherd, J. T., P. M. Vanhoutte. 1985. Spasm of the coronary arteries: causes and consequences (the scientist's viewpoint). Mayo Clin. Proc. **60:** 33–46.
56. Hladovec, J. & F. De Clerck. 1981. Protection by flunarizine against endothelial cell injury *in vivo*. Angiology **32:** 448–462.
57. Furchgott, R. F. & J. V. Zawadzki. 1980. The obligatory role of endothelial cells in the relaxation of arterial smooth muscle by acetylcholine. Nature **288:** 373–376.
58. Cohen, R. A., J. T. Shepherd & P. M. Vanhoutte. 1983. Inhibitory role of the endothelium in the response of isolated coronary arteries to platelets. Science **221:** 273–274.
59. Houston, D. S., J. T. Shepherd & P. M. Vanhoutte. 1985. Adenine nucleotides, serotonin and endothelium-dependent relaxations to platelets. Am. J. Physiol. **248:** H389–H395.
60. Henry, P. D. & K. I. Bentley. 1981. Suppression of atherogenesis in cholesterol-fed rabbit treated with nifedipine. J. Clin. Invest. **68:** 1366–1369.
61. Rouleau, J. L., W. W. Parmley, J. Stevens, J. Wikman-Coffelt, R. Sievers, R. W. Mahley, R. J. Havel & W. Brecht. 1983. Verapamil suppresses atherosclerosis in cholesterol-fed rabbits. J. Am. Coll. Cardiol. **1:** 1453–1466.
62. Blumlein, S. L., R. Sievers, P. Kidd & W. W. Parmley. 1984. Mechanism of protection from atherosclerosis by verapamil in the cholesterol-fed rabbit. Am. J. Cardiol. **54:** 884–889.
63. Betz, E., H. Hämmerle & T. Strohschneider. 1985. Inhibition of smooth muscle cell proliferation and endothelial permeability with flunarizine in vitro and in experimental atheromas. Res. Exp. Med. **185:** 325–340.
64. Ginsburg, R., K. Davis, M. R. Bristow, K. Mckennett, S. R. Kodsi, M. E. Billingham & J. S. Schroeder. 1983. Calcium antagonists suppress atherogenesis in aorta but not in the intramural coronary arteries of cholesterol-fed rabbits. Lab. Invest. **49:** 154–158.
65. Hugenholtz, P. G. & P. Lichtlen. 1986. On a possible role for calcium antagonists in atherosclerosis. A personal view. Eur. Heart J. **7:** 546–559.
66. Kazda, S., B. Garthoff, H. P. Krause & K. Schlossmann. 1982. Cerebrovascular effects of the calcium antagonistic dihydropyridine derivative nimodipine in animal experiments. Arzneim.-Forsch./Drug Res. **32:** 331–338.
67. Wauquier, A., D. Ashton & G. H. C. Clincke. Brain ischemia as a target for Ca^{2+} entry blockers. Ann. N.Y. Acad. Sci. (This volume.)
68. Favalli, L., E. Lanza, A. Rozza Dionigi, G. Assogna, D. Goggi & G. Ricevuti. 1985.

Flunarizine, cerebral blood flow and reversion of experimental atherosclerosis in rabbit. Drugs Exp. Clin. **11**(12): 845–850.
69. GELMERS, H. J. 1982. Effect of nimodipine (Bay e 9736) on postischaemic cerebrovascular reactivity, as revealed by measuring regional cerebral blood flow (rCBF). Acta Neurochir. **63:** 283–290.
70. AUER, L. M., Z. ITO, A. SUZUKI & H. OHTA. 1982. Prevention of symptomatic vasospasm by topically applied nimodipine. Acta Neurochir. **63:** 297–302.
71. VAN NUETEN, J. M., P. A. J. JANSSEN, W. DE RIDDER & P. M. VANHOUTTE. 1982. Interaction between 5-hydroxytryptamine and other vasoconstrictor substances in the isolated femoral artery of the rabbit; effect of ketanserin (R 41 468). Eur. J. Pharmacol. **77:** 281–287.
72. DE LA LANDE, I. S., V. A. CANNELL & J. C. WATERSON. 1966. The interaction of serotonin and noradrenaline on the perfused artery. Br. J. Pharmacol. **28:** 255–272.
73. KUBO, T. & C. SU. 1983. Effects of serotonin and some other neurohumoral agents on adrenergic neurotransmission in spontaneously hypertensive rat vasculature. Clin. Exp. Hypertension **A5**(9): 1501–1510.
74. LUNDBERG, J. M., L. TORSSELL, A. SOLLEVI, J. PERNOW, E. THEODORSSON NORHEIM, A. ÄNGGARD & B. HAMBERGER. 1985. Neuropeptide Y and sympathetic vascular control in man. Regul. Pept. **13:** 41–52.
75. EDVINSSON, L. 1985. Characterization of the contractile effect of neuropeptide Y in feline cerebral arteries. Acta Physiol. Scand. **125:** 33–41.
76. VAN ZWIETEN, P. A. 1986. Differentiation of calcium entry blockers into calcium channel blockers and calcium overload blockers. Eur. Neurol. **25** (Suppl. 1): 57–67.
77. VANHOUTTE, P. M. 1981. Differential effects of calcium entry blockers on vascular smooth muscle. *In* New Perspectives on Calcium Antagonists. Clinical Physiology Series. G. B. Weiss, Ed.: 109–121. American Physiological Society. Washington, D.C.
78. VANHOUTTE, P. M. & R. PAOLETTI. 1987. The WHO classification of calcium-antagonists. Trends Pharmacol. Sci. **8:** 4–5.
79. JONKMAN, F. A. M., H. W. G. M. BODDEKE & P. A. VAN ZWIETEN. 1986. Protective activity of calcium entry blockers against ouabain intoxication in anesthetized guinea pigs. J. Cardiovasc. Pharmacol. **8:** 1009–1013.
80. SJOGREN, A., L. EDVINSSON & A. OTTOSSON. 1986. Vasomotor responses of isolated human coronary arteries to magnesium, nitroglycerin and verapamil: a comparison with coronary arteries from cat and rat. Acta Pharmacol. Toxicol. **59:** 195–203.
81. DI PERRI, T., F. L. PASINI, M. GUERRINI, R. CAPPELLI & S. PECCHI. 1984. Treatment of peripheral obliterative arterial disease with calcium-entry blocker drugs. *In* Atherosclerosis and Cardiovascular Disease. S. Lenzi & G. C. Descovich, Eds.: 107–126. MTP Press Limited. Lancaster, England.

Antagonists and Activators at Calcium Channels

Effects in the Gastrointestinal Tract

MICHAEL SPEDDING

Syntex Research Center
Research Park
Riccarton
Edinburgh EH14 4AS, Scotland

This article will briefly cover some of the effects of calcium antagonists on the gastrointestinal (GI) tract and the question of whether selective agents may be developed for the Ca^{2+} channels involved in GI function (secretion/motility/blood flow). The effects of exogenous Ca^{2+} channel activators will be described in GI muscle, and the question of whether endogenous Ca^{2+} channel activators exist will be addressed. However, the article will concentrate on the interaction of drugs with voltage-operated Ca^{2+} channels (VOCs; L-channels) which are sensitive to the classical calcium antagonists.[1]

SMOOTH MUSCLE

Voltage-operated Ca^{2+} channels contribute to contractility in GI smooth muscle. The relative contribution of VOCs to a given effect varies, depending on the tissue and the activation conditions. The taenia smooth muscle of the guinea pig cecum has spontaneous Ca^{2+} spikes, the frequency of which is augmented by stretch and controls the degree of endogenous tone (FIGURE 1).[2]

This preparation has little sarcoplasmic reticulum and depends to a large extent on Ca^{2+} influx. Thus, abolition of VOC activity markedly reduces contractility (FIGURE 1), even though membrane potential is unchanged.

However, the smooth muscle from the taenia represents one end of a spectrum, in that other activation mechanisms may predominate in tissues where slow waves of depolarization are especially important in synchronizing contractility. In the guinea pig these slow waves are not susceptible to calcium antagonists (verapamil;[3] diltiazem;[4] FIGURE 2), but the Ca^{2+} spikes which are superimposed on the depolarization are abolished. This is shown in the work of Ishikawa *et al.*(FIGURE 2) where diltiazem inhibited selectively only the electrical components mediated by VOCs. Thus, a substantial component of the electrical activity in GI smooth muscle may be resistant to calcium antagonists. In this respect, few of the clinically used calcium antagonists cause marked side effects in the GI tract,[5] with the exception of verapamil which causes constipation. However, verapamil is a rather nonselective agent, with high affinity for α_1-receptors[6] and 5-hydroxytryptamine ($5HT_2$) receptors,[7] and it is not established that the inhibitory effects of verapamil in the GI tract relate simply to effects on VOCs. Nevertheless, gallopamil, a close analogue of verapamil, has been shown to inhibit slow waves in dog stomach,[8] which might imply species differences, but rather high concentrations of gallopamil (10 μM) were used. The mechanisms of slow wave generation and propagation are controversial, and, while the slow waves are

Ca^{2+} dependent but usually insensitive to calcium antagonists, they may involve cyclic changes in ion pumping mechanisms or perhaps activation of a different type of Ca^{2+} channel. In this respect phorbol esters, which activate protein kinase C, can induce rhythmic activity in smooth muscle[9,10] and activate Ca^{2+} channels which may be resistant to the "classical" calcium antagonists.[9,10]

However, it is likely that the VOCs responsible for spike activity in the GI tract are similar to VOCs in other smooth muscle, in that inhibitory potency of antagonists in K^+-depolarized taenia is very well correlated with hypotensive activity in cardiovascular preparations[11] (also unpublished observations), and GI smooth muscle can be used to predict affinity in vascular smooth muscle. Nevertheless, there are considerable

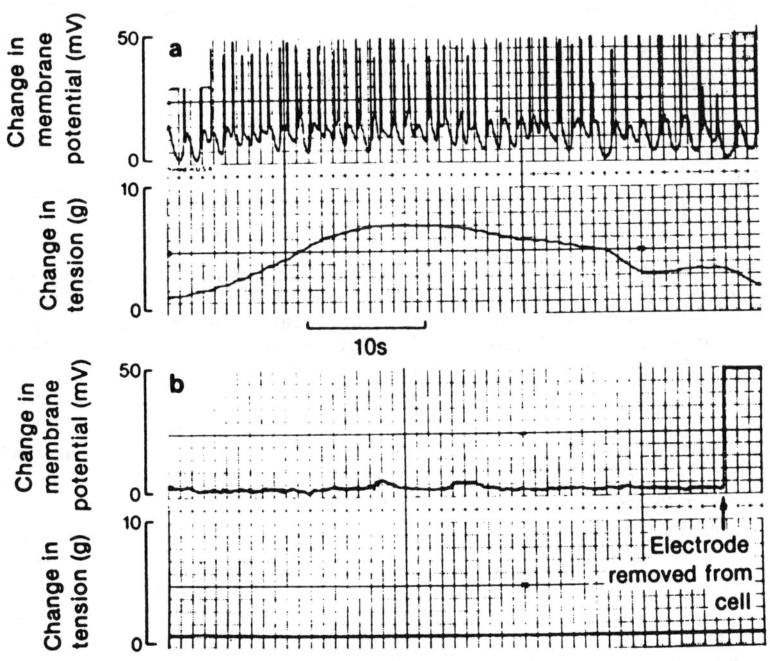

FIGURE 1. Ca^{2+} spikes in taenia smooth muscle from the guinea pig cecum. Note that spontaneous contractility is related to increased spike frequency (upper panel). Abolition of Ca^{2+} spike activity relaxes the tissue (lower panels). In this experiment, 2-2′-pyridylisatogen tosylate was used to block the Ca^{2+} spikes. (Reproduced from Reference 2 with permission.)

differences between VOCs in smooth muscle and those in nervous tissue[12] and skeletal muscle[13] with respect to their sensitivity to calcium antagonists.

If VOCs in the smooth muscle of blood vessels and the GI tract are similar, is it then possible to use calcium antagonists for gastrointestinal applications without concomitant cardiovascular effects? There are a large number of variables that influence the susceptibility of a tissue to calcium antagonists as a class (TABLE 1), one of the most important being the cellular membrane potential and frequency of Ca^{2+} spike potentials.[14-16] Most calcium antagonists bind with high affinity to the inactivated state of the channel, which is favored in depolarized states, but have low affinity

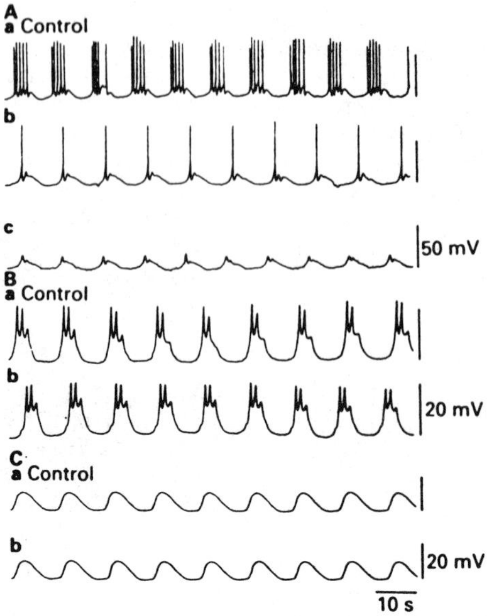

a: Control
b: Diltiazem

FIGURE 2. Effects of diltiazem on spontaneous electrical response recorded from circular smooth muscle cells of guinea pig antrum. A. Inhibition of Ca^{2+} spike potentials by 1 μM diltiazem after 7 (b) and 20 (c) minutes incubation. B. Resistance of slow waves with abortive spike potentials to 10 μM diltiazem. C. Resistance of slow waves to 10 μM diltiazem. (Reproduced from Reference 4 with permission.)

for the resting state in hyperpolarized cells.[14–16] Thus cells that are depolarized with repetitive Ca^{2+} spikes are most susceptible to the antagonists, and pathological conditions inducing such effects are prime indications for therapy with calcium antagonists. In this respect, patients with irritable bowel syndrome have excessive spike potential activity in the colon, with exagerated colonic contractions in response to food and intestinal distension; the excess spike activity and associated contractility may be treated with verapamil or nifedipine, without concomitant inhibition of ongoing slow wave activity.[17,18] Achalasia and other esophageal disorders may be similarly sensitive to this class of drugs (see Reference 5 for a review).

Is it therefore possible to develop calcium antagonists that are selective for the GI tract? This is more difficult to envisage, but the variables that influence the tissue selectivity of calcium antagonists are listed in TABLE 2. The site of action of a calcium antagonist within the Ca^{2+} channel is a particularly important determinant of the profile of a given calcium antagonist, and there appear to be three main classes of

TABLE 1. Variables Affecting the Susceptibility of a Tissue to Calcium Antagonists

1. Number and type of Ca^{2+} channels.
2. Relative contribution of Ca^{2+} channels to final response.
3. Membrane potential and frequency of Ca^{2+} channel activation.
4. Criticality of blood supply for expression of response: effects of antagonist on tissue blood flow.

TABLE 2. Variables Affecting the Tissue Selectivity of a Calcium Antagonist

1. Site of action within the Ca^{2+} channel (FIGURE 3).
2. Use dependence and membrane potential dependence of block.
3. Physicochemical properties (lipophilicity, pKa).
4. Activator/antagonist ratio may vary between tissues.
5. Metabolism.
6. Additional effects (α, 5HT receptor antagonism, etc.).

compound with different tissue selectivities.[16] The subclasses of compounds can be readily differentiated by a variety of simple pharmacological tests[16] (TABLE 3).

Nevertheless, it is unlikely that any of these compounds have any real selectivity for the GI tract. Verapamil, as mentioned above, causes constipation in some patients which may even lead to fecal impaction[19] at doses used for cardiovascular therapy. It has been reported that loperamide, an agent used to treat diarrhea, is a calcium antagonist with selectivity for the GI tract.[20] This compound shows how the variables in TABLE 2 can be exploited, leading to a drug with selectivity for the GI tract. Loperamide is rapidly metabolized by the liver, resulting in the fact that little of the compound reaches the peripheral circulation. Loperamide has affinity for opioid receptors which results in inhibition of motility[21] and at higher concentrations has marked calcium-antagonistic effects ($pA_2 7$).[21] Both effects may contribute to effectiveness against diarrhea.[20,22] The calcium-antagonistic effects of loperamide are reversed by calcium channel activators (FIGURE 3).

SECRETION

The role of VOCs in secretory responses in the GI tract is more complex than is the case in smooth muscle. Whereas secretion of some hormones, such as insulin, is

TABLE 3. Differentiation of Three Calcium Antagonist Subgroups in Gastrointestinal Smooth Muscle

	Bay K 8644[a]	Salicylate[b]	Contractile Proteins[b]	Selectivity for VOCs[c]
Dihydropyridines	Competitive reversal	No effect	−	++++
Verapamil, Diltiazem, Diclofurime	Noncompetitive reversal	Reversal	−	++
Lidoflazine, Pimozide, Prenylamine, Fendiline, Cinnarizine, Flunarizine, Perhexiline, Bepridil	No reversal	Potentiation	+	−

[a] Protocol as in Reference 40.
[b] Protocol as in Reference 16.
[c] Protocol as in References 16 and 42.

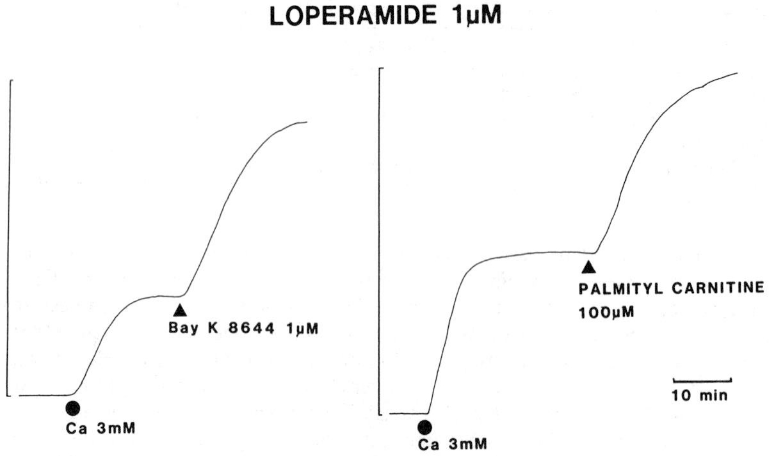

FIGURE 3. Reversal of the inhibitory effects of loperamide (1 μM for 30 minutes) on Ca^{2+} (3 mM) induced contractions in K^+-depolarized taena preparations from the guinea pig cecum. Vertical bars represent the contractile effects of 3 mM Ca^{2+} prior to exposure to loperamide.

dependent on VOC activity and can be inhibited by calcium antagonists and augmented by activators of VOCs,[23] the roles of VOCs in acid secretion in the stomach and in fluid secretion and absorption in the intestine are controversial.

Acid secretion from parietal cells in isolated stomach preparations has been shown to be Ca^{2+} dependent, in that secretion is reduced in low Ca^{2+} and augmented in high Ca^{2+} solutions.[24,25] However, control of the K^+/H^+ transporter via VOCs must be indirect. Indeed, a study of free cytosolic Ca^{2+}, using quin 2, in dog parietal cells showed that cytosolic Ca^{2+} increased in response to cholinergic stimuli but not to histamine; gastrin had intermediate effects.[26] Sewing and Hannemann showed that verapamil and gallopamil inhibit gastric acid secretion from parietal cells but concluded that the concentrations required (10 μM) interacted with the proton transporter and not with VOCs.[27,28] Verapamil does not inhibit gastric acid secretion in man at clinically used doses,[29,30] although gastrin-stimulated secretion may be inhibited.[31] It is therefore unlikely that presently available calcium antagonists will be of use in controlling gastric acid secretion. Nevertheless, high doses of calcium antagonists, which affect cardiovascular parameters, inhibit gastric acid secretion and may even be selective against certain secretagogues. Thus, the different subclasses of calcium antagonist have selective interactions with histamine- or pentagastrin-evoked gastric acid secretion in the rat[32] (FIGURE 4). Direct selective effects of these agents on the parietal cells should not be inferred from these experiments, because the nonspecific vasodilator hydralazine also inhibited gastric acid secretion, albeit nonselectively. As gastric acid secretion is critically dependent on mucosal blood flow, the changes in secretion could be secondary to vasodilatory effects; the calcium antagonists and hydralazine might be expected to have very complicated effects on mucosal blood flow. In addition to direct vasodilator effects, falls in systemic blood pressure would cause reflex alterations in autonomic outflow which would *reduce* GI blood flow and acid secretion. Thus effects of calcium antagonists on gastric acid secretion *in vivo* will be complex.

Ileal and colonic water absorption may be increased by verapamil and nifedipine, and Donowitz *et al.* have claimed that VOCs in the ileal basolateral membrane and colonic apical membrane control Na^+, Cl^-, and water absorption.[33] These studies are consistent with the known GI side effects of verapamil (see above) and suggest a role for calcium antagonists in the treatment of diarrhea.[33] Loperamide also inhibits fluid secretion by inhibiting Ca^{2+} entry.[22] Furthermore verapamil reversed the Na^+, Cl^-, and water secretion into the jejunum induced by an infusion of 5-HT in conscious dogs.[35] The authors indicated that verapamil might be useful in the treatment of carcinoid syndrome. In contrast, direct effects of calcium antagonists on Ca^{2+} transport across the duodenum have only been demonstrated with high, nonspecific, concentrations.[34]

ACTIVATORS

Dihydropyridines may interact with their binding site in the Ca^{2+} channel with very high affinity; binding to the channel can induce a conformational change, in that the binding of other ligands ([^{3}H] verapamil, [^{3}H] diltiazem) is modified allosterically and the state of the channel may change.[1] Although apparently binding at a single site, dihydropyridines can act both as antagonists and activators of VOCs, depending on the structure of the dihydropyridine. Indeed, some dihydropyridine structures have the ability to both activate and inactivate VOCs, with the enantiomers having opposite effects.[36,37] Thus, the enantiomers of Bay K 8644 (methyl, 1,4-dihydro 2,6-dimethyl-3-nitro-4-(2 trifluoromethylphenyl-pyridine-5-carboxylate) and of PN 202-791 (isopropyl 4-(2,1,3-benzoxazidol-4-yl)-1,4-dihydro-2,6-dimethyl-5-nitro-3-pyridine-carboxylate) augment or antagonize Ca^{2+}-induced contractions in K^+-depolarized taenia preparations (FIGURE 5). The enantiomers antagonize each other with the equilibrium effect being that of the racemate. There is such an excellent correlation between affinity for the dihydropyridines in binding and functional assays in intestinal smooth

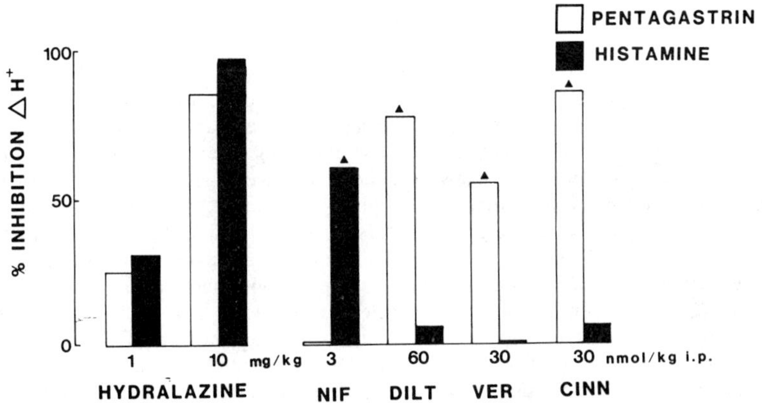

FIGURE 4. Inhibition of gastric acid secretion evoked by histamine (100 mg/kg intraperitoneally) or pentagastrin (20 μg/kg subcutaneously) in conscious rats after treatment with hydralazine, nifedipine (NIF), verapamil (VER), diltiazem (DILT), or cinnarizine (CINN); i.p. indicates a significant difference between the inhibition of histamine- or pentagastrin-evoked stimuli. (Data recalculated from Reference 30.)

muscle that there is little doubt that both assays represent direct effects at the Ca^{2+} channel.[38]

Channel activators can be used as tools to define the site of action of antagonists. Bay K 8644 competitively reverses the inhibitory effects of nifedipine in GI smooth muscle, under conditions of constant K^+ depolarization.[39] The inhibitory effects of verapamil and diltiazem which bind to sites allosterically linked to the dihydropyridine site are reversed noncompetitively. Loperamide seems to resemble verapamil and diltiazem (FIGURE 3). In complete contrast, the effects of group III calcium antagonists (cinnarizine, flunarizine, bepridil, etc.) are resistant to Bay K 8644,[40] indicating either that these antagonists "trap" VOCs in a state that is not accessible to the activator, or that the drugs act at other sites.[16,42] The same interactions occur between these drugs in the heart[41] as occur in GI smooth muscle.

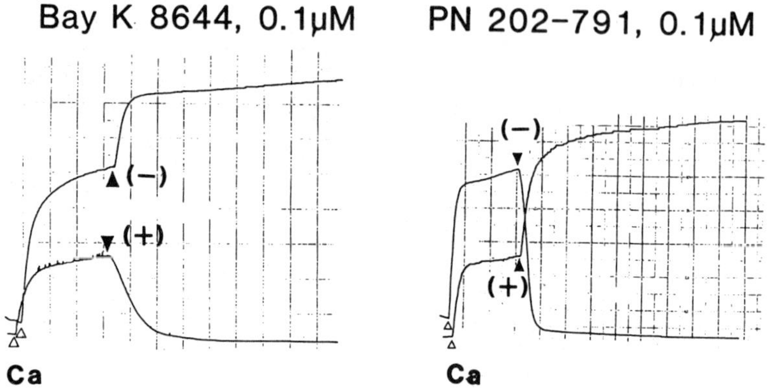

FIGURE 5. Effects of the enantiomers of Bay K 8644 and PN 202-791 on contractions of K^+-depolarized taenia preparations from the guinea pig cecum, induced by Ca^{2+} (100 μM).

ENDOGENOUS ACTIVATORS

The critical determinant of the activity of VOCs in the cardiovascular system and the GI tract is membrane potential and perhaps surface charge (FIGURES 1 and 2).[16] Indirect modulation of activity may occur following channel phosphorylation or interactions with G proteins.[43] However, there are several sites on VOCs with high affinity for exogenous substances (nifedipine, verapamil) for which there are no endogenous ligands. Nevertheless activators of VOCs with little selectivity may be expected to be toxic[16] and perhaps to contribute to certain pathological situations. In this respect, jejunal smooth muscle from rats infected with nematodes (*Nippostrongylus brasiliensis*) resembles smooth muscle treated with Bay K 8644.[44] In other pathological situations, endogenous lipid metabolites may activate VOCs.

Long chain acyl groups are transported in the form of acyl carnitine into mitochondria for β-oxidation. β-Oxidation of lipids cannot continue during ischemic conditions leading to a buildup of acyl carnitines in the cytosol and associated membranes, particularly the sarcolemma.[45,46] Acyl carnitines have detergent properties and change membranal properties, but they also selectively increase Ca^{2+} current in the heart.[47] In K^+-depolarized smooth muscle from the GI tract, palmityl carnitine has been shown to resemble the dihydropyridine Ca^{2+} channel activator Bay K 8644 in that both drugs increase the sensitivity of the tissues to Ca^{2+}, without interfering with the ability of the tissues to relax.[48,49] Furthermore palmityl carnitine, like Bay K 8644, has selective interactions with the different classes of calcium antagonist (TABLE 3),[48,49] with the inhibitory effects of verapamil being the most susceptible. The calcium antagonist effects of loperamide are also reversed by palmityl carnitine (FIGURE 3). Neither Bay K 8644 nor palmityl carnitine reverses the inhibitory effects of flunarizine or cinnarizine.[48,49] These findings, which are corroborated by ligand binding studies, argue for a more selective effect in the Ca^{2+} channel than if palmityl carnitine were acting as a simple detergent. Studies in rat cerebral cortex[48,49] show that palmityl carnitine has higher affinity in inhibiting [^{3}H]verapamil binding (IC_{50} 42 μM) than [^{3}H]diltiazem or [^{3}H]nitrendipine binding. Furthermore positive inotropic effects of palmityl carnitine in embryonic chick heart cells resemble those of Bay K 8644,[50] and palmityl carnitine reversed the inhibitory effects of verapamil and nisoldipine over precisely the same concentration range as it inhibited the binding of [^{3}H]verapamil and [^{3}H]nitrendipine in rat cortex. Nevertheless, although these effects point to a selective effect on the VOC subunit to which verapamil binds, it must be borne in mind that this site is very susceptible to local changes in pH and surface charge;[16] palmityl carnitine may not interact directly with the site in the same way as verapamil does.

There is therefore considerable evidence that palmityl carnitine, in concentrations that occur in myocardial sarcolemma during ischemia, resembles Bay K 8644 in causing activation of Ca^{2+} channels. Acyl carnitines may therefore exacerbate ischemic damage, at least in the heart. It is unclear to what extent acyl carnitines accumulate in the GI tract during ischemia, although they can clearly contract depolarized GI smooth muscle.

It must be recognized, however, that acyl carnitines have several other effects, in addition to any affinity for VOCs. Palmityl carnitine can have biphasic effects on protein kinase C activation[51] and inhibit Na^+/K^+ ATPase and Ca^{2+} ATPases.[52,53] Activation of VOCs in blood vessels may be augmented by effects in the endothelium, as acyl carnitines reduce release of endothelial-derived relaxant factor (EDRF).[54] It is therefore likely that acyl carnitines may modulate several cellular metabolic events.

SUMMARY

Most calcium antagonists have relatively minor effects in the gastrointestinal (GI) tract; the factors influencing drug selectivity are reviewed. Voltage-dependent Ca channels (VOCs) in GI smooth muscle appear to be essentially similar to those in the cardiovascular system in their sensitivity to calcium antagonists. However, selective conditions for channel activation may allow antagonists to be selective in certain disease conditions. Indirect effects on blood flow may be crucial to certain parameters (e.g., acid secretion). Activators of VOCs have similar effects in vascular and GI smooth muscle. Some endogenous activators of VOCs may exist and evidence for control of VOC activity by lipid metabolites is indicated. Acyl carnitines may function as endogenous activators of VOCs.

ACKNOWLEDGMENTS

I thank Miss H. Ross and Miss A. Stewart for typing the manuscript.

REFERENCES

1. HESS, P., J. B. LANSMAN, B. NILIUS & R. W. TSIEN. 1986. Calcium channel types in cardiac myocytes: modulation by dihydropyridines and β-adrenergic stimulation. J. Cardiovasc. Pharmacol. 8(Suppl. 9): S11–S21.
2. SMALL, R. C. & M. SPEDDING. 1978. The effects of 2-2′-pyridylisatogen tosylate on the electrical activity of smooth muscle of the isolated taenia caeci of the guinea-pig. Br. J. Pharmacol. **63:** 408P.
3. GOLENHOFEN, K. & E. LAMMEL. 1972. Spontaneous suppression of some components of spontaneous activity in various types of smooth muscle by iproveratril (verapamil). Pfluger's Arch. **331:** 233–243.
4. ISHIKAWA, S., K. KOMORI, T. NAGAO & H. SUZUKI. 1985. Effects of diltiazem on electrical responses evoked spontaneously or by electrical stimulation in the antrum smooth muscle cells of the guinea-pig stomach. Br. J. Pharmacol. **86:** 789–797.
5. TRAUBE, M. & R. S. MCCALLUM. 1984. Calcium channel blockers and the gastrointestinal tract. Am. J. Gastroenterol. **79:** 892–896.
6. MOTULSKY, H. J., M. D. SNAVELY, R. J. HUGHES & P. A. INSEL. 1983. Interaction of verapamil and other calcium channel blockers with α_1- and α_2-adrenergic receptors. Circ. Res. **52:** 226–231.
7. TAYLOR, J. E. & F. V. DEFEUDIS. 1985. Inhibition of [^{3}H]spiperone binding to 5-HT_2 receptors of rat cerebral cortex by the calcium antagonists verapamil and D600. Eur. J. Pharmacol. **106:** 215–216.
8. EL-SHARKAWY, T. Y., K. G. MORGAN & J. H. SZURSCEWSKI. 1978. Intracellular electrical activity of canine and human gastric smooth muscle. J. Physiol. **279:** 291–307.
9. SPEDDING, M. Interaction of phorbol esters with Ca^{2+} channels in smooth muscle. Br. J. Pharmacol. (In press.)
10. GLEASON, M. M. & S. F. FLAIM. 1986. Phorbol ester contracts rabbit thoracic aorta by increasing intracellular calcium and by activating calcium influx. Biochem. Biophys. Res. Commun. **138:** 1362–1369.
11. SPEDDING, M. 1982. Differences between the effects of calcium antagonists in the pithed rat preparation. J. Cardiovasc. Pharmacol. **4:** 973–979.
12. SPEDDING, M. & D. N. MIDDLEMISS. 1985. Central effects of calcium-antagonists. Trends Pharmacol. Sci. **6:** 309–310.
13. BEAN, B. P. 1986. Calcium channels in skeletal muscle: what do they do? Trends Neurochem. Sci. **8:** 535–536.
14. BEAN, B. P. 1984. Nitrendipine block of cardiac calcium channels: high affinity binding to the inactivated state. Proc. Nat. Acad. Sc. USA. **81:** 6388–6392.
15. SANGUINNETTI, M. C. & R. S. KASS. 1984. Voltage-dependent block of calcium channel current in the calf cardiac Purkinje fibre by dihydropyridine calcium channel antagonists. Circ. Res. **55:** 336–348.
16. SPEDDING, M. 1985. Activators and inactivators of Ca^{++} channels: new perspectives. J. Pharmacol. Paris **16:** 319–343.
17. NARDUCCI, F., M. A. PELLI & A. VENDOVELLI. 1983. Effects of nifedipine on human colonic myoelectric activity after stimulation by eating or edrophonium. Gastroenterology **84:** 1256.
18. BLUME, M., M. SCHUSTER & H. TUCKER. 1983. Effect of nifedipine on colonic motility in the irritable bowel syndrome. Gastroenterology **84:** 1109.
19. WARD, D. J., J. W. WARD & W. GRIFFO. 1982. Intravenous calcium for fecal impaction secondary to verapamil. N. Engl. J. Med. **307:** 1709–1710.
20. REYNOLDS, I. J., R. J. GOULD & S. H. SNYDER. 1984. Loperamide: blockade of calcium channels as a mechanism for antidiarrheal effects. J. Pharmacol. Exp. Ther. **231:** 628–632.
21. VAN NEUTEN, J. M., P. A. J. JANSSEN & J. FONTAINE. 1974. Loperamide (R 18553), a novel type of antidiarrheal agent. Arzneim. Forsch. **24:** 1641–1645.
22. CHANG, E. B., D. R. BROWN, N. S. WANG & M. FIELD. 1984. Loperamide selectively inhibits peptide-induced Cl secretion and calcium entry in the gut. Gastroenterology **86:** 1044.

23. LEBRUN, P. & I. ATWATER. 1985. Effects of the calcium channel agonist, Bay K 8644, on electrical activity in mouse pancreatic B-cells. Biophys. J. **48:** 919–930.
24. KASBEKAR, D. K. & H. CHUGANI. 1976. Role of calcium ions in in-vitro gastric acid secretion. *In* Gastric Hydrogen Ion Secretion. D. K. Kasbekar, G. Sachs & W. S. Rehm, Eds.: 187–211. Dekkar. New York, NY.
25. LOGSDON, C. D. & T. E. MACHEN. 1981. Involvement of extracellular calcium in gastric stimulation. Am. J. Physiol. **241:**G365–G375.
26. MUALLEM, S. & G. SACHS. 1984. Changes in cytosolic free Ca^{2+} in isolated parietal cells. Differential effects of secretagogues. Biochim. Biophys. Acta **805:** 181–185.
27. SEWING, K. F. & H. HANNEMANN. 1983. Calcium channel antagonists verapamil and gallopamil are powerful inhibitors of gastric acid secretion in isolated and enriched guinea pig parietal cells. Pharmacology **27:** 9–14.
28. SEWING, K. F. 1984. Antisecretagogues and parietal cells. Agents Actions **14:** 319–324.
29. AADLAND, E. & A. BERSTAD. 1983. Effect of verapamil on gastric secretion in man. Scand. J. Gastroenterol. **18:** 969–971.
30. LEVINE, R. A., S. PETOKAS, A. STARR & R. E. EICH. 1983. Effect of verapamil on basal and pentagastrin-stimulated gastric acid secretion. Clin. Pharm. Ther. **34:** 399–403.
31. KIRKEGAARD, P., J. CHRISTIANSEN, B. PETERSEN & P. SKOVOLSEN. 1982. Calcium and stimulus-secretion coupling in gastric fundic mucosa. Scand. J. Gastroenterology **17:** 533–638.
32. BOUCLIER, M. & M. SPEDDING. 1985. Differential effects of calcium channel antagonists on histamine and pentagastrin stimulated gastric acid secretion in the rat. Agents Actions **16:** 491–495.
33. DONOWITZ, M., S. LEVIN, G. POWERS, G. ELTA, P. COHEN & H. CHENG. 1985. Ca^{2+} channel blockers stimulate ileal and colonic water absorption. Gastroenterology **89:** 858–866.
34. FAVUS, M. J. & E. ANGEID-BACKMAN. 1985. Effects of $1,25(OH)_2D_3$ and calcium channel blockers on cecal calcium transport in the rat. Am. J. Physiol. **248:** G676–G681.
35. ZINNER, M. J., D. MCFADDEN, D. SHERLOCK & B. M. JAFFE. 1986. Verapamil reversal of serotonin-induced jejunal secretion of water and electrolytes in awake dogs. Gastroenterology **90:** 515–519.
36. HOF, R. P., U. T. RUEGG, A. HOF & A. VOGEL. 1985. Stereoselectivity at the calcium channel: opposite action of the enantiomers of a 1,4-dihydropyridine. J. Cardiovasc. Pharmacol. **7:** 689–693.
37. FRANCKOWIAK, G., M. BECHEM, M. SCHRAMM & G. THOMAS. 1985. The optical iosmers of the 1,4 dihydropyridine Bay K 8644 show opposite effects on Ca channels. Eur. J. Pharmacol. **114:** 223–226.
38. BOLGER, G. T., P. GENGO, R. KLOCKOWSKI, E. LUCHOWSKI, H. SIEGEL, R. A. JANIS, A. M. TRIGGLE & D. J. TRIGGLE. 1983. Characterization of binding of the Ca^{++} channel antagonist [^{3}H] nitrendipine to guinea-pig ileal smooth muscle. J. Pharmacol. Exp. Ther. **225:** 291–309.
39. SPEDDING, M. 1985. Competitive interactions between Bay K 8644 and nifedipine in K^+-depolarized smooth muscle: a passive role for Ca^{2+}? Naunyn-Schmiedeberg's Arch. Pharmacol. **328:** 464–466.
40. SPEDDING, M. & C. BERG. 1984. Interactions between a "calcium channel agonist," Bay K 8644, and calcium antagonists differentiate calcium antagonist subgroups in K^+-depolarized smooth muscle. Naunyn-Schmiedeberg's Arch. Pharmacol. **328:** 69–75.
41. BODDEKE, H. W. G. M., J. B. HEYNIS, B. WILFFERT & P. A. VAN ZWIETEN. A study on the mechanism of negative inotropy of some calcium entry blockers in isolated guinea-pig hearts. Br. J. Pharmacol. (In press.)
42. GRIMA, M., J. SCHWARTZ, M. O. SPACH & J. VELLY. 1986. Antiaginal arylalkylamines and sodium channels: [^{3}H]-batrachotoxin-A-20-α-benzoate and [^{3}H]-tetracaine binding. Br. J. Pharmacol. **89:** 641–646.
43. HOLZ, G. G. IV, S. G. RANE & K. DUNLOP. 1986. GTP-binding proteins mediate transmitter inhibition of voltage-dependent calcium channels. Nature **319:** 670–672.
44. FOX-ROBICHAUD, A. E. & S. M. COLLINS. 1986. Altered calcium-handling properties of jejunal smooth muscle from the nematode-infected rat. Gastroenterology **91:** 1462–1469.

45. IDELL-WENGER, J. A., L. W. GROTYOHANN & J. R. NEELY. 1978. Coenzyme A and carnitine distribution in normal and ischemic hearts. J. Biol. Chem. **253:** 4310–4318.
46. KNABB, M. T., J. E. SAFFITZ, O. B. CORR & B. E. SOBEL. 1986. The dependence of electrophysiological derangements on accumulation of endogenous long-chain acylcarnitine in hypoxic neonatal rat myocytes. Circ. Res. **58:** 230–240.
47. INOUE, D. & A. J. PAPPANO. 1983. L-Palmitylcarnitine and calcium ions act similarly on excitatory ionic currents in avian ventricular muscle. Circ. Res. **52:** 625–634.
48. MIR, A. K. & M. SPEDDING. 1986. Palmityl carnitine, a lipid metabolite produced in ischaemia, activates Ca^{++} channels in smooth muscle. Br. J. Pharmacol. **88:** 381P.
49. SPEDDING, M. & A. K. MIR. 1987. Direct activation of Ca^{2+} channels by palmityl carnitine, a putative endogenous ligand. Br. J. Pharmacol **92:** 457–468.
50. DUNCAN, G., L. PATMORE & M. SPEDDING. 1986. Positive inotropic effects of palmitoyl carnitine on embryonic chick heart cell aggregates. Br. J. Pharmacol. **89:** 757P.
51. WISE, B. C. & J. F. KUO. 1983. Modes of inhibition by acylcarnitines, adriamycin and trifluoperazine of cardiac phospholipid-sensitive calcium-dependent protein kinase. Biochem. Pharmacol. **32:** 1259–1265.
52. ADAMS, R. J., D. W. COHEN, S. GUPTE, J. D. JOHNSON, E. T. WALLICK, T. WANG & A. SCHWARTZ. 1979. In vitro effects of palmitylcarnitine on cardiac plasma membrane Na,K-ATPase and sarcoplasmic reticulum Ca^{2+}-ATPase and Ca^{2+} transport. J. Biol. Chem. **254:** 12404–12410.
53. PITTS, B. J. R., C. A. TATE, W. B. VAN WINKLE, K. M. WOOD & M. L. ENTMAN. 1978. Palmityl carnitine inhibition of the calcium pump in cardiac sarcoplasmic reticulum: a possible role in myocardial ischaemia. Life Sci. **23:** 391–402.
54. BIGAUD, M. & M. SPEDDING. 1986. Inhibition of the effects of endothelial-derived relaxant factor (EDRF) in aorta by palmityl carnitine. Br. J. Pharmacol. **89:** 540P.

Effects of Calcium "Antagonists" on Vertebrate Skeletal Muscle Cells[a]

L. A. HELLAND, J. R. LOPEZ,[b] S. R. TAYLOR,[c]
G. TRUBE,[d] AND L. A. WANEK

Department of Pharmacology
Mayo Foundation
Rochester, Minnesota 55905

INTRODUCTION

Dantrolene is well known as a relaxant that acts directly on vertebrate skeletal muscle. Action potential propagation along the length of a fiber is not markedly affected by dantrolene, which led to the suggestions that the spread of activation inward from the surface may also be unaltered and the locus of block may be the intracellular Ca^{2+}-release mechanism.[1] Several pieces of evidence are consistent with this idea. Isolated membranes of sarcoplasmic reticulum (SR) possess a class of sites that bind dantrolene with high affinity and contain a small conductance Ca^{2+} channel that is blocked by dantrolene.[2–4] The release of calcium from SR vesicles, but not the rate of uptake, is diminished by dantrolene,[5] and Ca^{2+}-induced contractions of mechanically skinned fibers are unchanged by dantrolene.[6]

However, the failure to change a surface action potential does not mean that action potentials in the transverse tubular (T) system are similarly unchanged. The influx of Ca^{2+} through fast calcium channels is responsible for a negligible portion of the total current in a normal action potential measured via a surface microelectrode; most voltage-activated calcium channels appear to be located in the T system.[7,8] One possible explanation for reduced twitch tension in dantrolene could be that the action potential does not penetrate as quickly or as deeply as normal in the T tubules.[9] We measured this microscopically, and also measured Ca^{2+} transients from intact fibers treated with dantrolene to confirm directly that the drug diminished release without affecting Ca^{2+} uptake.

Among muscle relaxants that act primarily in the central nervous system, benzodiazepines are reported to increase the force of twitch contraction.[10,11] But the benzodiazepine receptors in a muscle fiber are evidently different from their receptors in the central nervous system (CNS).[12] Some evidence indicates that benzodiazepines modulate Ca^{2+} channel activity, although the details of the possible interaction are not well defined.[13] Whereas the connections between benzodiazepine action in the CNS and the inhibition by gamma-aminobutyric acid (GABA) are well established, the role

[a]Supported by grants from the National Institutes of Health (NS 22369; CA 42286), the National Science Foundation (DMB-8503964), and USV Pharmaceutical Corporation.
[b]Present affiliation: Instituto Venezolano de Investigaciones Cientificas (IVIC), Centro de Biofisic y Bioquimica, Apartado 1827, Caracas 101, Venezuela.
[c]To whom correspondence should be addressed.
[d]Present affiliation: Max-Planck-Institute fur Biophysikalische Chemie, Karl-Friedrich-Bonhoeffer-Institut, Postfach 2841, D-3400 Gottingen-Nikolausberg, Federal Republic of Germany.

of GABA in peripheral tissues is poorly understood.[14,15] Hence we compared the effects of the benzodiazepine chlordiazepoxide with GABA, the GABA derivative baclofen, and also examined the effects of other compounds known to antagonize Ca-dependent excitation-contraction coupling.

In addition to the compounds mentioned above, we tested the "vascular selective" calcium antagonist flordipine,[16] and nylidrin, which is a relaxant for a variety of isolated smooth muscle preparations.[17] Meprobamate is among the compounds once used as centrally acting muscle relaxants, and we included this in our comparison.[18] We also tested D-600, which is reported to potentiate frog skeletal muscle contraction,[19] and procaine, which can potentiate twitches, calcium release, and contractile activity.[20–22]

Shorter reports of some of this work have been published.[23–25]

METHODS

Single fibers were isolated intact from leg muscles (tibialis anterior or semitendinosus) of the frog *Rana temporaria.* The fibers were mounted on the stage of an inverted microscope with one tendon gripped by fine forceps and the other attached to a force transducer. Glass micropipettes with a few drops of aequorin in aqueous solution were used to inject each fiber at several locations with the calcium-sensitive photoprotein. The fibers were stimulated with brief electric field pulses (0.1–1.0 msecond duration) to induce action potentials and enable us to monitor changes in intracellular Ca^{2+} and contractile force. Additional details of the methods, including the bathing solutions, have already been described.[26] All the aequorin experiments were conducted at 15°C with the fibers held just taut at slack length. Slack length corresponded to an average striation spacing of about 2.1 to 2.2 μm.

An integrated imaging system (Microtex Corporation, Cambridge, Mass.), based on a photodiode array sensor, 12 bit per pixel acquisition system, high-resolution display processor and monitor, and microVAX II host computer, was used to record microscopic changes in the muscle cells. FIGURE 1 shows a muscle fiber at rest. The original image was made with an immersion objective lens (×100; NA = 1.30; focal length = 1.9 mm). The image was projected onto a two-dimensional self-scanned sensor array, 128 × 128 picture elements (pixels), suspended from the wall, several feet above the fiber and microscope objective mounted on an air suspension table.

Because we could subtract stray light with our digital imaging system, we could use high numerical aperture objectives to illuminate the array and achieve a very shallow depth of field and excellent spatial resolution.[27,28] Some of the new possibilities in experimental biology that are resulting from this combination of light microscopy and digital computers are described in another publication of the Academy.[29]

We used a dc powered xenon lamp to achieve a steady level of illumination. Once a fiber was positioned beneath the objective the intermediate image was focused with an eyepiece and the position of the array was adjusted until the cross-hairs of the eyepiece were centered on the monitor. Then the eyepiece was removed and the intermediate image formed by the objective was focused via the monitor.

The upper left hand panel in FIGURE 1 shows an image of a resting fiber taken at 100 frames per second with an exposure time of a few milliseconds for each frame. The speed at which we could take full frames was not as fast as one can achieve with a cine-camera. Hence the array size was progressively reduced in software until we got a steady display of partial frames as the framing rate was increased. We used framing rates of 500 per second or greater to record the changes during single twitches. Each twitch was preceded by a few hundred seconds of rest.[26] The exposure time for each partial frame was about 500 microseconds or less. When the framing rate was still not high enough to obtain images without partially blurred features we could improve the images in several ways. We cooled the cell to slow down movements. In addition, the images were enhanced by way of digital processing software and hardware. For example, the images were filtered to emphasize selectively either the myofibrils or the

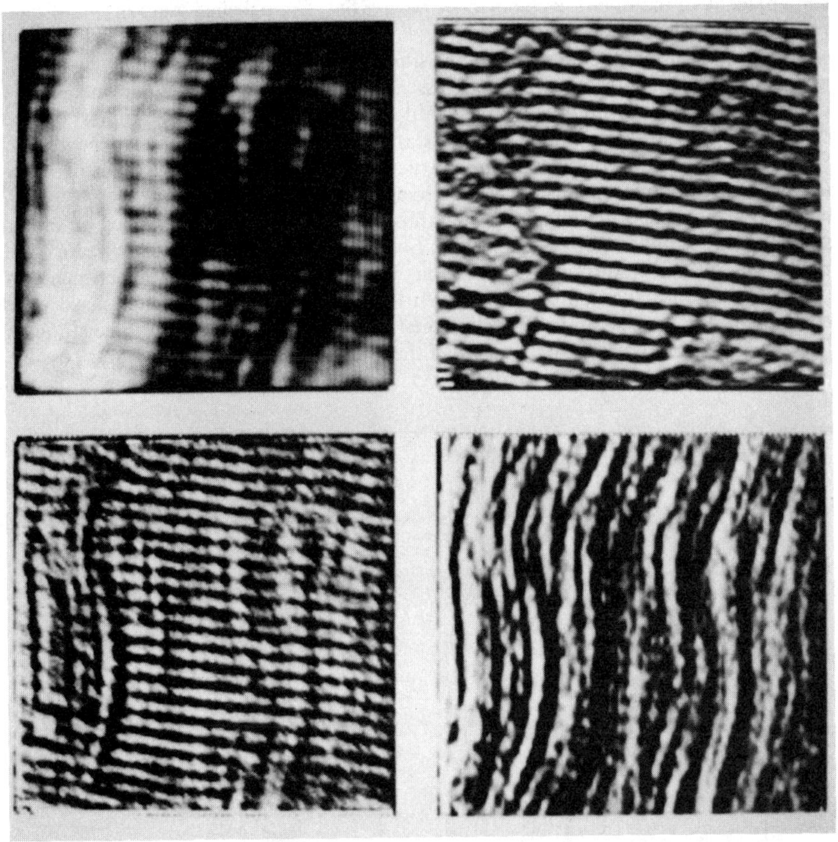

FIGURE 1. The image of a slightly compressed, resting skeletal muscle fiber before and after digital processing. The top left-hand panel shows the original image and the remaining panels show the same image convolved with different edge operators.[42] The time lag between the onset of straightening of myofibrils at either edge of an image and myofibrils in the center was among the features that are more easily measured after these operations.

striation pattern (FIGURE 1). The detection of motion (myofibrils straightening; striation spacing changing) could be enhanced by taking the difference image of consecutive frames. The stationary structures canceled out almost completely leaving only the moving features displayed on a uniform background.

Muscle fibers were mounted on a layer of freshly prepared silicone elastomer (Sylgard). The cell was pinned firmly against the substrate while bathed with Ringer solution. The tendon at one end was then released and, without lifting the major portion of the cell from the Sylgard, nudged towards the other tendon still held firmly. A portion of the cell membrane near the moving tendon usually resisted sliding along the Sylgard, particularly at points where the broadest cross-sectional dimension of the cell contacted the substrate. Moving one tendon no more than a few millimeters caused the myofibrils in the part of the cell not pressed against the Sylgard to be pushed into waves. Wavy myofibrils could also be produced by gently pressing on the portion of the cell adjacent to the microscope objective with a flat, fire-polished glass disc and then moving the tendons closer togther.

Wavy fibrils were first observed in the study that found striation spacings in resting and isometrically contracting fibers are essentially the same.[30] The significance of this observation was not fully exploited until much later.[31] Detailed studies of the development, characteristics, and significance of wavy myofibrils have now been reported. Wavy myofibrils are the only intrinsic criterion by which inactive or partially active areas can be recognized within a stimulated muscle fiber.[32,33]

Two fire-polished glass pipettes containing silver wires were positioned on either side of the fiber underneath the objective. Both wires served as cathodes to reduce the movement of a fiber during a contraction. In addition, most of the experiments in which the lag in activation between the surface and the center were measured were conducted at about 9°C to further slow the time course of movement.[31] The stimulus was timed to occur during the first third of the fourth frame. In this way it was possible

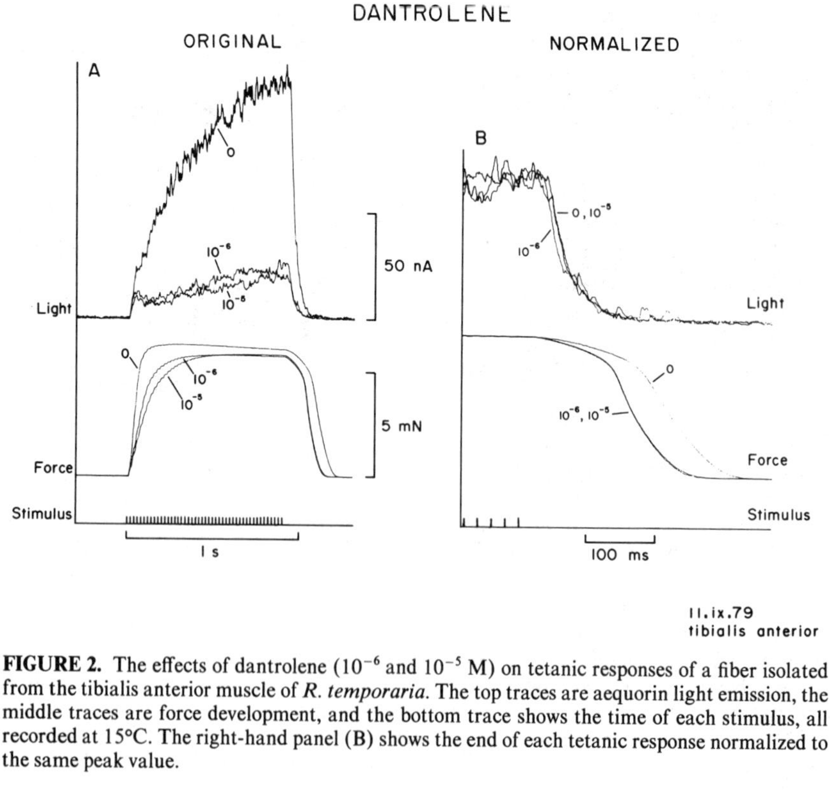

FIGURE 2. The effects of dantrolene (10^{-6} and 10^{-5} M) on tetanic responses of a fiber isolated from the tibialis anterior muscle of *R. temporaria.* The top traces are aequorin light emission, the middle traces are force development, and the bottom trace shows the time of each stimulus, all recorded at 15°C. The right-hand panel (B) shows the end of each tetanic response normalized to the same peak value.

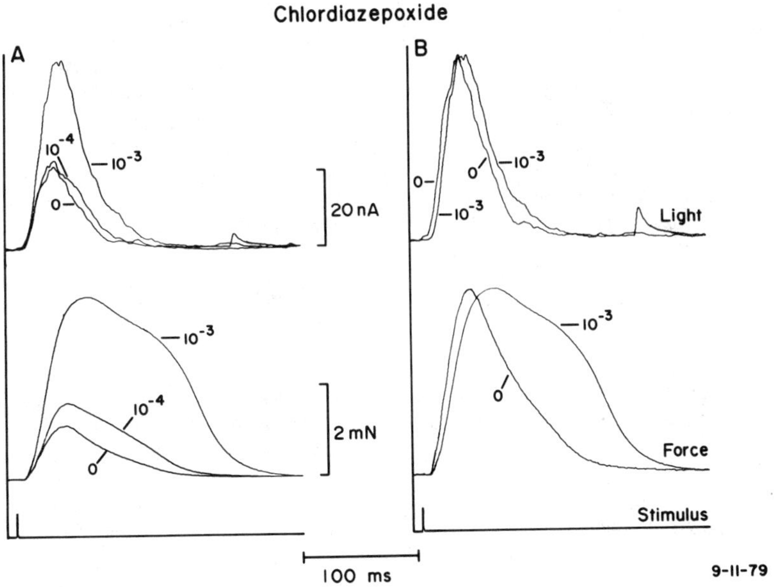

FIGURE 3. The potentiating effects of chlordiazepoxide (10^{-4} and 10^{-3} M) on twitch responses of a fiber isolated from the tibialis anterior of *R. temporaria*. The traces are positioned as described in the legend to FIGURE 2. Temperature is 15°C.

to detect the onset of straightening in fibrils in the outer parts of a fiber and count the number of frames before fibrils at the center straightened.

RESULTS

Dantrolene did not increase the time lag between activation of the superficial myofibrils and those at the center, as measured by the period between straightening of myofibrils near the edge of an image and straightening of fibrils at the center.[31] The action potential evidently spread as quickly and as deeply along the transverse tubular system as it does in the absence of dantrolene. The fact that the surface action potential is unchanged by dantrolene was not by itself sufficient evidence to rule out this possibility until now.

We also monitored calcium transients in single fibers injected with aequorin to explore further the idea that dantrolene reduces Ca^{2+} release from the SR. The left-hand side (A) of FIGURE 2 shows the effects of dantrolene on Ca^{2+} transients and force development recorded simultaneously during tetanic stimulation. Dantrolene markedly depressed intracellular Ca^{2+} transients in either a twitch or a tetanus although the effects on the plateau of tetanic force were small compared with the effects on active force as it rose towards its maximum. The decaying phases of the same records are shown on the right-hand side (B) on an expanded time scale. All light and force signals in panel B have been normalized to facilitate a comparison of the rates of decay. The rate of disappearance of Ca^{2+} from the cytoplasm is unchanged in the presence of dantrolene, and the compound evidently reduces calcium release in intact skeletal muscle without detectably changing uptake by the SR.

FIGURE 3 shows the effect of chlordiazepoxide on twitch responses of fibers treated in the same manner. It is evident from the normalized records (B) that the time course of both the cytoplasmic Ca^{2+} transient and twitch force after a single shock were shifted to a slightly later time by 10^{-3} M chlordiazepoxide. This effect can be explained by the fact that the upstroke of the action potential was slowed and its duration was prolonged (not shown). Concentrations less than 5×10^{-5} M, however, did not detectably influence action potentials, Ca^{2+} transients, or force development.

Baclofen, D-600, flordipine, GABA, meprobamate, and nylidrin produced effects similar to those of chlordiazepoxide. Their potency, however, was different, with the order from weakest to most potent as follows:

$$\text{baclofen} < \text{flordipine} < \text{meprobamate} < \text{chlordiazepoxide}$$

$$< \text{GABA} < \text{D-600} < \text{nylidrin}$$

Procaine (FIGURE 4) also enhanced calcium transients and potentiated force in single fibers as might be expected from the fact that it also prolongs the action potential.[34] At concentrations up to 10^{-4} M, however, the time course of Ca^{2+} transients during a twitch was changed very little, as is evident from the normalized, superimposed records in FIGURE 4B. The rate of Ca^{2+} removal after a tetanus was slightly slowed by procaine (panel D). Higher concentrations of this local anesthetic could not be tested reproducibly because they usually decreased excitability.

DISCUSSION

Voltage-activated Ca^{2+} channels seem to be localized primarily in the membranes of the transverse tubular system of skeletal muscle.[7] Calcium channels that are activated fast enough that they might operate in twitch contractions can be observed in intact fibers under certain experimental conditions. But their activity is short lived, perhaps because intracellular components are changed under the conditions that permit their detection.[7] Sodium channels, on the other hand, are present in lesser density in the T system,[35] and their diminished number or function might account for reduced twitch force under some circumstances.[9] Hence the minor changes in the surface action potential caused by dantrolene could not, prior to now, be assumed to be minor also in the T system.

The absence of an effect of dantrolene on the inward spread of activation is consistent with at least two possibilities: (1) dantrolene does not affect fast calcium current in the T system; (2) fast calcium current plays no direct role in twitch contractions.[8] The first possibility cannot be evaluated from our microscopic evidence alone. But cadmium, nifedipine, and D-600, all of which block both fast and slow calcium currents in frog skeletal muscle, actually potentiate twitch force.[7,19,36–39] Furthermore, removing substantial amounts of extracellular Ca^{2+} inhibits both fast and slow calcium currents in frog muscle, but has no detectable effect on either calcium transients or force in twitches.[26] It seems improbable, therefore, that the effects of dantrolene (FIGURE 2) are related to inhibition of voltage-gated calcium channels in the the T system.

Calcium channels have also been demonstrated in membranes of the sarcoplasmic reticulum, and major advances in understanding the pharmacology of excitation-contraction coupling have resulted from the implementation of technqiues to record Ca^{2+} channel currents from isolated membranes of the SR.[4,40,41] However, differences between the native environment of the channels and the experimental conditions,

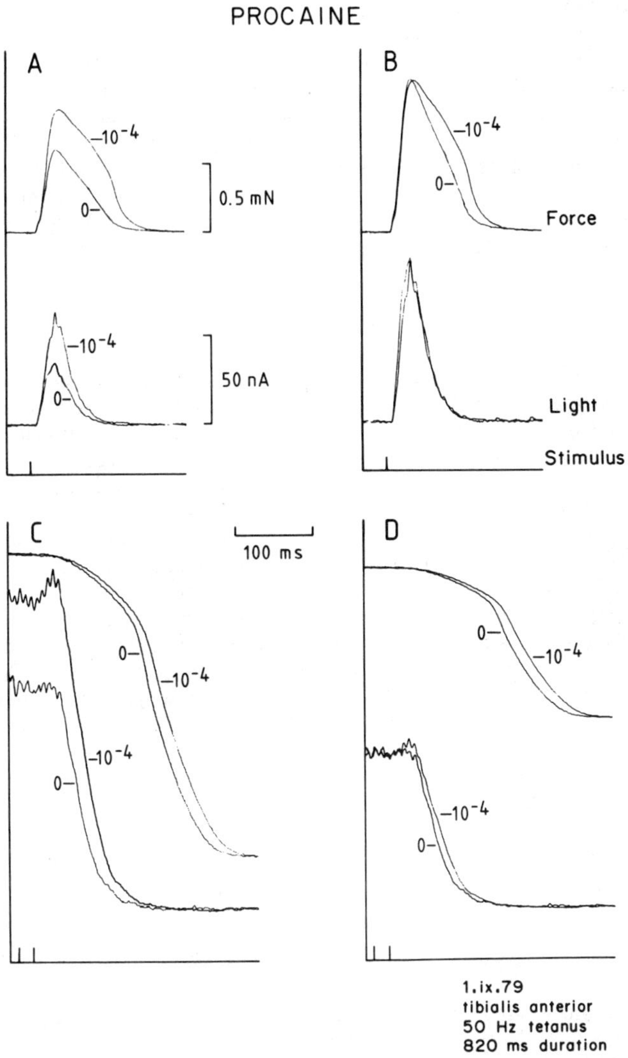

FIGURE 4. The potentiating effects of procaine (10^{-4} M) on responses of a fiber isolated from the tibialis anterior muscle of *R. temporaria*. Panel A shows the effects of twitch responses where both aequorin light emission and peak force are potentiated. The same records are shown normalized to their peak values in panel B. Panel C shows the end of the tetanic responses elicited from the same fiber. Aequorin light emission is larger in procaine. The plateau of tetanic force is not significantly changed. However, the rate of fall of force is slowed in procaine, which is consistent with the idea that Ca^{2+} release is enhanced by procaine in both twitch and tetanic responses. Panel D shows the tetanic responses normalized to the same peak value.

questions about the purity of isolated subunits, and a lack of knowledge as to what represents a complete and functional channel introduce uncertainties into the interpretation of these results. Such questions were avoided in the present experiments by monitoring drug- and Ca^{2+}-dependent changes from isolated *intact* muscle fibers.

Dantrolene has been shown to suppress calcium release from isolated vesicles of SR and to block the conductance of calcium channels in purified SR membranes studied with patch-clamp techniques.[5,41] SR Ca^{2+} channels in skeletal muscle are not blocked by some calcium antagonists even in relatively high concentrations.[4,39] Hence our comparison of dantrolene with other compounds confirms that so-called Ca^{2+} antagonists not only fail to block Ca^{2+} release in intact fibers, they actually enhance release and potentiate contractions. Dantrolene produced the opposite effects and is the only substance thus far reported to have such specific effects in intact skeletal muscle.

SUMMARY

Clinically potent skeletal muscle relaxants are used primarily for their effects on the central nervous system. But they also have direct effects on muscle contraction that possibly involve Ca^{2+} channels. We compared the effects of dantrolene, an agent known to have a direct action on vertebrate skeletal muscle, with other substances used as (1) relaxants and (2) antagonists of Ca-dependent excitation-contraction coupling. Isolated intact frog muscle cells were injected with the photoprotein aequorin, and membrane potential changes, intracellular Ca^{2+} transients, and contractile force were measured. Dantrolene (10^{-8} to 10^{-5} M) decreased the amplitude of Ca^{2+} transients, did not affect their rates of decay, and reduced contractile force. We also used an integrated digital-imaging system to record microscopic changes, namely, active shortening in myofibrils and changes in striation spacing. Dantrolene did not increase the time between contraction in myofibrils near the surface compared with myofibrils near the center of a cell. Hence dantrolene does not suppress Ca^{2+} transients by disturbing current flow in the transverse tubular system. Each of the following actually increased Ca^{2+} transients and contractile force evoked by action potentials: baclofen (10^{-7} to 10^{-5} M) < flordipine (10^{-6} M) < meprobamate (10^{-7} to 10^{-3} M) < chlordiazepoxide (10^{-5} to 5×10^{-4} M) < procaine (10^{-5} to 5×10^{-4}) < GABA (10^{-5} M) < D-600 (10^{-6} M) < nylidrin (10^{-5} M)—in order of increasing potency. Ca^{2+} channels in the sarcoplasmic reticulum of intact skeletal muscle are evidently inhibited by dantrolene but not by Ca^{2+} antagonists.

ACKNOWLEDGMENTS

We acknowledge gifts of compounds from Abbott Laboratories, Geigy Pharmaceuticals, Hoffmann-La Roche, Inc., Knoll AG, Pfizer Pharmaceuticals, G.D. Searle and Company, USV Pharmaceutical Corporation, and Wallace Laboratories. We are indebted to L. F. Wussow for preparing the figures and the manuscript, and to A. Isaacson for criticizing the manuscript.

REFERENCES

1. Ellis, K. O. & S. H. Bryant. 1972. Excitation-contraction uncoupling in skeletal muscle by dantrolene sodium. Naunyn-Schmiedebergs Arch. Pharmacol. **274:** 107–109.
2. Sengupta, C., U. A. Meyer & E. Carafoli. 1980. Binding of dantrolene sodium to muscle intracellular membranes. FEBS Lett. **117:** 37–38.

3. DANKO, S., & N. IKEMOTO. 1984. Dantrolene Na binding sites involved in inhibition of calcium release from SR *in vitro*. Biophys. J. **45:** 319a.
4. SUAREZ-ISLA, B. A., C. OROZCO, P. F. HELLER & J. P. FROEHLICH. 1986. Single calcium channels in native sarcoplasmic reticulum membranes from skeletal muscle. Proc. Nat. Acad. Sci. USA **83:** 7741–7762.
5. VAN WINKLE, W. B. 1976. Calcium release from skeletal muscle sarcoplasmic reticulum: site of action of dantrolene sodium? Science **193:** 1130–1131.
6. BROCKLEHURST, L. 1975. Dantrolene sodium and "skinned" muscle fibres. Nature **254:** 364.
7. AVILA-SAKAR, A. J., G. COTA, R. GAMBOA-ALDECO, J. GARCIA, M. HUERTA, J. MUNIZ & E. STEFANI. 1986. Skeletal muscle Ca^{2+} channels. J. Muscle Res. Cell Motil. **7:** 291–298.
8. BEAN, B. P. 1986. Calcium channels in skeletal muscle: what do they do? Trends Neurol. Sci. **9:** 535–536.
9. KOTSIAS, B. A., R. A. VENOSA & P. HOROWICZ. 1984. Denervated frog skeletal muscle: some electrical and mechanical properties. Pflügers Arch. **400:** 262–268.
10. OETLIKER, H. 1970. Action of chlordiazepoxide on contractile mechanism in single fibres of frog muscle. Experientia **26:** 682.
11. DEGROOF, R. C., C. P. BIANCHI, & S. NARAYAN. 1980. The effect of diazepam on tension and electrolyte distribution in frog muscle. Eur. J. Pharmacol. **66:** 193–199.
12. KHAN, A. R. 1983. Diazepam receptor in frog muscle fibres. Acta Physiol. Scand. **118:** 95–96.
13. RAMPE, D. & D. J. TRIGGLE. 1986. Benzodiazepines and calcium channel function. Trends Pharmacol. Sci. **7:** 461–464.
14. WU, J.-Y., C.-T., LIN, H. LIN, Y. XU, J.-W. LIU, B. H. HWANG & S. C. WEI. 1986. Immunochemical characterization and immunohistochemical localization of glutamate decarboxylase and GABA transaminase in peripheral tissues. *In* GABAergic Mechanisms in the Mammalian Periphery. S. L. Erdö & N. G. Bowery, Eds.: 19–34. Raven Press. New York, N.Y.
15. ERDÖ, S. L. 1986. GABA receptor binding sites in peripheral tissues of mammals. *In* GABAergic Mechanisms in the Mammalian Periphery. S. L. Erdö & N. G. Bowery, Eds.: 77–86. Raven Press. New York, N.Y.
16. SMITH, R. D., D. V. ROMANO, B. LOEV, T. P. PRUSS & P. S. WOLF. 1982. Comparison of the calcium antagonism and negative inotropic effects of flordipine (F) and nifedipine (N) in isolated canine vascular tissue and cat papillary muscle preparations. Pharmacologist **24:** 137.
17. WOLF, P. S., C. JOSEPOVITZ, C. GERACI & P. CERVONI. 1977. The alpha adrenoreceptor blocking effects of nylidrin. Pharmacologist **19:** 147.
18. LUDWIG, B. J. & J. R. POTTERFIELD. 1971. The pharmacology of propanediol carbamates. Adv. Pharmacol. Chemother. **9:** 173–240.
19. MARWAHA, J. & R. C. TREFFERS. 1980. Actions of a calcium antagonist, the D-600, on electrical and mechanical properties of frog skeletal muscle. Prog. Neuro-psychopharmacol. **4:** 145–152.
20. SANDOW, A., A. ISAACSON & H. PREISER. 1964. Potentiation of the twitch by eserine and imidazole. Fed. Proc. **23:** 366.
21. ISAACSON, A. & A. SANDOW. 1967. Quinine and caffeine effects on ^{45}Ca movements in frog sartorius muscle. J. Gen. Physiol. **50:** 2109–2128.
22. ISAACSON, A., M. J. HINKES & S. R. TAYLOR. 1970. Contracture and twitch potentiation of fast and slow muscles of the rat at 20 and 37°C. Am. J. Physiol. **218:** 33–41.
23. LOPEZ, J. R., L. A. HELLAND, L. A. WANEK, R. RÜDEL & S. R. TAYLOR. 1979. Calcium transients in skeletal muscle are not necessarily antagonized by muscle "relaxants." Biosphys. J. **25:** 119a.
24. TAYLOR, S. R., J. R. LOPEZ & H. H. SHLEVIN. 1979. Calcium movements in relation to muscle contraction. Proc. West. Pharmacol. Soc. **22:** 321–326.
25. TRUBE, G., J. R. LOPEZ, L. A. WANEK & S. R. TAYLOR. 1980. Effects of the local anesthetic procaine on E-C coupling in frog skeletal muscle. Fed. Proc. **39:** 580.
26. BLINKS, J. R., R. RÜDEL & S. R. TAYLOR. 1978. Calcium transients in isolated amphibian skeletal muscle fibres: detection with aequorin. J. Physiol. **277:** 291–323.

27. Allen, R. D., N. S. Allen & J. L. Travis. 1981. Video-enhanced contrast, differential interference contrast (AVEC-DIC) microscopy: a new method capable of analyzing microtuble-related motility in the reticulopodial network of *Allogromia laticollaris*. Cell Motil. **1:** 291–302.
28. Allen, R. D. & N. S. Allen. 1983. Video-enhanced microscopy with a computer frame memory. J. Microscopy **129:** 3–17.
29. Somlyo, A. P. 1986. Recent advance in electron and light optical imaging in biology and medicine. Ann. N.Y. Acad. Sci. **483:** 1–469.
30. Huxley A. F. & R. Niedergerke. 1958. Measurement of the striations of isolated muscle fibres with the interference microscope. J. Physiol. **144:** 403–425.
31. Gonzalez-Serratos, H. 1971. Inward spread of activation in vertebrate muscle fibres. J. Physiol. **212:** 777–799.
32. Brown, L. M., H. González-Serratos & A. F. Huxley. 1984. Structural studies of the waves in striated muscle fibres shortened passively below their slack length. J. Muscle Res. Cell Motil. **5:** 273–292.
33. Brown, L. M., H. González-Serratos & A. F. Huxley. 1984. Sarcomere and filament lengths in passive muscle fibres with wavy myofibrils. J. Muscle Res. Cell Motiol. **5:** 293–314.
34. Falk, G. 1961. Electrical activity of skeletal muscle. *In* Biophysics of Physiological and Pharmacological Actions: 259–279. Publication no. 69 of the American Association for the Advancement of Science, Washington, D.C.
35. Jaimovich, E., R. A. Venosa, P. Shrager & P. Horowicz. 1976. The density and distribution of tetrodotoxin receptors in normal and "detubulated" frog sartorius muscle. J. Gen. Physiol. **67:** 399–412.
36. Sandow, A. & A. Isaacson. 1966. Topochemical factors in potentiation of contraction. J. Gen. Physiol. **49:** 937–961.
37. Griffiths, P. J. & S. R. Taylor. 1982. The effects of calcium blockade on contraction in skeletal muscle fibres. J. Muscle Res. Cell Motil. **3:** 512.
38. Gonzalez-Serratos, H., R. Valle-Aguilera, D. A. Lathrop & M. C. Garcia. 1982. Slow inward calcium currents have no obvious role in muscle excitation-contraction coupling. Nature **298:** 292–294.
39. McClesky, E. W. 1985. Calcium channels and intracellular calcium release are pharmacologically different in frog skeletal muscle. J. Physiol. **361:** 231–249.
40. Smith, J. S., R. Coronado & G. Meissner. 1986. Single channel measurements of the calcium release channel from skeletal muscle sarcoplasmic reticulum. Activation by Ca^{2+} and ATP and modulation by Mg^{2+}. J. Gen. Physiol. **88:** 573–588.
41. Suárez-Isla, B. A. & V. Irribarra. 1987. Calcium channels in heavy sarcoplasmic reticulum membranes from the frog. Biophys. J. **51:** 351a.
42. Ballard, D. H. & C. M. Brown. 1982. Computer Vision. Prentice-Hall, Inc. Englewood Cliffs, N.J.

The Effect of Calcium Channel Antagonists on Peripheral Neurones[a]

RICHARD J. MILLER, DOUGLAS A. EWALD,
AARON P. FOX, LANE D. HIRNING,
EDWIN W. McCLESKEY,[b,c] TERESA M. PERNEY,
MICHAEL STUREK,[d] STANLEY A. THAYER,
RICHARD W. TSIEN,[b] AND MARY W. WALKER

Department of Pharmacological and Physiological Sciences
University of Chicago
947 East 58th Street
Chicago, Illinois 60637

[b]*Department of Physiology*
Yale University School of Medicine
333 Cedar Street
New Haven, Connecticut 06510

INTRODUCTION

The identification of high-affinity binding sites for dihydropyridines (DHPs) in the brain stimulated a search for effects of these and other organic Ca^{2+} antagonists on neuronal tissue.[1,2] Indeed, discovery of such effects could lead to novel therapeutic applications for these agents. Initially Ca^{2+} channel antagonists were not reported to have many effects on neurones and the question arose as to whether DHP binding sites in the nervous system really represented functional voltage-sensitive Ca^{2+} channels (VSCC).[3] For example, DHPs were reported to be ineffective in blocking evoked neurotransmitter release suggesting that they did not block VSCC in nerve terminals.[3,4] However, it has now become abundantly clear that DHP-sensitive VSCC do exist both in the central[5] and peripheral nervous systems.[6–8] In addition to DHP-sensitive VSCC, other types of Ca^{2+} channels also exist which are insensitive to DHPs and related agents.[5–8] Owing to their accessibility, peripheral neurones have been important systems for examining the properties and functions of the multiple types of VSCC. We shall summarize these studies briefly here. Extensive reviews of VSCC in neurones can be found elsewhere.[9,10]

SENSORY NEURONES

VSCC in sensory neurones have been more intensively studied than in any other type of vertebrate neurone. Thus, neuronal VSCC were first described in frog dorsal

[a]Supported by Public Health Service Grants DA-02121 and DA-02575 and MH-40165 to R.J.M. and HL-13306 and NS-24067 to R.W.T. and grants from Miles Pharmaceutical Inc.
[c]Present affiliation: Department of Physiology, Washington University School of Medicine, St. Louis, Mo. 63110.
[d]Present affiliation: Department of Physiology, University of Missouri School of Medicine, Columbia, Mo. 65212.

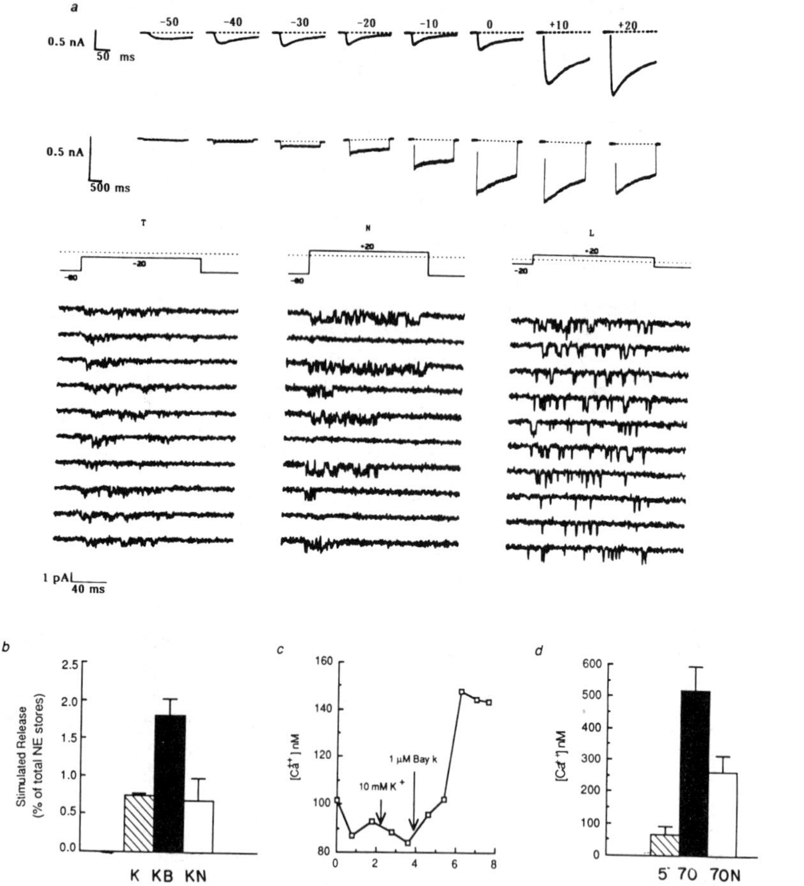

FIGURE 1. (**A**) The upper and middle traces illustrate Ca^{2+} currents in whole cell voltage-clamp recordings from a chick DRG neuron and a rat SCG neuron, respectively. In the upper trace, the holding potential was −100 mV; and in the middle trace, −90 mV. Test potentials are indicated above. External solution contained 135 mM tetraethylammonium chloride, 10 mM Hepes, 0.2 mM tetrodotoxin, and 10 mM $CaCl_2$ (upper) or 10 mM $BaCl_2$ (middle). Internal solution contained 100 mM CsCl, 10 mM Cs EGTA, 5 mM $MgCl_2$, 40 mM Hepes, 2 mM adenosine triphosphate, pH 7.3. The bottom traces illustrate the three types of unitary Ca^{2+} channel activity in cell-attached patch recordings from a chick DRG neuron with Ba^{2+} as the charge carrier. Patch pipettes contained 110 mM $BaCl_2$, 10 mM Hepes, 200 nM tetrodotoxin, pH 7.4. The cell resting potential was zeroed with an external solution containing 140 mM K^+ EGTA, 10 mM Hepes, 1 mM $MgCl_2$, pH 7.4. (Data from Reference 10 and unpublished observations.) (**B**) Release of norepinephrine from cultures of rat SCG neurons. Diagonal striped bar (K), release evoked by elevated K^+ (70 mM); black bar (KB), release evoked by elevated K^+ with BAY K8644 (10^{-6} M); open bar (KN), release evoked by elevated K^+ with nitrendipine (10^{-6} M). (**C**) Ca^{2+} uptake into a single SCG neuron measured with fura-2 microspectrofluorimetry. Note the augmenting effect of BAY K8644. (**D**) Uptake of Ca^{2+} into SCG neurons. Diagonal striped bar (5), $[Ca^{2+}]_i$ in 5 mM K^+; black bar (70), $[Ca^{2+}]_i$ in 70 mM K^+; open bar (70N) $[Ca^{2+}]_i$ in 70 mM K^+ with nitrendipine (10^{-6} M).

root ganglion cells (DRG) by Koketsu and his colleagues.[11,12] Sensory neurone action potentials show clear "shoulders" or "inflexions" that are mediated by Ca^{2+} currents.[9] In normal physiological medium these are more often observed in neurones from young or embryonic animals.[13] However, even with neurones from adult animals, Ca^{2+}-based action potentials can be easily observed following the suppression of Na^+ and K^+ currents. The properties of VSCC in DRG cells as studied using voltage clamp and patch clamp paradigms are now fairly well defined. Nowycky *et al.* established that chick DRG cells *in vitro* possessed three separate types of VSCC.[7,14,15] The contributions of these separate types of VSCC to the whole cell Ca^{2+} current (I_{Ca}) can be seen in FIGURE 1. From a relatively depolarized holding potential of about −40 mV, depolarizing voltage steps elicit an I_{Ca} that shows little tendancy to inactivate over several hundreds of mseconds. This component of the I_{Ca} has been designated "L." Depolarizing steps from negative holding potentials elicit a transient I_{Ca} designated T which reaches a maximum at about −30 mV. Stronger depolarizations elicit a second phase of inactivating current ("N type"). Thus, the N current is like the T type in that it is inactivating but similar to the L type in its voltage range of activation. Using the on-cell patch paradigm, Nowycky *et al.* were able to demonstrate the three VSCC types underlying these whole cell currents (FIGURE 1). The properties of these L, T,

TABLE 1. Properties of Multiple Calcium Channels Found in Chick Dorsal Root Ganglion Neurones

	Channel Type		
Property	T	N	L
Activation range (10 mM Ca)	Positive to −70 mV	Positive to −10 mV	Positive to −10 mV
Inactivation range	−100 to 60 mV	>−100 to −40 mV	−60 to 10 mV
Approximate single-channel conductance	9 pS	13 pS	25 pS
Cd^{2+} block	Weak; IC_{50} 100 μM	Strong; IC_{50} 10 μM	Strong; IC_{50} 10 μM
ω-CgTx block	Weak	Strong	Strong
DHP modulation	No	No	Yes

and N channels are summarized in TABLE 1. These properties are consistent with those of the whole cell currents discussed. VSCC with properties similar to T and L have been described in a variety of other cell types. Various combinations of N, L, and T have been found in other types of neurones (see below).[9] Of particular interest is the observation that in DRG cells as in other cases, the L channel can be powerfully modulated by dihydropyridines (DHPs) and other types of organic VSCC blockers. BAY K8644, for example, causes a large increase in the open times of single L channels and thus greatly increases the size of the corresponding portion of the whole cell current.[8] VSCC antagonists such as nitrendipine are able to block the sustained portion of the whole cell Ca^{2+} current. However the degree of block is critically dependent on the holding potential.[9] It has been suggested that DHP antagonists interact preferentially with L channels in an inactivated state favored by depolarized holding potentials ("Modulated receptor hypothesis").[31] Thus, under the appropriate circumstances nitrendipine will reduce the magnitude of the DRG L current. However, it is interesting to note that even when the voltage dependence of the block is taken into account, neuronal Ca^{2+} currents seem somewhat resistant to blockade by DHP antagonists in comparison to cardiac muscle for example. This fact would not be predicted from ligand binding studies.[14] The time and voltage dependences of the effects of DHP antagonists on neuronal L currents also help to explain the effects of these agents on the duration of the DRG action potential. Thus, although BAY K8644 can be shown to produce large increases in the duration of the DRG Ca^{2+} spike, blocking effects of nitrendipine have been much harder to demonstrate.[16]

The existence of three separate types of VSCC in DRG cells raises the important question as to which of these channel types provides the Ca^{2+} that triggers the release of neurotransmitters. In order to answer this question we investigated the release of substance P from DRG neurones *in vitro* (FIGURE 2). Release of this peptide can be evoked by field stimulation or by depolarizing the cells with elevated $[K^+]_0$.[16,17] Both of these procedures lead to the activation of VSCC. Release can also be elicited by capsaicin, the pungent algesic principle of hot peppers[18] (FIGURE 2). Capsaicin produces a large influx of Ca^{2+} into DRG cells by bypassing normal VSCC or other pathways.[18] Release induced by depolarization can be enhanced by DHP agonists, but release induced by capsaicin remains unaltered[6,17] (FIGURE 2). When cells are depolarized by raising $[K^+]_0$ the subsequent release of substance P has been reported to be substantially or completely blocked by Ca^{2+} channel antagonists such as nitrendipine or D-600. Release induced by field stimulation on the other hand is resistant to block by nitrendipine for the reasons elaborated above.[6,16] Thus, long-term depolarization using high $[K^+]$ presumably allows L channels to enter the inactivated state for a sufficient period of time to allow them to interact with DHP antagonists. This paradigm allows us to distinguish clearly the type of VSCC that participates in transmitter release—in this case predominantly the L type. The predominant role of L channels in mediating substance P release from DRG cells is unusual as in many other instances neurotransmitter release appears to be subserved by N channels[9,10] (see below). Furthermore, when release is evoked from slices of adult rat dorsal horn, DHPs

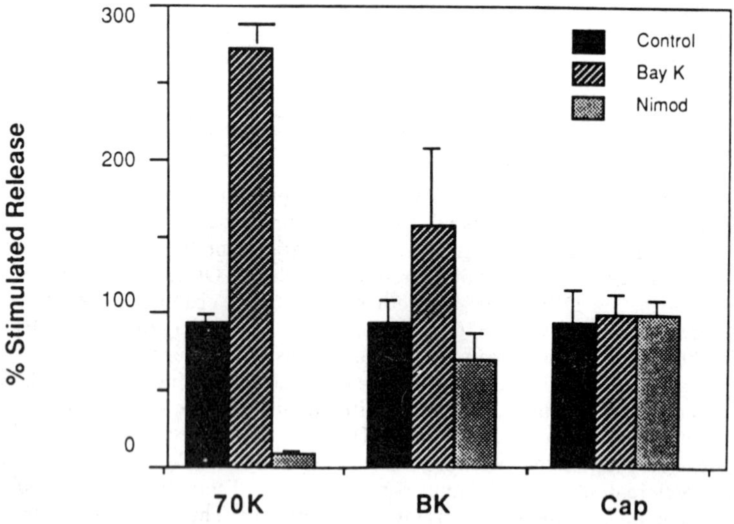

FIGURE 2. DHP sensitivity of substance P release. Pharmacology of evoked release of substance P from dorsal root ganglion neurones from neonatal rats *in vitro* (n = 6–12). BK, bradykinin (10^{-7} M); Cap, capsaicin (10^{-6} M); Nimod, nimodipine (10^{-6} M); Bay K, BAY K8644 (10^{-6} M).

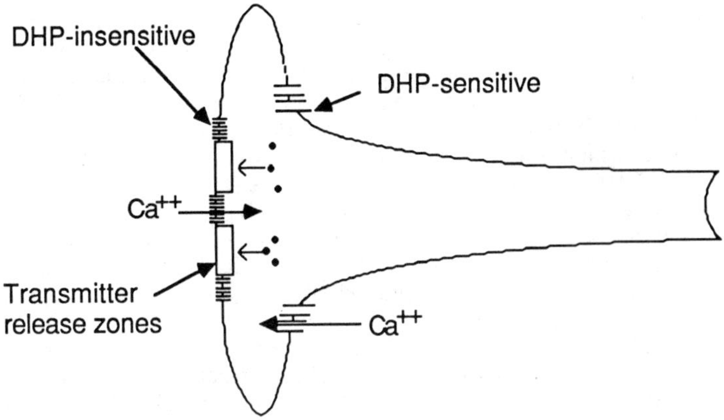

FIGURE 3. Hypothetical arrangement of dihydroyridine (DHP) sensitive (L) and DHP-sensitive (N) type calcium channels in a nerve terminal.

are much less effective (Perney and Miller, unpublished observations). It may be therefore that the L-channel-mediated release observed *in vitro* is of developmental significance.

It is also interesting to note that the release of substance P from DRG cells can be blocked by a number of different neurotransmitters including norepinephrine (α_2), gamma-aminobutyric acid (GABA) (B), dynorphin, neuropeptide Y (NPY), and adenosine.[9,19,20] The mechanism of this block appears to involve the direct inhibition of Ca^{2+} current, rather than other possibilities such as modification of K^+ currents. It is not yet clear whether N, L, or T currents are modulated by the neurotransmitters in question. From the above discussion, however, it would seem likely that L currents would be blocked and indeed this has been shown to be the case in some studies, although block of N currents may also occur.[9,17,20] The molecular mechanism by which the Ca^{2+} current is modulated is unknown. One possibility however is that it involves the participation of protein kinase C (PKC). Thus, diacylglycerol (DAG) analogues and phorbol esters have been shown to block L currents in DRG cells.[21] Moreover, removal of PKC from DRG cells by down regulation appears to abolish the blocking effects of norepinephrine and NPY for example (Ewald and Miller, unpublished observations). It has also been shown that both DRG N and L currents can be modulated by stable analogues of GTP introduced into the cell with a patch pipette.[22] In addition the effects of norepinephrine and other neurotransmitters can be blocked by pretreatment of DRG cells with pertussis toxin. These observations indicate that a G protein such as Gi or Go may be involved in the receptor/channel transduction mechanism.[23] G proteins have been shown to mediate the receptor-induced breakdown of membrane inositol phospholipids,[24] consistent with a role for the DAG/PKC system.

SYMPATHETIC NEURONES

Ca^{2+} spikes can be readily recorded from sympathetic neurones from a number of different species.[9] Ca^{2+} currents from whole cell voltage clamp recordings of rat superior cervical ganglion (SCG) neurones *in vitro* can be seen in FIGURE 1.

Depolarizing steps from a holding potential of −90 mV reveal no Ca^{2+} current up to −50 mV suggesting the absence of T channels in these cells. However strong depolarizations reveal the presence of a Ca^{2+} current with decaying and sustained phases comparable with the N and L currents of the DRG cell (see above). Moreover, nitrendipine depresses the sustained but not the transient phase of the current under the appropriate conditions. This suggests that SCG cells possess DHP-sensitive L currents and DHP-insensitive N currents but that T currents are absent. This hypothesis is substantiated by studies of single channels. Two types of channels can be observed. The smaller of these has a slope conductance of 11 pS and the larger of 27 pS—close to the values for N and L channels in DRG cells. In addition, openings of the larger channel type are greatly lengthened by BAY K8644 and suppressed by nitrendipine.

As with DRG cells, we also investigated which VSCC participated in neurotransmitter release from these cells (FIGURE 1). ^{3}H-Norepinephrine preaccumulated by SCG neurones *in vitro* could be released by depolarizing stimuli such as raising $[K^+]_0$ (FIGURE 1). Release could be blocked by Cd^{2+} or in Ca^{2+}-free medium.[6] In contrast to the situation in DRG cells, however, nitrendipine even at high concentrations only slightly inhibited release. The L channel agonist BAY K8644 clearly enhanced release and this enhancement could be reversed by nitrendipine or other DHP antagonists.[6] Thus, it seems as though L channels do not normally participate in release unless they are induced to do so by using BAY K8644. We considered the possibility that raising $[K^+]_0$ was an insufficient stimulus for the activation of L channels in SCG neurones. Therefore, we analyzed the depolarization-induced influx of Ca^{2+} directly into SCG neurones using fura-2 microspectrofluorimetry. FIGURE 1 shows that upon raising $[K^+]_0$, $[Ca^{2+}]_i$ in the cell bodies of SCG neurones rises from about 10^{-7} M to about 6×10^{-7} M. This increase in $[Ca^{2+}]_i$ could be partially inhibited by nitrendipine (approximately 50%) at concentrations that failed to block norepinephrine release. It seems therefore that when SCG neurones are depolarized by raising $[K^+]_0$, Ca^{2+} does indeed flow into the cells via both N and L channels. In order to explain these data we might hypothesize that VSCC in SCG nerve terminals are organized in the manner suggested in FIGURE 3.[10] It may be that N channels are preferentially localized or "clustered" around zones of neurotransmitter release. Normally Ca^{2+} entering via a particular channel will have a limited sphere of influence due to the neurone's internal buffering mechanisms. Thus, normally the release system will not sense Ca^{2+} entering via L channels as they are not in an advantageous position. However, under the influence of BAY K8644 so much Ca^{2+} now enters via L channels that the buffering system is overwhelmed and this Ca^{2+} may now start to participate in stimulus/secretion coupling. One prediction of this model is that although neurotransmitter release is not blocked by nitrendipine, SCG nerve terminals should contain L channels. FIGURE 4 demonstrates that application of BAY K8644 to the cell bodies of SCG neurones reveals the presence of L channels consistent with the electrophysiological data. It can also be seen that similar applications of BAY K8644 to axonal processes extending from SCG cell bodies also reveal the presence of L channels. Therefore, L channels appear to exist in both the cell bodies and terminals of SCG neurones. This rules out their absence from nerve terminals as a reason for the lack of effect of nitrendipine on neurotransmitter release. In recent studies utilizing bullfrog sympathetic neurones *in vitro,* Lipscombe *et al.* have also reported both N and L type VSCC openings in on-cell patches derived from cell bodies, axonal processes, and growth cones.[25]

Ca^{2+} currents in SCG neurones can also be inhibited by a variety of substances including norepinephrine (α_2), acetylcholine (muscarinic), adenosine, and prostaglandin E_1 (PGE_1). As N channels play a major role in stimulus/secretion coupling in these cells, it would be interesting if the N currents were the major target for neurotransmit-

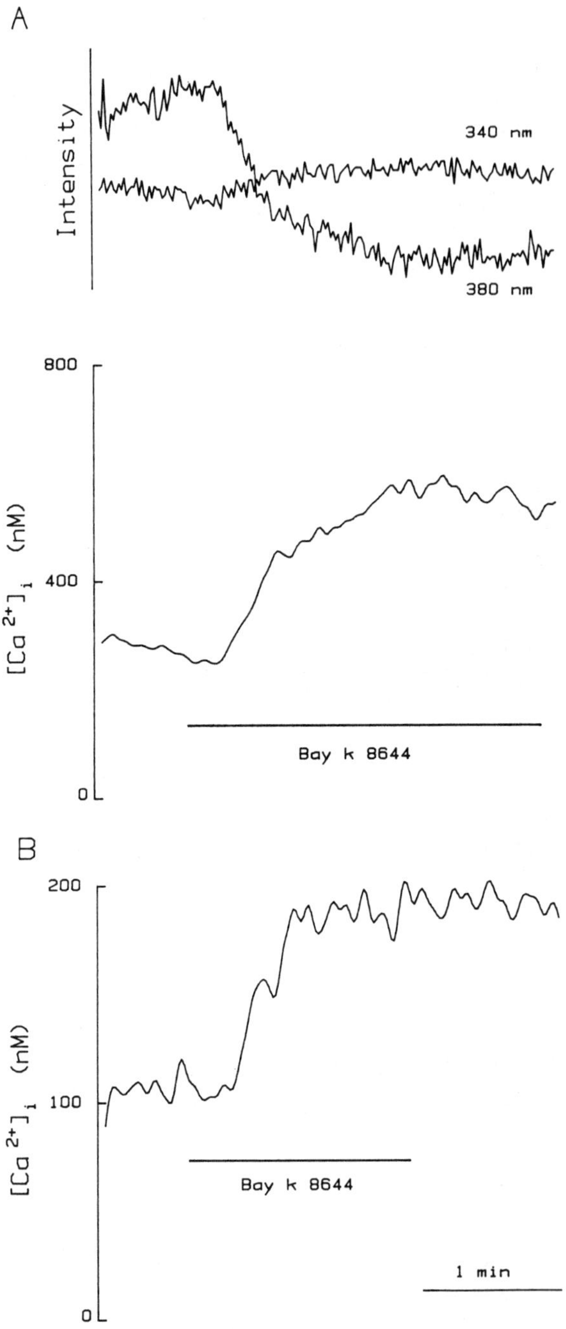

FIGURE 4. BAY K8644–induced increases in $[Ca^{2+}]_i$ in SCG neurons. 1 μM BAY K8644 was perfused onto a soma (A) or process (B) of a sympathetic neuron during the time indicated by the horizontal bar. Cells were loaded for 1 hour in 2 μM fura-2 AM, washed, mounted in the chamber of a microfluorimeter, and bathed in HEPES buffered Hank's solution pH 7.45 containing 10 mM K^+. The excitation wavelength was alternated between 340 and 380 nm at a frequency of 60 Hz. The average fura-2 fluorescence for each wavelength was determined each second as shown in the upper portion of A for the soma. $[Ca^{2+}]_i$ was calculated from the ratio of these two intensities.

ter-induced modulation. Galvan and Adams studied the inhibition of rat sympathetic neurone Ca^{2+} current by norepinephrine.[26] However, it is not completely clear in these studies which portion of the current is being blocked. On the other hand, a recent study by Wanke *et al.* clearly shows that muscarine selectively inhibits the inactivating (N type) portion of the Ca^{2+} current in rat SCG neurones.[27] This inhibition appears to be mediated through a G protein but does not seem to utilize cAMP or DAG as a second messenger. Thus, the mechanism of Ca^{2+} current inhibition in these cells seems to differ from that described above for DRG cells.

OTHER PERIPHERAL NEURONES

Relatively little is known about the Ca^{2+} currents in other types of peripheral neurones or their sensitivity to Ca^{2+}-channel-modulating drugs such as DHPs. In the enteric ganglia, however, Ca^{2+} currents recorded from neurones of the rat myenteric plexus *in vitro* reveal N and L type currents. In preliminary studies, it appears as though some portion of the Ca^{2+} current in myenteric neurones can be blocked by nitrendipine (Hirning, Sturek, and Miller, unpublished observations). Furthermore, portions of the current can also be blocked by norepinephrine or dynorphin. Recently it has been shown that there are two components of the Ca^{2+} current in motor neurones.[28] Interestingly, Atchison and O'Leary have found that, as in SCG neurones, evoked release of the neurotransmitter (acetylcholine) from motor neurones is resistant to blockade by DHP antagonists but is enhanced by BAY K8644.[29]

CONCLUSIONS

The above discussion indicates that VSCC that are sensitive to DHPs and related agents do appear to exist in several types of peripheral neurones. The physiological roles of these VSCC may vary according to the cell type and possibly the stage of neuronal development. Under the appropriate conditions, however, these VSCC can be made to participate in neurotransmitter release mechanisms. Furthermore, they may also be the targets for neurotransmitter-induced modulation which may play an important role in presynaptic inhibition and other phenomena. The difference in the pharmacology of substance P and norepinephrine release is interesting. Peptides (e.g., substance P) and small molecules (e.g., norepinephrine) are found to be localized in different types of secretory vesicles, even within the same nerve terminal.[30] One might speculate therefore that the difference we have observed could be related to the different types of neurotransmitters we have so far investigated.

REFERENCES

1. GLOSSMANN, H., D. R. FERRY, A. GOLL, J. STRIESSNIG & M. SCHOBER. 1985. J. Cardiol. Pharm. **6:** S608–S621.
2. JANIS, R. A., P. BELLEMANN, J. G. SARMIENTO & D. J. TRIGGLE. 1985. The dihydropyridine receptors. *In* Cardiovascular Effects of Dihydropyridine Ca^{2+} Channel Antagonists and Agonists. A. Fleckenstein & C. van Breemen, Eds.: 140–156. Springer-Verlag. Berlin, FRG.
3. MILLER, R. J. & S. B. FREEDMAN. 1984. Life Sci. **34:** 1205–1221.
4. NACHSHEN, D. A. & M. P. BLAUSTEIN. 1979. Mol. Pharmacol. **16:** 579–586.
5. THAYER, S. A., S. W. MURPHY & R. J. MILLER. 1986. Mol. Pharmacol. **30:** 505–509.

6. PERNEY, T. M., L. D. HIRNING, S. E. LEEMAN & R. J. MILLER. 1986. Proc. Nat. Acad. Sci. USA **83:** 6656–6659.
7. NOWYCKY, M. C., A. P. FOX & R. W. TSIEN. 1985. Nature **316:** 440–443.
8. NOWYCKY, M. C., A. P. FOX & R. W. TSIEN. 1985. Proc. Nat. Acad. Sci. USA **82:** 2178–2182.
9. MILLER, R. J. Calcium channels in neurones. *In* Structure and Physiology of the Slow Inward Calcium Channel. D. J. Triggle & J. C. Venter, Eds. Receptor Biochem Methodol. **7.** Plenum Press. New York, N.Y. (In press.)
10. MILLER, R. J. 1987. Science **235:** 46–52.
11. KOKETSU, K., J. A. CERF & S. NISHI. 1959. J. Neurophysiol. **22:** 177–194.
12. KOKETSU, K., S. NISHI & H. C. SOEDA. 1963. Nature **200:** 786–787.
13. SPITZER, N. C. 1979. Annu. Rev. Neurosci. **2:** 363–397.
14. MCCLESKEY, E. W., A. P. FOX, D. FELDMAN & R. W. TSIEN. 1986. J. Exp. Biol. **124:** 177–190.
15. FOX, A. P., M. C. NOWYCKY & R. W. TSIEN. J. Physiol. (In press.)
16. RANE, S. G., G. G. HOLZ & K. DUNLAP. Pflugers Arch. (In press.)
17. HOLZ, G. G., K. DUNLAP & R. M. KREAM. J. Neurosci. (In press.)
18. BEVAN, S. J., I. F. JAMES, H. P. RANG, J. WINTER & J. N. WOOD. The mechanism of action of capsaicin—a sensory neurotoxin. *In* Neurotoxins and Their Pharmacological Implications. Raven Press. New York, N.Y. (In press.)
19. MUDGE, A. W., S. E. LEEMAN & G. FISCHBACH. 1979. Proc. Nat. Acad. Sci. USA **76:** 526–530.
20. HOLZ, G. G., R. M. KREAM & K. DUNLAP. J. Neurosci. (In press.)
21. RANE, S. G. & K. DUNLAP. 1986. Proc. Nat. Acad. Sci. USA **83:** 184–188.
22. SCOTT, R. H. & A. C. DOLPHIN. 1986. Neurosci. Lett. **69:** 59–64.
23. HOLZ, G. G., S. RANE & K. DUNLAP. 1986. Nature **319:** 670–672.
24. MAJERUS, P. W., T. M. CONNOLLY, H. DECKMYN, T. S. ROSS, T. E. BROSS, H. ISHII, V. S. BANSAL & D. B. WILSON. 1986. Science **234:** 1519–1526.
25. LIPSCOMBE, D., M. POENIE, H. REUTER, R. Y. TSIEN & R. W. TSIEN. 1987. Biophys. J. **51:** 227a.
26. GALVAN, M. & P. R. ADAMS. 1982. Brain Res. **244:** 135–144.
27. WANKE, E., A. FERRONI, A. MALGAROLI, B. AMBROSINI, T. POZZAN & J. MELDOLESI. 1987. Proc. Nat. Acad. Sci. USA **84:** 4313–4317.
28. PENNER, R. & F. DRYER. 1986. Pflugers Arch. **406:** 190–197.
29. ATCHISON, W. D. & S. M. O'LEARY. (Submitted.)
30. DE CAMILLI, P. & P. GREENGARD. 1986. Biochem. Pharmacol. **35:** 4349–4357.
31. HILLE, B. 1984. Ionic Channels of Excitable Membranes. Sinauer Press. Sunderland, Mass.

Do Dihydropyridine-Sensitive Calcium Channels Play a Role in Neurosecretion in the Central Nervous System?

TIMOTHY J. TURNER AND STANLEY M. GOLDIN

Department of Biological Chemistry and Molecular Pharmacology
Harvard Medical School
25 Shattuck Street
Boston, Massachusetts 02115

Using patch clamp recording methods in primary cultures of autonomic ganglia, Tsien and co-workers identified three distinct types of Ca currents,[1] based on distinct biophysical and pharmacological properties. The channels that mediate these currents (identified as L, N, and T channels) are presumed to have different roles in regulating neuronal activity. Only one of these types, the L channel, is sensitive to blockade by dihydropyridine (DHP) antagonists. The patch clamp recordings were obtained from cell bodies, and do not directly reflect the electrical activity of the nerve terminals. The inaccessibility of nerve terminals to direct electrophysiological measurements complicates determination of the role of each type of Ca channel in regulating neurosecretion. This article discusses the results of alternative approaches which employ brain nerve terminal preparations (synaptosomes) to study Ca channel–mediated neurosecretion. By direct measurement of the pharmacological properties of depolarization-stimulated Ca uptake and neurotransmitter release from synaptosomes, the Ca channel classes controlling neurosecretion can in principle be identified.

The nerve terminal, or synaptic bouton, is relatively sensitive to shear due to the structure of neurons. Homogenization of brain tissue results in cleavage of the nerve terminal from the axon and allows severed terminals to seal off into vesicles. Synaptosomes, i.e., fractions of the homogenate highly enriched in nerve terminals, are then separated from the remaining material through differential centrifugation, which separates these vesicles based on their size and density.[2]

Blaustein and colleagues first demonstrated that synaptosomes had functional properties expected of nerve terminals.[3-5] Through the use of a dicarbocyanine dye, a fluorescent probe for membrane potentials, it was shown that these vesicles maintain an inside-negative membrane potential. The synaptosomal membrane potential depends on Na/K ATPase activity, since it can be abolished by ouabain. When the potassium gradient is diminished by exposing synaptosomes to elevated concentrations of KCl, the membrane potential is also diminished, indicating that it is sensitive to the diffusion potential for K^+. When synaptosomes are loaded with radiolabeled neurotransmitters or their precursors, exposure to KCl concentrations that depolarize the membrane cause an increase in the rate of release of these radiolabeled compounds. Release is dependent, in part, upon the presence of calcium in the external solution. Furthermore, KCl depolarizations cause an increase in the rate of synaptosomal $^{45}Ca^{2+}$ accumulation. These results are consistent with synaptosomal neurosecretion mediated by Ca influx through voltage-sensitive Ca channels.

Nachshen and Blaustein reported that K^+-stimulated Ca uptake by synaptosomes was insensitive to blockade by dihydropyridines, and only weakly sensitive to blockade by other organic antagonists such as D600 at concentrations >10 μM.[6] This was initially interpreted to indicate that neuronal Ca channels are relatively insensitive to organic Ca antagonists. However, the results of subsequent radioligand binding studies stimulated reexamination of the pharmacology of synaptosomal Ca channels.

The radiolabeled DHP ^{3}H-nitrendipine has been used to demonstrate that brain homogenates contain a high-affinity receptor that is very similar to the DHP binding site identified in heart and smooth muscle.[7] This receptor is fairly concentrated in brain, and autoradiography suggests that the receptor is located in regions of synaptic contact, although this method cannot resolve presynaptic from postsynaptic membranes.[8] The presence of DHP binding sites in regions of synaptic contact leads to the hypothesis that L-type Ca channels are in some way involved in neurotransmission.

One possible explanation for the discrepancy between the results of radioligand binding assays and the DHP insensitivity of synaptosomal Ca uptake was that processes other than Ca channels may mediate K-stimulated Ca entry. Synaptosomal membranes also contain an Na/Ca exchange activity,[9] which in theory could play such a role. This process exchanges three Na^+ for each Ca^{2+}, and hence is electrogenic.[10] Under resting conditions, Na/Ca exchange uses the combined driving forces of electrostatic field and concentration gradient of Na^+ to extrude Ca^{2+} against its large electrochemical gradient. Because Na/Ca exchange is electrogenic, it is also sensitive to the electrostatic field. Depolarization of the membrane can reverse the direction of transport, leading to net Ca uptake.

In order to examine the contribution of Na/Ca exchange to depolarization-stimulated Ca uptake, we performed parallel experiments in the absence of external Na^+, using choline as a substitute[11] (FIGURE 1). In the presence of external Na^+, the basal rate of Ca uptake is stimulated two- to threefold by KCl depolarization. The difference between basal and depolarized uptake is the net depolarization-dependent Ca uptake. This uptake is biphasic, with a rapid, terminating phase and a slow, persistent phase, thus replicating the observations of Nachshen.[12] In the absence of external Na^+, the net depolarization-dependent Ca uptake reaches a plateau within 1 second that is constant for at least 20 seconds. Thus, removing external Na^+ resolves the time course of Ca uptake into a rapid phase that terminates, eliminating the slow, persistent phase. The depolarization-stimulated uptake was tested further by measuring Ca uptake after predepolarization. Synaptosomes were depolarized with elevated KCl in the presence of a normal concentration of Ca in the uptake buffer, but with no $^{45}Ca^{2+}$. These depolarized synaptosomes were incubated for 15 seconds prior to exposure to $^{45}Ca^{2+}$. As illustrated, this procedure resulted in nearly total inactivation of the net depolarization-stimulated uptake, indicating that the uptake process inactivates within 15 seconds. These results are consistent with the fast, terminating phase of Ca uptake being mediated by voltage-sensitive Ca channels, and the slow, persistent phase being mediated by Na/Ca exchange. This has since been confirmed by other laboratories.[13,14]

Based on the above, it seemed reasonable that possible DHP sensitivity of synaptosomal Ca channels could have been masked by Na/Ca exchange. When we measured depolarization-stimulated Ca uptake in the presence of nifedipine, we therefore tried to improve the signal that might be produced by $^{45}Ca^{2+}$ entry through a Ca channel by making our uptake measurements more rapidly (as in FIGURE 1), thus reducing the contribution of Na/Ca exchange to net uptake.

We observe an inhibition of net Ca uptake of about 30% at concentrations of nitrendipine in the 1–10 μM range. The conclusion drawn from these experiments is that a portion of the rapid, transient phase of Ca uptake is sensitive to blockade by DHP in the micromolar range, while a majority of it is not, as previously reported.[11] These observations are consistent with Ca uptake being mediated by both DHP-

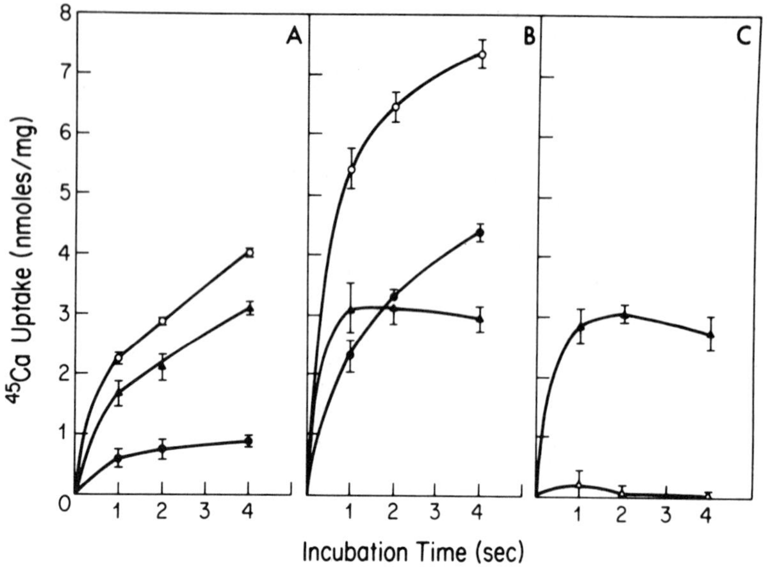

FIGURE 1. (A) Time course of $^{45}Ca^{2+}$ uptake by synaptosomes in basal (filled circles) and depolarizing (open circles) buffers containing NaCl (>95 mM). The net depolarization-stimulated Ca uptake (triangles) is the difference between basal and stimulated uptake. (**B**) Same as A, but choline Cl was substituted for NaCl ([Na] < 50 μM). (C) Synaptosomes were suspended in choline-substituted buffer containing elevated [K^+] (open triangles) or normal 5 mM K^+ (closed triangles) for 15 seconds. At that time, both samples were adjusted to a [K^+] of 60 mM, and $^{45}Ca^{2+}$ was added to measure the time course of uptake. Error bars denote standard error of measurement.

sensitive and -insensitive classes of Ca channels. However, the magnitude of K^+-stimulated Ca uptake in choline-containing buffer was subject to a time-dependent decline that was unaccounted for in our previous measurements of DHP sensitivity of Ca uptake and norepinephrine release. This systematic error led us to believe that DHPs were much more potent than in fact they are, and when this error is accounted for we do not observe dihydropyridine effects in the submicromolar concentration range.

There have been several other reports of dihidropyridine effects on the functional properties of synaptosomes (TABLE 1). Middlemiss and Spedding reported that submicromolar concentrations of Bay K 8644 could augment K-evoked serotonin release from cortical brain slices.[15] The augmented release was blocked by 1 μM nifedipine. Woodward and Leslie obtained similar results in synaptosomes, with a modest augmentation by 1 nM Bay K 8644 of K^+-stimulated Ca uptake and dopamine release that is blocked by 10 nM nimodipine.[16] Nordstrom *et al.* reported that nimodipine at concentrations at or exceeding 1 μM blocks up to 40% of synaptosomal Ca uptake.[17] They observed a 50% inhibition by nimodipine of acetylcholine release evoked by either field stimulation or elevated KCl concentrations. Interestingly, they observe up to a twofold increase in dopamine release in the presence of nimodipine. Rane *et al.* report an inhibitory effect of 0.1 μM DHP on Ca currents in cultured dorsal root ganglia.[18] They observe a 40% inhibition of substance P release by 5 μM nimodipine only when KCl is used as a stimulus, but not when field stimulation is employed. Thayer *et al.* employed microspectrofluorimetry of single cells using the Ca indicator dye Fura2 to image intracellular [Ca] transients resulting from KCl depolarization.[19] They found that the [Ca] transient could be blunted by 1 μM nitrendipine. The magnitude of this effect varies from region to region, but all regions examined showed some degree of dihydropyidine sensitivity.

However, even when measures are taken to minimize the contribution of Na/Ca exchange, many investigators do not observe effects of DHP on synaptosomal Ca uptake, even at supramicromolar DHP levels. Suszkiw used a quench-flow method to measure Ca uptake in the presence and absence of Na, but found no evidence for DHP-sensitivity.[13] Reynolds *et al.* found no evidence for effects of DHP agonists or antagonists on Ca uptake;[20] however, they did observe that omega-conotoxin (wCgTx), a marine snail peptide toxin, produced a potent blockade of 50% of Ca uptake and norepinephrine release. wCgTx produces a persistent blockade of both the L- and N-type Ca channels.[21] in sensory neurons. Because Reynolds *et al.* saw inhibition by wCgTx and not by DHP, they concluded that the N channel is involved in synaptosomal Ca uptake and norepinephrine release, and that the role of the L channel in the central nervous system (CNS) is undefined.

DHP sensitivity of Ca uptake is the distinguishing characteristic of L-type channel activity. The observation that wCgTx can block a portion of synaptosomal Ca uptake in the absence of DHP effects has led many to believe that only N-type channels

TABLE 1. Effects of Dihydropyridines in Central Nervous System Preparations

Authors	Results
Brown *et al.*, 1984[22]	Nimodipine inhibits cell body Ca currents by 50% in hippocampal slices and primary cultures.
Thayer *et al.*, 1985[19]	Nitrendipine inhibits K^+-stimulated Ca transients in primary cultures by 30–80%, depending on brain region examined.
Middlemiss & Spedding, 1985[15]	Bay K 8644 augments K^+-stimulated serotonin release in cortical slices; augmentation blocked by nifedipine.
Turner & Goldin, 1985[11]	Nifedipine and nitrendipine block K^+-stimulated Ca uptake in synaptosomes by 30–50%.
Nordstrom *et al.*, 1986[17]	Nimodipine blocks K^+-stimulated Ca uptake and acetylcholine release from synaptosomes by 30–50%. Nimodipine augments dopamine release by 120%.
Woodward & Leslie, 1986[16]	Bay K 8644 augments K^+-stimulated Ca uptake in synaptosomes; augmentation blocked by nimodipine.
White & Bradford, 1986[23]	Bay K 8644 augments K^+-stimulated Ca uptake and amino acid release from synaptosomes. Nimodipine inhibits Ca uptake.
Nachshen & Blaustein, 1979[6]	No effect of DHP on synaptosomal Ca uptake.
Ebstein & Daly, 1982[24]	No effect of DHP on K^+-stimulated catecholamine release from synaptosomes.
Daniell *et al.*, 1983[25]	No effect of DHP on K^+-stimulated Ca uptake in synaptosomes.
Crebba & Karobath, 1986[26]	No effect of DHP on K^+-stimulated transients in internal Ca concentration in synaptosomes.
Suszkiw *et al.*, 1986[13]	No effect of DHP on K^+-stimulated Ca uptake in synaptosomes using quenched-flow rapid mixing techniques.
Reynolds *et al.*, 1986[20]	No effect of DHP antagonists or agonists on Ca uptake or release of serotonin or norepiniephrine. wCgTx blocks 50% of K^+-stimulated Ca uptake, 30–40% of serotonin and norepinephrine release.

mediate neurosecretion, and that the L-type channel is not directly involved. However, as pointed out in TABLE 1, there are reports in the literature supporting the notion of DHP-sensitive Ca flux in nerve terminals. Is it possible that blockade of L-type channels in the CNS depends on conditions that are different from those required in smooth muscle, and that the reports where DHP effects are observed reflect the necessary conditions? One line of evidence supporting this possibility is the "use dependence" of DHP block of Ca currents observed in cardiac muscle,[27-29] pituitary cells,[30] and sensory neurons.[18] These experiments indicate that DHP block is both time and voltage dependent, and that long periods of depolarization are necessary to achieve maximal block of Ca currents. Because the assay for Ca uptake in most synaptosomal work involves a single KCl depolarization, such use dependence would not ordinarily develop. In this regard, Middelmiss and Spedding examined the DHP sensitivity of the release process by measuring K^+-evoked overflow of ^{3}H-5-hydroxytryptamine (5HT) from cortical slices in a two-stimuli protocol by comparing release in the second pulse to that in the first pulse.[15] Under these conditions, submicromolar concentrations of the DHP agonist Bay K8644, added after the first pulse, augment K^+-stimulated 5HT overflow in the second pulse; the augmented release was blocked by micromolar concentrations of nifedipine. Our own recent results (unpublished) using a rapid superfusion system to measure ^{3}H-gamma-aminobutyric acid (GABA) release indicate that DHP sensitivity becomes significant only after three pulses of KCl stimulation. Under these conditions, GABA release is blocked 50% by 1 μM nimodipine, and is blocked >90% by 0.3 μM wCgTx; these agents had no significant effect on GABA release in the first pulse.

In conclusion, a number of investigators have found evidence for both dihydropyridine-sensitive and -insensitive pathways mediating synaptosomal calcium uptake and neurosecretion. DHP blockade of Ca channels in the nerve terminal may depend on specific conditions, such as repetitive depolarization, not employed in many synaptosomal studies. Thus the lack of DHP sensitivity *in vitro* does not necessarily exclude a significant role for L-type calcium channels in mediating neurosecretion. Indirect evidence, such as the correlation between DHP binding site density and the magnitude of the rapid phase of synaptosomal K^+-stimulated Ca uptake in various brain regions,[31] supports continued examination of this issue.

REFERENCES

1. NOWYCKY, M. C., A. P. FOX & R. W. TSIEN. 1985. Nature **316:** 440–443.
2. WHITTAKER, V. P. 1969. *In* Handbook of Neurochemistry. A. Lajtha, Ed. **2:** 327–364. Plenum Press. New York, N.Y.
3. BLAUSTEIN, M. P. & J. M. GOLDRING. 1975. J. Physiol. **247:** 589–615.
4. BLAUSTEIN, M. P. 1975. J. Physiol. **247:** 617–655.
5. BLAUSTEIN, M. P. & C. J. OBORN. 1975. J. Physiol. **247:** 657–686.
6. NACHSHEN, D. A. & M. P. BLAUSTEIN. 1979. Mol. Pharmacol. **16:** 579–586.
7. GOULD, R. J., K. M. M. MURPHY & S. H. SNYDER. 1984. Mol. Pharmacol. **25:** 235–241.
8. GOULD, R. J., K. M. M. MURPHY & S. H. SNYDER. 1982. Eur. J. Pharmacol. **81:** 517–519.
9. GILL, D. L., E. F. GROLLMAN & L. D. KOHN. 1981. J. Biol. Chem. **256:** 184–192.
10. REEVES, J. P. & C. C. HALE. 1984. J. Biol. Chem. **259:** 7733–7739.
11. TURNER, T. J. & S. M. GOLDIN. 1985. J. Neurosci. **5:** 841–849.
12. NACHSHEN, D. A. & M. P. BLAUSTEIN. 1980. J. Gen. Physiol. **79:** 1065–1087.
13. SUSZKIW, J. B., M. E. O'LEARY, M. M. MURAWSKY & T. WANG. 1986. J. Neurosci. **6:** 1349–1357.
14. RAMPE, D., J. FERRANTE & D. TRIGGLE. 1986. Dev. Brain Res. **29:** 189–192.

15. MIDDLEMISS, D. N. & M. SPEDDING. 1987. Nature **314:** 94–96.
16. WOODWARD, J. J. & S. W. LESLIE. 1986. Brain Res. **370:** 397–400.
17. NORDSTROM, O., S. BRAESCH & T. BARTFAI. 1986. Acta Physiol. Scand. **126:** 115–121.
18. RANE, S. G., G. G. HOLZ & K. DUNLAP. 1987. Pflugers Arch **409:** 361–366.
19. THAYER, S. A., S. N. MURPHY & R. J. MILLER. 1986. Mol. Pharmacol. **30:** 505–509.
20. REYNOLDS, I. J., J. A. WAGNER, S. H. SNYDER, S. A. THAYER, B. M. OLIVERA & R. J. MILLER. 1986. Proc. Nat. Acad. Sci. USA **83:** 8804–8807.
21. MCCLESKEY, E. W., A. P. FOX, D. H. FELDMAN, L. J. CRUZ, B. M. OLIVERA, R. W. TSIEN & D. YOSHIKAMI. 1986. Proc. Nat. Acad. Sci. USA **84:** 4327–4331.
22. BROWN, D. A., A. CONSTANTI, R. J. DOCHERTY, M. GALVAN, B. GAHWILER, & J. V. HALLIWELL. 1984. IUPHAR: 343–348.
23. WHITE, E. J. & H. F. BRADFORD. 1986. Biochem. Pharmacol. **35:** 2193–2197.
24. EBSTEIN, R. P. & J. W. DALY. 1982. Cell. Mol. Neurobiol. **2:** 205–213.
25. DANIELL, L. C., E. M. BARR & S. W. LESLIE. 1983. J. Neurochem. **41:** 1455–1459.
26. CREBA, J. A. & M. KAROBATH. 1986. Biochem. Biophys. Res. Commun. **134:** 1038–1047.
27. BEAN, B. P. 1984. Proc. Nat. Acad. Sci. USA **81:** 6388–6392.
28. SANGUINETTI, M. C. & R. S. KASS. 1984. Circ. Res. **55:** 336–348.
29. SANGUINETTI, M. C., D. S. KRAFTE & R. S. KASS. 1986. J. Gen. Physiol. **88:** 369–392.
30. COHEN, C. J. & R. T. MCCARTHY. 1987. J. Physiol. **387:** 195–225.
31. SKATTEBOL, A. & D. J. TRIGGLE. J. Neurochem. (In press.)

Calcium Entry and Activation of Endocrine Cells

WILLY J. MALAISSE

Laboratory of Experimental Medicine
Brussels Free University
115 Boulevard de Waterloo
B-1000 Brussels, Belgium

INTRODUCTION

The facilitated influx of Ca^{2+} into endocrine cells may represent a major, albeit not the sole, determinant of the secretory response of these cells to suitable secretagogues. Both calcium agonists and antagonists have been widely used to document the role of calcium entry in the stimulation of hormonal release. In the present account, the process of glucose-stimulated insulin release will serve as the leading model to illustrate the influence of these pharmacological agents upon Ca^{2+} fluxes and hormone secretion.

In dealing with the effect of calcium agonists and antagonists upon pancreatic B-cell function, two apparently distinct concepts will be emphasized. The classical concept that stimulation of insulin release often results, in part at least, from the opening of calcium channels will be first briefly discussed. Thereafter, however, attention will be drawn to the fact that calcium antagonists may also affect biochemical and biophysical variables in pancreatic islet cells by mechanisms distinct from the blockade of calcium channels. This, in turn, will lead to the provocative proposal that the entry of calcium into islet cells might be mediated, to a limited extent, by native ionophores.

FACILITATION OF INSULIN RELEASE BY ORGANIC CALCIUM AGONISTS

The view that an increase in the cytosolic activity of Ca^{2+} may act as a trigger for insulin release was first postulated in the light of the findings that insulin release induced by D-glucose and other secretagogues is abolished in the absence of extracellular Ca^{2+},[1-3] and that a rise in extracellular Ca^{2+} concentration may provoke insulin release even in the absence of glucose.[4,5] It was later established that D-glucose indeed increases cytosolic Ca^{2+} activity in normal islet cells.[6] None of these observations, however, informs on the modality of Ca^{2+} entry into the islet cells.

In the first two studies dealing with the effects of organic calcium agonists upon insulin release from isolated islets,[7,8] it was shown that both BAY K 8644 [methyl 1,4-dihydro-2,6-dimethyl-3-nitro-4-(2-trifluoromethylphenyl)-pyridine-5-carboxylate] and CGP 28392 (4-[2-(difluoromethoxyphenyl]-1,4,5,7-tetrahydro-2-methyl-5-oxo-furo[3,4-b]pyridine-3-carboxylic acid ethylester) were unable to cause a sustained enhancement of basal insulin release as measured in islets incubated either in the absence of exogenous nutrient or at a low concentration of D-glucose (2.8 mM). Both agents, however, caused an increase in insulin output at higher concentrations of D-glucose (5.6 mM or more). In relative terms, such an increase was most marked at intermediate glucose concentrations in the 5.6 to 11.1 mM range. Actually, CGP 28392 failed to affect significantly insulin release at a higher glucose level (16.7 mM). These findings are consistent with the knowledge that the prevailing effect of these calcium agonists is to prolong the mean open time of calcium channels.

The secretory response to these pharmacological agents was dose related, in the 0.2 to 22.0 μM range in the case of BAY K 8644 and the 1.0 to 50.0 μM range in the case of CGP 28932. Incidentally, both agents, when used at higher concentrations (approximately 0.1 mM for BAY K 8644 and 0.5 mM for CGP 28392), inhibited glucose-stimulated insulin release and ^{45}calcium net uptake, suggesting that these drugs may also display a property similar to that of organic calcium antagonists.

The stimulation, or at least enhancement, of insulin release by either BAY K 8644 or CGP 28392 coincided with an increased net uptake of ^{45}Ca by the islets and, in a perifusion system, with an increase in ^{45}Ca efflux from the perifused islets. The latter increase did not occur when the islets were perifused in the absence of extracellular Ca^{2+}, suggesting that it corresponded to a process of exchange between influent ^{40}Ca and effluent ^{45}Ca. Incidentally, the perifusion model also documented that the secretory response to the calcium agonists represents a virtually immediate phenomenon.

The two organic calcium agonists protected insulin release against the inhibitory action of organic calcium antagonists (e.g., nifedipine or verapamil). This suggests that there exists, in the B cell, a regulatory site located at or near the calcium channel and that occupation of this site by specific dihydropyridines may either gate or block the transmembrane flux of Ca^{2+} into the cell.

Further studies have confirmed, and extended, these original observations,[9–11] suggesting the view that the entry of Ca^{2+} into islet cells by gated calcium channels represents an efficient modality for stimulation of insulin release.

In considering the latter conclusion, two remarks need to be underlined. First, it should be realized that the use of organic calcium agonists (and antagonists) does not represent the sole approach to the study of calcium channels in islet cells. As a matter of fact, the participation of calcium channels in the entry of the cation into islet cells is supported by an array of other observations, especially those dealing with the bioelectrical activity of intact B cells and the characterization of ionic channels by the patch clamp technique.

Second, it should be kept in mind that the facilitated entry of Ca^{2+} into the cell does not represent the sole modality for stimulation or potentiation of insulin release. In this respect, several other modalities could be mentioned. Thus, an increase in cytosolic Ca^{2+} activity may result, in addition to the facilitated entry of Ca^{2+} into the cell, from an intracellular redistribution of Ca^{2+} between organelle-bound and cytosolic pools.[12–14] Moreover, according to a current view, some second messengers, e.g., cyclic AMP, may exert little effect upon cytosolic Ca^{2+} activity and, instead, enhance insulin release by sensitizing and/or increasing the response to Ca^{2+} of the effector system for insulin release.[15] Last, it is conceivable that certain secretagogues, such as the tumor-promoting phorbol ester 12-*O*-tetradecanoyl-phorbol-13-acetate, provoke insulin release without initiating electrical activity in the B cell but by causing activation of protein kinase C.[16–18]

INHIBITION OF INSULIN RELEASE BY ORGANIC CALCIUM ANTAGONISTS

Organic calcium antagonists, such as verapamil, gallopamil, and nifedipine, are potent inhibitors of insulin release.[19–21] The relative extent of inhibition in insulin release depends on such variables as the type and concentration of the secretagogue(s) used to stimulate the islet cells, the concentration of the calcium antagonist, the respective order of administration of the secretagogue and antagonist, and the extracellular concentration of Ca^{2+}. In this respect, only a few examples will be briefly considered here.

The relative magnitude of the inhibitory effect of verapamil upon glucose-stimulated insulin release is enhanced at subnormal calcium concentration and decreased when the Ca^{2+} concentration is raised.[22,23] More precisely, an increase in Ca^{2+} concentration (e.g., from 1.0 to 2.0 mM) shifts to the right the regression line relating the relative extent of inhibition in insulin output to the concentration of verapamil (ranged on a logarithmic scale).

Theophylline, which enhances glucose-stimulated insulin release, protects, in part at least, the B cell against the inhibitory action of verapamil. This could reflect the fact that theophylline, possibly as a result of its capacity to increase the islet content in cyclic AMP, compensates for the verapamil-induced reduction in Ca^{2+} inward flux into the B cell.[22,23]

The presence of extracellular Ca^{2+} is not a prerequisite for disclosing an inhibitory action of verapamil upon insulin release. For instance, in the isolated perfused rat pancreas, verapamil (8 μM) markedly inhibits insulin release evoked, in the nominal

TABLE 1. Effect of Organic Calcium Antagonists upon ^{45}Ca Net Uptake by Pancreatic Islets

D-Glucose	Nil	16.7 mM
Verapamil (10.0 μM)	47.2 ± 4.9 (43)[a]	71.5 ± 3.1 (66)
Gallopamil (4.0 μM)	44.5 ± 5.6 (10)	66.7 ± 4.2 (10)
Suloctidil (5.0 μM)	58.3 ± 7.5 (16)	81.5 ± 3.9 (15)
Nifedipine (1.0 μM)	41.7 ± 6.7 (23)	74.4 ± 3.2 (13)

[a]Mean values for ^{45}Ca net uptake over 90 minutes incubation are expressed in percent of the mean control value found within the same experiment at the same concentration of D-glucose, and are shown together with the standard error of the mean and number of individual observations (in parentheses).

absence of Ca^{2+} and even in the presence of EGTA (1.0 mM), by the administration of Ba^{2+}. Verapamil also causes a dramatic inhibition of $^{133}Ba^{2+}$ net uptake by isolated islets.[24]

As a rule, organic calcium antagonists fail to exert any obvious effect upon glucose utilization and oxidation by isolated islets and fail to interfere with glucose-dependent functional events other than insulin release. For instance, verapamil fails to affect the stimulant action of D-glucose upon proinsulin biosynthesis.[25]

The inhibition of insulin release by organic calcium antagonists coincides with a decrease in glucose-stimulated ^{45}Ca net uptake.[20,21,25] Verapamil fails to suppress the early inhibition by D-glucose of ^{45}Ca outflow from prelabeled islets perifused in the presence of extracellular Ca^{2+}. This inhibitory effect of D-glucose upon ^{45}Ca outflow is better seen and quite sustained when the islets are perifused in the absence of extracellular Ca^{2+}; in this case also, verapamil or gallopamil fails to affect the inhibitory action of the hexose. Verapamil, however, causes a dose-related decrease of the glucose-induced secondary rise in effluent radioactivity, the latter rise reflecting the stimulant action of the hexose upon Ca^{2+} entry into the islet cells.[20,25]

A detailed analysis of the dose-action relationship for the inhibitory effect of verapamil upon both ^{45}Ca efflux and insulin release from islets stimulated by either a rise in the extracellular concentration of D-glucose or the administration of other secretagogues (e.g., hypoglycemic sulfonylureas or arginine) led us to postulate the existence of distinct modalities of Ca^{2+} influx into the pancreatic B cell.[26–28] For instance, it was proposed that the B cell may be equipped with two populations of calcium channels that differ in their sensitivity towards verapamil and possibly their voltage dependency.[26–28]

These considerations do not exhaust all that could be mentioned about the effects of organic calcium antagonists on islet cell function, but are hopefully sufficient to indicate that the use of the latter agents indeed allowed documentation of the significance of calcium channels in islet physiology. In this respect, it should be mentioned that organic calcium antagonists were also used in the study of hormonal secretion, e.g., glucagon release,[29,30] by non-B islet cells.

UNTOWARD EFFECTS OF ORGANIC CALCIUM ANTAGONISTS

Although the bulk of evidence supports the view that the inhibition of insulin release by calcium antagonists indeed results from the blockade of calcium channels, some effects of these drugs upon islet cells seem to be unrelated to the latter blockade. Three examples of such "untoward" effects will be mentioned here.

In the first instance, we observed that verapamil (0.1 mM) decreases the output of lactic acid from islets incubated in the presence of 16.7 mM D-glucose, whereas the utilization of D-[5-^{3}H]glucose and the oxidation of D-[U-^{14}C]glucose were both unaffected. We then became aware that verapamil failed to affect the total production of lactic acid, but caused its retention within the islet cells.[25]

In the second instance, it was found that verapamil (1 to 20 μM), like the cobalt ion (2.5 mM), provokes a rapid, sustained, and dose-related decrease in ^{86}Rb efflux from prelabeled islets perifused in the absence of D-glucose.[31] At variance with the inhibitory action of verapamil upon insulin release, the decrease in ^{86}Rb outflow not only persisted in the absence of extracellular Ca^{2+} and presence of EGTA but was also not abolished by an increase in extracellular Ca^{2+} concentration from 1.0 to 5.0 mM.[31] Hence, it was proposed that the calcium antagonist reduces K^+ conductance by a direct effect on K^+ channels, rather than by decreasing the intracellular Ca^{2+} concentration.

Last, and most importantly, it was consistently seen that organic calcium antagonists severely inhibit ^{45}Ca net uptake, as measured after extensive washing of the islets in order to remove contaminating extracellular $^{45}Ca^{2+}$, by islets incubated in the absence of exogenous nutrient.[20,21,25,32,33] As a matter of fact, the relative extent of the inhibitory action of organic calcium antagonists upon ^{45}Ca net uptake is more marked in glucose-deprived islets than in glucose-stimulated islets (TABLE 1). Verapamil also causes a dose-related decrease in basal ^{45}Ca fractional outflow rate from prelabeled islets perifused in the absence of glucose.[26] Since no electrical activity is recorded in glucose-deprived pancreatic B cells, it is tempting to conclude that organic calcium antagonists interfere with a bioelectrically silent modality of Ca^{2+} entry into the islet cells. It should be kept in mind, however, that the pancreatic islets contain not solely insulin-producing cells, but also non-B endocrine cells.

INHIBITION BY CALCIUM ANTAGONISTS OF IONOPHORE-MEDIATED CALCIUM TRANSLOCATION

The findings just outlined led us to investigate whether calcium antagonists are able to interfere with the process of ionophore-mediated Ca transport. The following observations indicate that such is indeed the case.

It was first observed that verapamil (8 to 81 μM) causes a dose-related inhibition of insulin release evoked by the ionophore A23187 in the isolated perfused rat pancreas.[34]

We then indicated that verapamil also inhibits the process of Ca translocation from an aqueous into an organic immiscible phase as mediated by the ionophore A23187.[35,36] Incidentally, the cobalt ion exerts a comparable inhibitory effect.[37] Organic calcium antagonists also inhibit ionophore-mediated translocation in the Pressman cell.[38,39]

In the two-phase bulk system, several factors modulate the relative magnitude of the inhibitory action of calcium antagonists upon ionophore-mediated Ca translocation. First, at a given concentration of a given ionophore, the extent of inhibition is variable with distinct antagonists. When the latter are structurally related, a significant rank correlation can be found between the ED_{50} for inhibition of Ca translocation and a Ca-dependent physiological process (e.g., guinea pig ileum contraction), respectively.[36,40] However, such is not the case for distinct antagonists of vastly different chemical structure, suggesting that the biological efficiency may be modulated by additional factors not operative in the artificial system.[40] Second, the relative magnitude of inhibition is tightly dependent on the antagonist/ionophore concentration ratio in the organic phase.[35,40] Third, the relative extent of inhibition in Ca translocation is tightly dependent on the concentration of Ca^{2+} in the aqueous phase.[36,40] In this respect, the situation in the artificial system resembles that found with living cells, in which case an increase in extracellular Ca^{2+} concentration protects the B-cell against the inhibitory action of organic calcium antagonists.[20,22] Last, at a fixed concentration of A23187 and gallopamil, the inhibition of Ca translocation is tightly dependent on the pH of the aqueous phase, being most marked at neutral pH and virtually abolished at pH values of 7.9–8.2.[41] Incidentally, conformational analysis of the protonated, but not neutral, form of gallopamil indicated the existence of different conformations with great mobility of the torsional angles and the ionized site of the molecule. Several of these conformers were characterized by an easily accessible cationic site and, hence, could be considered as most suitable for interaction with the calcium-binding site of ionophore systems.[41]

Verapamil, gallopamil, and suloctidil also inhibit the calcium exchange-diffusion process mediated by the ionophore bromolasalocid in liposomes of variable fluidity.[42] This inhibitory effect is dose related in the 0.1–0.5 mM range. Taken as a whole, these observations lend support to the view that the inhibitory action of calcium antagonists upon calcium-dependent functional processes may be attributable to a primary interference with the process of Ca transport across cell membranes, as mediated by either native ionophores or calcium channels.[26,43] In distinguishing between the latter two modalities of calcium transport, it should be kept in mind that ionophores may themselves be arranged to form ionic channels.[44]

IONOPHORE-MEDIATED CALCIUM TRANSPORT

The view that native ionophores might participate in the transport of calcium across living membranes may help, at least as a model, to understand a number of specific features encountered in the study of ionic fluxes in intact cells, as illustrated by the following considerations.

The efficiency of calcium transport by ionophores in the Pressman cell is affected by the Ca^{2+} concentration of each aqueous phase.[38] The translocation of a trace amount of $^{45}Ca^{2+}$ added to one chamber is increased when the concentration of $^{40}Ca^{2+}$ is increased in the other chamber. Such a situation may thus serve as a model for processes of calcium-calcium exchange or even calcium-stimulated calcium release, e.g., from intracellular organelles.[38,45]

If the ionophore under study is able to transport both monovalent and divalent cations, as is the case with the ionophore Br-X537A, a process of Na-Ca countertransport can be simulated in the Pressman cell.[46,47] It is conceivable, therefore, that such a countertransport process is indeed mediated by native ionophores. Incidentally, monovalent ions may also directly affect the handling of calcium by ionophoretic systems that specifically transport divalent cations.[48]

Distinct ionophores, when placed together in an organic phase, may cause a greater translocation of calcium than expected from a mere summation of the individual effects of each ionophore. Such a synergism was first documented in the case of the ionophores A23187 and Br-X537A.[49,50] The simultaneous presence of the two ionophores not only resulted in a synergistic increase in calcium translocation, but also dramatically altered the influence of environmental factors (e.g., Na^+ concentration) upon the ionophoretic response. The nuclear magnetic resonance spectrum obtained when the complexation of Ca^{2+} occurred in the presence of both ionophores differed strikingly from the individual spectra obtained with the A23187-Ca and Br-X537A-Ca complexes, indicating that the two ionophores are able to form hybrid complexes with Ca^{2+}.[50] A comparable situation was documented in the case of the interaction between A23187 and the hypoglycemic sulfonylurea gliclazide.[51] Hypoglycemic sulfonylureas also act synergistically with phospholipids such as phosphatidic acid and phosphatidylserine in causing calcium translocation in a two-phase bulk system.[52] The conformation analysis of a hybrid Ca^{2+} complex with both gliquidone and phosphatidylserine revealed configurations suitable for Ca^{2+} transport across a hydrophobic domain. These findings suggest that exogenous agents and/or native ionophores may act synergistically in mediating calcium transport across biological membranes. Thus, the formation of both homologous and hybrid calcium complexes[49,50] may condition the efficiency of the ionophoretic process. Moreover, in the case of certain agents, e.g., hypoglycemic sulfonylureas, the existence of Ca^{2+} complexes with distinct stoichiometries may, together with other factors such as the relative ability of the drug to be inserted into the phospholipid domain,[53] condition the efficiency of the biological response.[54]

The ionophoretic capacity of X537A is affected when the ionophore is converted to its dihydroderivative.[55] Oxidized glutathione (GSSG), but not reduced glutathione (GSH), inhibits the process of calcium translocation into an organic immiscible phase as mediated by either X537A or ionophoretic material extracted from pancreatic islets.[56] These findings raise the possibility that a change in cytosolic redox state, as observed in glucose-stimulated islet cells,[57,58] may alter the participation of native ionophores in the transport of cations across the B cell plasma membrane.[43,55]

In liposomes, the efficiency of ionophore-mediated calcium exchange diffusion is dramatically affected by a change in the viscosity of the liposomal matrix, as achieved by a change in either the lipid composition of the liposomes[59,60] or temperature.[61] Under these conditions, a comparison between either the results obtained with ionophores binding Ca in a 1/1 and 2/1 stoichiometry[59,60,62] or the rates of ^{45}Ca and ^{22}Na exchange diffusion[61] indicated that the membrane viscosity influences both the lateral and transverse mobility of the ionophores. Hence, environmental factors that affect the fluidity of cell membranes could exert a modulatory role upon the efficiency of ion transport as mediated by native ionophores. For instance, this could be the case in islets stimulated by D-glucose. The hexose indeed causes a rapid and dose-related decrease in the membrane viscosity of pancreatic endocrine cells.[63] At a glucose concentration of 16.7 mM, the estimated viscosity was 15 ± 3% lower than basal value (2.01 ± 0.12 P).

Exogenous agents, devoid of significant ionophoretic activity, are capable of modulating the efficiency of ionophore-mediated exchange diffusion in liposomes. For instance, both tumor-promoting and biologically inactive phorbol esters may affect the process of A23187-mediated calcium exchange diffusion in multilamellar liposomes formed of different types of lipids and incubated at variable temperatures.[64,65] Under suitable experimental conditions, the effect of phorbol esters upon calcium ionophoresis is observed despite unchanged viscosity of the liposomes and parallels their biological potency as either tumor promoter or insulin secretagogue.[64,65] The latter situation is probably accounted for by side-to-side interaction, e.g., between phorbol esters and phospholipids.[66,67] Since biologically active phorbol esters display a suitable conformation for insertion in phospholipid monolayers,[68,69] and indeed bind to artificial membranes,[70] these findings suggest that a change in ionophoresis may participate in the insulin secretory response to biologically active phorbol esters,[71,72] together with the activation of protein kinase C.[17]

Taken as a whole, all these observations, which are not exhaustive, duly illustrate, in my opinion, that the process of ionophore-mediated calcium transport, if it were to occur in living cells at the intervention of native ionophores in a manner comparable to that characterized in artificial membranes, could conceivably be modulated by a number of environmental factors and hence, in a teleological perspective, displays a sufficient versatility to participate in the physiological regulation of ionic fluxes.

NATIVE IONOPHORES IN PANCREATIC ISLETS

The experimental data so far reviewed in this account point to the possible participation of distinct modalities in the transfer of Ca^{2+} across living membranes. Needless to say, the two different pathways under consideration here, namely, the flux of Ca^{2+} through open channels and its transport by ionophores, do not exclude alternative modalities such as the active pumping of Ca^{2+} by suitable Ca^{2+}-responsive ATPases, which were indeed identified in islet cells.[73–75] Nevertheless, the question comes to mind whether islet cell membranes are indeed equipped with native ionophores. Our contribution to this field is summarized below.

In 1979, we first observed that a chloroform/methanol extract of pancreatic islets stimulates the translocation of ^{45}Ca from an aqueous into an organic immiscible phase. This ionophoretic activity, which was derived mainly from membrane-rich subcellular fractions, displayed several features in common with that of A23187 in the same artificial model. Thus, the phenomenon of calcium translocation caused by either the islet extract or the antibiotic ionophore represents a power function of the concentration of ionophoretic material, is saturable at high calcium concentration, is affected by the concentration of Na^+ and H^+ in the aqueous phase, and is inhibited by suloctidil, the latter inhibitory effect being antagonized by calcium itself.[76]

In further work, we used the islet extract as a model for the process of Na-Ca countertransport and its inhibition in response to the conversion of nutrient secretagogues to their acidic metabolites. The native ionophores extracted from the islets were indeed found able to transport Ca^{2+} from one aqueous medium into another across an organic immiscible phase. In the presence of a K^+, Na^+, Li^+, or H^+ gradient, Ca^{2+} was transported against its own concentration gradient from the medium of low monovalent-cation concentration to the opposite medium. Once again, the transport of Ca^{2+} was abolished by the organic calcium antagonist suloctidil.[39]

With the above information in mind, several questions can be raised. The first obvious question relates to the chemical identity of these native ionophores. With the limited amount of material extracted from the islets, we have so far only been able to show that the phospholipid fraction accounts for 62.0 ± 8.5% of the integrated amount of Ca^{2+} translocated by the different lipids separated from the islet extract by thin-layer chromatography.[77] Since the amount of lipids present in each fraction was not measured, these results do not provide information on the specific ionophoretic activity or affinity for Ca^{2+} of different islet lipids.

Second, it should be underlined that, in the studies so far summarized in this report, the material extracted from the islets was placed in suitable organic solvents and, hence, could move freely in the organic phase. The question remained, therefore, whether the ionophoretic capacity of the islet extract could still be disclosed when the latter is incorporated in artificial bilayer membranes. Three procedures were used to tackle the latter question. As a first approach, vesicles were prepared, by sonication, from the islet material and incubated at 37°C in a Tris-HCl buffer containing NaCl (120 mM) and $^{45}CaCl_2$ (0.07 mM). The initial rate of ^{45}Ca uptake averaged 7.0 ± 1.1 fmol/minute per islet equivalent, and happened to coincide with the value found in intact cells incubated, in the absence of D-glucose, at the same low Ca^{2+} concentration.[78] In the second procedure, the islet extract was inserted in liposomes formed from dipalmitoylphosphatidylcholine and cholesterol and found to increase the rate of ^{45}Ca outflow from liposomes prelabeled with ^{45}Ca.[78] In this respect, the islet extract acted synergistically with the ionophore A23187. Last, the islet material also augmented the Ca^{2+} conductance of a glycerol monoleate bilayer.[78] These findings support the view that the material extracted from the islets may participate in the transport of Ca^{2+} across the phospholipid domain of living membranes in their intact bilayer organization.

None of these findings unambiguously proves the participation of native ionophores in the transport of ions in intact islet cells. If such a participation were to be established, it should be considered whether a change in either the amount or intrinsic properties of native ionophores is involved in the delayed regulation of insulin release by ontogenic, nutritional, and/or endocrine factors.[79] For instance, we recently observed that the ionophoretic activity of islet extracts is higher in lactating than nonlactating rats, at least when expressed relative to the number of extracted islets.[80] Hence, it is conceivable that such a change accounts, together with other factors (e.g., a depletion of endogenous calcium islet content), for the functional differences found in isolated islets removed from lactating and nonlactating rats, respectively.[80,81]

CONCLUSION

The introduction of both calcium agonists and antagonists has helped to foster the concept that Ca^{2+} entry into endocrine cells through gated channels represents an essential, albeit not the sole, determinant of the increase in cytosolic Ca^{2+} activity and subsequent stimulation of hormonal release evoked by suitable secretagogues in endocrine cells. However, the influence of calcium antagonists upon ionic fluxes in intact cells has also led to the suggestion that passive cationic fluxes are not mediated solely through channels, but also conceivably by native ionophores. I realize that more work is required to assess the true contribution of distinct modalities to the overall and bidirectional fluxes of Ca^{2+} across cell membranes both in resting and stimulated cells. Likewise, further investigation should aim at the identification of native molecules with high specific ionophoretic activity. In these and other respects, some of the concepts defended in this review may well appear unwise or at least premature. But would it not be equally unwise to ignore the participation of ionophoretic processes in membrane physiology?

REFERENCES

1. Grodsky, G. M. & L. L. Bennett. 1966. Cation requirements for insulin secretion in the isolated perfused pancreas. Diabetes **15:** 910–913.
2. Milner, R. D. G. & C. N. Hales. 1967. The role of calcium and magnesium in insulin secretion from rabbit pancreas stimulated *in vitro*. Diabetologia **3:** 47–49.
3. Malaisse, W. J., G. Brisson & F. Malaisse-Lagae. 1970. The stimulus-secretion coupling of glucose-induced insulin release. I. Interaction of epinephrine and alkaline earth cations. J. Lab. Clin. Med. **76:** 895–902.
4. Devis, G., G. Somers & W. J. Malaisse. 1975. Stimulation of insulin release by calcium. Biochem. Biophys. Res. Commun. **67:** 525–529.
5. Devis, G., G. Somers & W. J. Malaisse. 1977. Dynamics of calcium-induced insulin release. Diabetologia **13:** 531–536.
6. Deleers, M., M. Mahy & W. J. Malaisse. 1985. Glucose increases cytosolic Ca^{2+} activity in pancreatic islet cells. Biochem. Int. **10:** 97–103.
7. Malaisse-Lagae, F., P. C. F. Mathias & W. J. Malaisse. 1984. Gating and blocking of calcium channels by dihydropyridines in the pancreatic B-cell. Biochem. Biophys. Res. Commun. **123:** 1062–1068.
8. Malaisse, W. J. & P. C. F. Mathias. 1985. Stimulation of insulin release by an organic calcium agonist. Diabetologia **28:** 153–156.
9. Malaisse, W. J., A. Sener & F. Malaisse-Lagae. 1985. Combined effects of a calcium-agonist and hypoglycemic or hyperglycemic sulfonamides upon insulin release. Res. Commun. Chem. Pathol. Pharmacol. **49:** 71–83.
10. Lebrun, P. & I. Atwater. 1985. Effects of the calcium channel agonist, BAY K 8644, on electrical activity in mouse pancreatic B-cells. Biophys. J. **48:** 919–930.
11. Henquin, J. C., W. Schmeer, M. Nenquin & H. P. Meissner. 1985. Effects of a calcium channel agonist on the electrical, ionic and secretory events in mouse pancreatic B-cells. Biochem. Biophys. Res. Commun. **131:** 980–986.
12. Brisson, G. R., F. Malaisse-Lagae & W. J. Malaisse. 1972. The stimulus-secretion coupling of glucose-induced insulin release. VII. A proposed site of action for adenosine-3′,5′-cyclic monophosphate. J. Clin. Invest. **51:** 232–241.
13. Brisson, G. R. & W. J. Malaisse. 1973. The stimulus-secretion coupling of glucose-induced insulin release. XI. Effects of theophylline and epinephrine on ^{45}Ca efflux from perifused islets. Metabolism **22:** 455–465.
14. Prentki, M. & C. B. Wollheim. 1984. Cytosolic free Ca^{2+} in insulin secreting cells and its regulation by isolated organelles. Experientia **40:** 1052–1060.
15. Malaisse, W. J. & F. Malaisse-Lagae. 1984. The role of cyclic AMP in insulin release. Experientia **40:** 1068–1075.
16. Malaisse, W. J., A. Sener, A. Herchuelz, A. R. Carpinelli, P. Poloczek, J. Winand & M. Castagna. 1980. Insulinotropic effect of the tumor promoter 12-*O*-tetradecanoyl-phorbol-13-acetate in rat pancreatic islets. Cancer Res. **40:** 3827–3831.
17. Hubinont, C., L. Best, A. Sener & W. J. Malaisse. 1984. Activation of protein kinase C by a tumor-promoting phorbol ester in pancreatic islets. FEBS Lett. **170:** 247–253.
18. Henquin, J. C., M. Nenquin, M. Bozem & W. Schmeer. 1986. Cyclic AMP and a phorbol ester amplify tolbutamide-induced insulin release by distinct mechanisms. Diabetologia **29:** 548A.
19. Devis, G., G. Somers, E. van Obberghen & W. J. Malaisse. 1975. Calcium antagonists and islet function. I. Inhibition of insulin release by verapamil. Diabetes **24:** 547–551.
20. Malaisse, W. J., G. Devis, D. G. Pipeleers & G. Somers. 1976. Calcium-antagonists and islet function. IV. Effect of D600. Diabetologia **12:** 77–81.
21. Malaisse, W. J. & A. C. Boschero. 1977. Calcium-antagonists and islet function. XI. Effect of nifedipine. Hormone Res. **8:** 203–209.
22. Somers, G., G. Devis, E. van Obberghen & W. J. Malaisse. 1976. Calcium-antagonists and islet function. II. Interaction of theophylline and verapamil. Endocrinology **99:** 114–124.
23. Malaisse, W. J., A. Herchuelz, J. Levy, G. Somers, G. Devis, M. Ravazzola, F. Malaisse-Lagae & L. Orci. 1975. Insulin release and the movements of calcium in

pancreatic islets. *In* Calcium Transport in Contraction and Secretion. E. Carafoli, F. Clementi, W. Drabikowski & A. Margreth, Eds.: 211–226. North-Holland Publishing Company. Amsterdam, Holland.

24. Somers, G., G. Devis, E. van Obberghen & W. J. Malaisse. 1976. Calcium-antagonists and islet function. VI. Effect of barium. Eur. J. Physiol. **365:** 21–28.
25. Malaisse, W. J., A. Herchuelz, J. Levy & A. Sener. 1977. Calcium-antagonists and islet function. III. The possible site of action of verapamil. Biochem. Pharmacol. **26:** 735–740.
26. Lebrun, P., W. J. Malaisse & A. Herchuelz. 1982. Evidence for two distinct modalities of Ca^{2+} influx into the pancreatic B-cell. Am. J. Physiol. **242:** E59–E66.
27. Lebrun, P., W. J. Malaisse & A. Herchuelz. 1982. Modalities of gliclazide-induced Ca^{2+} influx into the pancreatic B-cell. Diabetes **31:** 1010–1015.
28. Herchuelz, A., P. Lebrun, A. C. Boschero & W. J. Malaisse. 1984. The mechanism of arginine-stimulated Ca^{2+} influx into the pancreatic B-cell. Am. J. Physiol. **246:** E38–E43.
29. Leclercq-Meyer, V., J. Marchand & W. J. Malaisse. 1978. The role of calcium in glucagon release. Studies with verapamil. Diabetes **27:** 996–1004.
30. Leclercq-Meyer, V., J. Marchand & W. J. Malaisse. 1979. The calcium dependency of glucagon release: its modulation by nutritional factors. Am. J. Physiol. **236:** E98–E104.
31. Lebrun, P., W. J. Malaisse & A. Herchuelz. 1981. Effect of calcium antagonists on potassium conductance in islet cells. Biochem. Pharmacol. **30:** 3291–3294.
32. Malaisse, W. J., A. Sener, G. Devis & G. Somers. 1976. Calcium-antagonists and islet function. V. Effect of R33711. Horm. Metab. Res. **8:** 434–438.
33. Malaisse, W. J. 1977. Calcium-antagonists and islet function. X. Effect of suloctidil. Arch. Int. Pharmacodyn. **228:** 339–344.
34. Somers, G., G. Devis & W. J. Malaisse. 1976. Analogy between native and exogenous ionophores in the pancreatic B-cell. FEBS Lett. **66:** 20–22.
35. Malaisse, W. J., G. Devis & G. Somers. 1977. Inhibition by verapamil of ionophore-mediated calcium translocation. Experientia **33:** 1035–1036.
36. Malaisse, W. J. 1979. Protective effect of calcium against the verapamil-induced inhibition of ionophore-mediated calcium translocation. Experientia **35:** 1578–1579.
37. Couturier, E. & W. J. Malaisse. 1980. Cobalt-induced inhibition of ionophore-mediated calcium translocation. IRCS Med. Sci. **8:** 72.
38. Couturier, E. & W. J. Malaisse. 1980. An ionophoretic model for the study of calcium-calcium exchange. J. Inorg. Biochem. **12:** 57–69.
39. Anjaneyulu, K., R. Anjaneyulu & W. J. Malaisse. 1980. The stimulus-secretion coupling of glucose-induced insulin release. XLIII. Na-Ca countertransport mediated by pancreatic islet native ionophores. J. Inorg. Biochem. **13:** 178–188.
40. Malaisse, W. J., G. Somers, I. Valverde & E. Couturier. 1981. Organic calcium-antagonists and calcium ionophores. Arzneimittelforschung **31**(I): 628–633.
41. Brasseur, R., M. Deleers & W. J. Malaisse. 1983. Conformational analysis of the calcium-antagonist gallopamil. Biochem. Pharmacol. **32:** 437–440.
42. Deleers, M., M. Mahy & W. J. Malaisse. 1982. Inhibition by calcium antagonists of ionophore-mediated calcium transport in liposomes. Eur. J. Pharmacol. **83:** 21–24.
43. Malaisse, W. J., A. Herchuelz, G. Devis, G. Somers, A. C. Boschero, J. C. Hutton, S. Kawazu, A. Sener, I. J. Atwater, G. Duncan, B. Ribalet & E. Rojas. 1978. Regulation of calcium fluxes and their regulatory roles in pancreatic islets. Ann. N.Y. Acad. Sci. **307:** 562–582.
44. Boheim, G., D. Janko, T. Leibfritz, T. Ooka, W. A. König & G. Jung. 1976. Structural and membrane modifying properties of suzukacillin, a peptide antibiotic related to alamethicin. Part B. Pore formation in black lipid films. Biochim. Biophys. Acta **433:** 182–199.
45. Scholler, Y., V. de Maertelaer & W. J. Malaisse. 1985. Mathematical modelling of stimulus-secretion coupling in the pancreatic B-cell. II. Calcium-stimulated calcium release. Comput. Programs Biomed. **19:** 119–126.
46. Malaisse, W. J. & E. Couturier. 1978. An ionophoretic model for Na-Ca counter transport. Nature **275:** 664–665.

47. MALAISSE, W. J., K. ANJANEYULU, R. ANJANEYULU & E. COUTURIER. 1980. Ionophore-mediated Ca^{2+} countertransport: role of Na^+, Li^+ or H^+ gradient. Mol. Cell. Biochem. **30:** 67–70.
48. COUTURIER, E., M. DELEERS & W. J. MALAISSE. 1980. Inhibition by sodium of ionophore-mediated calcium translocation. Cell Calcium **1:** 171–179.
49. COUTURIER, E., M. DELEERS & W. J. MALAISSE. 1980. Synergism between two distinct ionophores in translocating calcium from an aqueous to an organic environment. Pharmacol. Res. Commun. **12:** 651–655.
50. DELEERS, M., M. GELBCKE & W. J. MALAISSE. 1981. Formation of hybrid complexes between Ca and the ionophores bromolasalocid (Br-X537A) and A23187. Proc. Nat. Acad. Sci. USA **78:** 279–282.
51. DELEERS, M., R. BRASSEUR, M. GELBCKE & W. J. MALAISSE. 1982. Homologous and hybrid calcium complexes of A23187 and hypoglycemic sulfonylureas: nuclear magnetic resonance and conformation analysis. J. Inorg. Biochem. **16:** 215–225.
52. DELEERS, M., P. GROGNET, M. MAHY, R. BRASSEUR & W. J. MALAISSE. 1983. Synergistic effect of hypoglycemic sulfonylureas and negative phospholipids on calcium transport: ionic and conformational aspects. Res. Commun. Chem. Pathol. Pharmacol. **41:** 407–424.
53. DELEERS, M. & W. J. MALAISSE. 1984. Binding of hypoglycaemic sulfonylureas to an artificial phospholipid bilayer. Diabetologia **26:** 55–59.
54. DELEERS, M., R. BRASSEUR & W. J. MALAISSE. 1983. Stoichiometry of calcium binding by hypoglycemic sulfonylureas. Res. Commun. Chem. Pathol. Pharmacol. **42:** 181–201.
55. MALAISSE, W. J., A. SENER, A. HERCHUELZ & J. C. HUTTON. 1979. Insulin release: the fuel hypothesis. Metabolism **28:** 373–386.
56. VALVERDE, I. & W. J. MALAISSE. 1980. Effects of reduced and oxidized glutathione upon calcium ionophoresis. IRCS Med. Sci. **8:** 191.
57. MALAISSE, W. J., F. MALAISSE-LAGAE & A. SENER. 1982. The stimulus-secretion coupling of glucose-induced insulin release. LIV. Effect of aminooxyacetate upon nutrient-stimulated insulin secretion. Endocrinology **111:** 392–397.
58. SENER, A., F. MALAISSE-LAGAE, S. P. DUFRANE & W. J. MALAISSE. 1984. The coupling of metabolic to secretory events in pancreatic islets. The cytosolic redox state. Biochem. J. **220:** 433–440.
59. DELEERS, M. & W. J. MALAISSE. 1980. Ionophore-mediated calcium exchange diffusion in liposomes. Biochem. Biophys. Res. Commun. **95:** 650–657.
60. DELEERS, M. & W. J. MALAISSE. 1980. Influence of membrane fluidity upon ionophore-mediated calcium transport in liposomes. Biomed. Res. **1:** 400–404.
61. DELEERS, M. & W. J. MALAISSE. 1982. Influence of membrane viscosity on the lateral and transverse mobility of carboxylic ionophores. Chem. Phys. Lipids **31:** 227–235.
62. DELEERS, M., E. COUTURIER & W. J. MALAISSE. 1981. Ionomycin-mediated calcium transport in rigid and fluid liposomes. Cell Calcium **2:** 159–171.
63. DELEERS, M., J. M. RUYSSCHAERT & W. J. MALAISSE. 1981. Glucose induces membrane changes detected by fluorescence polarization in endocrine pancreatic cells. Biochem. Biophys. Res. Commun. **98:** 255–260.
64. DELEERS, M., M. CASTAGNA & W. J. MALAISSE. 1981. Phorbol esters parallel effects on tumor promotion, insulin release and calcium ionophoresis. Cancer Lett. **14:** 109–114.
65. DELEERS, M. & W. J. MALAISSE. 1982. Influence of phorbol esters on ionophore-mediated calcium exchange-diffusion in liposomes. Chem. Phys. Lipids **31:** 1–11.
66. DELEERS, M., F. DEFRISE-QUERTAIN, J. M. RUYSSCHAERT & W. J. MALAISSE. 1981. Interaction of phorbol esters with lipid bilayers: thermotropic changes in fluorescence polarization, phase transition and calcium ionophoresis. Res. Commun. Chem. Pathol. Pharmacol. **34:** 423–439.
67. DELEERS, M., J. M. RUYSSCHAERT & W. J. MALAISSE. 1982. Interaction between phorbol esters and phospholipid in a monolayer model membrane. Chem. Biol. Interact. **42:** 271–278.
68. DELEERS, M., R. BRASSEUR, J.-M. RUYSSCHAERT & W. J. MALAISSE. 1983. Conformational analysis of phorbol esters at a simulated membrane-water interface. Biophys. Chem. **17:** 313–319.
69. BRASSEUR, R., M. DELEERS, J.-M. RUYSSCHAERT & W. J. MALAISSE. 1983. Conforma-

tional analysis of mixed monolayers of phorbol ester and phospholipid. Biochem. Int. **7:** 71–78.
70. DELEERS, M. & W. J. MALAISSE. 1982. Binding of tumor-promoting and biologically inactive phorbol esters to artificial membranes. Cancer Lett. **17:** 135–140.
71. MALAISSE, W. J., P. LEBRUN, A. HERCHUELZ, A. SENER & F. MALAISSE-LAGAE. 1983. Synergistic effect of a tumor-promoting phorbol ester and a hypoglycemic sulfonylurea upon insulin release. Endocrinology **113:** 1870–1873.
72. MALAISSE, W. J. & M. DELEERS. 1984. Interaction of phorbol esters with lipid monolayers and bilayers. Colloids Surfaces **10:** 257–268.
73. FORMBY, B., K. CAPITO, J. EGEBERG & B. C. J. HEDESKOV. 1976. Ca-activated ATPase activity in subcellular fractions of mouse pancreatic islets. Am. J. Physiol. **230:** 441–448.
74. CAPITO, K., B. FORMBY & C. J. HEDESKOV. 1980. Ca-ATPases in pancreatic islets. Horm. Metab. Res. Suppl. **10:** 50–55.
75. OWEN, A., A. SENER & W. J. MALAISSE. 1983. Stimulus-secretion coupling of glucose-induced insulin release. LI. Divalent cations and ATPase activity in pancreatic islets. Enzyme **29:** 2–14.
76. VALVERDE, I. & W. J. MALAISSE. 1979. Ionophoretic activity in pancreatic islets. Biochem. Biophys. Res. Commun. **89:** 386–395.
77. DIERYCK, P., J. WINAND & W. J. MALAISSE. 1981. Ionophoretic activity of lipids extracted from pancreatic islets. IRCS Med. Sci. **9:** 190.
78. DELEERS, M., M. MAHY & W. J. MALAISSE. 1982. Calcium ionophoresis by pancreatic islet extracts in model membranes. Biochem. Int. **4:** 47–57.
79. MALAISSE, W. J. 1972. Hormonal and environmental modification of islet activity. *In* Handbook of Physiology. D. F. Steiner & N. Freinkel, Eds. **1**(Chapter 14): 237–260. American Physiological Society. Washington, D.C.
80. HUBINONT, C. J. & W. J. MALAISSE. 1987. Lactation-induced changes in calcium handling by rat pancreatic islets. J. Dev. Biol. **9:** 31–39.
81. HUBINONT, C. J., S. P. DUFRANE, P. GARCIA-MORALES, I. VALVERDE, A. SENER & W. J. MALAISSE. 1986. Influence of lactation upon pancreatic islet function. Endocrinology **118:** 687–694.

Is the Felodipine-Resistant Component of the Alpha-Adrenergic Responses in Portal Vein Due to Inhibition of Ca^{2+} Extrusion through the Na^+/Ca^{2+} Exchanger?

B. JOHANSSON, B. LJUNG, AND A. NILSSON

Cardiovascular Research Laboratories
AB Hässle
S-431 83 Mölndal, Sweden

Felodipine in nanomolar concentrations inhibits action potentials in the smooth muscle of the rat portal vein. This leads at about 30 nM to abolition of both spontaneous myogenic activity and phasic contractions induced by norepinephrine or sympathetic nerve stimulation. However, a minor component of the contractile response to strong α-adrenergic stimulation remains even at micromolar levels of felodipine.[1] This component is dependent on extracellular Ca^{2+} as indicated by its rapid elimination in nominally Ca^{2+}-free medium.

Contractile responses independent of action potentials or tonic depolarization can be induced in the portal vein by low extracellular Na^+, and these effects are totally resistant to inhibition by felodipine and other calcium antagonists in micromolar concentrations.[2] It is considered that these contractions to low Na^+, which depend on extracellular Ca^{2+}, are the result of "reversed Na^+/Ca^{2+} exchange," and the findings then indicate that the Na^+/Ca^{2+} exchanger is not affected by Ca^{2+} antagonists.

A possible explanation for the felodipine-resistant component of the adrenergic responses could be that α-adrenoceptor activation under normal ionic conditions inhibits Ca^{2+} extrusion by the Na^+/Ca^{2+} exchanger. In that case norepinephrine would be expected to relax contractions evoked by reversed Na^+/Ca^{2+} exchange in the presence of felodipine. We tested this hypothesis but found that norepinephrine actually caused further and enhanced contraction when applied during a "low Na^+ contracture" (FIGURE 1).

It can be concluded, therefore, that the felodipine-resistant adrenergic response is not due to inhibition of Ca^{2+} efflux through the Na^+/Ca^{2+} exchanger, but probably to stimulated release of intracellular Ca^{2+} or enhanced influx of extracellular Ca^{2+} through pathways not associated with generation of action potentials. The latter mechanism is indicated by the sensitivity of the response to reduction in extracellular Ca^{2+} concentration.

REFERENCES

1. LJUNG, B., M. NORDLANDER & B. JOHANSSON. 1987. Felodipine sensitivity in vivo and in vitro of activation pathways in vascular smooth muscle. J. Cardiovasc. Pharmacol. **10**(Suppl. 1): S89–S95.
2. JOHANSSON, B. & P. HELLSTRAND. 1987. Contractures induced by reversed Na^+/Ca^{2+} exchange in rat portal vein: effects of calcium antagonists. J. Cardiovasc. Pharmacol. **10**(Suppl. 1): S75–S81.

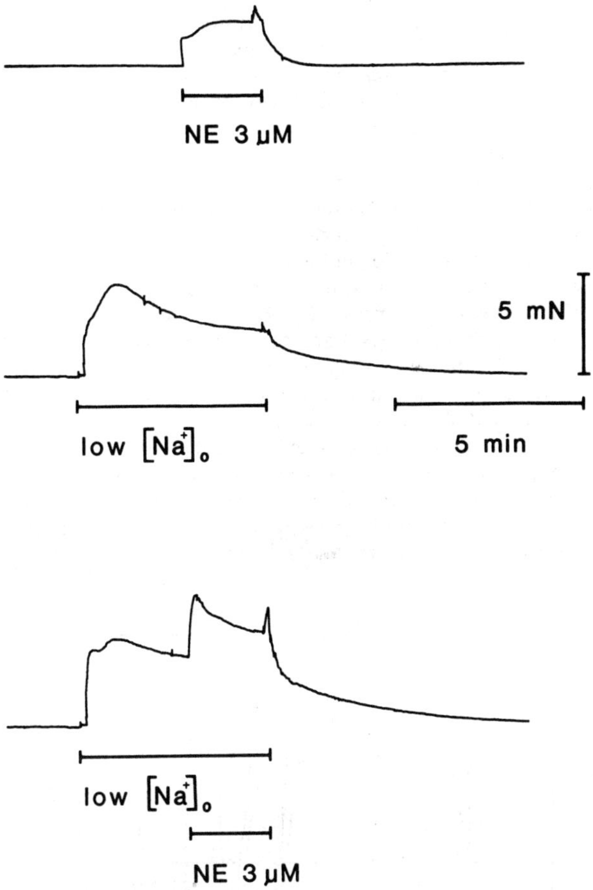

FIGURE 1. Contractile responses of rat portal vein exposed to 1 μM felodipine. Spontaneous activity is abolished by the calcium antagonist, but a small response to 3 μM norepinephrine remains (top tracing). Also contracture evoked by "reversed Na^+/Ca^{2+} exchange" through exposure to low extracellular Na^+ (17 mM) is resistant to felodipine (middle tracing). Norepinephrine causes further increase in contractile force when applied during the low-Na^+ response (bottom tracing).

Nisoldipine Enhances Capillary Recruitment in the Heart

PAUL F. McDONAGH

Department of Physiology
School of Medicine
Texas Tech University Health Sciences Center
Lubbock, Texas 79430

Calcium entry blockers increase myocardial blood flow. However little information exists on the effects of these agents on transport and exchange at the level of the coronary capillary. This study was performed to examine the effects of nisoldipine (Bay k 5552) on capillary perfusion in the heart. In the heart and skeletal muscle, all the blood flow is nutritional, that is, no significant anatomical arteriovenous (A-V) shunts exist. The total blood flow per gram (Q) then equals the product of the number of perfused capillaries per gram (N_p) and the average blood flow per capillary (Q_c). Under physiologic conditions N_p may be less than the total anatomical capillary density (N_t). Duran *et al.* found, in the heart, that N_p/N_t was roughly 0.5.[1] We found, in skeletal muscle, that N_p/N_t was less than 0.5.[2] Thus, a physiologic capillary "reserve" may exist which can be recruited when the need arises. Any intervention then that increases total organ flow (Q) may do so by increasing N_p, Q_c, or both. Increases in N_p will clearly facilitate blood-tissue solute exchange. However, increases in Q_c may either enhance or hinder transcapillary solute exchange depending on the physicochemical nature of the solute.

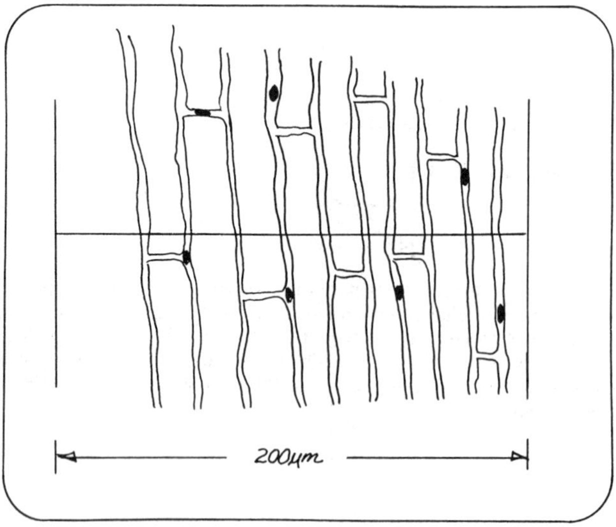

FIGURE 1. Measurement of red-cell-perfused coronary capillarity. On videotape playback, the number of red-cell-perfused capillaries crossing a 200 μm raster line was counted.

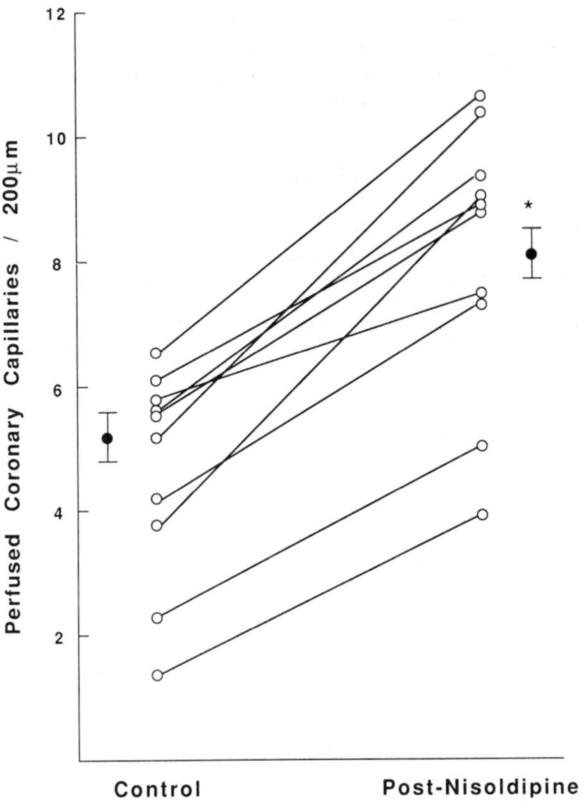

FIGURE 2. Capillarity response to nisoldipine. Perfused coronary capillarity was measured before and after a 0.2 μg injection of nisoldipine.

To directly visualize the coronary microcirculation, adult rat hearts were perfused and isolated as described previously.[3] Coronary capillary fields on the epicardial surface of the left ventricle were illuminated with a fluorescence microscope and videotaped with a low-light-level closed-circuit television system. While viewing and videotaping each coronary capillary field at 520× (specimen to monitor) magnification, a 0.2 μg dose of nisoldipine was injected into the perfusion line. On video playback, we counted the number of red-cell-perfused capillaries crossing a 200 μm raster line, before nisoldipine injection and again during the maximum flow response (FIGURE 1). We also visualized the red cell velocities and the distribution of velocities before and after nisoldipine injection.

FIGURE 2 is a plot of the individual perfused capillary results obtained in this study. In every case, nisoldipine injection caused an increase in total flow and an increase in the number of perfused coronary capillaries. The mean increase in flow was 66%, and the mean increase in perfused capillarity was 76%. From direct observations, it appeared that this agent caused a more homogeneous microvascular perfusion. That is, each field was more evenly perfused both in terms of perfused capillarity and in terms of red cell velocity.

The results indicate that a capillary reserve exists in our isolated heart model. This reserve can be recruited with the calcium blocker nisoldipine. The observed changes in capillarity and red cell velocity after nisoldipine support the hypothesis that vasodilation improves the homogeneity of perfusion in the heart.

REFERENCES

1. DURAN, W. N., T. H. MARSICANO & R. W. ANDERSON. 1977. Capillary reserve in isometrically contracting dog hearts. Am. J. Physiol. **232**(2): H276–H281.
2. MCDONAGH, P. F., R. W. GORE & S. D. GRAY. 1982. Perfused capillary surface area in postural and locomotor skeletal muscle. Microvasc. Res. **24:** 142–157.
3. MCDONAGH, P. F., A. T. NIVEN & D. ROBERTS. 1984. Direct visualization of the coronary microcirculation for pharmacologic and physiologic studies. Microvasc. Res. **28:** 180–196.

Role of Calcium Channels in the Rat Esophageal Tunica Muscularis Mucosae[a]

S. E. OHIA, Y. D. CHEUNG, D. BIEGER, AND C. R. TRIGGLE

Faculty of Medicine
Memorial University of Newfoundland
St. John's, Newfoundland, Canada A1B3V6

In the rat esophageal tunica muscularis mucosae (TMM), tetrodotoxin (TTX) insensitive field-stimulation-evoked relaxations (FSR), under conditions of induced tone with muscarinic receptor agonists, have been shown to be highly sensitive, indeed more sensitive than the contractile response, to inhibition by Ca^{2+} channel antagonists (CATs).[1] This action appears to be exerted directly on the smooth muscle cell,[2] and similarly TMM can be relaxed with the Ca^{2+} ionophore, A23187. A role for Ca^{2+} and Ca^{2+} channels in mediating not only contraction but also relaxation is thus inferred. This hypothesis was further tested by examining $^{45}Ca^{2+}$ uptake and [^{3}H]-nitrendipine binding in the TMM. For the former studies, tissues were incubated in Tyrode solution containing $^{45}Ca^{2+}$. The effects of a 2 minute exposure to a muscarinic agonist (CD, 0.3 μM), KCl (80 mM), and ionophore A23187 (1 μM) were determined in the absence or presence of a 20 minute exposure to the CATs.

TABLE 1. Effect of (+)PN-200 110 (10 nM) on Ionophore A23187 (1 μM) Stimulated $^{45}Ca^{2+}$ Uptake in Rat Esophageal Tunica Muscularis Mucosae[a]

Segment	$^{45}Ca^{2+}$ Uptake (μmol/kg wet weight) Basal	A23187	A23187 + PN-200 110	n
Proximal	345.2 ± 13.4	471.0 ± 24.8	480.2 ± 14.5	6
Distal	424.6 ± 24.9	602.7 ± 40.8	608.6 ± 45.9	6

[a]Values are mean ± standard error of the mean; n = number of tissues, two tissues per animal.

Uptake of $^{45}Ca^{2+}$ in the TMM was significantly lower ($p < 0.01$) in the proximal than in the distal segments (TABLE 1). CD, KCl, and A23187 produced significant increases ($p < 0.05$) in the uptake of $^{45}Ca^{2+}$ in both proximal and distal segments (FIGURE 1). Verapamil and the 1,4-dihydropyridine (DHP) nifedipine counteracted the enhancement of $^{45}Ca^{2+}$ uptake by CD and KCl in a concentration-dependent manner (TABLE 2). The uptake of $^{45}Ca^{2+}$ induced by A23187 was, however, unaffected by (+)PN-200 110 (10 nM) (TABLE 1).

A low capacity and high affinity [^{3}H]-nitrendipine saturable binding site was identified in TMM membranes and interestingly, an apparently unsaturable component was also detected (FIGURE 2). The high-affinity site demonstrated stereoselectiv-

[a]Supported by the Medical Research Council of Canada.

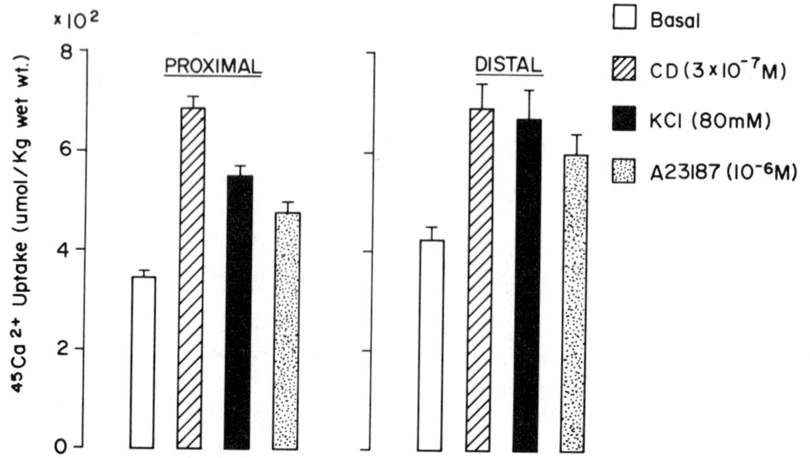

FIGURE 1. Effects of *cis*-2-methyl-4-dimethylaminoethyl-1,3 dioxolane methiodide (CD), KCl, and A23187 on $^{45}Ca^{2+}$ uptake in proximal and distal segments of rat esophageal tunica muscularis mucosae. Increases in $^{45}Ca^{2+}$ uptake produced by these agents were statistically significant ($p < 0.05$). ($n = 6$).

ity for (+)PN-200 110 ($K_i = 0.064$ nM) as compared to the (−)enantiomer ($K_i = 14.98$ nM). In contrast, the phenylalkylamine D-600 only caused incomplete (60%) displacement at 10^{-4} M.

$^{45}Ca^{2+}$ uptake stimulated by KCl was more susceptible to blockade by the CATs than that induced by CD, suggesting the coexistence of both voltage-operated channels (VOCs) and receptor-operated channels (ROCs) in the TMM. In contrast with the guinea pig intestinal smooth muscle,[3] the influx of $^{45}Ca^{2+}$ stimulated by A23187 in the TMM was not sensitive to inhibition by Cats. Results from the DHP radioligand binding experiment suggest that Ca^{2+} channels in the TMM possess properties similar to those observed in other tissues such as the guinea pig ileum[4] and brain.[5]

The questions of whether both the high- and low-affinity [^{3}H]-nitrendipine sites have pharmacological functions and whether the same Ca^{2+} channel facilitates both relaxation and contraction of esophageal smooth muscle require further investigation.

TABLE 2. Comparison of Potency of Nifedipine and Verapamil in Inhibiting KCl and *cis*-2-Methyl-4-dimethylaminoethyl-1,3 Dioxolane Methiodide (CD) Stimulated $^{45}Ca^{2+}$ Uptake in Rat Esophageal Tunica Muscularis Mucosae[a]

		IC_{50}		
Agent	Segment	Nifedipine (nM)	Verapamil (μM)	*n*
KCl	Proximal	0.15	0.36	6
	Distal	0.13	0.43	6
CD	Proximal	12.9	2.26	6
	Distal	10.0	2.08	6

[a] IC_{50} = concentration of Ca^{2+} channel antagonist producing 50% inhibition of $^{45}Ca^{2+}$ uptake activated by KCl (80 mM) and CD (0.3 μM); n = number of tissues, two tissues per animal.

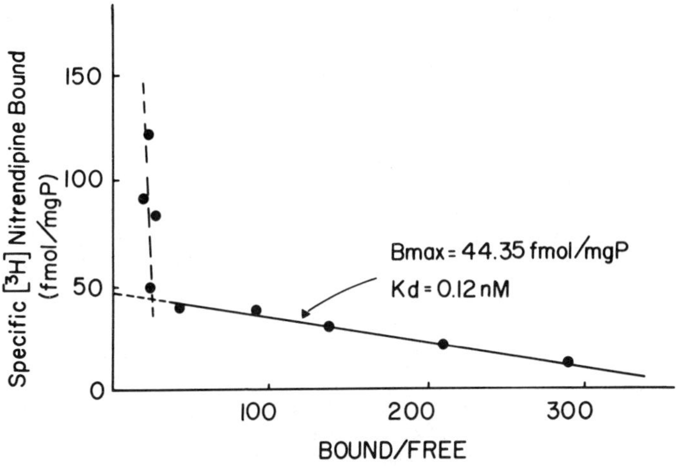

FIGURE 2. Scatchard plot of [^{3}H]-nitrendipine binding to rat esophageal tunica muscularis mucosae. Rat esophageal TMM membranes (40–80 μg protein) were incubated at 23°C with [^{3}H]-nitrendipine (0–12 nM) for 45–60 minutes. Specific binding was defined as that displaceable by 10 μM nifedipine. Data presented are from a representative experiment (n = 4) performed in triplicate, yielding a K_D of 0.09 ± 0.01 nM and a B_{max} of 44 ± 0.2 fmol/mg protein.

REFERENCES

1. AKBARALI, H. I., D. BIEGER & C. R. TRIGGLE. 1986. J. Physiol. **381:** 49–63.
2. AKBARALI, H. I., D. BIEGER & C. R. TRIGGLE. 1987. Can. J. Physiol. Pharmacol. **65:** 23–29.
3. ROSENBERGER, L. B. & D. J. TRIGGLE. 1979. Can. J. Physiol. Pharmacol. **57:** 348–358.
4. BOLGER, G. T., P. GENGO, R. KLOCKOWSKI, E. LUCHOWSKI, H. SIEGEL, R. A. JANIS, A. M. TRIGGLE & D. J. TRIGGLE. 1983. J. Pharmacol. Exp. Ther. **225:** 291–309.
5. GLOSSMANN, H. & D. R. FERRY. 1983. Drug Dev. Evaluation **9:** 63–98.

PN 200-110, a Calcium Antagonist with High Potency and Selectivity for Vascular Smooth Muscle

URS T. RÜEGG, GÜNTER SCHOLTYSIK, NIGEL S. COOK, ARNOLD VOGEL, AND ROBERT P. HOF

Preclinical Research
Sandoz Limited
4002 Basel, Switzerland

Calcium entry through voltage-sensitive calcium channels (VSCC) can be modulated by calcium entry blockers (CEBs) and activators. Classically, this modulation is measured indirectly, i.e., by the measurement of inhibition of KCl induced contraction by a calcium channel blocker. Alternatively, uptake of $^{45}Ca^{2+}$ into tissue such as aortic rings can be measured.

We have recently described a cell line derived from rat aortic smooth muscle that responds to depolarization with an increased $^{45}Ca^{2+}$ uptake.[1] This increase is sensitive to blockade by inorganic as well as organic calcium antagonists and can be used for the direct study of the pharmacology of the VSCC in smooth muscle. FIGURE 1 illustrates such a finding. The potencies in inhibiting $^{45}Ca^{2+}$ uptake into KCl-depolarized cells correlate very well with the inhibition of contraction of KCl-constricted rabbit aortic rings.[2] As can be seen (FIGURE 1) the dihydropyridine PY 108-068 (darodipine) is about 100 times more potent than the phenylalkylamine verapamil. PN 200-110 (LOMIR) is a dihydropyridine containing an assymmetric carbon.[3] The two enantio-

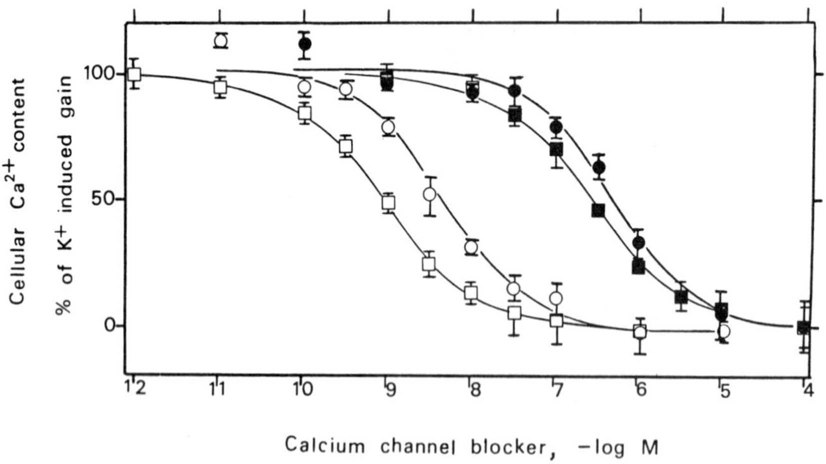

FIGURE 1. Effect of calcium entry blockers on $^{45}Ca^{2+}$ uptake into smooth muscle cells. Cells in culture were depolarized with 55 mM KCl and $^{45}Ca^{2+}$ uptake was studied as described.[1,2] Filled circles, verapamil; open circles, darodipine (PY 108-068); filled squares, (−)PN 200-110; open squares, (+)PN 200-110. Mean ± standard error of the mean for $n = 4$.

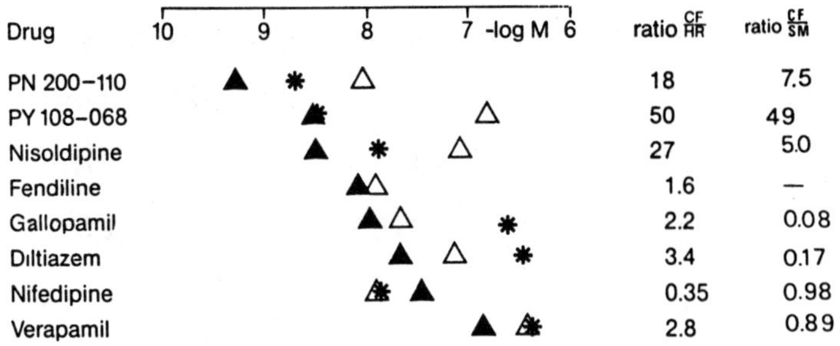

FIGURE 2. Comparative effects of calcium entry blockers on heart and smooth muscle; logarithmic scale. Open triangles are the EC_{25} values for the negative inotropic effect on paced guinea pig left atria; filled triangles reflect EC_{25} values for the negative chronotropic effect on spontaneously beating guinea pig right atria. Experiments were performed as described;[5] each concentration-response curve was for $n = 6$. The asterisks indicate the IC_{50} values determined by inhibition of $^{45}Ca^{2+}$ uptake into smooth muscle cells as in FIGURE 1. The ratios give an indication of the chronoselectivity (CF, contractile force; HR, heart rate) and of the selectivity for smooth muscle (SM) for each of the compounds tested.

mers of this compound showed an about 300-fold difference in their potency in blocking Ca^{2+} uptake, (+)PN 200-110 being the most potent compound (FIGURE 1). A similar difference in potency has been found *in vivo*.[4]

Myocardial cells also contain VSCC, some of which are also affected by CEBs. Blockade leads to a decrease in myocardial contractility and to a negative chronotropic effect. Some of the typical CEBs were tested for these properties on isolated atria from guinea pig hearts as described.[5] The values obtained for decreases in heart rate and in contractile force were compared to the inhibition of $^{45}Ca^{2+}$ entry into smooth muscle cells (FIGURE 2). The selectivity ratios shown on the right of FIGURE 2 indicate that there are large differences between the tissue sensitivity to different CEBs. The dihydropyridines exhibit a similar potency in their effects on heart rate and smooth muscle contraction, whereas diltiazem, verapamil, and D-600 are more effective modulators of cardiac function. The most selective CEB with respect to smooth muscle is PY 108-068,[5] followed by PN 200-110 which shows a potent chronotropic effect in addition to its action on smooth muscle (cf. ratios in FIGURE 2).

Although these drugs are thought to interact with the same type of calcium channel their differences in tissue selectivity, as reported here, suggest that either the interaction with the binding site is dependent on voltage and, possibly, on the kinetics of the gating process of the channel or that several channel types exist to varying degrees in different tissues which are affected to a greater or lesser extent by CEBs.

REFERENCES

1. RÜEGG, U. T., V. M. DOYLE, J.-F. ZUBER & R. P. HOF. 1985. Biochem. Biophys. Res. Commun. **130:** 447–453.
2. RÜEGG, U. T., V. M. DOYLE & R. P. HOF. 1985. J. Hypertension **3**(Suppl. 3): S57–S59.
3. HOF, R. P., G. SCHOLTYSIK, R. LOUTZENHISER, H. J. VUORELA & P. NEUMANN. 1984. J. Cardiovasc. Pharmacol. **6:** 399–406.
4. HOF, R. P., A. HOF, U. T. RÜEGG, N. S. COOK & A. VOGEL. 1986. J. Cardiovasc. Pharmacol. **8:** 221–226.
5. HOF, R. P. & G. SCHOLTYSIK. 1983. J. Cardiovasc. Pharmacol. **5:** 176–183.

Calcium Antagonist Enantiomers Discriminate between Vascular and Myocardial Calcium Channels in the Retrogradely Perfused Rat Heart

F. TH. M. VAN AMSTERDAM, M. HAAS,
AND J. ZAAGSMA

Department of Pharmacology and Therapeutics
University of Groningen
A. Deusingln 2
9713 AW Groningen, the Netherlands

Stereoselectivity at calcium-antagonist-sensitive sites can provide us with much information about the interaction of this large group of drugs and about the sites themselves. Differences in stereoisomers of verapamil and congeners were reported for smooth and cardiac muscle contraction with 10- to 100-fold potency differences.[1,2] This was also found for dihydropyridine calcium antagonists in radioligand binding studies; the two enantiomers of recently developed calcium agonists were even found to have functionally opposite, agonistic and antagonistic, activities.[3]

In this study, we compared the dose-dependent effects of the stereoisomers of verapamil (VER), gallopamil (D600), desmethoxyverapamil (D888), and bepridil (BEP) on the coronary flow and the left ventricular pressure (LVP) in the retrogradely perfused rat heart, paced at 300 beats per minute. In addition, the time courses of onset

TABLE 1. pEC_{50} Values and Stereoselectivity Factors of the Enantiomers of Verapamil, Gallopamil, D-888, and Bepridil for Coronary Flow Increase and Negative Inotropic Activity in the Langendorff Perfused Rat Heart

	Coronary Flow		Ratio	Left Ventricular Pressure	
	$EC_{50}(+)/EC_{50}(-)$	pEC_{50}	EC_{50} LVP / EC_{50} Flow	pEC_{50}	$EC_{50}(+)/EC_{50}(-)$
(+)-BEP	0.23 <	6.76	12.6	5.66	> 0.37
(−)-BEP		6.13	7.9	5.23	
(+)-VER	2.45 <	7.31	43.6	5.67	> 31.6
(−)-VER		7.70	3.4	7.17	
(+)-D600	3.3 <	7.12	15.8	5.92	> 56.2
(−)-D600		7.64	0.93	7.67	
(+)-D888	19.9 <	7.21	4.5	6.56	> 61.7
(−)-D888		8.51	1.45	8.35	

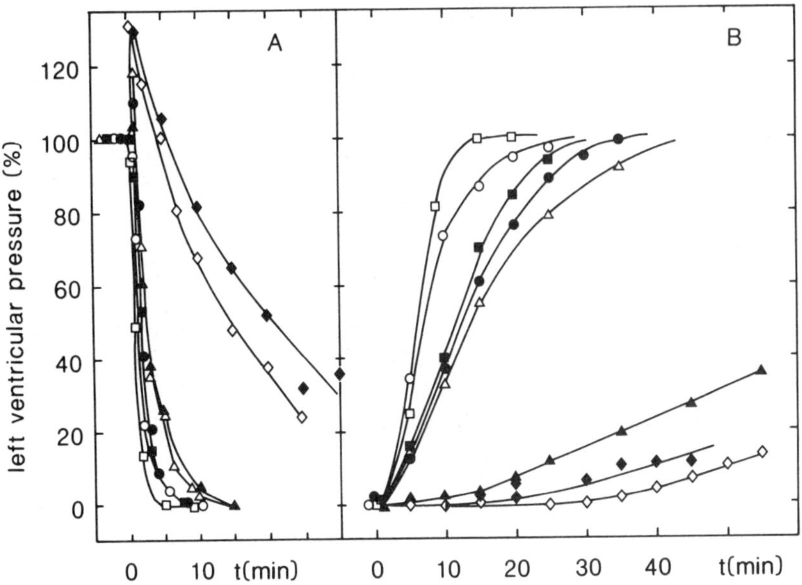

FIGURE 1. Time courses of onset and recovery of negative inotropic activity of 30 nM (−)- and 10 μM (+)-verapamil (filled and open circles, respectively), 30 nM (−)- and 10 μM (+)-D600 (filled and open squares, respectively), 30 nM (−)- and 1 μM (+)-D888 (filled and open triangles, respectively), and 10 μM (−)- and 3 μM (+)-bepridil (filled and open diamonds, respectively).

and recovery of these effects were studied at equipotent dosages for coronary flow increase and for LVP depression.

Dose-effect curves revealed high stereoselectivity ratios (sr's) for LVP depression of 62 (D888), 56 (D600), and 32 (VER) in favor of the (−)-enantiomers. For coronary flow increase, the sr's were much lower (20, 3.3, and 2.5, respectively; TABLE 1). Comparison of the coronary vascular and the myocardial effects revealed a high vasoselectivity in the (+)-enantiomers, in contrast to the (−)-enantiomers, which surprisingly were almost equipotent on the vascular and myocardial isochannels. It therefore appears that the distomeric (+)-isomers show the same vascular preference as the dihydropyridines[4] and might have a similar voltage-dependent potency, whereas the eutomeric (−)-isomers can block both isochannels equipotently despite the different resting states. BEP, with the (+)-enantiomer being more potent, showed sr values for LVP depression and for coronary flow increase of 2.7 and 4.3, respectively (TABLE 1).

Clear differences in onset and offset velocities were found as well. At equipotent concentrations, coronary flow increase showed identical, fast onset and recovery kinetics for all eight enantiomers, whereas LVP kinetics were slower and markedly different for the enantiomers of each drug (FIGURE 1). The $t_{1/2}$ values for the recovery of the LVP depression were 6.2, 7.1, and 13.8 minutes for the (+)-enantiomers of D600, VER, and D888, respectively. The (−)-enantiomers of the same drugs showed considerably slower recovery values of 11.8, 12.5, and 70 minutes, respectively. Bepridil was slowest in onset and offset, the more potent isomer having the higher $t_{1/2}$ for LVP recovery as with the verapamil congeners.

The kinetic results provide additional information about the differences between the coronary vascular and the myocardial isochannels. The former is rapidly accessible for all types of calcium antagonists (cf. Reference 4), whereas the latter isochannel, being less accessible for more hydrophobic drugs, presumably has its "verapamil" site associated with the inner mouth of the channel.

Furthermore, the differences in recovery of LVP depression between each pair of verapamil type enantiomers suggest that the recovery rate may directly reflect dissociation from the myocardial isochannel verapamil site.

REFERENCES

1. ANGUS, J. A. & R. M. BRAZENOR. 1983. J. Cardiovasc. Pharmacol. **5:** 321–328.
2. RASCHACK, M. & K. ENGELMANN. 1983. Adv. Myocardiol. **4:** 505–512.
3. FRANCKOWIAK, G., M. BECHEM, M. SCHRAMM & G. THOMAS. 1985. Eur. J. Pharmacol. **114:** 223–226.
4. VAN AMSTERDAM, F. TH. M., M. HAAS & J. ZAAGSMA. 1987. J. Cardiovasc. Pharmacol. **9:** 570–577.

The Mode of Action of Dihydropyridines in Vascular Smooth Muscle

Correlated Binding and Mechanical Studies

M. WIBO AND T. GODFRAIND

Laboratory of General Pharmacodynamics and Pharmacology
Catholic University of Louvain
Avenue E. Mounier, 73
B 1200 Brussels, Belgium

Calcium entry blockers of the 1,4-dihydropyridine type are increasingly used as antianginal and antihypertensive agents. With the aim of better defining their mode of action in vascular smooth muscle, we performed correlated binding and mechanical

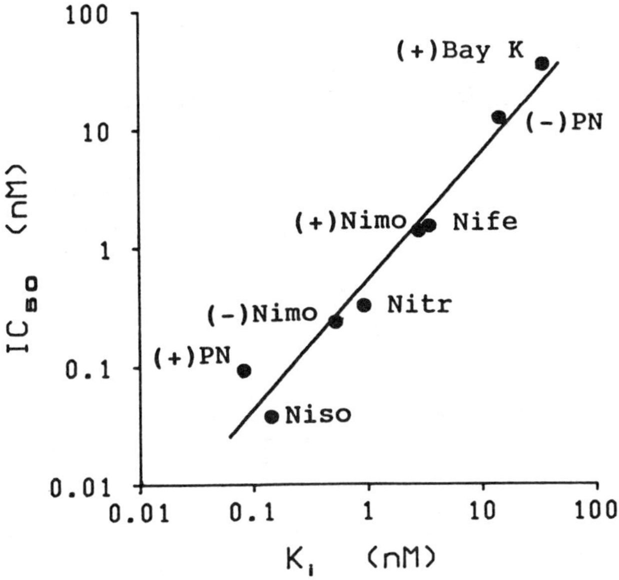

FIGURE 1. Correlation between data from binding and mechanical studies on rat aortic tissue. In binding studies, microsomal fractions from rat aorta were incubated for 60 minutes at 37°C in Tris-buffered medium (see Reference 1) containing 0.12 nM [^{3}H]-(+)PN 200-110, in the presence of various concentrations of (+)PN 200-110, nisoldipine, (−)nimodipine, nitrendipine, (+)nimodipine, nifedipine, (−)PN 200-110, or (+)Bay K 8644. Nonspecific binding was measured in the presence of 1 μM nifedipine. Measurement of bound radioligand and estimation of K_i values were made as described by Godfraind and Wibo.[1] Mechanical studies were carried out as described by Godfraind.[2] Aortic rings were preincubated with drug for 90 minutes before stimulation by a solution containing 100 mM KCl. Inhibitory effects were measured 35 minutes after switching to the high-KCl solution (see FIGURE 2, inset), and IC_{50} values were determined from log concentration/inhibition curves.

studies on rat aortic tissue. Dihydropyridine binding sites were characterized in membrane fractions using [^{3}H]-(+)PN 200-110 [isopropyl 4-(2,1,3-benzoxadiazol-4-yl)-1,4-dihydro-5-methoxycarbonyl-2,6-dimethyl-3-pyridinecarboxylate]. Only one class of sites was detected in saturation experiments (K_D 0.1 nM, 37°C), as well as in kinetic experiments (k_{-1} 0.052 min^{-1}; k_{+1} 0.61 nM^{-1} × min^{-1}). Binding sites were concentrated in microsomal fractions (343 ± 21 fmol/mg protein, n = 8) in accordance with their putative plasmalemmal localization. K_i values were determined in

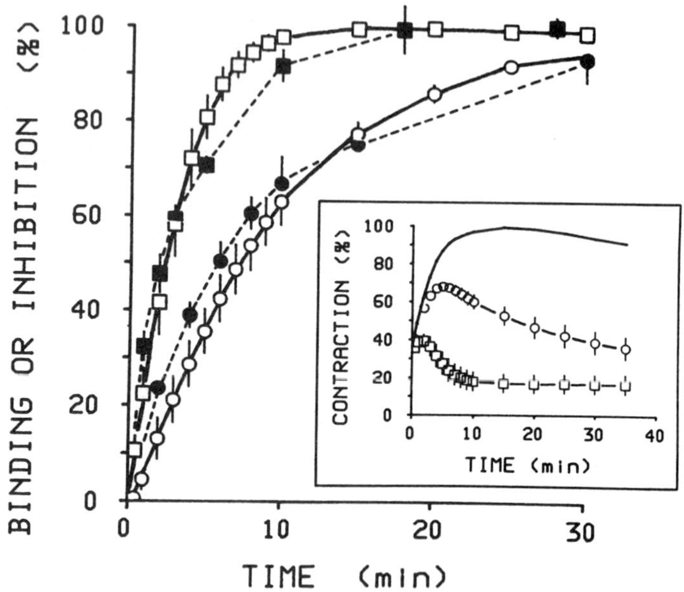

FIGURE 2. Comparison between kinetics of [^{3}H]-(+)PN 200-110 association to its specific binding site in isolated membranes and kinetics of inhibition by (+)PN 200-110 of KCl-evoked contraction of aortic rings. The time course of specific [^{3}H]-(+)PN 200-110 binding (dashed line) was measured at two concentrations of radioligand: 0.1 nM (filled circles) and 0.38 nM (filled squares); results (means from three determinations, standard error indicated by vertical bars) are expressed as the percentage of the maximal binding at each concentration. Inhibition of the mechanical response (solid line) by 0.1 nM (open circles) and 0.3 nM (open squares) (+)PN 200-110 was followed as a function of time after initiation of KCl depolarization. Results (means from four rings, standard error indicated by vertical bars) are expressed as the percentage of inhibition at 35 minutes. These inhibition curves were constructed from the graphs shown in the inset, which give the mechanical responses to KCl depolarization of control aortic rings (upper curve) and rings treated with 0.1 nM (open circles) or 0.3 nM (open squares) (+)PN 200-110.

binding competition experiments for a series of eight dihydropyridines, including enantiomers of PN 200-110 and nimodipine (see FIGURE 1).

In parallel studies, we determined the potencies of the same dihydropyridines as inhibitors of the contraction of aortic rings evoked by KCl depolarization. Rings were preincubated for 90 minutes with dihydropyridines before stimulation by 100 mM KCl, and contractions were followed for 35 minutes.[2] We observed a nearly 1:1 correlation between the concentrations that inhibited mechanical responses (at 35 minutes) by 50% (IC_{50}) and K_i values obtained in binding studies (FIGURE 1). Furthermore, despite extensive preincubation with (+)PN 200-110 before KCl depolarization, the inhibitory effect of this drug developed only gradually, and the kinetics of the development of inhibition were similar to the kinetics of [^{3}H]-(+)PN 200-110 binding to isolated membranes (FIGURE 2).

These results indicate that the dihydropyridine binding sites detected in membrane fractions from rat aorta can be identified with the receptor sites for dihydropyridine calcium entry blockers in depolarized ring preparations. They suggest also that depolarization of vascular smooth muscle increases the affinity of calcium channels for dihydropyridine inhibitors, thereby allowing them to bind to the channels, and to block them, at low concentrations.

REFERENCES

1. GODFRAIND, T. & M. WIBO. 1985. Subcellular localization of [^{3}H]-nitrendipine binding sites in guinea-pig ileal smooth muscle. Br. J. Pharmacol. **85:** 335–340.
2. GODFRAIND, T. 1983. Actions of nifedipine on calcium fluxes and contraction in isolated rat arteries. J. Pharmacol. Exp. Ther. **224:** 443–450.

Calcium Channels in Smooth Muscle[a]

T. GODFRAIND

Catholic University of Louvain
Laboratory of General Pharmacodynamics and Pharmacology
U.C.L. 7350
Emmanuel Mounier Avenue, 73
B-1200 Brussels, Belgium

The sodium theory of conduction of excitation in nerve[1] proposed by Hodgkin and Huxley in 1952 has prompted investigations on ionic channels in various excitable tissues including smooth muscles.[2] A first indication of the existence of gated calcium channels was reported in 1953 by Fatt and Katz, who found calcium-dependent action potentials in crustacean muscle fibers.[3] In this presentation, I would like to examine the experimental evidence showing the existence of calcium channels in the pericellular membrane of the smooth muscles. In addition, I would like to discuss the factors intrinsic and extrinsic to the smooth muscle cell that modulate the function of the channels.[4]

Several experimental protocols have been proposed in order to characterize by which mechanisms extracellular calcium could be translocated in order to activate the contractile machinery of the smooth muscle. The various methodologies have included contraction measurement, electrical activity recordings using sucrose gap microelectrodes for direct records of action potentials, and measurement of currents during voltage clamp and patch clamp studies. Measurements of unidirectional calcium fluxes in relation to cellular activation have also been performed. The use of calcium antagonists and of calcium agonists has also contributed greatly to the understanding of the mechanisms of activation and of the role of calcium channels.[4]

CALCIUM MOVEMENTS AND CONTRACTION

Estimation of unidirectional calcium fluxes in smooth muscle requires appropriate methodologies. As initially shown by Weiss and Goodman and by van Breemen and his colleagues, lanthanum allows the delineation of intra- and extracellular pools of calcium because it does not penetrate the cell and displaces calcium from its extracellular binding sites.[5,6] In vascular smooth muscle only one-tenth of the total calcium content is intracellular; therefore, when the tissue is bathed in ^{45}Ca-containing physiological solution, changes of its specific activity are obscured by the large fraction of extracellular calcium bound on the external surface of the smooth muscle cells and on connective tissue. We have developed a method allowing measurements in rat aorta of changes in the specific activity of the lanthanum-resistant calcium fraction once the tissue is incubated in radioactive solution.[7] In resting conditions, the specific activity of intracellular calcium defined as the lanthanum-resistant calcium fraction increases with the duration of incubation in radioactive solution and reaches a plateau after one or two hours, when inward and outward movements become equal. However, the initial rate of uptake of ^{45}Ca may be taken as reflecting an inward flux—as, when the

[a]This work has been supported by FRSM grant 3.9006.87.

intracellular fraction is completely loaded, the initial rate of ^{45}Ca loss after transfer to nonradioactive solutions depends mainly on outward movement.

Calcium influx rate under resting conditions is about 0.014 and 0.03 pmol $\times$ $cm^{-2} \times second^{-1}$ respectively in rat aorta[7] and in rabbit aorta.[5] This calcium influx has been termed passive Ca leak, because it is thought to occur through pathways that differ from those involved in calcium influx evoked by stimulating agents. Indeed most of this calcium influx is resistant to calcium entry blockers that block stimuli-dependent calcium influx.[4]

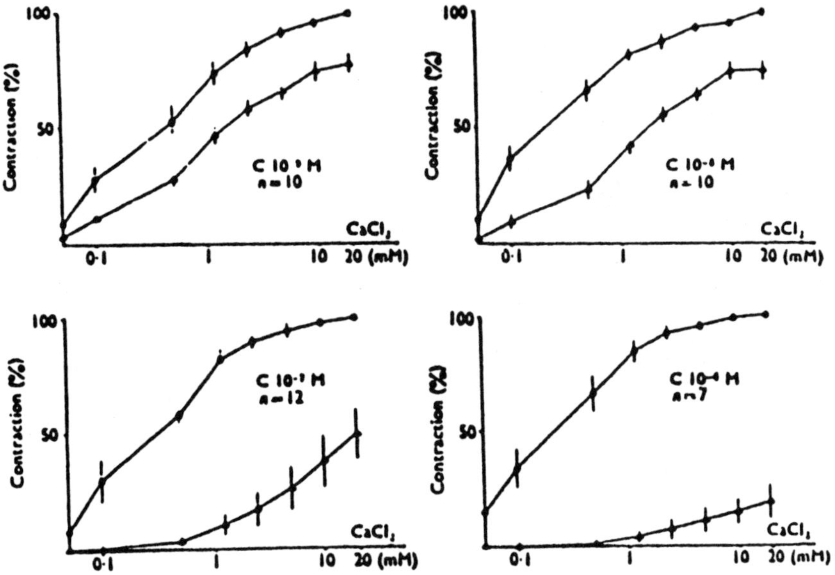

FIGURE 1. Effect of cinnarizine on contractions evoked by Ca^{2+} in K^+-depolarized rabbit mesenteric arteries. Arterial preparations were preincubated in Ca^{2+}-free physiological solution, depolarized in Ca^{2+}-free KCl-rich solution, and then further incubated with increasing Ca^{2+} concentrations. Cumulative concentration-effect curves were obtained before (circles) and after (triangles) addition of cinnarizine (C) at the concentrations indicated. Responses are expressed in percentage of maximal contraction evoked before addition of cinnarizine. The inhibitory effect of cinnarizine is observed at concentrations as low as 1 nM and resembles the action of antagonists in receptor studies. In view of this similarity, the term "calcium antagonist" was suggested to describe the action of cinnarizine. (Reproduced from Reference 19, with permission.)

Changes in the calcium concentration of the perfusing fluid do not usually affect the contractile state of smooth muscle at rest. As initially reported by Edman and Schild in isolated rat uterus,[8] the picture is quite different once stimulation occurs with KCl depolarization and with acetylcholine. For instance, in preparations immersed in solutions where NaCl is replaced by an appropriate concentration of KCl, the cell membrane is depolarized and a change in its permeability to Ca^{2+} is observed. This may be demonstrated by a calcium-dependent increase in tone of the muscle preparation; this increase is a function of the calcium concentration in the external medium. This observation has been repeated in various smooth muscles,[9] including vascular smooth muscle (FIGURE 1). A more direct demonstration of such changes in calcium permeability may be obtained when ^{45}Ca fluxes are measured.

As FIGURE 2 illustrates for rat aorta, norepinephrine stimulation and KCl depolarization evoke a nearly 20-fold increase in the rate of calcium influx. There is a major difference between the two stimuli as shown by net ^{45}Ca uptake at steady state. Indeed, norepinephrine does not influence net ^{45}Ca uptake, whereas the net uptake is much higher in KCl-depolarized aortas. This observation is in agreement with the existence of receptor-operated calcium channels (ROCs) and of potential operated calcium channels (POCs), as proposed in 1979 by Bolton[10] and by van Breemen.[5] A third type of calcium channel has been postulated by Bevan and co-workers, the

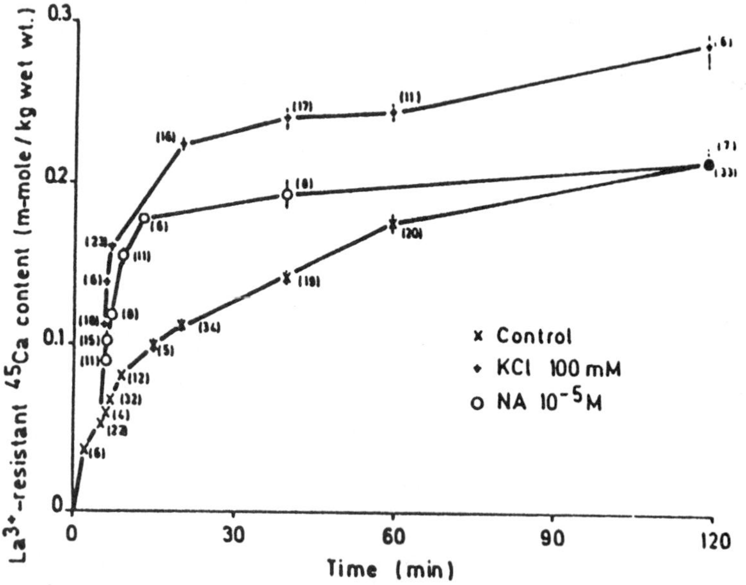

FIGURE 2. Effect of norepinephrine (10^{-5} M) (NA) and of K^+ depolarization (KCl 100 mM) on $^{45}Ca^{2+}$ influx in rat aorta. Ordinate: $^{45}Ca^{2+}$ content of the La^{3+}-resistant Ca^{2+} fraction expressed in mmol/kg wet weights. Abscissa: time in radioactive solution for controls and treated arteries. The number of determinations is given on the graph. Vertical bars represent standard error of the mean (SEM). (Data from Reference 27.)

stretch-operated calcium channels (SOCs).[11] These authors have supported their view by several functional observations. It is first interesting to note that this functional recognition of three types of calcium channels is in agreement with the existence of three main categories of excitation; electrical, related to membrane depolarization by conducted potentials or by neurotransmitters; pharmacomechanical, related to activation by transmitters without cell membrane depolarization; and mechanical, induced by stretches causing or not causing depolarization. Among experimental evidences favoring a distinction between ROCs and POCs is the observation reported by Meisheri, Hwang, and van Breemen that maximal ^{45}Ca influxes stimulated in rabbit aorta by norepinephrine and high KCl solution are additive.[12]

There is obviously an information gap between the above classification of calcium channels and the identification of functional Ca channels in isolated cells using the patch clamp technique. Tsien and his co-workers have reported distinct types of POCs in cultured sensory neurones of the chick dorsal root ganglion and in mammalian cardiac cells.[13] In cardiac cells, they have found two types of unitary conductance with different kinetic features, which can be attributed to the opening of two distinct calcium channels—the T type and the L type; only the latter are sensitive to dihydropyridines. In chick dorsal root ganglion cells, a third type of conductance (N type) has been identified. Recent observations made in vascular smooth muscles by Bean *et al.*,[14] Worley *et al.*,[15] and Droogmans *et al.*[16] using the patch clamp technique have established the existence of voltage-controlled calcium channels selective for divalent cations over monovalent cations. Worley *et al.* have identified two conductance levels, 8 pS and 15 pS, that are similar to those reported for calcium channels from heart muscle.[15] The electrophysiological properties of calcium channels seem similar in heart and smooth muscle, as well as their response to agonist and antagonist dihydropyridines. Worley *et al.* pointed out that in excised patches, both Ca channel types in vascular smooth muscle function for hours without loss of Ca channel activity when Ca channels in heart patches become nonfunctional[15]; therefore, metabolic regulation of Ca channels may be different in the two tissues. In addition, their physiological regulation may be different, owing to the lower membrane potential of smooth muscle cell as compared to cardiac cell. The existence of different voltage-operated calcium channels in smooth muscle membrane does not prove the existence of ROCs, POCs and SOCs, but it does not disprove it at all. Therefore, on the basis of the actual information, it is better to keep than to disclose this distinction.

CALCIUM MOVEMENTS AND RELAXATION

In the resting state, the cytosolic calcium concentration is probably not higher than 100 nM, and the ratio of extracellular to intracellular Ca^{2+} exceeds 10,000. Upon stimulation, the cytosolic Ca^{2+} rises, partly as a result of an influx of extracellular Ca^{2+}, and partly following the mobilization of internal Ca^{2+} stores, to reach about 10 μM. To restore the low resting cytosolic Ca^{2+} and to maintain Ca^{2+} homeostasis, the cell uses Ca^{2+} transport systems that are able to operate against large electrochemical gradients. Such systems have been demonstrated in the plasma membrane and in intracellular organelles, mainly the endoplasmic (sarcoplasmic) reticulum.

There are two main mechanisms allowing "uphill" Ca^{2+} transport. The first relies on the direct utilization of energy from ATP (Ca^{2+} transport ATPase), and the second uses the Na^+ electrochemical potential to drive the extrusion of Ca^{2+} in exchange for Na^+ entry (Na^+-Ca^{2+} exchange). ATP-dependent Ca^{2+} pumps with different properties are present in the plasma membrane and the endoplasmic reticulum. Their identification in smooth muscle has relied mainly on cell fractionation techniques, including the digitonin shift method.[17] The plasma membrane Ca^{2+} pump is activated by calmodulin, which acts mainly by enhancing the affinity of the pump for Ca^{2+}. In smooth muscle, the Ca^{2+} transport capacity of the Na^+-Ca^{2+} exchange system and its Ca^{2+} affinity seem to be distinctly lower than those of the plasmalemmal Ca^{2+} transport ATPase in contrast to the heart sarcolemma where the transport capacity of the exchanger is much higher than that of the Ca^{2+} pump (FIGURE 3).[17,18]

THE INTERACTION OF CALCIUM MODULATORS WITH POCs

As defined elsewhere,[4] calcium modulators are those pharmacological agents that interfere with gating of the calcium channels of pericellular membrane evoked by depolarization or receptor activation. FIGURE 1 shows the effect of cinnarizine on the contraction evoked by calcium in isolated rabbit mesenteric arteries. Isolated arteries were first depolarized by immersing them in a Ca^{2+}-free solution containing 100 mM KCl. Addition of Ca^{2+} to the depolarized solution evokes an increase in tension that is concentration dependent. In the presence of cinnarizine, concentration-dose effect curves were displaced to the right and their maximum was progressively depressed. The inhibitory effect is typical of that observed with other calcium entry blockers[4] and resembles the action of antagonists in receptor studies. In view of this similarity, the term "calcium antagonist" was suggested in 1968 to describe the action of cinnarizine.[19] Like cinnarizine, nifedipine inhibits the entry of calcium in depolarized smooth muscle cell; this is shown in FIGURE 4. When the concentration of nifedipine is varied, there is a close correlation between inhibition of contraction and of ^{45}Ca entry. That this action is related to specific receptor sites for nifedipine is indicated by a close

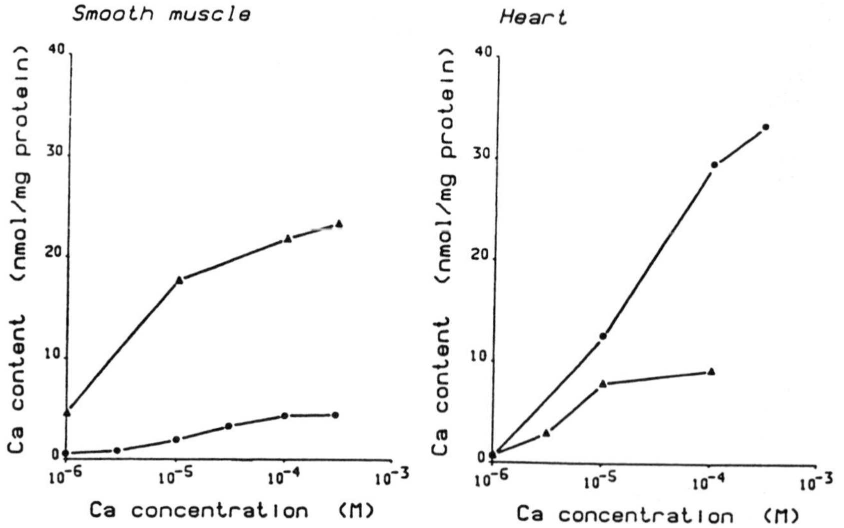

FIGURE 3. Comparison between ATP-dependent (triangles) and Na-Ca exchange dependent (circles) transport of calcium in plasma membrane of smooth and cardiac muscle.[24]

similarity between IC_{50} values obtained on intact tissue and K_i values measured in microsomal preparations, an observation confirmed with several other dihydropyridines.[4] Using the digitonin shift method, which allows characterization of an activity associated with the plasma membrane, Godfraind and Wibo (see Reference 4) have shown that those specific receptors sites are located on the plasmalemmal membrane of the smooth muscle cell. There is some evidence that the specific receptor sites for dihydropyridines are on Ca channels.

In cultured cells from rat aorta, Mras and Sperelakis have reported Ca-dependent action potentials when the cells were treated by 10 mM tetraethylammonium; those spikes are blocked by calcium entry blockers.[20] In taenia coli of the guinea pig, histamine evokes action potentials, and Morel, Hardy, and Godfraind have shown that they are amplified by the Ca agonist BAY K8644,[21] an action antagonized by nifedipine (FIGURE 5). In patch clamp studies of smooth muscles as discussed above,[21]

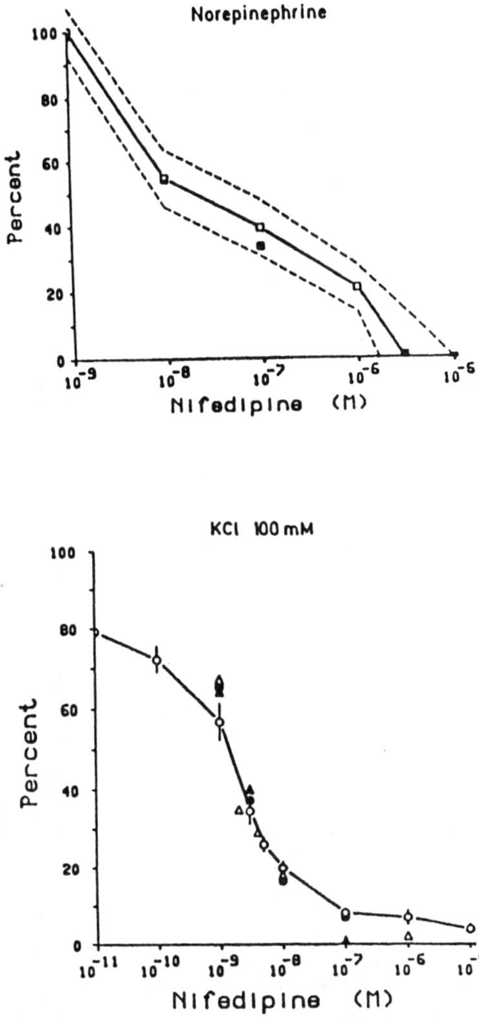

FIGURE 4. Upper panel: depression by nifedipine of norepinephrine-evoked ^{45}Ca influx (filled squares) and contraction (open squares) in rat aorta. Ordinate: nifedipine-sensitive component in percentage of the maximum. Each point is the mean calculated from at least five experiments. SEMs are shown by the dashed lines. Lower panel: nifedipine-induced depression of K-depolarization-evoked ^{45}Ca influx and contraction in rat aorta and mesenteric artery. Aorta contraction (open circles); aorta corrected ^{45}Ca influx (open triangles); mesenteric artery contraction (filled circles); and mesenteric artery ^{45}Ca influx (filled triangles). Each point is the mean of at least six determinations. SEMs are shown for contractions. (Data from Reference 35.)

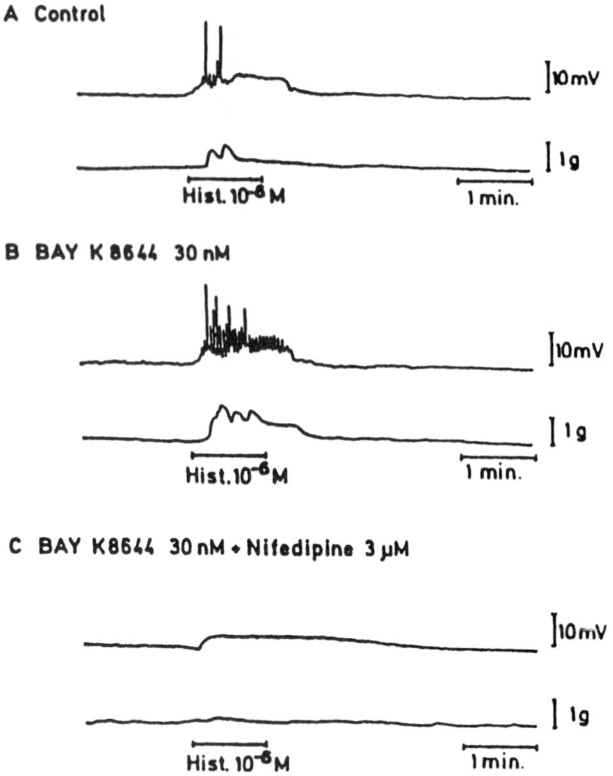

FIGURE 5. Electrical (upper trace) and mechanical (lower trace) responses of guinea pig taenia coli evoked by histamine 10^{-6} M, applied for 1 minute. (A) Control record. (B) Potentiation of the responses to histamine by Bay K 8644. Responses were obtained after 30 minutes perfusion with Krebs physiological solution containing Bay K 8644 30 nM. (C) Depression of the mechanical and electrical responses to histamine by nifedipine 10^{-6} M. Nifedipine 10^{-6} M was added to the perfusion medium in the continuous presence of Bay K 8644 30 nM. A, B, and C were obtained from the same muscle preparation. (Data from Reference 21.)

Ca conductance was elicited by BAY K8644 and this action was blocked by nisoldipine. FIGURE 6 shows the time course of the contractions of rat mesenteric artery evoked by KCl and by norepinephrine, before and after treatment with flunarizine 3×10^{-8} M. It is quite obvious that the pattern of inhibition of the contraction depends on the stimulus. The inhibition of norepinephrine-evoked contraction is unchanged during the 30 minute stimulation in the presence of flunarizine.[22] On the other hand, with KCl, the inhibition develops gradually being maximum after about 15 minutes. As FIGURE 7 illustrates, several potent dihydropyridines show the same time-dependent pattern of inhibition of KCl-evoked contractions, which could be reproduced in successive contractions, separated by a resting period of 30 minutes in physiological solution in the presence of drug. This time dependency is not observed with less potent drugs such as (−)PN 200-110 and (+)BAY K 8644, the antagonist enantiomer of BAY K 8644. As illustrated by us in another paper in this volume with (+)PN 200-110, the kinetics of inhibition during depolarization are similar to the kinetics of binding to isolated membranes.[23] This suggests that depolarization induces a conformation of calcium channels with increased affinity for dihydropyridines and that this high-affinity form is similar to that found in isolated membranes. This hypothesis has been examined in isolated rat mesenteric arteries by Morel and Godfraind, who have observed that the specific binding of (+)PN 200-110 was increased after prolonged depolarization when compared to binding in arteries bathed in physiological solution.[24] Both in polarized and depolarized arteries, specific binding was fitted by one hyperbolic curve, indicating a one-to-one binding to one class of sites. Maximum binding capacity was unchanged while apparent K_D was significantly lower in depolarized than in polarized arteries (respectively 44 ± 2 and 200 ± 20 pM); these binding data are consistent with the observations obtained in mechanical studies. These results indicate that calcium channels in vascular smooth muscle are modulated by membrane potential in a way similar to that reported for cardiac muscle by Bean[25] and by Reuter.[26]

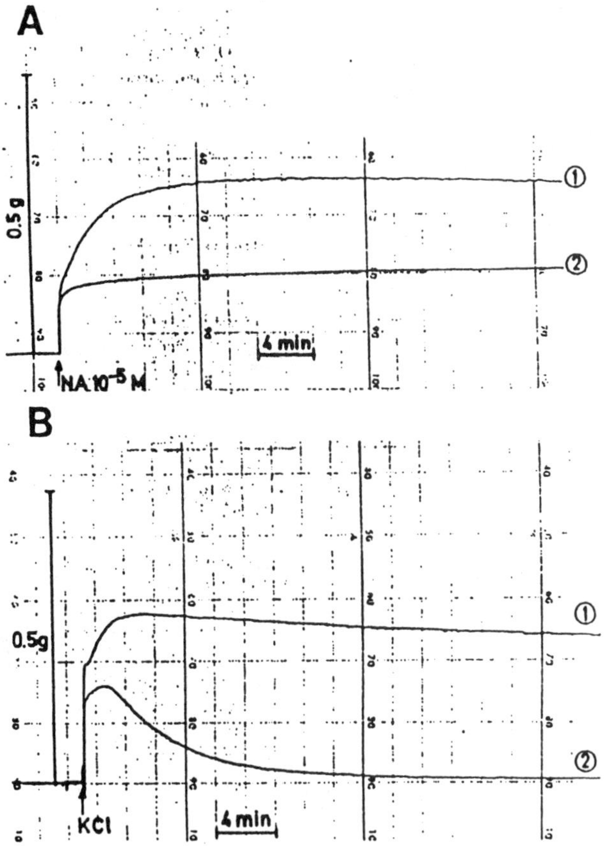

FIGURE 6. Typical experiments showing the effect of flunarizine (3×10^{-8} M) on norepinephrine (10^{-5} M) (A) or K-depolarizing solution (B) induced contraction of rat superior mesenteric artery. Control curve (1), curve in presence of flunarizine 90 minutes preincubated (2). (Data from Reference 22.)

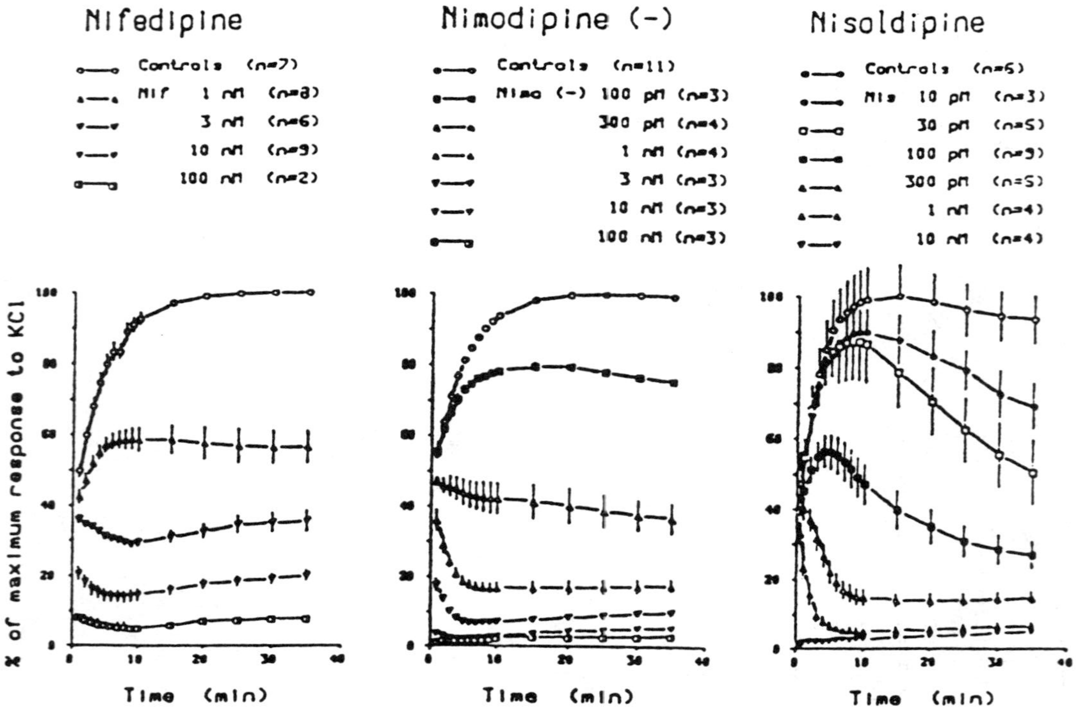

FIGURE 7. Time course of the contraction of rat aorta evoked by K depolarization before (control) and after 90 minutes preincubation with various concentrations of one of the dihydropyridines indicated on the graph. Note time-dependent inhibition mainly observable with nisoldipine. (Data from Reference 36.)

THE INTERACTION OF CALCIUM MODULATORS WITH ROCs

Let us now consider the effects of calcium entry blockers on responses to agonists, in particular norepinephrine and related sympathomimetics. As illustrated in FIGURE 8, nifedipine inhibits the contraction of rat aorta evoked by norepinephrine in a noncompetitive manner. Micromolar concentrations of nifedipine that completely blocked contraction evoked by depolarization reduce by only about 50% the maximal contraction evoked by the agonist in rat aorta. Godfraind has shown that the nifedipine-sensitive part of the contraction is attributable to an influx of Ca^{2+} and that

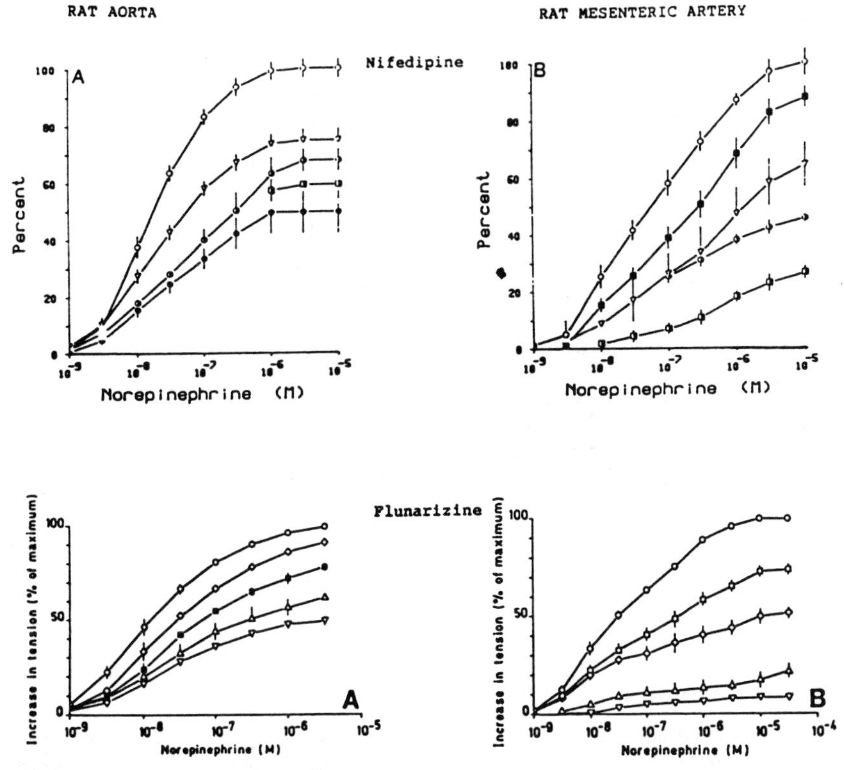

FIGURE 8. Upper panel: the effect of nifedipine on norepinephrine-induced contractions of rat aorta (A) and of rat superior mesenteric artery (B). Each graph shows concentration-effect curves obtained in the absence (open circles) and in the presence of various concentrations of nifedipine—2×10^{-9} M (filled squares); 10^{-8} M (open triangles); 10^{-7} M (half filled circles); 10^{-6} M (half filled squares); and 3×10^{-6} M (filled circles). Each curve is the mean of at least five experiments. SEM is indicated. The preparations were preincubated for 90 minutes in the presence of nifedipine. Lower panel: the effect of flunarizine on norepinephrine-induced contractions of rat aortae (A) and of rat superior mesenteric arteries (B). Each graph shows concentration-effect curves obtained in the absence (open circles) and in the presence of various concentrations of flunarizine—10^{-8} M (open squares); 3×10^{-8} M (open diamonds); 10^{-7} M (filled squares); and 3×10^{-6} M (open triangles). Each curve is the mean of at least five experiments. SEM is indicated. The preparations were preincubated for 90 minutes in the presence of flunarizine.

the potency of nifedipine as inhibitor of this influx is about 10-fold less than its potency as inhibitor of the Ca^{2+} entry induced by KCl depolarization.[35] As shown in FIGURE 9, high concentrations of other calcium entry blockers such as flunarizine or D600 also leave about 50% of the contraction unaffected.[27] A contraction of a similar magnitude is also evoked by norepinephrine in aortic preparations maintained for 10 minutes in a Ca^{2+}-free medium (while this treatment completely abolishes the mechanical response

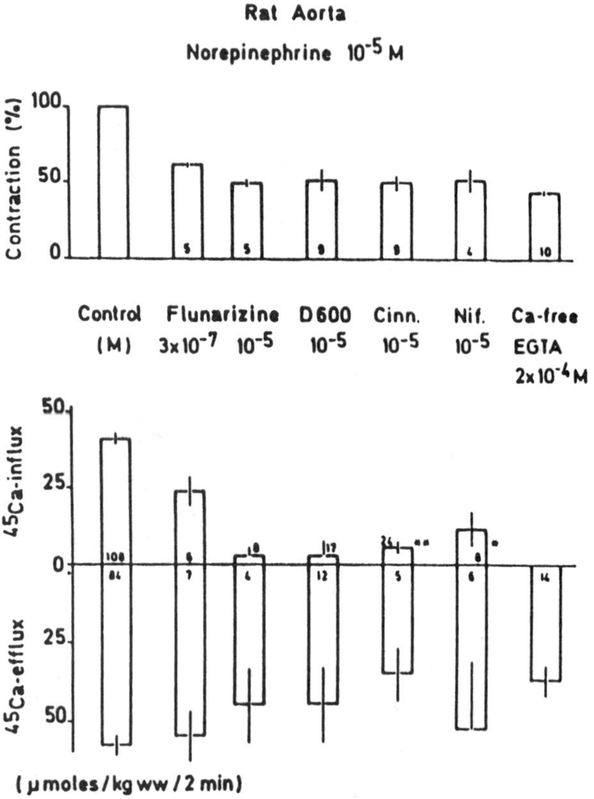

FIGURE 9. Effect of calcium entry blockers and of Ca^{2+}-free medium on contraction (top) and ^{45}Ca influx and efflux (bottom) evoked by norepinephrine (10 μM) in rat isolated aorta. Tissues were preincubated with blockers for 90 minutes, or with EGTA for 5 minutes, before addition of norepinephrine. Contractions are expressed as the percentage of the contraction induced in the absence of drug (control). Numbers in columns, number of determinations; vertical bars, SE. Cinn., cinnarizine; Nif., nifedipine. (Reproduced from Reference 27 with permission.)

to K^+ depolarization). Thus, we may conclude that calcium entry blockers block only that part of the contraction that depends on an influx of Ca^{2+} through receptor-operated channels. The other part, which persists after removal of extracellular Ca^{2+}, can be attributed to a mobilization of Ca^{2+} from internal stores, probably in the endoplasmic reticulum. It is likely that alpha-adrenoceptor activation induces an increased hydrolysis of phosphatidylinositol biphosphate in the plasma membrane, and that inositol 1,4,5-trisphosphate serves as a messenger from the plasma membrane to the endoplasmic reticulum and triggers the release of Ca^{2+} from this organelle.[28]

The effect of calcium entry blockers on agonist-evoked contractions may be substantially different in other arteries. For example, in rat mesenteric artery, less than 25% of the contraction evoked by norepinephrine is resistant to nifedipine and to flunarizine.[4] In rabbit aorta, calcium entry blockers are slightly effective on norepinephrine-induced contractions,[6] probably because these contractions are less dependent on extracellular Ca^{2+} in this tissue than they are in rat aorta. It has been reported that, in rabbit small mesenteric vessels, diltiazem is more potent as an inhibitor of agonist- than of K^+-induced contractions and ^{45}Ca influx.[29]

As previously shown in several studies in our laboratory, the dose-effect curves for inhibition of norepinephrine-evoked calcium influx and contraction are superimposed,[4] suggesting that the reduction of the noradrenaline effect on muscle tone was due to blockade of agonist-dependent ^{45}Ca entry that is specifically sensitive to blockers. As FIGURE 9 illustrates, at maximum effective concentration of several calcium entry blockers, part of the noradrenaline-dependent influx (10% to 15%) was resistant to blockade. This indicates that the contraction resistant to calcium entry blockers may be supported by this resistant calcium influx. However, in view of the presence of a large contraction in calcium-free medium, it is most likely that calcium may also originate from inside the cell to support the contraction resistant to calcium entry blockers. This is confirmed by the observation that norepinephrine evokes a release of calcium from arteries in calcium-free solution; this release is resistant to nifedipine and related drugs. FIGURE 9 also shows that the release of calcium evoked in physiological solution is barely affected by calcium entry blockers and therefore indicates that internal calcium release also occurs in the presence of extracellular calcium.

Yamamoto, Hwang, and van Breemen have shown in rabbit aorta that the agonist dihydropyridine BAY K 8644 could still produce contraction and increase calcium influx in tissue maximally stimulated by norepinephrine.[30] Those effects are blocked by an antagonist dihydropyridine ineffective against norepinephrine. The authors suggest that the additional contraction is due to POC—but not to ROC—activation.

ENDOTHELIUM MODULATES GATING OF ROCs

Endothelium plays a major role in vascular relaxation.[31] Removal of endothelium enhances the contractile response of rat aorta to alpha-adrenoceptor agonists. This enhanced response is highly sensitive to inhibition by calcium entry blockers.[32] This indicates that it is related to increased calcium entry during agonist stimulation. Experiments were designed in order to examine whether endothelium modulation of contraction was related to calcium channel gating during stimulation by norepinephrine and K depolarization. The effects of endothelium removal, of methylene blue, and of the lipid-soluble analogue of cyclic GMP, 8-bromo-cyclic GMP, were investigated on Ca influx and on contractile responses.[32]

As FIGURE 10 illustrates, removal of endothelium enhanced the contractile response to norepinephrine 10^{-8} M. The contractile force developed by aorta rings without endothelium was sixfold higher than the force developed by preparations with endothelium present ($p < 0.01$). A similar amplification of the response was observed in preparations pretreated with methylene blue 3×10^{-6} M during 10 minutes ($p < 0.01$). Treatment of aorta without endothelium by 8-bromo-cyclic GMP (10^{-4} M) reduced the contractile response to norepinephrine ($p < 0.01$) (FIGURE 11). Removal of endothelium evoked a small but significant increase of ^{45}Ca entry in unstimulated preparations. FIGURE 10 shows that norepinephrine-dependent ^{45}Ca entry was twofold higher in preparations without endothelium than in preparations with endothelium ($p < 0.01$). Pretreatment during 30 minutes of the preparations containing endothelium by methylene blue 3×10^{-6} M also enhanced norepinephrine-dependent ^{45}Ca entry ($p < 0.01$). Pretreatment of preparations without endothelium by 8-bromo-cyclic GMP 0.1 mM, during 30 minutes, resulted in a reduction of norepinephrine-dependent ^{45}Ca entry close to the level found in preparations with endothelium preserved ($p < 0.01$).

These observations show that vascular endothelium controls both ^{45}Ca entry and contraction evoked by norepinephrine. Removal of endothelium and inhibition of

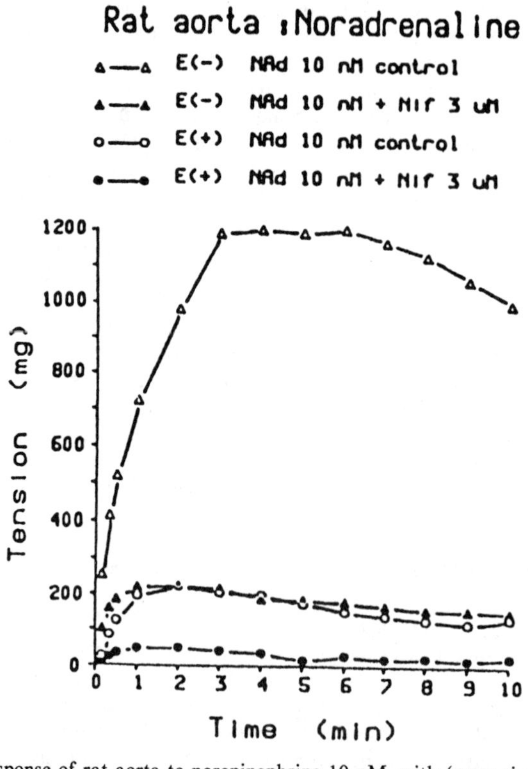

FIGURE 10. Response of rat aorta to norepinephrine 10 nM, with (open circles) and without (open triangles) endothelium: inhibition by nifedipine 3 μM. (Data from Reference 36.)

guanylate cyclase by methylene blue increased these responses. Increase in cellular cyclic GMP, a result of treatment with 8-bromo-cyclic GMP, allowed the observation, in preparations without endothelium, of responses close to those observed in preparations with endothelium. Experimental results reported in FIGURE 11 indicate that the gating of receptor-operated Ca channels by norepinephrine is sensitive to the presence of EDRF and to the cellular content in cyclic GMP. Those experimental observations show that endothelium modulates the response of vascular smooth muscle to alpha-adrenoceptor agonists. This modulation is related to changes in alpha-agonist efficacy and it changes the mode of antagonism of the alpha-1 antagonist prazosin, an effect

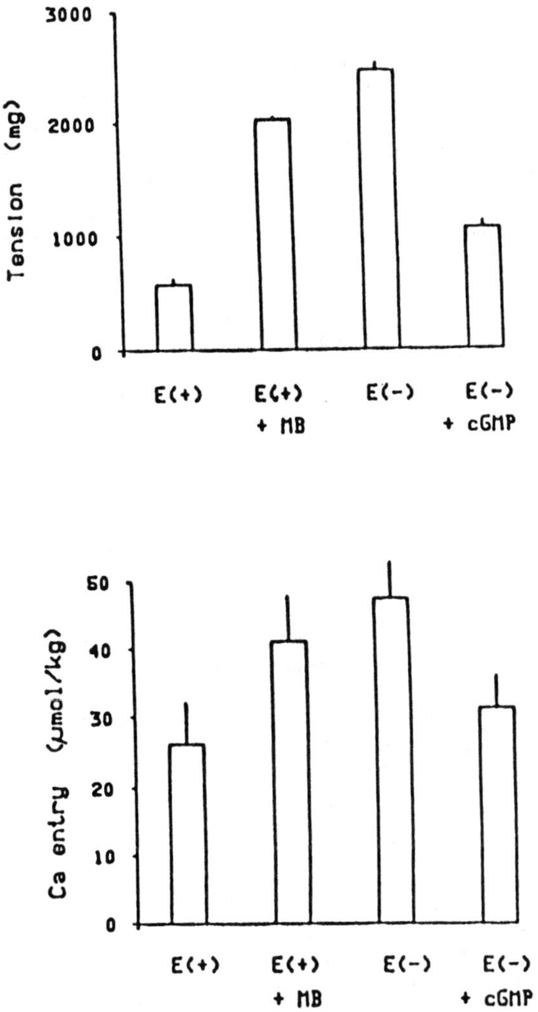

FIGURE 11. Upper panel: tonic contractile force (expressed in mg) developed by rings of rat aorta stimulated by norepinephrine 10^{-8} M. Each value is the mean of 6 determinations; SE is indicated on the graph: E(+), preparations with endothelium intact; E(+) + MB, preparations with endothelium intact pretreated with methylene blue during 10 minutes before adrenaline; E(−), preparations where endothelium was removed; E(−) + cGMP, preparations where endothelium was removed after pretreatment with cyclic GMP 0.1 mM during 30 minutes before noradrenaline. Lower panel: ^{45}Ca influx (expressed in μmol/kg wet weight) in preparations treated by norepinephrine 10^{-8} M during 2 minutes; each value is the mean of 12 determinations; SE is indicated on the graph; symbols: see above. (Data from Reference 32.)

attributed to change in receptor reserve that affects agonists action. This change in receptor reserve appears to be related to suppression of the inhibitory effect of EDRF(s) on the gating of adrenoceptor-operated calcium channels.[33]

CONCLUDING REMARKS

As already pointed out above, some uncertainty is still prevalent concerning similarities and differences of ROCs and POCs, although it is well demonstrated that there are different POCs in pericellular membranes with different sensitivities to membrane potential. The activation of receptors evokes in many tissues both a release of intracellularly bound calcium and the opening of ROCs. The former action is related to the stimulation of inositol phospholipid metabolism to produce IP_3, responsible for the release of intracellular calcium. Recently another inositol phosphate, IP_4, has been shown to regulate cellular calcium,[34] probably by opening of calcium channels. This concept is very promising but it needs further evaluation. Nevertheless, it is attractive to consider the hypothesis of a modulation of calcium channels in vascular smooth muscles by regional factors such as EDRFs (stimulating guanylate cyclase) having an effect opposite to vasoconstrictor agonists (stimulating inostol phospholipid metabolism).

ACKNOWLEDGMENT

I thank M. Wibo for reading the manuscript.

REFERENCES

1. HODGKIN, A. L. & A. F. HUXLEY. 1952. J. Physiol. **115:** 473–496.
2. BULBRING, E., A. F. BRADING, A. W. JONES & T. TOMITA, Eds. 1981. Smooth Muscle: an Assessment of Current Knowledge. Edward Arnold Ltd. London, England.
3. FATT, P. & B. KATZ. 1953. J. Physiol. **120:** 171–204.
4. GODFRAIND, T., R. MILLER & M. WIBO. 1986. Pharmacol. Rev. **38:** 321–416.
5. WEISS, G. B. & F. R. GOODMAN. 1969. J. Pharmacol. Exp. Ther. **169:** 46–55.
6. VAN BREEMEN, C., C. CAUVIN, A. JOHNS, P. LEIJTEN & H. HAMAMOTO. 1986. Fed. Proc. **45:** 2746–2751.
7. GODFRAIND, T. 1976. J. Physiol. London **260:** 21–35.
8. EDMAN, K. A. P. & H. O. SCHILD. 1962. J. Physiol. London **161:** 424–441.
9. VAN NUETEN, J. M. 1969. Eur. J. Pharmacol. **6:** 286–293.
10. BOLTON, T. B. 1979. Physiol. Rev. **59:** 606–718.
11. BEVAN, J. A., R. D. BEVAN, J. J. HWA, M. P. OWEN, F. M. TAYO & R. J. WINQUIST. 1982. Calcium intrinsic (myogenic) vascular tone. *In* Calcium Modulators. T. Godfraind, A. Albertini & R. Paoletti, Eds.: 125–132. Elsevier Biomedical Press. Amsterdam, Holland.
12. MEISHERI, K. D., O. HWANG & C. VAN BREEMEN. 1981. J. Membr. Biol. **59:** 19–25.
13. TSIEN, R. W. 1983. Annu. Rev. Physiol. **45:** 341–358.
14. BEAN, B. P., M. STUREK, A. PUGA & K. HERMSMEYER. 1986. Circ. Res. **59:** 229–235.
15. WORLEY, J. F., J. W. DEITMER & M. T. NELSON. 1986. Proc. Nat. Acad. Sci. USA **83:** 5746–5750.
16. DROOGMANS, G. & G. CALLEWAERT. 1986. Pflügers Arch. **406:** 259–265.
17. MOREL, N. & T. GODFRAIND. 1982. Arch. Int. Pharmacodyn. Ther. **258:** 319–321.
18. GODFRAIND, T., N. MOREL & M. WIBO. 1986. Scand. J. Clin. Lab. Invest. **46**(Suppl. 180): 29–40.

19. GODFRAIND, T. & A. KABA. 1969. Br. J. Pharmacol. **35:** 354P–355P.
20. MRAS, S. & N. SPERELAKIS. 1981. Eur. J. Pharmacol. **71:** 13–19.
21. MOREL, N., J. P. HARDY & T. GODFRAIND. Eur. J. Pharmacol. (Submitted.)
22. GODFRAIND, T. & D. DIEU. 1981. J. Pharmacol. Exp. Ther. **217:** 510–515.
23. WIBO, M. & T. GODFRAIND. Ann. N.Y. Acad. Sci. (This volume.)
24. MOREL, N. & T. GODFRAIND. J. Pharmacol. Exp. Ther. (In press.)
25. BEAN, B. P. 1984. Proc. Nat. Acad. Sci. USA **81:** 6388–6392.
26. REUTER, H., H. PORZIG, S. KOKUBUN & B. PROD'HOM. 1985. J. Gen. Physiol. **86:** 5A–6A.
27. GODFRAIND, T. & R. C. MILLER. 1983. Circ. Res. **52:** 81–91.
28. SOMLYO, A. V., M. BOND, A. P. SOMLYO & A. SCARPA. 1985. Proc. Nat. Acad. Sci. USA **82:** 5231–5235.
29. CAUVIN, C. & C. VAN BREEMEN. 1985. J. Cardiovasc. Pharmacol. **7:** S4–S10.
30. YAMAMOTO, H., O. HWANG & C. VAN BREEMEN. 1984. Eur. J. Pharmacol. **102:** 555–557.
31. FURCHGOTT, R. F. & J. V. ZAWADZKI. 1980. Nature **288:** 373–376.
32. GODFRAIND, T. 1986. Eur. J. Pharmacol. **126:** 341–343.
33. ALOSACHIE, I. & T. GODFRAIND. 1986. Br. J. Pharmacol. **89:** 525–532.
34. HOUSLAY, M. D. 1987. Trends Biochem. Sci. **12:** 1–2.
35. GODFRAIND, T. 1983. J. Pharmacol. Exp. Ther. **224:** 443–450.
36. GODFRAIND, T. 1986. Acta Pharmacol. Toxicol. **58**(Suppl. II): 5–30.

Calcium Transients in Smooth Muscle[a]

KATHLEEN G. MORGAN, ARLENE BRADLEY,[b]
AND TIA T. DEFEO

Charles A. Dana Research Institute
and Harvard Thorndike Laboratory
Department of Medicine
Harvard Medical School
Beth Israel Hospital
330 Brookline Avenue
Boston, Massachusetts 02215

INTRODUCTION

The importance of calcium in the generation and maintenance of tone in vascular smooth muscle has been acknowledged for many years; however, this is largely based on indirect experiments and analogy to skeletal and cardiac muscle. Many investigators have observed a dependence of contractile force on the presence of extracellular calcium although exceptions have been reported where contractions occur in the absence of extracellular calcium.[1] This latter phenomenon is sometimes referred to as "pharmacomechanical coupling." Similarly, calcium influx studies have demonstrated a partial correlation between influx of calcium and strength of contraction.[2,3] Data from chemically skinned smooth muscle preparation have demonstrated, more directly, a dependence of the contractile apparatus on ionized calcium levels (for example, see Reference 4). However, it is well recognized that the process of chemical skinning can cause the loss of calmodulin and other regulatory components of the contractile apparatus; thus, there has been a need for the development of an application of calcium indicator technology to smooth muscle. Although this developmental stage has not yet been completed, significant gains have been achieved in the past seven or eight years which will be described below.

CHOICE OF CALCIUM INDICATOR IN SMOOTH MUSCLE

At the time of this writing, the majority of the published studies performed to directly measure cytoplasmic ionized calcium levels ($[Ca^{2+}]_i$) in vascular smooth muscle have been performed with the photoprotein aequorin; however, in the last year there has been a tremendous expansion of the calcium indicator field as the result of the introduction of fura-2 and indo-1, fluorescent indicators that can be readily loaded into smooth muscle cells and that produce signals that can be recorded on commercially available apparatus. A detailed comparison of the relative advantages and disadvantages of luminescent indicators versus fluorescent indicators in smooth muscle has been presented elsewhere,[5,6] but the two points to be emphasized here are (1) there

[a]Supported in part by National Institutes of Health Grant HL31704 and an Established Investigatorship to KGM.

[b]Present affiliation: Cardiovascular Division, Harper Hospital, Wayne State University, 3990 John R., Detroit, Mich. 48201.

is no "perfect" calcium indicator available and (2) we continue to be biased toward the use of aequorin as an indicator of $[Ca^{2+}]_i$ in intact smooth muscle (even though fluorescent indicators may offer advantages in studies on subcellular imaging). There are two main reasons for our bias: (1) aequorin is a well-established $[Ca^{2+}]_i$ indicator for which the limitations of interpretation that must be placed on the signals are well established; and (2) aequorin's nonlinear properties may be necessary in order to detect the very small changes in calcium that appear to accompany tonic contractions in vascular smooth muscle.

CORRELATIONS BETWEEN CALCIUM AND FORCE

It appears that the simplest correlation between $[Ca^{2+}]_i$ and force occurs in the case of contractures induced by low concentrations of potassium. FIGURE 1 shows typical simultaneously recorded $[Ca^{2+}]_i$ and force profiles from a ferret aorta in response to increasing doses of potassium. At each concentration, relatively parallel, monotonic increases in $[Ca^{2+}]_i$ and force are observed. One has to keep in mind that this is a multicellular preparation where there could be minor temporal differences as a

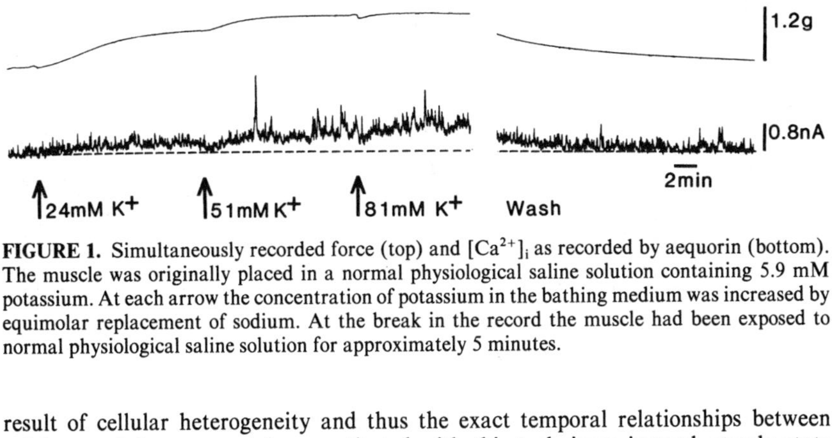

FIGURE 1. Simultaneously recorded force (top) and $[Ca^{2+}]_i$ as recorded by aequorin (bottom). The muscle was originally placed in a normal physiological saline solution containing 5.9 mM potassium. At each arrow the concentration of potassium in the bathing medium was increased by equimolar replacement of sodium. At the break in the record the muscle had been exposed to normal physiological saline solution for approximately 5 minutes.

result of cellular heterogeneity and thus the exact temporal relationships between calcium and force cannot be quantitated with this technique; instead, steady state relationships should be emphasized. It should be noted from this figure, that, at the higher doses of potassium (i.e., above 51 mM), further increases in $[Ca^{2+}]_i$ (as indicated by aequorin) are observed, even though further increases in force are not detected. A similar phenomenon was previously reported for ferret portal vein.[7] These results suggest that some calcium regulatory site associated with the contractile apparatus has been saturated at the $[Ca^{2+}]_i$ achieved with 51 mM potassium depolarization.

When these aequorin signals are translated into absolute calcium concentrations, $[Ca^{2+}]_i$-force curves can be obtained,[8] such as that shown in FIGURE 2. A number of assumptions are included in the quantitation of aequorin signals, as is true of the calibration of any calcium indicator. With respect to aequorin, the critical assumptions are (1) that $[Ca^{2+}]_i$ is uniform throughout the cytoplasmic space (since aequorin will cause a magnification of any focal areas of high $[Ca^{2+}]_i$ and cause them to appear to dominate the "average" signal) and (2) $[Mg^{2+}]_i$ is assumed to be 0.5 mM. This is an important assumption because the luminescence-$[Ca^{2+}]$ curve is shifted to the right by increasing $[Mg^{2+}]_i$ in the physiologic range. The first assumption is probably relatively safe to make for a steady state potassium contracture, since it seems unlikely that large cytoplasmic gradients could be maintained in small, 2–5 micron diameter, cells for the time courses described here (on the order of 5–10 minutes). This assumption becomes much more questionable in the case of spikelike signals seen with other agonists in smooth muscles and in striated muscle in response to electrical stimulation. The second assumption is more controversial. Until recently, there were no direct measurements of $[Mg^{2+}]_i$ in smooth muscle. However, recent NMR smooth muscle studies do indicate that $[Mg^{2+}]_i$ ranges around 0.5 mM.[9]

Keeping these limitations in mind, the calcium-force curves generated by this

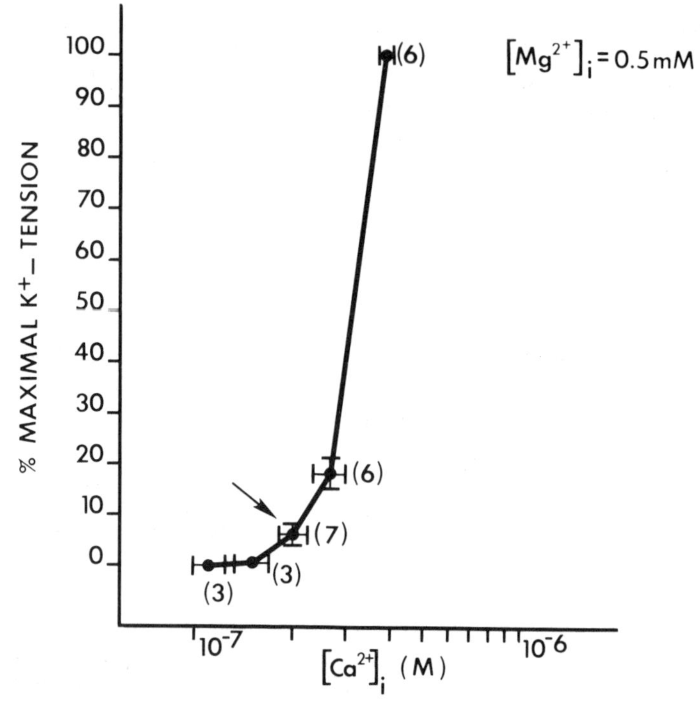

FIGURE 2. Calcium-force curve from aequorin-loaded intact ferret portal vein at 35°C. The arrow indicates the unstimulated muscle in normal physiological saline solution. (Reprinted from Reference 8 with permission.)

method are rather interesting. A small amount of intrinsic tone is observed in the ferret portal vein under resting conditions, but depletion of extracellular calcium to the extent that $[Ca^{2+}]_i$ is lowered to 100 nM removes all active tone from the muscle. Although, for technical reasons, only a limited number of points on the calcium-force curve can be obtained in an individual muscle, it is obvious that the curve shows an extreme steepness. Moving up the curve from the fully relaxed muscle to the fully contracted muscle appears to require only doubling or tripling of resting $[Ca^{2+}]_i$. Comparing the aequorin results to skinned smooth muscle preparations is difficult because of the tremendous diversity of results that have been obtained in the various types of skinned muscles. The $[Ca^{2+}]_i$ threshold obtained with aequorin compares reasonably well with the same parameter estimated from some skinned muscle experiments, but the slope is generally much less steep in the skinned preparations.[10–12] However, when very fresh muscles are used with only short incubation times in the skinning solutions, it may be possible to produce curves of increased slope.[13] It is also generally acknowledged that chemical skinning of smooth muscle is a traumatic process which can result in the loss of calmodulin or other calcium regulatory substances, which could cause a rightward shift or a change in the slope of the calcium-force relationship. It is of interest that the calcium dependence of myosin light chain phosphorylation and also of myosin ATPase activation has been reported to be similarly more steep than the Ca-force relationship in most chemically skinned smooth muscles.[14] Additionally, a report using the fluorescent indicator fura-2 has appeared indicating relatively similar results to the aequorin results.[15]

At 22°C, resting $[Ca^{2+}]_i$ is 1.8×10^{-7}M in the ferret portal vein, which has little resting tone, and 2.7×10^{-7}M in the ferret aorta, which has considerable resting tone.[8] These are "reasonable" values since they are slightly higher than values reported for striated muscle,[5] which does not have intrinsic tone, and similar values are now being reported with fluorescent indicators in isolated smooth muscle cells.[16]

If these $[Ca^{2+}]_i$-force curves are taken as valid, then the question arises as to the mechanism of this steepness and the identity of the calcium binding site (or sites) involved. It is generally thought that activation of myosin light chain kinase by calcium and calmodulin is a requirement for most contractions of smooth muscle. One could try to compare the $[Ca]_i$-force curves to what is known about the calcium sensitivity of myosin light chain kinase; however, myosin light chain kinase has been reported to be positively cooperative with regard to $[Ca^{2+}]$, indicating that the enzyme could be activated by small changes in $[Ca^{2+}]_i$ with the mechanism acting like "an on-off switch."[17] However, it is very difficult to determine an overall apparent K_d for the system with respect to $[Ca^{2+}]$ since the actual $[Ca^{2+}]_i$ required for activation depends not only upon the free calmodulin concentrations but also on the ratio of the calmodulin concentration to the concentration of the enzyme.[17] The concentration of myosin light chain kinase in smooth muscle is approximately 0.5-1 μM,[18–20] but the calmodulin concentration is difficult to estimate since there will be competition for binding to calmodulin binding proteins other than myosin light chain kinase. Kamm and Stull have suggested that, in tracheal smooth muscle, there is sufficient calmodulin in the intact muscle to fully activate myosin light chain kinase and based on these assumptions have suggested a theoretical $[Ca^{2+}]_i$-activation curve for the system that would be far to the right of the $[Ca^{2+}]_i$-force curve we have measured with aequorin in our vascular smooth muscles.[21] Obviously these sorts of measurements need to be obtained directly, in the same tissue.

AGONIST-INDUCED VARIATION IN THE RELATIONSHIP BETWEEN CALCIUM AND FORCE

Although the calcium profile during a potassium contracture generally parallels the force profile very closely, in actuality, the first calcium transients to be recorded during vascular smooth muscle contractions showed considerable dissociation between $[Ca^{2+}]_i$ and force.[22] An example of this sort of dissociation is shown in FIGURE 3, where the $[Ca^{2+}]_i$ and force recordings to two different agonists recorded in the same ferret portal vein are shown at the same gain. Again, the $[Ca^{2+}]_i$ profile more or less parallels the force profile in response to potassium depolarization, but in response to phenylephrine, there is a transient large elevation in $[Ca^{2+}]_i$ during the development of the tonic

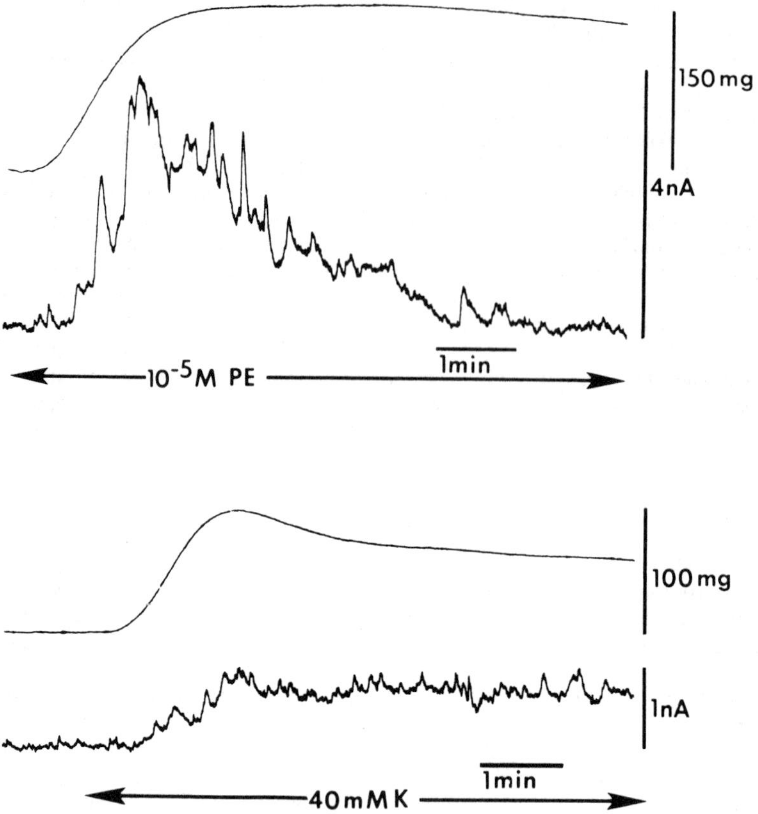

FIGURE 3. Effect of phenylephrine (PE) and a potassium depolarization on force (top) and light (bottom) in an aequorin-loaded ferret portal vein strips. Both sets of traces from the same muscle. (Reprinted from Reference 7 with permission.)

contraction followed by a fall of $[Ca^{2+}]_i$ back to a near-basal plateau level during tone maintenance.

We have seen many similar examples of spikelike initial elevations followed by lower plateau levels of $[Ca^{2+}]_i$ in the presence of several different agonists in different types of smooth muscle.[8,23,24] But, since this is not the "expected" $[Ca^{2+}]_i$ profile, the challenge has been to demonstrate that this is not an artifact of a new methodology but, rather, an accurate reflection of the intracellular events. Of particular concern is the possibility that the magnifying properties of aequorin might artifactually produce the initial spike by magnifying a relatively unimportant focal $[Ca^{2+}]_i$ signal or, alternatively, that the fall in $[Ca^{2+}]_i$ after the spikelike elevation is due to consumption of aequorin. The latter argument is easier to disprove, simply because these responses are reproducible. We have also produced essentially identical responses to phenylephrine and potassium in single individual enzymatically isolated smooth muscle cells loaded with a fluorescent indicator[25] (which is linear in response to $[Ca^{2+}]_i$ and would be less likely to magnify a focal signal).

We have been particularly intrigued with the fact that, in the steady state, the amount of force maintained per unit elevation in $[Ca^{2+}]_i$ differs in the presence of different agonists. For example, in FIGURE 3, the steady state force/calcium ratio is much greater than the steady state force/calcium ratio in the presence of potassium depolarization.

We have seen extreme examples where contractions can occur in the absence of any convincing change in intracellular $[Ca^{2+}]_i$. Two examples are the $PGF2_\alpha$-induced contraction of the hog coronary artery[23] and the phorbol ester–induced contraction of the ferret aorta.[26] An example of the former is shown in FIGURE 4. This illustration demonstrates the largest change in $[Ca^{2+}]_i$ we have seen in response to $PGF2_\alpha$ and compares it to the increase in $[Ca^{2+}]_i$ during a contraction of much lesser magnitude produced by potassium. Although the potassium causes a significant elevation in $[Ca^{2+}]_i$, $PGF2_\alpha$ produces a much larger contraction with no convincing sustained increase in $[Ca^{2+}]_i$.

The finding of the occurrence of contractions in the virtual absence of any change in $[Ca^{2+}]_i$ has suggested to us that there may be calcium-independent pathways. However, when we have pursued these possibilities we have found that, in the rat aorta, even when no detectable increase in $[Ca^{2+}]_i$ occurs during the development of a phorbol ester–induced contraction, if $[Ca^{2+}]_i$ is made to decrease far enough below baseline, the magnitude of the contraction does decrease.[26] Thus, the process appears to be calcium dependent, in that a calcium-force curve could be drawn, but the curve would be shifted to the left of the normal curve. The cause of the apparent change in $[Ca^{2+}]_i$ sensitivity is, at the present time, unknown.

Many investigators have hypothesized, for many reasons, that there is a "second system," i.e., a calcium regulatory system other than myosin light chain kinase; and many have postulated that this second system has a relatively high sensitivity to $[Ca^{2+}]_i$. Our results with phorbol esters have led us to postulate (as have others) that the "second system" might involve protein kinase C.[27–29] A useful way to think of smooth muscle, with the information that we currently have available, is that it *might* be "a two-kinase system" as is illustrated in FIGURE 5. Others have shown that increased myosin light chain kinase activity and the consequent increased phosphorylation of the myosin light chains result in an increased V_{max} of the muscle.[30] The role of the spikelike elevations of $[Ca^{2+}]_i$ we have observed with some agonists may be to increase maximal cross-bridge cycling velocities or to "prime" the system and to serve a sort of trigger function to initiate muscle contraction. Then protein kinase C may play a role by phosphorylating another regulatory protein which causes the maintenance of tension in the presence of a much lower $[Ca^{2+}]_i$. Consistent with this idea, many of the agonists that we have observed to produce high steady state force/calcium

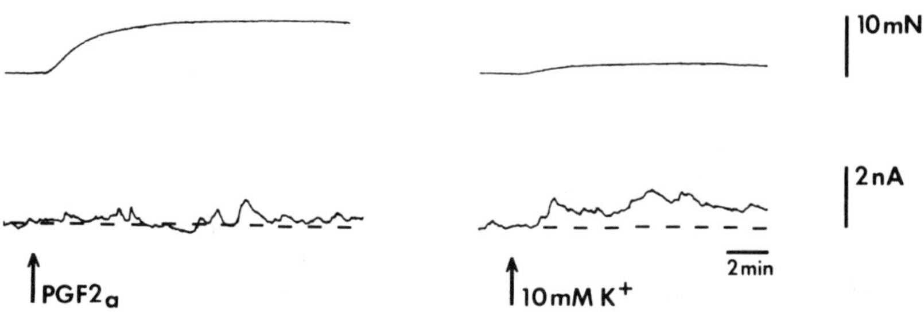

FIGURE 4. Two sets of traces from the same coronary artery, force (top) and light (bottom). (Reprinted from Reference 23 with permission.)

ratios are also agents that either have been shown to increase polyphosphoinositide turnover or have been shown directly to increase diacylglycerol levels, suggesting an activation of protein kinase C,[29,31,32] such that its calcium requirement is lowered to the range of resting calcium levels. The main problem with this hypothesis is that we do not know the identity of the pertinent protein that protein kinase C phosphorylates. There are a number of putative actin-binding proteins that have been speculated to play a role in tone maintenance. The one about which we know the most is caldesmon which is an inhibitory actin-binding protein. When Ca calmodulin is bound to caldesmon the inhibition is reversed.[33,34] Thus, this could provide a feasible "second system." There are, however, many other possibilities. Caldesmon itself is also phosphorylated by a calmodulin and a calcium-dependent kinase,[34] and there are other actin-binding proteins that have been suggested, such as desmin and filamin, some of which have also been reported to be phosphorylated by protein kinase C.[35,36]

RELEVANCE TO CALCIUM CHANNEL BLOCKERS

There have been isolated reports of the effects of calcium channel blockers to inhibit vascular smooth muscle by mechanisms other than preventing calcium influx. However these reports remain controversial, particularly with respect to the likelihood that they occur in physiologic concentrations, or even in therapeutic concentrations. It has been well documented in many different vascular muscles that the contraction in response to potassium depolarization will be blocked by blocking influx through the voltage-dependent calcium channels, and similarly many, but not all, agonist-induced contractions require calcium influx. However, it has been postulated that the voltage-dependent calcium channel which is preferentially blocked by the calcium channel blockers is only one mode of influx of calcium and that there are voltage-independent

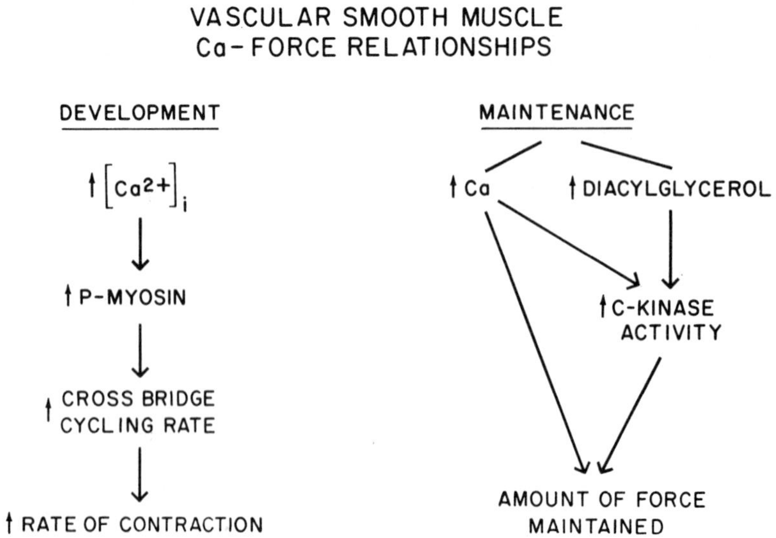

FIGURE 5. Hypothetical scheme describing smooth muscle as a "two kinase system." See text for details.

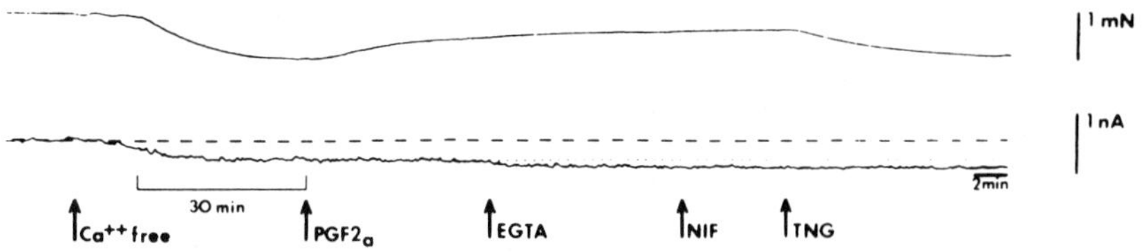

FIGURE 6. Simultaneously recorded force (top) and light (bottom) recordings from a hog coronary artery. (Reprinted in part from Reference 23 with permission.) See text for details.

or "receptor-operated channels" also present in vascular smooth muscle.[37] Additionally, we have shown that contractions can occur in vascular smooth muscle by virtue of a change in the sensitivity of the contractile apparatus to calcium with no necessary change in the actual $[Ca^{2+}]$ in the cytoplasm.[26] In these cases it might be expected that calcium channel blockers would not be effective in reversing the contractions.

An example of a situation where a calcium channel blocker is not effective in relaxing a contraction is shown in FIGURE 6. This recording is from an aequorin-loaded hog coronary artery.[23] The initial maneuver was to switch from a normal physiological saline solution to a calcium-free physiological saline solution. This causes a decrease in the level of intrinsic tone of the preparation, and, interestingly, this is accompanied by, and possibly caused by, a drop in $[Ca^{2+}]_i$ below the original position of resting $[Ca^{2+}]_i$ (as indicated by the dashed line). After more than 30 minutes equilibration in calcium-free physiological saline solution, $PGF2_\alpha$ is added to the bath and this causes a contraction of the muscle in the absence of any detectable change in $[Ca^{2+}]_i$. That we were not below the level of detection of aequorin was demonstrated by the fact that the addition of EGTA to further lower the extracellular $[Ca^{2+}]$, and consequently $[Ca^{2+}]_i$, did cause a detectable decrease in the aequorin signal. The addition of nifedipine at a subsequent point in time did not cause any further detectable decrease in intracellular calcium and, more importantly, did not cause any drop in tone. In contrast, the addition of nitroglycerine was effective in decreasing the generated tone. Since $[Ca^{2+}]_i$ would be expected to be very low at this point, the fact that no fall in calcium was detected with nitroglycerin has to be viewed with caution. At that point we might well have been below the level of detection of $[Ca^{2+}]$ with aequorin. However, there must be some difference in the mechanism of action of nitroglycerine that allows it to be effective in inhibiting these contractions which do not seem to require an increase in $[Ca^{2+}]_i$. Results like this are suggestive that nitroglycerine might be an agent that is effective against the "second system."

ACKNOWLEDGMENTS

The authors acknowledge the helpful critical review of the manuscript by M. J. Jiang, and secretarial assistance of S. E. Reynolds.

REFERENCES

1. DEVINE, C. E., A. V. SOMLYO & A. P. SOMLYO. 1972. Sarcoplasmic reticulum and excitation-contraction coupling in mammalian smooth muscle. J. Cell. Biol. **52:** 690–718.

2. VAN BREEMEN, C. 1977. Calcium requirement for activation of intact aortic smooth muscle. J. Physiol. **272:** 317–329.
3. VAN BREEMEN, C., B. R. FARINAS, R. CASTEELS, P. GERBA, F. WUYTACK & R. DETH. 1973. Factors controlling cytoplasmic Ca^{2+} concentration. Phil. Trans. R. Soc. London Ser. B **265:** 57–71.
4. ENDO, M., T. KITAZAWA, S. Y. YAGI, M. INDO & Y. KAKUTA. 1977. Some properties of chemically skinned smooth muscle fibers. *In* Excitation-Contraction Coupling in Smooth Muscle. R. Casteels, T. Godfraind & J. Ruegg, Eds.: 199–209. Elsevier. Amsterdam, Holland.
5. BLINKS, J. R., W. G. WIER, P. HESS & F. G. PRENDERGAST. 1982. Measurement of Ca^{2+} concentrations in living cells. Prog. Biophys. Mol. Biol. **40:** 1–114.
6. MORGAN, K. G. & F. V. BROZOVICH. Intracellular calcium levels and arterial smooth muscle. *In* Essential Hypertension and Calcium: Calcium Ions, Calcium Channels, Calcium Agonists and Antagonists. K. Aoki & E. D. Frohlich, Eds. Academic Press. New York, N.Y. (In press.)
7. MORGAN, J. P. & K. G. MORGAN. 1984. Stimulus-specific patterns of intracellular calcium levels in smooth muscle of the ferret portal vein. J. Physiol **351:** 155–167.
8. DEFEO, T. T. & K. G. MORGAN. 1985. Calcium-force relationships as detected with aequorin in two different vascular smooth muscles of the ferret. J. Physiol. **369:** 269–282.
9. KUSHMERICK, M. J., P. F. DILLON, R. A. MEYER, T. R. BROWN, J. M. KRISANDA & H. L. SWEENEY. 1986. ^{31}P NMR spectroscopy, chemical analysis and free Mg^{2+} of rabbit bladder and uterine smooth muscle. J. Biol. Chem. **261:** 14420–14430.
10. PETERSON, J. W. 1982. Rate-limiting steps in the tension development of freeze-glycerinated vascular smooth muscle. J. Gen. Physiol. **79:** 437–452.
11. RUEGG, J. C. & R. J. PAUL. 1982. Vascular smooth muscle; calmodulin and cyclic AMP-dependent protein kinase alter calcium sensitivity in porcine carotid skinned fibers. Circ. Res. **50:** 394–399.
12. ITOH, T., H. KURIYAMA & H. UENO. 1983. Mechanisms of the nitroglycerine-induced vasodilation in vascular smooth muscle of the rabbit and pig. J. Physiol. **343:** 233–252.
13. HOAR, P. E., W. G. L. KERRICK & P. S. CASSIDY. 1979. Chicken gizzard: relation between calcium-activated phosphorylation and contraction. Science **204:** 503–506.
14. SOBIESZEK, A. 1977. Ca-linked phosphorylation of a light chain of vertebrate smooth muscle myosin. J. Biochem. **73:** 477–483.
15. WILLIAMS, D. A., K. E. FOGARTY & F. S. FAY. 1986. Maximum cell shortening in single smooth cells requires only small transient changes in cytosolic Ca^{2+}. J. Gen. Physiol. **88:** 61a.
16. WILLIAMS, D. A., K. E. FOGARTY, R. Y. TSIEN & F. S. FAY. 1985. Calcium gradients in single smooth muscle cells revealed by the digital imaging microscope using Fura-2. Nature **318:** 558–561.
17. STULL, J. T., M. H. NUNNALLY & C. H. MICHNOFF. 1986. Calmodulin-dependent protein kinases. Enzymes **17:** 113–166. (Academic Press. New York, N.Y.)
18. ADELSTEIN, R. S. & E. EISENBERG. 1980. Regulation and kinetics of the actin-myosin-ATP interaction. Annu. Rev. Biochem. **49:** 921–956.
19. ADELSTEIN, R. S. & C. B. KLEE. 1981. Purification and characterization of smooth muscle myosin light chain kinase. J. Biol. Chem. **256:** 7501–7509.
20. WALSH, M. P., S. HINKINS, I. L. FLINK & D. J. HARTSHORNE. 1982. Bovine stomach myosin light chain kinase: purification, characterization and comparison with the turkey gizzard enzyme. Biochemistry **21:** 6890–6896.
21. KAMM, K. E. & J. T. STULL. 1985. The function of myosin and myosin light chain kinase phosphorylation in smooth muscle. Annu. Rev. Pharmacol. Toxicol. **25:** 593–620.
22. MORGAN, J. P. & K. G. MORGAN. 1982. Vascular smooth muscle: the first recorded Ca^{2+} transients. Pflugers Arch. **395:** 75–77.
23. BRADLEY, A. B. & K. G. MORGAN. 1986. Alterations in cytoplasmic calcium sensitivity during porcine coronary artery contractions as determined by aequorin. J. Physiol. **385:** 437–448.
24. MORGAN, K. G. & M. J. JIANG. 1986. Measurement of cytoplasmic Ca^{2+} during tonic and phasic contractions of mammalian smooth muscle. Excerpta Med.: 109–123.

25. DeFeo, T. T. & K. G. Morgan. 1986. A comparison of two different indicators: quin 2 and aequorin in isolated single cells. Pflugers Arch. **405:** 77–79.
26. Jiang, M. J. & K. G. Morgan. 1986. Intracellular Ca^{++} levels in phorbol ester induced contractions of ferret aorta. Biophys. J. **49:** 188a.
27. Rasmussen, H., J. Forder, I. Kojima & A. Scriabine. 1984. TPA-induced contraction of isolated rabbit vascular smooth muscle. Biochem. Biophys. Res. Commun. **122:** 775–784.
28. Danthuluri, N. R. & R. C. Deth. 1984. Phorbol ester–induced contraction of arterial smooth muscle and inhibition of alpha-adrenergic response. Biochem. Biophys. Res. Commun. **125:** 1103–1109.
29. Nishizuka, Y. 1984. The role of protein kinase C in cell surface signal transduction and tumor promotion. Nature **308:** 693–698.
30. Dillon, P. F., M. O. Aksoy, S. P. Driska & R. A. Murphy. 1981. Myosin phosphorylation and the crossbridge cycle in arterial smooth muscle. Science **211:** 495–497.
31. Williamson, J. R., R. H. Cooper, S. K. Joseph & A. P. Thomas. 1985. Inositol triphosphate and diacylglycerol as intracellular second messengers in liver. Am. J. Physiol. **248:** 203–216.
32. Griendling, K. K., S. E. Rittenhouse, T. A. Brock, L. K. Ekstein, M. A. Gimbrone & R. W. Alexander. 1986. Sustained diacylglycerol formation from inositol phospholipids in angiotension II–stimulated vascular smooth muscle cells. J. Biol. Chem. **261:** 5901–5906.
33. Clark, T., P. K. Ngai, C. Sutherland, U. Groschel-Stewart & M. P. Walsh. 1986. Vascular smooth muscle caldesmon. J. Biol. Chem. **261:** 8026–8035.
34. Marston, S. B. & W. Lehman. 1985. Caldesmon is a Ca^{2+}-regulatory component of native smooth muscle thin filaments. Biochem. J. **231:** 517–522.
35. Small, J. V., D. O. Fust & J. DeMey. 1986. Localization of filamin in smooth muscle. J. Cell. Biol. **102:** 210–220.
36. Park, S. & H. Rasmussen. 1986. Carbachol-induced protein phosphorylation changes in bovine tracheal smooth muscle. J. Biol. Chem. **261:** 15734–15739.
37. Bolton, T. B. 1979. Mechanisms of action of transmitters and other substances on smooth muscle. Physiol. Rev. **59:** 656–718.

The Effects of Ca^{2+} Antagonists on Isolated Rat and Rabbit Mesenteric Resistance Vessels[a]

What Determines the Sensitivity of Agonist-Activated Vessels to Ca^{2+} Antagonists?

CYNTHIA CAUVIN,[b] MAITE TEJERINA,[c]
OK HWANG,[d] MIEKO KAI-YAMAMOTO,[d]
AND CORNELIS VAN BREEMEN[d]

[b]*Division of Preclinical Research*
Sandoz, Limited
CH-4002 Basel, Switzerland

[c]*Faculty of Medicine*
Coordinated Department of Pharmacology
School of Medicine
City University
28040 Madrid, Spain

[d]*Department of Pharmacology*
University of Miami School of Medicine (R-189)
Miami, Florida 33101

INTRODUCTION

The phenomena that underlie the selective effects of organic Ca^{2+} antagonists in inhibiting vascular smooth muscle preferentially over other tissues and in selectively inhibiting certain vascular smooth muscles and certain modes of activation over others have been extensively studied and reviewed.[1–4] Although considerable progress has been made in the characterization of the voltage dependence of Ca^{2+} antagonist potency in Ca^{2+} channel blockade,[5–7] and of use or frequency dependence of Ca^{2+} antagonist blockade,[1,6,8] many observations relating to Ca^{2+} antagonist selectivity remain unexplained. We present in this paper a summary of the observations we have made over the last five years in the study of the effects of Ca^{2+} antagonists on peripheral resistance vessels from the mesenteric vasculature of rabbit and rat. We will attempt to relate these observations to those of others, who are approaching the questions pertaining to Ca^{2+} antagonist selectivity through the study of Ca^{2+} currents in single cells or single Ca^{2+} channels. Finally, we will reiterate a hypothesis, which remains to be directly tested, that the Ca^{2+} antagonist sensitivity of agonist-activated Ca^{2+} entry into vascular smooth muscle depends on the extent to which the agonist mobilizes intracellular Ca^{2+}.[2,9–11]

[a]Supported by the National Institutes of Health (HL 30412 and 29467) and the Florida Affiliate of the American Heart Association. The work was performed at the University of Miami.

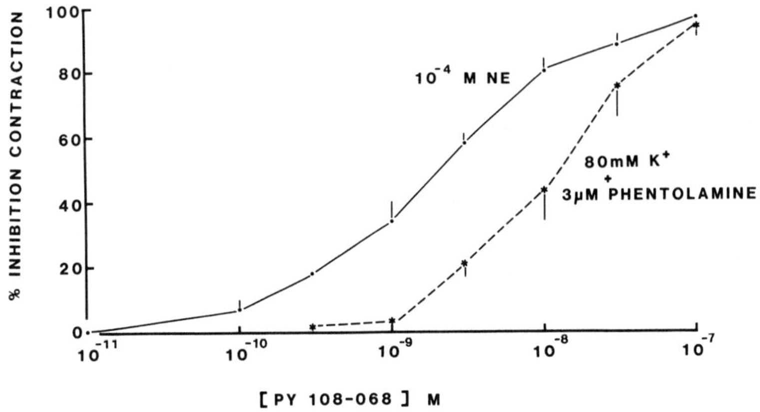

FIGURE 1. Inhibition by PY 108-068 of maximal norepinephrine (NE) induced and high K^+ (80 mM) induced tension in rabbit mesenteric resistance vessels (ca. 200 μm, i.d.; $n \geq 4$).

METHODS

The tension and ^{45}Ca influx measurements done in rabbit aorta[12] and in rabbit[13] and rat[14–16] mesenteric resistance vessels have been described elsewhere in detail and will not be repeated here.

RESULTS AND DISCUSSION

Rabbit Vessels

FIGURES 1 through 5 show the concentration response curves for inhibition of maximum norepinephrine (NE) induced and 80 mM K^+-induced tension in the isolated rabbit aorta and mesenteric resistance vessels by PY 108-068, nisoldipine, oxodipine, D600, and diltiazem. Inhibition of stimulated ^{45}Ca influx (measured during

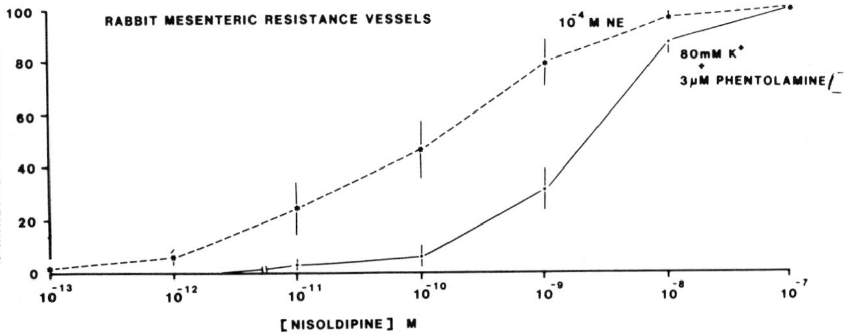

FIGURE 2. Inhibition by nisoldipine of maximal norepinephrine (NE) induced and high K^+ (80 mM) induced tension in rabbit mesenteric resistance vessels (ca. 200 μm, i.d.; $n \geq 4$).

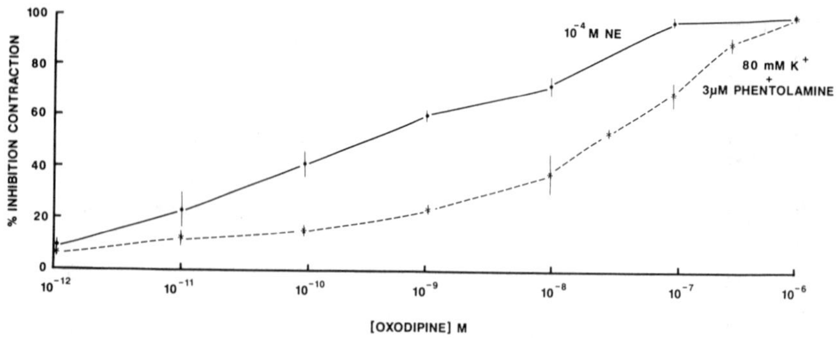

FIGURE 3. Inhibition by oxodipine of maximal norepinephrine (NE) induced and high K^+ (80 mM) induced tension in rabbit mesenteric resistance vessels (ca. 200 μm, i.d.; $n \geq 4$).

the first 90 seconds of activation) closely parallels inhibition of tension in the mesenteric resistance vessels by diltiazem (FIGURE 5).

The profile of the tension responses differs quite markedly between NE and high K^+ activation in these vessels. The high-K^+-induced tension is characterized by a rapid phasic response (which peaks during the first minute of activation), followed by a steadily declining tension response (in the presence of 3 μM phentolamine), which is quite variable in its rate of decline. The NE-induced tension, on the other hand, is characterized by a rapid phasic response (which peaks during the first 10–20 seconds of activation), following by a gradually increasing tonic response, which reaches a steady state level within approximately 3–5 minutes. Hence, the time at which inhibition of maximum contraction is measured is different for high K^+ and NE activation. This difference may be, in part, responsible for the observation that the Ca^{2+} antagonists are all more potent in inhibiting NE- than high-K^+-induced maximum tension responses (see TABLE 1 for IC_{50}s). Nonetheless, stimulated ^{45}Ca

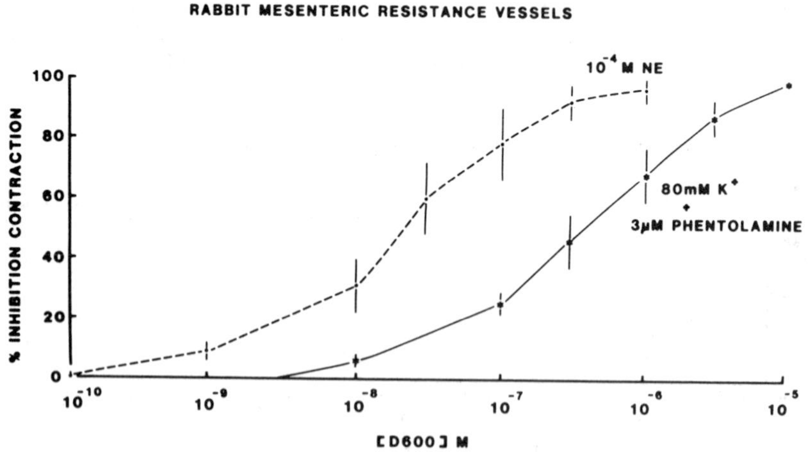

FIGURE 4. Inhibition by D600 of maximal norepinephrine (NE) induced and high K^+ (80 mM) induced tension in rabbit mesenteric resistance vessels (ca. 200 μm, i.d.; $n \geq 4$).

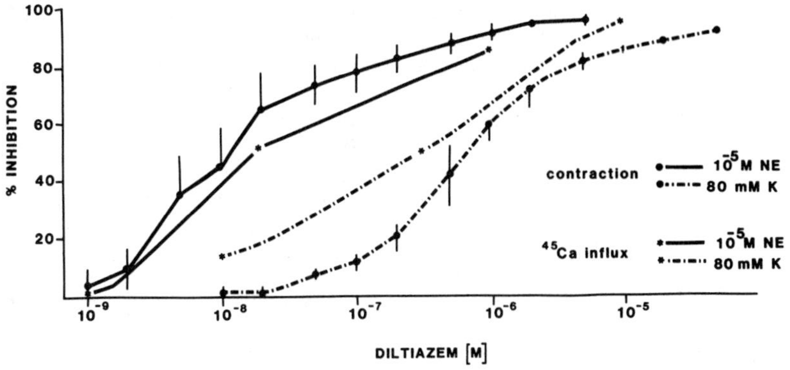

FIGURE 5. Inhibition by diltiazem of norepinephrine (NE) induced and 80 nM K^+-induced contractions and stimulated ^{45}Ca influx in rabbit mesenteric resistance vessels. Each point on contraction curves represents the mean ± SEM for 4–5 experiments. Each point on ^{45}Ca influx curves represents the mean for at least 3 tissues each from 3 to 4 rabbits. Standard errors of mean ^{45}Ca influx values were in all cases less than 10% of the mean.

influx has been measured for NE and high K^+ only during the first 90 seconds of activation. FIGURE 5 shows that the ^{45}Ca influx stimulated by NE is also more sensitive to diltiazem inhibition than is that stimulated by 80 mM K^+. Hence, it is more likely that the Ca^{2+} entry processes activated by the two agents are differentially sensitive to Ca^{2+} antagonists.

Recent studies of Ca^{2+} currents in single cells from rat mesenteric artery[7] and single Ca^{2+} channels in rabbit mesenteric arteries[17] (first-generation branches) have shown that there are two types of voltage-sensitive Ca^{2+} channels in these vessels. In voltage-clamped single cells of the rat mesenteric artery, one type of channel is activated by small depolarizations and inactivates quickly, while the other type is activated by stronger depolarizations and inactivates more slowly.[7] The slower of these two channels was found to have voltage-dependent sensitivity to nitrendipine. The nitrendipine K_D for the resting state of this channel was estimated to be ~200 nM, while that for the inactivated state of the channel was calculated to be ~0.5 nM (the nitrendipine sensitivity of the faster Ca^{2+} channel was not carefully assessed in this

TABLE 1. IC_{50}s-Inhibition of Maximum Contraction[a]

	Rabbit Aorta		Rabbit Mesenteric Resistance Vessels	
	80 mM K^+	10^{-5} M NE	80 mM K^+	10^{-4} M NE
Nisoldipine	2×10^{-9} M	$>10^{-3}$ M	2×10^{-9} M	10^{-10} M
PY108-068	10^{-10} M	$\gg 10^{-3}$ M	2×10^{-8} M	2×10^{-9} M
Oxodipine	3×10^{-9} M	$>10^{-7}$ M	3×10^{-8} M	3×10^{-10} M
D600	2×10^{-7} M	$>10^{-3}$ M	3×10^{-7} M	2×10^{-8} M
Diltiazem	5×10^{-7} M	$>10^{-3}$ M	6×10^{-7} M	10^{-8} M

[a]The values at which the Ca^{2+} antagonists inhibited maximum contractions by 50% (IC_{50}s) were obtained from graphs of concentration–mean response curves. In the aorta, maximum responses to 80 mM K^+ and NE are reached after approximately 10 minutes. In the mesenteric resistance vessels, the maximum response to high K^+ occurs within about 1 minute, while that to NE occurs within about 5 minutes.

study). In the rabbit mesenteric artery, two types of single Ca^{2+} channels (one with a slope conductance of 8 pS and the other 15 pS) have also been identified in cell-attached membrane patches; however, both types appear to require fairly strong depolarizations for activation, and both are sensitive to inhibition by nisoldipine.[17] At 50 nM, nisoldipine was found to reduce the average current through both channels by 95%, which very closely agrees with the inhibition of peak 80 mM K^+-induced tension in the rabbit mesenteric resistance vessels (FIGURE 2) and in the rabbit aorta (TABLE 1). The other two dihydropyridines presently studied (PY 108-068 and oxidipine) display an interesting difference from nisoldipine in that they are less potent in inhibiting maximum high-K^+-induced tension in the resistance vessels than in the aorta. This difference may be related to differences between the two vessels in the activation of the two hypothesized voltage-sensitive Ca^{2+} channels by 80 mM K^+ and/or to differential affinities of these two types of Ca^{2+} channels for the various dihydropyridines.

The differences between the rabbit aorta and mesenteric resistance vessels with respect to Ca^{2+} antagonist sensitivity during high K^+ depolarization are relatively minor as compared to the differences between the sensitivities of the two vessel types to Ca^{2+} antagonists during agonist-induced contraction with NE, when there are differences in the range of 3 to 7 orders of magnitude. These differences are assuredly due, at least in part, to the relatively greater contribution of intracellular Ca^{2+} release, which is not inhibited by the Ca^{2+} antagonists, to NE-induced contraction in the rabbit aorta as compared to that in the mesenteric resistance vessels.[18] FIGURE 6 shows the responses of the small vessels to NE after various preincubation times in Ca^{2+}-free medium. After only 5 minutes in Ca^{2+}-free medium, addition of 10^{-4} NE gives only about 10% of the contraction it would give in Ca^{2+}-containing medium (see FIGURE 6); a similar procedure in the rabbit aorta would give about 80% of the control contraction in Ca^{2+}-containing medium.[20,21] The half-time ($t_{1/2}$) of loss of the Ca^{2+} store that supports tension in the absence of extracellular Ca^{2+} is about 5 minutes in the resistance vessels (see FIGURE 6), while it is about 35 minutes in the aorta.[19,20]

The differences in Ca^{2+} antagonist sensitivities of agonist-induced contractions between the aorta and the mesenteric resistance vessels are not, however, solely due to the differential dependence of the two types of vessels upon extracellular Ca^{2+} for agonist-induced tension; the ^{45}Ca influx maximally stimulated by NE in the resistance vessels is also approximately four orders of magnitude more sensitive to diltiazem inhibition than is that in the aorta.[13] One difference between the two vessels which may alter Ca^{2+}-antagonist sensitivity during NE activation is that the resistance vessels depolarize (from ~ -58 mV to ~ -30 mV) in response to NE, while the rabbit aorta does not depolarize (from its resting potential of ~ -52 mV). One might, therefore, hypothesize that NE acts in the resistance vessels to open slow Ca^{2+} channels,[7] perhaps similar to "L"-type Ca^{2+} channels identified in cardiac muscle as having high affinity for Ca^{2+}-antagonists.[5,21] This hypothesis is refuted, however, by the following observations: (1) NE stimulation of ^{45}Ca influx and tension development are virtually the same in resistance vessels previously depolarized (to ~ -20 mV) with 80 mM K^+ as they are in normally polarized vessels;[13] (2) the depolarization associated with NE-induced tension can be prevented by diltiazem;[13] and (3) the sensitivity of NE-induced tension and stimulated ^{45}Ca influx to diltiazem is not voltage dependent. FIGURE 7 shows that the 50% maximally effective concentration (EC_{50}) of diltiazem is the same in inhibiting ^{45}Ca influx whether it is induced by a 25% of maximal concentration of NE (i.e., 3×10^{-6} M, which depolarizes the vessels to ~ -43 mV) or by a 100% effective NE concentration (i.e., 10^{-4} M which depolarizes the vessels to ~ -30 mV). Moreover, the work of Worley *et al.* in cell-attached patches of first-branch rabbit mesenteric arterial cells indicates that both types of Ca^{2+} channels identified in this tissue (i.e., 8 pS and 15 pS) only activate at pulse potentials positive to −40 mV (from a holding potential of −75 mV), and that further altering the pulse potential to −25 mV (from a holding potential of −75 mV) increases the percentage of pulses that activate Ca^{2+} channels to ~50%.[17] FIGURE 8 shows that, while these observations[17] correlate well with the coupling of voltage and tension changes induced by depolarizing K^+ media in the rabbit mesenteric resistance vessels, approximately 50% of NE-induced tension occurs

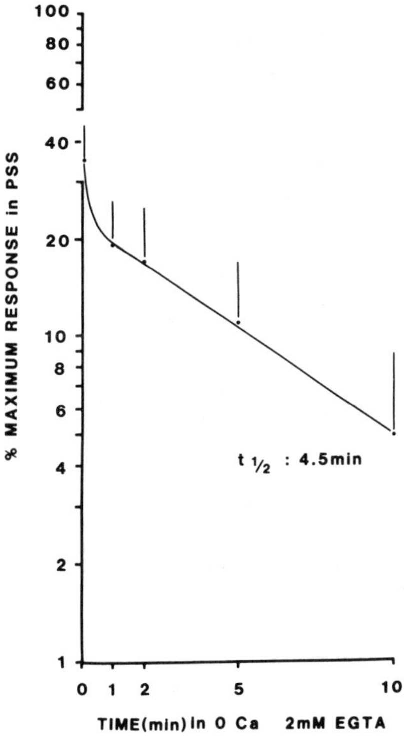

FIGURE 6. The time course of decline in the magnitude of norepinephrine (10^{-4} M) induced contractions in Ca^{2+}-free medium (0 Ca, 2 mM EGTA). The vessels were preincubated in the Ca^{2+}-free medium for varying periods of time (0, 1, 2, 5, 10 minutes) prior to application of NE. After the transient contraction induced by NE, it was washed out in the same medium for 2 minutes, then the vessels were reequilibrated in normal Ca^{2+} (1.5 mM) containing (PSS) for 5 minutes to replace the Ca^{2+} mobilized by NE in the Ca^{2+}-free medium. The time for which it took for the response to decline to half its value during the monoexponential phase of decline ($t_{1/2}$) was 4.5 minutes ($n = 5$).

at membrane potentials more negative than −40 mV. Moreover, the coupling of NE-stimulated ^{45}Ca influx and membrane potential is similar to that of tension and membrane potential.[13] Hence ~50% of NE-stimulated ^{45}Ca influx in the resistance vessels occurs at membrane potentials at which the reported voltage-sensitive Ca^{2+} channels in this tissue are not activated.[17] It could still be suggested that NE acts on voltage-sensitive Ca^{2+} channels, but by altering them in such a way that (1) their

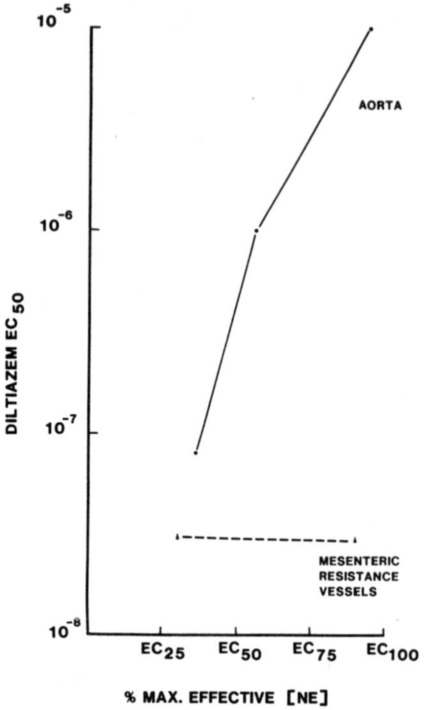

FIGURE 7. The half maximally effective diltiazem concentration (ordinate) in inhibiting ^{45}Ca influx stimulated by the various percent maximally effective concentrations of norepinephrine (abscissa) in isolated rabbit aorta and mesenteric resistance vessels. (Reprinted from Reference 13 with permission.)

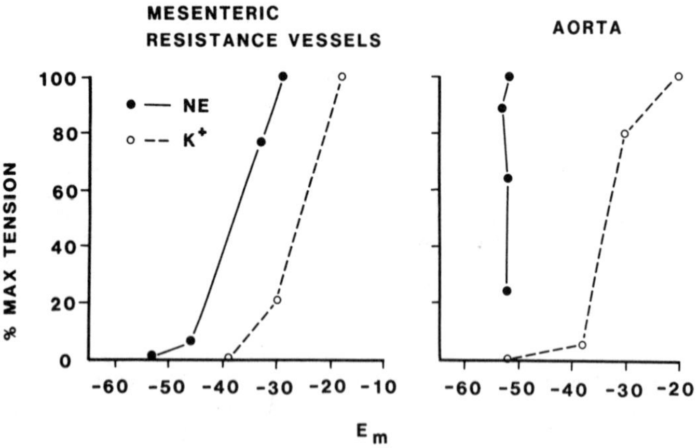

FIGURE 8. Voltage-tension coupling for NE (10^{-7}, 10^{-6}, 10^{-5}, and 10^{-4} M) induced and high K^+ (20, 40, and 80 mM) induced tension in the rabbit aorta and mesenteric resistance vessels. (Reprinted from Reference 13 with permission.)

voltage dependence is shifted to more negative membrane potentials for activation; (2) voltage dependence of Ca^{2+} antagonist blockade of the channels is negated; and (3) their affinity for Ca^{2+} antagonists is increased.

It could alternatively be hypothesized that NE activates a different type of channel altogether, perhaps a nonspecific cation channel analogous to that activated in cells of the guinea pig ileum by acetylcholine.[22] Such a channel may be the hypothesized receptor-operated channel.[23,24] If NE were to activate a nonspecific receptor-operated cation channel at membrane potentials more negative than −40 mV and to open additional voltage-sensitive Ca^{2+} channels at membrane potentials more positive than −40 mV, and if these various channels were to have different affinities for Ca^{2+} antagonists, one might predict that concentration response curves for Ca^{2+} antagonist inhibition of activation by 10^{-4} M NE (which depolarizes to ~−30 mV) may exhibit properties consistent with multiple sites of Ca^{2+} antagonist action. Simple inspection of these curves (see FIGURES 1–5) suggests that the ranges of effective Ca^{2+} antagonist

TABLE 2. IC_{50}s: Percent Inhibition of Tension and Stimulated ^{45}Ca Influx

	80 mM K^+	NE (10^{-4} M)
Tension		
PN 200-110:		
WKY	$2.5 \pm 1.5 \times 10^{-8}$ M	$3.4 \pm 0.9 \times 10^{-9}$ M
SHR	$2.8 \pm 1.3 \times 10^{-8}$ M	$3.3 \pm 1.8 \times 10^{-8}$ M
Nisoldipine:		
WKY	$1.2 \pm 0.9 \times 10^{-8}$ M	$1.6 \pm 0.6 \times 10^{-10}$ M
SHR	$1.1 \pm 0.4 \times 10^{-8}$ M	$2.2 \pm 0.3 \times 10^{-9}$ M[a]
Stimulated ^{45}Ca Influx		
PN 200-110:		
WKY	—	$2.3 \pm 5.9 \times 10^{-11}$ M
SHR	—	$1.0 \pm 0.9 \times 10^{-10}$ M
Nisoldipine:		
WKY	—	$7.6 \pm 1.7 \times 10^{-14}$ M
SHR	—	$1.9 \pm 0.9 \times 10^{-9}$ M[a]

[a]Indicates significant difference from WKY ($p < 0.05$). IC_{50} = concentration of dihydropyridine that produced 50% inhibition of tension or stimulated ^{45}Ca influx (100% inhibition occurred when the response in the presence of the dihydropyridine equaled the basal response, i.e., that in the absence of a stimulating agent).

concentrations is quite broad for inhibition of NE (but not high K^+) activation. These curves (FIGURES 1–3) have been fitted by computer to two site of action models with the following K_is for the dihydropyridines [± standard error of the mean (SEM)]:

PY 108-068	$2.0 \pm 1.0 \times 10^{-11}$ M	
	$2.9 \pm 0.6 \times 10^{-9}$ M	($r^2 > 0.99$)
nisoldipine	$6.0 \pm 0.6 \times 10^{-13}$ M	
	$4.3 \pm 3.6 \times 10^{-10}$ M	($r^2 > 0.99$)
oxodipine	$1.3 \pm 0.4 \times 10^{-11}$ M	
	$2.4 \pm 1.3 \times 10^{-8}$ M	($r^2 > 0.99$)

It seems likely, therefore, that NE activates more than one Ca^{2+}-antagonist-sensitive Ca^{2+} entry mechanism in the rabbit mesenteric resistance vessels.

Rat Vessels

We have also examined the inhibition of tension and stimulated ^{45}Ca influx for NE- and 80 mM K^+-induced activation of mesenteric resistance vessels from spontaneously hypertensive rats (SHR) and their normotensive control Wistar-Kyoto rats (WKY). TABLE 2 gives the values for IC_{50}s of nisoldipine and PN 200-110 inhibition of NE- and high-K^+-induced tension and of NE-stimulated ^{45}Ca influx. Inspection of the concentration response curves for these two dyhydropyridines (FIGURES 9–12) again

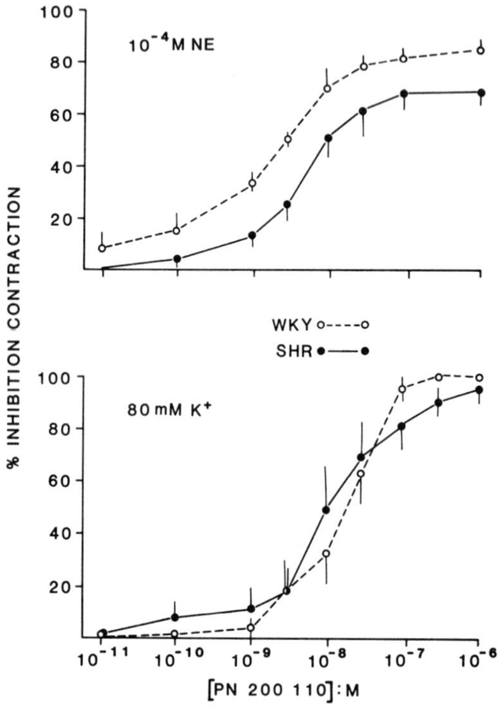

FIGURE 9. Concentration-response curves for PN 200-110 inhibition of 10^{-4} M NE (top) and 80 mM K^+ (bottom) induced tension in SHR ($n = 5$) and WKY ($n = 5$) mesenteric resistance vessels. The curves for inhibition of NE-induced tension are significantly different when the two strains are compared.

indicates broad concentration ranges for their effects on NE-stimulated tension and ^{45}Ca influx, a pattern similar to that seen in the rabbit mesenteric resistance vessels. It is interesting to note that the WKY vessels are more sensitive to Ca^{2+} antagonist inhibition than are the SHR vessels. This difference is not apparently related to differences in resting membrane potential or in NE-induced changes in membrane potential between the two groups.[25] It may, however, be related to their different rates of loss of Ca^{2+} from the NE-releasable intracellular store. In experiments similar to that shown in FIGURE 6, the $t_{1/2}$ for decline of NE-induced tension after preincubation

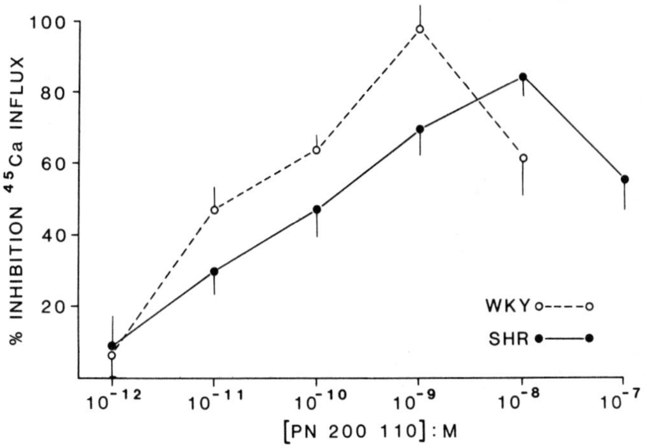

FIGURE 10. Concentration-response curves for PN 200-110 inhibition of 10^{-4} M NE stimulated ^{45}Ca influx in SHR and WKY mesenteric resistance vessels. The curves for WKY and SHR are significantly different. Each data point represents at least 2 tissues from each of at least 5 animals from each strain.

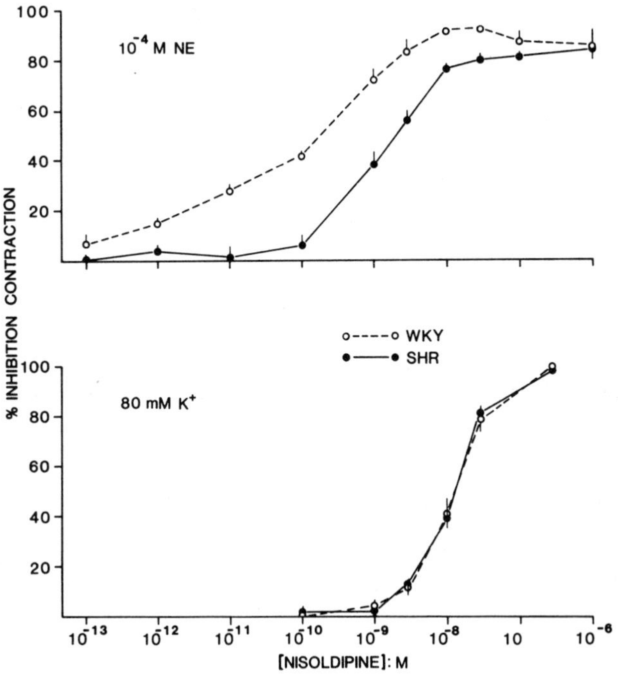

FIGURE 11. Concentration-response curves for nisoldipine inhibition of 10^{-4} M NE (top) and 80 mM K^+ (bottom) induced tension in SHR ($n = 5$) and WKY ($n = 5$) mesenteric resistance vessels. The curves for nisoldipine inhibition of NE-induced tension are significantly different when the two strains are compared.

in Ca^{2+}-free medium is ~5 minutes in the WKY vessels, but is ~9 minutes in the SHR vessels.

We have observed, therefore, in rabbit aorta and mesenteric resistance vessels, and in SHR and WKY mesenteric resistance vessels, an inverse relationship between Ca^{2+} antagonist sensitivity (in inhibiting ^{45}Ca influx or Ca^{2+}-influx-mediated tension) of NE-induced activation and the extent to which NE causes the release of intracellular Ca^{2+} stores. A similar inverse relationship has been described in the rabbit aorta, wherein ^{45}Ca influx stimulated by low concentrations of NE, which release little intracellular Ca^{2+}, is far more sensitive to Ca^{2+} antagonist (nisoldipine, D600, and diltiazem) inhibition than that stimulated by higher concentrations, which release a substantial quantity of intracellular Ca^{2+}.[9–11] (see FIGURE 7 for diltiazem data.) These observations support, but unfortunately do not prove, the following hypothesis: the release of intracellular Ca^{2+} by NE decreases the Ca^{2+} antagonist affinity for the Ca^{2+} channels (or perhaps for the proposed receptor-operated cation channels). Direct evidence in support of this hypothesis has been impossible to obtain from ^{45}Ca flux

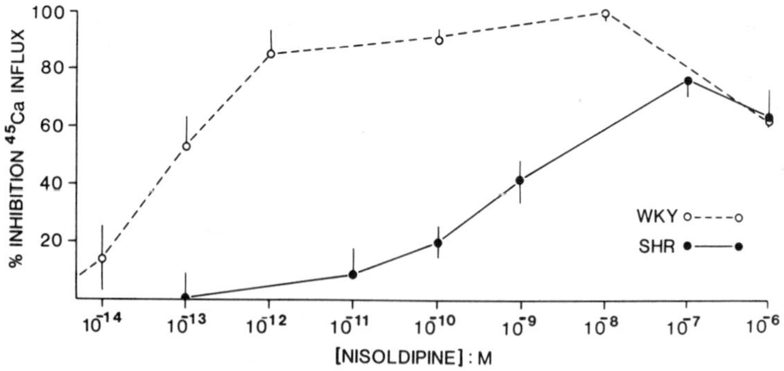

FIGURE 12. Concentration-response curves for nisoldipine inhibition of 10^{-4} M NE stimulated ^{45}Ca influx in SHR and WKY mesenteric resistance vessels. The curves for WKY and SHR are significantly different. Each data point represents at least 2 tissues from each of at least 5 animals from each strain.

experiments,[9–11] and may be equally difficult to obtain from Ca^{2+} current measurements. Two plausible theoretical schemata are as follows: (1) norepinephrine releases membrane-bound Ca^{2+}, perhaps Ca^{2+} bound to channel molecules themselves, that may be crucial for inactivation of the channels; when these Ca^{2+} binding sites are unoccupied, the channels do not inactivate and, hence, have lower affinity for Ca^{2+} antagonists; and (2) norepinephrine activates some second messenger system which mediates release of intracellular Ca^{2+}; some mediator in this system may affect channel molecules, decreasing their affinity for Ca^{2+} antagonists. As IP_3 has been identified as a second messenger in the release of intracellular Ca^{2+}, perhaps one of the phosphoinositides may be a candidate for the mediator in scheme 2.

ACKNOWLEDGMENT

Thanks to Maria Martinez for typing the manuscript.

REFERENCES

1. GODFRAIND, T., R. MILLER & M. WIBO. 1986. Calcium antagonism and calium entry blockade. Pharmacol. Rev. **38:** 321–416.
2. CAUVIN, C., R. LOUTZENHISER & C. VAN BREEMEN. 1983. Mechanisms of Calcium Antagonist-induced vasodiation. Annu. Rev. Pharmacol. Toxicol. **23:** 373–396.
3. CAUVIN, C. & C. VAN BREEMEN. 1986. Calcium entry blockers. *In* Handbook of Hypertension: Pathophysiology of Hypertension-Cartiovascular Aspects. A. Zanchetti & R. Tarazi, Eds. **7:** 375–407. Elsevier Science Publishers. Amsterdam, Holland.
4. CAUVIN, C. & C. VAN BREEMEN. 1987. Vascular effects of Ca^{2+} antagonists. ISI Atlas of Science: Pharmacology **1:** 13–19.
5. HESS, P., J. B. LANSMAN & R. W. TSIEN. 1984. Different modes of Ca channel gating behaviour favoured by dihydropyridine Ca agonists and antagonists. Nature **311:** 538–544.
6. KASS, R. S., M. C. SANGUINETTI, P. B. BENNETT, B. E. COPLIN & D. S. KRAFTE. 1985. Voltage-dependent modulation of cardiac Ca-channels by dihydropyridines. *In* Cardiovascular Effects of Dihydropyridine-Type Calcium Antagonists and Agonists. A Fleckenstein, C. van Breemen, R. Gross & F. Hoffmeister, Eds.: 198–215. Springer-Verlag. Berlin, FRG.
7. BEAN, B. P., M. STUREK, A. PUGA & K. HERMSMEYER. 1986. Calcium channels in muscle cells isolated from rat mesenteric arteries: modulation by dihydropyridine drugs. Circ. Res. **59:** 229–235.
8. VAN BREEMEN, C., C. CAUVIN, H. YAMAMOTO & A. ZSCHAUER. 1987. Vascular smooth muscle calcium channels. J. Cardiovasc. Pharmacol. **10** (Suppl. X): S10–S15.
9. CAUVIN, C. & C. VAN BREEMEN. 1985. Different calcium entry mechanisms along the arterial tree. J. Cardiovasc. Pharmacol. **7:** S4–S10.
10. CAUVIN, C., S. LUKEMAN, J. CAMERON, K. MEISHERI, H. YAMAMOTO & C. VAN BREEMEN. 1984. Theoretical bases for vascular selectivity of Ca^{2+} antagonists. J. Cardiovasc. Pharmacol. **6:** S630–S638.
11. CAUVIN, C. & VAN BREEMEN. 1985. Effects of Ca^{2+} antagonists on isolated rabbit mesenteric resistance vessels as compared to rabbit aorta. *In* Cardiovascular Effects of Dihydropyridine-Type Calcium Antagonists and Agonists. A. Fleckenstein, C. van Breemen, R. Gross & F. Hoffmeister, Eds.: 259–269. Springer-Verlag. Berlin, FRG.
12. MEISHERI, K., O. HWANG & C. VAN BREEMEN. 1981. Evidence for two separate Ca^{2+} entry pathways in smooth muscle plasmalemma. J. Membr. Biol. **59:** 19–25.
13. CAUVIN, C., S. LUKEMAN, J. CAMERON, O. HWANG & C. VAN BREEMEN. 1985. Differences in norepinephrine activation and diltiazem inhibition of Ca^{2+} channels in isolated rat aorta and mesenteric resistance vessels. Circ. Res. **56:** 822–828.
14. CAUVIN, C. 1986. Increased Ca^{2+} entry and increased contractions in isolated mesenteric resistance vessels from spontaneously hypertensive rats. *In* New Therapy of Ischaemic Heart Disease and Hypertension. P. R. Lichtlen, Ed.: 225–231. Elsevier Science Publishers. Amsterdam, Holland.
15. CAUVIN, C., O. HWANG, M. YAMAMOTO & C. VAN BREEMEN. 1987. Effects of dihydropyridines on tension and ^{45}Ca influx in isolated mesenteric resistance vessels from spontaneously hypertensive rats. Am. J. Cardiol. **59:** 116B–122B.
16. CAUVIN, C., C. GELBAND & C. VAN BREEMEN. 1987. ^{45}Ca fluxes in isolated rat mesenteric resistance vessels. J. Cardiovasc. Pharmacol. **10** (Suppl. I): S44–S48.
17. WORLEY, J. F. III, J. W. DEITMER & M. T. NELSON. 1986. Single nisoldipine-sensitive calcium channels in smooth muscle cells isolated from rabbit mesenteric artery. Proc. Nat. Acad. Sci. USA **83:** 5746–5750.
18. CAUVIN, C., K. SAIDA & C. VAN BREEMEN. 1983. Extracellular Ca^{2+} dependence and diltiazem inhibition of contraction in rabbit conduit arteries and mesenteric resistance vessels. Blood Vessels **21:** 23–31.
19. DETH, R. & C. VAN BREEMEN. 1977. Agonist-induced release of intracellular Ca^{2+} in the rabbit aorta. J. Membr. Biol. **30:** 363–380.
20. LEIJTEN, P. & C. VAN BREEMEN. 1984. The effects of caffeine on the noradrenaline-sensitive calcium store in rabbit aorta. J. Physiol. **357:** 327–339.

21. NOWYCKY, M. C., A. P. FOX & R. W. TSIEN. 1985. Three types of neuronal calcium channel with different calcium agonist sensitivity. Nature **316:** 440–444.
22. BENHAM, C. D., T. B. BOLTON & R. J. LANG. 1985. Acetylcholine activates an inward current in single mammalian smooth muscle cells. Nature **316:** 345–347.
23. VAN BREEMEN, C., P. AARONSON & R. LOUTZENHISER. 1979. Na^{+}, Ca^{2+} interactions in mammalian smooth muscle. Pharmacol. Rev. **30:** 167–208.
24. BOLTON, T. B. 1979. Mechanisms of action of transmitters and other substances on smooth muscle. Physiol. Rev. **3:** 606–718.
25. MULVANY, M. J. 1986. Altered vascular calcium metabolism as a possible cause of increased blood pressure in essential hypertension. *In* Essential Hypertension: Ca^{2+} Mechanisms and Treatment. K. Aoki, Ed.: 51–65. Springer-Verlag. Tokyo, Japan.

Receptor Subtypes Involved in the Action of Calcium Entry Blockers

P. A. VAN ZWIETEN[a] AND P. B. M. W. M. TIMMERMANS[b]

[a]*Division of Pharmacotherapy*
University of Amsterdam
Academic Medical Center
Meibergdreef 15
1105 AZ Amsterdam, the Netherlands

[b]*E.I. du Pont de Nemours & Company Inc.*
Medical Products Department
Experimental Station, E400-4257
Wilmington, Delaware 19898

INTRODUCTION

After the recognition that the pharmacological activities of calcium entry blockers (CEB) are mediated by specific calcium channels in the membranes of cardiac and vascular smooth muscle cells, the necessity was felt to subdivide the calcium channels into potential (voltage) operated and receptor operated channels (POC and ROC, respectively).[1-3] It seems likely that the CEB predominantly act at the level of POC, and the evidence for a substantial influence of these drugs on ROC is limited and not generally accepted. However, evidence has been accumulating since the beginning of the 1980s that a relevant interaction occurs between CEB and α-adrenoceptors on vascular smooth muscle. The discovery of this subtle interaction between CEB and α-adrenoceptors has shed some new light upon the relevance of ROC for the pharmacological activities of the CEB. Our interest in the interaction between CEB and α-adrenoceptor-mediated vasoconstriction was aroused by the following experimental findings.

The stimulation of both α_1- and α_2-adrenoceptors in a postsynaptic position causes vasoconstriction and hence an increase in total peripheral resistance and arterial blood pressure. However, the profile of vasoconstriction mediated by either of the two subtypes is somewhat different, as reflected by a different time course of the constriction and by different dose-response curves for the α_1- and α_2-adrenoceptor agonists. These discrepancies prompted us to study the process of vasoconstriction, triggered by both α_1- and α_2-adrenoceptor subtypes in more detail, in particular with respect to the role of extracellular calcium ions involved in the contractile process. Before dealing with these investigations, we shall present a brief survey of the modern subclassification of α-adrenoceptors.

CLASSIFICATION OF α-ADRENOCEPTORS

α-Adrenoceptors can be divided in the α_1- and α_2-subtypes.[4-11] This subclassification is based upon the affinity of selective agonists and antagonists for these two subtypes, whereas the subdivision into presynaptic and postsynaptic (pre- and postjunctional) α-adrenoceptors defines the localization with respect to the synapse.

Presynaptic receptors are located on the sympathetic nerve ending, whereas postsynaptic receptors occur on the target organ, such as a blood vessel. Noradrenaline and adrenaline are nonselective agonists, that is, they stimulate α_1- and α_2-adrenoceptors equally well. Similarly, classical α-adrenoceptor blockers, like for instance phentolamine, are nonselective compounds that antagonize both α_1- and α_2-adrenoceptors.[10,11]

Presynaptic α-adrenoceptors are almost exclusively of the α_2-subtype, as judged by their affinity for selective α_2-receptor agonists and antagonists.[12–14] However, both α_1- and α_2-adrenoceptors occur in comparable numbers at postsynaptic sites. Stimulation of presynaptic α_2-adrenoceptors reduces the release of endogenous noradrenaline from the nerve ending. Stimulation of postsynaptic α_1- and α_2-adrenoceptors by their respective agonists causes vasoconstriction.[14] In a series of recent experiments in human subjects, both in normotensive volunteers and in hypertensive patients, it could be shown that the stimulation of both postsynaptic α_1- and α_2-adrenoceptors causes

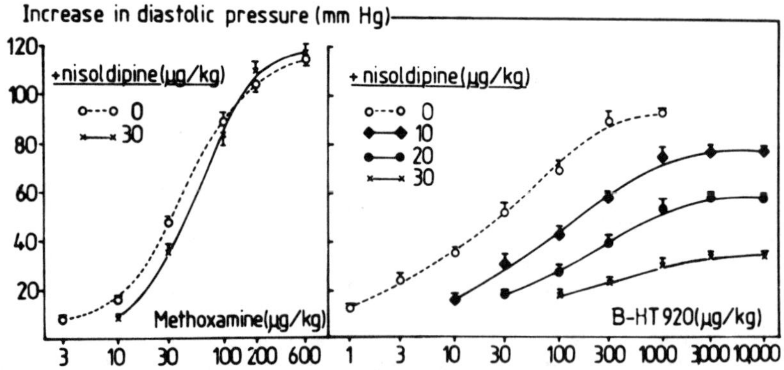

FIGURE 1. Effect of the calcium entry blocker nisoldipine on the pressor effects elicited by excitation of postsynaptic α_1- and α_2-adrenoceptors, respectively. Experiments were performed on pithed rats. Selective stimulation of α_1-adrenoceptors was obtained following injection of methoxamine, that of α_2-adrenoceptors following administration of the experimental compound B-HT 920. Nisoldipine markedly depresses the pressor responses induced by α_2-adrenoceptor stimulation, whereas the rise in pressure due to stimulation of α_1-adrenoceptors is virtually unaffected by nisoldipine. Data from Van Meel *et al.*[21] (For details, see text.)

constriction of the vessels in the forearm, as reflected by reduced perfusion by means of a plethysmographic technique.[15–20]

We wondered whether the contractile process in smooth muscle cells, occurring after stimulation of either α_1- and α_2-adrenoceptors subtypes, would differ in the involvement of calcium movements. Accordingly, dose-response curves were made for vasoconstrictor effects *in vivo* as reflected by the rise in diastolic blood pressure in pithed rat preparations and in similar preparations from other animal species.

The rise in blood pressure, reflecting constriction of the precapillary arterioles (resistance vessels) occurred more rapidly upon selective stimulation of postsynaptic α_1-adrenoceptors than upon stimulation of postsynaptic α_2-adrenoceptors. Not only the rate of rise in blood pressure but also the course of the dose-response characteristics was different: as a rule, the dose-response curve reflecting the pressor effect due to α_1-stimulation was steeper and achieved a higher maximum than that resulting from

α_2-adrenoceptor excitation (FIGURE 1), at least in pithed rats, cats, and rabbits. It is well known that *in vitro* it is extremely difficult to demonstrate the vasoconstrictor response to α_2-adrenoceptor stimulation. For this reason, we mainly performed *in vivo* studies concerning the α_2-effect. However, α_1-adrenoceptor-mediated vasoconstriction was also studied *in vitro* (see below).

INFLUENCE OF CALCIUM ENTRY BLOCKERS ON α_2-ADRENOCEPTOR-MEDIATED VASOCONSTRICTION

Differences in the contractile process following the stimulation of two α-receptor subtypes were further accentuated when the influence of CEB pretreatment was investigated. It drew our attention that the response to α_2-receptor activation was obviously sensitive to CEB, whereas such a sensitivity was much less pronounced in the case of α_1-adrenoceptor-mediated vasoconstriction (see subsequent paragraphs). An example of this differential influence of CEB is shown in FIGURE 1. As visualized in FIGURE 1, a marked and dose-dependent shift and flattening of the dose response with B-HT 920, a selective α_2-agonist, were observed after pretreatment with nisoldipine. This finding was substantiated with several α-adrenoceptor agonists, CEB, and other animal species in a series of confirmatory experiments (FIGURE 2). Moreover, we also demonstrated that the impairing effect of the CEB on α_2-adrenoceptor-triggered vasoconstriction was directly dependent upon the degree of calcium entry blockade induced by each individual drug (CEB) investigated. As reported in Reference 21, the effect of the CEB on α_2-adrenoceptor-mediated vasoconstriction was expressed and quantified by means of pD'_2 values (*in vivo*). Conversely, the degree of calcium entry blockade calcium antagonistic activity was assessed in isolated rabbit aorta strips, in which contraction was provoked by means of potassium deplorization. The degree of inhibition of this effect by CEB is considered to be a measure for calcium antagonistic activity, which can be quantified by means of pD'_2 values (*in vitro*). As shown in FIGURE 3 a linear and highly significant correlation appears to exist between pD'_2 (*in vivo*) and pD'_2 (*in vitro*), strongly suggesting that the blunting of α_2-adrenoceptor-mediated vasoconstriction by the CEB is directly related to the calcium entry blockade induced by these drugs.

After the initial series of experiments with a limited number of classical CEB and α_2-adrenoceptor stimulants, several newer and less current examples of both series of compounds were included into the study. Similar results were obtained as with the classical compounds and in all cases the CEB appeared to impair the vasoconstriction induced by the stimulation of postsynaptic α_2-adrenoceptors in the smooth muscle of resistance vessels. Accordingly, the increase in diastolic pressure brought about by the selective α_2-receptor agonists B-HT 920, B-HT 933 (azepexole), xylazine, UK-14, 304, M-7, TL-99, and DP-6,7-ADTN appeared to be invariably sensitive to impairment by nifedipine.[22]

Evidence has been presented suggesting that this susceptibility of α_2-adrenoceptor-triggered vasoconstriction to impairment by blockade of the calcium inward flux occurs independently of the nature, potency, or efficacy (intrinsic activity) of the α_2-adrenoceptor agonist used. This statement is supported by our demonstration that nifedipine exerted a similar inhibitory potency towards the increase in diastolic pressure of the partial agonist of the postjunctional vascular α_2-adrenoceptors, B-HT 958, as compared to the full agonist B-HT 920.[23] The experimentally established interaction between vascular postsynaptic α_2-adrenoceptor and CEB may be explained adequately by the following hypothesis.

Stimulation of vascular postsynaptic α_2-adrenoceptors in resistance vessels by an

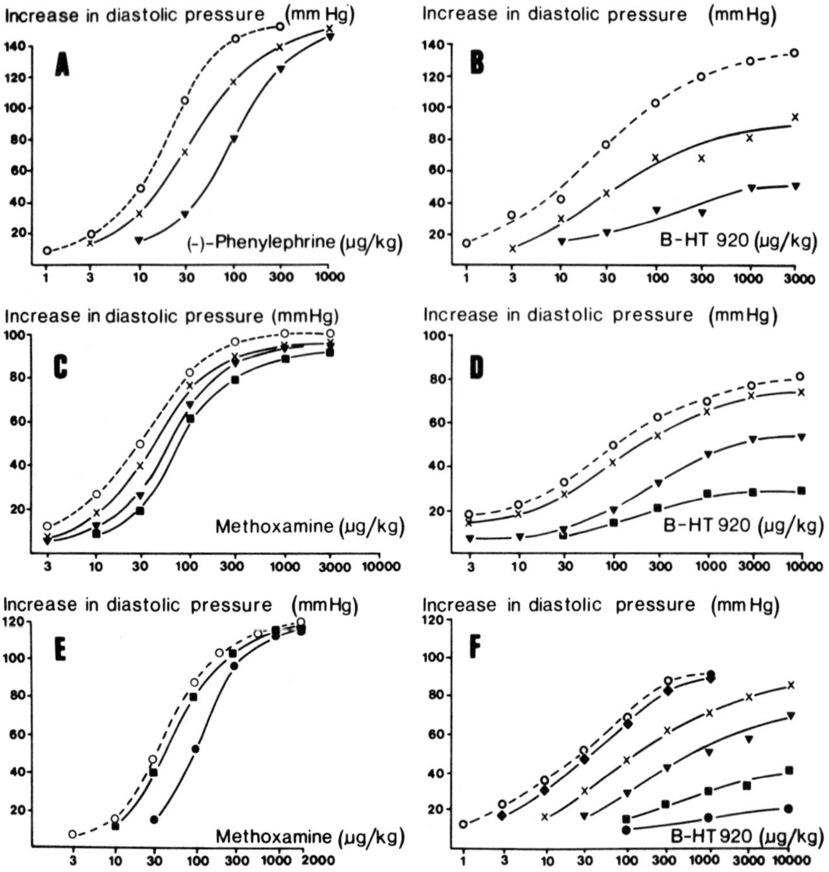

FIGURE 2. Increase in diastolic pressure (mm Hg) of pithed cats (A and B), ganglion-blocked vagotomized rabbits (C and D), and pithed normotensive rats (E and F), induced by intravenous (−)-phenylephrine and methoxamine (α_1-antagonist) and B-HT 920 (selective α_2-agonist) 15 minutes after saline treatment (open circles) or after various doses of the calcium entry blocker nifedipine (diamonds, 10; crosses, 30; triangles, 100; squares, 300; and filled circles, 100 μg/kg intravenously). Symbols represent mean values of 5–6 individual experiments.

agonist opens calcium channels in the smooth muscle membrane. The influx of extracellular calcium is a prerequisite for the vasoconstriction process which is triggered by the formation of the α-agonist–receptor complex. Calcium entry blockers and also disodium edetate inhibit the calcium influx and hence prevent the process of vasoconstriction, whereas the formation of the agonist-receptor complex remains unimpaired. This hypothesis is visualized in FIGURE 4.

Further support for the aforementioned hypothesis was obtained in recent experiments with the calcium promoter (calcium agonist) Bay K 8644 as discussed in the subsequent paragraph.

INTERACTION BETWEEN THE CALCIUM ENTRY PROMOTER BAY K 8644 AND α_2-RECEPTOR-INDUCED VASOCONSTRICTION

The dihydropyridine derivative Bay K 8644 has been reported to enhance the calcium influx through the specific membrane channels into the cells.[24] This calcium agonistic drug allowed us to further substantiate the hypothesis developed to explain the interaction between CEB and α_2-adrenoceptor-mediated vasoconstriction. The experiments, performed in pithed rats and published elsewhere in full detail,[25] may be summarized as follows.

Intravenous administration of the selective α_2-adrenoceptor agonist B-HT 920 elicited a dose-dependent increase in diastolic pressure which was dose-dependently enhanced by the calcium entry promoter Bay K 8644 (0.1 and 1 mg/kg, respectively). As shown in FIGURE 5, Bay K 8644 induced a parallel leftward shift of the log-dose response curve to B-HT 920, whereas the maximal pressure effect was increased.

A similar enhancement, although quantitatively different between the various agents, was obtained when the influence of Bay K 8644 on the pressor responses to other α_2-adrenoceptor stimulants like DP-6, 7-ADTN, TL-99, and B-HT 958 was studied. The enhancing effect of Bay K 8644 on α_2-adrenoceptor-induced vasoconstriction was even more pronounced after initial pretreatment with the CEB nifedipine. These results indicate that the calcium entry promoter Bay K 8644 behaves with respect to α_2-adrenoceptor-induced vasoconstriction as a mirror image of a CEB. As a whole, the experimental findings are in accordance with the concept of antagonism between Bay K 8644 and CEB at the level of calcium channels.

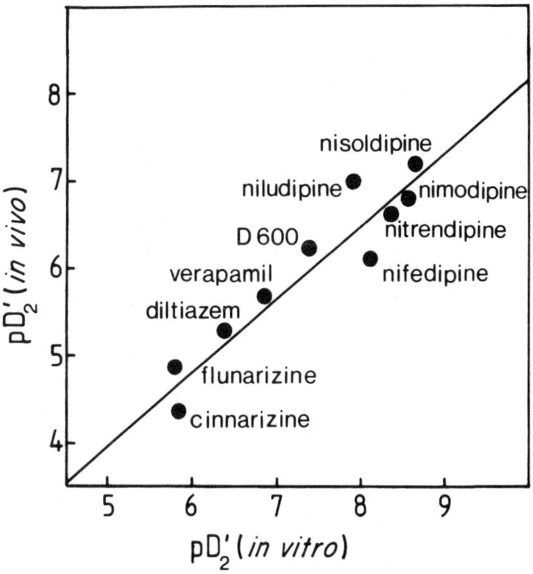

FIGURE 3. Relationship between the inhibitory activities of calcium entry blockers on K^+-induced contractions of rabbit thoracic aorta strips, and α_2-adrenoceptor-induced vasopressor responses in the pithed rat. Data from Van Meel *et al.*[21]

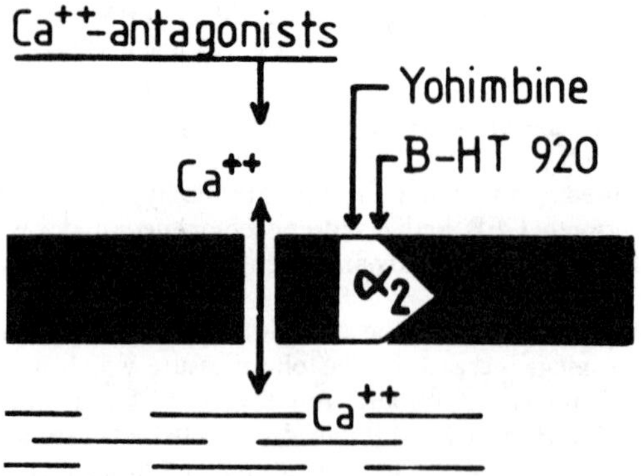

FIGURE 4. Schematic representation of the hypothesis by which stimulation of α_2-adrenoceptors in the vascular wall will lead to vasoconstriction. The formation of the α_2-adrenoceptor–agonist complex is accompanied by influx of extracellular calcium ions, which is sensitive to calcium entry blockers. (For details see text.)

INFLUENCE OF CALCIUM ENTRY BLOCKERS ON VASOCONSTRICTION MEDIATED BY α_1-ADRENOCEPTORS

In an early series of experiments we found that vasoconstriction triggered by α_1-adrenoceptor stimulants such as cirazoline, methoxamine, phenylephrine, and amidephrine was relatively insensitive or even completely resistant to inhibition by CEB.[26–29] For methoxamine this phenomenon is shown in FIGURE 1. In that early stage of investigation we incorrectly assumed that α_1-adrenoceptor-triggered vasoconstriction was invariably less sensitive to CEB than α_2-induced constriction. However, more recent experiments by our group have shown that the vasoconstriction induced by a few particular but selective α_1-adrenoceptor agonists is significantly impaired by pretreatment with CEB.[29–31] The most prominent example of this group of α_1-agonists is the experimental compound Sgd 101/75 (2-[2-methylindazol-4-imino]-imidazolidine · HCl).[31] The rise in blood pressure induced by this compound in pithed normotensive rats and cats was selectively inhibited by the CEB nifedipine.[29] In this respect Sgd 101/75 appears to be different from other α_1-adrenoceptor agonists (see above) which elicit vasoconstriction resistant to impairment by calcium entry blockade.

In vitro, mainly α_1-adrenoceptors are demonstrable and it is hardly possible to induce vasoconstriction by stimulation of α_2-adrenoceptors. For this and other reasons we also studied the influence of CEB on rat isolated aorta preparations. The experimental details and results are reported in Reference 32. Similarly as observed in the pithed rat preparation, imidazolidine–α_1-adrenoceptor agonists caused contractions of the aorta which proved markedly sensitive to CEB. Conversely, most phenylethylamine-like α_1-adrenoceptor agonists caused contraction which proved resistant to CEB pretreatment, with the exception of cirazoline. Accordingly, *in vivo* (pithed rat) and *in vitro* (aorta) data are in satisfactory accordance.

From the vast body of experimental data we concluded that α_1-adrenoceptor-induced vasoconstriction is associated with and or caused by:

1. Influx of extracellular calcium ions; this process is sensitive to CEB;
2. The release of calcium ions from intracellular stores, a process uninfluenced by CEB.

The ratio between phenomena 1 and 2 can be imagined to vary, dependant on the vascular tissue or the particular α-adrenoceptor agonist involved. Accordingly, the sensitivity of α_1-adrenoceptor-mediated vasoconstriction to blockade by CEB depends on the question as to which degree both mechanisms of calcium mobilization contribute to the overall contraction process and varies between vascular tissues and α_1-adrenoceptor agonists.

It has been recently shown by Timmermans *et al.* that phenoxybenzamine enhances the potency of CEB to inhibit the pressor effects to α_1-adrenoceptor agonists in pithed rats.[33] These findings could be confirmed in rat perfused hindquarters[34] and in rat isolated aorta preparations.[35] A reduction of the number of α_1-adrenoceptors per se does not alter the relative contribution of both mechanisms involved in the vasoconstriction triggered by α_1-adrenoceptor stimulation. It has been speculated[33] that phenoxybenzamine selectively interferes with the calcium influx independent process, thus unmasking the residual calcium-influx-sensitive mechanism. A mechanism at the level of the α-adrenoceptor complex seems unlikely, since α-adrenoceptor antagonists do not discriminate between calcium-sensitive and -insensitive processes.[36] The mechanism of the interaction of phenoxybenzamine remains unknown at present.

CONCLUSIONS

The sensitivity of α_2-adrenoceptor-mediated vasoconstriction to CEB appears to be a very general phenomenon, which can readily be demonstrated for a variety of α_2-receptor stimulants and CEB in several animal species, including man. The major body of evidence for this concept has been obtained *in vivo,* but under particular

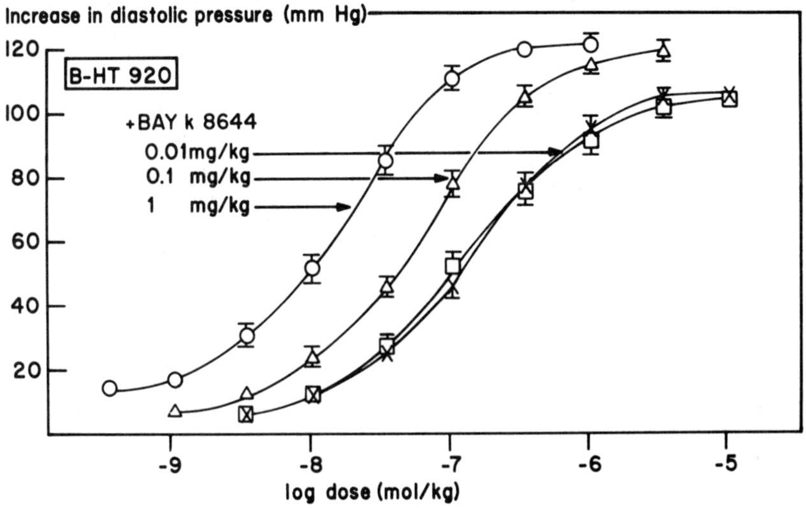

FIGURE 5. Log dose-response curves for the maximal increase in diastolic pressure elicited by intravenous administration of B-HT 920 in pithed normotensive rats. Pressor responses were obtained after intraarterial pretreatment (−15 minutes) with the vehicle of Bay K 8644 (crosses) or various doses of Bay K 8644. Symbols represent mean values ± standard error of the mean (n = 6). Data from Wilffert *et al.*[25]

experimental conditions it can also be demonstrated *in vitro*. The concept of a calcium influx accompanying the formation of the α_2-agonist receptor complex was substantiated by recent studies with the calcium entry promoter Bay K 8644, the latter compound showing a mirror image when compared to the CEB.

Vasoconstrictor processes triggered by α_1-adrenoceptor stimulation appear to involve both intracellular release of calcium and the influx of extracellular calcium ions. The ratio between intracellular and transmembranous events is strongly dependent upon the type of agonist and the preparation used. This ratio can be influenced by phenoxybenzamine which may interfere with the release of intracellular calcium, thus enhancing the importance of extracellular calcium flowing into the cell, causing a more elevated sensitivity to CEB.

The experiments on α_1-adrenoceptor vasoconstriction do not necessarily point towards a division of α_1-adrenoceptors into different subtypes. However, it seems likely that each α_1-adrenoceptor agonist interacts in its own individual way with the receptor. "Full" α_1-adrenoceptor agonists, such as phenylephrine, methoxamine, cirazoline, and amidephrine, are capable of triggering both processes of Ca^{2+} utilization, whereas vasoconstriction to "partial" α_1-adrenoceptor agonists, such as Sgd 101/75, has to rely more heavily on the influx of extracellular Ca^{2+}.[37]

SUMMARY

A survey is given of the interaction between α-adrenoceptor-triggered vasoconstriction and the influx of extracellular calcium ions. This problem was investigated by studying the influence of calcium entry blockers (CEB) on the vasoconstriction induced by several types of α_2- and α_1-adrenoceptor agonists both *in vivo* and *in vitro*. In addition, experiments were performed with the calcium entry promoter Bay K 8644. α_2-Adrenoceptor-triggered vasoconstriction is invariably accompanied by an influx of extracellular calcium ions which substantially contributes to the initiation of vascular smooth muscle contraction. This concept is a very general phenomenon, which holds for a variety of α_2-adrenoceptor agonists and CEB, *in vivo* and *in vitro*, and in different animal species.

The α_1-adrenoceptor-induced vasoconstriction appears to be caused both by the release of intracellular calcium and by the transmembranous influx of intracellular calcium. The ratio between both processes is very different, depending upon the type of α_1-adrenoceptor agonist and on the experimental preparation used. It has been speculated that this ratio can be influenced by phenoxybenzamine.

REFERENCES

1. CAVERO I. & M. SPEDDING. 1983. Calcium antagonists: a class of drugs with a bright future. Part I. Cellular calcium homeostasis and calcium as a coupling messenger. Life Sci. **33:** 2571–2581.
2. SPEDDING, M. & I. CAVERO. 1983. Calcium antagonists: a class of drugs with a bright future. Determination of basic pharmacological properties. Life Sci. **35:** 575–587.
3. REUTER, H. 1985. Calcium movements through cardiac cell membranes. Med. Res. Rev. **5:** 427–440.
4. BERTHELSEN, S. & W. A. PETTINGER. 1977. A functional basis for classification of α-adrenergic receptors. Life Sci. **21:** 595–606.
5. STARKE, K. 1981. α-Adrenoceptor subclassification. Rev. Physiol. Biochem. Pharmacol. **88:** 199–236.
6. TIMMERMANS, P. B. M. W. M. & P. A. VAN ZWIETEN. 1981. The postsynaptic α_2-adrenoceptor. J. Auton. Pharmacol. **1:** 171–175.

7. McGrath, J. C. 1982. Evidence for more than one type of α-adrenoceptor. Biochem. Pharmacol. **31:** 467–484.
8. Timmermans, P. B. M. W. M. & P. A. van Zwieten. 1982. α_2-Adrenoceptors: classification, localization, mechanisms and targets for drugs. J. Med. Chem. **25:** 1389–1401.
9. van Zwieten, P. A. & P. B. M. W. M. Timmermans. 1984. Central and peripheral α-adrenoceptors. Pharmacological aspects and clinical potential. Adv. Drug. Res. **13:** 209–254.
10. Timmermans, P. B. M. W. M. & P. A. van Zwieten: 1984. α-Adrenoceptor antagonists. *In* Handbook of Hypertension. P. A. van Zwieten, Ed. **3:** 239–248. Elsevier Scientific Publications. Amsterdam, Holland.
11. Langer S. Z., K. Starke & M. L. Dubocovich, Eds. 1979. Presynaptic Receptors. Pergamon Press. Oxford, England
12. Paton, D. M., 1979. The release of catecholamines from adrenergic neurones. Pergamon Press. Oxford, England
13. van Zwieten, P. A. & P. B. M. W. M. Timmermans. 1980. Recent advances in the classification of α-adrenoceptors. Pharm. Weekbl. Sci. Ed. **115:** 1669–1676.
14. Timmermans, P. B. M. W. M., A. de Jonge, M. J. M. C. Thoolen, B. Wilffert & P. A. van Zwieten. 1984. Quantitative relationships between α-adrenergic activity and binding activity of α-adrenoceptor agonists and antagonists. J. Med. Chem. **27:** 447–452.
15. Jie, K., P. van Brummelen, P. Vermeij, P. B. M. W. M. Timmermans & P. A. van Zwieten. 1984. Identification of vascular postsynaptic α_1- and α_2-adrenoceptors in man. Circ. Res. **54:** 447–452.
16. Jie, K., P. van Brummelen, P. Vermeij, P. B. M. W. M. Timmermans & P. A. van Zwieten. 1984. Effects of exogenous adrenaline and noradrenaline on postsynaptic α_1- and α_2-adrenoceptors in man. J. Hypertension **2**(Suppl 3): 119–121.
17. van Brummelen, P., K. Jie, P. B. M. W. M. Timmermans & P. A. van Zwieten. 1984. Postjunctional alpha-adrenoceptors in man. Bibl. Cardiol. No. **38:** 270–276.
18. van Brummelen, P., K. Jie & P. A. van Zwieten. 1986. α-Adrenergic receptors in human blood vessels. Br. J. Clin. Pharmacol. **21:** 33S–39S.
19. Jie, K., P. van Brummelen, P. Vermij, P. B. M. W. M. Timmermans & P. A. van Zwieten. 1986. Alpha$_1$- and alpha$_2$-adrenoceptor mediated vasoconstriction in the human forearm of normotensive and hypertensive subjects. J. Cardiovasc. Pharmacol. **8:** 190–196.
20. Jie, K., P. van Brummelen & P. A. van Zwieten. 1986. α-Adrenoceptors in blood vessels of the human forearm. Prog. Pharmacol. **6:** 39–45.
21. van Meel, J. C. A., R. Toward, S. Kazda, P. B. M. W. M. Timmermans & P. A. van Zwieten. 1983. Correlation between the inhibitory activities of calcium entry blockers on vascular smooth muscle contraction in vitro after K^+-depolarisation and in vivo after α_2-adrenoceptor stimulation. Naunyn-Schmiedeberg's Arch. Pharmacol. **322:** 34–37.
22. Timmermans, P. B. M. W. M., M-J. Mathy, M. J. M. C. Thoolen, A. de Jonge, B. Wilffert & P. A. van Zwieten. 1984. Invariable susceptibility to blockade by nifedipine of vasoconstriction to various α_2-adrenoceptor agonists in pithed rats. J. Pharm. Pharmacol. **36:** 772–775.
23. Wilffert, B., P. N. M. van Heiningen, M-J. Mathy, H. D. Batink, A. de Jonge, M. J. M. C. Thoolen, P. B. M. W. M. Timmermans & P. A. van Zwieten. 1984. Lack of relationship between intrinsic activity and susceptibility of pressor responses to blockade by nifedipine among the α_2-adrenoceptor agonists B-HT 920 and B-HT 958. Naunyn-Schmiedeberg's Arch. Pharmacol. **327:** 90–92.
24. Schramm, M., G. Thomas, R. Toward & G. Franckowiak. 1983. Activation of calcium channels by novel 1,4-dihydropyridines. A new mechanism for positive inotropics or smooth muscle stimulants. Arzneim.-Forsch. **33:** 1268–1272.
25. Wilffert, B., P. N. M. van Heiningen, M-J. Mathy, A. de Jonge, M. J. M. C. Thoolen, P. B. M. W. M. Timmermans & P. A. van Zwieten. 1984. Interactions between the putative calcium entry promotor Bay K 8644 and pressor responses produced by α_1- and α_2-adrenoceptor agonists in the pithed normotensive rat. Naunyn-Schmiedeberg's Arch. Pharmacol. **328:** 76–82.
26. Timmermans, P. B. M. W. M., M. J. M. C. Thoolen, A. de Jonge, B. Wilffert & P. A.

VAN ZWIETEN. 1985. Calcium entry- and α-adrenoceptor-induced vasoconstriction in vivo and in vitro. *In* Alpha-Adrenoceptor Blockers in Cardiovascular Diseases. H. Refsum & O. D. Mjos, Eds.: 30–50. Churchill Livingstone. London & New York.
27. VAN ZWIETEN, P. A., P. B. M. W. M. TIMMERMANS, M. J. M. C. THOOLEN, B. WILFFERT & A. DE JONGE. 1985. Calcium dependency of vasoconstriction mediated by α_1- and α_2-adrenoceptors. J. Cardiovasc. Pharmacol. 7(Suppl. 6): S113–S120.
28. TIMMERMANS, P. B. M. W. M., A. T. CHIN & M. J. M. C. THOOLEN. Calcium handling in vasoconstriction to stimulation of *alpha*-1 and *alpha*-2 adrenoceptors. Can. J. Physiol. Pharmacol. (In press.)
29. TIMMERMANS, P. B. M. W. M., M-J. MATHY, B. WILFFERT, H. O. KALKMAN, M. J. M. C. THOOLEN, A. DE JONGE, J. C. A. VAN MEEL & P. A. VAN ZWIETEN. 1983. Differential effect of calcium entry blockers on α_1-adrenoceptor-mediated vasoconstriction *in vivo*. Naunyn-Schmiedeberg's Arch. Pharmacol. **324:** 239–245.
30. TIMMERMANS, P. B. M. W. M., M. J. M. C. THOOLEN, M-J. MATHY, B. WILFFERT, A. DE JONGE & P. A. VAN ZWIETEN. 1983. Sgd 101/75 is distinguished from other selective α_1-adrenoceptor agonists by the inhibition of its pressor responses by calcium blockade and vasodilatation in pithed rats and cats. Eur. J. Pharmacol. **96:** 187–192.
31. MATHY, M-J., M. J. M. C. THOOLEN, P. B. M. W. M. TIMMERMANS & P. A. VAN ZWIETEN. 1983. Sgd 101/75: cardiovascular effects in various animal preparations; interactions with vascular postjunctional α_1- and α_2-adrenoceptors. Br. J. Pharmacol. **81:** 255–262.
32. BECKERINGH, J. J., M. J. M. C. THOOLEN, A. DE JONGE, B. WILFFERT, P. B. M. W. M. TIMMERMANS & P. A. VAN ZWIETEN. 1984. Differential effects of the calcium entry blocker D 600 on contraction of rat and guinea-pig aortas elicited by alpha-1 adrenoceptor agonists. J. Pharmacol. Exp. Ther. **29:** 515–522.
33. TIMMERMANS, P. B. M. W. M., M. J. M. C. THOOLEN, M-J. MATHY, B. WILFFERT, A. DE JONGE & P. A. VAN ZWIETEN. 1985. Effects of the irreversible α-adrenoceptor antagonists phenoxybenzamine and benextramine on the effectiveness of nifedipine in inhibiting α_1- and α_2-adrenoceptor mediated vasoconstriction in pithed rats. Naunyn-Schmiedeberg's Arch. Pharmacol. **329:** 404–413.
34. KORSTANJE, C. 1986. Cardiovascular α-adrenoceptors in the rat. Ph.D. Thesis. University of Amsterdam. Amsterdam, Holland.
35. BECKERINGH, J. J. 1986. Alpha-1 adrenoceptor mediated vasoconstriction and calcium utilization in preparations of the rat, guinea-pig and rabbit. Ph.D. Thesis. University of Amsterdam. Amsterdam, Holland.
36. KORSTANJE, C., B. WILFFERT, A. DE JONGE, M. J. M. C. THOOLEN, P. B. M. W. M. TIMMERMANS & P. A. VAN ZWIETEN. 184. Calcium-influx-dependent and -independent α_1-adrenoceptor-mediated processes of vasoconstriction *in vivo* do not operate via different α_1-adrenoceptor subtypes. J. Cardiovasc. Pharmacol. **6:** 1102–1108.
37. CHIU, A. T., M. J. M. C. THOOLEN & P. B. M. W. M. TIMMERMANS. 1986. Ca^{2+}-utilization in the constriction of rat aorta to full and partial *alpha*-1 adrenoceptor agonists. J. Pharmacol. Exp. Ther. **238:** 224–231.

The Relationship of Receptor Reserve and Agonist Efficacy to the Sensitivity of α-Adrenoceptor-Mediated Vasopressor Responses to Inhibition by Calcium Channel Antagonists

ROBERT R. RUFFOLO, JR. AND ANDREW J. NICHOLS

Department of Pharmacology
Smith Kline and French Laboratories (L-522)
709 Swedeland Road
Swedeland, Pennsylvania 19479

INTRODUCTION

The interaction between calcium channel antagonists and α-adrenoceptors, particularly in the vasculature, has been the subject of intense research and controversy. Over the last few years, views on the mechanisms of these interactions have changed and been modified in the light of new experimental data. Many of the data obtained concerning the interaction of calcium channel antagonists with α-adrenoceptors appear to be conflicting, and at first sight are not amenable to a single unifying hypothesis. However, recent studies on the processes that link α-adrenoceptor activation to changes in calcium ion fluxes and vascular smooth muscle contraction shed new light on the mechanisms by which calcium channel antagonists interact with α-adrenoceptors.

VASCULAR α-ADRENOCEPTORS AND CALCIUM CHANNEL ANTAGONISTS

It is now known that postjunctional vascular α_1- and α_2-adrenoceptors coexist in the arterial and venous circulations, and that both α-adrenoceptor subtypes mediate vasoconstriction (see Reference 1). van Meel *et al.* first demonstrated that α_2-adrenoceptor-mediated pressor responses in pithed rats were selectively inhibited by calcium channel antagonists, whereas pressor responses mediated by α_1-adrenoceptors were resistant to blockade by calcium channel antagonists.[2] These results suggested that an influx of extracellular calcium ions was necessary for α_2-adrenoceptor-mediated arteriolar vasoconstriction, and that α_1-adrenoceptor-mediated vasoconstriction resulted primarily from the mobilization of intracellular stores of calcium. The primary role of extracellular calcium ions in α_2-adrenoceptor-mediated vasoconstriction was subsequently confirmed *in vitro* in both arterial[3] and venous[4] preparations. Furthermore, the α_2-adrenoceptor agonist B-HT 920 has been shown to induce the influx of $^{45}Ca^{2+}$, and this process is inhibited by the calcium channel antagonists verapamil and nifedipine.[5] This same α_2-adrenoceptor agonist does not induce the release of intracellular calcium.[6] As such, it has become generally accepted that vasoconstriction mediated by α_2-adrenoceptors is invariably susceptible to inhibition by calcium channel antagonists, and is therefore thought to be mediated exclusively by an influx of extracellular calcium.[7]

Although pressor responses mediated by postjunctional vascular α_1-adrenoceptors were initially thought to be resistant to inhibition by calcium channel antagonists,[2] it was subsequently established that this is not the case for all α_1-adrenoceptor agonists. Thus, St 587, Sgd 101/75, and (−)-dobutamine were found to produce α_1-adrenoceptor-mediated pressor responses in pithed rats that were highly sensitive to inhibition by calcium channel blockers.[8,9] Moreover, in isolated arterial tissues *in vitro,* vasoconstriction evoked by α_1-adrenoceptor activation was oftentimes found to be sensitive to inhibition by calcium channel blockers.[10] In rat aorta, α_1-adrenoceptor-mediated vasoconstrictor responses induced by Sgd 101/75 are highly sensitive to inhibition by calcium channel antagonists.[11] In this respect, rat aorta is thought to be similar to pithed rat in the sensitivity of α_1-adrenoceptor-mediated vasoconstrictor responses to inhibition by calcium channel antagonists. It is obvious, therefore, that the sensitivity of α_1-adrenoceptor-mediated vasoconstrictor responses to inhibition by calcium channel antagonists can vary with the agonist used and the tissue studied. Studies of $^{45}Ca^{2+}$ influx in a variety of tissues have invariably demonstrated that α_1-adrenoceptor activation produces an influx of extracellular calcium ions which is utilized in the production of the contractile response.

RECEPTOR NUMBER, AGONIST EFFICACY, AND SENSITIVITY TO CALCIUM CHANNEL ANTAGONISTS

The relationship between α_1-adrenoceptor occupancy and vasoconstriction has been studied extensively *in vitro.* Full α_1-adrenoceptor agonists generally have nonlinear relationships between α_1-adrenoceptor occupancy and response in most arterial blood vessels, and most full agonists (e.g., norepinephrine, epinephrine, phenylephrine, and cirazoline) produce half-maximal vasoconstrictor response at approximately 10% α_1-adrenoceptor occupancy in large blood vessels such as rat aorta.[12] Because of the difficulty in obtaining α_2-adrenoceptor-mediated contractile responses in arterial blood vessels *in vitro,* no comparison between α_1- and α_2-adrenoceptor occupancy-response relationships has been made.

On the other hand, α_2-adrenoceptor-mediated arterial vasoconstriction can be readily studied *in vivo,* where comparisons between the occupancy-response relationships for α_1- and α_2-adrenoceptor-mediated vasoconstriction have been made. Irreversible alkylation of postjunctional vascular α_1-adrenoceptors with phenoxybenzamine *in vivo* results in marked rightward shifts in the vasopressor dose-response curves to α_1-adrenoceptor agonists at degrees of α_1-adrenoceptor alkylation that do not result in depression of the maximum vasopressor response. In contrast, inactivation of a similar proportion of the α_2-adrenoceptor population with phenoxybenzamine is associated with significant depression of the maximum vasopressor response and only small rightward shifts in the dose-response curves to α_2-adrenoceptor agonists.[8,13,14] These results are highly suggestive of a more favorable relationship between receptor occupancy and response for α_1-adrenoceptors relative to α_2-adrenoceptors, and are consistent with the notion that a larger receptor reserve exists in the arterial circulation for α_1-adrenoceptors than for α_2-adrenoceptors.[14]

This differential pattern between α_1- and α_2-adrenoceptor-mediated vasoconstrictor responses following alkylation of vascular α-adrenoceptors was analyzed further in the pithed rat using cirazoline as an α_1-adrenoceptor agonist and B-HT 933 as an α_2-adrenoceptor agonist.[14] Cirazoline demonstrated a hyperbolic relationship between the maximum pressor effect obtained and the fraction of α_1-adrenoceptors remaining available for interaction with cirazoline after irreversible alkylation of a portion of the α_1-adrenoceptor pool with phenoxybenzamine, suggesting highly favorable coupling between α_1-adrenoceptor occupation and vasoconstriction, and possibly the existence of a large α_1-adrenoceptor reserve. In marked contrast, for the α_2-adrenoceptor agonist B-HT 933, a linear relationship was found to exist between the maximum pressor response obtained and the proportion of intact α_2-adrenoceptors available for interaction with the agonist,[14] a situation characteristic of a system that is less favorably coupled and one that lacks a receptor reserve.[15] These differences resulted from a 5- to 10-fold more favorable occupancy-response relationship for the α_1-adrenoceptor-mediated vasoconstrictor effects of cirazoline than for the α_s-adrenoceptor-mediated effects of B-HT 933.[14] This apparent large difference in the coupling between α_1- and α_2-adrenoceptor activation and arterial vasoconstriction may explain the differential effects that calcium entry blockers have on α_1- and α_2-adrenoceptor-mediated vasopressor effects *in vivo*.[8] Similar results to those described above have also been reported in venous tissue,[16,17] and it is now abundantly clear that the relationship between α-adrenoceptor occupancy and response is much more favorable for α_1-adrenoceptors than for α_2-adrenoceptors in both arterial and venous vascular smooth muscle.

Those α_1-adrenoceptor agonists whose responses are sensitive to inhibition by calcium channel antagonists in pithed rats (e.g., St 587, Sgd 101/75, and dobutamine) are partial agonists, whereas those agonists that are resistant to calcium channel antagonists (e.g., cirazoline, phenylephrine, and methoxamine) are full agonists. There are no full agonists whose responses are sensitive to inhibition by calcium channel antagonists, and there are no partial agonists whose responses are resistant to calcium channel antagonists. However, when α_1-adrenoceptor number is reduced by pretreatment with phenoxybenzamine or benextramine, such that there is no longer a receptor reserve for full α_1-adrenoceptor agonists, the pressor responses of these full agonists become sensitive to inhibition by calcium channel antagonists,[8] as expected according to receptor theory.[8] Similarly, it has also been shown using the canine saphenous vein, in which there exists a larger reserve for α_1-adrenoceptors than for α_2-adrenoceptors,[17] that responses to the α_2-adrenoceptor agonist B-HT 920 are sensitive to inhibition by calcium channel antagonists, whereas those produced by full α_1-adrenoceptor agonists are relatively resistant.[5] As is the case *in vivo,* partial α_1-adrenoceptor agonists are highly sensitive to inhibition by calcium channel antagonists, and, after elimination of the α_1-adrenoceptor reserve, even the responses mediated by full α_1-adrenoceptor agonists are sensitive to inhibition by calcium channel blockers.[5] Likewise, pressor responses to the full α_1-adrenoceptor agonist methoxamine are insensitive to functional antagonism by the nonspecific vasodilator nitroprusside at a dose that noncompetitively blocks the vasoconstrictor response to the α_2-adrenoceptor agonist B-HT 933. In contrast, after the removal of the α_1-adrenoceptor reserve with phenoxybenzamine, the vasoconstriction produced by methoxamine becomes equally sensitive as that produced by B-HT 933 to functional antagonism by vasodilators.[18] A similar phenomenon has also been observed in the pithed rat after functional antagonism by nitroprusside and hydralazine.[19] These phenomena can be explained in the simplest terms by the influence of receptor number and agonist efficacy on the differential sensitivity of a full agonist and a partial agonist to a reduction in the efficiency of receptor-effector coupling caused by a noncompetitive antagonist, such as a calcium entry blocker.[8] These interpretations do not necessarily support the contention that α_1- and α_2-adrenoceptors utilize different calcium pools to elicit a response, or that full and partial α_1-adrenoceptor agonists interact at different sites on the α_1-adrenoceptor to produce vasoconstriction, as has been proposed.[9]

Timmermans *et al.* have suggested that the effects of calcium channel antagonists on α_1-adrenoceptor-mediated responses can be explained by the existence of two α_1-adrenoceptors, or two distinct sites on one α_1-adrenoceptor, which possess different sensitivities to phenoxybenzamine and calcium channel antagonists.[9] These authors have proposed that one receptor (or site) is linked to intracellular calcium release and is highly sensitive to inhibition by phenoxybenzamine but is relatively insensitive to calcium channel antagonists, whereas the other α_1-adrenoceptor (or site) possesses the inverse properties and is linked to the translocation of extracellular calcium. In this scheme, full agonists can activate both sites, which renders them sensitive to calcium channel antagonists only after removal of the phenoxybenzamine-sensitive site, whereas partial agonists can only activate the site that is sensitive to calcium channel antagonists, which makes them sensitive to inhibition by calcium channel antagonists under normal conditions. The major problem with this hypothesis is that there exists no pharmacologic evidence to support the notion of two α_1-adrenoceptors, or two sites on one α_1-adrenoceptor, possessing differential sensitivities to phenoxybenzamine and calcium channel antagonists.

RELATIONSHIP BETWEEN α_1-ADRENOCEPTOR ACTIVATION AND CALCIUM TRANSLOCATION

It is now becoming obvious that the relationship between α_1-adrenoceptor activation and the subsequent translocation of calcium leading to vascular smooth contraction is complex. Heaslip and Rahwan have shown that the vasoconstrictor response to norepinephrine in rat aorta produced in calcium-free medium, which is mediated exclusively by the release of intracellular calcium,[20] is associated with little or no α_1-adrenoceptor reserve.[21] Thus, it would appear that despite there being a large receptor reserve for the total α_1-adrenoceptor-mediated contractile response of rat aorta to norepinephrine, there is little or no receptor reserve for the component of the response that is dependent upon intracellular calcium release. This observation has been confirmed in studies of intracellular calcium release in which it has been shown that norepinephrine is less potent at inducing intracellular calcium release than at producing contraction in rat aorta, and that the partial agonist Sgd 101/75 has little, if any, effect on intracellular calcium release.[11] Despite there being little or no receptor reserve for the release of intracellular calcium, this response has a relatively high capacity since the maximum response of rat aorta to the full agonist norepinephrine is reduced by only approximately 30% when extracellular calcium influx is totally abolished by nifedipine, and where the residual response must depend solely on intracellular calcium.[11] If there is little or no receptor reserve for the release of intracellular calcium, or for that component of the vasoconstrictor response produced by intracellular calcium release, but there is a large α_1-adrenoceptor reserve for the *total* response, then there must exist a receptor reserve for that component of the vasoconstrictor response that is dependent upon the influx of extracellular calcium. This is supported by the finding that Sgd 101/75 is a partial agonist in rat aorta with respect to the final contractile response, but is a full agonist for the α_1-adrenoceptor-mediated influx of extracellular calcium.[11] Furthermore, the full agonists, norepinephrine and phenylephrine are more potent at producing calcium influx than at producing contraction in rat aorta. Since the intracellular calcium release component has a high maximum capacity, the extracellular component must have a relatively low capacity. This is supported by the observation that Sgd 101/75, which utilizes mainly extracellular calcium,[11] produces a maximum response in rat aorta of only approximately 40% of the norepinephrine response. Thus, it appears that the component of the α_1-adrenoceptor-mediated response in vascular smooth muscle that is critically dependent upon the influx of extracellular calcium has a high efficiency of coupling, and is therefore hyperbolic with respect to α_1-adrenoceptor occupancy. This causes there to be a significant receptor reserve for the component of the α_1-adrenoceptor-mediated vasoconstrictor response that is dependent upon extracellular calcium, whereas the intracellular component has a low efficiency of coupling, leading to a low or nonexistent receptor reserve.

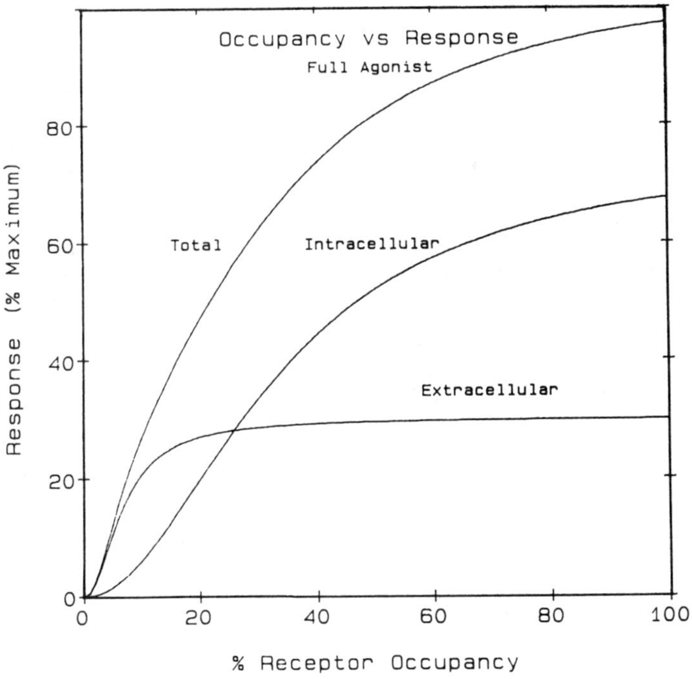

FIGURE 1. Theoretical occupancy-response relationships for the intracellular and extracellular components of the total response to a full α_1-adrenoceptors angonist.

A NOVEL HYPOTHESIS TO EXPLAIN THE INFLUENCE OF RECEPTOR NUMBER AND AGONIST EFFICACY ON SENSITIVITY TO CALCIUM CHANNEL ANTAGONISTS

The different occupancy-response relationships for the two calcium fluxes that underly α_1-adrenoceptor-mediated vasoconstriction can be used to formulate a novel hypothesis to explain the complex relationship between receptor number, agonist efficacy, and receptor reserve, on one hand, to the sensitivity to calcium channel antagonists on the other. Using experimental results relating to occupancy-response relationships for α_1- and α_2-adrenoceptors, it is possible to employ the basic concepts of receptor theory to explain the noncompetitive interaction that exists between calcium channel antagonists and α-adrenoceptors. The relationship between the overt pharmacologic response produced by an agonist to the biological stimulus, S, generated by the agonist-receptor interaction is defined as follows:[22,23]

$$S = \epsilon[R_t]y \tag{1}$$

where ϵ is the intrinsic efficacy of the agonist, $[R_t]$ is the total receptor concentration, and y equals receptor occupancy which is derived from the mass-law relationship involving both the agonist-receptor dissociation constant and the concentration of agonist. The final response, R, is related to the biologic stimulus by the following logistic relationship:[24]

$$R = \frac{R_{max} S^n}{S^n + \beta^n} \tag{2}$$

where n is the coupling state and β is the efficiency of coupling between occupancy and response. Using these equations that relate agonist concentration to receptor stimulus, and the relationship between stimulus and response as described above, as well as our knowledge of the differences that exist between the receptor-effector coupling of the intracellular and extracellular components of the α_1-adrenoceptor-mediated response (see above), it is possible to construct occupancy-response relationships and theoretical dose-response curves for the total α_1-adrenoceptor-mediated vasoconstrictor response

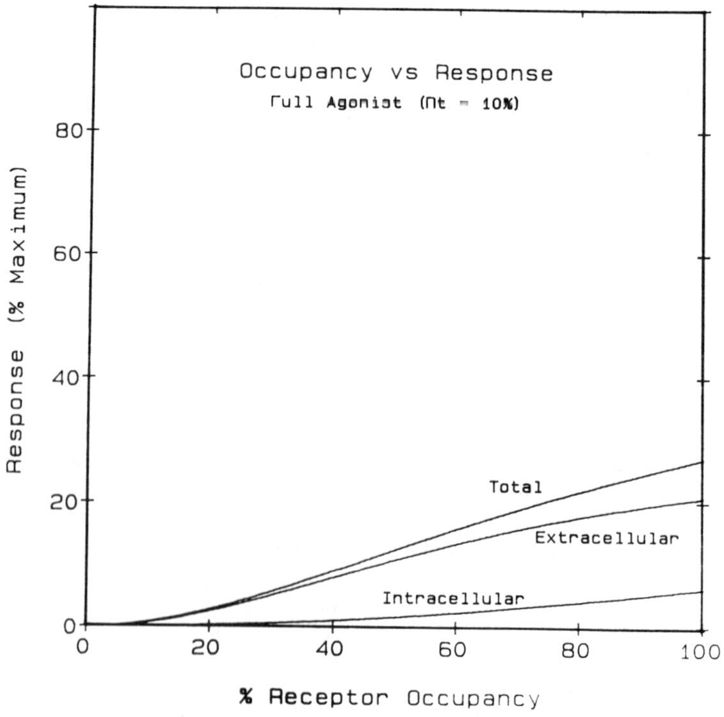

FIGURE 2. Theoretical occupancy-response relationships for a full α_1-adrenoceptor agonist after removal of 90% of the receptors.

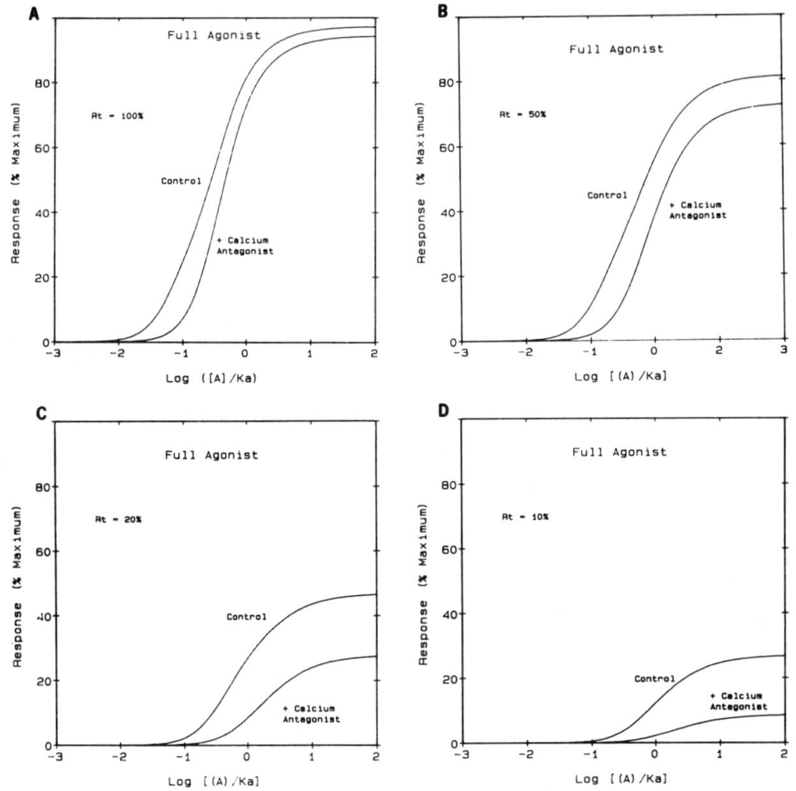

FIGURE 3. Theoretical log dose-response curves showing the effect of a calcium channel antagonist on the response to a full α_1-adrenoceptor agonist whose receptor reserve has been progressively reduced by a reduction in R_t from 100% to 10% (A–D).

based on the individual intracellular and extracellular calcium components. Furthermore, we can simulate the effect of calcium channel antagonists on the log dose-response curves to full and partial α_1-adrenoceptor agonists, and determine what effect changes in receptor number, as would occur upon irreversible alkylation with phenoxybenzamine, and agonist efficacy have on the inhibitory effects of calcium channel antagonists.

As indicated above, evidence suggests that there is either a low or no α_1-adrenoceptor reserve for that component of the vasoconstrictor response mediated by intracellular calcium,[11] and that this response must have a relatively high capacity since the maximum response of rat aorta to the full α_1-adrenoceptor agonist norepinephrine is reduced by only approximately 30% when extracellular calcium influx is totally abolished by nifedipine.[11] By inference, the extracellular calcium component, which must be associated with a significant receptor reserve, can have only a low capacity. The coupling between α_1-adrenoceptor occupancy and the translocation of extracellular calcium is approximately fivefold more efficient than the coupling between α_1-adrenoceptor occupancy and the mobilization of intracellular calcium based on the results of Chiu *et al.*[11] Using this information, we can model the

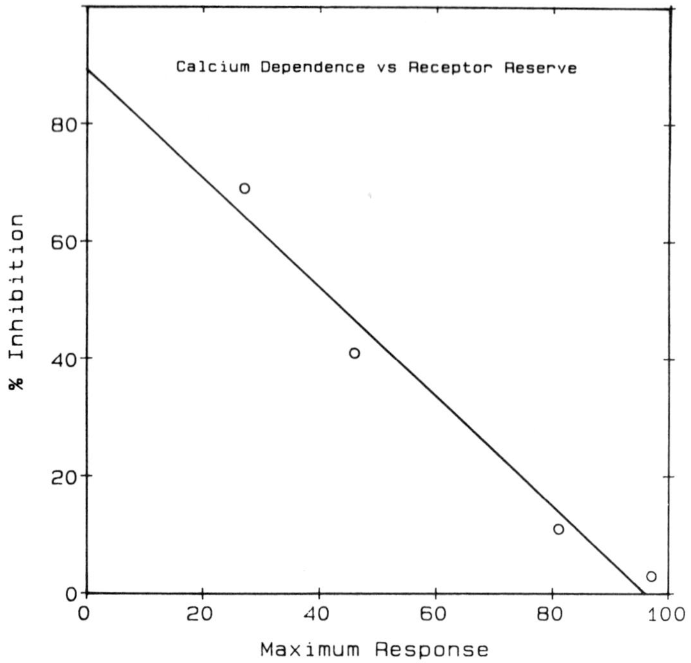

FIGURE 4. Correlation between the maximum response elicited by a full α_1-adrenoceptor agonist after progressive removal of the receptor reserve, and the percentage reduction in the maximum response produced by a calcium channel antagonist, obtained from the data presented in FIGURE 3.

occupancy-response relationships and dose-response curves for the intracellular and extracellular processes as they relate to vasoconstrictor responses mediated by α_1-adrenoceptors.

In the modeling, it is assumed that a single agonist interacts with a single receptor site of given receptor density ($[R_t]$), and thus the intrinsic efficacy of the agonist (ϵ) must be the same for both calcium processes since they are triggered by the same receptor activation. The difference in the maximum response of the two processes is modeled simply by assigning different maximum response values in accord with experimental observations.[11] The different occupancy-response relationships for the intracellular and extracellular processes cannot arise from differences in agonist efficacy for the two processes, since the agonist interacts with only one receptor site. Therefore, the different occupancy-response relationships for those components of the α_1-adrenoceptor-mediated response resulting from the intracellular and extracellular calcium fluxes are modeled by the difference in the efficiency of coupling (β) between the two calcium processes, and recent experimental evidence suggests that the difference in coupling between α_1-adrenoceptor activation and extracellular and intracellular calcium mobilization is three- to fivefold, with the extracellular process being most efficient.[11] Assuming that the maximum vasoconstrictor response (R_{max}) for the extracellular process accounts for only approximately 30% of the total response, a good fit of the model describing a full agonist to the experimental data is obtained with the following parameters: for both the intracellular and extracellular processes,

$\epsilon = 3.0$, $[R_t] = 1.0$, $n = 2$; these parameters are the same for both processes because they relate to the interaction of the drug with the receptor. For the extracellular process, $R_{max} = 30\%$, and the efficiency of coupling is high, as indicated by a low absolute value of β (i.e., $\beta = 0.2$). For the intracellular process, $R_{max} = 70\%$, and the efficiency of coupling is low, as indicated by a higher absolute value of β (i.e., $\beta = 1$) (see Reference 24 for explanation of the term β). The difference in efficiency of coupling for the two processes is assumed to be fivefold, which is consistent with experimental observations.[11] The total response was obtained by computer-assisted addition of the two individual components, each component being based on Equations 1 and 2.

FIGURE 1 shows the occupancy-response relationships obtained for the vasoconstrictor response mediated by a full α_1-adrenoceptor agonist. It can be seen that the extracellular response has a low maximum (30%), but the half-maximal response for this process is achieved with approximately 7% receptor occupation, and is therefore considered to be highly coupled. In contrast, the intracellular response has a relatively high maximum (70%), with the half-maximal response occurring when approximately 40% of the α_1-adrenoceptors are occupied, consistent with a lower degree of coupling. Thus, the total response represents a hyperbolic occupancy-response relationship, with the half-maximal response being produced by 20% receptor occupation, consistent with

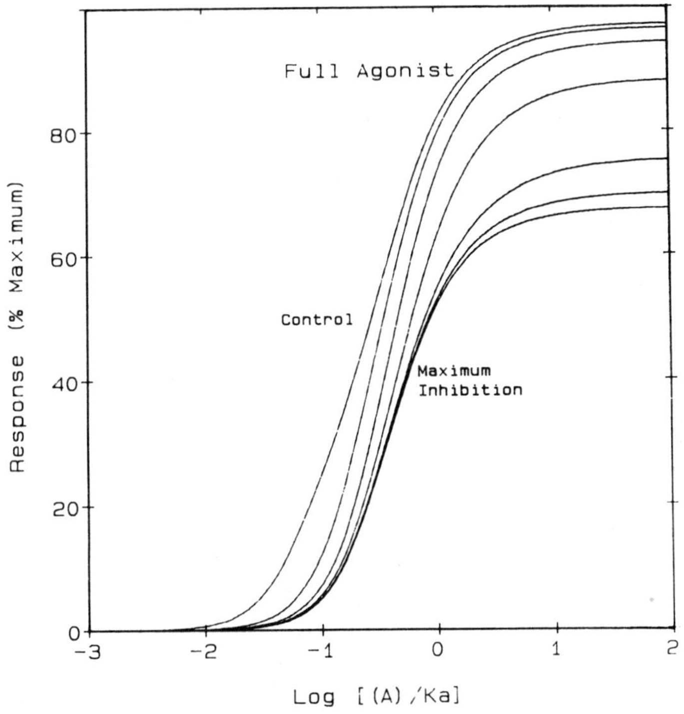

FIGURE 5. Theoretical log dose-response curves showing the effect of varying degrees of reduction in the efficiency of coupling of the extracellular process, β, from 0.2 to 0.5, 1.0, 2.0, 5.0, 10, and 100, showing the maximal inhibition obtainable for a full α_1-adrenoceptor agonist with complete removal of the extracellular process.

experimental observations.[12] When receptor number is reduced by alkylation (i.e., reducing $[R_t]$ in Equation 1), the intracellular component (FIGURE 2) of the response is reduced to a much greater extent than the extracellular component as a result of the much lower efficiency of coupling for the intracellular process. Thus, the total response will be more sensitive to inhibition by calcium channel antagonists as receptor number is lowered, a prediction that is also borne out by experimental observation.[8] Furthermore, not only is a greater proportion of the response mediated by extracellular calcium influx as receptor number is reduced, but the extracellular component itself will become more sensitive to inhibition as its own receptor reserve is reduced.[15] Thus, as receptor number is decreased (i.e., as $[R_t]$ is reduced in Equation 1), the degree of inhibition produced by calcium channel antagonists (which will decrease the efficiency of coupling of the extracellular process, and this is modeled by increasing β in Equation 2 by fivefold) is increased, as has been reported previously in pithed rat.[8] The effect of calcium channel antagonists on the log dose-response curves to a full agonist with different levels of receptor alkylation is shown in FIGURE 3. It can clearly be seen that as receptor number is reduced, the calcium channel antagonist produces an increasingly greater inhibition of the response (FIGURE 3). Ruffolo *et al.* reported an identical effect in the pithed rat, and further showed that there was an inverse linear relationship between the maximum response to the full α_1-adrenoceptor agonist following phenoxybenzamine treatment (which is dependent upon receptor number) and the degree to which the residual response was inhibited by the calcium channel antagonist.[8] When

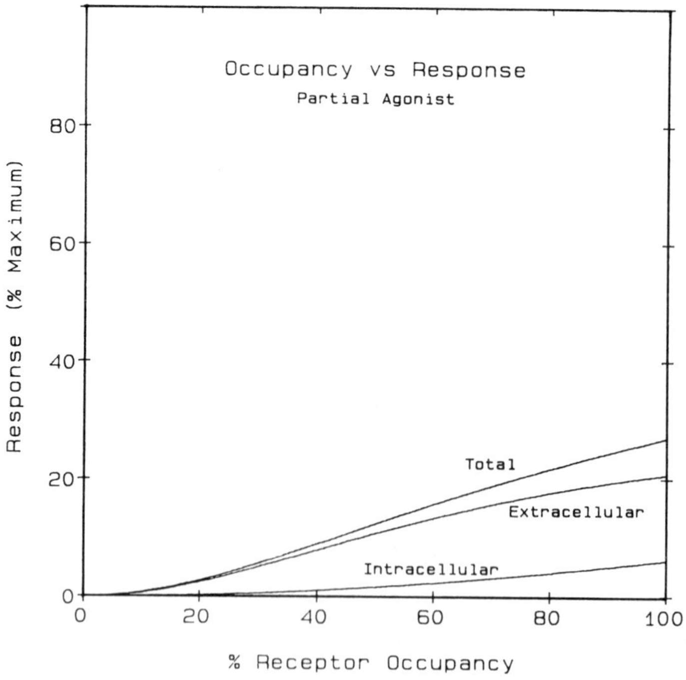

FIGURE 6. Theoretical occupancy-response curves for the intracellular and extracellular components of the total response to a partial α_1-adrenoceptor agonist with an intrinsic efficacy, E, equal to 10% of that for the full agonist.

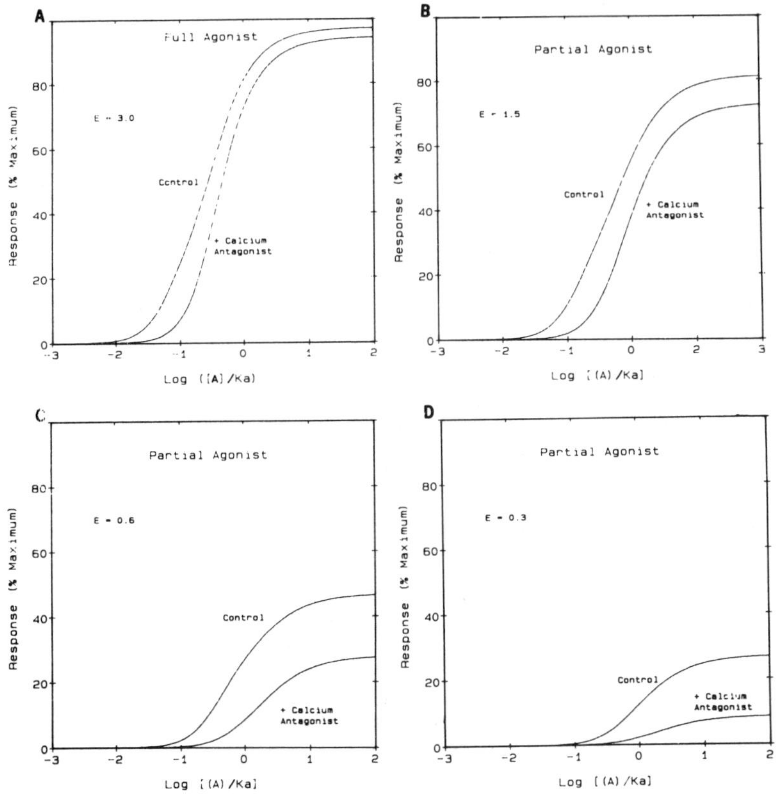

FIGURE 7. Theoretical log dose-response curves showing the effect of a calcium channel antagonist on the response to a series of α_1-adrenoceptor agonists with intrinsic efficacies (E) varying from 3.0 to 0.3 (A–D).

the results of the modeling in FIGURE 3 are analyzed in the same way, it is found that there is, indeed, an inverse linear relationship between the maximum response remaining after partial receptor alkylation and the percentage inhibition produced by calcium channel antagonists (FIGURE 4). In addition, this model predicts that there will be a limited 30% inhibition of the response to a full α_1-adrenoceptor agonist (in the absence of receptor alkylation) by calcium channel antagonists, and this is associated with a threefold rightward shift in the log dose-response curve (FIGURE 5). In this regard, too, the model is compatible with experimental observations *in vitro* and *in vivo* where a calcium channel antagonist produces a 15–30% reduction in the maximum response of a full α_1-adrenoceptor agonist, with a three- to fivefold rightward shift in the ED_{50}. Thus, the modeling can account for the effect of receptor reserve on the sensitivity to calcium channel antagonists, and the existence of a limited degree of inhibition of a full agonist by a calcium channel antagonist in the normal state. Furthermore, the model acknowledges the existence of two sources of calcium available for the production of a response, yet does not require assuming that one agonist interacts with two sites on one receptor, or two distinct α_1-adrenoceptors, as proposed by Timmermans *et al.*,[9] for which no experimental support exists.

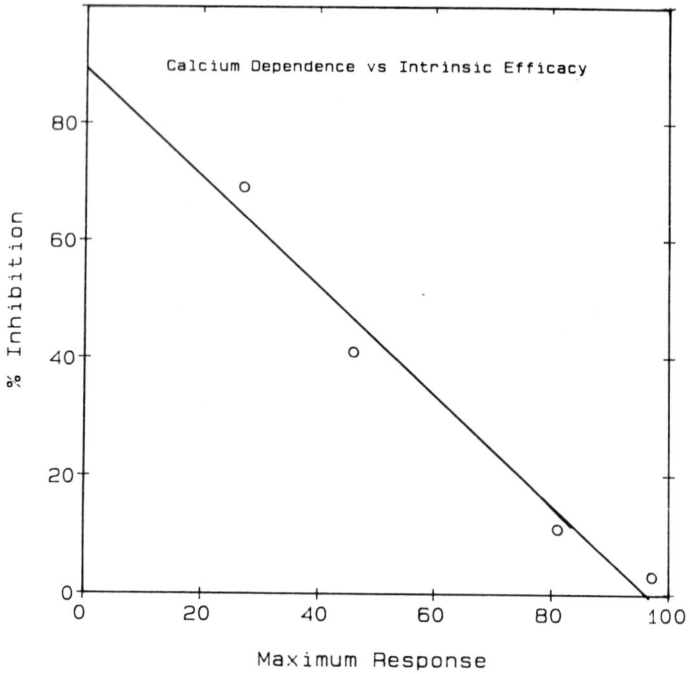

FIGURE 8. Correlation between the maximum response produced by a series of α_1-adrenoceptor agonists with varying intrinsic efficacies, and the percentage inhibition of the maximum response produced a calcium channel antagonist, obtained from the data presented in FIGURE 7.

To model a partial agonist, the intrinsic efficacy of the agonist (ϵ) is reduced in Equation 1 as receptor theory would predict. The effect of this change is shown in FIGURE 6 where the intrinsic efficacy of the partial agonist is reduced 10-fold (i.e., ϵ = 0.3). The most striking effect of this reduction in intrinsic efficacy is the almost complete elimination of the intracellular process, with only a small reduction in the extracellular process. Again, this prediction is supported by experimental evidence.[11] The reason for this differential effect on the two responses lies in the difference in the efficiency of coupling between α_1-adrenoceptor activation and intracellular and extracellular calcium utilization. Because the component of the response that is dependent on extracellular calcium has a high efficiency of coupling and a large receptor reserve, and the intracellular component has a low efficiency of coupling and a small (or no) receptor reserve, it is apparent from FIGURE 6 that, in contrast to the full agonist (FIGURE 1) where the intracellular response predominates, the response to the partial agonist is almost exclusively dependent upon the extracellular process, and this results simply from reducing ϵ in the model. Furthermore, the total occupancy-response relationship is nearly linear for the partial agonist, and this is also observed experimentally for partial agonists.[12]

Over a range of intrinsic efficacies from 3.0 to 0.3, the relative importance of the extracellular component increases with decreasing efficacy, and the total occupancy-response relationship, based on the intracellular and extracellular components, approaches linearity, both of these factors being supported by experimental observations. Furthermore, as agonist efficacy decreases, the ability of a calcium channel antagonist to inhibit the response of the partial agonist (modeled by decreasing the coupling efficiency of the extracellular process by reducing β in Equation 2) will increase (FIGURE 7) due to the increasing dependence on extracellular calcium that occurs as intrinsic efficacy decreases (FIGURE 6), as predicted by the model. In fact, the effect that agonist efficacy has on the sensitivity to inhibition by calcium channel antagonists should be the same as that produced by a reduction in receptor number, since the stimulus is proportional to both the intrinsic efficacy and receptor number (see Equation 1), and this, in fact, has been reported.[8] As a result, the model predicts an inverse linear relationship between intrinsic activity (which is dependent upon intrinsic efficacy) and the degree to which the response is inhibited by calcium channel antagonists, as is shown in FIGURE 8. This has also been observed experimentally in the pithed rat[8] and rat aorta.[11] Furthermore, as intrinsic efficacy decreases, it is predicted that the maximum inhibition of the response that can be produced by a calcium channel antagonist is increased, as is observed in the pithed rat[9] and rat aorta,[11] and this is a direct result of a decreased role of intracellular calcium and the porportionally greater role of extracellular calcium that occurs as intrinsic efficacy is decreased (see FIGURES 6 and 8).

It is readily apparent that the receptor model described herein can predict all the observed interactions between α_1-adrenoceptor agonists and calcium channel antagonists. There exists other important information that can be learned from this modeling

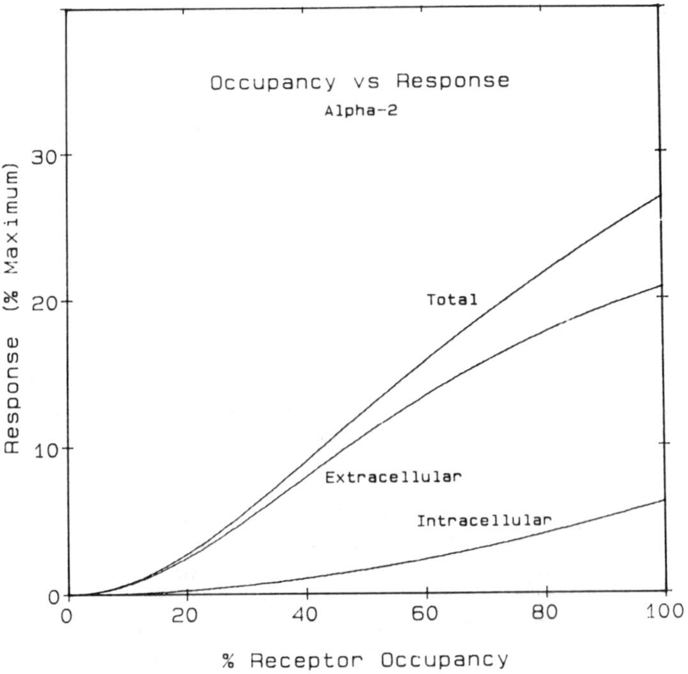

FIGURE 9. Theoretical occupancy-response relationships for an α_2-adrenoceptor agonist with efficiency of coupling, β, of the intracellular and extracellular responses 10-fold lower than those for the α_1-adrenoceptor agonist shown in FIGURE 1.

regarding the role of intracellular and extracellular calcium in relation to the intrinsic efficacy of an agonist. Chiu *et al.* have proposed that full agonist activity requires mobilization of both intracellular and extracellular calcium processes via activation of two distinct processes,[11] possibly as a result of an interaction with two sites on the α_1-adrenoceptor.[9] Furthermore, they propose that partial agonist activity can result from activation of only one of the processes alone. In support of their argument, Chiu *et al.* have shown that the partial α_1-adrenoceptor agonist Sgd 101/75 is a full agonist for extracellular calcium influx without producing any discernible intracellular calcium release.[11] Furthermore, they predict that it is possible for an agonist to work by release of intracellular calcium alone, although such an agonist has never been identified. Our

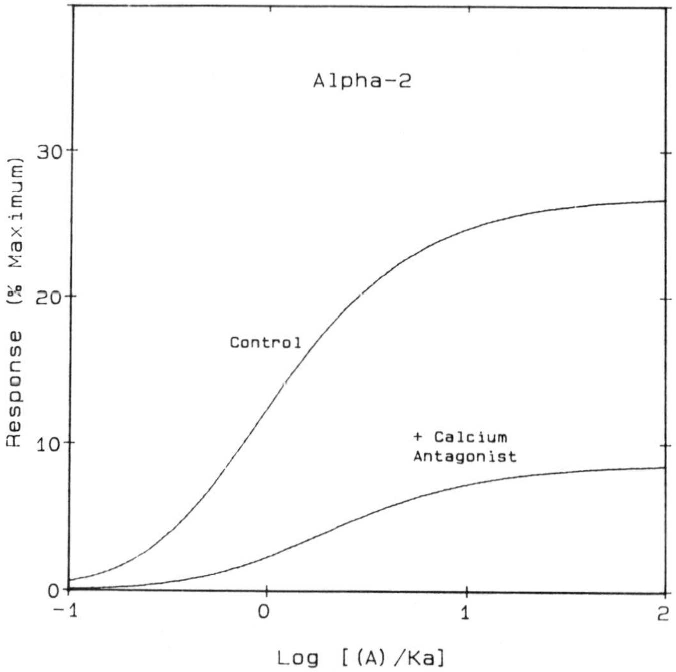

FIGURE 10. Theoretical log dose-response curves showing the effect of a calcium channel antagonist on the response to an α_2-adrenoceptor agonist.

model shows that a full agonist may indeed activate both processes, and that a weak partial agonist may activate only the extracellular process. Furthermore, our model predicts that a partial agonist cannot work solely via the release of intracellular calcium. It is purely the intrinsic efficacy of the agonist that determines the degree and extent of activation of both processes, and thus determines the intrinsic activity of the agonist and its sensitivity to inhibition by calcium channel antagonists. The existence of two different sites on the α_1-adrenoceptor, as proposed by Timmermans *et al.*,[9] which has never been proven, is not a requirement of this model.

Finally, using this model, it becomes apparent why α_2-adrenoceptor agonists are invariably sensitive to inhibition by calcium channel antagonists. Assuming that the utilization of intracellular and extracellular calcium for the α_2-adrenoceptor-mediated vasoconstrictor process is identical to that for the α_1-adrenoceptor-mediated process, by factoring into the model the known 5- to 10-fold lower coupling that exists between α_2-adrenoceptor occupancy and response relative to the α_1-adrenoceptor occupancy-response relationship,[14,16] which amounts to increasing the β-factor by 5- to 10-fold, the relative proportion of the intracellular component decreases and the extracellular component increases (FIGURE 9), such that a nearly complete dependence on extracellular calcium results. Blockade of α_2-adrenoceptor-mediated vasoconstriction by a calcium channel antagonist (which increases the β component further in the extracellular process only) is expected to be nearly complete by the model (FIGURE 10). These predictions are entirely consistent with the extreme sensitivity of α_2-adrenoceptor-mediated pressor responses to inhibition by calcium channel antagonists.

REFERENCES

1. RUFFOLO, R. R., JR. 1985. Distribution and function of peripheral α-adrenoceptors in the cardiovascular system. Pharmacol. Biochem. Behav. **22:** 827–833.
2. VAN MEEL, J. C. A., A. DE JONGE, H. O. KALKMAN, B. WILFFERT, P. B. M. W. M. TIMMERMANS & P. A. VAN ZWIETEN. 1981. Organic and inorganic calcium antagonists reduce vasoconstriction *in vivo* mediated by postsynaptic α_2-adrenoceptors. Naunyn-Schmiedeberg's Arch. Pharmacol. **316:** 288–293.
3. MEDGETT, I. C. & M. A. S. RAJANAYAGAM. 1984. Effects of reduced calcium ion concentration and of diltiazem on vasoconstrictor responses to noradrenaline and sympathetic nerve stimulation in rat isolated tail artery. Br. J. Pharmacol. **83:** 889–898.
4. COOKE, J. P., T. J. RIMELE, N. A. FLAVAHAN & P. M. VANHOUTTE. 1985. Nimodipine and inhibition of α-adrenergic activation of the isolated canine saphenous vein. J. Pharmacol. Exp. Ther. **234:** 598–602.
5. MATTHEWS, W. D., K. F. JIM, J. P. HIEBLE & R. M. DEMARINIS. 1984. Postsynaptic α-adrenoceptors on vascular smooth muscle. Fed. Proc. **43:** 2923–2928.
6. JIM, K. F. & W. D. MATTHEWS. 1985. Role of extracellular calcium in contractions produced by activation of postsynaptic α_2-adrenoceptors in canine saphenous vein. J. Pharmacol. Exp. Ther. **234:** 161–165.
7. TIMMERMANS, P. B. M. W. M., M. J. MATHY, M. J. M. C. THOOLEN, A. DE JONGE, B. WILFFERT & P. A. VAN ZWIETEN. 1984. Invariable susceptibility to blockade by nifedipine of vasoconstriction to various α_2-adrenoceptor agonists in pithed rats. J. Pharm. Pharmacol. **36:** 772–775.
8. RUFFOLO, R. R., JR., E. L. MORGAN & K. MESSICK. 1984. Possible relationship between receptor reserve and the differential antagonism of *alpha*-1 and *alpha*-2 adrenoceptor-mediated pressor responses by calcium channel antagonists in the pithed rat. J. Pharmacol. Exp. Ther. **230:** 587–594.
9. TIMMERMANS, P. B. M. W. M., M. J. M. C. THOOLEN, M. J. MATHY, B. WILFFERT, A. DE JONGE & P. A. VAN ZWIETEN. 1985. Effects of the irreversible α-adrenoceptor antagonists phenoxybenzamine and benextramine on the effectiveness of nifedipine in inhibiting α_1- and α_2-adrenoceptor mediated vasoconstriction in pithed rats. Naunyn-Schmiedeberg's Arch. Pharmacol. **329:** 404–413.
10. VAN BREEMEN, C. & B. SIEGEL. 1980. The mechanism of α-adrenergic activation of the dog coronary artery. Circ. Res. **46:** 426–429.
11. CHIU, A. T., D. E. MCCALL, M. J. M. C. THOOLEN & P. B. M. W. M. TIMMERMANS. 1986. Ca^{++} utilization in the constriction of rat aorta to full and partial *alpha*-1 adrenoceptor agonists. J. Pharmacol. Exp. Ther. **238:** 224–231.
12. RUFFOLO, R. R., JR., E. L. ROSING & J. E. WADDELL. 1979. Receptor interactions of imidazolines. I. Affinity and efficacy for *alpha*-adrenergic receptors. J. Pharmacol. Exp. Ther. **209:** 429–436.
13. HAMILTON, C. A., J. L. REID & D. J. SUMNER. 1983. Acute effects of phenoxybenzamine

on α-adrenoceptor responses *in vivo* and *in vitro;* relation of *in vivo* pressor responses to the number of specific adrenoceptor binding sites. J. Cardiovasc. Pharmacol. **5:** 868–873.

14. RUFFOLO, R. R., JR., & E. L. YADEN. 1984. Existence of spare α_1-adrenoceptors, but not α_2-adrenoceptors, for respective vasopressor effects of cirazoline and B-HT 933 in the pithed rat. J. Cardiovasc. Pharmacol. **6:** 1011–1019.
15. RUFFOLO, R. R., JR. 1982. Important concepts of receptor theory. J. Auton. Pharmacol. **2:** 277–295.
16. RUFFOLO, R. R., JR. & R. L. ZEID. 1985. Relationship between *alpha*-adrenoceptor occupancy and response for the *alpha*-1 adrenoceptor agonist, cirazoline, and the *alpha*-2 adrenoceptor agonist, B-HT 933, in canine saphenous vein. J. Pharmacol. Exp. Ther. **235:** 636–643.
17. FLAVAHAN, N. A. & P. M. VANHOUTTE. 1986. *Alpha*-1 and *alpha*-2 adrenoceptor: response coupling in canine saphenous and femoral veins. J. Pharmacol. Exp. Ther. **238:** 131–138.
18. LEW, M. J. & J. A. ANGUS. 1985. α_1- and α_2-adrenoceptor mediated pressor responses: are they differentiated by calcium antagonists or by functional antagonism? J. Cardiovasc. Pharmacol. **7:** 401–408.
19. PEDRINELLI, R. & R. C. TARAZI. 1985. Calcium entry blockade by nitrendipine and *alpha*-adrenergic responses *in vivo:* comparison with noncalcium entry blocker vasodilators in absence and presence of phenoxybenzamine pretreatment. J. Pharmacol. Exp. Ther. **233:** 636–642.
20. HEASLIP, R. J. & R. G. RAHWAN. 1983. Norepinephrine-induced contractions of the rat aorta in the absence of extracellular calcium. II. Effects of calcium antagonists. Gen. Pharmacol. **14:** 505–512.
21. HEASLIP, R. J. & R. G. RAHWAN. 1983. Norepinephrine-induced contractions of the rat aorta in the absence of extracellular calcium. I. Effects of α-adrenoceptor blockers. Gen. Pharmacol. **14:** 497–503.
22. STEPHENSON, R. P. 1956. A modification of receptor theory. Br. J. Pharmacol. **11:** 379–393.
23. FURCHGOTT, R. F. 1966. The use of β-haloalkylamines in the differentiation of receptors and in the determination of dissociation constants of receptor-agonist complexes. Adv. Drug Res. **3:** 21–55.
24. KENAKIN, T. P. 1984. The classification of drugs and drug receptors in isolated tissues. Pharmacol. Rev. **36:** 165–222.

Poster Paper

Arguments Against the Role of Receptor Reserve as a Determinant of the Sensitivity of α_1-Adrenoceptor-Mediated Pressor Responses to Inhibition by Ca^{2+} Entry Blockers in the Pithed Rat

PIETER B. M. W. M. TIMMERMANS AND
MARTIN J. M. C. THOOLEN

Division of Cardiovascular Diseases
Medical Products Department
E.I. du Pont de Nemours & Company Inc.
Experimental Station, E400/4257
Wilmington, Delaware 19898

The effects of the irreversible antagonist of α_1-adrenoceptors, phenoxybenzamine, on the effectiveness of nifedipine to inhibit the increase in diastolic pressure to the selective α_1-adrenoceptor full agonist, phenylephrine, were quantified in pithed normotensive rats.

In a dose-dependent fashion, nifedipine [intraarterially (ia), −15 minutes] maximally shifted the log dose–pressor response curve to intravenous (iv) phenylephrine fivefold to the right, amounts of 1 and 3 mg/kg being equieffective (FIGURE 1). Phenoxybenzamine (3–1000 μg/kg, iv, −60 minutes) enhanced the effectiveness of nifedipine, expressed as −log ID_{50} (ID_{50}: dose in mol/kg for 50% reduction of maximum pressor response), to inhibit the vasopressor response to phenylephrine. FIGURE 2 shows the effect of pretreatment with 100 μg/kg of phenoxybenzamine. The potentiating action of phenoxybenzamine was already demonstrable at a low dose of 3 μg/kg, which by itself had no influence on the log dose–pressor response curve to phenylephrine. This effect was also clearly limited, inasmuch as the −log ID_{50} values of nifedipine determined following treatment with 0.1 (6.03 ± 0.17), 0.3 (6.08 ± 0.13), and 1 mg/kg (6.01 ± 0.09) of phenoxybenzamine were identical and similar to the value reported for nifedipine against α_2-adrenoceptor-mediated vasoconstriction in pithed rats (6.11 ± 0.09).[7] Infusion of vasopressin to counteract the vasodilatory action of nifedipine did not affect this inhibitory potency compared to its effectiveness quantified under the conditions of reduced baseline diastolic pressure.

The interaction pattern of nifedipine with respect to its inhibition of the increase in diastolic pressure to phenylephrine and other selective α_1-adrenoceptor agonists,[7] as well as the dissociation between irreversible α_1-adrenoceptor blockade of phenoxybenzamine and its potentiation of nifedipine's inhibitory effect, combined with the absence of an inverse relationship between the magnitude of the maximum pressor response and the sensitivity to inhibition by nifedipine, leads us to dismiss the hypothesis[2–6] that α_1-adrenoceptor reserve plays a principal role in determining the susceptibility of α_1-adrenoceptor-mediated pressor responses to inhibition by Ca^{2+} entry blockers. The resistance of the pressor effects of various α_1-adrenoceptor agonists in pithed rats to inhibition by Ca^{2+} entry blockers is in full agreement with the results of numerous studies *in vitro* showing that vasoconstriction to α_1-adrenoceptor stimulation is

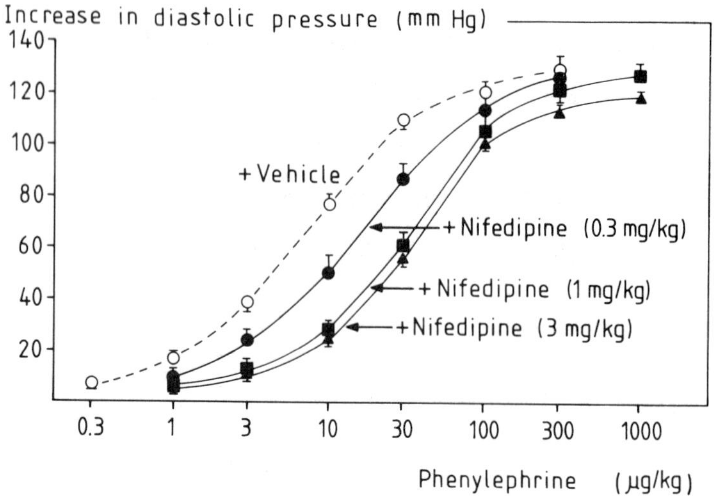

FIGURE 1. Log dose-response curves with respect to absolute increments in diastolic pressure produced by phenylephrine injected iv to pithed normotensive rats 15 minutes after ia pretreatment with various doses of nifedipine. Symbols represent mean values ± standard error of the mean (SEM) ($n = 6$–7).

governed by a transmembraneous Ca^{2+} influx, which is sensitive to inhibition by Ca^{2+} entry blockers and/or an intracellular release of Ca^{2+}, which is insensitive to blockade by these drugs (see Reference 1).

This study also shows that restoration of the baseline diastolic pressure with vasopressin did not change the profound inhibitory action of nifedipine. This result

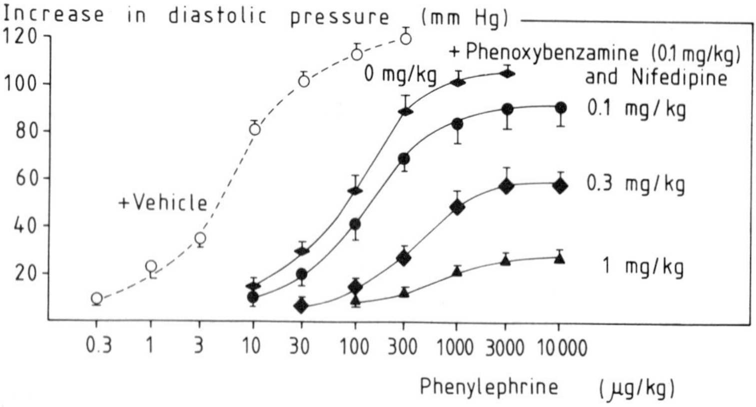

FIGURE 2. Log dose-response curves with respect to absolute increments in diastolic pressure produced by phenylephrine injected iv to pithed normotensive rats 1 hour after iv treatment with phenoxybenzamine (0.1 mg/kg) and 15 minutes after ia pretreatment with various doses of nifedipine. Symbols represent mean values ± SEM ($n = 6$–7).

does not support the suggestion that functional antagonism exerted by nifedipine plays a major role.[4,5]

We submit that it is appropriate to explain the differential inhibitory effect of Ca^{2+} entry blockers on vasconstriction to the various α-adrenoceptor agonists by the differential degree to which their response relies on an influx of extracellular Ca^{2+}, rather than attributing these differences to differential degrees of receptor reserve of the α-adrenoceptor stimulants and/or functional antagonism exerted by the Ca^{2+} channel blocker.

REFERENCES

1. CAUVIN, C., R. LOUTZENHISER & C. VAN BREEMEN. 1983. Annu. Rev. Pharmacol. Toxicol. **23:** 373.
2. COOKE, J. P., T. J. RIMELE, N. A. FLAVAHAN & P. M. VANHOUTTE. 1985. J. Pharmacol. Exp. Ther. **234:** 597.
3. JIM, K. F., R. A. MACIA & W. D. MATTHEWS. 1986. J. Pharmacol. Exp. Ther. **238:** 89.
4. LEW, M. J. & J. A. ANGUS. 1985. J. Cardiovasc. Pharmacol. **7:** 401.
5. PEDRINELLI, R. & R. C. TARAZI. 1985. J. Pharmacol. Exp. Ther. **233:** 636.
6. RUFFOLO, R. R., E. L. MORGAN & K. MESSICK. 1984. J. Pharmacol. Exp. Ther. **230:** 537.
7. TIMMERMANS, P. B. M. W. M., M. J. M. C. THOOLEN, M. J. MATHY, B. WILFFERT, A. DE JONGE & P. A. VAN ZWIETEN. 1985. Naunyn-Schmiedeberg's Arch. Pharmacol. **329:** 404.

Ca^{2+} Antagonists and Vascular Disease

PAUL M. VANHOUTTE

Department of Physiology and Biophysics
Mayo Clinic and Mayo Foundation
Rochester, Minnesota 55905

The free intracellular concentration of the activator ion Ca^{2+} is controlled by a number of energy-dependent processes among which are those preventing its entry or seeking its active removal, as exaggerated amounts of Ca^{2+} are toxic. Of the processes allowing increases of cytoplasmic Ca^{2+} concentrations in vascular cells, the most important is the opening of Ca^{2+} channels, which can be inhibited pharmacologically by a heterogeneous class of compounds called the Ca^{2+} antagonists (FIGURE 1).[15,18] These drugs affect vascular function, particularly under pathological conditions, which may explain why they are beneficial in the treatment of vascular disease. The present essay discusses this hypothesis and summarizes several similar attempts, to which the readers are referred for details and references.[4–7,11–17,19,20,22,23]

PHARMACOLOGY

Vascular Smooth Muscle

The organic calcium entry blockers (cinnarizine, diltiazem, flunarizine, nifedipine, nimodipine, and verapamil) inhibit smooth muscle contraction by blocking calcium influx through gated channels (FIGURE 2).[8] In the presence of these drugs the inhibition of potassium-stimulated calcium influx in various vascular smooth muscle preparations is highly correlated with the inhibition of the contraction.

When comparing the responses of vascular smooth muscle preparations from different species and/or anatomical origin, a wide range of sensitivity to a variety of vasoactive agents is observed. These include the Ca^{2+} antagonists. Indeed, major differences in potency are seen among the individual Ca^{2+} antagonists in various vascular smooth muscle preparations. These can be related to differences in calcium influx pathways and multiple states and/or types of calcium channels. In general, the Ca^{2+} antagonists are more selective for potential- over receptor-operated channels. Thus, the ability of a given vasoconstrictor agonist to induce membrane depolarization (and thereby activate the potential-operated channel, which is more sensitive to calcium entry blockade) is an important factor influencing the ability of a Ca^{2+} antagonist to inhibit the contractile response in various blood vessels.

Autonomic Nerves

At very high concentrations Ca^{2+} antagonists may affect the release of norepinephrine. However, it is generally accepted that this is not a major component of their vasodilator properties.

Endothelial Cells

Adherence

In the animal, Ca^{2+} antagonists reduce the desquamation of endothelial cells triggered by a number of stimuli. Whether or not this action helps to explain the protective effect of calcium antagonists against atherosclerosis is not demonstrated, albeit likely.

Release of Vasoactive Factors

The endothelial cells can release a vasodilator substance (endothelium-derived relaxing factor, EDRF).[1,2,21] Although an increase in cytoplasmic concentration of Ca^{2+} is pivotal in the production of this endothelium-derived relaxing factor, under most circumstances its release does not involve the influx of Ca^{2+} through channels that are sensitive to Ca^{2+} antagonists. Experiments in isolated coronary arteries of the dog suggest that the action of Ca^{2+} antagonists and endothelium-derived relaxing factor(s) is synergistic in favoring relaxation of vascular smooth muscle (FIGURE 3).

Endothelial cells also release substances (endothelium-derived contracting factors, EDCFs) that cause contraction of the underlying smooth muscle. One of the substances is a product of cyclooxygenase. The other type of endothelium-derived contracting factor, which is not a metabolite of arachidonic acid, is released under hypoxic conditions in a variety of blood vessels.[3,9,10] Although endothelium-dependent hypoxic contractions are readily inhibited by Ca^{2+} antagonists, this probably is due to an action of these compounds on vascular smooth muscle rather than the endothelial cells (FIGURE 4).

PATHOPHYSIOLOGY

Hypertension

No single derangement is responsible for the increased systemic vascular resistance in essential hypertension. The arterioles develop myogenic tone; this phenomenon depends highly upon the influx of extracelllular calcium. In certain isolated blood vessels, spontaneous myogenic contractions dependent on availability of extracellular calcium can also be observed. They presumably result from spontaneous depolarization of the cell membrane, which then opens calcium channels. The degree of myogenic activity is dependent on the distension imposed upon the blood vessel wall in part because progressive distension causes depolarization of the cell membrane, bringing it closer to threshold for spontaneous action potentials. This relation helps to explain the maintenance of blood flow despite variations of arterial blood pressure (autoregulation). Ca^{2+} antagonists inhibit the myogenic activity of isolated blood vessels with varying potencies, with the dihydropyridines being the most potent. Because the myogenic tone of the arterioles also depends upon the entry of extracellular calcium, it is not suprising that the Ca^{2+} antagonists, which are the most potent inhibitors of this spontaneous activity in the isolated blood vessels, also cause the greatest decrease in peripheral vascular resistance in the intact organism, and hence are the most likely candidates as antihypertensive agents.

VERAPAMIL

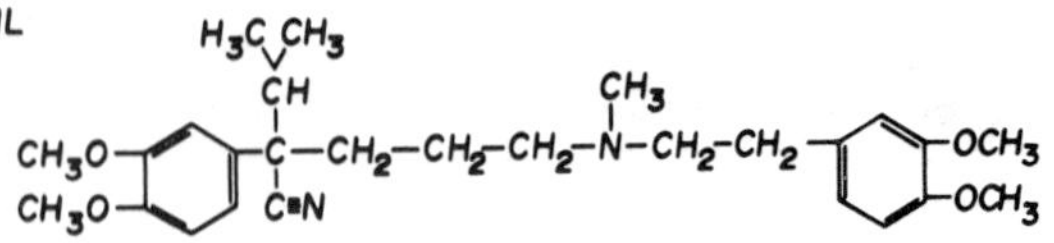

NIFEDIPINE

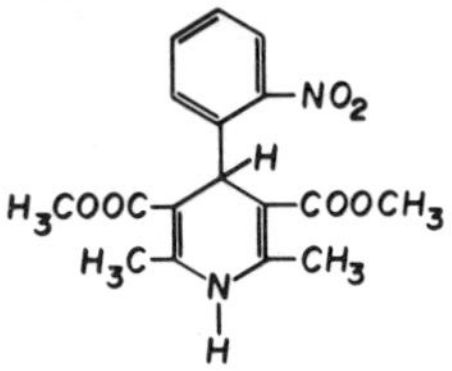

DILTIAZEM

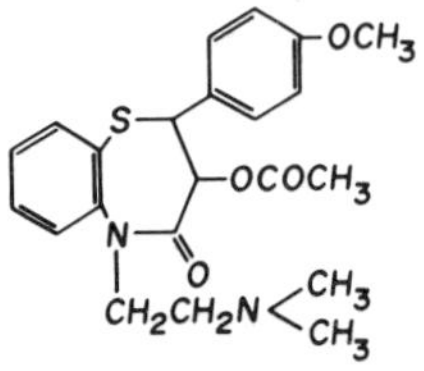

FLUNARIZINE

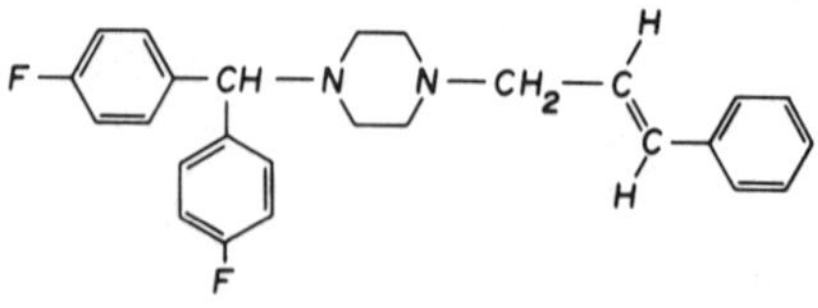

FIGURE 1. Chemical structure of the major Ca^{2+} entry blockers.

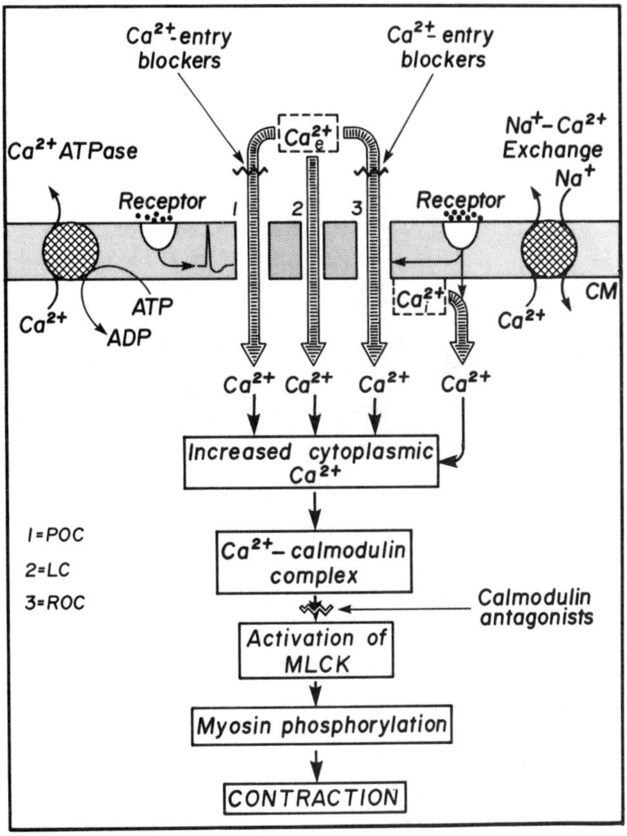

FIGURE 2. Calcium-dependent regulation of contractile activity in vascular smooth muscle. Cytoplasmic calcium (Ca^{2+}) levels are increased by Ca^{2+} influx through potential-operated Ca^{2+} channels (1, POC), a passive Ca^{2+} "leak" pathway (2, LC) (Ca^{2+} entry that occurs under resting conditions), and receptor-operated Ca^{2+} channels (3, ROC). Receptor occupation by a specific agonist (●) may also induce release of Ca^{2+} from intracellular storage sites or may depolarize ( ) the cell membrane and activate the potential-operated channel. Calcium activates myosin light chain kinase (MLCK) by binding to calmodulin. Activated myosin light chain kinase catalyzes the phosphorylation of myosin which increases actin-myosin interactions resulting in contraction. Cytoplasmic Ca^{2+} levels are reduced through the operation of cell membrane pumps, including Ca^{2+}-ATPase (far left) and a Na^+/Ca^{2+} countertransport (far right), that promote Ca^{2+} efflux. ⁓ = inhibited by the Ca^{2+} entry blockers. ⁓ = inhibited by hydrophobic compounds including pimozide and trifluoperazine. (Reproduced from Reference 4, by permission.)

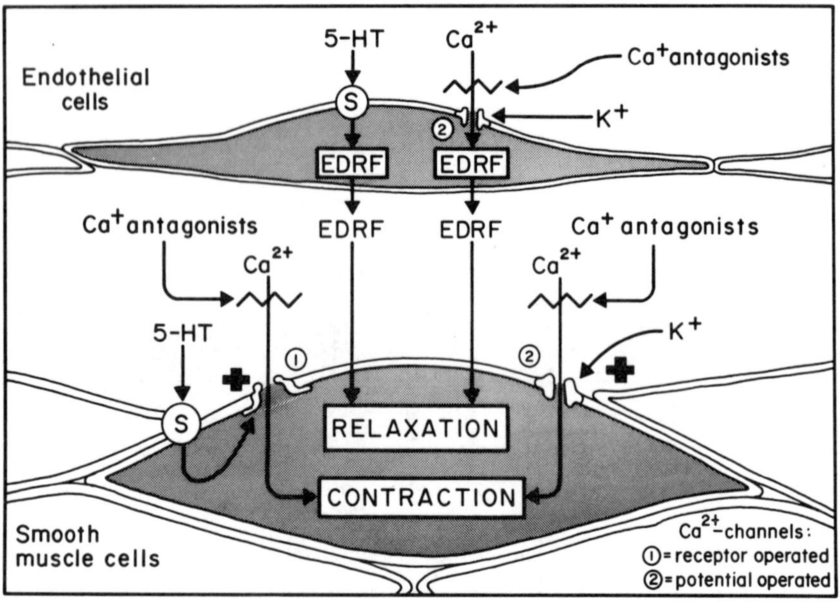

FIGURE 3. Summary of the effects of Ca^{2+} antagonists on endothelial cells and smooth muscle in large canine coronary arteries. EDRF = endothelium-derived relaxing factor(s); 5-HT = 5-hydroxytryptamine; S = serotonergic receptor.

Ischemia

Whenever the cardiovascular system fails to meet the demands of an individual tissue, cellular intoxication follows. The pathophysiological consequences of ischemia are remarkably similar in different tissues (heart, brain, limbs). Since in most components of the cardiovascular system Ca^{2+} profoundly modulates cellular function, the ability of Ca^{2+} antagonists to prevent exaggerated entry of the ion helps to explain why they restore the balance between the oxygen demands of and the blood supply to ischemic tissues.

Myocardial Ischemia

The beneficial effects of Ca^{2+} antagonists in the treatment of angina pectoris can be explained pharmacodynamically by the reduction in the amount of cardiac work or the improvement in perfusion of ischemic areas of the myocardium or both (FIGURE 5). It is impossible to dissociate the actions of these drugs on the myocardium from those on vascular smooth muscle of the coronary and peripheral blood vessels.

Work of the Heart. The Ca^{2+} antagonists reduce cardiac work by causing dilatation of the systemic veins and thus reducing the preload of the ventricles. They affect mainly the splanchnic veins, which are a dynamic controller of the return of blood to the right atrium. Cutaneous veins appear to be less sensitive, which ensures little interference with the thermoregulatory and orthostatic adjustments of the peripheral venous system. By inhibiting the myogenic tone of the precapillary vessels and decreasing their responsiveness to vasoconstrictor substances, the calcium antagonists reduce the afterload of the left ventricle; this is most pronounced for substances such as verapamil and nifedepine

In vitro, all Ca^{2+} antagonists have a negative inotropic effect; however, important differences exist between the individual compounds in that regard. Furthermore, in the intact organism, the negative inotropic effect of Ca^{2+} antagonists such as nifedepine can be counteracted by reflex increases in sympathetic drive to the heart.

The negative chronotropic properties of the Ca^{2+} antagonists vary, depending mainly on their propensity to depress the generation and conduction of impulses in the specialized tissues of the heart and the reflex adjustment of sympathetic tone they induce.

Coronary Perfusion. Provided their effect on diastolic pressure is not marked, the Ca^{2+} antagonists can theoretically improve coronary perfusion to the ischemic areas of the heart by (1) decreasing heart rate and thus prolonging the diastolic filling time; (b) reducing wall tension by improving relaxation of the myocardium and decreasing external load—this may be particularly important in anoxic regions where Ca^{2+} antagonists prevent the rigor of the myocardial cells due to exaggerated accumulation of intracellular Ca^{2+}; (c) dilating coronary resistance vessels—the Ca^{2+} antagonists would have to preferentially dilate the ischemic regions to avoid a circulatory "steal

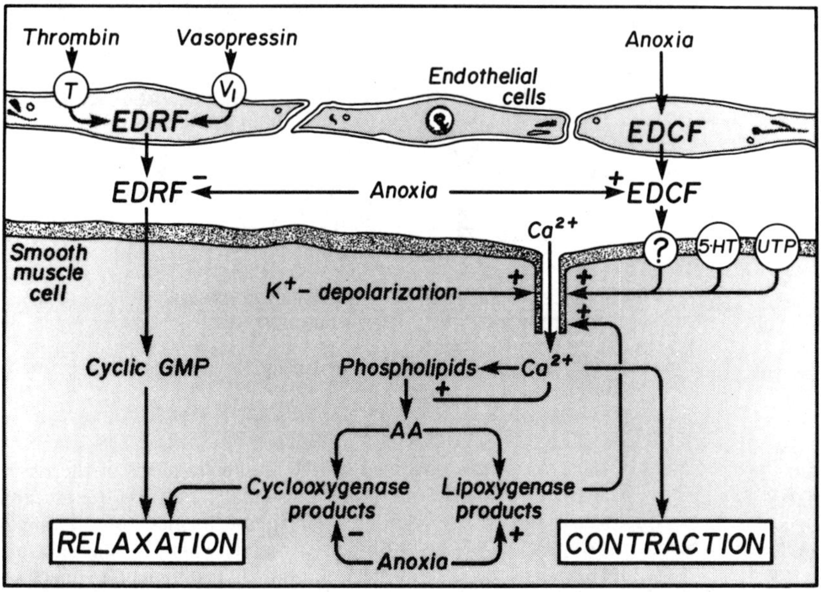

FIGURE 4. Possible effects of anoxia on events in endothelial and smooth muscle cells which may explain anoxic contractions of canine cerebral arteries. Certain interactions are derived from work on systemic or coronary smooth muscle. AA, arachidonic acid; EDCF, endothelium-derived contracting factor(s); EDRF, endothelium-derived relaxing factor(s); GMP, guanylate 3′,5′-monophosphate; 5-HT, serotonergic receptor; UTP, receptor for uridine triphosphate; T, thrombin receptor; V_1, V_1 vasopressinergic receptor; ?, unknown action; +, facilitation; −, inhibition. (Reproduced from Reference 3, by permission.)

phenomenon;" data in isolated coronary arteries suggest that conditions mimicking tissue ischemia (particularly the combination of a low P_{O_2} with high extracellular concentrations of K^+) cause contraction of coronary vascular smooth muscle, a response inhibited by Ca^{2+} antagonists; (d) antagonizing coronary vasospasm. Although the cause of coronary spasm is unknown, the clinical evidence that Ca^{2+} antagonists can prevent it is convincing. *In vitro* work on large coronary arteries demonstrates that these compounds inhibit contraction caused by several possible mediators of coronary vasospasm or by ergonovine, which is used diagnostically to induce coronary spasm.

Peripheral Tissues

Provided the pressure generated by the heart is sufficient, the amount of blood delivered to each tissue will depend on the resistance that its blood vessels offer. The

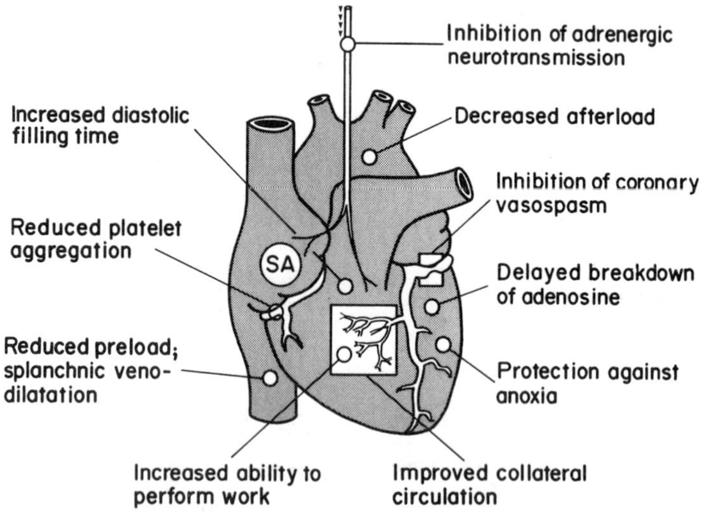

FIGURE 5. Effects of Ca^{2+} entry blockers that help explain their beneficial effects in the treatment of angina pectoris.

degree of opening of the arterioles is governed by the metabolic needs of the tissues surrounding them. There is no evidence that under abnormal conditions the precapillary resistance vessels lose the ability to dilate in response to metabolic demands. Hypoxia of peripheral tissues and of the brain occurs mainly when the diameter of a large artery is reduced and if the collateral circulation is insufficient to meet the demands of the tissue. If the restriction of the blood flow to an organ is due solely to mechanical obstruction, no beneficial effect can be predicted from Ca^{2+} antagonists. However, obstruction can be due to spasm of the vascular smooth muscle of the arterial wall. Indeed, most arteries contain substantial amounts of smooth muscle which react strongly to vasoconstrictor substances released by nerves, endothelial cells, or aggregating platelets. In all arterial smooth muscle studied so far, Ca^{2+} entry blockers are potent inhibitors of the contractile responses evoked by these vasoconstrictor substances (FIGURE 6).

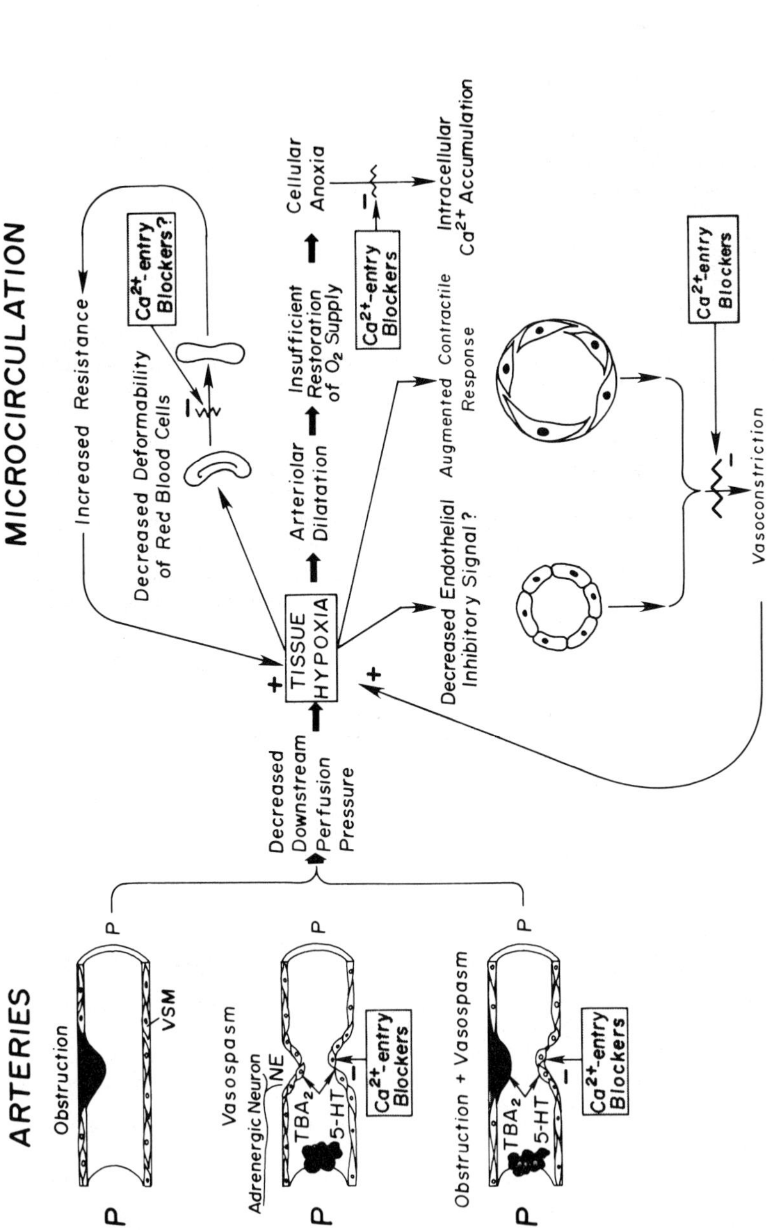

FIGURE 6. The events leading to and maintaining tissue ischemia, with indication of the possible sites of action of Ca^{2+} entry blockers; P = blood pressure; VSM = vascular smooth muscle; 5-HT = 5-hydroxytryptamine. (Reproduced from Reference 16, by permission.)

The viscosity of the blood helps to determine the resistance to flow; hyperviscosity may be one of the factors in peripheral vascular disease. The viscosity of the blood is determined in part by the deformability of the red and white blood cells; this deformability is of critical importance at the microcirculatory level, where these cells travel through capillaries with a diameter smaller than their own. Metabolic deprivation markedly reduces blood cell deformability, which increases the apparent viscosity of the blood and, thus, the resistance to flow, and reduces proper oxygenation of the tissues. Certain Ca^{2+} antagonists can reduce the viscosity of hypoxic blood; this could explain, in part, a beneficial effect on peripheral vascular insufficiency (FIGURE 6).

CONCLUSIONS

The therapeutic effects of Ca^{2+} antagonists in cardiovascular disease can be related to their effects on the function of the contractile cells located in the heart and the vascular wall; their effects on the endothelium and the formed elements of the blood are still a matter of discussion. Even if the direct interference of these agents with the contractile process in cardiac and vascular muscle cells fails to restore an appropriate blood flow to ischemic areas, they will prevent the exaggerated influx of extracellular Ca^{2+} during and after the ischemic episodes. Hence, they protect the cells against some of the most deleterious effects of oxygen-deprivation and the most damaging events in the early stages of reperfusion; this has been documented both in the myocardium and in the brain. The inhibitory effect of Ca^{2+} antagonists on the desquamation of endothelial cells and that of platelet aggregation will reduce the release of vasoconstrictor substances (such as serotonin or thromboxane A_2 which may contribute to vasospasm) but will also slow the progression of the atherosclerotic process.

ACKNOWLEDGMENTS

I wish to thank Mr. Robert Lorenz for preparing the illustrations and Mrs. Cindy Camrud for typing the manuscript.

REFERENCES

1. FURCHGOTT, R. F. 1983. Role of the endothelium in responses of vascular smooth muscle. Circ. Res. **53:** 557–573.
2. FURCHGOTT, R. F. 1984. The role of the endothelium in responses of vascular smooth muscle to drugs. Annu. Rev. Pharmacol. Toxicol. **24:** 175–197.
3. KATUSIC, Z. S. & P. M. VANHOUTTE. 1986. Anoxic contractions in isolated canine cerebral arteries: contribution of endothelium-derived factors, metabolites of arachidonic acid, and calcium entry. J. Cardiovasc. Pharmacol. **8:** S97–S101.
4. RIMELE, T. J. & P. M. VANHOUTTE. 1984. Differential effects of calcium entry blockers on vascular smooth muscle. Int. Angiol. **3:** 17–23.
5. SHEPHERD, J. T. & P. M. VANHOUTTE. 1985. Circulation in tissues with obstructive arterial disease. *In* Calcium Entry Blockers and Tissue Protection. T. Godfraind, P. M. Vanhoutte, S. Govoni & R. Paoletti, Eds.: 107–116. Raven Press. New York, N.Y.
6. VANHOUTTE, P. M. 1981. Calcium entry blockers and cardiovascular failure. Fed. Proc. **40:** 2882–2887.
7. VANHOUTTE, P. M. 1981. Differential effects of calcium entry blockers on vascular smooth muscle. *In* New Perspectives on Calcium Antagonists. G. B. Weiss, Ed.: 109–121. The American Physiological Society. Washington, D.C. (Clinical Physiology Series).

8. VANHOUTTE, P. M. 1982. Calcium entry blockers and vascular smooth muscle. Circ 65(Suppl. I): I-11–I-19.
9. VANHOUTTE, P. M. 1982. Hypoxia and tissue perfusion. *In* Cerebral Hypoxia in the Pathogenesis of Migraine. F. C. Rose & W. K. Amery, Eds.: 3–11. Pitman Press. London, England.
10. VANHOUTTE, P. M. 1982. Effects of calcium entry blockers on tissue hypoxia. J. Cereb. Blood Flow Metab. **2:**(Suppl. 1): S-42–S44.
11. VANHOUTTE, P. M. 1983. Hypoxia, tissue perfusion and potential role of vasodilator drugs. Symp. Front. Pharmacol. **3:** 97–102.
12. VANHOUTTE, P. M. 1984. Introductory remarks: calcium entry blockers in vascular disease. Int. Angiol. **3:** 5–7.
13. VANHOUTTE, P. M. 1985. Calcium entry blockers and peripheral vascular disease. *In* Calcium Entry Blockers and Tissue Protection. T. Godfraind, P. M. Vanhoutte, S. Govoni & R. Paoletti, Eds.: 195–202. Raven Press. New York, N.Y.
14. VANHOUTTE, P. M. 1985. Calcium-entry blockers, vascular smooth muscle and hypertension. Am. J. Cardiol. **55:** 17B–23B.
15. VANHOUTTE, P. M. 1987. The expert committee of the World Health Organization on classification of calcium antagonists: the viewpoint of the rapporteur. Am. J. Cardiol. **59:** 3A–8A.
16. VANHOUTTE, P. M. Ca^{2+} antagonists: what are they and what do they do? *In* Drugs in Intensive Medicine. P. Lawin & G. Thieme, Eds. Verlag Stuttgart. New York. N.Y. (In press.)
17. VANHOUTTE, P. M. & R. A. COHEN. 1983. Calcium entry blockers and cardiovascular disease. Am. J. Cardiol. **52:** 99A–103A.
18. VANHOUTTE, P. M. & R. PAOLETTI. 1987. Classification of calcium antagonists. The viewpoint of the expert committee of the World Health Organization. Trends Pharmacol. Sci. **8:** 4–5.
19. VANHOUTTE, P. M. & T. J. RIMELE. 1983. Effects of calcium entry blockers on isolated blood vessels. Prog. Pharmacol. **5:** 23–36.
20. VANHOUTTE, P. M., T. J. RIMELE & T. W. ROOKE. 1984. Calcium entry and the contraction of vascular smooth muscle. Adv. Cyclic Nucleotide Protein Phosphorylation Res. **17:** 569–573.
21. VANHOUTTE, P. M., G. M. RUBANYI, G. M. MILLER & D. S. HOUSTON. 1986. Modulation of vascular smooth muscle contraction by the endothelium. Annu. Rev. Physiol. **48:** 307–320.
22. VAN NUETEN, J. M. & P. M. VANHOUTTE. 1981. Calcium entry blockers and vasospasm. *In* Vasodilatation. P. M. Vanhoutte & I. Leusen, Eds.: 459–468. Raven Press. New York, N.Y.
23. VAN NUETEN, J. M. & P. M. VANHOUTTE. 1981. Calcium entry blockers and vascular smooth muscle heterogeneity. Fed. Proc. **40:** 2862–2865.

Calcium Antagonists and Low Density Lipoprotein Receptors

R. PAOLETTI, F. BERNINI, R. FUMAGALLI,
M. ALLORIO, AND A. CORSINI

Institute of Pharmacological Sciences
University of Milan
Via Andrea del Sarto 21
I-20129 Milan, Italy

INTRODUCTION

A line of evidence indicates that compounds with calcium channel blocking activity (CA) interfere with the metabolism of low density lipoproteins (LDL) in the cells of the arterial wall and peripheral tissues.[1–4] This interference appears to be directed on different steps of the intracellular pathway of LDL-receptor-mediated catabolism.

Among others, verapamil has been reported to inhibit the degradation of LDL by human fibroblasts, thus preventing the feedback modulation of cholesterol biosynthesis normally associated with LDL cholesterol uptake in the cells.[1] Such an effect has been proposed to be mediated by an inhibition of LDL degradation in the lysosomes, owing to the lysosomotropic property of these drugs, and not related to their activity on intracellular calcium.[2] More recently Stein and collaborators have shown that verapamil only delays LDL degradation and that the increase of LDL uptake cannot be explained on the basis of accumulation of undegraded LDL in the cells.[3] In fact, after six hours of incubation the amount of LDL endocytosed by human fibroblasts (uptake plus degradation) was stimulated by verapamil.[3] This effect of verapamil involves an enhancement of LDL binding to the cell membrane via an increased number of specific receptors and no modification of the affinity.[3] Studies with cycloheximide and α-amanitin[3,4] and direct evaluation by ^{35}S-methionin incorporation[5] clearly demonstrated that the effect of verapamil involves DNA transcription and synthesis of new receptors. However, the possibility that verapamil may act also by increasing the receptor recycling cannot be ruled out.

Recently an expert committee of the World Health Organization has classified CA into six subtypes based on their pharmacological activities.[6] We have evaluated compounds of four types: type I (verapamillike), type II (nifedipinelike), and type III (diltiazem), which are all selective for the slow calcium channels; among the nonselective (types IV, V, and VI), the type IV flunarizine has been tested. Our data indicate that all compounds tested of classes I and III increased the receptor-mediated uptake of LDL by normal fibroblasts in culture, while the drugs of type II and IV were inactive. CA were also effective in fibroblasts obtained from a hypercholesterolemic type IIa heterozygous patient and in the hepatoma cell line HepG2, but not in receptor-negative fibroblasts from homozygous hypercholesterolemic subjects.

MATERIALS AND METHODS

Eagle's minimum essential medium (F-11), fetal calf serum (FCS), trypsin-EDTA (1 ×), penicillin (10,000 U/ml), streptomycin (10 mg/ml) tricine buffer (1 M, pH

7.4), HEPES (1 M, pH 7.4), and nonessential amino acids (100 ×) were purchased from GIBCO (Madison, Wis.); disposable culture flasks and petri dishes were from Corning Glassworks (Corning, N.Y.), filters from Millipore (Bedford, Mass.). Sodium ^{125}I-iodide, carrier free in 0.1 N NaOH was purchased from Amersham (Amersham, United Kingdom).

Verapamil, ronipamil, anipamil (Knoll AG, Ludwigshafen, Federal Republic of Germany), Bay K 8644, nifedipine (Bayer, Leverkusen, FRG) and nitrendipine (Miles, Ill.) were dissolved in ethanol; D600 (Gallopamil HCl—Knoll AG, Ludwigshafen, FRG), flunarizine HCl (Janssen, Beerse, Belgium), diltiazem HCl (Lusofarmaco, Milan, Italy) α-amanitin (Boehringer, Mannheim, FRG), heparin sodium salt and cycloheximide (Sigma St. Louis, Mo.) were dissolved in distilled water before assay.

Cell Culture

Human skin fibroblasts (HSF) were grown from explants of skin biopsies obtained from normolipidemic clinically healthy individuals, and from type IIa hyperlipoproteinemic heterozygous and homozygous patients, selected on a clinical and biochemical basis.

Cells were grown in monolayers at 37°C in a humidified atmosphere of 95% air, 5% CO_2 in F-11 medium supplemented with 10% FCS, nonessential amino acid solution (1%, v:v). penicillin (100 U/ml), streptomycin (100 μg/ml), tricine buffer (20 mM, pH 7.4), $NaHCO_3$ (24 mM). For all experiments, cells were seeded in 60 mm plastic petri dishes (2.5×10^5 cells) and used six days after plating.

The established human hepatoma cell line HEP G2 was obtained from American Type Culture Collection (Rockville, MD. USA). The cells were grown in monolayers with the addition to the medium of 0.11 g/l of sodium pyruvate. For all experiments cells were seeded in 60 mm plastic dishes ($0.5–0.7 \times 10^6$ cells) and used six days after plating.

Lipoproteins and Lipoprotein-Deficient Serum

LDL (d = 1.019–1.063 g/ml) were prepared from the plasma of clinically healthy normolipidemic volunteers by sequential preparative ultracentrifugation.[7]

Lipoproteins were iodinated with ^{125}I by the McFarlane monochloride procedure[8] as modified for lipoproteins[9] and exhaustively dialyzed at 4°C against 0.15 M NaCl, 0.3 mM EDTA, pH 7.4[10].

The final specific activity varied between 100 and 200 cpm/ng of LDL protein. Lipoprotein-deprived serum (LPDS) was prepared by ultracentrifugation of pooled human sera at d =1.25, 40,000 rpm in 50.2 Ti Beckman rotor for 72 hours.[11]

Binding, Internalization, and Degradation of ^{125}I-LDL

Confluent cells were preincubated for 24 hours at 37°C in a medium containing 5% human LPDS in the presence of CA at the concentrations indicated in figures and tables.

The corresponding solvents were added to control cell dishes. Then 10 μg/ml of ^{125}I-LDL proteins were added to the medium and the incubation was continued for a further four hours at 37°C. Cell viability, assessed by tripan blue exclusion, was greater than 95% at the drug concentrations used.

The cell surface binding of ^{125}I-LDL was determined at 37°C as heparin-releasable radioactivity.[12] Fibroblast monolayers were then digested in 0.1 N NaOH to measure LDL internalization[13] and protein content.[14] For total uptake (binding + internalization) of LDL, cell monolayers were directly digested in 0.1 N NaOH. The aspecific LDL binding, internalization, and total uptake were evaluated in the presence of a 50-fold excess of unlabeled LDL. LDL degradation was measured from the accumulation of noniodide trichloroacetic acid–soluble ^{125}I in the incubation medium in excess of that occurring in the absence of cells.[10] Uptake and degradation of ^{125}I-LDL by cultured Hep G2 were determined as described for HSF.

RESULTS

The data reported in TABLE 1 show the effect of different CA on receptor-mediated catabolism of LDL in human fibroblasts. It can be observed that only the CA of types I and III were effective on this cellular function. Under our experimental conditions, verapamil, anipamil, ronipamil, and diltiazem were the most potent agents in stimulating the LDL uptake. In the presence of these compounds (10 μM), the amounts of LDL bound and internalized by the cells were increased between 1.5 and 2 times above the control value. In contrast, neither the dihydropyridine derivatives nor the piperazinelike compound flunarizine significantly affected LDL uptake.

TABLE 1. Effect of Calcium Antagonists on ^{125}I-LDL Catabolism by Human Skin Fibroblasts[a]

Type	Compounds	μM	Uptake[b]	Degradation[b]
I	Verapamillike			
	Verapamil	10	145.0 ± 0.9[f]	132.0 ± 3.1[c]
	Gallopamil	10	130.0 ± 10.9[c]	59.2 ± 12.6[c]
	Ronipamil	10	189.4 ± 12.3[f]	105.8 ± 7.4
	Anipamil	1	97.7 ± 3.5	113.3 ± 12.6
		5	129.5 ± 9.8[c]	89.7 ± 6.7
		10	171.2 ± 7.8[f]	47.5 ± 10.6[d]
II	Nifedipine-like			
	Nifedipine	10	103.0 ± 8.4	96.8 ± 7.4
		100	89.5 ± 7.3	113.0 ± 8.1
	Nitrendipine	10	119.4 ± 6.1	101.6 ± 17.7
		100	106.0 ± 6.9	72.6 ± 17.9
III	Diltiazem	10	141.7 ± 12.9[e]	85.0 ± 8.1
IV	Flunarizine	10	97.1 ± 16.7	97.5 ± 3.7

[a]Confluent monolayers were preincubated for 24 hours at 37°C in a medium supplemented with 5% LPDS in the presence or absence of the indicated drugs. After addition of ^{125}I-LDL (10 μg LDL protein/ml), cells were incubated at 37°C for a further 4 hours. LDL uptake and degradation were determined as described in Materials and Methods. Values are means ± SD of three determinations.

[b]Percent of Control.

[c]$p < 0.05$.

[d]$p < 0.02$.

[e]$p < 0.01$.

[f]$p < 0.001$.

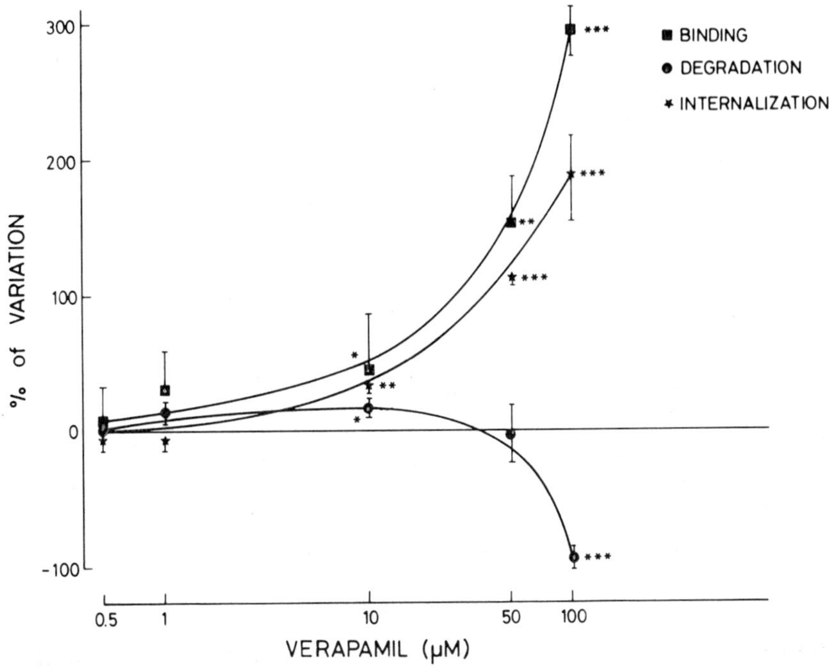

FIGURE 1. Effect of verapamil on the binding, internalization, and degradation of ^{125}I-LDL by normal human skin fibroblasts. Cells were preincubated for 24 hours in a medium supplemented with 5% LPDS and increasing concentrations of the drug; 10 μg of ^{125}I-LDL protein/ml were then added and the incubation was carried out at 37°C for a further 4 hours. Each point represents the mean ± standard deviation (SD) of triplicate determinations; *p < 0.05; **p < 0.01; ***p < 0.001.

The effect of verapamil in increasing LDL binding and internalization was dose dependent, as reported in FIGURE 1. A biphasic effect was observed when LDL degradation was considered; 10 μM verapamil increased LDL degradation, while higher concentrations proved to be inhibitory (FIGURE 1).

The effect of verapamil was also investigated in fibroblasts obtained from a type IIa heterozygous hypercholesterolemic patient (FIGURE 2). In these cells the stimulatory effect of the drug on specific LDL uptake was more pronounced compared to normal cells; cellular degradation of these lipoproteins was stimulated at concentrations up to 50 μM. Also the stimulatory effect of diltiazem on LDL uptake was dose dependent in both normal and heterozygous cells (TABLE 2), while degradation was only slightly affected at all the concentrations tested. TABLE 2 also reports the lack of effect of verapamil and diltiazem on LDL uptake and degradation in receptor-negative cells.

To investigate whether the stimulating effect of verapamil and diltiazem on LDL uptake involved a *de novo* synthesis of LDL receptors, these drugs were tested in the presence of cycloheximide, an inhibitor of protein synthesis, or α-amanitin, an inhibitor of RNA polymerase A2.[15] Data in Table 3 show that these inhibitors completely prevented the effect of both CA on LDL uptake by the cells.

The effect of verapamil has been tested in the human hepatoma cell line Hep G2.

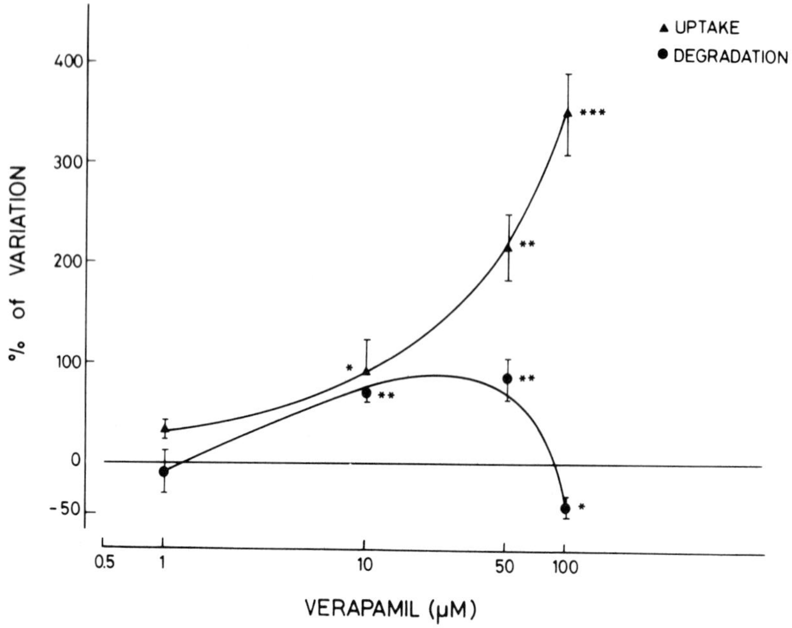

FIGURE 2. Effect of verapamil on the uptake and degradation of ^{125}I-LDL by heterozygous human skin fibroblasts. Experimental conditions as in FIGURE 1. Each point represents the mean ± SD of triplicate dishes; *$p < 0.05$; **$p < 0.01$; ***$p < 0.001$.

TABLE 2. Effect of Calcium Antagonists on ^{125}I-LDL Catabolism by Human Fibroblasts[a]

Fibroblasts	μM	Uptake[b]	Degradation[b]
Normal			
Diltiazem	10	131.4 ± 11.7[c]	78.5 ± 5.5[c]
	50	174.1 ± 22.7[d]	88.0 ± 14.0
	100	232.2 ± 11.8[e]	67.5 ± 9.0[d]
Heterozygous			
Diltiazem	10	115.1 ± 24.6	73.9 ± 7.6
	50	147.6 ± 8.7[c]	95.8 ± 12.6
	100	250.0 ± 56.3[c]	98.3 ± 5.0
Homozygous			
Verapamil	100	125.0 ± 37.5	106.2 ± 50.0
Diltiazem	100	105.0 ± 7.5	103.1 ± 59.4

[a]Experimental conditions as in TABLE 1. Each point represents the mean ± SD of three determinations.

[b]Percent of control.

[c]$p < 0.05$.

[d]$p < 0.02$.

[e]$p < 0.001$.

These cells are considered a valuable model for hepatic handling of LDL.[16,17] The data reported in FIGURE 3 show the effect of verapamil and diltiazem on uptake and degradation of radioactive LDL in these cells. Both drugs stimulated LDL uptake in a dose-dependent manner, but less effectively than in fibroblasts. Degradation was not affected or slighly reduced.

DISCUSSION

Verapamil, a calcium antagonist, is reported to increase the catabolism of LDL by different types of cells in culture. This effect is directed specifically to the receptor-mediated endocytosis of this lipoprotein family.[3]

Calcium-antagonistic activity is displayed by a heterogeneous group of compounds, with different chemical structures, tissue specificities, pharmacological effects, clinical profiles, and modes of action.[18–20]

TABLE 3. Effect of Cycloheximide and α-Amanitin on the Calcium-Antagonist-Induced Catabolism of LDL by Human Skin Fibroblasts[a]

Compounds	Uptake[b]	Degradation[b]
Verapamil 50 μM	277.6 ± 23.8[e]	100.0 ± 19.9
Cycloheximide 500 μM	22.8 ± 7.1[d]	ND
Verapamil + cycloheximide	66.0 ± 11.5[c,f]	ND
Diltiazem 50 μM	207.1 ± 21.6[d]	109.6 ± 16.1
Diltiazem + cycloheximide	27.1 ± 5.7[d,f]	ND
α-Amanitin 5 μg/ml	27.6 ± 4.1[d]	41.3 ± 14.3[c]
Diltiazem + α-amantin	37.4 ± 9.4[d,f]	55.1 ± 2.6[c]

[a]Experimental conditions as in TABLE 1. ND = not detectable.
[b]Percent of Control.
[c]$p < 0.05$.
[d]$p < 0.01$.
[e]$p < 0.001$.
[f]Not significant vs. cycloheximide or α-amanitin.

Our results demonstrate that the stimulating activity of verapamil on LDL uptake by human fibroblasts is shared by all the verapamillike (type I) compounds tested and by the structurally unrelated benzothiazepine diltiazem (type III) and that this effect depends on the concentration of drugs in the incubation media.

Verapamil and diltiazem are also effective in fibroblasts cultured from a type IIa heterozygous hypercholesterolemic patient, in the hepatoma cell line Hep G2, but not in receptor-negative fibroblasts, confirming the specificity of both drugs on the receptor-mediated mechanisms for LDL catabolism.

In contrast to CA of types I and III, the dihydropyridines (type II) and flunarizine (type IV) were inactive.

The latter data may suggest that the stimulating effect observed with CA of types I and III may not be mediated by their effect on calcium transport. This hypothesis is supported by the relatively high concentrations needed for the stimulating effect. It has been observed that verapamil and diltiazem share the properties to be bases and to accumulate in the lysosomes where they inhibit LDL degradation.[2] These properties are also displayed by another class of compounds structurally unrelated to CA, the beta-adrenoceptor antagonists,[21] which stimulate the LDL receptor activity in human fibroblasts.[22,23] However, the effect on degradation alone cannot explain the increase of the receptor activity. A simple accumulation of undegraded LDL in the lysosomes would not lead to an increase of the total endocytosed LDL. The interruption of the feedback mechanism due to a lack of release of free cholesterol from LDL would not explain the increase of receptor synthesis in cells incubated in a medium depleted of LDL.

High concentrations of verapamil and diltiazem interfere with intracellular calcium by mechanisms other than the interaction with the calcium channels.[24] It is possible that the regulation of LDL receptors elicited by CA is mediated by a change of

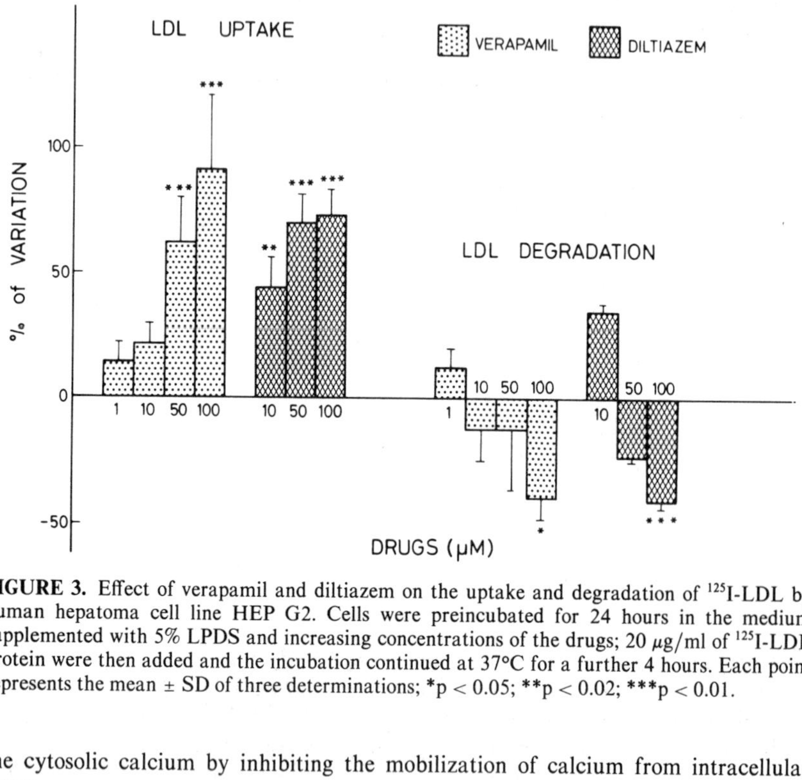

FIGURE 3. Effect of verapamil and diltiazem on the uptake and degradation of ^{125}I-LDL by human hepatoma cell line HEP G2. Cells were preincubated for 24 hours in the medium supplemented with 5% LPDS and increasing concentrations of the drugs; 20 μg/ml of ^{125}I-LDL protein were then added and the incubation continued at 37°C for a further 4 hours. Each point represents the mean ± SD of three determinations; *$p < 0.05$; **$p < 0.02$; ***$p < 0.01$.

the cytosolic calcium by inhibiting the mobilization of calcium from intracellular stores.

Also propranolol, a lipophilic beta-adrenoceptor antagonist stimulating LDL uptake in fibroblasts, is reported to interfere with intracellular calcium.[25]

Studies with the calcium ionophore A 23187 and phorbol esters suggest an involvement of intracellular calcium and protein kinase C in the regulation of receptor-mediated catabolism of LDL.[26,27] In our laboratory, concentrations of ionophore A 23187 as low as 50 nM drastically antagonized both basal and verapamil-induced LDL receptor activity.

All together, these findings suggest that intracellular calcium may play a major role in the regulation of LDL receptor activity, and leave open the possibility that CA stimulation of LDL receptors is mediated by a decrease in intracellular calcium.

Recently organic calcium antagonists have been reported to act favorably on the formation and regression of atherosclerotic lesions in cholesterol-fed rabbits. Such an effect is exerted without any interference with the concentrations of plasma lipids.[28-30] The relationship between the effect of CA in stimulating LDL receptors *in vitro* and the antiatherosclerotic effect demonstrated *in vivo* should be clarified.

The concentrations of CA effective on the expression of LDL receptors are not achieved *in vivo,* and this would explain why plasma cholesterol levels are not affected by CA treatment. On the other hand, CA may reach concentrations in membranes up to 20 times higher than in plasma.[24] Since the plasma concentration of cholesterol is regulated mainly by the liver,[31] it is possible that the sensitivity of the hepatocytes to CA is different from that of cells of the arterial wall.

In our experiments, for instance, CA were less effective in stimulating LDL receptor activity in the hepatoma cells than in fibroblasts.

Stein *et al.* propose that the stimulation of receptor-mediated uptake of LDL might promote the transfer of LDL cholesteryl ester from the arterial interstitium to the intracellular catabolic compartment.[3]

Increase of calcium in the arterial wall is implicated in the pathogenesis of atherosclerosis. The data obtained with the calcium ionophore A 23187 indicate that the increase of calcium in the cellular compartments of the arterial wall may decrease the receptor-mediated metabolism of LDL, thus generating a metabolic imbalance between the intracellular and extracellular space within the arterial wall. Since CA have an opposite effect on LDL metabolism than A 23187, they may exert a significant antiatherosclerotic activity by restoring the receptor-mediated LDL metabolism of the arterial wall, impaired by calcium accumulation.

SUMMARY

The effect of different calcium antagonists on receptor-mediated LDL catabolism by human cells in culture was investigated.

The calcium antagonists have been recently classified in six types, based on their pharmacological activities. The three types selective for the slow calcium channels (types I, II, and III), and the nonselective type IV have been investigated in respect to LDL metabolism.

Calcium antagonists of type I (verapamil-related compounds) and type III (diltiazem) induce an increase of receptor-mediated uptake of human LDL. In contrast, calcium antagonists of type II (nifedipine-related compounds) and type IV (flunarizine) are inactive. Verapamil and diltiazem stimulate LDL receptor activity in normal fibroblasts, in fibroblasts obtained from a hypercholesterolemic type IIa heterozygous patient, in the human hepatoma cell line HepG2, but not in receptor-negative cells.

The stimulatory effect depends on drug concentrations in the culture medium.

Cycloheximide and α-amanitin prevent the stimulating effect of calcium antagonists on LDL uptake.

The possible mechanisms of this action of calcium antagonists and the relationship between the *in vitro* stimulation of LDL receptor activity and the *in vivo* inhibition of lipid deposition in the arterial wall elicited by calcium antagonists are discussed.

Calcium antagonists may exert part of their antiatherosclerotic activity by counteracting the inhibition of receptor-mediated lipid metabolism induced by calcium deposition in the cellular components of the arterial walls.

ACKNOWLEDGMENTS

We are grateful to Miss Agnese Granata for expert technical assistance and to Miss Simona Scattolon for her help in preparing this manuscript.

REFERENCES

1. RANGANATHAN, S., J. A. K. HARMONY & R. L. JACKSON. 1982. Biochem. Biophys. Res. Commun. **107:** 217–224.
2. RANGANATHAN, S. & R. L. JACKSON. 1984. Biochem. Pharmacol. **33:** 2377–2382.
3. STEIN, O., E. LEITERSDORF & Y. STEIN. 1985. Arteriosclerosis **5:** 35–44.
4. CORSINI, A., A. GRANATA, R. FUMAGALLI & R. PAOLETTI. 1986. Pharmacol. Res. Commun. **18:** 1–15.
5. FILIPOVIC, I. & E. BUDDECKE. 1986. Biochem. Biophys. Res. Commun. **136:** 845–850.
6. VANHOUTTE, P. M. & R. PAOLETTI. 1987. Trends Pharmacol. Sci. **8:** 4–5.
7. DE LALLA, O. F. & J. W. GOFMAN. 1954. Methods Biochem. Anal. **1:** 459–478.
8. MCFARLANE, A. S. 1958. Nature **182:** 53.
9. BILHEIMER, D. W., S. EISEMBERG & R. I. LEVY. 1972. Biochim. Biophys. Acta **260:** 212–221.
10. GOLDSTEIN, J. L. & M. S. BROWN. 1974. J. Biol. Chem. **249:** 5153–5162.
11. BROWN, M. S., S. E. DANA & J. L. GOLDSTEIN. 1974. J. Biol. Chem. **249:** 789–796.
12. GOLDSTEIN, J. L., S. K. BASU, G. Y. BRUNSCHEDE & M. S. BROWN. 1976. Cell **7:** 85–95.
13. STEIN, O., D. B. WEINSTEIN, Y. STEIN & D. STEINBERG. 1976. Proc. Nat. Acad. Sci. USA **73:** 14–18.
14. LOWRY, O. H., N. J. ROSEBROUGH, A. L. FARR & R. J. RANDALL. 1951. J. Biol. Chem. **193:** 265–275.
15. TSAI, S. Y., M. J. TSAI & B. W. O'MALLEY. 1981. Proc. Nat. Acad. Sci. USA **78:** 879–883.
16. DASHTI, N., G. WOLFBAUER, E. KOREN, B. B. KNOWLES & P. ALAUPOVIC. 1983. Arteriosclerosis **3:**498a.
17. ILLINGWORTH, D. R., S. LINDSEY & F. C. HAGEMENAS. 1984. Exp. Cell Res. **155:** 518–526.
18. NAYLER, G. W. & J. D. HOROWITZ. 1983. Pharmacol. Ther. **20:** 203–262.
19. SPEDDING, M. 1985. Trends Pharmacol. Sci. **6:** 109–114.
20. VAN ZWIETEN, P. A. 1985. Arzneim-Forsch. Drug Res. **35:** 298–301.
21. CRAMB, G. 1986. Biochem. Pharmacol. **35:** 1365–1372.
22. GHISELLI, G., F. BERNINI, R. MUSANTI & R. FUMAGALLI. 1981. Biochem. Biophys. Res. Commun. **103:**1060–1068.
23. BERNINI, F., A. CORSINI, M. ALLORIO, R. MUSANTI & R. FUMAGALLI. Pharmacology **34:** 225–232.
24. JANIS, R. A. & A. SCRIABINE. 1983. Biochem. Pharmacol. **32:** 3499–3507.
25. NOACK, E., M. KURZMACK, S. VERJOVSKI-ALMEIDA & G. INESI. 1978. J. Pharmacol. Exp. Ther. **206:** 281–288.
26. MAZIÈRE, J. C., C. MAZIÈRE, L. MORA, J. CARDETTE & J. POLONOVSKI. 1984. FEBS **177:** 76–80.
27. MAZIÈRE, J. C., C. MAZIÈRE, L. MORA, M. AUCLAIR, S. GOLDSTEIN & J. POLONOVSKI. 1986. FEBS **195:** 135–139.
28. ROULEAU, J. L., W. W. PARMLEY, J. STEVENS, J. WIKMAN-COFFELT, R. SIEVERS, R. W. MAHLEY & R. J. HAVEL. 1983. J. Am. Coll. Cardiol. **1:** 1453–1460.
29. GINSBURG, R., K. DAVIS, M. R. BRISTOW, K. MCKENNET, S. R. KODSI, M. E. BILLINGHAM & J. SCHROEDER. 1983. Lab. Invest. **49:** 154–158.
30. BLUMLEIN, S. L., R. SIEVERS, P. KIDD & W. W. PARMLEY. 1984. Am. J. Cardiol. **54:** 884–889.
31. BILHEIMER, D. W., G. L. GOLDSTEIN, S. M. GRUNDY, T. E. STARZL & M. S. BROWN. 1984. N. Engl. J. Med. **311:** 1658–1664.

The Effect of Calcium Antagonists on Intimal Cell Proliferation in Atherogenesis[a]

EBERHARD BETZ

Institute of Physiology (I)
University of Tübingen
Gmelinstrasse 5
D-7400 Tübingen, Federal Republic of Germany

In the past, various techniques have been developed for the production of atheromas in animal experiments. The most frequently used method is the feeding of rabbits or monkeys with an atherogenic diet, e.g., 1% or 2% cholesterol in the chow. With this technique it is difficult to predict the site of the initial atheroma and it is therefore not easy to investigate the sequence of reactions during atherogenesis. By means of mechanical or thermal lesions of the endothelial lining, reactions in the vessel wall are induced, which resemble some forms of human atherosclerosis. The lesion causes adherence of platelets on areas denuded of endothelium, and proliferation of the underlying media cells into the intima. However, it is difficult to quantify and standardize this type of lesion.

In order to quantify and standardize the plaque development for studying the actions of various calcium antagonists on the growth of atherosclerotic plaques, we have developed a method of producing atheromas that fulfills the following conditions:

1. It makes it possible to obtain a quantitative measure of the relation between stimuli and reaction of the vessel wall in the form of a dose/response curve.
2. The morphology of the experimentally produced atheroma is similar to a human atheroma and the endothelial lining is not destroyed.
3. The production of the atheroma requires only a short time so that the relation between stimulus and response is clear. Moreover, in this model, each stage of the development of an atheroma can be controlled.
4. It is possible to choose the site in the artery system where a plaque is to be induced.
5. The model allows insight into the mechanism of antiatherogenic therapy, its quantitative analysis, and comparison of the action of various drugs.

Earlier experiments in rabbits[1–3] and in monkeys[1] have indicated that administration of calcium antagonists reduces the formation of lipid deposits in artery walls. Such antiatherogenic effects were obtained with diphosphonates,[4] lanthanum,[2] nifedipine,[5,6] and verapamil.[7,8] Fleckenstein has demonstrated that calcium antagonists were very effective in inhibiting vitamin D–induced calcium deposition in vessel walls.[9,10] However, the mechanisms by which calcium antagonists inhibit atherogenesis have not been so intensively investigated. Calcium participates in numerous reactions of the

[a]Supported by the Bundesministerium für Forschung und Technologie (0318846A).

intracellular metabolism. It also plays a role in the transport of substances across cell membranes and participates in the metabolism of the extracellular materials. In atherogenesis, the effects of calcium antagonists on migration and proliferation of cells in the intima are particularly interesting since these are the very components of atherogenesis that lead to stenoses of the arteries. Cell migration and proliferation involve calcium-dependent intracellular as well as membrane reactions. Calcium enters cells through the cell membranes by various mechanisms. The calcium binding sites on cell membranes are partially proteins that form the so-called calcium channels. The transport of calcium through channels depends on transmitters and on the membrane potential. Some channel proteins exhibit more than one single binding site for calcium antagonists so that different types of calcium antagonists can adhere at the same time on a single channel protein.[11] Within the smooth muscle cells there is a broad spectrum of enzymes whose activities are influenced by calcium or by calcium-activated calmodulin. Direct quantification of the effects of calcium antagonists on the development of atheromas in humans is scarcely possible within a reasonable period of time. Despite considerable progress in the last years, angiographic and sonographic techniques do not give such a high resolution of the vessel wall structures that allows slight changes of vessel wall thickenings to be measured with a precision necessary for the control of drug actions. The recommendations of certain substances as antiatherogenic drugs, therefore, were made to a great degree on the basis of epidemiological studies of occlusive diseases of arteries, postmortem histological studies of artery walls, and analyses of various blood constituents. Within the past few years, an important experimental basis for the secondary prophylaxis of human atherogenesis has been established. These experiments also included the use of calcium antagonists for the prevention of atherosclerosis.

Atherogenesis as such is multifactorial.[12–16] The most important processes leading to formation of atheromas are:

1. Increased permeability of the arterial endothelium for macromolecules, e.g., lipoproteins.
2. Invasion of white blood cells (granulocytes and monocytes) into the intima.
3. Migration of smooth muscle cells (SMC) from the inner layer of the media into the subendothelial space (intima).
4. Mitotic division of these cells in the intima (proliferation) and as a consequence stenoses of the arteries.
5. Formation of abundant matrix material (collagen, elastin, glycosaminoglycans) by the intimal myocytes.
6. Increased endocytosis of lipids by mononuclear cells and SMC, formation of foam cells in hyperlipidemic animals.
7. If the thickness of the proliferate exceeds a certain limit, necrotic regions develop within the plaque with calcium deposition and mineralization of the matrix materials.

A model exhibiting these characteristics is the induction of an atheroma in a carotid artery by stimulating the artery wall with weak electrical currents in rabbits, either fed normal chow or a diet with 1% cholesterol. To assess the therapeutic value of calcium antagonists, a group of animals were treated with the drugs which were either added to their food pellets or given by subcutaneous injection. An 8 mm long section of the carotid artery wall was stimulated with impulses of 100 μA lasting for 15 mseconds/impulse and at a frequency of 10 Hz. The results of a single stimulation period or of daily repeated stimulations were then measured over a period of maximally

4 weeks. In the experiments with chronically implanted electrodes, the painless stimulation periods lasted 30 minutes in the morning and 15 minutes in the afternoon (for details of the techniques see Reference 17). Two days after the onset of the stimuli, it was observed that granulocytes, monocytes, and smooth muscle cells invaded the subendothelial space beneath the anode. The amount of smooth muscle cells increased in subsequent days due to additional migrations from the underlying media as well as mitotic division of the SMC within the intimal proliferate. The number of granulocytes, however, decreased again in the course of a few days. The relative number of macrophages also decreased in this type of a plaque to about 5% of all cells in the proliferate. The remaining amount of macrophages within the plaques was higher in hypercholesterinemic animals (about 15–20%).

Since the proliferating cells arrange themselves in layers with extracellular matrix material in the form of lamellae between the various layers it is easy to count the number of cell layers. The maximal number, usually found beneath the anode region, is a quantitative measure of the proliferative response after a four week period of repeated stimulations. In the controls, the plaque development showed only moderate standard deviations in the number of cell layers, so that this type of plaque production was taken as a standardized model of atherogenesis.[17] If the animal received a drug in its chow or by subcutaneous injection, the effect of the drug on the plaque development can be controlled histologically after the period of treatment and compared with the plaque sizes of untreated animals.

In animal models it is difficult to ascertain whether (1) a drug exerts its effect via a toxic action, (2) the drug inhibits only the SMC proliferation or also the growth of other cells; and (3) the drug action on the plaque formation is direct or indirect. These questions can be answered by analyzing the drug effects on cultures of cells from the artery walls. Supplementary studies of the effects of calcium antagonists on cultures of vascular SMC and of fibroblasts of rabbits facilitate the evaluation of these problems and the distinction between the actions of the various types of calcium antagonists. The techniques of the cultivation of SMC and fibroblasts have been described elsewhere in detail.[18] In the following sections the effects of some calcium antagonists on endothelial permeability, plaque growth, and cell cultures will be described.

ENDOTHELIAL PERMEABILITY

In order to study the influence of calcium antagonists on the permeation of macromolecules through the endothelium of stimulated and nonstimulated carotid artery walls, a carotid artery wall in anesthetized rabbits was stimulated with weak DC impulses (0.1 mA, 15 mseconds/imp, 10 Hz) for maximally 45 minutes. Six minutes before termination of the stimulation period, 10,000 U horseradish perixodase/kg body weight (40,000 dalton, pH 7.2) was infused intravenously within 3 minutes. The stimulated and the contralateral unstimulated carotid arteries were then perfusion fixed and the perioxidase reaction products were stained with the method of Forssmann[19] (for details see Reference 20). In order to quantify the amount of reaction products of peroxidase within the intima, a densitometric technique was established. The accumulation of peroxidase reaction products in the intima was analyzed under five different experimental conditions: (1) without stimulation, (2) immediately after stimulation, (3) 1 hour after stimulation, (4) 5 hours after stimulation, and (5) immediately after stimulation in animals that received a calcium antagonist either prior to or during the stimulation.

RESULTS OF THE PERMEABILITY STUDY

In unstimulated arteries a small amount of peroxidase permeated through the endothelial lining into the intima via interendothelial clefts. Small quantities were also found in intracellular vesicles of the endothelial cells. Immediately after stimulation, there was a massive uptake of horseradish peroxidase beneath the anode in contrast to only a small increase in uptake beneath the cathode. After a period of only one hour following stimulation, the uptake decreased towards normal levels and five hours later, there was no difference between the stimulated and nonstimulated artery when perodixase was administered six minutes prior to the fixation of the vessel.

Administration of calcium antagonists inhibited the uptake of peroxidase as is shown in FIGURE 1. The various concentrations of the drugs showed different degrees of inhibition. We could not use equimolar concentrations because of the marked differences in the effects of the substances on systemic blood pressure.

The analysis of the electron microscopic pictures showed that the preponderant amount of peroxidase reached the subendothelial space via intercellular clefts and that calcium antagonists blocked this route of transport. The number of intracellular vesicles filled with peroxidation products, however, was also smaller in the animals treated with calcium antagonists. In an earlier study it was demonstrated that calcium antagonists also inhibited the uptake of ruthenium red into endothelial cells in stimulated arteries.

EFFECTS OF CALCIUM ANTAGONISTS ON THE GROWTH OF ATHEROMAS

In the model described, the cell proliferation occurred almost exclusively beneath the anode. The endothelial lining was not destroyed and remained in place during the four week period of daily repeated stimulations. FIGURE 2 shows a typical plaque after stimulation over four weeks in a rabbit that received 1% cholesterin in its chow. The plaques contain smooth muscle cells and about 15% macrophages. In the animals that received normal food the number of macrophages was considerably smaller (2–5%). FIGURE 3 depicts the effect of three different calcium antagonists. Both flunarzine and verapamil inhibited the growth of the plaque whereas nimodipine did not show this effect. Analyses of the concentrations of nimodipine in the blood revealed that the bioavailability of the substance was so low that even the administration of 90 mg of nimodipine/kg body weight per day did not have any effect on SMC proliferation.

The effects of the drugs on the lipid concentrations were moderate and were not entirely inhibiting. However, high doses of 30 mg flunarizine/kg body weight per day led to inhibition of the uptake of lipoids into the plaques despite high concentrations of cholesterol in the serum (above 1000 mg/100 ml serum).

CELL CULTURES

Vascular smooth muscle cells were obtained from explants of media tissue of thoracic aortas of rabbits. After a 14 day incubation of the explants the proliferating myocytes were subcultured. The cultures were found to be void of mycoplasms.

Fibroblasts were obtained from subcutaneous tissue of the same animals. Pieces of tissue (2 mm^2) were pressed to the bottom of culture flasks. After addition of 3 ml growth medium, the primary cultures were incubated under 5% CO_2. Two weeks later,

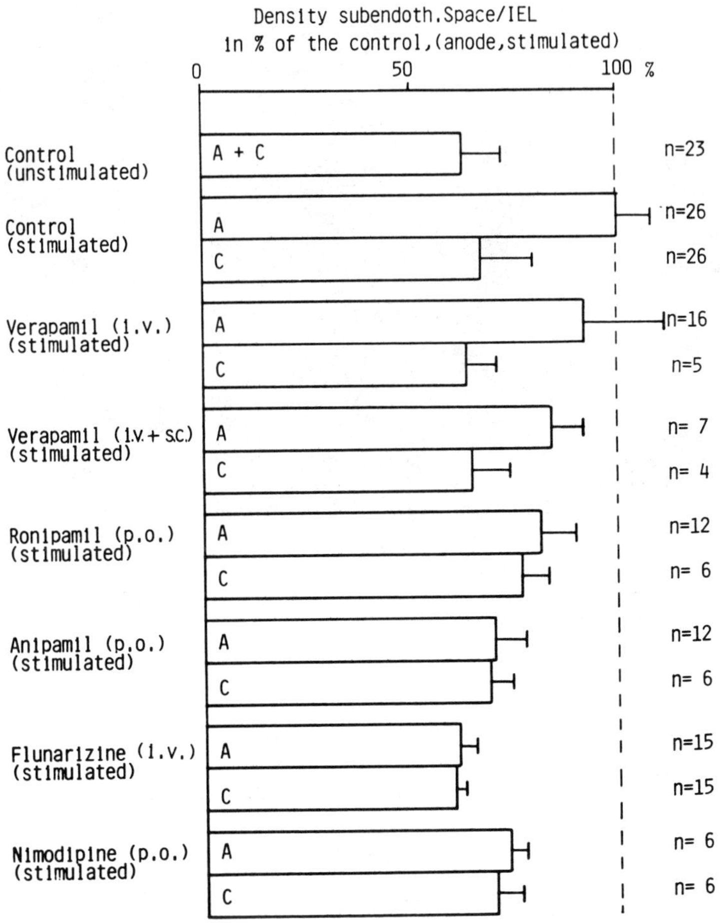

FIGURE 1. The effect of various calcium antagonistic substances on the permeability of unstimulated and stimulated carotid arteries. The amounts of peroxidase reaction products are measured with a microdensitometer. The density index, i.e., the quotient of the density of the subendothelial space and the density of the internal elastic lamina (IEl), was used as a relative measure of the uptake of the peroxidase. In the subanodal region of the stimulated untreated artery the index has the highest value, which is set to 100%. The other indices are referred to this value. As can be seen from the unstimulated control some peroxidase penetrated also through the endothelium of normal arteries. The various drugs were applied as follows. Verapamil: either 0.5 mg/kg b.wt. applied intravenously in the form of an infusion during the 30 minute period of stimulation or 1 mg/kg b.wt. subcutaneously 30 minutes prior to the onset of stimulation and additionally 0.5 mg/kg b.wt. in a continuous infusion during the whole stimulation period. Ronipamil: oral application starting 3 days before peroxidse administration. Dose: 46.6 mg/kg b.wt. per day. The last dosis was applied 6 hours prior to the stimulation. Anipamil: same application and same dosages as with ronipamil. Flunarizine: 4 mg/kg b.wt. intravenously 20 minutes prior to the stimulation period. Nimodipine: intravenous infusion of 1 $\mu g \times kg^{-1} \times minute^{-1}$ during the whole time of stimulation. As can be seen all calcium antagonists reduce the endothelial permeability for peroxidase of stimulated arteries. A = anode side, C = cathode side, p.o. = per os, i.v. = intravenously.

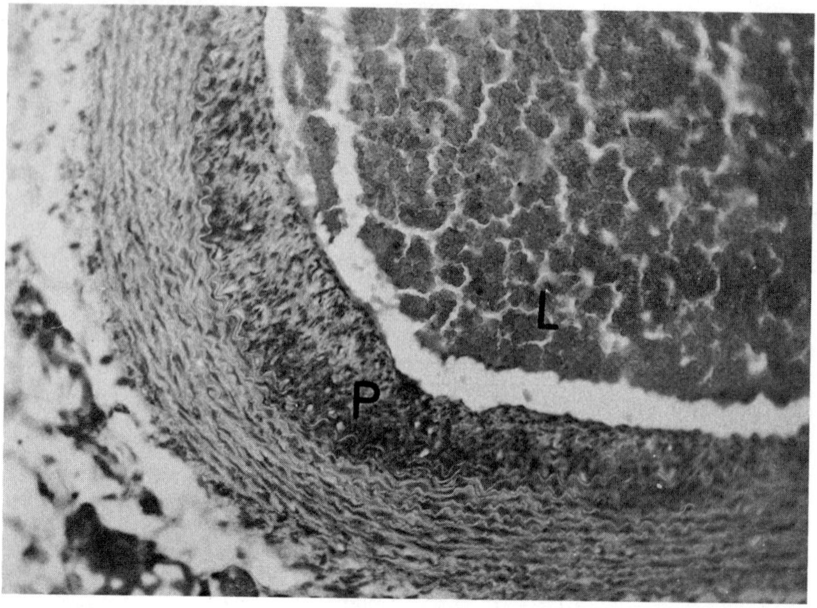

FIGURE 2. Typical atheroma in the carotid artery beneath the anode 4 weeks after the onset of daily repeated local transmural stimulations of the carotid artery wall of a rabbit. Duration of the stimulation periods: 30 minutes in the morning, 15 minutes in the afternoon. L = lumen, P = proliferate. Magnification: 600×.

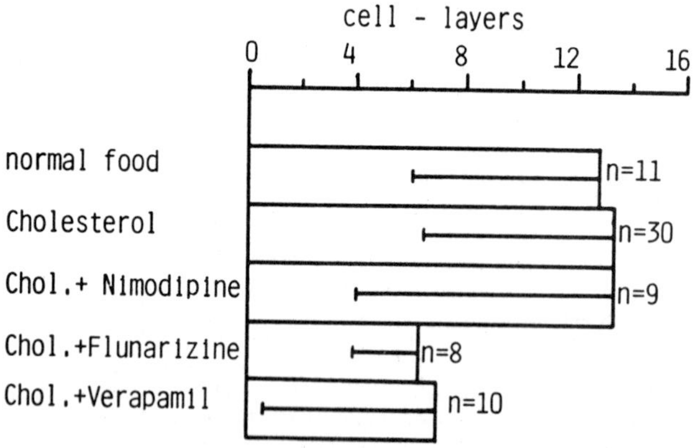

FIGURE 3. The effect of three calcium antagonistic substances on the development of an intimal proliferation beneath the stimulated region. All animals received a diet with 1% cholesterol. During the experiments which lasted 28 days each, the carotid arteries of the rabbits were stimulated twice daily with electrical impulses of 0.1 mA, 10 msecond/impulse, 10 Hz. Stimulation time 30 minutes in the morning, 15 minutes in the afternoon. The number of cell layers is a measure of the thickness of the proliferate. Verapamil, flunarizine, and nimodipine were added to the food pellets so as to guarantee an even uptake. Verapamil was additionally injected subcutaneously twice daily. Oral doses (daily) of the calcium antagonists/kg b.wt.: nimodipine 90 mg/kg, flunarizine 10 mg/kg, verapamil 21.5 mg/kg plus 2 × 1 mg verapamil/kg subcutaneously.

the proliferated cells were harvested. Details concerning the culture media and procedures are described elsewhere.[20]

The effect of calcium antagonists added to the culture media was measured after four passages. Besides the mass cultures, clone cultures were also established and analyzed. FIGURE 4 depicts the effects of various concentrations of flunarizine on the growth of mass cultures and fibroblasts. FIGURE 5 demonstrates the reactions of the cultures to nimodipine, and FIGURE 6 the effects of verapamil. By comparing the results it becomes evident that flunarizine and nimodipine inhibited the growth of the cultures whereas with verapamil no significant difference between the controls and the treated cells was found (t-test).

With clone cultures similar results were obtained. Flunarizine and nimodipine inhibited the growth of clones in a dose-dependent manner. With verapamil only a moderate inhibition could be seen. Comparisons of flunarizine and nimodipine showed that concentrations of nimodipine above 10^{-5} mol/l caused toxic effects whereas flunarizine did not show a toxic reaction in the same doses. The effect of flunarizine on endothelial cells was also tested. It could be seen that the growth of endothelial cells was inhibited in a similar way as that of SMC. Finally, the effect of verapamil on primary cultures of SMC was tested and it was found that in this type of cell cultures the inhibitory effects of the drug on SMC growth was already significant at concentrations as low as 10^{-6} mol/l.

DISCUSSION

Only a limited number of calcium antagonists have been tested with respect to their antiatherogenic effects. A number of studies including our own have demonstrated that some calcium antagonists have an inhibitory effect on a decisive component of stenosing arteries, namely, SMC proliferations within the intima. In the present experiments, flunarizine and verapamil inhibited proliferations in doses that are assumed to be tolerable in patients.

The systemic effects of the substances used in the experiments differ. Flunarizine caused only a slight decrease in blood pressure whereas the same concentrations of nimodipine led to a substantial reduction in arterial blood pressure. Verapamil had an intermediary effect. Oral administation of 1–30 mg flunarizine/kg body weight per day inhibited in a dose-dependent manner the proliferation of cells in the intima. Verapamil had an inhibitory effect only when administered both orally and via subcutaneous injection, and only in hypercholesterinemic animals. The suppression of SMC growth in a stimulated artery region of normally fed animals was not significant.

Oral administration of nimodipine in the rabbit did not cause inhibition of cell growth due to a first pass effect which prevented sufficient concentration of the drug in the blood. In man the concentration of the drug in the blood is considerably higher at the same doses per kg body weight. The administration of low amounts of calcium antagonists did not lead to any decrease in serum cholesterol. High doses of flunarizine, however, led to a reduction of the lipid deposits in the stimulated region of the arteries. The permeation of peroxidase through the endothelial lining was inhibited with all calcium antagonists investigated. However, the degree of inhibition differed depending on the doses used. Drastic differences in the actions of the three calcium antagonists were observed in cell cultures. Nimodipine showed toxic effects in doses higher than 10^{-5} mol/l. Verapamil inhibited only primary cultures when used in concentrations of 10^{-5} mol/l and the same concentation of flunarizine had unequivocal inhibitory effects on SMC cultures, fibroblast cultures, and cultures of endothelial cells. Toxic effects

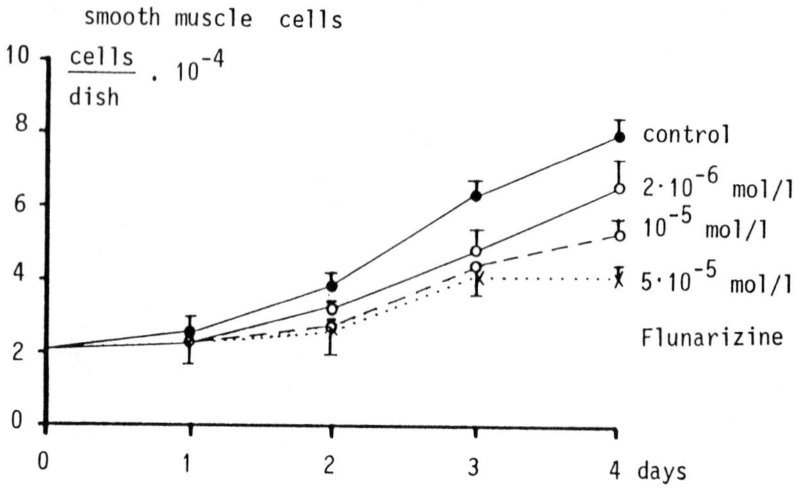

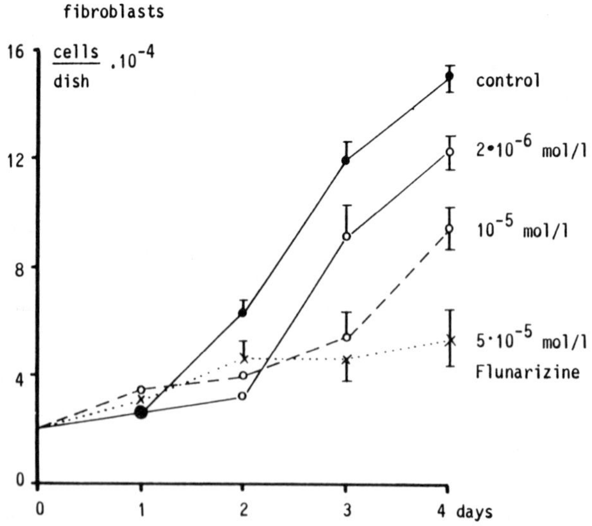

FIGURE 4. Dose-dependent inhibition of the proliferation in mass cultures containing flunarizine of vascular myocytes (top) and fibroblasts of rabbits (bottom). The counted number of cells/dish multiplied with 10^{-4} is the value on the ordinate. Example: if 10^5 cells were counted, its multiplication with the factor 10^{-4} gives the value 10 on the ordinate.

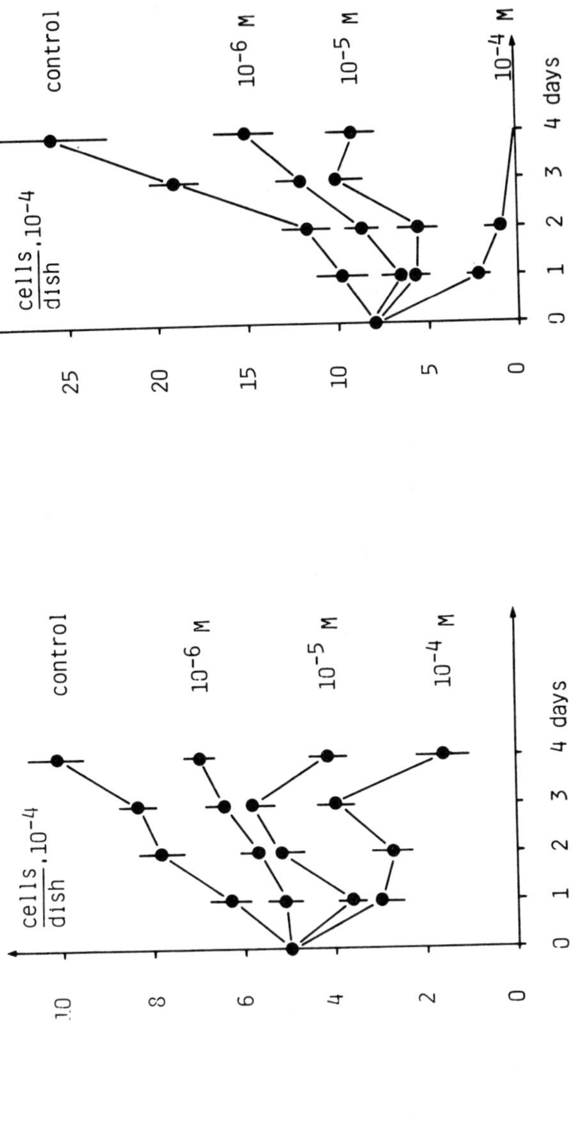

FIGURE 5. The effect of nimodipine on cultures of vascular smooth muscle cells of rabbits (left) and cultures of fibroblasts of rabbits (right).

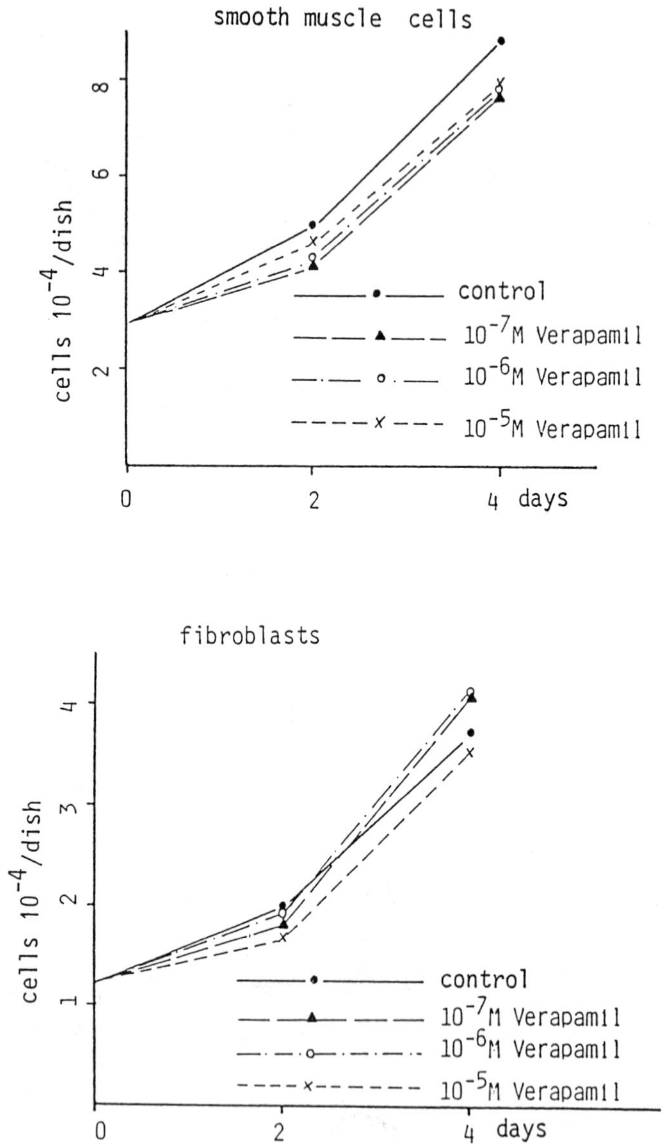

FIGURE 6. The effect of various concentrations of verapamil on cultures of rabbit vascular smooth muscle cells (top) and cultures of fibroblasts (bottom).

were not seen with more than 10^{-5} mol/l of flunarizine. These differences seem to indicate that the drugs inhibit growth via different mechanisms and that the serum concentrations of the drugs depend also on other factors besides the concentrations in the food. Stoclet *et al.* showed that flunarizine changes the rate of calcium entry into cells and also inhibits calmodulin.[21] The latter effect is not seen with verapamil. In unpublished studies we observed that typical calmodulin antagonists such as chlorpromazine or calmidazolium inhibited the growth of cell cultures considerably when they were added to the culture medium in concentrations of more than 10^{-6} mol/l. Cellular damage could be seen with calmidazolium when used in concentrations of 10^{-5} mol/l.

From these experimental studies one can conclude that some calcium antagonists counteract atherogenesis. Whether the experimental data are of such high significance as to justify their being recommended for a secondary prophylaxis of human atherosclerosis is still controversial. There are differences in the rate of the development in experimentally produced plaques and the spontaneous development of human atherosclerosis. However, in bypassed vessels or after percutaneous angioplasty the speed of reocclusion by intimal proliferation may be as rapid as in the experiments demonstrated here. Also there is little experience with high doses of these drugs administered over long periods of time and with regard to possible side effects during this time. The inhibitory effect on endothelial cells is an undesired side effect. In spite of the side effects the results from the experiments seem to justify a more extensive therapeutic study in groups of patients.

ACKNOWLEDGMENTS

The author wishes to thank Dr. Kling, Dr. Hämmerle, and Dr. Strohschneider for their help and advice.

REFERENCES

1. Kramsch, D. M., C. T. Chan, A. J. Aspen & H. Wells. 1978. Prevention and therapy of induced atherosclerosis in rabbits and monkeys. *In* State of Prevention and Therapy in Human Arteriosclerosis and in Animal Models. W. H. Hauss, R. W. Wissler & R. Lehmann, Eds.: 153–172. Westdeutscher Verlag. Opladen, FRG.
2. Kramsch, D. M., A. J. Aspen & C. S. Apstein. 1980. Suppression of experimental atherosclerosis by the Ca^{++}-antagonist lanthanum. J. Clin. Invest. **65:** 967–981.
3. Kramsch, D. M., A. J. Aspen & L. J. Rozler. 1981. Atherosclerosis: prevention by agents not affecting abnormal levels of blood lipids. Science **213:** 1511–1512.
4. DeOlivera, J. M. 1969. The effect of pyridinol carbamate on experimental atherosclerosis. *In* Atherogenesis. T. Shimamoto & F. Numano. 53. Excerpta Medica Foundation. Amsterdam, Holland.
5. Henry, P. D. & K. I. Bentley. 1981. Suppression of atherogenesis in cholesterol-fed rabbit treated with nifedipine. J. Clin. Invest. **68:** 1633–1639.
6. Stender, S., I. Stender, B. Nordestgaard, & K. Kjeldsen. 1984. No effect of nifedipine on atherogenesis in cholesterol-fed rabbits. Arteriosclerosis **4:** 389–394.
7. Blumlein, S. L., R. Sievers, P. Kidd & W. W. Parmley. 1984. Mechanism of protection from atherosclerosis by verapamil in the cholesterol-fed rabbit. Am. J. Physiol. **54:** 884–889.
8. Rouleau, J. L., W. W. Parmley, J. Stevens, J. Wikman-Coffelt, R. Sievers, R. W. Mahley, R. J. Havel & W. Brecht. 1983. Verapamil suppresses atherosclerosis in cholesterol-fed rabbits. Am. J. Coll. Cardiol. **1:** 1453–1460.
9. Fleckenstein, A. 1983. History of calcium antagonists. Circ. Res. **52:** 3–16.

10. FLECKENSTEIN, A. 1984. Calcium antagonism: history and prospects for a multifaceted pharmacodynamic principle. *In* Calcium Antagonists and Cardiovascular Disease. L. H. Opie, Ed.: 9–28. Raven Press. New York, N.Y.
11. GLOSSMANN, H., A. GOLL, M. ROMBUSCH & D. R. FERRY. 1985. Molecular pharmacology of Ca^{2+} channels: receptor binding studies. *In* Nimodipine, Pharmacological and Clinical Properties. E. Betz, K. Deck & F. Hoffmeister, Eds.: 57–73. Schattauer-Verlag. Stuttgart & New York.
12. FUCHS, U. 1977. Sucmicroscopy of the Arterial Vascular Wall. Exp. Pathol. Suppl. 2. (VEB Gustav Fischer, Jena.)
13. JELLINEK, H. 1974. Arterial Lesions and Arteriosclerosis. Plenum Press. London & New York.
14. ROSS, R. & J. A. GLOMSET. 1976. The pathogenesis of Atherosclerosis. N. Engl. J. Med. **295:** 420–425.
15. WISSLER, R. W. & D. VESSELINOVITCH. 1977. Animal models of regression. *In* Atherosclerosis. G. Schettler, Y. Gotho, Y. Hata & G. Klose, Eds. **4:** 377–385. Springer-Verlag. Berlin, Heidelberg & New York.
16. WHITTINGTON-COLEMAN, P. J. & O. CARRIER. 1970. Effects of agents altering vascular calcium in experimental atherosclerosis. Atherosclerosis **12:** 15–26.
17. BETZ, E. & H. HÄMMERLE. 1984. Arterienwandproliferate und Zellkulturen als Indikatoren für Hemmstoffe der Atherogenese. Funkt. Biol. Med. **3:** 146–55.
18. HÄMMERLE, H. 1984. Vergleich von Wirkungen einzelner Pharmaka auf die Proliferation von Gefäßmuskelzellen in vivo und in vitro. *In* Gefäßwandelemente in vivo und in vitro. H. Fischer & E. Betz. Eds.: 43–57. Wiss. Verlagsgesellschaft mbH. Stuttgart, FRG.
19. FORSSMANN, W. G. 1969. A method for in vivo diffusion tracer studies combining perfusion fixation with intravenous tracer injection. Histochemie **20:** 277–286.
20. BETZ, E., H. HÄMMERLE & T. STROHSCHNEIDER. 1985. Inhibition of smooth muscle cell proliferation and endothelial permeability with flunarizine in vitro and in experimental atheromas. Res. Exp. Med. **185:** 325–340.
21. STOCLET, J. C., C. LUGNIER, A. FOLLENIUS, J. M. SCHEFTEL & D. GERARD. 1985. Calmodulin and calcium regulation: effect of antagonists. *In* Calcium Entry Blockers and Tissue Protection. T. Godfraind, P. M. Vanhoutte, S. Govoni & R. Paoletti, Eds.: 31–40. Raven Press. New York, N.Y.

Calcium Antagonists as Antiatherogenic Agents

PHILIP D. HENRY

Baylor College of Medicine
The Methodist Hospital
Section of Cardiology
6535 Fannin (F-905)
Houston, Texas 77030

INTRODUCTION

Experimental studies published over the past 30 years demonstrate that pharmacological manipulations influencing calcium metabolism may modify the progression of atherosclerosis. In this paper, we briefly review the evidence that agents with calcium-chelating and calcium-antagonistic effects may suppress atherogenesis in animals fed high-fat diets.

CALCIUM CHELATING (ANTICALCIFYING) AGENTS

EDTA (Ethylenediaminetetraacetic Acid, Edetic Acid, Versene)

EDTA, a tetracarboxylic acid compound that chelates Ca^{2+} and other metallic ions, inhibits the formation of apatite crystals *in vitro* and *in vivo* ("anticalcifying effect"). Treatment of occlusive arterial disease with EDTA has been advocated since the early fifties, but this therapy has never been evaluated in a controlled clinical trial. Experimental data on possible antiatherosclerotic effects of EDTA are limited. Boyle, McCann, and collaborators showed that treatment of cholesterol-fed rabbits with MgEDTA suppressed the deposition of defatted solids, total lipid, collagen, and elastin within the aortic wall.[1,2] The treatment had no effect on the hypercholesterolemic response to the diet. Therefore, it appeared that suppression of atherogenesis was not related to a hypocholesterolemic effect. The authors suggested that transient hypocalcemia induced by EDTA injections stimulated the release of parathyroid hormone, an effect thought to suppress mineralization and deposition of matrix proteins in arterial walls. The weakness of the studies by Boyle and collaborators[1,2] is that appropriate statistical evaluations of the data were not presented.

Diphosphonates

Diphosphonates are pyrophosphoric acid analogues that have been extensively studied for their inhibitory effects on apatite crystal formation and dissolution *in vitro* and *in vivo*. Ethane-1-hydroxy-1, 1-diphosphonic acid (EHDP) has been repeatedly reported to suppress atherosclerosis in rabbits and monkeys (*Macaca fascicularis*) fed high-fat diets.[3–9] In none of these studies did EHDP reduce serum cholesterol or triglycerides.[4,8]

Thiophene Compounds

Like EDTA and EHDP, thiophene carboxylic acid derivatives bind Ca^{2+} and inhibit apatite crystal formation *in vitro* and *in vivo*. Chan, Wells and Kramsch treated cholesterol-fed rabbits with different thiophene carboxylic acid derivatives and demonstrated that some of these agents effectively suppressed the deposition within the aortic wall of total and free cholesterol, triglyceride, calcium, collagen, and elastin without, however, influencing hypercholesterolemia.[10]

METALLIC IONS

Effects of metal ions (Mg^{2+}, Sr^{2+}, Ba^{2+}, La^{3+}, Co^{2+}, Ni^{2+}, Cu^{2+}, Zn^{2+}, Cd^{2+}) on calcium-dependent biochemical reactions are complex, and studies on the effects of these ions on atherosclerosis in man and in experimental animals have yielded contradictory results (for a review, see Reference 11). Unlike anionic agents that bind (chelate) Ca^{2+}, cations compete for extra- or intracellular calcium binding sites. Fleckenstein and collaborators[12] and Schraven *et al.* [13] have reported that $Mgcl_2$ suppressed calcium uptake by the aorta of vitamin D–intoxicated rats with acute hypercalcemia. In rabbits[14,15] and in *Macaca fascicularis*[8] fed high-fat diets. treatment with trivalent lanthanum ($LaCl_3$) has suppressed atherosclerosis quantitated by planimetry of sudanophiliic lesions and measurements of aortic matrix proteins.

CALCIUM ANTAGONISTS (CALCIUM CHANNEL BLOCKERS)

Dihydropyridine Derivatives

Nifedipine,[16–19] nicardipine,[18] isradipine (PN 200-110),[20,21] and nisoldipine[22] have been reported to reduce atherosclerosis in cholesterol-fed rabbits. In our initial study, aortic sudanophilic lesions, aortic total cholesterol, and aortic tissue calcium were reduced by 57%, 39%, and 32% in treated compared to untreated rabbits.[16] In the study by Willis *et al.*, nifedipine suppressed stainable lesions and cholesterol in aortic walls by 59% and 69%.[18] In the reports by Henry[16] and Willis,[18] nifedipine was administered in high doses (13 and 80 mg/kg daily). In our second study with isradipine, we used a low dosage (0.15 mg/kg twice daily) which proved likewise effective.[20] In a preliminary report, Vesselinovitch, Mullan, Wissler, and Davis found that nifedipine suppressed atherosclerosis of the carotid artery of Rhesus monkeys fed a cholesterol/coconut oil/butter diet.[23] In studies with rabbits and monkeys cited above, antiatherosclerotic effects were not associated with changes in plama lipid and lipoprotein patterns, although Willis *et al.* observed that nicardipine, but not nifedipine, reduced the cholesterol concentration by 42% in the $d < 1.006$ g/ml fraction.[18]

In two studies, dihydropyridine calcium blockers were reported not to influence atherosclerosis in cholesterol-fed rabbits.[24,25] In the study by Naito *et al.* sudanophilic lesions covering the aorta were approximately 5 to 10 times less extensive than those generally reported in the literature, and in two untreated control groups the extent of the lesions differed by more than 300%,[24] a variation among cholesterol-fed controls that should make the demonstration of therapeutic effects virtually impossible. In the other study, Stender *et al.* appeared to have had difficulties in administering oral nifedipine capsules to their rabbits.[25] Stender *et al.*[25] misquoted our work,[16] claiming that our measurements of aortic lipids were unduly low (our values, expressed in their units, are in fact slightly higher than theirs).

Verapamil and Derivatives

Rouleau *et al.*[26] and Blumlein *et al.* [27] demonstrated in cholestrol-fed rabbits that parenteral verapamil in doses producing detectable drug levels (0.5 and 1.5 mg/kg daily) suppressed the development of aortic lesions without exerting a hypocholesterolemic effect. Stender *et al.* confirmed that verapamil [daily dose 2 mg/kg subcutaneously (sc) plus 16 mg/kg per os (po)] reduced atherosclerosis in rabbits fed a 2% cholesterol diet and found lower cholesterol concentrations in the thoracic aorta of treated compared to untreated animals (29 vs. 43 μmol/g wet weight).[28] Anipamil, a derivative of verapamil, has been likewise found to reduce atherosclerosis in cholesterol-fed rabbit.[29–31]

Diltiazem

Ginsburg *et al.* demonstrated that diltiazem (103 mg/kg orally daily) suppressed aortic atherosclerosis in rabbits receiving a 2% cholesterol diet.[15] Sugano *et al.* treated cholesterol-fed rabbits with parenteral diltiazem [50 mg/rabbit intraperitoneally (ip) daily] and nearly completely suppressed the development of aortic lesions (lesion area as a percent of total area 27% in untreated and 0.7% in treated rabbits.).[32] An unusual feature of Sugano's study is that diltiazem produced significant reductions in plasma total cholesterol, very low density lipoprotein (VLDL) cholesterol, low density lipoprotein (LDL) cholesterol, and high density lipoprotein (HDL) cholesterol. Naito *et al.* found that diltiazem (210 mg/rabbit daily admixed to the diet) exerted no antisclerotic effects in cholesterol-fed rabbits,[24] but as mentioned above lesions in untreated controls were excessively variable and unusually small in this study.

Flunarizine

Ginsburg *et al.*[15] and Betz *et al.*[33] showed that flunarizine inhibits the formation of atherosclerotic lesions in cholestrol-fed rabbits.

HYPERCALCEMIC AGENTS

The experimental production of calcific arterial lesions with large doses of irradiated ergosterol (Vigantol) dates back to the 1920s.[34,35] Subsequently, vitamin D preparations have been often used as adjuncts to atherogenic diets. Fleckenstein and collaborators demonstrated in rats that verapamil protects against vascular calcinosis induced by massive doses of vitamin D_3.[36] Hyperparathyroidism has been associated with increased atherosclerosis in experimental animals and in man.[37,38] Accelerated atherosclerosis occurring with vitamin D intoxication, hyperparathyroidism, and chronic hemodialysis are often complicated by arterial hypertension, which may contribute to the vascular injury. Hypercalcemic states resulting in vascular calcinosis are associated with generalized metastatic calcifications, which is not part of commonly occurring forms of atherosclerosis including Mönkeberg's type of arteriosclerosis.

Effects of catecholamines are mediated in part by stimulating cellular calcium uptake, and catecholamine-induced cell necrosis may be associated with prominent accumulations of calcium. It is of interest that a variety of antiadrenergic interventions (reserpine, guanethidine, propanolol, sympathectomy) appear to suppress atherogenesis in rabbits[39–42] and monkeys[23,43] fed high-fat diets.

MECHANISM OF ACTION

Effects on Arterial Pressure

Arterial pressure is a risk factor of atherosclerosis and increases in arterial pressure are known to accelerate atherogenesis in cholesterol-fed rabbits.[44] We have therefore considered the possibility that calcium antagonists, effective antihypertensive agents, exert their antiatherogenic effects by reducing arterial pressure.[16] In our first study high doses of nifedipine evoked only small transient decreases in pressure, and in our second study with low doses of isradipine hypotensive effects were not demonstrable.[16,20] Similarly, Blumlein *et al.* concluded that antiatherosclerotic effects of verapamil in rabbits were not related to hypotensive effects.[27] Theoretically, calcium antagonists could influence atherogenesis by fluid-mechanical mechanisms not detected by measurements of central (aortic) pressure. Such mechanisms include pulse pressures, secondary flow patterns, and vasa vasorum flow.

Effects on Circulating Lipoproteins and Lipids

In most studies with calcium-chelating or calcium-antagonistic agents detailed analyses of lipoproteins were not reported. Therefore, although most authors observed no changes in major plasma lipids and lipoproteins, an action on unmeasured lipoprotein classes cannot be ruled out. In addition, postprandial lipoprotein patterns after a standard lipid administration were not evaluated. Calcium antagonists have been used extensively worldwide in patients with arterial disease and dyslipoproteinemias, and thus far these agents have not been shown to produce alterations in major lipoprotein classes.

As mentioned above, in two studies with cholesterol-fed rabbits, hypolipidemic effects were observed. Willis *et al.* found that large doses of nicardipine (80 mg/kg daily) reduced cholesterol concentration in the $d < 1.006$ g/ml fraction,[18] and Sugano *et al.* found that diltiazem decreased total plasma cholesterol and cholesterol in major lipoprotein fractions (VLDL, LDL, HDL).[32] Ginsburg *et al.*[15] and Naito *et al.*[24] have however observed no hypocholesterolemic effects with diltiazem and nicardipine. Of interest is the report by Ohata *et al.*, who found that nicardipine (10–100 mg/kg daily) produced in rats dose-dependent decreases in total plasma cholesterol and LDL cholesterol, and dose-dependent increases in HDL_2 cholesterol.[45]

Effects on Lipoprotein Uptake and Metabolism

Stein *et al.* have reported that verapamil (10–50 μM) may increase the uptake and degradation of human ^{125}I-LDL by human skin fibroblasts and bovine aortic endothelial and smooth muscle cells in culture.[46] Incubation of fibroblasts with 50 μM verapamil for 24 hours appeared to increase ^{125}I-LDL binding and uptake by augmenting the number of receptors. Verapamil did not influence LDL uptake of receptor-deficient cells from subjects with homozygous familial hypercholesterolemia. Paoletti *et al.* presented evidence at this symposium that verapamil may induce the *de* novo synthesis of Apo-B,E receptors.[47] In the context of receptor-mediated effects, it is of interest that atherosclerosis in Watanabe rabbits, an animal with an inherited LDL-receptor defect, has thus far not been reported to respond to treatment with calcium antagonists (nifedipine).[19,48]

Recently, Etingin and Hajjar demonstrated that in smooth muscle cells cultured from arteries of egg-fed rabbits, incubation for one week with ~ 0.3 μM nifedipine promoted the loss of cholesterol ester from the lipid-laden cells.[49] Saito *et al.* observed that in rabbit aortic smooth muscle cells in culture, nifedipine (up to 146 mM!) did not influence binding or degradation of ^{125}I-LDL.[50] They found that nifedipine blocked esterification of ^{3}H-cholesterol in a concentration-dependent manner with concentrations ranging between 14 and 58 μM. Over a same range of concentrations, nifedipine inhibited cholesterol synthesis from ^{14}C-acetate. In our laboratories, we have repeatedly attempted over the past five years to demonstrate that dihydropyridine derivatives and diltiazem influence receptor-dependent uptake of human LDL by human skin fibroblasts and rabbit alveolar macrophages in culture. With the use of nonanesthetic drug concentrations (up to 1 μM), effects on binding or uptake could not be demonstrated (in press).

Recently, Heider and collaborators showed that isradipine (PN 200-110) (10–100 mM) reduced cholesterol ester accumulation by smooth muscle in culture in a dose-dependent manner.[21] In addition, the drug (1–50 μM) inhibited the incorporation of ^{14}C-proline into matrix proteins.

With the exception of the experiments by Etingin and Hajjar,[49] reports on lipoproteins and lipid metabolism cited above appear to involve high to extremely high drug concentrations.

Effects on Cell Migration and Cell Proliferation

Nakao *et al.* showed that nicardipine over a low range of concentrations (0.1–10 nM) inhibited the 12-HETE (arachidonate metabolite) induced migration of rat aortic smooth muscle in culture.[51]

Van Valen *et al.* described that treatment of rats with isradipine (PN 200-110; 1 mg/kg daily) reduced the proliferative lesions developed by balloon-injured carotid arteries.[52] Betz and collaborators showed that treatment of rabbits with flunarizine[33] or anipamil[31] inhibited proliferative lesion formation produced in carotid arteries by local electric stimulation and cholesterol feeding. These antiproliferative effects were associated with a reduction in the atherosclerotic endothelial hyperpermeability as assessed by *in vivo* permeation of horseradish peroxidase (M_r 40000).[31,33] Lenke and Müller, producing atherosclerotic lesions in rabbits by cholesterol feeding and/or local electric stimulation of the carotid artery,[30] confirmed the effects of anipamil reported by Betz *et al.*[31]

Effects on Cell Necrosis

Experimental and clinical studies support the concept that cell necrosis in foam cell lesions might play an important role in atheroma formation.[53–58] There is increasing evidence that calcium antagonists may exert cell protective effects in syndromes associated with "calcium overload" and cell necrosis.[59] Therefore, antiatherogenic effects of these agents might be related to a nonspecific cell-protective (antinecrotic) action. We have previously reviewed the evidence that an atherogenic lipid (high-cholesterol) environment might produce membrane changes apt to promote net calcium uptake by cells.[59] As mentioned above, agents that may stimulate calcium uptake such as catecholamines and vitamin D may accelerate atherogenesis. Accordingly, antiatherosclerotic effects of calcium antagonists and antiadrenergic agents (β-blockers) might be mediated in part by common mechanisms of action.

CONCLUSION

Agents with calcium-chelating and calcium-channel-blocking effects have been shown to inhibit the development of atherosclerotic lesions in rabbits and monkeys fed high-fat diets. Although the mechanisms of action of these different agents have not been established, current evidence indicates that they do not act by reducing circulating lipids and lipoproteins. Experiments in several laboratories are under way to determine whether calcium antagonists may promote the regression of atherosclerotic lesions.

Multicenter clinical trials designed to examine the question of whether calcium antagonists might exert antiatherosclerotic effects in man have been initiated. What would make calcium antagonists attractive for the treatment of atherosclerosis is that they have a relatively low toxicity and that they are already extensively used for the treatment of ischemic syndromes. Since calcium antagonists do not appear to act predominantly by reducing circulating lipids, their effects might be additive to that of hypolipidemic interventions.

SUMMARY

Pharmacological manipulations of calcium metabolism in animals fed high-fat diets may slow the progression of atherosclerosis. Agents with calcium-chelating (diphosphonic acid and thiophene carboxylic acid derivatives) or calcium-channel-blocking properties (dihydropyridine derivatives, verapamil and its derivatives, diltiazem) have been demonstrated to suppress atherogenesis in rabbits and monkeys. The antiatherosclerotic effects appear to occur in the absence of hypolipidemic effects. The mechanisms of action of the structurally unrelated drugs remain to be elucidated.

REFERENCES

1. LACSON, T., D. S. MCCANN & A. J. BOYLE. 1966. Effects of MgEDTA on the mucopolysaccharide metabolism in the atherosclerotic aorta. J. Atheroscler. Res. **6:** 277–282.
2. WARTMAN, A., T. L. LAMPE, D. S. MCCANN & A. J. BOYLE. 1967. Plaque reversal with MgEDTA in experimental atherosclerosis: elastin and collagen metabolism. J. Atheroscler. Res. **7:** 331–341.
3. FLEISCH, H. A., R. G. G. RUSSELL, S. BISAZ & R. C. MÜHLBAUER. 1970. The inhibitory effect of phosphonates on the formation of calcium phosphate crystals in vitro and on aortic and kidney calcification in vivo. Eur. J. Clin. Invest. **1:** 12–18.
4. ROSENBLUM, I. Y., L. FLORA & R. EISENSTEIN. 1975. The effect of disodium ethane-1-hydroxy-1, 1-diphosphonate (EHDP) on a rabbit model of athero-arteriosclerosis. Atherosclerosis **22:**411–424.
5. POTOKAR, M. & M. SCHMIDT-DUNKER. 1978. The inhibitory effect of new diphosponic acids on aortic and kidney calcification in vivo. Atherosclerosis **30;** 313–320.

6. KRAMSCH, D. M. & C. T. CHAN. 1978. The effect of agents interfering with soft tissue calcification and cell proliferation on calcific fibrous-fatty plaques in rabbits. Circ. Res. **42:** 562–571.
7. HOLLANDER, W., J. PADDOCK, S. NAGRAJ, M. COLOMBO & B. KIRKPATRICK. 1979. Effects of anticalcifying and antifibrotic drugs on pre-established atherosclerosis in the rabbit. Atherosclerosis **33:** 111–123.
8. KRAMSCH, D. M., A. J. ASPEN & L. J. ROZLER. 1981. Atherosclerosis: prevention by agents not affecting abnormal levels of blood lipids. Science **213;** 1511–1512.
9. KUNITOMO, M., K. TAKAOKA, J. MATSUMOTO, H. IWAI & Y. BANDO. 1983. Experimental induction of atherosclerosis in guinea pigs fed a cholesterol, vitamin D_2–rich diet. Folia Pharmacol. Japon. **81:** 275–283.
10. CHAN, C. T., H. WELLS & D. M. KRAMSCH. 1978. Suppression of calcific fibrous-fatty plaque formation in rabbits by agents not affecting elevated serum cholesterol levels. Circ. Res. **43:**115–125.
11. MERTZ, W. 1982. Trace minerals and atherosclerosis. Fed. Proc. **41:** 2807–2812.
12. JANKE, J., B. HEIN, P. PACHINGER, O. LEDER & A. FLECKENSTEIN. 1972. Hemmung arteriosklerotischer Gefässprozesse durch prophylaktische Behandlung mit $MgCl_2$, KCl und organischen Ca^{++}-Antagonisten (Quantitative Studien mit Ca^{45} bei Ratten). *In* Vascular Smooth Muscle. E. Betz, Ed.: 71–72. Springer-Verlag. Berlin, FRG.
13. SCHRAVEN, E., D. TROTTNOW & R. E. NITZ. 1983. Inhibition of vitamin D_3–induced vascular calcification by carbocromen. *In* Advances in Myocardiology. E. Chazov, V. Saks & G. Rona, Eds. **4:** 263–267. Plenum Medical Book Company. New York & London.
14. KRAMSCH, D. M., A. J. ASPEN & C. S. APSTEIN. 1980. Suppression of experimental atherosclerosis by the Ca^{++}-antagonist lanthanum. J. Clin. Invest. **65:** 967–981.
15. GINSBURG, R., K. DAVIS, M. R. BRISTOW, K. MCKENNETT, S. R. KODSI, M. E. BILLINGHAM & J. S. SCHROEDER. 1983. Calcium antagonists suppress atherogenesis in aorta but not in the intramural coronary arteries of cholesterol-fed rabbits. Lab. Invest. **49**(2): 154–158.
16. HENRY, P. D. & K. I. BENTLEY. 1981. Suppression of atherogenesis in cholesterol-fed rabbit treated with nifedipine. J. Clin. Invest. **68:** 1366–1369.
17. PANAGIOTOPOULOS, S. & W. G. NAYLER. 1984. Calcium antagonists and the suppression of atherosclerosis. J. Mol. Cell. Cardiol. **16:** xiv.
18. WILLIS, A. L., B. NAGEL, V. CHURCHILL, M. A. WHYTE, D. L. SMITH, I. MAHMUD & D. L. PUPPIONE. 1985. Antiatherosclerotic effects of nicardipine and nifedipine in cholesterol-fed rabbits. Arteriosclerosis **5:** 250–255.
19. WATANABE, N., Y. ISHIKAWA, J. MUKODANI, N. MIYAZAKI, M. TSUKITANI, S. TAKANO, R. OKAMOTO, Y. WATANABE & H. FUKUZAKI. 1985. Nifedipine suppresses arteriosclerosis in cholesterol-fed rabbits but not in WHHL-rabbits. Circulation **72:** III-281.
20. HABIB, J. B., C BOSSALLER, S. WELLS, C. WILLIAMS, J. D. MORRISETT & P. D. HENRY. 1986. Preservation of endothelium-dependent vascular relaxation in cholesterol-fed rabbit by treatment with the calcium blocker PN 200110. Circ. Res. **58:** 305–309.
21. WEINSTEIN, D. B. & J. G. HEIDER. 1987. Antiatherogenic properties of calcium antagonists. Am. J. Cardiol. **59:** 163B–172B.
22. FRONEK, K. Effect of nisoldipine on diet-induced atherosclerosis in rabbits. Ann. N.Y. Acad. Sci. (This volume.)
23. VESSELINOVITCH, D., J. F. MULLAN, R. W. WISSLER, H. R. DAVIS & T. BRIDENSTINE. 1986. Carotid atherogenesis inhibited by sympathectomy, propranolol and nifedipine in Rhesus monkeys. Arteriosclerosis **6:** 561a.
24. NAITO, M., F. KUZUYA, K. ASAI, K. SHIBATA & N. YOSHIMINE. 1984. Ineffectiveness of Ca^{2+}-antagonists nicardipine and diltiazem on experimental atherosclerosis in cholesterol-fed rabbits. Angiology **35:** 622–627.
25. STENDER, S., I. STENDE, B. NORDESTGAARD & K. KJELDSEN. 1984. No effect of nifedipine on atherogenesis in cholesterol-fed rabbits. Arteriosclerosis **4:** 389–394.
26. ROULEAU, J. L., W. W. PARMLEY, J. STEVENS, J. WILKMAN-COFFELT, R. SIEVERS, R. W. MAHLEY & R. J. HAVEL. 1983. Verapamil suppresses atherosclerosis in cholesterol-fed rabbits. J. Am. Coll. Cardiol. **1**(6): 1453–1460.

27. Blumlein, S. L., R. Sievers, P. Kidd & W. W. Parmley. 1984. Mechanism of protection from atherosclerosis by verapamil in the cholesterol-fed rabbit. Am. J. Cardiol. **54:** 884–889.
28. Stender, S., H. Ravn, M. Haugegaard & K. Kjeldsen. 1986. Effect of verapamil on accumulation of free and esterified cholesterol in the thoracic aorta of cholesterol-fed rabbits. Atherosclerosis **61:** 15–23.
29. Catapano, A. L., F. M. Maggi & U. Cicerano. The antiatherosclerotic effect of anipamil in cholesterol-fed rabbits. Ann. N.Y. Acad. Sci. (This volume.)
30. Lenke, D. & C. D. Muller. 1987. Inhibition of experimentally induced atherosclerosis by anipamil. Paper presented at the International Symposium on Calcium Antagonists, New York, N.Y., February 10–13.
31. Betz, E. & D. Kling. The effect of calcium antagonists on intimal cell proliferation in atherogenesis. Ann. N.Y. Acad. Sci. (This volume.)
32. Sugano, M., Y. Nakashima, T. Matsushima, K. Takahara, M. Takasugi, A. Kuroiwa& O. Koide. 1986. Suppression of atherosclerosis in cholesterol-fed rabbits by diltiazem injection. Arteriosclerosis **6:** 237–241.
33. Betz, E., H. Hammerle & T. Strohschneider. 1985. Inhibition of smooth muscle cell proliferation and endothelial permeability with flunarizine in vitro and in experimental atheromas. Res. Exp. Med. **185:** 325–340.
34. Kreitmaier, H. & T. Moll. 1928. Hypervitaminose durch grosse Dosen von Vitamin D. Muench. Med. Wochenschr. (MMW) **75:** 637–639.
35. Schiff, A. 1930. Die durch Vigantol erzeugbaren Gefassveranderungen und ihre Ruckbildungsfahigkeit im Tierversuch. Arch. Pathol. Anat. **278:** 62–83.
36. Fleckenstein, A. 1983. Calcium Antagonism in Heart and Smooth Muscle: 272–279. John Wiley & Sons, Inc. New York, N.Y.
37. Strevel, R. F. & B. M. Wagner. 1969. Experimental tissue calcification. Arch. Pathol. **87:** 93–99.
38. Roberts, W. C. & B. F. Waller. 1983. Chronic hypercalcemia as a risk factor for coronary atherosclerosis. Cardiovasc. Rev. Rep. **4:** 1275–1280.
39. Whittington-Coleman, P. J. & O. Carrier, Jr. 1970. Effects of agents altering vascular calcium in experimental atherosclerosis. Atherosclerosis **12:** 15–24.
40. Whittington-Coleman, P. J., O. Carrier, Jr. & P. H. Douglas. 1973. The effects of propranolol on cholesterol-induced atheromatous lesions. Atherosclerosis **18:** 373–345.
41. Spence, J. D., D. G. Perkins, R. L. Kline, M. A. Adams & M. D. Haust. 1984. Hemodynamic modification of aortic atherosclerosis. Atherosclerosis **50:** 325–333.
42. Chobanian, A. V., P. Brecher & C. Chan. 1985. Effects of propranolol on atherogenesis in the cholesterol-fed rabbit. Circ. Res. **56:** 755–762.
43. Kaplan, J. R., S. B. Manuck, T. B. Clarkson, M. R. Adams & K. W. Weingand. 1986. Effects of propranolol HCL on behaviorally induced atherosclerosis in hyperlipoproteinemic monkeys. Arteriosclerosis **6:** 545.
44. Bretherton, K. N., A. J. Day & S. L. Skinner. 1977. Hypertension-accelerated atherogenesis in cholesterol-fed rabbits. Atherosclerosis **27;** 79–87.
45. Ohata, I., N. Sakamoto, K. Nagano & H. Maeno. 1984. Low density lipoprotein–lowering and high density lipoprotein–elevating effects on nicardipine in rats. Biochem. Pharmacol. **33:** 2199–2205.
46. Stein, O., E. Leitersdorf & Y. Stein. 1985. Verapamil enhances receptor-mediated endocytosis of low density lipoproteins by aortic cells in culture. Arteriosclerosis **5:** 35–44.
47. Paoletti, R., F. Bernini, R. Fumagalli, M. Allorio & A. Corsini. Calcium antagonists and low density lipoprotein receptors. Ann. N.Y. Acad. Sci. (This volume.)
48. Van Niekerk, J. L. M., T. H. Hendriks, H. H. M. De Boer & A. Van't Laar. 1984. Does nifedipine suppress atherogenesis in WHHL rabbits? Atherosclerosis **53:** 91–98.
49. Etingin, O. R. & D. P. Hajjar. 1985. Nifedipine increases cholesteryl ester hydrolytic activity in lipid-laden rabbit arterial smooth muscle cells. J. Clin. Invest. **75:** 1554–1558.
50. Saito, Y., Y. Fujiyama, K. Shirai & S. Yoshida. 1983. Effect of nifedipine on lipid metabolism in smooth muscle cells. *In* Proceedings of the 6th International Adalat® Symposium. New Therapy of Ischaemic Heart Disease and Hypertension. P. R. Lichtlen, Ed.: 479–483. Excerpta Medica. Amsterdam, Holland.

51. NAKAO, J., I. HIDEKI, T. OOYAMA, W. CHANG & S. MUROTA. 1983. Calcium dependency of aortic smooth muscle cell migration induced by 12-L-hyroxy-5,8,10,14-eicosatetraenoic acid. Atherosclerosis **46:** 309–319.
52. VAN VALEN, R. G., R. W. DEACON, C. FARLEY, M. K. MELDEN, M. F. UHL, R. N. SAUNDERS & D. A. HANDLEY. 1985. Antiproliferative effect of calcium channel blockers PN 200-110 and PY 108-068 in the rat carotid model of balloon catheterization. Fed. Proc. **44:** 737.
53. KIM, K. M. 1976. Calcification of matrix vesicles in human aortic valve and aortic media. Fed. Proc. **35:** 156–162.
54. THOMAS, W. A., J. M. REINER, R. A. FLORENTIN, K. T. LEE & W. M. LEE. 1976. Population dynamics of arterial smooth muscle cells v. cell proliferation and cell death during initial 3 months in atheroslcerotic lesions induced in swine by hypercholesterolemic diet and intimal trauma. Exp. Mol. Pathol. **24:** 360–374.
55. STARY, H. C. 1977. Arterial cell injury and cell death in hypercholesterolemia and after reduction of high serum cholesterol levels. Prog. Biochem. Pharmacol. **14:** 241–247.
56. TRACY, R. E., V. T. TOCA, C. R. LOPEZ, G. E. KISSLING & K. DEVANEY. 1983. Fibrous intimal thickening and atheronecrosis of the thoracic aorta in coronary heart disease. Lab. Invest. **48:** 303–312.
57. STARY, H. C. 1983. Structure and ultrastructure of the coronary artery intima in children and young adults up to age 29; and Macrophages in coronary artery and aortic intima and in atherosclerotic lesions of children and young adults up to age 29. *In* Atherosclerosis VI. F. G. Schettler, *et al.*, Eds.: 82–86; 462–466. Springer Verlag. Berlin, FRG.
58. FRANK A. S., W. T. FRANCO & A. S. DAOUD. 1985. Effect of ethane-1-hydroxy-1, 1-diphosphonate (EHDP) on necrosis of the atheroma. Arteriosclerosis **5:** 527a.
59. HENRY, P. D. 1985. Atherosclerosis, calcium, and calcium antagonists. Circulation **72:** 456–459.

Protection of Arterial and Arteriolar Wall Structure by Specific Calcium Antagonists[a]

M. FREY, J. ZORN, A. FLECKENSTEIN, AND G. FLECKENSTEIN-GRÜN[b]

Study Group for Calcium Antagonism
Physiological Institute
University of Freiburg
Hermann-Herder-Strasse 7
7800 Freiburg, Federal Republic of Germany

INTRODUCTION

The large scope of cardiovascular calcium-antagonistic drug responses is based upon one and the same fundamental mechanism of action: calcium antagonists inhibit transmembrane calcium influx into myocardium, cardiac pacemakers, and vasculature.[1–6,8,25] Thus, calcium antagonists interfere with many Ca^{2+}-dependent physiological or pathophysiological phenomena. Calcium antagonists:

1. Counteract myocardial hypercontractile disorders and prevent structural damage produced by myocardial calcium overload.
2. Damp excessive automaticity of nomotopic and, particularly, ectopic cardiac pacemakers as well as reentry activity.
3. Relax vascular and intestinal smooth muscle so that spasms are neutralized.
4. Moreover, they provide anticalcinotic vascular protection—at least in animal experiments.

The present article concentrates particularly on this latter topic.

RESULTS

Calcium Overload—a Decisive Factor in the Development of Myocardial Necroses and Arteriosclerotic Vascular Lesions

Apart from their various physiological functions, the endogenous calcium ions in myocardium, smooth musculature, and other organs (kidney, liver, brain cells) can adopt the role of malignant "killers" if the cellular calcium metabolism runs out of control and the calcium levels in the cytoplasm increase to several times the normal value.

As we have already shown in 1968, heart muscle fibers undergo severe alterations,

[a]The studies were supported by grants from the Federal Ministry for Scientific Research and Technology, Bonn, Federal Republic of Germany.
[b]To whom correspondence should be addressed.

finally resulting in necrotization, as soon as free calcium ions penetrate excessively through the sarcolemma membrane into the myoplasm so that the capacities of the calcium binding or extrusion processes become overpowered (FIGURE 1).[7] The crucial event in the development of such lesions is high-energy phosphate deficiency which results from (1) excessive consumption of ATP due to supernormal activation of calcium-dependent intracellular ATPases; and (2) insufficient ATP resynthesis in consequence of calcium-induced functional and structural impairment of the mitochondria. Overstimulation of calcium-activated phospholipases probably plays a key role in mitochondrial disintegration.

In addition, Ca overload stimulates specific proteases that digest the contractile myofibrils. However, by interference with excessive calcium influx, calcium antagonists can preserve myocardial integrity.[5,8–13,18]

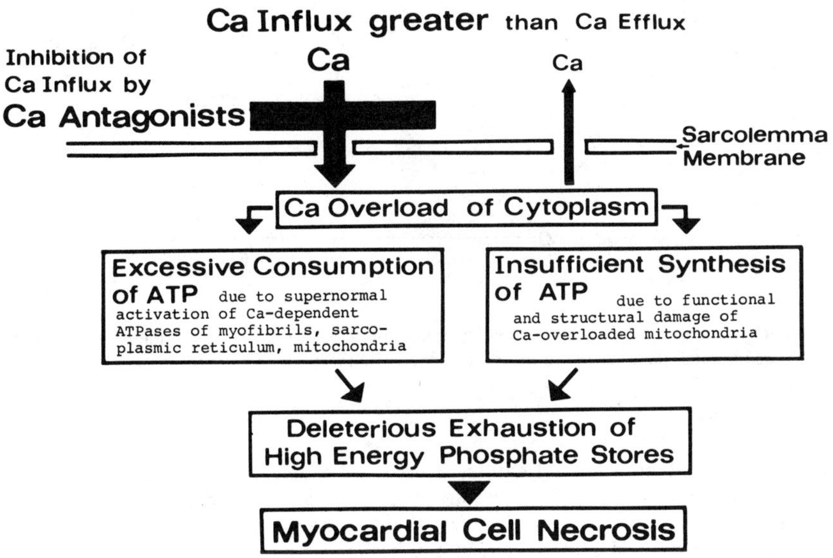

FIGURE 1. Scheme of myocardial necrotization produced by intracellular Ca^{2+} overload and of cardioprotection with Ca^{2+} antagonists.[5]

Inspired by these results on Ca^{2+} overload of the myocardium, our interest has focused since 1970 on the pathogenetic consequences of excessive calcium uptake in arterial smooth muscle cells, and on the vascular protection that various calcium antagonists can provide.[14] Obviously, augmentation of arterial wall cholesterol and Ca^{2+} overload are latent precursors of manifest arteriosclerosis. FIGURE 2 represents observations of Max Bürger published in 1939 which show consistent increases in the cholesterol and calcium contents of senescent human aortas over an age span from 10 to 70 years.[15] In spite of this correspondency, pathologists, in their search for the origin of arteriosclerosis, have put weight for more than 50 years nearly exclusively on the causative role of the accumulation of lipids, whereas the simultaneous calcinosis has mostly been considered a phenomenon of secondary importance. But the present experimental data clearly show that arterial Ca^{2+} overload is by no means a negligible factor.

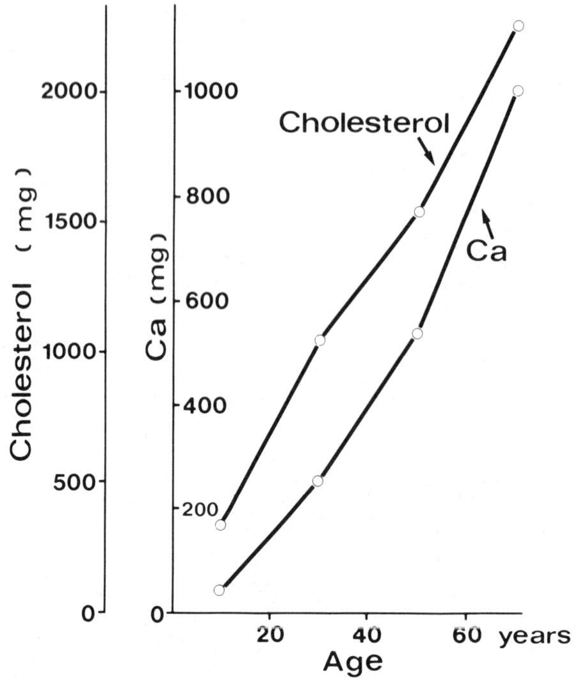

FIGURE 2. Human aortic wall: age-dependent increases in Ca^{2+} and cholesterol contents, expressed in mg/100 g dry tissue. (Reproduced from Reference 15 with permission.)

To obtain more detailed data about the age-dependent changes in calcium and magnesium content of normal human arteries, we have examined arterial wall tissue that mostly originated from forensic autopsies covering the whole life span from 1 to 90 years. The analyses were carried out on the descending branch of the left coronary artery, the superior mesenteric artery, the basilar artery, and aortic tissue.[5,16–19] All artery segments with visible plaques were discarded. In fact, the ageing process of human arteries is reflected in a spectacular augmentation of their calcium content. In contrast, the Mg^{2+} concentration does not dramatically change. As shown in FIGURE 3, the wall of the human aorta contains approximately 100 times more calcium at an age of 80 to 90 years than at an age of below 10 years.

FIGURE 4 is based on the analysis of arteries of more than 700 persons, partially healthy individuals, partially patients with severe risk factors such as uncontrolled diabetes, excessive smoking, or hypertension. As indicated by the dashed horizontal line, the upper tolerable limit of arterial calcium accumulation is in the range of approximately 100 to 300 mmol calcium per kg dry arterial wall tissue. Obviously, spontaneous age-induced calcium accumulation is a continuously developing process which starts many years before dramatic degrees of arterial calcinosis are reached. But at an age of 60 to 70 years, the situation becomes critical, and the structural integrity of the arterial walls is more and more jeopardized. In this context, our comparative analytical data from the arterial tissue of severe diabetics, heavy smokers, and hypertensive individuals are of particular interest, because these risk factors accelerate the natural age-dependent process of spontaneous arterial calcium accumulation so that—for instance in uncontrolled diabetics—the development of arterial calcinosis and its pathological consequences may be anticipated by 25 years.[18,19] Also in heavy smokers the evidence of premature arterial Ca^{2+} accumulation was overwhelming in our studies, whereas human hypertension was associated with arterial Ca^{2+} overload of lesser severity.

Experimental Hypertension

Antihypertensive and Life-Prolonging Effects of Calcium Antagonists

As to the risk factor hypertension, we have carried out extensive experimental observations in hypertensive rats, partially in spontaneously hypertensive Okamoto rats (SHRs), partially in sodium chloride–loaded salt-sensitive Dahl rats.[5,17–23] To visualize the antihypertensive effects of calcium antagonists, we treated spontaneously hypertensive rats over 18 to 20 months with daily oral doses. The therapy was started at an age of 1 month. As can be seen from the upper curve in FIGURE 5, hypertensive Okamoto rats that were not given a calcium antagonist showed an increase in blood pressure of nearly 100% within 4 months, that is to say, up to almost 230 millimeters of mercury. In contrast, Okamoto rats treated with suitable calcium antagonists (in this

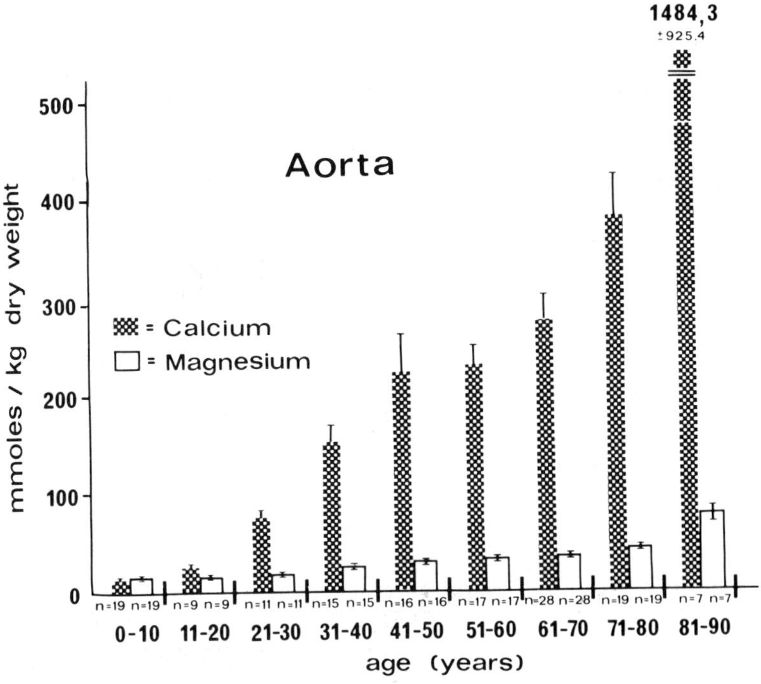

FIGURE 3. Progressive arterial Ca^{2+} overload and increase in the ratio Ca:Mg with advanced age in human aortas ($n = 141$). The preparations mostly originated from autopsies of traffic victims. Only artery segments without visible plaques were analyzed using atomic absorption spectrometry. (Data from Reference 16, see Reference 17.)

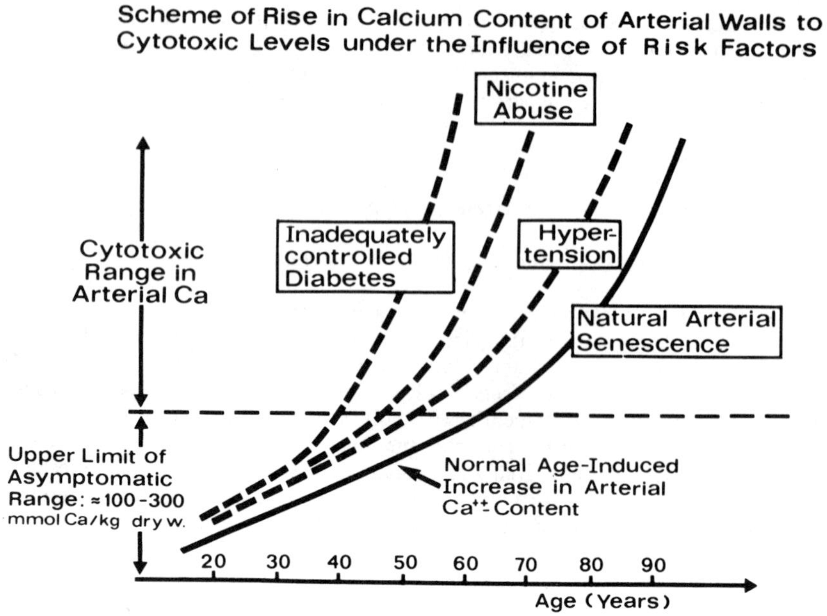

FIGURE 4. Acceleration of natural age-dependent arterial calcium accumulation in humans by inadequately controlled diabetes, heavy cigarette smoking, and hypertension. Estimation on the basis of analytical data obtained on the arteries of a total of 712 humans.[19]

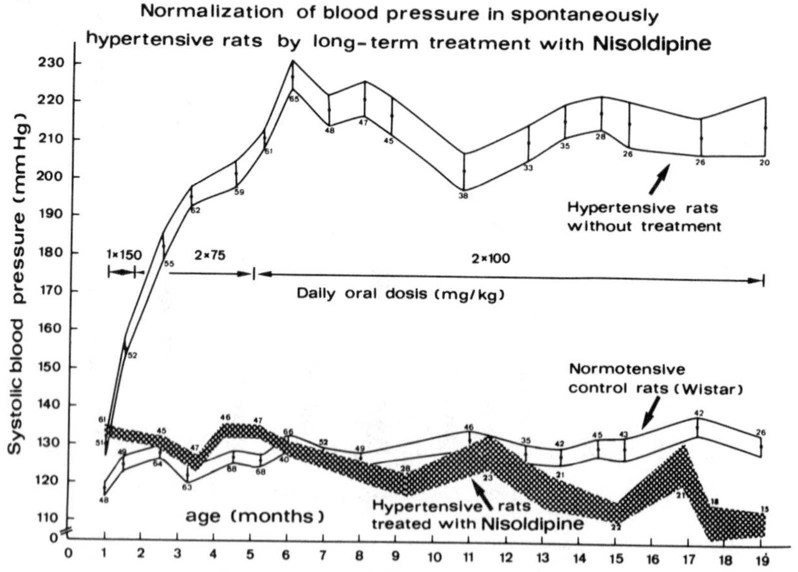

FIGURE 5. Normalization of systolic arterial blood pressure of rats suffering from spontaneous hypertension (Okamoto rats, SHRs) by chronic oral administration of nisoldipine over 18 months. Treatment began at an age of 1 month and lasted until the 19th month.[23]

case nisoldipine) behaved like normotensive control Wistar rats of the same age. Identical results were obtained with the use of nifedipine, nitrendipine, nimodipine, felodipine, and verapamil.[5,17–23] Salt-sensitive Dahl rats fed with an NaCl-rich diet for 2 months behaved, in principle, like SHRs: They also developed severe hypertension and responded promptly with a fall of blood pressure almost to control level as soon as the antihypertensive Ca^{2+} antagonists, previously tested in SHRs, were applied.[21]

Needless to say, the best criterion of the therapeutic value of an antihypertensive treatment consists of its capacity to improve life expectancy. In fact, suitable calcium antagonists can prolong the life span of Okamoto rats considerably. As already reported,[21] less than 20% of the untreated hypertensive Okamoto rats reached an age of 21 months, whereas more than 65% of these animals were still alive at this time if they were protected with verapamil added to the standard diet.

Even more dramatic results were obtained in further studies in which we used hypertensive salt-sensitive Dahl rats. If these animals were fed a diet with 8% NaCl, only 20% of them survived a 2½ month period. But if nitrendipine was administered daily with a stomach tube, in addition to the NaCl-rich diet, the life expectancy increased enormously: then 100% of the rats were still alive after an 8½ month period of salt loading. Even after 10½ months on the salt-rich regimen, 37.5% of the rats were still in good condition (FIGURE 6).

Fundamental Pathogenic Consequences of Arterial and Arteriolar Calcium Overload in Hypertensive Rats; Functional and Structural Vascular Protection with Calcium Antagonists

What are the reasons for the early death of hypertensive Okamoto rats and salt-sensitive Dahl rats if they are not protected by a prophylactic long-term treatment with calcium antagonists? Hypertension per se is certainly not the crucial factor. But there are many observations that stress the high pathogenic importance of generalized calcium overload of the arteriolar and arterial vasculature in hypertensive rats. This calcium overload has far-reaching consequences because both vascular function and structure are seriously impaired. As a matter of fact, calcium overload produces vasoconstriction in the systemic arterioles, and thereby increases flow resistance so that arterial blood pressure goes up. However, in addition, calcium overload progressively destroys the arteriolar wall structure, as can be seen from the appearance of arteriolar microaneurysms. Furthermore, the larger arteries are also heavily affected by excessive calcium accumulation, since the calcium-overloaded arterial walls develop arteriosclerosis. But with the help of calcium antagonists, not only calcium-dependent arteriolar spasms and structural lesions, but also the arteriosclerotic alterations of the larger arteries could be prevented.

Observations on Arterioles. Concerning the influence of calcium antagonists on systemic arteriolar tone and the formation of microaneurysms, our results are based upon an ophthalmoscopic examination of the ocular fundus of many thousands of rat eyes. As already known from observations by Takahashi, the calibers of the retinal arterioles diminish in spontaneously hypertensive rats during the period of progressive blood pressure elevation.[24] As to the normal aspect of the retinal blood vessels in normotensive control Wistar rats, the veins are normally about twice as large as the arterioles. However this ratio always changes profoundly as soon as the Okamoto rats develop hypertension. In fact, *pari passu* with the increase in blood pressure, the arterioles of the ocular fundus exhibit progressive constriction. After fully developed hypertension, parts of the arterioles may even escape the ophthalmoscopic examina-

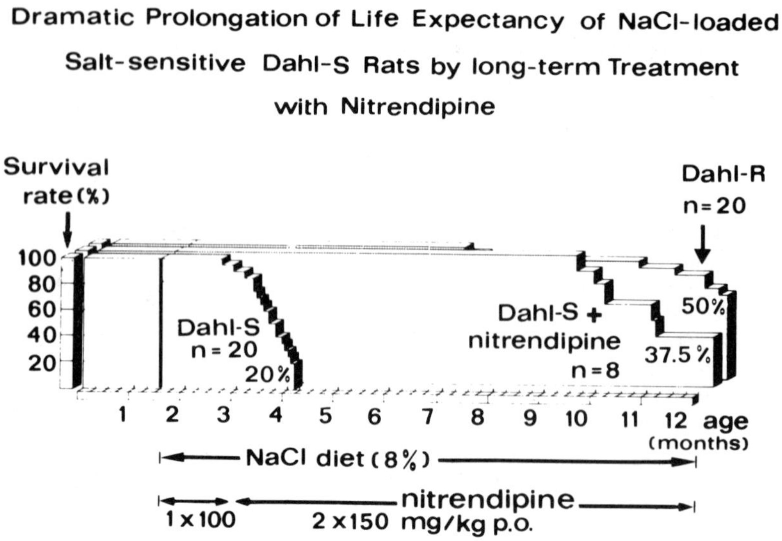

FIGURE 6. Increase in the survival rate of NaCl-loaded (8% NaCl diet) salt-sensitive Dahl rats (Dahl-S) by chronic administration of nitrendipine. Without nitrendipine treatment, only 20% of the Dahl-S rats survived the NaCl-rich diet for 2½ months. Under the influence of the Ca^{2+} antagonist nitrendipine, however, 100% of the NaCl-loaded Dahl-S rats were still alive after 8½ months; 37.5% of them even tolerated the salt-rich regimen for 10½ months. Dahl-R rats which are resistant to NaCl loading served as controls.

tion, because they become invisible due to severe spasm and ischemia. If however, calcium antagonists such as verapamil, diltiazem, and nifedipine (or other Ca^{2+}-antagonistic 1,4-dihydropyridine compounds) are applied, the retinal arterioles respond with an almost immediate relaxation, and the blood pressure goes down.

In the eyes of untreated hypertensive Okamoto rats, apart from uniform spastic arteriolar constriction, multiple microaneurysms appear after some months. However, also these structural alterations do not occur if the Okamoto rats or salt-sensitive Dahl rats are subjected to a long-term calcium antagonist treatment (at a dose level that keeps the blood pressure at normal). Or more precisely, our ophthalmoscopic photographs revealed an incidence of aneurysmlike arteriolar caliber irregularities of about 75 to 85% in the ocular fundus of 18- and 20-month-old *hypertensive Okamoto rats* that had not received a calcium antagonist treatment. In contrast, all these severe arteriolar structure changes could be totally prevented in the overwhelming majority of eyes by long-term administration of the Ca antagonists nitrendipine, nisoldipine, or verapamil.[19–23] In the ocular fundus of *salt-sensitive Dahl rats,* the development of arteriolar aneurysms amounted to 100% after feeding them with an 8% NaCl-containing diet for 2½ months. On the other hand, calcium antagonists such as anipamil[21] or nitrendipine protected these eyes with 100% efficacy. Our ophthalmoscopic results were depicted elsewhere more in detail.[20–23]

Observations on Arteries. As we have found nearly 10 years ago, the development of spontaneous hypertension in Okamoto rats is reflected in a highly significant increase in the Ca content of the walls of larger arteries such as aorta and mesenteric artery. For instance, without calcium antagonist treatment, the mesenteric artery of Okamoto rats accumulates great amounts of calcium so that, finally, after 20 months, the calcium concentration in the proximal part is 3 to 4 times higher than normal whereas the augmentation of the calcium content in the distal part of the mesenteric artery branches is up to 20-fold.

If, however, nifedipine, nisoldipine, nitrendipine, nimodipine, or verapamil[18–23] were administered for 20 months to the Okamoto rats in a dose that prevented hypertension, the aortic and mesenteric calcium contents remained completely or almost completely at normal, as documented in FIGURE 7 with the use of nisoldipine.

As already noted, the calcium-overloaded arteries of untreated Okamoto rats or salt-sensitive Dahl rats develop calcinotic and sclerotic lesions. Particularly in the mesenteric arteries, spectacular alterations develop. Thus untreated 18- to 20-month-old hypertensive Okamoto rats regularly exhibit enormous increases in the diameter of the distal mesenteric artery branches, as well as excessive tortuosity, local thrombosis, calcific incrustations, arteritis nodosa, and ischemic alterations of the gut.[19–23] In salt-sensitive NaCl-loaded hypertensive Dahl rats, the arterial destruction proceeds still much faster. Here, practically all abdominal arteries were affected after 2½ months of a sodium-rich diet (FIGURE 8A). In contrast, chronic treatment of Okamoto rats or of salt-sensitive Dahl rats with suitable calcium antagonists that kept calcium content and blood pressure at normal also preserved the integrity of the arterial and arteriolar structures (FIGURE 8B).

We could further concretize these findings[19–23] on the distal branches of the

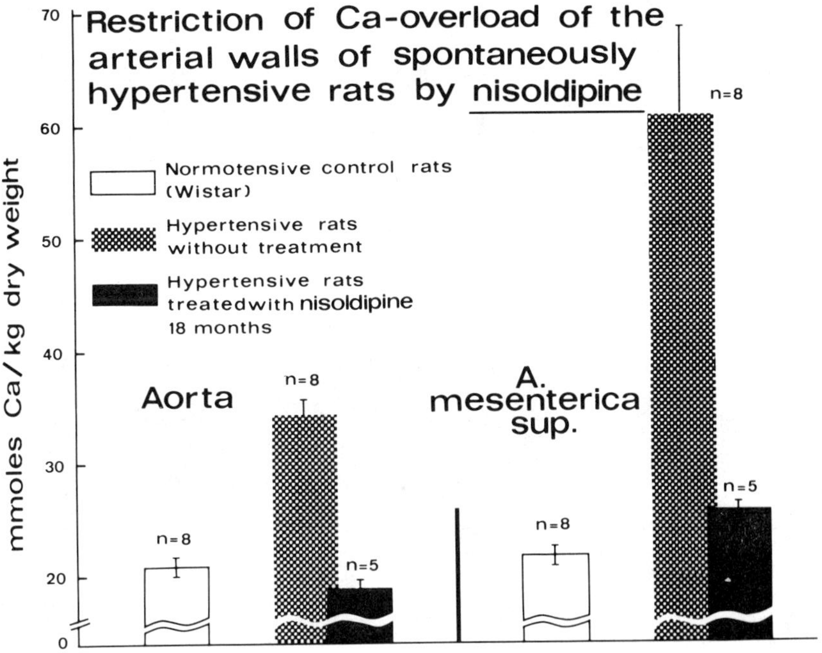

FIGURE 7. Chronic treatment of spontaneously hypertensive Okamoto rats (SHRs) with nisoldipine during 18 months (beginning at an age of 1 month; dose as in FIGURE 5) prevents not only the excessive rise in arterial blood pressure, but also the increase in Ca^{2+} content of the arterial walls (aorta, mesenteric artery).[23]

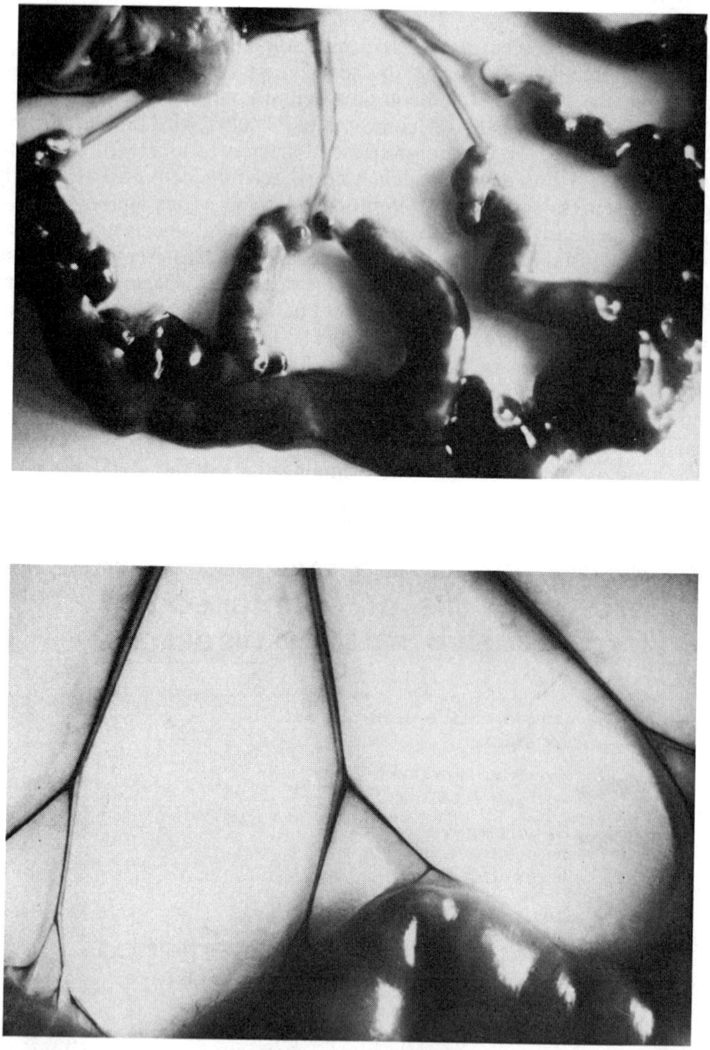

FIGURE 8. Prevention by nitrendipine of severe destruction of the terminal branches of the mesenteric artery of salt-sensitive Dahl rats, receiving 8% NaCl in the diet. (A) Without prophylactic administration of Ca^{2+} antagonists, all NaCl-loaded salt-sensitive Dahl rats (n =20) developed the same type of severe mural damage and thromboembolism in the distal sections of the mesenteric artery within 2½ months. (B) Nitrendipine, given in the same daily oral doses as in FIGURE 6 together with the NaCl-rich diet, not only neutralized hypertension, but also provided dramatic protection of arterial integrity.

mesenteric artery also in extensive histological studies. Thus an enormous proliferation and a calcification of media cells were the most regular phenomena in *untreated hypertensive Okamoto rats*. At an advanced age of 18–20 months, luminal obliterations and calcified thrombi also occurred quite frequently. In the mesenteric arteries of *salt-sensitive Dahl rats*, after a salt-rich diet (8% NaCl over 2½ months), spotlike calcium precipitates were dispersed over the enlarged vascular media.[21] Simultaneously, pronounced endothelial lesions, Ca^{2+}-and lipid-containing intimal plaques, and lining of the luminal side of the arterial wall with a layer of fibrin were typical findings. There is a strong correspondence of this type of vascular alterations with the arteriosclerotic intima lesions in humans.

Antiarteriosclerotic Protection by Calcium Antagonists in Nonhypertensive Rats

It should be emphasized in this context that the Ca^{2+} overload-induced vascular damage associated with hypertension is only *one* special type of calcium-induced

TABLE 1. Types of Arterial Calcinosis Studied in Experiments on Rats

Types	Effective Ca Antagonists Examined
1. Intoxication with dihydrotachysterol (AT10) or vitamin D_3[5;14;19;20;29–32]	Verapamil, diltiazem
2. Hereditary spontaneous hypertension[5;17;19–23;29–33] (Okamoto rats; SHRs)	Nifedipine, nisoldipine, nitrendipine, nimodipine, amlodipine, verapamil
3. NaCl-sensitive hypertension (Dahl-S rats[21])	Nitrendipine, anipamil
4. Advanced age[30;31]	Verapamil
5. Alloxan diabetes[5;29–31]	Verapamil
6. Chronic oral administration of nicotine[34]	Nifedipine, verapamil, diltiazem
7. Combined administration of vitamin D_3 + nicotine[35]	Diltiazem, verapamil

structural impairment, whereas in other disease models of vascular sclerosis, excessive arterial Ca^{2+} accumulation may also occur at absolutely normal blood pressure levels. TABLE 1 summarizes our pertinent observations carried out since 1971 on a total of approximately 50,000 rats. Here, high doses of dihydrotachysterol and vitamin D_3 as well as the well-known risk factors such as advanced age, alloxan-diabetes, and nicotine (particularly if administered together with vitamin D_3 or dihydrotachysterol) also enhanced noxious arterial calcium uptake in the absence of consistent blood pressure changes. However again, calcium antagonists provided also in these cases spectacular arterial protection against calcium-induced structural damage. The calcium antagonists used for this purpose are shown in the right column of TABLE 1.

Evidently, calcium antagonists possess a wide scope of fundamental anticalcinotic properties. Instead of operating superficially as blood pressure cosmetics, they seem to act simultaneously on the common pathogenic roots of both hypertension and sclerotic vascular injury, i.e., calcium overload. In all probability, vascular calcium overload will be accompanied by hypertension if the most peripheral sections of the systemic circulation (small distal artery branches and arterioles, i.e., the resistance vessels) are a major place of excessive calcium intrusion.

CONCLUDING REMARKS

The classical indication for calcium antagonists has hitherto been coronary heart disease. However, our present experimental data as well as many clinical observations, now encourage a broader use of calcium antagonists also for antihypertensive and vasoprotective purposes.[19–23,26–28] So we are expecting that in the near future, the long-term application of calcium antagonists against hypertension and against Ca^{2+}-dependent arterial or arteriolar destruction will become another therapeutical "hit."

As to further research on the pathogenesis of arteriosclerosis, concomitant attempts should be made to elucidate the "missing link" between the disorders of calcium and lipid metabolism. However it is to be noted that arteriosclerosis in humans is not a uniform disease, and also in animal models different morphological types are discernible. Thus the predominant media calcinosis, producible in rats with overdoses of vitamin D_3 or dihydrotachysterol, closely resembles the special Mönckeberg-type of calcific arteriosclerosis in man. On the other hand, in hypertensive rats, the morphology of the arterial lesions corresponds more to the common type of human arteriosclerosis. Nevertheless, even here, there are clear differences between the arteriosclerotic changes in Okamoto rats (SHRs) and in hypertensive NaCl-loaded salt-sensitive Dahl rats. In SHRs, the arterial media cells proliferate more than in hypertensive Dahl rats whereas the intimal lesions are less pronounced. Conversely, as shown on the mesenteric arteries of Dahl rats, this type of arteriosclerosis is characterized by a relatively early development of arteriosclerotic intima plaques with endothelial desquamation and fibrin deposition, initiating thromboembolism. Nevertheless in all these different subtypes of arteriosclerosis, calcium overload seems to be the common denominator. This is the new message that the ubiquitous vasoprotective actions of calcium antagonists have provided.

REFERENCES

1. FLECKENSTEIN, A. 1964. Die Bedeutung der energiereichen Phosphate für Kontraktilität und Tonus des Myocards. Verh. Deutsch. Ges. Inn. Med **70**(Kongress): 81–99.
2. FLECKENSTEIN, A. 1970/71. Specific inhibitors and promoters of calcium action in the excitation-contraction coupling of heart muscle and their role in the prevention or production of myocardial lesions. *In* Calcium and the Heart. P. Harris & L. Opie, Eds.: 135–188. Academic Press. London & New York.
3. GRÜN, G. & A. FLECKENSTEIN. 1972. Die elektro-mechanische Entkoppelung der glatten Gefässmuskulatur als Grundprinzip der Coronardilatation durch 4-(2′-Nitrophenyl)-2,6-dimethyl-1,4-dihydropyridin-3,5-dicarbonsäure-dimethylester (Bay a 1040, Nifedipin). Arzneim. Forsch. (Drug Res.) **22:** 334–344.
4. FLECKENSTEIN, A. 1983. History of calcium antagonists. Am. Heart Assoc. Monogr. No. **95:** 3–16.
5. FLECKENSTEIN, A. 1983. Calcium Antagonism in Heart and Smooth Muscle—Experimental Facts and Therapeutic Prospects. John Wiley Publishing Company. New York, Chichester, Brisbane, Toronto & Singapore.
6. FLECKENSTEIN-GRÜN, M. FREY & A. FLECKENSTEIN. 1984. Calcium antagonists: mechanisms and therapeutic uses. Trends Pharmacol. Sci. **5:** 283–286.
7. FLECKENSTEIN, A. 1968. Myokardstoffwechsel und Nekrose. *In* Proceedings VI. Symposium der Deutschen Gesellschaft für Fortschritte auf dem Gebiet der Inneren Medizin

über "Herzinfarkt und Schock." L. Heilmeyer & H. J. Holtmeier, Eds.: 94–109. Georg Thieme Verlag. Stuttgart, FRG.
8. FLECKENSTEIN, A. 1968. Experimental heart failure due to disturbances in high-energy phosphate metabolism. *In* Proceedings of the V European Congress of Cardiology, Athens, Greece, Sept. 1968: 255–269.
9. FLECKENSTEIN, A. 1968. Experimentelle Pathologie der akuten und chronischen Herzinsuffizienz. Verh. Dtsch. Ges. Kreislaufforsch. **34** (Tagung): 15–34.
10. FLECKENSTEIN, A. 1971. Neuere Ergebnisse zur Physiologie, Pharmakologie und Pathologie der elektromechanischen Koppelungsprozesse im Warmblütermyokard. *In* Vorträge der Erlanger Physiologentagung 1970. W. D. Keidel & K. H. Plattig, Eds.: 13–52. Springer Verlag. Berlin, Heidelberg & New York.
11. FLECKENSTEIN, A., J. JANKE, H. J. DÖRING & O. PACHINGER. 1973. Ca overload as the determinant factor in the production of catecholamine-induced myocardial lesions. *In* Recent Advances in Studies on Cardiac Structure and Metabolism. Cardiomyopathies. E. Bajusz & G. Rona, Eds. **2:** 455–466. University Park Press. Baltimore, Md.
12. FLECKENSTEIN, A., J. JANKE, H. J. DÖRING & O. LEDER. 1974. Myocardial fiber necrosis due to intracellular Ca overload—a new principle in cardiac pathophysiology. *In* Recent Advances in Studies on Cardiac Structure and Metabolism. Myocardial Biology. N. S. Dhalla, Ed. **4:** 563–579. University Park Press. Baltimore, Md.
13. FLECKENSTEIN, A., J. JANKE, H. J. DÖRING & O. LEDER. 1975. The key role of Ca in the production of noncoronarogenic myocardial necroses. *In* Recent Advances in Studies on Cardiac Structure and Metabolism. Pathophysiology and Morphology of Myocardial Cell Alterations. A. Fleckenstein & G. Rona Eds. **6:** 21–32. University Park Press. Baltimore, London & Tokyo.
14. JANKE, J., B. HEIN, O. PACHINGER, O. LEDER & A. FLECKENSTEIN. 1972. Hemmung arteriosklerotischer Gefässprozesse durch prophylaktische Behandlung mit $MgCl_2$, KCl und organischen Ca^{++}-Antagonisten (quantitative Studien mit Ca^{45} bei Ratten). *In* Vascular Smooth Muscle. E. Betz, Ed.: 71–72. Springer Verlag, Berlin, Heidelberg & New York.
15. BÜRGER, M. 1939. Die chemischen Altersveränderungen an Gefässen. Z. Neurol. Psychiatr **167:** 273–280.
16. FLECKENSTEIN, A., G. FLECKENSTEIN-GRÜN, J. JANKE & M. FREY. 1977. Kardiovaskuläre Grundwirkungen der Ca^{++}-Antagonisten und deren therapeutischer Wert in Kombination mit Herzglykosiden. Zeitschr. Präklin. Geriatr. **7:** 269–284.
17. FLECKENSTEIN-GRÜN, G. & A. FLECKENSTEIN. 1981. Calcium antagonism, a basic principle in vasodilation. *In* Calcium Antagonism in Cardiovascular Therapy: Experience with Verapamil. A. Zanchetti & D. M. Krikler, Eds.: 30–48. Excerpta Medica. Amsterdam, Oxford & Princeton.
18. FLECKENSTEIN, A. 1985. Calcium antagonism in heart and vascular smooth muscle. Med. Res. Rev. **5:** 395–425.
19. FLECKENSTEIN, A., M. FREY & G. FLECKENSTEIN-GRÜN. 1984/86. Antihypertensive and arterial anticalcinotic effects of calcium antagonists. Am. J. Cardiol. **57:** 1D–10D.
20. FLECKENSTEIN, A., M. FREY, J. ZORN & G. FLECKENSTEIN-GRÜN. 1985. Experimental basis of the long-term therapy of arterial hypertension with calcium antagonists. Am. J. Cardiol. **56:** 3H–14H.
21. FLECKENSTEIN, A., G. FLECKENSTEIN-GRÜN, M. FREY, & J. ZORN. 1987. Future directions in the use of calcium antagonists. Am. J. Cardiol. **59:** 177B–187B.
22. FLECKENSTEIN, A., M. FREY, J. ZORN & G. FLECKENSTEIN-GRÜN. 1985/86. Antihypertensive, anticalcinotische und antiarteriosklerotische Effekte von Calcium-Antagonisten. Model-Experimente an spontan-hypertensiven Ratten (SHR). *In* Calcium-Antagonisten in der Hochdrucktherapie. European Bayotensin-Symposium. A. Distler, Ed.: 3–24. Schattauer Verlag. Stuttgart & New York.
23. FLECKENSTEIN, A., M. FREY, J. ZORN & G. FLECKENSTEIN-GRÜN. 1985. Interdependence of antihypertensive, anticalcinotic and antiarteriosclerotic effects of calcium antagonists—model experiments on spontaneously hypertensive rats. *In* Cardiovascular Effects of Dihydropyridine-Type Calcium Antagonists and Agonists. Bayer-Symposium IX. A. Fleckenstein, C. van Breemen, R. Gross & F. Hoffmeister, Eds.: 480–499. Springer Verlag. Berlin, Heidelberg, New York & Tokyo.

24. TAKAHASHI, S. 1972. On the fundus of spontaneously hypertensive rats. *In* Spontaneous Hypertension. Its Pathogenesis and Complications. K. Okamoto, Ed.: 160–165, Igaku Shoin Ltd. Tokyo, Japan. Springer. Berlin, Heidelberg & New York.
25. FLECKENSTEIN, A. 1977. Specific pharmacology of calcium in myocardium, cardiac pacemakers, and vascular smooth muscle. Annu. Rev. Pharmacol. Toxicol. **17:** 149–166.
26. KIYOMOTO. A. 1979. Antihypertensive effects of diltiazem in rats. *In* New Drug Therapy with a Calcium Antagonist, Diltiazem. R. J. Bing, Ed.: 112–125. Excerpta Medica. Amsterdam & Princeton.
27. LARAGH, J. H. 1984. Proceedings of a Symposium on Calcium Metabolism and Calcium Channel Blockers for Understanding and Treating Hypertension. Am. J. Med. **77**(Suppl. 6B): 1–23.
28. BÜHLER, F. R., L. HULTHEN, W. KIOWSKI & P. BOLLI. 1982. Greater antihypertensive efficacy of the calcium channel inhibitor verapamil in older and low renin patients. Clin. Sci. (Suppl. I).
29. FLECKENSTEIN, A. 1984. Calcium antagonism: history and prospects for a multifaceted pharmacodynamic principle. *In* Calcium Antagonists and Cardiovascular Disease. L. H. Opie, Ed.: 9–28, Raven Press. New York, N.Y.
30. FLECKENSTEIN, A., M. FREY & G. FLECKENSTEIN-GRÜN. 1983. Protection by calcium antagonists against experimental arterial calcinosis. *In* Secondary Prevention of Coronary Heart Disease. K. Pyörälä, E. Rapaport, K. König, G. Schettler & C. Diehm, Eds.: 109–122. G. Thieme Verlag. Stuttgart & New York.
31. FLECKENSTEIN, A., M. FREY & O. LEDER. 1983. Prevention by calcium antagonists of arterial calcinosis. *In* Drug Development and Evaluation—New Calcium Antagonists—Recent Developments and Prospects. A. Fleckenstein, K. Hashimoto, M. Herrmann, A. Schwartz & L. Seipel, Eds.: 15–31, Gustav Fischer Verlag. Stuttgart & New York.
32. FLECKENSTEIN, A., M. FREY & H. V. WITZLEBEN. 1983. Vascular calcium overload—a pathogenetic factor in arteriosclerosis and its neutralization by calcium antagonists. *In* New Therapy of Ischemic Heart Disease and Hypertension. M. Kaltenbach & H. N. Neufeld, Eds.: 36–52. Excerpta Medica. Amsterdam, Oxford & Princeton.
33. WITZLEBEN, H. V., M. FREY., J. KEIDEL & A. FLECKENSTEIN. 1980. Normalisierung des Bluthochdrucks bei spontan hypertensiven Ratten durch eine Langzeitbehandlung mit den Ca-Antagonisten Verapamil oder Nifedipin. Therapiewoche **30:** 7895.
34. FREY, M., A. FLECKENSTEIN & G. FLECKENSTEIN-GRÜN. 1984. Prevention of nicotine-induced Ca overload of the arterial walls of rats by oral long-term administration of calcium antagonists. Pflügers Arch. Eur. J. Physiol. **400**(Suppl): R25.
35. FREY, M., A. FLECKENSTEIN & G. FLECKENSTEIN-GRÜN. 1984. Acute arterial calcinosis by simultaneous administration of nicotine plus vitamin D_3. Preventive action of diltiazem. Naunyn-Schmiedeberg's Arch. Pharmacol. **325**(Suppl): R43.

Pathophysiology of Cardiomyocytes[a]

M. BORGERS, L. VER DONCK, AND G. VANDEPLASSCHE

Laboratory of Cell Biology
Department of Life Sciences
Janssen Pharmaceutica
Turnhoutseweg, 30
B-2340 Beerse, Belgium

INTRODUCTION

The use of isolated cardiomyocytes in experimental cardiovascular research has become increasingly popular in the past years. Investigations on isolated cell systems provide several advantages. The homogeneity of the population makes it possible to evaluate the characteristics of the individual cells in the absence of external influences, i.e., cells are not subjected to neuronal modulation; interactions between the myocyte and the microvasculature and mechanical influences of neighboring tissues are eliminated. Another important advantage of isolated cardiomyocytes is their suitability for electrophysiological studies. In contrast to the multicellular preparations, in which it is very difficult to obtain adequate potential control, voltage clamp studies can easily be performed on individual cardiomyocytes. Finally, isolated cells may provide excellent material for biochemical analysis and subcellular fractionation studies.

On the other hand, experimental methods using isolated cells are not devoid of shortcomings. The proteolytic enzymes used during isolation may have altered some of the sarcolemmal components and may therefore influence certain cell functions. One must also keep in mind that removing cells from their natural habitat creates an experimental condition that may be profoundly different from the *in vivo* situation. For example, the bathing medium of isolated cells represents an infinite space in contrast to the limited extracellular space in the intact myocardium in which metabolic end products and ions diffuse. Under certain conditions this may result in intracellular concentrations of ions and metabolites that are different between *in vitro* and *in vivo* situations. It is evident that experimental conditions using isolated cells can be validated only be demonstrating their homology with the tissue of origin. Discrepancies between *in vivo* and *in vitro* situations are inevitable, but they do not necessarily invalidate the model.

Discussing the homology of the *in vivo* and *in vitro* situation, it is obvious that adult cardiomyocytes are closer to the adult heart than are embryonic cells. The latter were, however, the first cardiac cells successfully isolated and accepted as a model system for studies of cellular cardiology.[1–3] Limitations of these cultured embryonic cells are that they do not show the functional and structural differentiations of adult tissue and that culturing conditions and contaminations of nonmuscle cells may influence cellular characteristics.[4,5]

The use of isolated adult cardiac cells during the earlier days of research was limited by the inability of the adult cells to remain viable in media containing physiological Ca^{2+} concentrations.[6,7] Following the initial work of Vahouny *et al.*,[8]

[a]This work is supported by a grant from the IWONL (Instituut tot Aanmoediging van het Wetenschappelijk Onderzoek in Nijverheid en Landbouw).

Powel and Twist succeeded for the first time in isolating Ca^{2+} tolerant adult cardiomyocytes.[9] Thereafter, adult cardiomyocytes were cultured successfully; however, they underwent a transition from rod-shaped to rounded cells within a period of a few days.[10,11] These transformed cells regained their myotypic structure in a manner that resembled the original development during cellular differentiation *in vivo*. The fully differentiated form was never regained. Another isolation procedure yielding a high number of Ca^{2+} tolerant cells was introduced by Piper *et al.*[12] Under these conditions, cells do not contract spontaneously and maintain their morphologic features and energetic stability up to one week in culture.

The latter method forms the basis of the majority of Ca^{2+} overload experiments reported in this paper. By the phenomenon of "Ca^{2+} overload" we mean that intracellular Ca^{2+} exceeds the Ca^{2+} sequestration capacity of the intracellular organelles whereby the cytosol becomes exposed to an amount of free Ca^{2+} resulting in irreversible hypercontracture and cell death.[13] Such a Ca^{2+} overload could be induced by exposing the cells to either severe hypoxia, high K^+, veratrine, ouabain, free-radical-generating systems, uncouplers of oxidative phosphorylation, charged amphiphiles, A 23187, or acylcarnitines. Furthermore, the effects of representative compounds of the different subclasses of Ca^{2+} antagonists have been investigated. These comprise drugs with high affinity for the slow Ca^{2+} channels (verapamil, nifedipine, nicardipine, diltiazem) and those with no or only slight affinity for the slow Ca^{2+} channels (flunarizine, cinnarizine, lidoflazine, mioflazine). The latter have been classified as compounds with no or only a slight affinity for the slow channel, in contrast to Ca^{2+} antagonists of the slow-channel-blocking type, because they do not shorten the Ca^{2+}-dependent plateau phase of the action potential,[14] exert no or only weak negative inotropic effects at high concentrations,[15,16] and do not counteract the enhanced contractility elicited by increasing concentrations of Ca^{2+} in electrically stimulated cardiac preparations.[15]

CHARACTERISTICS OF ISOLATED ADULT RAT CARDIOMYOCYTES

In the herein described experiments, in which Ca^{2+} antagonists have been evaluated, we used cells either directly after isolation[13] or after short culturing periods.[17] The employed isolation procedure yielded 70–80% rod-shaped Ca^{2+} tolerant and 20–30% rounded Ca^{2+} intolerant myocytes. The cells were then plated on petri dishes and since only intact rod-shaped cells can attach to the dish, a population of almost 100% rod-shaped cells was obtained.[13] Criteria such as dye exclusion, ultrastructural Ca^{2+} cytochemistry, morphology, and electrical excitability were used to judge cell viability.

Trypan blue dye was excluded by 99% of the rod-shaped myocytes, indicating a good preservation of sarcolemmal integrity. Electronmicroscopic observations have indicated that isolated cells retain the essential structural features of undissociated myocardial cells.[12,18–20] The myocytes showed numerous parallel myofibrils, separated by rows of mitochondria that contain the typical osmiophilic granules. Also all other cellular features appeared to be well preserved and within normal ranges. The cells exhibited an intact sarcolemma, and the irregular intercalated disk areas appeared as a microvillar border. The only slight morphological modifications found were a discontinuous external coat of the glycocalyx and swelling of the transverse (T) tubules. Ca^{2+} localization was assessed with the phosphate pyroantimonate method (PPA), as described by Borgers *et al.*[21] With this technique Ca^{2+} deposits, possibly bound to acidic phospholipids,[22] were almost exclusively confined to the sarcolemma, sarcolemma-derived vesicles, T tubules, and intercalated disks (FIGURE 1). Internalized vacuoles, most probably derived from the intercalated disks, showed deposits as well. It is noteworthy that these short-term cultured myocytes exhibit the same pattern of Ca^{2+} deposits as in the intact myocardium, even though they usually lack the outer lamina of the glycocalyx. Myocytes incubated in the absence of extracellular Ca^{2+} (0.1 mM EGTA) showed a similar pattern of Ca^{2+} deposition. The formation of sarcolemmal Ca^{2+} deposits is completely prevented by La^{3+} (FIGURE 2), suggesting that the Ca^{2+} pool, visualized by PPA, may belong to an exchangeable pool possibly involved in excitation-contraction coupling. This is in agreement with observations made by Langer that the ability of a series of cations (La^{3+}, Ca^{2+}, Mg^{2+} Mn^{2+}) to uncouple excitation from contraction was the same as their ability to displace Ca^{2+} from sarcolemmal sites.[23,24]

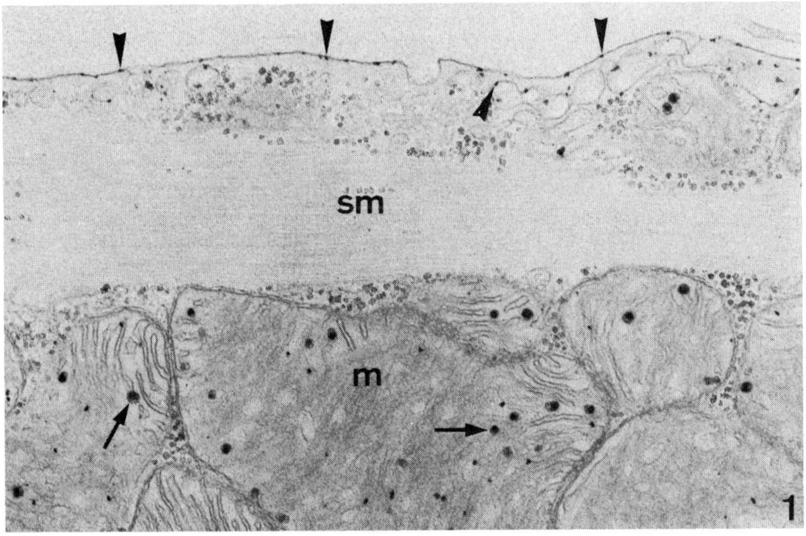

FIGURE 1. Part of a Ca^{2+}-tolerant rod-shaped cardiomyocyte showing normal subcellular organelles: sarcomeres (sm) and rows of mitochondria (m) containing osmiophilic intramatricial granules (arrows) are longitudinally arranged in this section. Glycogen particles are abundantly present. Small electrondense particles (arrowheads) representing Ca^{2+} deposits are associated with the cytoplasmic face of the sarcolemma and sarcolemma-derived vesicles. Mitochondria are free of Ca^{2+} precipitate. 41310×.

In contrast to the *in vivo* situation where myocytes are continuously contracting, the rod-shaped isolated cells were mechanically inactive and showed no spontaneous contractions even in the presence of Ca^{2+} concentrations as high as 10 mM. This is not so surprising since isolated cells are separated from the activity of spontaneous depolarizing pacemaker cells. The response to electrical field stimulation of the otherwise quiescent cells suggests that these cells have retained their electrophysiological integrity.[25,26] In our experiments myocytes were stimulated at 2 Hz with a pulse duration of 10 mseconds and a voltage ranging between 0 and 99.

The number of synchronously contracting myocytes increased with increasing voltage, and a maximum of nearly 100% contracting cells was obtained at about 80 V. When Ca^{2+} ions were complexed by EGTA, cells could no longer be stimulated. This

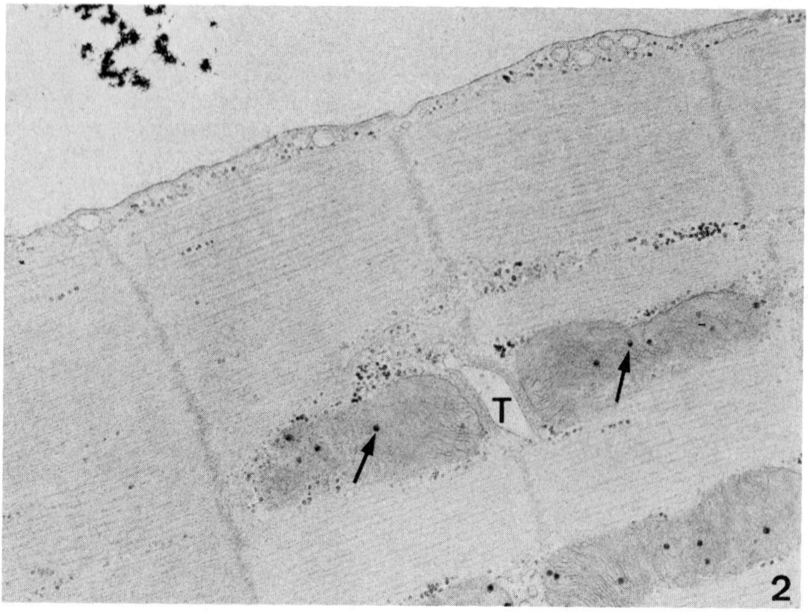

FIGURE 2. Cardiomyocytes after exposure to 1 mM $LaCl_3$ for 5 minutes. The cell is in a relaxed state and mitochondria appear normal. The sarcolemma, T tubuli (T), and sarcolemma-derived vesicles are devoid of Ca^{2+} deposits. Osmiophilic intramatricial granules (arrows) are still present. La^{3+} precipitate is seen outside the cell (left top corner). 27115×.

picture of electrical excitability changed after preincubation of the myocytes with Ca^{2+} antagonists (TABLE 1). Most drugs tested at 10^{-5} M severely inhibited the electrical excitability of the myocytes. At 10^{-6} M a clear difference was observed among the Ca^{2+} antagonists tested. Those with no or only slight affinity for the slow channels (cinnarizine, flunarizine, lidoflazine, and mioflazine) only slightly interfered with the electrical excitability of the myocytes. On the other hand, the typical slow channel blockers profoundly inhibited the excitability of the myocytes, with the exception of diltiazem. This inhibitory effect was most pronounced with the dihydropyridines

TABLE 1. Electrical Excitability of Isolated Cardiomyocytes Incubated with Ca^{2+} Antagonists

Drug (10^{-6} M)	Percent Excitable Cardiomyocytes
Solvent	100
Cinnarizine	87
Flunarizine	62
Lidoflazine	84
Mioflazine	95
Verapamil	46
Nifedipine	2
Nicardipine	5
Diltiazem	95

(nifedipine, nicardipine) and correlates well with the negative inotropic effect of these drugs.[27,28] Cheung *et al.* obtained analogous results with verapamil and nifedipine in paced cardiomyocytes under hypoxic conditions.[29] The protective effect seen with these drugs was attributed to depressed cellular contractile activity. In our experiments, diltiazem had no effect on the electrical excitability of the rod-shaped cells in spite of its known negative inotropic effects *in vivo*. This discrepancy may be due, at least in part, to the fact that the negative inotropic effects of diltiazem only appear at temperatures above 30°C (maximal at 37°C),[25] whereas our experiments were performed at room temperature.

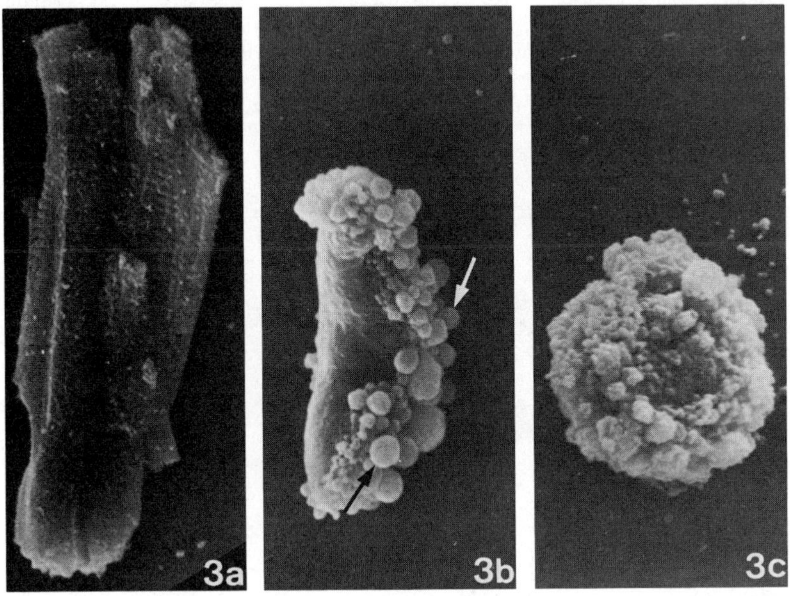

FIGURE 3. Scanning electron micrographs showing the characteristic stages of cardiomyocyte shape changes. 785×. (a) Ca^{2+} tolerant rod-shaped cardiomyocyte with cross striations and "Treppe-like" organized intercalated disks; (b) intermediate stage of shape changes showing a partially contracted cardiomyocyte with formation of large surface blebs (arrows); (c) final stage of shape changes represented by a round hypercontracted cell.

INDUCTION OF HYPERCONTRACTURE BY PATHOLOGICAL STIMULI

Upon exposure to various stimuli the quiescent cardiomyocytes (FIGURE 3a) started to contract vigorously, followed by sarcomere shortening and bleb formation (FIGURE 3b). Eventually, cells rounded up as a consequence of irreversible contracture (FIGURE 3c). These shape changes indicate a loss of viability and represent a state of Ca^{2+} overloading.[13,14,18] TABLE 2 summarizes the various stimuli and experimental conditions employed to induce shape changes. The number of cells (expressed as a percentage of the initial number of rod-shaped cells) that underwent hypercontracture due to the various aggressions is presented in TABLE 2. Each stimulus induced alterations at the cellular level that might be of importance under various pathological *in vivo* conditions.

Intracellular Na^+ and Ca^{2+} overload was induced using veratrine, an alkaloid that prolongs the open state of the Na^+ channel.[30] This resulted in hypercontracture of almost all rod-shaped cells within five minutes. This phenomenon was Ca^{2+} mediated since omission of the extracellular Ca^{2+} entirely prevented rounding up of the cells. The mechanism by which veratrine stimulates Ca^{2+} influx has been discussed earlier.[13]

Ca^{2+} overload due to cardiac glycoside intoxication is often observed in clinical situations.[31,32] The dose range in which these drugs exert a positive inotropic effect is quite small and is close to the toxic dose that induces myocardial dysfunction and eventually cardiac failure.[32] When tested at the cellular level, ouabain did not induce changes in the quiescent myocytes even with concentrations up to 10^{-4} M. However, incubation of electrically stimulated cardiomyocytes for 20 minutes in the presence of 10^{-4} M ouabain resulted in rounding up of nearly all myocytes (TABLE 2).

Free-radical-induced damage has been reported in a variety of pathological conditions in many tissues.[33–35] A role for oxygen free radicals as mediators of tissue

TABLE 2. Pathological Stimuli to Induce Shape Changes in Isolated Cardiomyocytes

Pathological Stimulus		Time of Exposure (minutes)	Percent Hypercontracted Cells after Stimulus
Na^+ and Ca^{2+} overload	100 μg/ml veratrine	5	97
Na^+-K^+-ATPase inhibition	1.10^{-4} M ouabain + electrical field stimulation	20	96
Oxygen free radicals	1.10^{-3} M hypoxanthine + 0.025 U/ml xanthine oxidase	60	99
	5.10^{-8} M rose bengal + 560 nm light	5	97
Charged amphiphiles	1.10^{-4} M polymyxin B	60	99
Acylcarnitine	8.10^{-6} M palmitoylcarnitine	15	99
DNP	2.10^{-4} M 2,4-dinitrophenol	12	99

damage during postischemic reperfusion of the heart has been implicated.[36–38] It was suggested that xanthine and hypoxanthine which are formed during ischemia react with molecular oxygen to produce superoxide anions. This reaction is catalyzed by xanthine oxidase which is formed during ischemia through conversion of xanthine dehydrogenase. The subsequent dismutation reaction of superoxide to hydrogen peroxide (H_2O_2), catalyzed by superoxide dismutase (SOD), is followed by a transformation of H_2O_2 to H_2O and O_2 by catalase or glutathion peroxidase.[38] Under pathological conditions the sequestration capacity of the latter enzymes is exceeded and the highly reactive hydroxyl radical is produced from H_2O_2. This induces a chain reaction of lipid peroxidation resulting in structural and functional damage of membranes.[36] To examine the effects of free radical damage at the cellular level, two different free-radical-generating systems have been used (TABLE 2). Firstly, as described by Burton *et al.*,[39] superoxide anion was generated by addition of hypoxanthine and xanthine oxidase to the cardiomyocytes, and after one hour incubation, typical shape changes were seen in nearly all cells. Secondly, singlet oxygen was produced by photoexcitation of rose bengal, a photosensitive dye that is excited to the triplet state upon exposure to a 560 nm light source.[40] Singlet oxygen, resulting from active quenching by molecular oxygen, initiates peroxidation of membranes.[41,42] This reaction, the so called "dye-sensitized photooxygenation," leads to hypercontracture of the cardiomyocytes within a few minutes. The same reaction, but at a much slower rate, was obtained by exposing cells incubated with rose bengal to daylight. The damage induced by both free-radical-generating systems could be prevented by catalase or a mixture of SOD and catalase, whereas SOD alone could not inhibit the hypercontracture. The metal-chelating agent desferrioxamine delayed the occurrence of hypercontracture in the first system but had no effects on shape changes induced by singlet oxygen.

Polymyxin B (PXB), a positively charged amphiphilic compound, is known to decrease sarcolemmal-bound Ca^{2+} probably by decreasing the number of negatively charged sites.[24,43] In view of the possible important role of sarcolemmal Ca^{2+} for cell viability, we examined the effects of PXB in isolated cardiomyocytes. After one hour incubation of the myocytes with 10^{-4} M PXB, hypercontracture was seen in almost all cells.

Acylcarnitines are known to accumulate in ischemic tissue and change the properties of cardiac cell membranes, thereby contributing to a decline in myocardial contractility, arrhythmias, and cell death.[44,45] When cardiomyocytes were incubated with one of the acylcarnitines (palmitoylcarnitine) shape changes were observed in the majority of cells within 15 minutes of exposure.

Inhibition of mitochondrial oxidative phosphorylation as achieved by the addition of dinitrophenol (DNP, 2.10^{-4} M) led to a slow transformation of the rod-shaped cells into square-shaped cells, eventually resulting in complete hypercontracture with the formation of peripheral blebs. This observation is in agreement with those of Ganote *et al.* in isolated hearts, where DNP was found to induce contraction.[46]

Apart from the pathological stimuli mentioned in TABLE 2, other aggressions investigated induced hypercontracture and Ca^{2+} overload. One of these was exposure of the cells to high extracellular K^+ concentrations to cause sustained depolarization. Cardiomyocytes indeed have been shown to undergo shape changes when incubated with 50 mM K^+.[14,18] Incubation of the cells with the Ca^{2+} ionophore A 23187 resulted in hypercontracture in the majority of the cells as a consequence of increased Ca^{2+} influx. In view of a highly variable day to day outcome, the A 23187 experiments were not further pursued.

Trials to induce a Ca^{2+} paradox situation in isolated cardiomyocytes, unlike in the whole heart, failed completely.[19] It might well be that the integrity of the sarcolemma of isolated cells is preserved during the Ca^{2+}-depletion period since no shifts in sarcolemmal Ca^{2+} could be demonstrated. This is in contrast with the observations on the intact isolated heart, in which cells that are sensitive to the paradox upon reintroduction of Ca^{2+} show a loss of sarcolemmal-bound Ca^{2+} at the end of the Ca^{2+} free period.[19] Intercellular relationships apparently play a dominant role in the Ca^{2+} paradox phenomenon.[47]

Relevant to the clinical pathology of cardiac ischemia are experiments where oxygen shortage and reoxygenation are imposed on cardiac cultures. Piper *et al.* reported a significant reduction in energy-rich phosphates during anoxia, correlating with increased lactate and cytosolic enzyme release.[48,49] These events take place during the first hour of anoxia, while shape changes in part of the cell population occur only during the second hour of anoxic incubation. Reoxygenation of the cells resulted in partial biochemical recovery up to 120 minutes of anoxia,[48] indicating that reversible membrane alterations were probably responsible for the biochemical findings reported above.

Most of the pathological stimuli mentioned were able to induce hypercontracture of the myocytes only in the presence of extracellular Ca^{2+}, suggesting that an enhanced transmembrane flux of Ca^{2+} is a prerequisite for the development of hypercontracture. Two exceptions were found where extracellular Ca^{2+} was not essential to induce shape changes. Such was the case after prolonged exposure to severe hypoxia in a Ca^{2+} free culture medium (results not shown). The absence of Ca^{2+} delayed rather than prevented hypercontracture. In experiments using DNP as an uncoupler of oxidative phosphorylation, shape changes occurred both in the presence and in the absence of extracellular Ca^{2+}. These observations correlate well with those of Ganote in isolated hearts.[46,50] Furthermore, they are in agreement with fluoroprobe measurements of intracellular Ca^{2+} concentrations in metabolically inhibited myocardial cells, showing no rise in intracellular Ca^{2+} levels during cell shortening.[51] Shape changes that occur during metabolic inhibition and prolonged hypoxia can likely be attributed to the very low ATP levels. It is known that cell shortening can occur under conditions of strongly reduced ATP levels in a manner independent of extracellular Ca^{2+}.[52,53] Cell shortening is most probably due to changes in the affinity of troponin-C for Ca^{2+} caused by low ATP levels.[54]

EFFECTS OF Ca^{2+} ANTAGONISTS

The similarity between effects of intracellular Ca^{2+} accumulation under ischemic conditions *in vivo* (e.g., References 55–57) and the effects of the pathophysiologic stimuli (TABLE 2) applied to isolated cardiac cells *in vitro* might suggest that pharmacological interventions that can counteract the damaging effects of Ca^{2+} overload *in vivo* might also affect shape changes induced by various pathophysiological stimuli *in vitro*. The effects of compounds belonging to different subclasses of Ca^{2+} antagonists in counteracting the shape changes induced by various pathological stimuli (TABLE 2) were investigated. The contact time with the drugs before the Ca^{2+} overload stimulus was kept at 30 minutes. The percentage of remaining rod-shaped cells after each stimulus was taken as a measure for protection afforded by the various drugs.

FIGURE 4 displays the effects of the Ca^{2+} antagonists against veratrine-induced shape changes in isolated myocytes. Lidoflazine, flunarizine, and cinnarizine were the most potent drugs providing protection from 10^{-7} M onward. Nicardipine and mioflazine were protective from 10^{-6} M onward whereas verapamil was protective only at the 10^{-5} M concentration. The other slow channel blockers nifedipine and diltiazem afforded no protection at any of the concentrations tested. Similar degrees of protection with these drugs have been reported previously in high-K^+ induced Ca^{2+} overload in isolated cardiomyocytes.[14] In view of these observations, it is likely that the Ca^{2+} responsible for the induction of these shape changes enters the cell through membrane domains other than the slow channels. It has been shown in neuroblastoma cells that veratrine, apart from prolonging the open state of Na^+ channels, also blocks the slow Ca^{2+} channels.[58] This supports the assumption that the Ca^{2+} influx induced after veratrine addition is not mediated through the slow channel. These as yet unidentified domains may be the preferred binding sites for the Ca^{2+} antagonists of the non-slow-channel type. The protective effects of nicardipine at 10^{-6} and 10^{-5} M and of verapamil at 10^{-5} M may be explained by an additional membrane stabilizing effect of these drugs at higher concentrations. Such a nonspecific membrane effect at high doses (membrane-stabilizing effect) has been suggested for both drugs.[28,59,60]

After exposure of electrically stimulated cells to ouabain, protective effects were observed with, on the one hand, flunarizine and cinnarizine and on the other hand, verapamil, nifedipine, and nicardipine (FIGURE 5a). This effect of the latter three drugs can most likely be explained by their inhibitory effect on the electrical excitability of isolated cells (TABLE 1). Interestingly, diltiazem showed no protection against ouabain-induced shape changes, which correlates well with the observation that this compound did not inhibit electrical excitability at room temperature (TABLE 1). Flunarizine and cinnarizine, which only minimally interfere with electrical excitability (TABLE 1) and do not have negative inotropic effects,[15,16] also afforded considerable protection against ouabain-induced shape changes. This is in agreement with the observations of Jonkman *et al.*, who reported protective effects of flunarizine against ouabain-induced arrhythmias in guinea pig hearts.[27] These data demonstrate that Ca^{2+} antagonists that are devoid of slow channel affinity can prevent intracellular Ca^{2+} overload due to digitalis intoxication, without interfering with the proper inotropic action of the cardiac glycoside.[27]

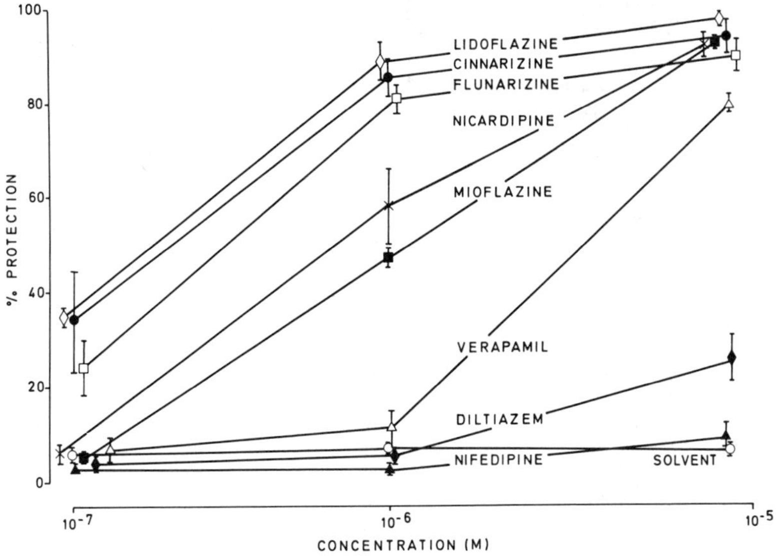

FIGURE 4. Protective effects by Ca^{2+} antagonists against veratrine-induced shape changes. The results show the percentage of remaining rod-shaped cardiomyocytes 5 minutes after veratrine addition [mean ± standard error of the mean (SEM), $n = 6$].

Free-radical-induced damage was also influenced by pretreatment with Ca^{2+} antagonists. Upon superoxide anion generation, moderate protection was seen with both slow channel and non-slow-channel blockers with the exception of mioflazine and nicardipine which afforded a higher degree of protection (FIGURE 5b). The protection with the different drugs against hypercontracture induced by singlet oxygen was different (FIGURE 5c). It is clear that under these conditions the non-slow-channel blockers were the most protective drugs. After incubation of the cells with PXB the shape changes were again prevented most effectively by Ca^{2+} antagonists with the least affinity for the slow channels (FIGURE 5d).

In conclusion, in most of the above-described experimental conditions, the stimulated Ca^{2+} entry is not mediated through the slow channels since the potent slow channel blockers are generally the least protective.

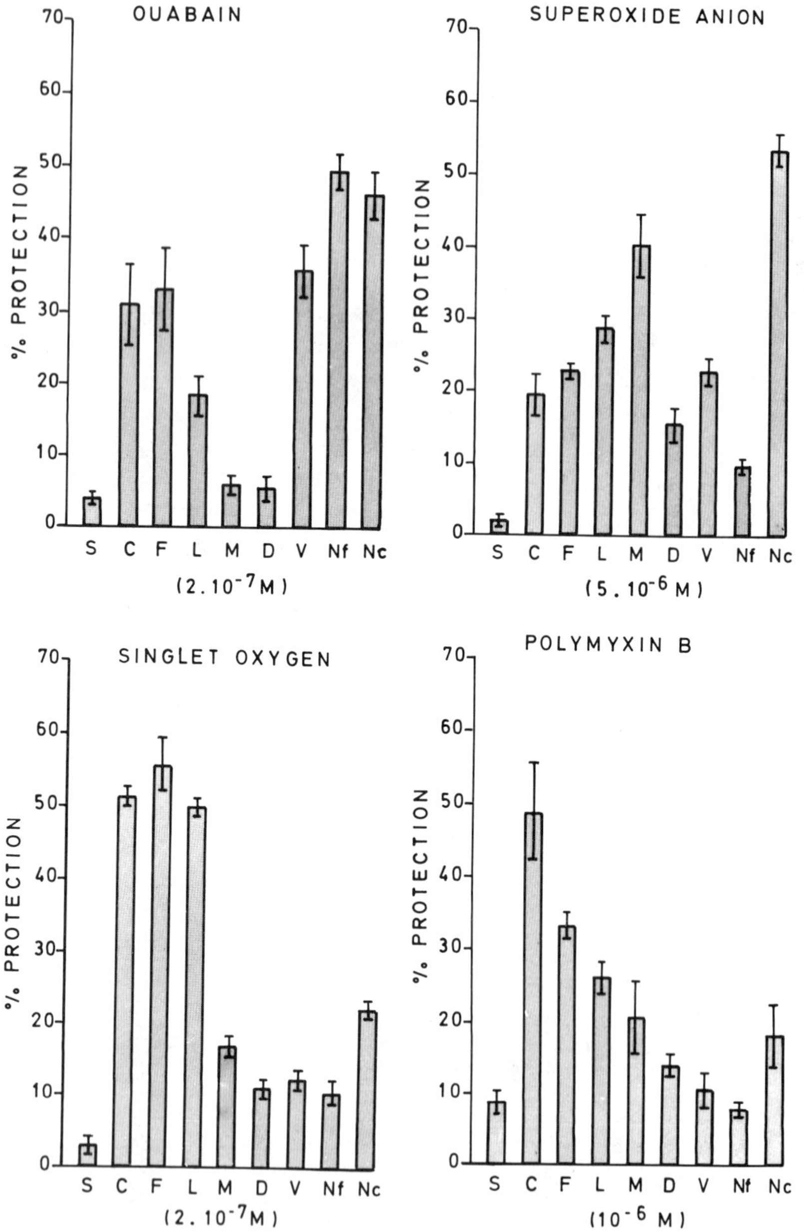

FIGURE 5. Protective effects of Ca^{2+} antagonists against shape changes induced by various pathological stimuli. The results show the percentage of remaining rod-shaped cardiomyocytes (i.e., percent protection): (a) effect of ouabain [drugs tested at 2.10^{-7} M (mean ± SEM, $n = 4$)]; (b) effect of superoxide anion [drugs tested at 5.10^{-6} M (mean ± SEM, $n = 6$)]; (c) effect of singlet oxygen [drugs tested at 2.10^{-7} M (mean ± SEM, $n = 5$)]; (d) effect of polymyxin B [drugs tested at 10^{-6} M (mean ± SEM, $n = 6$)]. Abbreviations: S = solvent; C = cinnarizine; F = flunarizine; L = lidoflazine; M = mioflazine; D = diltiazem; V = verapamil; Nf = nifedipine; Nc = nicardipine.

Hypercontracture induced by inhibition of mitochondrial respiration by DNP or the addition of palmitoylcarnitine could not be prevented by any of the Ca^{2+} antagonists. This is not too surprising in the case of DNP since contracture was induced independent of Ca^{2+} influx. The dose of palmitoylcarnitine used in our experiments induced disruption of the sarcolemma as displayed in the electron microscope (see below). Such discontinuities would enable extracellular Ca^{2+} to enter the cell freely. This type of structural damage due to fatty acid accumulation in ischemic myocardial tissue has also been reported in a review by Katz and Messineo.[61] Such a structural damage is not likely to be antagonized by any type of drug.

The results with the various Ca^{2+} antagonists in each experiment were subjected to an average linkage cluster analysis to detect relationships between the varying degrees

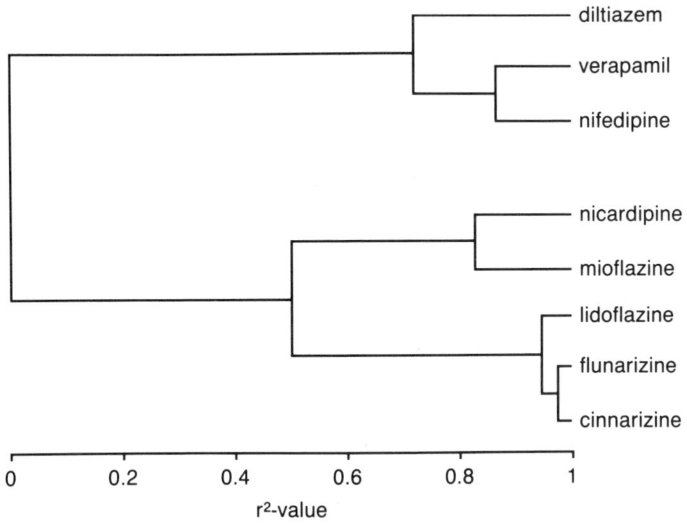

FIGURE 6. Results of the average linkage cluster analysis performed on results obtained with the Ca^{2+} antagonists in the experiments with veratrine, ouabain, superoxide anion, singlet oxygen, and polymyxin B. The horizontal axis represents the square of the correlation coefficient (r^2 value) found for the relationship between effects of drugs or groups of drugs in the various experiments in this study. The r^2 value for a given relationship can be derived from this graph by extrapolating the verticle line, relating two drugs or groups with each other, to the r^2 axis.

of protection obtained by all drugs against the pathophysiological stimuli described above. The results of this analysis are presented in FIGURE 6 and show the degree of similarity between individual drugs or groups of drugs. The degree of similarity is expressed as the square of the correlation coefficient for each similarity. This figure clearly demonstrates that (1) the results obtained with cinnarizine, flunarizine, and lidoflazine are highly correlated ($r^2 = 0.95$); (2) the structurally unrelated mioflazine and nicardipine act rather similarly; (3) the latter are related to the first group to some extent ($r^2 = 0.50$); (4) both of the above groups do not show any correlation with the slow channel blocking drugs verapamil, nifedipine, and diltiazem ($r^2 = 0$).

The reason why mioflazine seems to diverge from the other diarylalkylpiperazines is not clear. A possible reason might be the different lipophilicity of this compound, whereby the adsorption to vial surfaces reduces the availability of mioflazine molecules

TABLE 3. Ca^{2+} Shifts after Pathophysiological Stimuli[a]

Experimental Condition	Rod-Shaped Cells				Rounded Cells			
			Mitochondria				Mitochondria	
	Percent	Sarcolemmal Ca^{2+}	Single Ca^{2+} Deposits	Ca^{2+} Clusters	Percent	Sarcolemmal Ca^{2+}	Single Ca^{2+} Deposits	Ca^{2+} Clusters
Control:								
1 mM Ca^{2+}	99	+	−	−	1	−	+	−
0.1 mM EGTA	99	+	−	−	1	−	+	−
Veratrine	3	±	−	−	97	−	±	−
Ouabain	4	−	−	−	96	−	±	±
O_2 radicals							−	−
Superoxide anion	1	±	−	−	99	−	+	+
Singlet O_2								
10′	88	++	−	−	12	−	+	−
25′	64	++	−	−	36	−	+	−[b]
40′	25	+	−	−	75	−	+	+[b]
75′	8	±	−	−	92	−	+	+[b]
90′	3	−	−	−	97	−	+	+[b]
Polymyxin B								
15′	74	±	−	−	26	−	+	+[b]
60′	3	−	±	−	97	−	+	+[b]
Acylcarnitine	1	±	−	−	99	−	±	−[c]
DNP								
3′	80	++	−	−	20	−	+	±[b]
12′	1	±	+	−	99	−	+	+[b]
Anoxia								
30′	95	++	±	−	5	++	++	−
60′	95	++	+	−	5	++	++	−
90′	80	++	+	−	20	++	++	−
120′	65	++	+	−	35	−	−	++[b]

[a]Observations apply to the majority of cells. Ca^{2+} deposits at the sarcolemma and in mitochondria are evaluated as absent (−), sparsely (±), moderately (+), or abundantly (++) present.
[b]Clumping of mitochondrial cristae.
[c]Disrupted sarcolemma.

in solution. This assumption is supported by the high degree of protection obtained with mioflazine in experiments where the drug was tested at high concentrations (e.g., in the veratrine, superoxide anion, and PXB experiments). Another unexpected finding concerns the divergence between the dihydropyridines nifedipine and nicardipine. The higher degree of protection of the latter may possibly be attributed to an additional membrane-stabilizing effect of this compound at high concentrations.

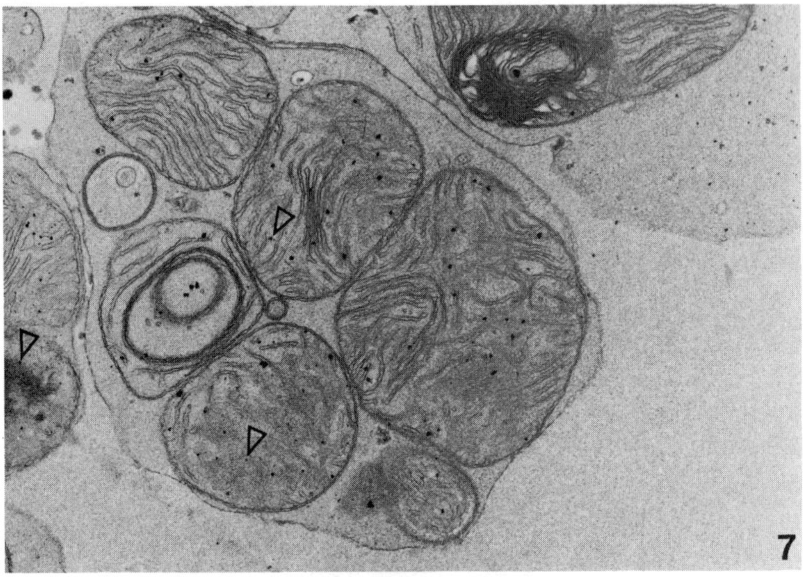

FIGURE 7. Part of a hypercontracted cell after exposure to veratrine, showing cytoplasmic blebs filled with mitochondria. Mitochondria already contain Ca^{2+} deposits (open arrowheads) whereas the sarcolemma is completely devoid of precipitate. 33277×.

ULTRASTRUCTURAL CHANGES AND Ca^{2+} SHIFTS INDUCED BY PATHOLOGICAL STIMULI: EFFECT OF Ca^{2+} ANTAGONISTS

Shape changes induced in isolated cardiomyocytes by the pathological stimuli mentioned coincide with changes in the pattern of Ca^{2+} deposition (TABLE 3). When cells become hypercontracted, all sarcolemmal Ca^{2+} deposits are lost and mitochondria accumulate single and/or clustered Ca^{2+} deposits. FIGURE 7 shows an example of a hypercontracted cell after veratrine addition, showing large cytoplasmic protrusions filled with mitochondria in which Ca^{2+} accumulated. The intermediate stages of shape changes, as can be observed in experiments with a rather slow rate of shape transformation (e.g., severe hypoxia), are characterized by an increase of Ca^{2+} deposits at the sarcolemma and in the mitochondria. This occurs already before marked cell shortening has taken place (FIGURE 9). Later on, with progressing contracture formation, the Ca^{2+} deposition in mitochondria increases further. Finally the sarcolemma loses all Ca^{2+} binding ability and clustering of Ca^{2+} within the mitochondrial matrices becomes a frequently observed phenomenon (FIGURE 10). The reason why the sarcolemma loses its ability to bind Ca^{2+} in progressing pathological

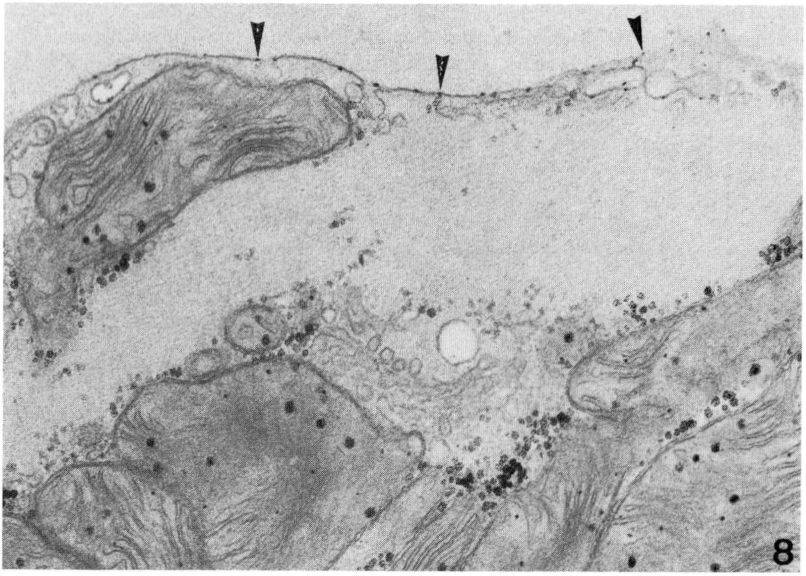

FIGURE 8. Mioflazine (10^{-6} M) pretreated cardiomyocyte after veratrine, showing preservation of sarcolemma-bound Ca^{2+} deposits (arrowheads). Mitochondria do not show precipitate. 43690×.

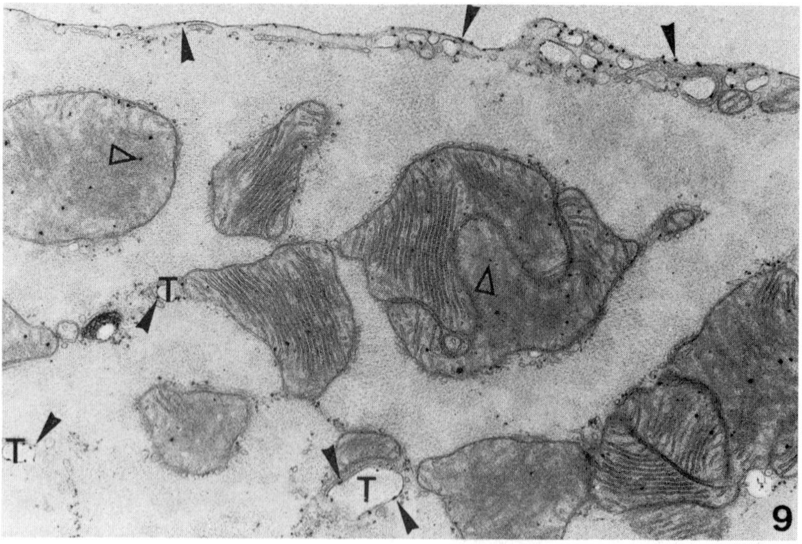

FIGURE 9. Rod-shaped cardiomyocyte after 60 minutes of anoxic incubation, showing an increased amount of Ca^{2+} precipitate (arrowheads) at the sarcolemma, T tubuli (T), and sarcolemma-derived vesicles. The mitochondria have lost their electron-dense granules and show accumulation of single Ca^{2+} deposits (open arrowheads). 22950×.

cell injury is not fully understood. The cytochemical demonstrable Ca^{2+} deposits at the sarcolemma of normal cells are believed to be related to the Ca^{2+} binding of anionic phospholipids.[22] A change in sarcolemmal composition could result in a decreased affinity of the acidic phospolipids for Ca^{2+} leading to increased cytosolic Ca^{2+} concentrations and Ca^{2+} overload. In recent experiments of global normothermic ischemia in dogs[62,63] and rabbits,[64] a loss of sarcolemma-associated Ca^{2+} has also been demonstrated in subendocardial areas (dog) and in the midmyocardium (rabbit) prior to reperfusion. Cells in these areas of the myocardium usually showed signs of irreversible damage upon reperfusion. This loss of sarcolemma-associated deposits was also observed in other experimental conditions: in isolated rat hearts after a period of

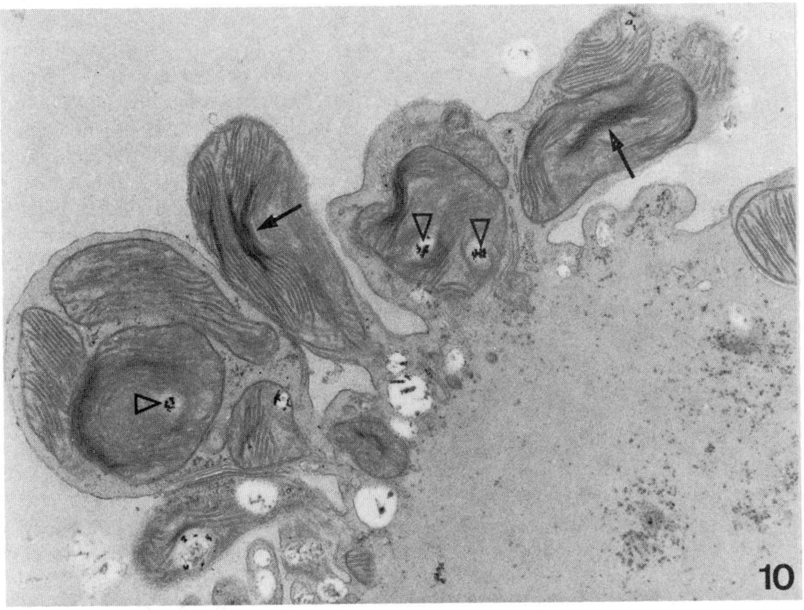

FIGURE 10. Irreversibly damaged cell after 120 minutes of anoxia showing disorganization of the contractile apparatus and formation of cytoplasmic blebs filled with mitochondria. These mitochondria display clustering of Ca^{2+} deposits (open arrowheads) and clumping of mitochondrial cristae (arrows). The sarcolemma is completely devoid of precipitate. 22950×.

Ca^{2+} free perfusion sufficient to elicit the "Ca^{2+} paradox";[19] in isolated cardiac myocytes after sustained depolarization with a high K^+ concentration; and in isolated rat hearts exposed to exhaustive stimulation with high doses of epinephrine and ouabain.[18] Under all these conditions, as with prolonged hypoxia, the myocardial cell finally becomes irreversibly injured. These results indicate that impairment of sarcolemmal Ca^{2+} binding reflects irreversible damage probably due to impaired cellular Ca^{2+} homeostasis.

Besides the occurrence of Ca^{2+} shifts, a marked disorganization of the mitochondrial substructure is displayed after some pathological stimuli. Abnormal clumping of mitochondrial cristae was most obvious after exposure to severe hypoxia, during singlet-oxygen-induced shape changes and after exposure to PXB or DNP. This characteristic morphological alteration is possibly related to the occurrence of lipid peroxidative reactions in metabolically malfunctioning mitochondria.[65]

Protected rod-shaped myocardial cells from drug-pretreated cultures show a pattern of sarcolemma-associated Ca^{2+} precipitate similar to control cells. FIGURE 8 shows a picture of a mioflazine (10^{-6} M) pretreated cell after veratrine challenge. Similar observations could be made on remaining rod-shaped cells treated with the various drugs that afforded protection against stimulated Ca^{2+} overload.

In another study, detailed analysis of Ca^{2+} shifts was made in a time-dependent way on anoxic cardiomyocytes with and without pretreatment with lidoflazine, one of the cardioprotective Ca^{2+} antagonists of the non-slow-channel type.[17,66] In this study, the pattern of distribution of Ca^{2+} deposits at the sarcolemma and in the mitochondria of the cultures was scored in function of the injury progressing with duration of anoxic incubation.[17] The lesion score (as detailed in the legend to FIGURE 11) indicates a pattern of Ca^{2+} deposition ranging from score 0 (no Ca^{2+} deposits in mitochondria and normal Ca^{2+} deposits at the sarcolemma), score 1 (slightly altered pattern), score 2 (moderately altered), score 3 (severely altered), to score 4 (severely altered pattern characterized by clustering of Ca^{2+} in mitochondria and total absence of sarcolemmal Ca^{2+}). The latter changes were interpreted as changes at the edge of irreversibility.[17] From FIGURE 11 it can be seen that a tendency towards recovery is present upon reoxygenation after up to 90 minutes of anoxia in solvent-treated cultures whereas reoxygenation after 120 minutes anoxia resulted in further deterioration. Statistical analysis (Jonckheere-Terpstra test for ordered alternatives)[67] revealed that increasing duration of anoxia was paralleled by increased damage. Lidoflazine-treated cultures, on the other hand, showed a less severe alteration in Ca^{2+} shifts, especially after 60 minutes of anoxia where recovery upon reoxygenation was very marked (FIGURE 11). It may be concluded from these results that anoxia-induced deleterious Ca^{2+} shifts are postponed in lidoflazine-treated cultures.

Data in the present and earlier studies show preservation of sarcolemma-bound Ca^{2+} with the non-slow-channel Ca^{2+} antagonists.[62,64,68,69] This suggests a protective effect at the level of the sarcolemma in the sense that the structural integrity of the membrane is preserved with retention of the membranes' capacity to bind Ca^{2+}. The weak degree of protection obtained with typical slow channel blockers against most of the pathological stimuli inducing Ca^{2+} overload corresponds well with the relative inability of this type of drug to antagonize Ca^{2+} overload during reperfusion of ischemic tissue.[70,71] All these observations suggest that in many of the pathological conditions mentioned, the bulk of Ca^{2+} that crosses the sarcolemma is not mediated through slow channels. This is supported by the fact that the diarylalkylpiperazines, which have no or only a very weak affinity for slow Ca^{2+} channels,[14–16] demonstrated superior protection compared with the slow channel blockers. The exact role that both groups of Ca^{2+} antagonists, which apparently behave so differently, may play in the prevention and therapy of cardiac pathology is unsolved at present but undoubtedly is an intriguing subject that will gain great attention in the years to come.

SUMMARY AND CONCLUSIONS

Isolated cardiomyocytes lend themselves very well to the quantification of pathological damage and to the determination of reversible versus irreversible changes. These single cells were used to study the cellular response to a variety of pathologic stimuli that impair structure and function. Degenerative alterations are accompanied by hyperactivation and irreversible rounding up of otherwise quiescent rod-shaped cells. Stereotypic degenerative changes and loss of sarcolemma-bound Ca^{2+} were seen

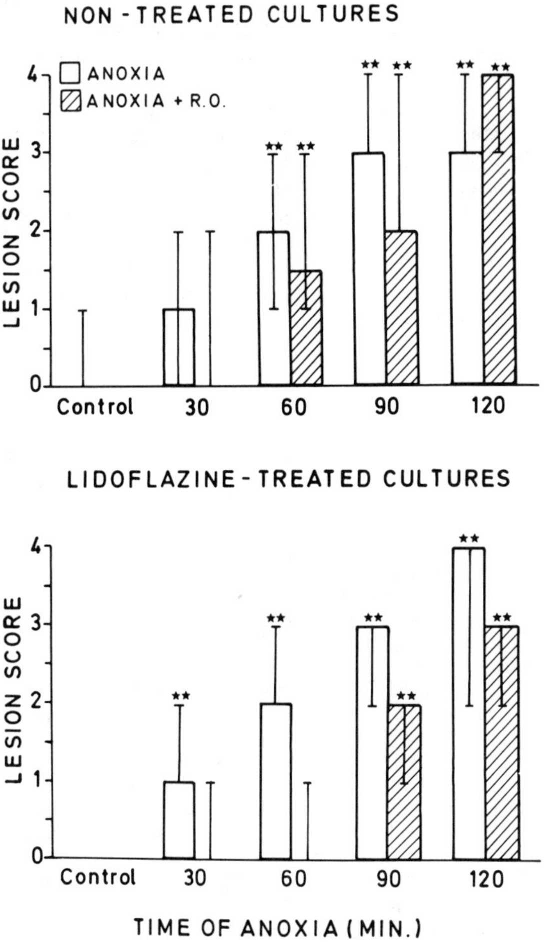

FIGURE 11. Pattern of Ca^{2+} distribution after various periods of anoxia [open columns in solvent (upper) and lidoflazine (5.10^{-6} M) (lower) treated cultures]. Anoxic periods followed by 30 minutes of reoxygenation (RO) are represented by hatched columns. Score 0. Normal pattern of distribution: moderate number of deposits along the sarcolemma and T tubules; no or occasional single deposits in mitochondria (as in FIGURE 1). Score 1 (slightly altered): slightly increased number of sarcolemmal and mitochondrial (single) deposits. Score 2 (moderately altered): marked increase in both sarcolemmal and mitochondrial (single) deposits (as in FIGURE 9). Score 3 (severely altered): mixture of (a) cells with marked increase in sarcolemmal deposits and single deposits in mitochondria; and (b) cells with complete absence of sarcolemmal deposits and the presence of clustered deposits in mitochondria. Predominance of (a). Score 4 (severely altered): as score 3 but predominance of (b) (as shown in FIGURE 10). The two-tailed Mann-Whitney U test[66] was used to determine statistical significance between normoxic controls and each of the anoxic groups, and to evaluate the effect of reoxygenation. $p < 0.01$ (**) was considered to indicate significant difference from control. Results are presented as median score and range ($n \geq 5$).

during prolonged severe hypoxia, exposure to either depolarizing concentrations of potassium, veratrine, acylcarnitines, cationic amphiphiles, free-radical-generating systems, cardiac glycosides, or uncouplers of oxidative phosphorylation. Since the presence of extracellular Ca^{2+} is a prerequisite to obtain cell degeneration in most of these aggressive insults and since cellular Ca^{2+} overload parallels the damage, we studied the influence of representative compounds of the various subclasses of Ca^{2+} antagonists: verapamil, nifedipine, nicardipine, and diltiazem (Ca^{2+} blockers with high affinity for cardiac slow Ca^{2+} channels), cinnarizine, flunarizine, lidoflazine, and mioflazine (Ca^{2+} blockers with no affinity for cardiac slow Ca^{2+} channels). The non-slow-channel-blocking drugs were generally superior in protection against the imposed insults suggesting that prevention of Ca^{2+} overload is not correlated with slow channel blockade. For the latter group of drugs, other (hitherto not elucidated) mechanisms of membrane-drug interactions seem to be responsible for the preservation of Ca^{2+} homeostasis during the induction of pathological Ca^{2+} influx.

REFERENCES

1. DE HAAN, R. L. & R. HIRAKOW. 1972. Synchronization of pulsation rates in cardiac myocytes. Exp. Cell. Res **70:** 214–220.
2. KASTEN, F. H. 1972. Rat myocardial cells in vitro: mitosis and differentiated properties. In vitro **8:** 128–150.
3. SPERELAKIS, N. 1978. Cultured heart cell reaggregated model for studying cardiac toxicology. Environ. Health Perspect. **26:** 243–267.
4. MARK, G. E., J. D. MACKNEY & F. F. STRASSER. 1967. Morphology and contractile behavior of cultured heart cells, and their response to various oxygen concentrations. *In* Factors Influencing Myocardial Contractility. R. D. Tanz, F. Kavaler & J. Roberts, Eds.: 301. Academic Press, Inc. New York, N.Y.
5. KURAMITSU, H. & I. HARARY. 1964. Studies in vitro on single beating rat heart cells. III. Enzyme changes and loss of specific function in culture. Biochem. Biophys. Acta **86:** 65–73.
6. SANFORD, P. D. & J. L. DRUMMOND. 1979. Surface morphology and cell size measurement of isolated rat cardiac myocytes. J. Mol. Cell. Cardiol. **11:** 423–433.
7. CUTILLETTA, A. F., M. C. AUMOUNT, A. C. NAG & R. ZAK. 1977. Separation of muscle and non muscle cells from adult rat myocardium: an application to the study of RNA polymerase. J. Mol. Cell. Cardiol. **9:** 399–407.
8. VAHOUNY, G., R. WEI, R. STARKWEATHER & C. DAVIS. 1970. Preparation of beating heart cells from adult rats. Science **167:** 1616–1618.
9. POWEL, T. & V. W. TWIST. 1976. A rapid technique for the isolation and purification of adult cardiac muscle cells having respiratory control and tolerance to calcium. Biochem. Biophys. **72:** 327–333.
10. JACOBSON, S. L. 1977. Culture of spontaneously contracting myocardial cells from adult rats. Cell Struct. Funct. **2:** 1–9.
11. NAG, A. C. & M. CHENG. 1981. Adult mammalian cardiac muscle cells in culture. Tissue Cell **13:** 515–523.
12. PIPER, H. M., I. PROBST, P. SCHWARTZ, J. F. HÜTTER & P. G. SPIECKERMAN. 1982. Culturing of calcium stable adult cardiac myocytes. J. Mol. Cell. Cardiol. **14:** 397–412.
13. VER DONCK, L., P. J. PAUWELS, G. VANDEPLASSCHE & M. BORGERS. 1986. Isolated rat cardiac myocytes as an experimental model to study calcium overload: the effect of calcium-entry blockers. Life Sci. **38:** 765–772.
14. BORGERS, M., F. DE CLERCK, J. VAN REEMPTS, R. XHONNEUX & J. VAN NUETEN. 1984. Selective blockade of cellular Ca^{2+} overload by flunarizine. Int. Angiol. **3:** 25–31.
15. VANHOUTTE, P. M. & J. M. VAN NUETEN. 1983. Lidoflazine. *In* New Drugs Annual: Cardiovascular Drugs. A. Scriabine. Ed.: 203–226. Raven Press, New York, N.Y.
16. VAN NUETEN, J. M. 1982. Selectivity of calcium entry blockers. *In* Calcium Modulators. T.

Godfraind, A. Albertini & R. Paoletti, Eds.: 119–208. Elsevier Biomedical Press. Amsterdam, Holland.

17. BORGERS, M. & H. M. PIPER. 1986. Calcium-shifts in anoxic cardiac myocytes. A cytochemical study. J. Mol. Cell. Cardiol. **18:** 439–448.
18. BORGERS, M., F. THONÉ & L. VER DONCK. 1985. Sarcolemma-bound calcium. Its importance for cell viability. Basic Res. Cardiol. **80**(Suppl. 1): 31–36.
19. BORGERS, M. & H. VAN BELLE. 1985. Intracellular Ca^{2+} shifts during the Ca^{2+} paradox. Basic Res. Cardiol. **80**(Suppl. 2): 25–30.
20. VAHOUNY, G., A. TAMBOLI, E. M. ALBERT, W. B WEGLECKI & A. M. SPANIER. 1985. Structural and functional characteristics of cardiac myocytes. Basic Res. Cardiol. **80**(Suppl. 1): 45–49.
21. BORGERS, M., F. THONÉ, A. VERHEYEN & H. E. D. J. TER KEURS. 1984. Localization of calcium in skeletal and cardiac muscle. Histochem. J. **16:** 295–309.
22. BOSKEY, A. L. & A. S. POSNER. 1982. Optimal conditions for Ca^{2+}-acidic-phospholipid-PO_4 formation. Calcif. Tissue Int. **34;** S1–S7.
23. LANGER, G. A. 1984. Calcium at the sarcolemma. J. Mol. Cell. Cardiol. **16:** 147–153.
24. LANGER, G. A. 1986. Role of sarcolemma bound calcium in regulation of myocardial contractile force. J. Am. Coll. Cardiol. **8:** 65A–68A.
25. KOCH, R. & H. M. PIPER. 1985. Optodektor-System zum Erfassen von Kontraktionen einzelner Herzmuskelzellen. Biomed. Tech. **30:** 7–8.
26. BARRIT, G. & M. LEE. 1985. Effects of electrical stimulation and an intracellular calcium chelator on calcium movement in suspension of isolated myocardial muscle cells. Cardiovasc. Res. **19:** 370–377.
27. JONKMAN, F. A. M., H. W. G. M. BODDEKE & P. A. VAN ZWIETEN. 1986. Protective activity of calcium entry blockers against ouabain intoxication in anesthetized guinea pigs. J. Cardiovasc. Pharmacol. **8:** 1009–1018.
28. NAKAYAMA, K., J. KURIHARA, Y. MIYAJIMA, K. ISHII & H. KATO. 1985. Calcium antagonistic properties of nicardipine, a dihydropyridine derivative assessed in isolated cerebral arteries and cardiac muscle. Arzneim.-Forsch./Drug. Res. **35:** 687–693.
29. CHEUNG, J. Y., A. LEAF & J. BONVENTRE. 1984. Mechanism of protection by verapamil and nifedipine from anoxic injury in isolated cardiac myocytes. Am. J. Physiol. **246:** C323–C329.
30. HONERJAGER, P. 1982. Cardioactive substances that prolong the open state of sodium channels. Rev. Physiol. Biochem. Pharmacol. **92:** 2–74.
31. LEE, K. S. & W. KLAUS. 1971. The subcellular basis for the mechanism of inotropic action of cardiac glycosides. Pharmacol. Rev. **23:** 193–261.
32. PILATI, C. E. & N. F. PARADISE. 1984. Ouabain induced mechanical toxicity: aberrations in left ventricular function, Ca^{2+} concentration and ultrastructure. Proc. Soc. Exp. Biol. Med. **175:** 342–350.
33. DEL MAESTRO, R. F. 1980. An approach to free radicals in medicine and biology. Acta. Physiol. Scand. **492**(Suppl.): 153–168.
34. ADKINSON, D., M. E. HÖLLWARTH, J. N. BENOIT, D. A. PARKS, J. M. MCCORD & D. N. GRANGER. 1986. Role of free radicals in ischemia-reperfusion injury to the liver. Acta Physiol. Scand. **548:** 101–108.
35. GRANGER, D. N., M. E. HÖLLWARTH & D. A. PARKS. 1986. Ischemia-reperfusion injury: role of oxygen derived free radicals. Acta Physiol. Scand. **548:** 47–63.
36. HESS, M. C., N. H. MANSON & E. OKABE. 1982. Involvement of free radicals in the pathophysiology of ischemic heart disease. Can. J. Physiol. Pharmacol. **60:** 1382–1389.
37. GAUDUEL, Y. & M. A. DUVELLEROY. 1984. Role of oxygen radicals in cardiac tissue due to reoxygenation. J. Mol. Cell. Cardiol. **16:** 459–470.
38. MCCORD, J. M. 1985. Oxygen derived free radicals in postischemic tissue injury. N. Engl. J. Med. **312:** 159–164.
39. BURTON, K. P., J. M. MCCORD & G. GHAI. 1984. Myocardial alterations due to free radical generation. Am. J. Physiol. **246;** H776–H783.
40. WATSON, B. D., W. D. DIETRICH, R. BUSTO, M. S. WACHTEL & M. D. GINSBERG. 1985. Induction of reproducible brain infarction by photochemically initiated thrombosis. Ann. Neurol. **17:** 497–504.

41. FOOTE, C. S. 1976. Photosensitisized oxidation and singlet oxygen: consequences in biological systems. *In* Free Radicals in Biology. W. A. Pryor, Ed. **2:** 85–134. Academic Press, Inc. New York, N.Y.
42. RAWLS, H. R. & P. J. VAN SANTEN. 1970. A possible role for singlet oxygen in the initiation of fatty acid autoxidation. J. Am. Oil Chem. Soc. **47;** 121–125.
43. BURT, J. M., C. J. DUENAS & G. A. LANGER. 1983. Influence of polymyxin B, a probe for anionic phospholipids on calcium binding and calcium and potassium fluxes of cultured cardiac cells. Circ. Res. **53:** 679–687.
44. CORR, P. B., R. W. GROSS & B. E. SOBEL. 1984. Amphipathic metabolites and membrane dysfunction in ischemic myocardium. Circ. Res. **55:** 140–154.
45. KNABB, M. T., J. E. SAFFITZ, P. B. CORR & B. E. SOBEL. 1986. The dependence of electrophysiological derangements on accumulation of endogenous long-chain acylcarnitine in hypoxic neonatal rat myocytes. Circ. Res. **58:** 230–240.
46. GANOTE, C. E., P. A. GRINWALD & W. G. NAYLER. 1984. 2,4-Dinitrophenol-(DNP)-induced injury in calcium-free hearts. J. Mol. Cell. Cardiol. **16:** 547–557.
47. FRANK, J. S., A. J. BRADY, S. FARNSWORTH & G. MOTTINO. 1986. Ultrastructure and function of isolated myocytes after calcium depletion and repletion. Am. J. Physiol. **250:** H265–H275.
48. PIPER, H. M., J. F. HÜTTER & P. G. SPIECKERMANN. 1984. Relation between enzyme release and metabolic changes in reversible anoxic injury of myocardial cells. Life Sci. **35:** 127–134.
49. PIPER, H. M., P. SCHWARTZ, J. F. HÜTTER & P. G. SPIECKERMANN. 1984. Energy metabolism and enzyme release of cultured adult rat heart muscle cells during anoxia. J. Mol. Cell. Cardiol. **16:** 995–1007.
50. GANOTE, C. E. 1984. Parallel temperature dependence of contracture associated enzyme release due to anoxia, 2,4-dinitrophenol, or caffeine and the Ca^{2+}-paradox. Am. J. Pathol. **116:** 94–106.
51. COBBOLD, P. H. & P. K. BOURNE. 1984. Aequorin measurements of free calcium in single heart cells. Nature **312:** 444–446.
52. HAWORTH, R. A., D. R. HUNTHER & H. A. BERKOFF. 1981. Contracture in isolated adult rat heart cells. Role of Ca^{2+}, ATP, and compartmentation. Circ. Res. **49:** 1119–1128.
53. MCCLELLAN, G., A. WEISBERG & S. WINEGRAD. 1983. Energy transport from mitochondria to myofibril by a creatin phosphate shuttle in cardiac cells. Am. J. Physiol. **245:** C423–C427.
54. BREMEL, R. D. & A. WEBER. 1972. Cooperation within actin filament in vertebrate skeletal muscle. Nature New Biol. **238:** 97–101.
55. JENNINGS, R. B. & K. A. REIMER. 1981. Lethal myocardial ischemic injury. Am. J. Cardiol. **102:** 241–255.
56. NAYLER, W., P. A. POOLE-WILSON & A. WILLIAMS. 1979. Hypoxia and calcium. J. Mol. Cell. Cardiol. **11:** 683–706.
57. SHINE, K. I. 1981. Ionic events in ischemia and anoxia. Am. J. Pathol. **102:** 256–261.
58. JACQUES, Y., C. FRELIN, P. VIGNE, G. ROMEY, M. PARJARI & M. LAZDUNSKI. 1981. Neurotoxins specific for the sodium channel stimulate calcium entry into neuroblastoma cells. Biochemistry **20:** 6219–6225.
59. SMITH, H. J. 1982. The need to redefine membrane stabilizing activity of beta-adrenergic receptor antagonists. J. Mol. Cell. Cardiol. **14:** 495–500.
60. BAKER, J. E. & D. J. HEARSE. 1983. Slow calcium channel blockers and the calcium paradox: comparative studies in the rat with seven drugs. J. Mol. Cell. Cardiol. **15:** 475–485.
61. KATZ, A. M. & F. C. MESSINEO. 1981. Lipid-membrane interactions and the pathogenesis of ischemic damage in the myocardium. Circ. Res. **48:** 1–16.
62. FLAMENG, W., R. XHONNEUX, H. VAN BELLE, M. BORGERS, A. VAN DE WATER, L. WOUTERS, J. WIJNANTS, F. THONÉ, P. VAN DAELE & P. A. J. JANSSEN. 1984. Cardioprotective effects of mioflazine during 1 h normothermic global ischemia in the canine heart. Cardiovasc. Res. **18:** 528–537.
63. BORGERS, M. 1983. The role of the sarcolemma-glycocalyx complex in myocardial cell function. *In* Factors Influencing the Course of Myocardial Ischemia. M. E. DeBakey & A. M. Gotto, Eds.: 55–65. Elsevier Science Publ. B.V. Amsterdam, Holland.

64. LIU, G.-S., M. BORGERS, R. XHONNEUX, P. VAN OVERLOOP, F. THONÉ, L. WOUTERS & L. LEIJSSEN. 1986. Evaluation of protective effects of lidoflazine and mioflazine in cardiac ischemia. Drug Dev. Res. **8:** 407–416.

65. VANDEPLASSCHE, G. & M. BORGERS. 1987. Ultrastructural characteristics of stunned myocardium. J. Mol. Cell. Cardiol. **19** (Suppl. III): 101.

66. PIPER, H. M. & M. BORGERS. 1986. Effect of lidoflazine on intracellular Ca^{2+}-localization in cardiac myocytes during anoxia. J. Mol. Cell. Cardiol. **18**(Suppl.): 217.

67. DANIEL, W. W. 1978. Applied Nonparametric Statistics. Houghton Mifflin Cir. Boston, Mass. (Monograph.)

68. BORGERS, M. 1985. Morphological assessment of tissue protection. *In* Calcium-Entry Blockers and Tissue Protection. T. Godfraind, P. M. Vanhoutte, S. Govoni & R. Paoletti, Eds.: 173–181. Raven Press. New York, N.Y.

69. BORGERS, M. & W. FLAMENG. 1984. Basic and clinical aspects of myocardial protection by calcium entry blockers. *In* Calcium-Entry Blockers in Cardiovascular and Cerebral Dysfunctions. T. Godfraind, A. Herman & D. Wellens, Eds.: 145–153. M. Nijhoff Publ. Amsterdam, Holland.

70. BOURDILLON, P. D. V. & P. A. POOLE-WILSON. 1982. The effects of verapamil, quiescence and cardioplegia on calcium exchange and mechanical function in ischemic rabbit myocardium. Circ. Res. **50:** 360–368.

71. POOLE-WILSON, P. A., D. P. HARDING, P. D. V. BOURDILLON & M. A. TONES. 1984. Calcium out of control. J. Mol. Cell. Cardiol. **16:** 175–187.

Metabolism of Arachidonic Acid

S. MONCADA AND E. A. HIGGS

The Wellcome Research Laboratories
Langley Court
Beckenham, Kent BR3 3BS, United Kingdom

INTRODUCTION

The 20-carbon fatty acid arachidonic acid (AA) is the most common fatty acid present in the phospholipids of mammalian cells and can be obtained by desaturation and chain elongation of dietary linoleic acid or directly from the diet. The metabolic products of 20-carbon fatty acids are known collectively as eicosanoids. They are made by all tissues except red blood cells and are released very easily by perturbation of cell membranes induced mechanically or by chemicals. The two main routes of metabolism of arachidonic acid are (a) the cyclooxygenase enzyme, which gives rise, via unstable endoperoxides, to the stable prostaglandins (PGs) D_2, E_2, and $F_{2\alpha}$ as well as the unstable products prostacyclin (PGI_2) and thromboxane A_2 (TXA_2) (FIGURE 1) and (b) the lipoxygenase enzymes, which give rise to hydroperoxy acids and leukotrienes (LTs) (FIGURE 2).

These arachidonic acid metabolites have potent and sometimes opposing activities in many biological systems, including platelet function, vascular smooth muscle activity, bronchopulmonary function, and gastrointestinal integrity.

CYCLOOXYGENASE METABOLISM OF ARACHIDONIC ACID

Arachidonic acid is metabolized by cyclooxygenase, which is ubiquitous in mammalian tissues, to form a number of products including TXA_2, prostacyclin, and the stable PGs E_2, D_2, and $F_{2\alpha}$ (see FIGURE 1). In 1974, Hamberg and Samuelsson isolated two cyclic endoperoxides, formed as intermediates in the transformation of AA to prostaglandins, thus proving that prostaglandin synthesis involved two stages, cyclooxygenation followed by isomerization or reductive cleavage of the endoperoxides.[1] The cyclic endoperoxides possess intrinsic biological activity as vasodilators and aggregators of platelets but they are unstable and are normally rapidly converted to other products.

Different tissues give rise to different arachidonate metabolites. The main cyclooxygenase product of AA in vascular tissue is prostacyclin,[2] which is a potent vasodilator and inhibitor of platelet aggregation. It is chemically unstable with a half-life of 2–3 minutes, breaking down to 6-oxo-$PGF_{1\alpha}$. The ability of the large vessel to synthesize prostacyclin is greatest at the intimal surface and progressively decreases towards the adventitia. Production of prostacyclin by cultured cells from vessel walls also shows that endothelial cells are the most active producers of prostacyclin (for review, see Reference 3).

Prostacyclin is a very potent endogenous inhibitor of platelet aggregation. This effect is short lasting *in vivo,* disappearing within 30 minutes of stopping an intravenous administration. Prostacyclin disperses platelet clumps *in vitro,* in various animal models of thrombus formation, and in the circulation of man. Prostacyclin inhibits platelet aggregation by stimulating adenylate cyclase, leading to an increase in cAMP levels in the platelets. In this respect it is much more potent than either PGE_1 or PGD_2 and its effect is longer lasting. Prostacyclin enhances Ca^{2+} sequestration in platelet membranes. Moreover, inhibitory effects on platelet phospholipase and platelet cyclooxygenase have been described (for references, see Reference 3). All these effects are related to its ability to increase cAMP in platelets. By inhibiting several steps in the activation of the AA metabolic cascade, prostacyclin exerts an overall control of platelet aggregability.

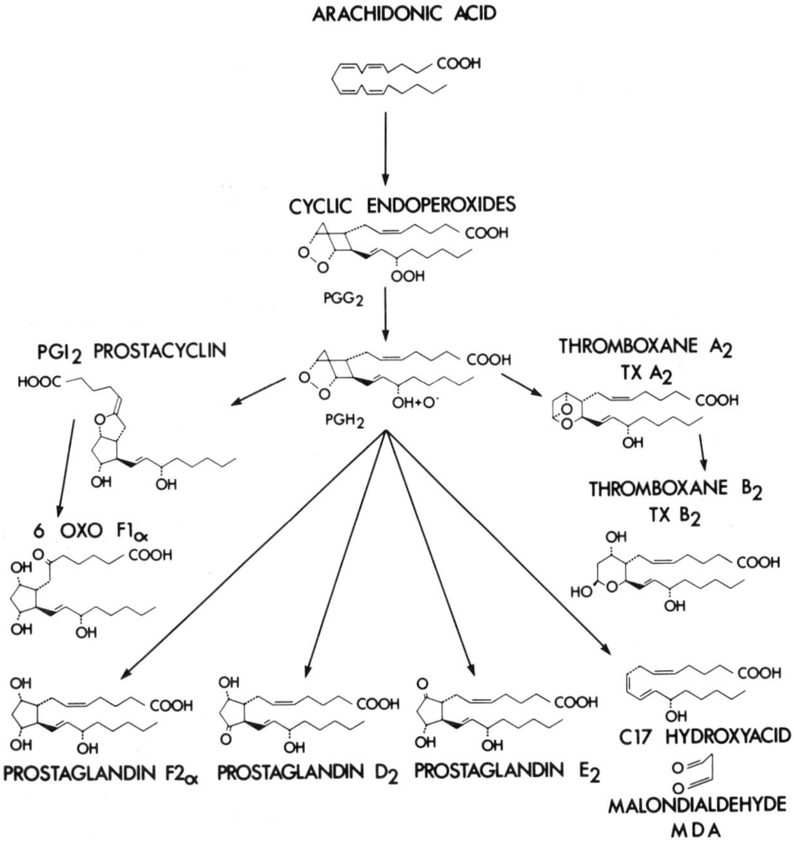

FIGURE 1. Cyclooxygenase pathway of arachidonic acid metabolism.

Prostacyclin is a strong hypotensive agent through vasodilation of all vascular beds studied, including the pulmonary and cerebral circulation.[4] Its other biological actions include enhancement of cholesterol ester metabolism and of fibrinolytic activity, as well as cytoprotective activity which has been demonstrated in platelets, in the gut, and in myocardial tissue (for review, see Reference 5). Many other tissues, apart from blood vessels, are now known to be capable of generating prostacyclin or its degradation product 6-oxo-$PGF_{1\alpha}$. The organs include lung, stomach, intestine, heart, kidney,

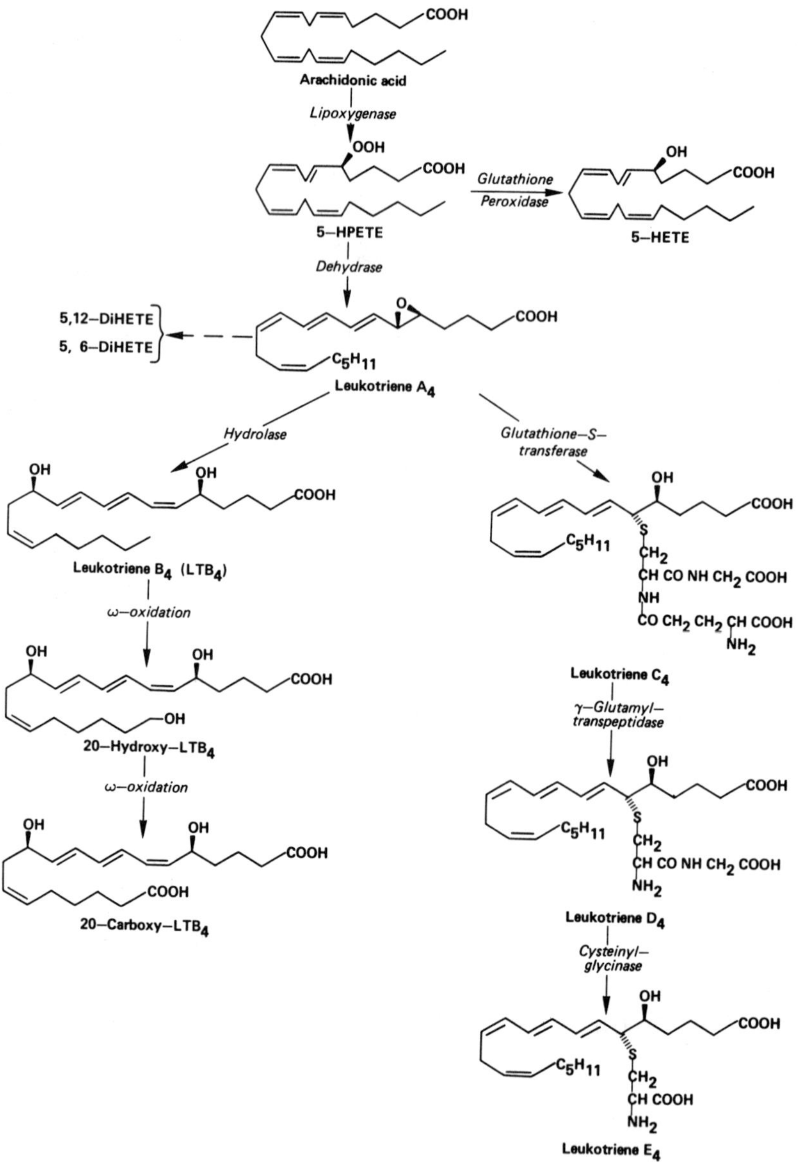

FIGURE 2. Lipoxygenase pathway of arachidonic acid metabolism.

uterus, cerebral cortex, eye, and serosal membranes such as pericardium, pleura, and peritoneum (for references, see Reference 6).

Platelets do not produce prostacyclin, and by far the major cyclooxygenase product of AA in platelets is TXA_2.[7] TXA_2 aggregates platelets and potently constricts vascular and airway smooth muscle (for review, see Reference 8). TXA_2, which breaks down to TXB_2, has a chemical half-life at body pH and temperature of 30 seconds, although the presence of albumin appears to stabilize the molecule. The reduction in cAMP levels brought about by many stimulators of platelet aggregation can be inhibited by thromboxane synthase inhibitors, thus suggesting that TXA_2 formation itself can decrease platelet cAMP and lead to aggregation.

The enzyme that synthesizes TXA_2 from PG endoperoxides was first localized in the high-speed particulate fraction of human and horse blood platelets. The enzyme has been solubilized and separated from the cyclooxygenase, and detailed studies of human and bovine platelet thromboxane synthase have been published. Separation of platelet membrane fractions suggests that the biosynthesis of thromboxane from AA is associated with intracellular membrane components of the dense tubular system (for references, see Reference 9).

Synthesis of TXA_2 has been demonstrated in certain vascular tissues, including rabbit pulmonary arteries, dog mesenteric arteries, and bovine cerebral arteries as well as human umbilical arteries and veins and saphenous veins (for references, see Reference 9). Porcine, bovine, and human aortic endothelial cells in culture are also capable of generating TXA_2, both from exogenous and endogenously released substrate. The role of TXA_2 generated by the vasculature is not clear, but its production may be particularly significant in certain pathological situations where prostacyclin production is impaired. Indeed, mesenteric arteries from diabetic dogs generate more TXA_2 than do vessels from normal control dogs.[10] Other cells and tissues in which TXA_2 synthesis has been detected include polymorphonuclear leukocytes (PMNs), macrophages, monocytes, fibroblasts, lungs, kidney, spleen, gastric mucosa, and inflammatory granuloma.[11] TXA_2 concentrations in inflammatory exudates increase in parallel with the accumulation of leukocytes in the early stages of inflammation, but the role of TXA_2 in inflammation remains to be defined.

The stable prostaglandins PGE_2, PGD_2, and $PGF_{2\alpha}$ are also produced by vascular tissue, by platelets, and by most other cells and tissues. Their numerous and diverse effects include the relaxation or contraction of many smooth muscles such as vascular, bronchial, tracheal, uterine, and gastrointestinal smooth muscle. Much evidence has now accumulated to indicate that PGE_2 plays a major role in the development of inflammatory erythema, edema and pain (for review, see Reference 12).

LIPOXYGENASE METABOLISM OF ARACHIDONIC ACID

In addition to the cyclooxygenase pathway, polyunsaturated fatty acids such as AA can be oxidized, via lipoxygenase enzymes, to form the corresponding hydroperoxides (see FIGURE 2). The first such enzyme was originally found in lung and platelets[13,14] and is responsible for the formation of lipid peroxides such as 12-hydroperoxyeicosatetraenoic acid (12-HPETE) and its degradation product 12-hydroxyeicosatetraenoic acid (12-HETE), which is a potent chemotactic agent for PMNs. Subsequently, a number of enzymes have been discovered that peroxidize AA in different positions. The most important of these is a 5-lipoxygenase, which occurs in PMNs.[15] The action of this enzyme results in the formation of a complex group of compounds known collectively as leukotrienes.

The first step of the 5-lipoxygenase pathway is the formation of 5-HPETE: this is converted either to the related monohydroxyeicosatetraenoic acid (5-HETE) or to a 5,6 epoxide, known as leukotriene A_4 (LTA_4). Leukotriene A_4 may itself be transformed either to 5,12-dihydroxyeicosatetraenoic acid, known as leukotriene B_4 (LTB_4), or to leukotriene C_4 (LTC_4); the latter is a glutathionyl derivative formed by the action of a glutathione-*S*-transferase. Leukotriene D_4 (LTD_4) is synthesized by the removal of glutamic acid from LTC_4, and LTE_4 results from the subsequent cleavage of glycine. The final step of these transformations produces LTF_4 by the reincorporation of γ-glutamic acid into the molecule to form a γ-glutamyl, cysteinyl derivative (see References 16 and 17).

Of the leukotrienes, LTB_4 is one of the most potent naturally occurring inducers of neutrophil chemotaxis both *in vitro* and *in vivo*. LTB_4 also induces leukocyte aggregation and release of lysosomal enzymes and is released during the inflammatory process in animals and man. LTB_4 promotes adherence of PMNs to endothelial cells by an effect on the endothelial cells, suggesting a physiological role for LTB_4 in PMN margination. LTB_4 also possesses potent calcium ionophore activity. For reviews of the pharmacology of leukotrienes see References 18–20.

The bronchoconstrictor mediator slow-reacting substance of anaphylaxis (SRS-A), discovered more than 40 years ago, is now known to be a mixture of LTC_4, LTD_4, and LTE_4. There is evidence to suggest that lipoxygenase activity is involved both in the generation of anaphylactic mediators and in the sensitization of smooth muscle to their contractile actions.[21,22]

The presence of a 5-lipoxygenase system and the production of leukotrienelike material have been demonstrated in vascular tissue. Leukotrienes C_4 and D_4 are powerful vasoconstrictors in the coronary and other vascular beds in several species, as well as in the microvasculature (for review, see Reference 23). It is interesting that the production of lipoxygenase products is greatest in the adventitia and decreases towards the intima, following a reverse pattern of production to that of prostacyclin (Piper, 1985, personal communication). The interaction between products of the two eicosanoid pathways in the vessel wall has yet to be investigated; however, it is possible that generation *in vivo* of lipoxygenase products in the vascular wall may contribute to pathological changes in blood vessel tone. Indeed, lipoxygenase products, such as 15-HPETE, are selective inhibitors of prostacyclin formation.[24]

An additional series of AA products in human neutrophils has recently been described.[25] These compounds contain conjugated tetraene structures, and, since they appear to arise from the interactions of multiple distinct lipoxygenase pathways, they have been given the name lipoxins. One of the series, lipoxin A, has been shown to be a potent releaser of lysosomal enzymes from human neutrophils. This action is accompanied by O_2^- generation, but, unlike LTB_4, lipoxin A does not aggregate the neutrophils.[26]

INHIBITORS OF ARACHIDONIC ACID METABOLISM

Aspirinlike Drugs

In 1971, Vane, using cell-free homogenates of lung tissue, showed that aspirin, sodium salicylate, or indomethacin caused a dose-dependent reduction in prostaglandin synthesis and proposed that this was the biochemical basis for the actions of aspirinlike drugs.[27] These drugs inhibit the cyclooxygenase step by preventing the abstraction of hydrogen from C-13 and, therefore, blocking peroxidation at C-11 or C-15. This action is highly specific, for similar abstraction and peroxidation reactions by lipoxygenases at other points in the the fatty acid molecule are not inhibited, so they do not prevent the formation of leukotrienes. Furthermore, cyclooxygenase inhibitors do not prevent the generation of prostaglandins from cyclic endoperoxides. The therapeutic efficacy of aspirinlike antiinflammatory drugs largely parallels their ability to inhibit cyclooxygenase.[12]

A consequence of the discovery of prostacyclin in 1976 has been the need to reassess the use of aspirin as an antithrombotic agent. Because aspirin prevents the production of the endoperoxide intermediates from which all the cyclooxygenase products of AA are formed, it can prevent not only production of TXA_2 in platelets but also production of prostacyclin in vascular tissue. Several important considerations have emerged in relation to aspirin. First, inhibition of the vascular cyclooxygenase—unlike the platelet cyclooxygenase which is inhibited by aspirin for the entire lifespan of the platelet—persists for a much shorter period because of the generation of a new enzyme. Second, the platelet cyclooxygenase appears to be more sensitive *in vitro* and *in vivo* than the vascular cyclooxygenase to the inhibitory action of aspirin.[28] Third, and most recently, studies using a deuterated aspirin analogue have shown that platelets passing through the gut capillaries while an oral dose of aspirin is undergoing presystemic hydrolysis can be exposed to higher concentrations of aspirin than platelets present in the peripheral circulation.[29] Thus, serum thromboxane levels are significantly reduced by orally administered aspirin prior to the drug's appearance in the systemic circulation where it can inhibit prostacyclin synthesis by systemic vascular endothelium.

During the past few years attempts have been made to titrate aspirin dosage down to find one that will achieve inhibition of TXA_2 formation in man without affecting prostacyclin production. This has been done by using doses as low as 20 mg/day, by "slow-release" administration of very low doses, or by using aspirin in combination with dipyridamole. Recent reports suggest that this may be difficult to achieve in practice, although the hypothesis is still being tested.[30–32] The problem with aspirin as a potential antithrombotic agent, however, lies not in the fact that the ideal regimen has not been found but in the fact that platelet aggregation is a complex mechanism in which several pathways are involved, only one of them depending on the release of TXA_2. Since we do not know which of the pathways is involved in platelet aggregation in the different pathophysiological entities that we aim to prevent, then the use of aspirin as a comprehensive antithrombotic agent is not justified. However, it is important to stress that, alongside many negative reports, aspirin has been shown in well-designed clinical trials to be effective in reducing the complications associated with artifical heart valves,[33,34] preventing strokes and death in patients with transient ischemic attacks,[35,36] and reducing the incidence of myocardial infarction and cardiac death in patients with unstable angina.[37]

Thromboxane Synthase Inhibitors

Theoretically, a selective inhibitor of thromboxane synthase should prove to be a superior antithrombotic agent to aspirin as it would allow continued prostacyclin formation by vessel walls or other cells either from their own endoperoxides or from those released from platelets. However, in some individuals, termed "nonresponders," platelet aggregation in response to AA is unaffected even after total inhibition of TXA_2 synthesis.[38] This may be because the net balance of AA products after thromboxane synthase inhibition varies between individuals, so that in nonresponders the effects of the proaggregatory metabolites (cyclic endoperoxides, any residual TXA_2, and possibly PGE_2) predominate over those of the antiaggregatory metabolites, prostacyclin and PGD_2.

The major types of selective thromboxane synthase inhibitor that have now been developed comprise imidazole and pyridine derivatives and structural analogues of endoperoxides and TXA_2. Selective inhibition of thromboxane synthesis has been demonstrated *in vitro* and *in vivo*. Thromboxane synthase inhibitors have been tested clinically in patients with Raynaud's syndrome[39] and with peripheral vascular disease.[40] Some benefical effects were observed, but the results were not conclusive. OKY-1581 was effective in reducing the severity of myocardial infarction in 11 patients,[41] and dazmegrel (UK 38485) has been reported to inhibit microalbuminuria in a small group of diabetic patients.[42]

The combination of a thromboxane synthase inhibitor with a TXA_2 antagonist that will also block endoperoxide activity may prove to be clinically useful.[43,44] An ideal compound should inhibit thromboxane formation and prevent the proaggregatory effects of the endoperoxides without affecting cyclooxygenase, prostacyclin synthase, and PGD_2-isomerase; nor should it antagonize the antiaggregatory effects of prostacyclin or PGD_2.

Lipoxygenase Inhibitors

Because of the increasing evidence for the involvement of leukotrienes in inflammatory responses, such as bronchoconstriction, chemotaxis, vascular permeability, and the sensitization of smooth muscle to the contractile actions of anaphylactic mediators, inhibitors of the lipoxygenase enzymes would be expected to be antiinflammatory agents.

Various acetylenic analogues of AA inhibit different lipoxygenases *in vitro,* but this type of compound is not active *in vivo.* Several compounds inhibit various lipoxygenases *in vitro.* These include nordihydroguaiaretic acid (NDGA), benoxaprofen, baicalein, esculetin, some flavonoids, and caffeic acid (for references, see Reference 45). There are, however, relatively few reports of lipoxygenase inhibitors with *in vivo* activity. In fact benoxaprofen, while inhibiting 5-lipoxygenase in isolated leukocytes,[46] has no effect on LTB_4 generation in acute experimental inflammation.[47]

The evidence to support the hypothesis that lipoxygenase inhibitors may have important therapeutic effects is confined, at present, to experiments with dual inhibitors of cyclooxygenase and lipoxygenase. The most studied of these is the pyrazoline BW755C.[12] BW755C and its analogue phenidone inhibit both pathways of AA metabolism in isolated platelets, lungs, and leukocytes (for reviews, see References 12 and 45).

In vivo BW755C, in common with dexamethasone, causes dose-dependent reductions in the concentrations of PGE_2 and LTB_4 in inflammatory exudates whereas aspirin, indomethacin, and flurbiprofen selectively reduce PGE_2.[48] Unlike indomethacin and the salicylates, BW755C does not enhance leukocyte migration at low doses but reduces edema, PGE_2 concentrations, and leukocyte numbers at the same dose.[49,50] The experimental compounds timegadine[51] and CBS-1108[52] also act as dual inhibitors *in vitro* and have a similar profile of antiinflammatory activity to BW755C. It is not known, however, if the activity of these compounds is associated with inhibition of LTB_4 *in vivo.*

The chemotactic-factor-induced increase in permeability of leukocyte membranes to calcium is prevented by NDGA,[53] and this may be because a lipoxygenase product is necessary for calcium influx. NDGA and BW755C also inhibit calcium-dependent responses of isolated smooth muscle,[54,55] and it is possible that effects on calcium movement may contribute to the inhibition of leukocyte migration by BW755C. This suggestion is supported by the observations that verapamil, a calcium channel blocker, inhibits chemotaxis *in vitro*[56] and leukocyte accumulation *in vivo.*[57] On the other hand, the concentrations of BW755C that are required to block calcium responses are high and the underlying mechanism with these doses may be unrelated to lipoxygenase inhibition. Furthermore, calcium-dependent degranulation of human PMNs is not dependent on the 5-lipoxygenation of AA.[58]

It is now apparent that leukocyte migration plays a key role in the development of a number of pathological conditions, such as rheumatoid arthritis, myocardial infarction, different forms of lung damage, and vascular disease. Thus, control of leukocyte accumulation may be an important therapeutic approach to limiting tissue damage. Inhibition of the lipoxygenase enzymes and hence of the production of some very potent agents chemotactic for leukocytes is one way in which such control may be achieved.

CONCLUSION

Arachidonic acid metabolites are active in a number of biological systems, thus inhibitors of their formation are potentially useful therapeutic agents. At present the aspirinlike drugs, which inhibit the cyclooxygenase pathway of AA metabolism, are used therapeutically as antiinflammatory agents and in the treatment of some vascular diseases. It is likely that the development of inhibitors of thromboxane synthase and of lipoxygenase inhibitors with activity *in vivo* will contribute significantly to the treatment available for a number of thrombotic disorders and inflammatory diseases.

REFERENCES

1. HAMBERG, M. & B. SAMUELSSON. 1974. Proc. Nat. Acad. Sci. USA **71:** 3400–3404.
2. MONCADA, S., R. GRYGLEWSKI, S. BUNTING & J. R. VANE. 1976. Nature **263:** 663–665.
3. MONCADA, S. 1982. Br. J. Pharmacol. **76:** 3–31.
4. DUSTING, G. J., K. M. MULLANE & S. MONCADA. 1986. Prostacyclin and vascular smooth muscle. *In* Handbook of Hypertension. A. Zanchetti & R. C. Tarazi, Eds. **7:** 408–426. Elsevier Science Publishers BV. Amsterdam, Holland.
5. MONCADA, S. 1985. Prostacyclin—discovery and biological importance. *In* Prostaglandins: Research and Clinical Update. G. L. Longenecker & S. W. Schaffer, Eds.: 1–39. Alpha Editions. Minneapolis, Minn.
6. DUSTING, G. J., S. MONCADA & J. R. VANE. 1982. Prostacyclin: its biosynthesis, actions and clinical potential. *In* Prostaglandins and the Cardiovascular System. J. A. Oates, Ed.: 59–106. Raven Press. New York, N. Y.
7. HAMBERG, M., J. SVENSSON & B. SAMUELSSON. 1975. Proc. Nat. Acad. Sci. USA **72:** 2994–2998.
8. WHITTLE, B. J. R. & S. MONCADA. 1983. Br. Med. Bull. **39:** 232–238.
9. BUNTING, S., S. MONCADA & J. R. VANE. 1983. Br. Med. Bull. **39:** 271–276.
10. STERIN-BORDA, L., A. M. FRANCHI, E. S. BORDA, E. DEL CASTILLO, M. F. GIMENO & A. L. GIMENO. 1984. Eur. J. Pharmacol. **103:** 211–221.
11. MONCADA, S. & J. R. VANE. 1979. Pharmacol. Rev. **30:** 293–331.
12. HIGGS, G. A., S. MONCADA & J. R. VANE. 1984. Ann. Clin. Res. **16:** 287–299.
13. HAMBERG, M., J. SVENSSON, T. WAKABAYASHI & B. SAMUELSSON. 1974. Proc. Nat. Acad. Sci. USA **71:** 345–349.
14. NUGTEREN, D. H. 1975. Biochim. Biophys. Acta **380:** 299–307.
15. BORGEAT, P., M. HAMBERG & B. SAMUELSSON. 1976. J. Biol. Chem. **251:** 7816–7820.
16. SAMUELSSON, B. 1983. Science **220:** 568–575.
17. HAMMARSTROM, S. 1983. Annu. Rev. Biochem. **52:** 355–377.
18. BRAY, M. A. 1983. Br. Med. Bull. **39:** 249–254.
19. LEWIS, R. A. & K. F. AUSTEN. 1984. J. Clin. Invest. **73:** 889–897.
20. HIGGS, G. A. & S. MONCADA. 1985. Drugs **30:** 1–5.
21. ADCOCK, J. J. & L. G. GARLAND. 1980 Br. J. Pharmacol.**69:** 167–169.
22. PATTERSON, R., J. J. PRUZANSKY & K. E. HARRIS. 1981. J. Allergy Clin. Immunol. **61:** 444–449.
23. PIPER, P. J., A. W. B. STANTON, L. J. MCLEOD, S. A. GALTON & L. G. LETTS. 1984. *In*

Proceedings, IUPHAR 9th International Congress of Pharmacology: 63–67. Macmillan Press. London, England.
24. Moncada, S., R. J. Gryglewski, S. Bunting & J. R. Vane. 1976. Prostaglandins **12:** 715–733.
25. Serhan, C. N., M. Hamberg & B. Samuelsson. 1984. Biochem. Biophys. Res. Commun. **118:** 943–949.
26. Serhan, C. N., M. Hamberg & B. Samuelsson. 1984. Proc. Nat. Acad. Sci. USA **81:** 5335–5339
27. Vane, J. R. 1971. Nature New Biol. **231:** 232–235.
28. Burch, J. W., N. L. Baenziger, N. Stanford & P. W. Majerus. 1978. Proc. Nat. Acad. Sci. USA **75:** 5181–5184
29. Pedersen, A. K. & G. A. FitzGerald. 1984. N. Engl. J. Med. **311:** 1206–1211.
30. Patrignani, P., P. Filabozzi & C. Patrono. 1982. J. Clin. Invest. **69:** 1366–1372.
31. FitzGerald, G. A., J. A. Oates, J. Hawiger, R. L. Maas, L. J. Roberts II, J. A. Lawson & A. R. Brash. 1983. J. Clin. Invest. **71:** 676–688.
32. Weksler, B. B., K. Tack-Goldman, V. A. Subramanian & W. A. Gay. 1985. Circulation **71:** 332–340.
33. Dale, J., E. Myhre, O. Storstein, H. Stormorken & L. Efskind. 1977. Am. Heart J. **94:** 101–111.
34. Altman, R., F. Boullon, J. Rouvier, R. Raca, L. de La Fuente & R. Favaloro. 1976. J. Thorac. Cardiovasc. Surg. **72:** 127–129.
35. Fields, W. S., N. A. Lemak, R. F. Frankowski & R. J. Hardy. 1977. Stroke **8:** 301–314.
36. The Canadian Cooperative Study Group. 1978. N. Engl. J. Med. **299:** 53–59.
37. Lewis, H. D., J. W. Davis, D. G. Archibald, W. E. Steinke, T. C. Smitherman, J. E. Doherty, H. W. Schnaper, M. M. Le Winter, E. Linares, J. M. Pouget, S. C. Sabharwal, E. Chesler & H. De Mots. 1983. N. Engl. J. Med. **309:** 396–403.
38. Bertele, V., A. Falanga, M. Tomasiak, C. Chiabrando, C. Cerletti & G. De Gaetano. 1984. Blood **63:** 1460–1466.
39. Belch, J. J. F., J. Cormie, P. Newman, M. McLaren, J. Barbenel, H. Capell, P. Lieberman, C. D. Forbes & C. R. M. Prentice. 1983. Br. J. Clin. Pharmacol. **15**(Suppl. 1): 113S–116S.
40. Raftery, A. T., S. Livesey & J. Forty. 1983. Br. J. Clin. Pharmacol. 15(Suppl. 1): 119S–121S.
41. Tada, M., S. Hoshida, T. Kuzuya, M. Inoue, T. Minamino & H. Abe. 1985. Int. J. Cardiol. **8:** 301–312.
42. Barnett, A. H., K. Wakelin, B. A. Leatherdale, J. R. Britton, A. Polak, J. Bennett, M. Toop, D. Rowe & K. Dallinger. 1984. Lancet **i:** 1322–1325.
43. Gresele, P., E. Van Houtte, J. Arnout, M. Deckmyn & J. Vermylen. 1984. Thromb. Haemostas. **52:** 364.
44. FitzGerald, G. A., I. A. G. Reilly & A. K. Pedersen. 1985. Circulation **72:** 1194–1201.
45. Moncada, S. 1986. Prospects for inhibition of leukotriene biosynthesis. *In* The Leukotrienes: Their Biological Significance. P. J. Piper, Ed.: 99–107. Raven Press. New York, N. Y.
46. Harvey, J., H. Parish, P. P. K. Ho, J. R. Boot & W. Dawson. 1983. J. Pharm. Pharmacol. **35:** 44–45.
47. Salmon, J. A., G. A. Higgs, L. Tilling, S. Moncada & J. R. Vane. 1984. Lancet **i:** 848.
48. Salmon, J. A., P. M. Simmons & S. Moncada. 1983. J. Pharm. Pharmacol. **35:** 808–813.
49. Hammarstrom, S. 1977. Biochim. Biophys. Acta. **487:** 517–519.
50. Jugdutt, B. I., G. M. Hutchins, B. H. Bulkley & L. C. Becker. 1980. Am. J. Cardiol. **46:** 74–82.
51. Ahnfelt-Ronne, I. & E. Arrigoni-Martelli. 1982. Biochem. Pharmacol. **31:** 2619–2624.
52. Bertez, C., M. Miguel, C. Coquelet, D. Sincholle & C. Bonne. 1984. Biochem. Pharmacol. **33:** 1757–1762.

53. NACCACHE, P. H., H. J. SHOWELL, E. L. BECKER & R. I. SHAAFI. 1979. Biochem. Biophys. Res. Commun. **89:** 1224–1230.
54. COPP, F. C., G. A. HIGGS, S. MONCADA & K. G. MUGRIDGE. 1983. Br. J. Pharmacol. **80:** 611P.
55. RIMELE, T. J. & P. M. VANHOUTTE. 1983. J. Pharmacol. Exp. Ther. **225:** 720–728.
56. ELFERINK, J. G. R. & M. DEIERKAUF. 1984. Biochem. Pharmacol. **33:** 35–39.
57. HIGGS, G. A., K. G. MUGRIDGE & S. MONCADA. 1985. Arachidonic acid metabolism and calcium flux. *In* Calcium Entry Blockers and Tissue Protection. T. Godfraind, P. M. Vanhoutte, S. Govoni & R. Paoletti, Eds.: 51–58. Raven Press. New York, N. Y.
58. SMITH, R. J., F. F. SUN, S. S. IDEN, B. J. BOWMAN, H. SPRECHER & J. C. MCGUIRE. 1981. Clin. Immunol. Immunopathol. **20:** 157–169.

A Potential Role of Calcium Ions in Early Ischemic and Reperfusion Arrhythmias

L. H. OPIE, W. A. COETZEE, S. C. DENNIS,
AND F. T. THANDROYEN

Ischemic Heart Disease Research Unit
of the Medical Research Council
Department of Medicine
University of Cape Town
Observatory 7925
South Africa

INTRODUCTION

The genesis of early ventricular ischemic arrhythmias is still not well understood. Among the factors thought to explain such arrhythmias is the loss of potassium from intracellular to extracellular sites in the ischemic zone, thereby causing conduction slowing and predisposing to reentrant arrhythmias. More recently, abnormal control of intracellular calcium ion movements has been proposed as also playing a role in the development of injury current in the genesis of ischemic ventricular arrhythmias.[10–13,63] We have systematically explored the role of Ca^{2+} by (1) using pharmacological probes to achieve inhibition of Ca^{2+} movements both at cell entry level and at the level of the sarcoplasmic reticulum; and (2) studying factors provoking or inhibiting calcium-related electrophysiological abnormalities such as delayed afterdepolarizations (DADs) and the transient inward current (i_{ti}), slow responses, and conduction slowing. Our electrophysiological data lead us to suggest that the effects of Ca^{2+} can be most clearly linked to a specific electrophysiological abnormality, namely, the provocation of DADs, in conditions where there is an adequate supply of energy available in the form of ATP. Thus abnormalities of intracellular Ca^{2+} control are more likely to be linked to reperfusion rather than to ischemic arrhythmias.

ROLE OF CALCIUM IONS DURING EARLY ISCHEMIC AND REPERFUSION ARRHYTHMIAS

Intracellular Calcium Ion Concentration during Early Myocardial Ischemia and Reperfusion

During myocardial ischemia there is some indirect evidence that excess accumulation of Ca^{2+} may occur in the cytosol. The evidence includes (1) the development of ischemic contracture within 10–20 minutes of the onset of ischemia apparently independently of the ATP levels;[5,6] (2) the attenuation of very early ischemic depolarization by calcium channel blockers;[12,73] and (3) measurements of Ca^{2+} concentration by Quin 2 in simulated ischemic damage.[45] None of this evidence is, however, conclusive. More positive are the preliminary data of Murphy *et al.*, where free cytosolic Ca^{2+} concentrations were measured in the perfused rat heart using fluorine nuclear magnetic resonance techniques with a special compound that undergoes a chemical shift upon binding to calcium.[46] The average level of internal calcium was about 6×10^{-7} M and it fell by about half during cardiac arrest, with a sharp rise in free calcium to 7×10^{-6} M during severe ischemia as now published in detail.[62] In contrast, the overall measured calcium content of the myocardium increases in (1) reperfusion damage[59] and (2) prolonged hypoxic-ischemic damage,[68] provided that there is some continued perfusion.

Evidence for a Role of Calcium Ions in Early Ischemic Ventricular Arrhythmias

Our first data related to the involvement of the β-adrenoceptor and cyclic AMP, both agents that increase the calcium current[57] in the regulation of the ventricular fibrillation threshold, or the occurrence of ventricular tachycardia or fibrillation following acute myocardial ischemia. These data[49] included (1) the rise of cyclic AMP in ischemic tissue associated with the onset of ventricular fibrillation in the baboon and pig models; (2) the dose-response curve linking increases in tissue cyclic AMP with the increase in the ventricular fibrillation threshold in the isolated rat heart model; (3) the shift of this dose-response curve to the right, and the delay in the rise of tissue cyclic AMP during β-adrenergic stimulation by the β-adrenergic antagonist agent atenolol; (4) the opposite effects on the dose-response curve obtained by theophylline, an inhibitor of phosphodiesterase; (5) the effect of addition of dibutyryl cyclic AMP (or of cyclic AMP plus theophylline) by decreasing the ventricular fibrillation threshold in the isolated rat heart; (6) the effect of coronary artery ligation in elevating tissue cyclic AMP and decreasing the fibrillation threshold in rat heart; and (7) the effect of infusions of dibutyryl cyclic AMP at the edge of experimental infarction in promoting arrhythmias.[55]

Although not all our findings can be explained by the proposed arrhythmogenic properties of cyclic AMP,[43] it was logical to search for a role of Ca^{2+} in early ventricular arrhythmias, because Ca^{2+} is a proposed third messenger of catecholamine stimulation.

Early Ischemic Ventricular Arrhythmias and Calcium Antagonists

There is considerable experimental evidence showing that calcium antagonists can prevent ventricular arrhythmias during acute myocardial ischemia.[10,12,13,35,54,63] However, due to the heterogeneity of the action of calcium antagonists and in particular to the possibility that they might have an antiischemic effect, the unanswered question is the mechanism of such protection by calcium antagonists. Thandroyen studied the effects of *dl*-verapamil and the enantiomers, $d(+)$ and $l(-)$ verapamil, as well as nifedipine, diltiazem, and tiapamil on the ventricular fibrillation threshold of the isolated rat heart (FIGURE 1). All these agents [except $d(+)$ verapamil, which is less active against calcium channels] were effective in elevating towards normal the ventricular fibrillation threshold which had been reduced by a combination of coronary ligation and adrenaline in the isolated rat heart. These data are compatible with a specific role for calcium antagonism in the prevention of early ischemic ventricular arrhythmias, as are the data of Curtis and Walker, since the $l(-)$ enantiomer is thought to be more active against the calcium channel and the $d(+)$ isomer more active against the sodium channel.[19] However, in some other experiments,[24,63] it would appear that the ventricular antiarrhythmic activity of verapamil may be due to inhibition of both calcium and sodium influx. It should be noted that tiapamil is a mixed sodium-calcium antagonist so that its antiarrhythmic effect may also be due to a combination of properties.[53]

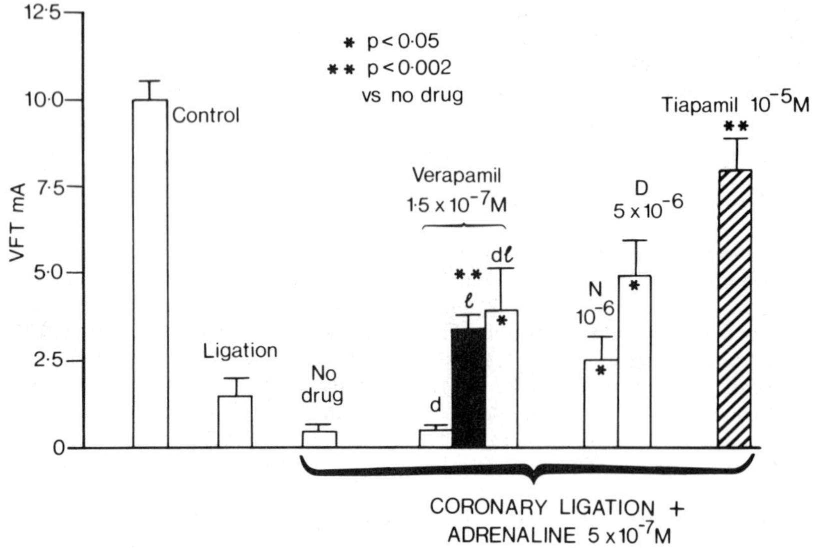

FIGURE 1. Effect of calcium antagonists on ventricular fibrillation threshold of rat heart. In an isolated rat heart preparation, coronary artery ligation decreases the ventricular fibrillation threshold (VFT), an effect further enhanced by the addition of adrenaline (5×10^{-7} M). The threshold reverts towards normal with verapamil and the *l*-form is more potent than the *d*-form. Other active agents are nifedipine (N) 10^{-6}M, diltiazem (D) 5×10^{-6} M, and tiapamil (T) 10^{-5} M. For methods and further discussion of the data with verapamil isomers, see References 50, 65, and 66. Note that the distinction between the *l*- and *d*-isomers of verapamil is only found in the presence of catecholamine stimulation.[63]

In large animal preparations such as the pig where ventricular fibrillation consistently develops after coronary artery ligation, Muller (unpublished observations) has shown that certain doses of the calcium antagonists verapamil and tiapamil are able to inhibit the development of ventricular fibrillation in the pig model. However, due to the complexity of the hemodynamic actions of calcium antagonists *in vivo* including a possible redistribution of coronary blood flow, these observations should not be taken as supporting a direct role of Ca^{2+} in early ventricular fibrillation.

We recognize that links between gross electrophysiological disturbances such as ventricular fibrillation and Ca^{2+} are only indirect, and chiefly the pointer to further work with more precise techniques. We have therefore increasingly come to rely on the examination of basic electrophysiological mechanisms that could be related to Ca^{2+} abnormalities.

Reperfusion Arrhythmias and Calcium Antagonists

The effects of calcium channel blockers on reperfusion arrhythmias are inconsistent. Nifedipine and diltiazem were found to be protective against reperfusion arrhythmias in the rat heart.[39,67] For the dog, more variable results were obtained. Some groups described protective effects of nifedipine and verapamil,[7,18] while others found nifedipine, diltiazem, and verapamil not to be protective.[47,60]

POSSIBLE ELECTROPHYSIOLOGICAL ROLE OF CALCIUM IN ISCHEMIC AND REPERFUSION ARRHYTHMIAS

There are a variety of mechanisms whereby calcium could cause or promote early ischemic or reperfusion ventricular arrhythmias.

Intracellular Calcium Oscillations and the Transient Inward Current

Rhythmical Internal Calcium Oscillations

The role of the sarcoplasmic reticulum in regulating calcium uptake and release has been emphasized by recent information showing that intracellular Ca^{2+} concentrations show small oscillations even at a subcellular level.[2,22] These oscillations are thought to be caused by an oscillatory release and uptake of calcium by the sarcoplasmic reticulum[30,31] with depolarization by the normal action potential "resetting" these calcium oscillations within the cell.

These Ca^{2+} movements are sensitive to *caffeine*, which appears to inhibit the calcium oscillations at the level of the sarcoplasmic reticulum. *Ryanodine*, another

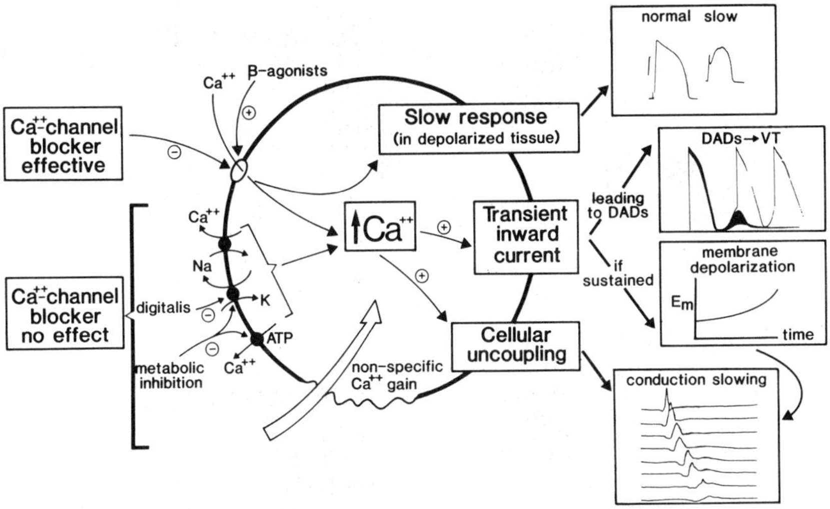

FIGURE 2. Cell Ca^{2+} and arrhythmias. Assuming that intracellular calcium does increase during ischemia (see text), there are a number of potential mechanisms by which the calcium current could be arrhythmogenic: (a) Ca^{2+} influx might elicit slow responses; (b) an additional increase in cytosolic Ca^{2+} could activate oscillatory inward current flow and precipitate DADs; (c) if the calcium activation of this inward current were sustained, then accelerated depolarization might increase injury current across the ischemic boundary and precipitate fibrillation; (d) through promoting depolarization and increasing the coupling resistance between cells, a raised cytosolic $[Ca^{2+}]$ might also slow conduction and increase the likelihood of reentry. Ca^{2+} channel blockers should be effective against the effects of a gain of intracellular Ca^{2+} resulting from enhanced Ca^{2+} entry through the calcium channel. However, these agents should not benefit the consequences of sodium pump or metabolic inhibition or nonspecific Ca^{2+} gain except by their antiischemic effect (see Reference 14).

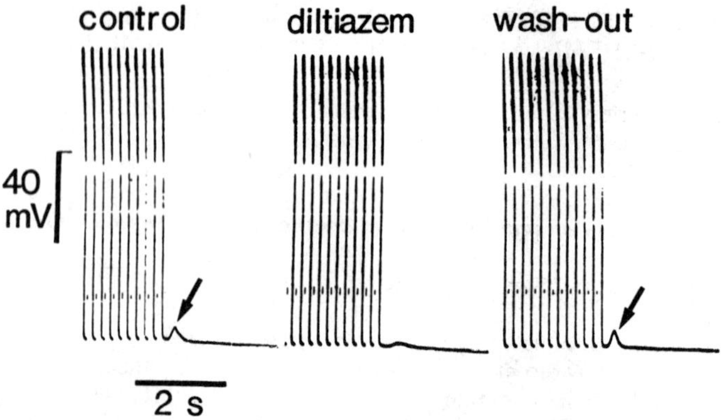

FIGURE 3. DADs were provoked using a train of rapid stimulation (35 pulses at a frequency of 5 Hz) in the presence of isoproterenol (3×10^{-7} M). Following the cessation of stimulation, a DAD is observed (arrow). Diltiazem (10^{-6} M) reduced the amplitude of the DAD within 20 minutes. The effect was reversible after 45 minutes. (Reproduced from Reference 14 with permission.)

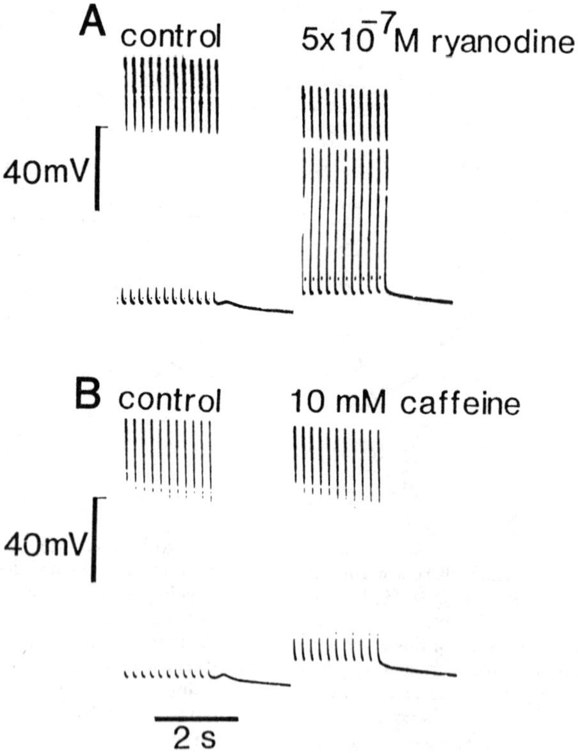

FIGURE 4. DADs produced by the same mechanism as in FIGURE 3 were also inhibited by ryanodine and caffeine. (From Reference 15 by permission.)

agent inhibiting sarcoplasmic reticulum Ca^{2+} fluxes, is also able to prevent these rhythmical oscillations.

Delayed Afterdepolarizations

Delayed afterdepolarizations are electrophysiological abnormalities caused by the rhythmical internal calcium oscillations described in the previous section. They can be evoked by a variety of conditions that induce intracellular calcium overload, including

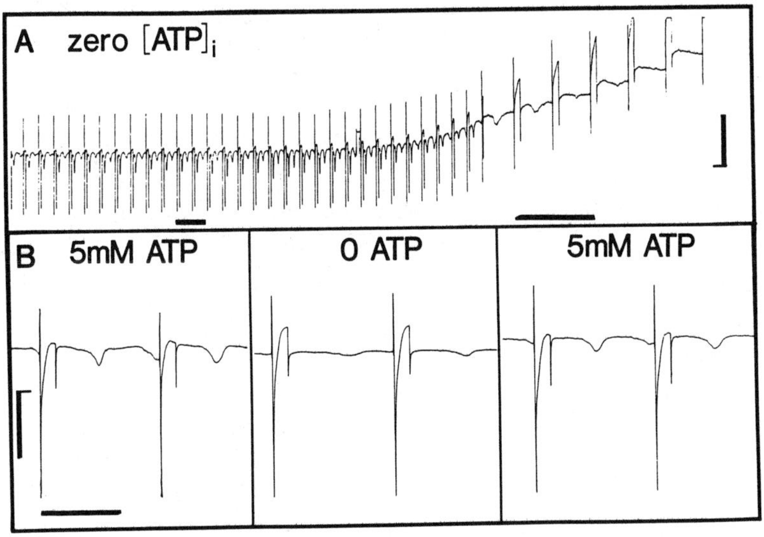

FIGURE 5. The effect of perfusion with ATP-free solution on the transient inward current in a guinea pig ventricular myocyte after a voltage step from −55 mV to 0 mV. The currents were measured using the whole cell clamp technique. A transient inward current was evoked 10 minutes after the start of the cell perfusion by exposing the cell to a Tyrode solution containing 0.54 mM K and 5.4 mM Ca. The transient inward current (arrow) was found while the cell was perfused by a pipette containing 5 mM ATP solution. In the middle panel, 10 minutes after perfusion with an ATP-free medium, the transient inward current has virtually disappeared. Then, after restoration of ATP, the transient inward current develops again. Note that the calcium current (in the same direction as transient inward current) is not affected by lack of ATP. Time calibration in 1 second and current calibration 0.5 nA. (From Reference 17 by permission.)

fast pacing, isoproterenol, dibutyryl cyclic AMP, and intracellular injection of calcium. Since calcium overload may occur both during ischemia and reperfusion, a reasonable hypothesis would be that delayed afterdepolarizations (DADs) could play a role in ischemic or reperfusion arrhythmias.

We found that DADs were abolished by simulated ischemia (increased extracellular potassium, high lactate, low pH, hypoxia).[17] Furthermore, DADs were abolished by hypoxia alone, or by the addition of 1 mM DNP or 2 mM CN^-. These findings are supported by Bhattacharyya and Vasalle, who also found digitalis-induced DADs to be abolished by metabolic inhibition.[3] On the basis of these results alone, the precise electrophysiological mechanism could not be resolved. The most likely explanation for the inhibitory effect of hypoxia on DADs was a reduced Ca^{2+} influx due to the associated action potential duration shortening. An alternative possibility was that intracellular energy metabolism could be directly involved in the genesis of DADs. To answer these questions we had to use the voltage clamp technique and study the current system underlying DADs, namely, the transient inward current.

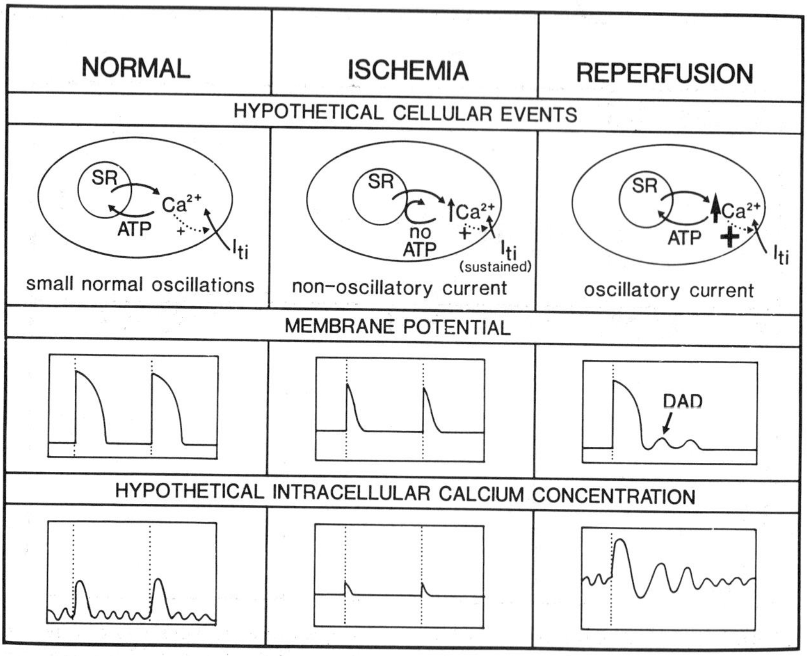

FIGURE 6. A possible sequence of events occurring in normal, ischemic, or reperfused myocardial cells. In each case a schematic representation of the myocardial cell and the sarcoplasmic reticulum is shown. In the lower panel, action potentials are illustrated along with the hypothetical changes of the intracellular Ca^{2+} concentration. Note that in severe ischemia although the internal cytosolic calcium rises, calcium flux in and out of the sarcoplasmic reticulum is inhibited and therefore oscillatory i_{ti} cannot develop. On the other hand, sustained inflow of current via i_{ti} leads to increasing depolarization which enhances the difference between ischemic and nonischemic zones and predisposes to arrhythmias. Note that in reperfusion when ATP becomes available and the Ca^{2+} fluxes in and out of the sarcoplasmic reticulum are resumed, an oscillatory i_{ti} can develop at a lower postulated intracellular Ca^{2+} concentration and that arrhythmias dependent on DADs may now be provoked. (From Reference 15 with permission.)

The Transient Inward Current

The mechanism underlying DADs is the calcium-induced transient inward current, T_i or i_{ti}. Thus rhythmical internal Ca^{2+} oscillations cause rhythmical switching on and off of i_{ti} and may thus predispose to any arrhythmias mediated by this current. The mechanism of the abolition of DADs by metabolic inhibition[17] was investigated in guinea pig ventricular myocytes under voltage clamp conditions.[14-16] Our data indicate

TABLE 1. Effects of Modulation of Ca^{2+} Ion Movements on Experimental Ventricular Arrhythmias in Heart[a]

Proposed Site of Inhibition	Inhibitor	Effect	Comment	Reference
1. Transsarcolemmal Ca^{2+} influx via slow channel	Ca^{2+} antagonist agents	Usually decrease ischemic ventricular arrhythmias	Nonspecific effects need evaluation (alpha receptor inhibition and/or effects on outward K^+ currents)	63 50 54 9
2. Cyclic AMP–induced phosphorylation of Ca^{2+} channel	Beta-adrenergic blocking agents	Usually decrease ischemic ventricular arrhythmias	Numerous other effects of beta-adrenergic blockade make interpretation difficult	44
3. $Alpha_1$-adrenergic receptor	Prazosin	Inhibits fall of ventricular fibrillation threshold induced by methoxamine; in regional ischemia; effects nonspecific	Alpha-adrenoceptors may play only a "secondary" role in regulation of calcium flux	4, 64
4. Phasic movement of calcium ions in and out of sarcoplasmic reticulum	Caffeine Ryanodine	1. Decrease of digitalis arrhythmias 2. Decrease of ischemic arrhythmias	1. Depression of myocardial contractile activity makes interpretation difficult 2. Ryanodine superior to caffeine—no mechanical effects	21 65, 66
5. Transient inward current	Lack of ATP, cyanide	Inhibition of current	Would explain inhibition of delayed afterdepolarization by lack of energy	17

[a]Modified from Reference 51 with permission.

that the blocking effect of metabolic inhibition on DADs cannot be explained solely as being secondary to changes induced in the K current as a result of ATP depletion nor to changes of i_{ca}. Rather, we show that ATP depletion by itself blocked i_{ti} probably by interfering with the Ca uptake of the sarcoplasmic reticulum, although a direct effect on the transport mechanism for i_{ti} could not be excluded.

The Possible Contribution of i_{ti} to Ischemic and Reperfusion Arrhythmias

The voltage clamp data indicate that i_{ti} is dependent on intracellular energy metabolism. These results suggest that i_{ti} is a less likely source of arrhythmias on the severely ischemic tissue, since energy metabolism is severely hampered under such conditions. The contribution of i_{ti} to ischemic arrhythmias cannot be excluded on these grounds. For example, Thandroyen *et al.* showed that ischemic arrhythmias were inhibited by caffeine and ryanodine[66]—both agents that reduce intracellular calcium oscillations and i_{ti}. The contribution of i_{ti} to arrhythmias during moderate ischemia, or arrhythmias originating in the normal side of the ischemic border, therefore has to be considered. Direct proof of the contribution of i_{ti} to ischemic arrhythmias thus remains to be achieved.

Delayed afterdepolarizations can occur during reoxygenation following a period of simulated ischemia,[14–16,23] thereby indirectly arguing for a role of calcium in reperfusion arrhythmias. These DADs upon reoxygenation are blocked by verapamil.[41] Further evidence for the involvement of DADs in reperfusion arrhythmias is that these arrhythmias are inhibited by ryanodine and caffeine in the isolated perfused rat heart.[64]

Calcium and the Injury Current

Injury current flowing between ischemic and nonischemic myocardium might be a possible source of ischemic arrhythmias.[28] Such injury currents will flow as a result of a potential difference between a depolarized ischemic area and a fully polarized nonischemic myocardium as demonstrated using the sucrose-gap technique.[33] In the latter study, a potassium gradient across a nonconducting sucrose medium (used to prevent the extracellular flow of current) led to partial depolarization and automaticity in the more polarized part of the preparation. The same phenomenon of depolarization-induced automaticity can be demonstrated by the constant current injection[34] or by blockade of the inward rectifier by barium.[42]

Calcium channel blockers might act by several mechanisms to reduce the depolarization-induced automaticity that is caused by the current of injury.[14–17] First, calcium channel blockers may decrease the size of the injury current by decreasing the area of the ischemic tissue or the severity of ischemia, thus lessening potassium loss by the ischemic tissue (an antiischemic effect). A second and possibly important action of calcium channel blockers, usually often overlooked, is as follows. Automaticity occurring at depolarized levels is partly due to the calcium current[25] and is influenced by changes in $[Ca]_o$.[32] Thus, the depolarization-induced automaticity occurring in normal tissue adjacent to the ischemic zone as a result of the flow of injury current may be inhibited by calcium channel blockers.

Calcium channel blockers could also be potentially effective in a third way. Early ischemic depolarization is not well understood—most seems to be K induced. However, the membrane potential (E_m) does not directly approach the potassium equilibrium potential (E_k) during early ischemia (Figure 2 of Reference 37), as would be expected for an increased potassium conductance resulting from the increased $[K]_o$. Thus a small component other than potassium might contribute to membrane depolarization during the very early stages of ischemia. With a sustained increase of intracellular calcium, for example, with calcium injection,[40] a steady-state inward current can be evoked. The mechanism of this current might be the same as for the "transient" inward current—in that case, the current would not be transient, since the fiber was not stimulated and therefore the calcium could not markedly fluctuate. Clusin *et al.* proposed that this current system might partly contribute to very early ischemic depolarization and thus to injury current, and that this component of ischemic depolarization can be blocked by calcium channel blockers to reduce injury current.[12,13]

Delayed Intraventricular Conduction Slowing

During myocardial ischemia, the conduction velocity of impulse propagation slows down and may predispose to ischemic arrhythmias.[38] The slowing of conduction might be caused mainly by two factors. An increase in $[K]_o$ will depolarize the membrane potential, moving into a range of potentials where the steady-state inactivation parameter decreases. The result will be a partly inactivated Na current, leading to a decreased rate of upstroke of the action potential (dV/dt) and thus a lower conduction velocity. Within a certain range of $[K]_o$, the upstroke of such a "depressed fast response" might actually consist of two phases, the first of which can be blocked by sodium channel blockers, and the second of which is increased by Mg^{2+} and isoproterenol, while it is blocked by calcium channel blockers.[1,61] Thus, if this were to be the mode of action of calcium channel blockers during myocardial ischemia, one would expect these agents to increase the severity of the slowing of conduction velocity caused by ischemia—precisely the opposite of the expected beneficial effect.

Another way that conduction velocity may be changed during myocardial ischemia is that the cable properties of the myocardium are altered by ischemia. Thus, hypoxia increases the internal longitudinal resistance (R_i).[27,69] This effect is also seen with increased cAMP,[70] increased $[Ca]_o$, or intracellular acidosis.[20] All these effects are probably mediated by an elevated cytosolic Ca^{2+}, since the junctional conductance is much more dependent on Ca_i than pH_i.[48] Under normoxic conditions, calcium channel blockers were reported to be ineffective in changing R_i.[56] These agents can, however, reduce conduction impairment in a model of ischemia (hypoxia, hyperkalemia, and acidosis) without affecting the membrane potential.[36]

Slow Response Action Potentials

Experimentally, it is possible to elicit "slow response" action potentials by the addition of catecholamines or other agents elevating cyclic AMP in the presence of elevated potassium concentrations.[1,8,58] Theoretically, because of the rise in external potassium and the release of catecholamines during ischemia,[26] the slow response may explain some aspects of ischemic arrhythmias, although the rate of conduction of ventricular arrhythmias is such that true slow responses are unlikely.[29] Nonetheless, it is difficult to exclude the possibility that slow response action potentials, by creating areas of extremely slow conduction, could predispose to the formation of reentry circuits which, in turn, could have a higher rate of conduction.

CONCLUSIONS

The possible role of Ca^{2+} in *ischemic* ventricular fibrillation was first revealed by the findings that verapamil could inhibit this arrhythmia in dogs. Verapamil is, however, a relatively nonspecific agent, also having sodium-blocking qualities especially at high concentrations. Further work on an isolated heart preparation has shown an antiarrhytmic effect of *l*-verapamil, *dl*-verapamil, nifedipine, diltiazem, and tiapamil. A possible role for Ca^{2+} influx in early ischemic arrhythmias is also supported by the data linking intracellular cyclic AMP with ventricular fibrillation. Nonetheless such arguments are essentially indirect. More convincing proof for the role of Ca^{2+} now comes from two sources. Firstly, there is increasing evidence that cytosolic Ca^{2+} concentrations may be enhanced in acute ischemia. Secondly, intracellular injections of calcium cause inward currents, which might predispose to the electrophysiological phenomena of DADs and the transient inward current (i_{ti}). In some circumstances, abnormal oscillations of Ca^{2+} early in myocardial ischemia could predispose to ventricular arrhythmias. Alternatively, a sustained rise in cytosolic Ca^{2+} concentration could provoke an inward depolarizing current, thereby increasing ischemic depolarization and the likelihood of currents between nonischemic and ischemic zones. However, because DADs are energy dependent and because i_{ti} is abolished by lack of ATP, it seems unlikely that the mechanism relating calcium to early ischemic arrhythmias is directly related to the formation of DADs, unless these were being formed in nonischemic or mildly ischemic or borderline tissue. The situation in the case of *reperfusion* arrhythmias seems more clear, and our results (see also Reference 23) suggest that DADs play an important role in this type of arrhythmia, thus more directly linking cytosolic calcium to reperfusion arrhythmias.

REFERENCES

1. ARITA, M., T. KIYOSUE, M. AOMINE & S. IMANISHI. 1983. Nature of "residual fast channel" dependent action potentials and slow conduction in guinea-pig ventricular muscle and its modification by isoproterenol. Am. J. Cardiol. **51:** 1433–1440.
2. BERLIN, J. R., M. B. CANNEL, W. F. GOLDMAN, W. J. LEDERER, E. MARBAN & W. G. WIER. 1986. Subcellular calcium inhomogeneity indicated by fura-2 develops with calcium overload in single rat heart cells. J. Physiol. **371:** 200P.
3. BHATTACHARYYA, M. L. & M. VASSALLE. 1981. The effect of metabolic inhibitors on strophanthidin-induced arrhythmias and contracture in cardiac Purkinje fibers. J. Pharmacol. Exp. Ther. **219:** 75–84.
4. BRALET, J. J-P. DIDIER, D. MOREAU, L. H. OPIE & L. ROCHETTE. 1985. Effect of alpha-adrenoceptor antagonists (phentolamine, nicergoline and prazosin) on reperfusion arrhythmias and noradrenaline release in perfused rat heart. Br. J. Pharmacol. **84:** 9–18.
5. BRICKNELL, O. L. & L. H. OPIE. 1978. Effects of substrates on tissue metabolic changes in the isolated rat heart during underperfusion and on release of lactate dehydrogenase and arrhythmias during reperfusion. Circ. Res. **43:** 102–115.
6. BRICKNELL, O. L., P. S. DARIES & L. H. OPIE. 1981. A relationship between adenosine triphosphate, glycolysis and ischaemic contracture in the isolated rat heart. J. Mol. Cell. Cardiol. **13:** 941–945.
7. BROOKS, W. W., R. L. VERRIER & B. LOWN. 1980. Protective effect of verapamil on vulnerability to ventricular fibrillation during myocardial ischemia and reperfusion. Cardiovasc. Res. **14:** 295–302.
8. CARMELIET, E. & J. VEREECKE. 1969. Adrenaline and the plateau phase of the cardiac action potential. Eur. J. Physiol. **313:** 300–315.
9. CLUSIN, W. T. 1983. Mechanism by which metabolic inhibitors depolarise cultured cardiac cells. Proc. Nat. Acad. Sci. USA **80:** 3865–3869.

10. CLUSIN, W. T., M. R. BRISTOW, D. S. BAIN, J. S. SCHROEDER, P. JAILLON, P. BRETT & D. C. HARRISON. 1982. The effects of diltiazem and reduced serum ionized calcium on ischemic ventricular fibrillation in the dog. Circ. Res. **50:** 518–526.
11. CLUSIN, W. T., M. BUCHBINDER & D. C. HARRISON. 1983. Calcium overload, "injury" current, and early ischaemic cardiac arrhythmias: a direct connection Lancet **i:** 272–274.
12. CLUSIN, W. T., M. BUCHBINDER, M. R. BRISTOW & D. C. HARRISON. 1984. Evidence for a role of calcium in the genesis of early ischemic cardiac arrhythmias. *In* Calcium Antagonists and Cardiovascular Disease. L. H. Opie, Ed.: 293–302. Raven Press. New York, N.Y.
13. CLUSIN, W. T., M. BUCHBINDER, A. K. ELLIS, D. S. KERNOFF, J. C. GIACOMINI & D. C. HARRISON. 1984. Reduction of ischemic depolarization by the calcium channel blocker diltiazem. Correlation with improvement of ventricular conduction and early arrhythmias in the dog. Circ. Res. **54:** 10–20.
14. COETZEE, W. A., S. C. DENNIS, L. H. OPIE & C. A. MULLER. 1987. Calcium channel blockers and early ischemic ventricular arrhythmias: electrophysiological versus anti-ischemic effects. J. Mol. Cell. Cardiol. **19** (Suppl. II): 77–97.
15. COETZEE, W. A., L. H. OPIE & S. SAMAN. Proposed role of energy supply in the genesis of delayed afterdepolarizations—implications for ischemic or reperfusion arrhythmias. J. Mol. Cell. Cardiol. (Suppl). (In press.)
16. COETZEE, W. A., G. BIERMANS, G. CALLEWAERT, J. VEREECKE, L. H. OPIE & E. CARMELIET. The effect of inhibition of mitochondrial energy metabolism on the transient inward current of isolated guinea-pig ventricular myocytes. J. Mol. Cell. Cardiol. (In press.)
17. COETZEE, W. A. & L. H. OPIE. 1987. The effects of components of ischemia and metabolic inhibition on delayed afterdepolarizations in guinea-pig papillary muscle. Circ. Res. **61:** 157–165.
18. COKER, S. J. & J. R. PARRATT. 1983. Nifedipine reduces arrhythmias but does not alter prostanoid release during coronary artery occlusion and reperfusion in anaesthetised greyhounds. J. Cardiovasc. Pharmacol. **5:** 406–417.
19. CURTIS, M. J. & M. J. A. WALKER. 1986. The mechanism of action of the optical enantiomers of verapamil against ischaemia-induced arrhythmias in the conscious rat. Br. J. Pharmacol. **89:** 137–147.
20. DE MELLO, W. C. 1982. Intercellular communication in cardiac muscle. Circ. Res. **51:** 1–9.
21. DI GENNARO M., P. CARBONIN & M. VASSALLE. 1984. On the mechanism by which caffeine abolishes the fast rhythms induced by cardiotonic steroids. J. Mol. Cell. Cardiol. **16:** 851–862.
22. EISNER, D. A. & M. VALDEOLMILLOS. 1986. A study of intracellular calcium oscillations in sheep cardiac Purkinje fibers measured at the single cell level. J. Physiol. **372:** 539–556.
23. FERRIER, G. R., M. P. MOFFAT & A. LUKAS. 1985. Possible mechanisms of ventricular arrhythmias elicited by ischemia followed by reperfusion. Circ. Res. **56:** 184–194.
24. GIACOMINI, J. C., R. H. ZOBRIST, D. ROOD, H. J. GORDON & K. M. GIACOMINI. 1984. Contribution of sodium channel blockade on the antifibrillatory effects of verapamil (Abstr). Circulation **70**(Suppl II): II-239.
25. HAUSWIRTH, O., D. NOBLE & R. W. TSIEN. 1909. The mechanism of oscillatory activity at low membrane potentials in cardiac Purkinje fibers. J. Physiol. **200:** 255–265.
26. HIRCHE, H., C. FRANZ, L. BOS, R. BISSIG, R. LANG & M. SCHRAMM. 1980. Myocardial extracellular K^+ and H^+ increase and noradrenaline release as possible causes of early arrhythmias following acute coronary artery occlusion in pigs. J. Mol. Cell. Cardiol. **12:** 579–593.
27. IKEDA, K. & M. HIRAOKA. 1982. Effects of hypoxia on passive electrical properties of canine ventricular muscle. Pflugers Arch. **393:** 45–50.
28. JANSE, M. J., F. J. L. VAN CAPELLE, H. MORSINK, *et al.* 1980. Flow of "injury" current and patterns of excitation during early ventricular arrhythmias in acute regional myocardial ischemia in isolated porcine and canine hearts. Circ. Res. **47:** 151–165.
29. JANSE, M. J., A. G. KLEBER, A. CAPUCCI, R. CORONEL & F. WILMS-SCHOPMAN. 1986.

Electrophysiological basis for arrhythmias caused by acute ischemia. Role of the subendocardium. J. Mol. Cell. Cardiol. **18:** 339–355.
30. KASS, R. S., W. J. LEDERER, R. W. TSIEN & R. WEINGARD. 1978. Role of calcium ions in transient inward currents and aftercontractions induced by strophanthidin in cardiac Purkinje fibers. J. Physiol. **281:** 187–208.
31. KASS, R. S., R. W. TSIEN & R. WEINGARD. 1978. Ionic basis of transient inward current induced by strophanthidin in cardiac Purkinje fibers. J. Physiol. **281:** 209–226.
32. KATZUNG, B. G. 1975. Effects of extracellular calcium and sodium on depolarization-induced automaticity in guinea-pig papillary muscle. Circ. Res. **37:** 118–127.
33. KATZUNG, B. G., L. M. HONDEGHEM & A. O. GRANT. 1975. Cardiac ventricular automaticity induced by current of injury. Pflugers Arch. **360:** 193–197.
34. KATZUNG, B. G. & J. A. MORGENSTERN. 1977. Effects of extracellular potassium on ventricular automaticity and evidence for a pacemaker current in mammalian ventricular myocardium. Circ. Res. **40:** 105–111.
35. KAUMANN, A. J. & P. ARAMENDIA. 1968. Prevention of ventricular fibrillation induced by coronary ligation. J. Pharmacol. Exp. Ther. **164:** 326–332.
36. KIMURA, S., J. S. CAMERON, P. L. KOZLOVSKIS, A. C. BASSETT & R. T. MYERBURG. 1985. Delayed afterdepolarizations and triggered activity induced in feline Purkinje fibres by alpha-adrenergic stimulation in the presence of elevated calcium levels. Circulation **70:** 1074–1082.
37. KLEBER, A. G. 1983. Resting membrane potential, extracellular potassium activity, and intracellular sodium activity during acute global ischemia in isolated perfused guinea-pig hearts. Circ. Res. **52:** 442–450.
38. KLEBER, A. G., M. J. JANSE, F. J. G. WILMS-SCHOPMAN, A. A. M. WILDE & R. CORONEL. 1986. Changes in conduction velocity during acute ischemia in ventricular myocardium of the isolated porcine heart. Circulation **73:** 189–198.
39. LUBBE, W. F., J. A. MCLEAN & T. NGUYEN. 1983. Antiarrhythmic actions of nifedipine in acute myocardial ischemia. Am. Heart J. **105:** 331–333.
40. MATSUDA, H. 1983. Effects of intracellular calcium injection on steady state membrane currents in isolated single ventricular cells. Pflugers Arch. **397:** 81–83.
41. MOHABIR, R., M. P. MOFFAT & G. R. FERRIER. 1983. Effects of verapamil and low Ca^{2+} on mechanisms of arrhythmia induced by conditions of ischemia and reperfusion. (abstr). Circulation **68**(Suppl. III): III–220.
42. MUGELLI, A., S. AMERINI. G. PIAZZESI & A. GIOTTI. 1983. Barium-induced spontaneous activity in sheep cardiac Purkinje fibers. J. Mol. Cell. Cardiol. **15:** 697–712.
43. MULLER, C. A., C. W. HAMM, F. T. THANDROYEN & L. H. OPIE. 1985. Tiapamil and verapamil prevent ventricular function during myocardial infarction in the porcine model. (abstr). J. Mol. Cell. Cardiol. **17:** 43.
44. MULLER, C. A., L. H. OPIE, C. W. HAMM, M. PEISACH & D. GIHWALA. 1986. Prevention of ventricular fibrillation by metoprolol in a pig model of acute myocardial ischaemia: absence of a major arrhythmogenic role for cyclic AMP. J. Mol. Cell Cardiol. **18:** 375–387.
45. MURPHY, E., R. JACOB & M. LIEBERMAN. 1985. Cytosolic free calcium in chick heart cells: its role in cell injury. J. Mol. Cell. Cardiol. **17:** 221–231.
46. MURPHY, E., C. STEENBERGEN & R. LONDON. 1986. Cytosolic free calcium measured by fluorine NMR in perfused rat heart. (Abstr). J. Mol. Cell. Cardiol. **18**(suppl. 1): 111.
47. NAITO, M., E. L. MICHELSON, J. J. KMETZO, E. KAPLINSKY & L. S. DREIFUS. 1981. Failure of antiarrhythmic drugs to prevent experimental reperfusion ventricular fibrillation. Circulation **63:** 70–79.
48. NOMA, A. & N. TSUBOI. 1987. Dependence of junctional conductance on proton, calcium and magnesium ions in cardiac paired cells of guinea-pig. J. Physiol. **382:** 193–211.
49. OPIE, L. H., C. MULLER, D. NATHAN, P. DARIES & W. F. LUBBE. 1980. Evidence for role of cyclic AMP as second messenger of arrhythmogenic effects of beta-stimulation. Adv. Cyclic Nucleotide Res. **12:** 63–69.
50. OPIE, L. H. & F. T. THANDROYEN. 1983. Calcium antagonists, ventricular fibrillation, and enzyme release in ischemic rat hearts. Fed. Proc. **42:** 2465–2469.
51. OPIE, L. H. & F. T. THANDROYEN. 1985. Multiple sites of modualtion of calcium ion movements in cardiac tissue: implications for early ischemic ventricular fibrillation. *In*

Membranes and Muscle. M. Berman, W. Gevers & L. H. Opie, Eds.: 279–289. IRL Press. Oxford, England.
52. Opie, L. H., E. P. Owen, S. C. Dennis. 1985. Glycolysis prevents ischemic contracture. (abstr). Circulation **72**(Suppl III): III–349.
53. Osterrieder, W. 1986. Inhibition of the fast Na^+ inward current by the Ca^{2+} channel blocker tiapamil. J. Cardiovasc. Pharmacol. **8:** 1101–1106.
54. Parratt, J. R. 1982. Inhibitors of the slow calcium current and early ventricular arrhythmias. *In* Early Arrhythmias Resulting from Myocardial Ischaemia. Ed J. R. Parratt, Ed.: 329–346. MacMillan. London, England.
55. Podzuweit, T., D. J. Els & B. C. Shanley. 1978. Catecholamine-cAMP induces arrhythmias in the infarcting pig heart. (abstr). J. Mol. Cell. Cardiol. **10**(Suppl 1): 77.
56. Pressler, M. L., V. Elharrer & J. C. Bailey. 1982. Effects of extracellular calcium ions verapamil and lanthanum on active and passive properties of canine cardiac Purkinje fibers. Circ. Res. **52:** 637–651.
57. Reuter, H. 1983. Calcium channel modulation by neurotransmitters, enzymes and drugs. Nature **301:** 569–574.
58. Schneider, J. A. & N. Sperelakis. 1975. Slow Ca^{2+} and Na^+ responses induced by isoproterenol and methylxanthines in isolated perfused guinea-pig hearts exposed to elevated K^+. J. Mol. Cell. Cardiol. **7:** 249–273.
59. Sharma, A. D., J. E. Saffitz, B. I. Lee, B. E. Sobel & P. B. Corr. 1983. Alpha-adrenergic-mediated accumulation of calcium in reperfused myocardium. J. Clin. Invest. **72:** 802–818.
60. Sheehan, F. H. & S. E. Epstein. 1982. Effects of calcium channel blocking agents on reperfusion arrhythmias. Am. Heart J. **103:** 973–978.
61. Spah, F. & A. Fleckenstein. 1979. Evidence of a new, preferentially Mg-carrying transport system besides the fast Na and the slow Ca channels in the excited myocardial sarcolemma membrane. J. Mol. Cell. Cardiol. **11:** 1109–1127.
62. Steenbergen, C., E. Murphy, L. Levy & R. E. London. 1987. Cytosolic free calcium concentration early in myocardial ischemia in perfused rat heart. Circ. Res. **60:** 700–707.
63. Thandroyen, F. T. 1982. Protective action of calcium channel antagonist agents against ventricular fibrillation in the isolated perfused rat heart. J. Mol. Cell. Cardiol. **14:** 21–32.
64. Thandroyen, F. T., M. G. Worthington, L. M. Higginson & L. H. Opie. 1983. The effect of alpha- and beta-adrenoceptor antagonist agents on reperfusion ventricular fibrillation and metabolic status in the isolated perfused rat heart. J. Am. Coll. Cardiol. **4:** 1056–1066.
65. Thandroyen, F. T., L. M. Higginson, L. H. Opie & E. Yon. 1986. The influence of verapamil and its isomers on vulnerability to ventricular fibrillation during acute myocardial ischemia and adrenergic stimulation in isolated rat heart. J. Mol. Cell. Cardiol. **18:** 645–649.
66. Thandroyen, F. T., J. McCarthy, K. P. Burton & L. H. Opie. Ryanodine and caffeine prevent ventricular arrhythmias during acute myocardial ischemia and reperfusion in rat heart. Circ. Res. (In press.)
67. Weishaar, R. E. & R. J. Bing. 1980. The beneficial effect of a calcium channel blocker, diltiazem, on the ischemic-reperfused heart. J. Mol. Cell. Cardiol. **12:** 993–1009.
68. Willerson, J. T., A. Mukherjee, K. Chien, C. Izquierdo & L. M. Buja. 1984. Calcium and acute myocardial infarction. *In* Calcium Antagonists and Cardiovascular Disease. L. H. Opie, Ed.: 257–268. Raven Press. New York, N.Y.
69. Wojtczak, J. 1979. Contractures and increase in internal longitudinal resistance of cow ventricular muscle induced by hypoxia. Circ. Res. **44:** 88–95.
70. Wojtczak, J. 1982. Influence of cyclic nucleotides on the internal longitudinal resistance and contracture in the normal and hypoxic mammalian cardiac muscle. J. Mol. Cell. Cardiol. **14:** 259.

Brain Ischemia as a Target for Ca^{2+} Entry Blockers

A. WAUQUIER, D. ASHTON, AND G. H. C. CLINCKE

Department of Neuropharmacology
Janssen Pharmaceutica
B-2340 Beerse, Belgium

In the group of cardiac arrest victims in which conventional cardiopulmonary resuscitation succeeds in restoring cardiac function, about 50% develop brain death and 10 to 40% of survivors suffer permanent brain damage.[1] The goal of therapy in cardiopulmonary *cerebral* resuscitation is the restoration of neurological function, and the absence of neurological damage postischemia.

Intensive research work in the last decade has revealed much of the pathophysiology of brain ischemia (for reviews, see References 2–4). This knowledge directly implicated Ca^{2+} movements across the plasmalemma in two critical stages of ischemic neuronal damage. Firstly, during the initial stages of ischemia, when the neuronal membrane depolarizes, Ca^{2+} leaves the extracellular space down its concentration gradient. This has been suggested to produce a rapid rise in free fatty acid concentration,[3,5,6] leading to uncoupling of oxidative phosphorylation,[7] tissue swelling,[8,9] and inhibition of synaptosomal amino acid uptake mechanism.[10] Secondly, in areas of the brain that are selectively vulnerable to maturational ischemic damage, dense Ca^{2+} deposits are found in necrotic neurons.[11] It was hoped that Ca^{2+} antigonists would prevent or reduce these two phenomena. In addition, Ca^{2+} antagonists as a group possess vasodilating or antivasoconstrictive effects; it was thus possible that these properties would improve the reduced cerebral blood flow (CBF) seen postischemia.

This three-pronged rationale was sufficient to instigate a widespread interest in the possibilities of using Ca^{2+} antagonists in models of ischemia. The intention of the present article is to review the literature on the use of Ca^{2+} antagonists in animal models of brain ischemia. For this purpose we have selected targets for therapy with reference to both pathophysiology and scientific approach. These targets include increase of postischemic CBF, reduction of neurological deficit, increase in survival, improvement of postischemic electroencephalogram (EEG) and evoked potentials, preservation of ion homeostasis, preservation of energy metabolites, reduction in brain edema, and increase in neuronal survival as judged histologically. These targets are different but overlapping criteria to judge the success of therapy. Studies will be considered in which the drug was given preinsult (protection, P) or postinsult (resuscitation, R). Ischemia is either global (G) or focal (F) depending upon whether the whole brain is involved or not. In both types of ischemia the insult can be complete (C) or incomplete (I) depending upon whether there is a complete cessation of flow. The effect of Ca^{2+} antagonists on each type of ischemia will be examined target by target in an attempt to bring current knowledge in this area into focus (TABLE 1).

CEREBRAL BLOOD FLOW

There is no cerebral function without (an adequate) CBF, and following ischemia, a prerequisite for the restoration of neuronal function is the reestablishment of CBF. However, the restoration of nutrient flow to the brain does not necessarily guarantee a favorable outcome, since much of the damage to the brain occurs in the postresuscitation phase. Nevertheless, reestablishing CBF is clearly a target for Ca^{2+} antagonists, because of their evident vasodilatory or antivasospastic actions.

There are only four different studies with flunarizine on CBF following GC ischemia. Flunarizine given intravenously (iv): at the dose of 0.1 mg/kg post–cardiac arrest in dogs restored CBF almost to control values, at least measured 6 hours postarrest.[12] Using the same CBF technique (sagital sinus venous outflow), Newberg *et al.*, failed to demonstrate an improved CBF in their canine model of GC ischemia,[13] produced by temporary ligation of venae cavae and aorta. Apart from the difference in model and the fact that there was no matched control group, they used an extremely low iv dose of flunarizine (6 μg/kg).

Measuring regional cortical CBF using the hydrogen clearance technique, Marrannes *et al.* found that flunarizine at the iv dose of 0.1 mg/kg significantly antagonized the decreased flow produced by vessel clamping in dogs.[14] This result confirmed and extended results previously obtained.[15] Finally, Deshpande and Wieloch found that in rats, in spite of an improved histological outcome, flunarizine either given per orally (po) at the dose of 40 mg/kg before the insult or iv at the dose of 0.1 mg/kg after the insult did not improve CBF as measured using ^{14}C-iodoantipyrine as tracer.[16]

Lidoflazine given at the dose of 1 mg/kg post–cardiac arrest in dogs ameliorated regional CBF as measured by a thermal dilution method.[17] However, when lidoflazine was given at the same dose in dogs in which GC was produced by aortic cross-clamping, it did not affect the reperfusion phenomenon (regional CBF measured with radiolabeled microspheres).[18]

In the three studies on GC (TABLE 1), nimodipine proved to increase CBF. In a rat study where GI was produced by common carotid artery occlusion combined with arterial hypotension, nimodipine (0.1 mg/kg) given before the induction of ischemia increased CBF (using autoradiographic techniques with ^{14}C-iodoantipyrine as the tracer), but in some brain regions there was a hypoperfusion while in others hyperperfusion was seen.

The results obtained with nimodipine on ischemia produced by medial cerebral artery (MCA) occlusion vary from zero to a positive effect (TABLE 1). These scattered results cannot be explained by differences in doses because in all studies the same doses (between 0.6 and 1 μg/kg per minute) were given as continuous infusions. Species differences do not offer an explanation either, because different results are obtained even with the same species and using the same technique for measuring CBF. However, the key to the problem might be in the treatment time. Thus, when nimodipine is given at a dose of 1 μg/kg per minute for 30 minutes before and for 30 minutes after the induction of MCA occlusion in rats, it effectively increased CBF.[19] When, however, the same amount of drug was given 5 minutes after the induction of the occlusion, it failed to modify the CBF pattern.[20]

Finally, in all studies except one, topical application of nimodipine to vessels displaying vasospasm due to cisternal application of autologous blood resulted in an antagonism of vasospasm. The results obtained with nifedipine, however, are inconsistent (TABLE 1).

In GC in dogs, verapamil 0.15 mg/kg iv given post–cardiac arrest improved CBF.[17] In dogs and cats subject to vasospasm, topical verapamil (0.1 mg/kg) dilated previously constricted cortical arteries.[21,22]

SURVIVAL

We could only find five studies in which survival was used as an experimental parameter.[23–27] In four studies, it was combined with a neurophysiological measure or a neurological deficit score.[23–25,27]

TABLE 1. Effects of Ca^{2+} Antagonists in Animal Models of Ischemia[a]

Drug	Type	Reference	Species	CBF	Neuro.	Surv.	Neuro-Physio.	Cell-Physio.	Histo.	Treatment
Nimodipine	GC	23	cat	·	·	+	EEG +	·	·	P*
		24	cat	+	·	+	EEG +	·	·	P*
		50	cat	+	·	·	·	·	·	P*
		28	dog	+	+	·	·	·	·	P*
		28	dog	+	0	·	·	energy	·	*R
		29	monkey	·	+	·	EEG 0	·	+	*R
	GI	40	gerbil	·	·	·	·	energy	·	P*
		35	rat	·	·	·	EEG +	energy	·	P*
		36	rat	+/−	·	·	EVP 0/EEG −	·	·	P*
		27	gerbil	·	−/0	−/0/+	·	·	·	P*
		27	gerbil	·	−/0	0/+	·	·	·	*R
		46	rat	·	·	·	·	·	0	*R
	FC	37	cat	0	·	·	EEG 0	·	·	*R
		45	baboon	0/+	·	·	·	ion/edema −	·	P*
		19	rat	+	·	·	·	·	+	P*
		44	baboon	+	·	·	·	ion/edema −	·	P*
		38	cat	0/+	·	·	EEG 0/+	·	0	P*
		20	rat	0	·	·	·	·	0	*R
	FI	51	dog	spasm +	·	·	·	·	·	*R
		52	cat	spasm +	·	·	·	·	·	*R
		53	dog	spasm +	·	·	·	·	·	*R
		54	monkey	spasm +/0	·	·	·	·	·	*R
		55	monkey	spasm −	·	·	·	·	·	*R
Nifedipine	FI	56	cat	spasm +	·	·	·	·	·	*R(T)
	FI	57	dog	spasm 0	·	·	·	·	·	*R
		58	dog	spasm −	·	·	·	·	·	*R
		59	dog	spasm +	·	·	·	·	·	P
Nicardipine	GI	11	rat	·	·	·	·	·	+	P*

Flunarizine	GC	60	rat	·	·	·	·	ions	·	P*
		34	cat	·	·	·	EEG/EVP 0	energy	·	*R
		26	rat	·	·	+	·	·	·	P*
		13	dog	0	0	·	·	energy	·	*R
		12	dog	+	+	·	EEG +	energy	·	*R
		31	dog	·	+	·	EEG +	·	·	*R
		14	dog	+	·	·	·	·	·	*R
	GI	60	rat	·	·	·	·	ions	·	P*
		43	rat	·	·	·	·	catechol.	+	P*
		11	rat	·	·	·	·	·	+	P*
		42	rat	·	·	·	·	catechol.	·	P*
		16,41	rat	0	·	·	·	energy	+	P*
		16,41	rat	0	·	·	·	energy	+	*R
		15	dog	+	·	·	EEG +	·	·	P*
		32	gerbil	·	+	·	·	·	·	*R
		47	rat	·	·	·	·	·	+	*R
		46	rat	·	·	·	·	·	+	*R
Lidoflazine	GC	18	dog	0	·	·	·	·	·	*R
		17	dog	+	·	·	·	·	·	*R
		33	dog	·	+	·	·	·	·	*R
Verapamil	GC	17	dog	+	·	·	·	·	·	*R
	GI	30	pig/baboon	·	0	·	·	·	·	*R
	FI	21	dog	spasm +	·	·	·	·	·	*R(T)
		22	cat	spasm +	·	·	·	·	·	*R(T)
Diltiazem	GI	11	rat	·	·	·	·	·	0	P*
HA 1004	FI	61	dog	spasm +	·	·	·	·	·	*R
HA 1077	FI	61	dog	spasm +	·	·	·	·	·	*R
PY 108-068	FC	25	rat	·	+	+	·	edema 0	·	*R

[a]Abbreviations used: CBF, cerebral blood flow; Neuro., neurological evaluation; Surv., survival; Neuro-Physio., neurophysiology; Cell-Physio., cell physiology; Histo., histology; G, global; F, focal; C, complete; I, incomplete; P, protection or pretreatment; R, resuscitation or posttreatment; +, indicates a positive effect; −, negative effect; 0, no effect; ·, not evaluated; MAP, mean arterial pressure.

The effect of Ca^{2+} antagonists on survival has been most frequently tested in GI models. Hermans *et al.* showed that iv pretreatment with 1 mg/kg of flunarizine enhanced recovery of the electrocardiogram (ECG), aortic pressure (AoP), and respiration from 5 consecutive 1 minute periods of ventricular fibrillation in the rat.[26] None of the treated animals died, in contrast to the 25% mortality in the control group. In two publications Hofmeister *et al.* present data on 7 minute neck-cuff ischemia in the cat.[23,24] Oral pretreatment with 1 mg/kg of nimodipine enhanced survival 24 hours after ischemia from 1 out of 10 in the control group to 9 out of 10 in the treated group. Fujisawa *et al.* tested two intraperitoneal (ip) doses (0.01 or 0.1 mg/kg) of nimodipine given before or after bilateral common carotid occlusion in the gerbil.[27] Significantly lower mortality rates were observed with the highest dose (0.1 mg/kg) when given before the occlusion or 20 to 30 minutes after the reperfusion. However, a low dose of nimodipine (0.01 mg/kg) increased mortality rates with a factor 5 when given before a 10 minute carotid occlusion. Chronic po treatment for 3 days with 300 μg/kg of a new dihydropyridine PY 108-068 resulted in higher survival rates in a microsphere emolization model of focal ischemia in the rat.[25]

NEUROLOGIC OUTCOME

We identified nine papers in which neurologic outcome was used as a parameter in a drug study. In all cases except one,[25] global ischemia was induced (TABLE 1).

Steen *et al.* reported that pretreatment with nimodipine improved neurologic status in dogs 48 hours after 10 minutes GC ischemia.[28] However, there was no significant improvement when the treatment (10 μg/kg followed by 1 μg/kg per minute for 2–3 hours) was started two minutes postischemia. The same group treated primates 5 minutes postischemia with a dose of 10 μg/kg followed by 1 μg/kg per minute for 10 hours.[29] In this study neurologic function 96 hours postischemia was significantly better in nimodipine-treated monkeys. Although both papers came from the same research unit, it is difficult to compare the results. Species, duration of insult, method to induce ischemia, neurologic evaluation list, and time of evaluation after ischemia are all at variance. Each of these elements may have contributed to the contradictory results from those two studies. Neurologic deficit was significantly higher when gerbils were treated with low doses (0.01 mg/kg) either before or after GI ischemia.[27] A similar negative result was seen when the high dose (0.1 mg/kg) was given 30 minutes after reperfusion. When longer periods of ischemia (15 or 20 minutes) were applied, neurologic deficits were similar in treated and control animals.

A single study reported that a high iv dose (0.7 mg/kg) of verapamil did not improve neurological outcome when given after variable times of brachiocephalic and subclavian clamping.[30]

Newberg *et al.* found no improvement of neurologic recovery when 6 μg/kg of flunarizine was given 10 minutes after resuscitation from GC induced by occlusion of ascending aorta and venae cavae.[13] In contrast Edmonds *et al.*[12] and Wauquier *et al*[31] reported a better neurological recovery 6 hours after a 10 minute cardiac arrest when dogs were treated with 0.1 mg/kg of flunarizine at the beginning of resuscitation. Improved outcome with this drug (1 mg/kg iv at reperfusion) was also observed after bilateral carotid occlusion (5 minutes) in the gerbil.[32] Winegar *et al.* found a significantly improved neurologic recovery in the first 12 hours after cardiac arrest (15 minutes) in dogs when the animals were treated iv with 1 mg/kg of lidoflazine.[33]

PY 108-068 was effective in a model of focal complete ischemia.[25] It almost normalized function in surviving rats after three days chronic treatment with 300 μg/kg po.

NEUROPHYSIOLOGY

EEG measurement is most frequently used to evaluate the functional recovery of the central nervous system (CNS). Evaluation ranges from timing of return of electrical activity[28] over qualitative scoring of graphoelements[23] to quantitative spectral analysis.[15]

In GC ischemia (10 minutes cardiac arrest), postischemic iv treatment with 0.1 mg/kg flunarizine resulted in both qualitative[12] and quantitative[31] improvement of cortical activity. In contrast, Hossmann *et al.* induced prolonged (1 hour) GC (clamping of the left subclavian, innominate, and both mammarian arteries).[34] Treatment with 0.1 mg/kg iv of flunarizine followed by continuous iv infusion of 0.1 mg/kg per hour during 3 hours did not enhance functional recovery from this extreme ischemia. Nimodipine pretreatment (1 mg/kg) improved EEG recovery in the cat,[23,24] in contrast to postischemic treatment (10 μg/kg + 1 μg/kg per minute) in primates where no significant differences in EEG return or in EEG pattern were found.[29]

In one study the effect of pretreatment with a single dose of flunarizine (0.1 mg/kg iv) was tested in a model of repeated (20 minutes) GI ischemia (clamping left subclavian and brachiocephalic artery).[15] This treatment improved EEG both during clamping and in the reperfusion phase. Pretreatment with nimodipine (10 μg/kg) and continuous infusion during ischemia (30 minutes) and postischemia with 1 μg/kg per minute enhanced EEG recovery.[35] In another experiment, a single bolus injection of 0.1 mg/kg before GI ischemia enhanced postischemic CBF but did not improve return of EEG activity or recovery of sensory responses.[36]

In focal ischemia induced by MCA occlusion, Date and Hossmann saw no effect of nimodipine treatment on the cat EEG.[37] Barnett *et al.*, who used a pretreatment, reported positive effects when MAP was kept above 90 mmHg, but not when MAP dropped below that value.[38]

CELLULAR PHYSIOLOGY AND BIOCHEMISTRY

Only one study is available with nimodipine in which biochemical variables were studied after GC ischemia.[28] In dogs subject to 10 minutes of temporary ligation of the aorta and venae cavae, nimodipine was given 2 minutes postischemia (10 μg/kg iv followed by 1 μg/kg per minute for 2–3 hours). No differences were found between control and treated animals after 120 minutes of reperfusion with respect to levels of phosphocreatine, ATP, glucose, or lactate. The CMR O_2 was significantly lower in the solvent and nimodipine treated groups as compared to untreated animals. This is therefore probably related to the solvent (15% ethanol, 15% polyethylene glycol). It should be pointed out that the authors compared data with a control group obtained 6 years previously.[39]

Four studies are available with flunarizine in this area. In the first study cats were subjected to 1 hour of GC global ischemia by vessel clamping, and then 3 hours of reperfusion.[34] Flunarizine was administered after 55 minutes of ischemia as an iv bolus (0.1 mg/kg) followed by 0.1 mg/kg per hour. Animals were sacrificed after 3 hours of recirculation. No differences were found between control and treated animals. However, despite the heroic length of the ischemia, recovery levels of ATP were good and brain levels of sodium, calcium, magnesium, and potassium were similar in the two groups.

Two studies are available using flunarizine in dogs: Newberg *et al.* used vessel clamping;[13] and Edmonds *et al.* used cardiac arrest.[12] In each case the duration of ischemia was 10 minutes. The Newberg study used 0.6 $\mu g/kg$ iv given 10 minutes after recirculation. The Edmonds study employed 0.1 mg/kg iv given 1 minute after resuscitation. In the study by Newberg *et al.*, flunarizine-treated dogs had significantly worse ATP, lactate, and glucose levels during recirculation.[13] However, the flunarizine-treated animals used for biochemical determinations developed pulmonary edema, while the animals given the same dose but used for neurological scoring did not. The two groups differed only in the anesthesia used, suggesting that the worsened biochemical recovery was not the result of flunarizine treatment but of the anesthesia. Furthermore, the Newberg *et al.* study[13] again uses controls from 6 years previously.[39] In the Edmonds *et al.* study, no significant differences were found between flunarizine and solvent treated animals with respect to blood chemistry;[12] however, 4 hours postresuscitation, CMR O_2 was 121 ± 43% of baseline in flunarizine-treated animals, and 37 ± 9% in control animals.

Again only flunarizine and nimodipine have been studied in GI ischemia. In the mongolian gerbil, where ischemia was induced by bilateral common carotid artery occlusion during 1, 2, or 5 minutes, animals were pretreated with 1 mg/kg nimodipine ip. Animals were killed after recirculation periods of 0, 1, or 5 minutes. In the nimodipine group ATP levels were significantly higher during ischemia, and after 5 minutes of recirculation they had higher glucose levels in cortex and striatum.[40] In rats exposed to 30 minutes of ischemia, induced by 4 vessel occlusion and mild hypotension, levels of ATP and free fatty acids were studied after administration of nimodipine (10 mg/kg iv preischemia, 1 mg/kg per minute during ischemia and recirculation). During the ischemic period, there were no differences in levels of ATP and free fatty acids between the nimodipine and the control group. After 120 minutes of recirculation, nimodipine-treated animals had significantly better ATP levels. The authors conclude that improvement of functional and metabolic recovery by nimodipine is due either to improvement of postischemic hypoperfusion or a direct action on metabolic processes during the reperfusion period.[35]

In the Lund model (2 vessel occlusion + hypotension), flunarizine was given at 0.1 mg/kg iv after 5 minutes of recirculation. After 15 minutes of recirculation, the level of ATP and the energy charge were lower in the flunarizine group. In addition, levels of arachidonic acid and total free fatty acids were increased in the flunarizine group. The authors concluded that significantly improved histological outcome after flunarizine was unrelated to changes in free fatty acids and energy metabolites.[16,41]

Two studies have examined the effects of flunarizine on transmitter release postischemia. Govoni *et al.* studied release from striatal slices made 1 hour after exposure of Levine rats to nitrogen gas.[42] K^+-stimulated dopamine release was increased in controls, but normalized by po pretreatment with 40 mg/kg of flunarizine. Met-enkephalin immunoreactivity release was reduced in controls but normal in flunarizine-treated animals. This suggests that flunarizine protects the brain from disturbed transmitter release postinsult. In a further study flunarizine pretreatment (40 mg/kg divided over 3 injections) was given to 7-day-old rat pups with unilateral carotid ligation + exposure to 2 hours of 8% O_2.[43] At the end of the hypoxic period striatal slices were prepared. Dopamine turnover was increased in hypoxic controls (DA/HVA ratio) by 8 to 20 times, but was normal in the flunarizine group and in animals from the solvent group. Thus, normalization of DA turnover was solvent dependent, but unrelated to the better histological recovery seen in the flunarizine group.[43]

In monkeys subject to MCA, nimodipine pretreatment (0.6 $\mu g/kg$ per minute continuously) increased the threshold levels of flow, at which disturbances of ion homeostasis and cortical edema developed. The authors concluded that nimodipine interferes with cellular energy metabolism and increases susceptibility to ischemic damage.[44,45]

PY 108-068 has been studied on MCA occlusion in cats. Continuous treatment with PY 108-868, 0.2 μg/kg per minute iv led to a significant progressive increase in P_{O_2} values within the infarct area.[25]

HISTOLOGY

The advantage of histological assessment is that it can provide a quantitative regional count of the numbers of necrotic nerve and glial cells following an ischemic period. In both animals and humans secondary maturational neuronal damage has been demonstrated; histological models therefore tend to require longer survival periods.

Nimodipine is the only Ca^{2+} antagonist studied in GC ischemia that has been assessed histologically.[29] Steen *et al.* demonstrated that in monkeys subject to 17 minutes of ischemia, nimodipine (10 μg/kg iv + 1 μg/kg per minute for 10 hours) given 5 minutes postischemia significantly improved global histopathology 96 hours postischemia.[29]

In the Lund model (two-vessel occlusion + hypotension), flunarizine has been shown to significantly reduce pyramidal cell damage in the hippocampus, when given as a protectant or as a resuscitant. Pretreatment with flunarizine 40 mg/kg orally 24 hours and 4 hours before ischemia reduced the number of acidophilic pyramidal cells in CA_1 from 91% to 52% and in CA_3 from 29% to 1%, after a one week recovery period.[16,41] In the same model flunarizine was given as a resuscitant 5 minutes after the ischemic period (0.1 mg/kg iv) and 8 and 24 hours later (40 mg/kg orally). A decrease of approximately 50% in the number of necrotic CA_1 pyramidal cells was shown in the hippocampus after a 1 week survival period.[16,41,46] This beneficial effect was not related to improvement of CBF during the period of delayed hypoperfusion.[16,41] Nimodipine given at the same doses and the same time intervals did not improve the histological outcome.[46] The authors of the last study suggest that either the poor outcome with nimodipine was a result of a pronounced decrease of MAP postischemia or that interference with postischemic changes in microcirculation are insufficient to provide improved structural outcome, i.e., direct cellular effects may be responsible for the improvement seen after flunarizine, but not with this dose of nimodipine.

Although it is not strictly a model of GI ischemia, the Levine model of hypoxic-oligemic encephalopathy has been widely used for histological assessment. In this preparation, the right carotid artery is ligated and animals are intermittently exposed to 100% nitrogen 4 hours later. Oral pretreatment with flunarizine (10, 20, and 40 mg/kg—4 hours), or nicardipine (40 mg/kg—1 hour) significantly reduced damage to parietal cortex after a 24 hour survival period. Lower doses of nicardipine (1 and 10 mg/kg) or diltiazem (40 mg/kg—1 hour) had no effect.[11,47] The authors again speculate that direct neuronal effects are necessary to achieve an improved histological outcome.[47]

Finally, flunarizine has also been tested in a Levine-type model in immature rat pups pretreated with flunarizine (30 mg/kg ip). In this model the cross-sectional area of the hemisphere ipsilateral to the carotid ligation was 15% smaller to the contralateral side in the solvent group, but only 1% smaller in the flunarizine group. The authors conclude that flunarizine has potent neuroprotective properties against morphologic brain injury from hypoxia/ischemia.[43]

In the MCA occlusion models of focal ischemia, nimodipine is the only Ca^{2+} antagonist tested thus far. In the rat, 1 μg/kg per minute of nimodipine was given for 30 minutes before and 30 minutes after MCA occlusion. Histological assessment revealed that 3 hours postocclusion, the volume and extent of ischemic damage was reduced in the periphery but not the core of the lesion.[19] In a further study by the same group, nimodipine was given at the same dose from 5 minutes postocclusion until sacrifice 4 hours later. No difference could be found with respect to the volume of irreversible ischemic damage in cortex, caudate nucleus, or the hemisphere as a whole. The authors suggest that once flow has fallen below the levels to initiate ischemic damage in the penumbra zone, nimodipine is unable to reverse the sequence of events leading to damage.[20] Lastly, nimodipine has been studied in cats exposed to MCA occlusion. Drug treatment, 0.1 mg /kg per minute, was started 15 minutes before occlusion and continued for 3½ hours until sacrifice. The authors divided the drug-treated animals into groups in which MAP was less than, or greater than, 90 mmHg. The low-pressure group did not fare better than controls. However, the high-pressure group demonstrated some improvement. Even so, histological examination of the percentage of ischemic grey matter revealed 27.8 ± 4 in controls and 23.3 ± 9 in the high-pressure nimodipine group. This difference was not significant.[38]

DISCUSSION

The Ca^{2+} antagonists are quite heterogenous with respect to their chemical formulae and their pharmacological profile, both *in vitro*[48] and *in vivo*.[49] This heterogeneity is also evident from the variability of the results obtained when reviewing their antiischemic action. Only about 50 studies could be found dealing with Ca^{2+} -antagonists in animal models of ischemia. Thus, most of the drugs have not been examined in all the different forms of ischemia. Whether a compound is given as a protectant or resuscitant may play a crucial role in determining outcome. Further, the severity of insult, dose, and survival time are also critical factors influencing outcome. For example, nimodipine given before MCA occlusion protects against the ensuring hypoperfusion.[19] However, given 5 minutes after MCA occlusion it had no positive effects.[20] Comparison between studies is further hampered by differences in evaluation techniques for the same target. For instance for neurological-deficit scoring systems, some authors use very detailed scoring systems,[33] while others only allow very crude grading where mortality is considered as a maximum deficit.[28]

The targets against which we have examined the effects of Ca^{2+} antagonists are to some extent hierarchical. Survival after an ischemic insult is of highest priority. From the five reviewed studies[14,23–26] it seems that preinsult treatment with Ca^{2+} antagonists enhances survival rates in both global and focal ischemia models, irrespective of the species used. Postinsult neurological deficit has been studied almost exclusively in global ischemia where in general some amelioration of neurlogical deficit was observed. The third most important target is limitation of the number of necrotic neurons postinsult. The majority of studies in which histological damage has been assessed after treatment with Ca^{2+} antagonists are positive. GI ischemia is the most widely studied. It is suggested that direct neuronal effects are necessary to achieve an improved histological outcome.[16,41,47]

It is generally assumed that normalization of postinsult CBF is a prerequisite for a favorable outcome. This is clearly the case in most of the studies involving vasospasm. In nearly all cases Ca^{2+} antagonists antagonized the spasm and restored flow. There are several examples in the presently reviewed studies where there is a dissociation between the results on CBF and the outcome. For example in the study by Deshpande and Wieloch pre- or posttreatment with flunarizine had no effect on CBF but improved histological outcome.[16,41] A far-reaching conclusion to be derived from the dissociation between CBF and histological outcome is that the posthypoperfusion phenomenon does not play a significant role in the pathogenesis of irreversible brain damage.[16] A conclusion along the same lines was formulated by Dean *et al.,* who found that lidoflazine did not alter CBF, and thus that there is no support for "perfusion preservation as a mechanism of amelioration of neurologic injury after ischemia."[18]

Recovery of EEG is generally correlated with improvement of CBF. Therefore, changes in EEG patterns cannot be considered as measurements of neuronal integrity, since changes in CBF are only poorly correlated with neurological or histological outcome.

In general, biochemical measures were made very soon after the insult. As yet there is no measured biochemical variable that correlates with outcome.

In conclusion, the presently reviewed studies make it obvious that in animal models some amelioration of the results of ischemia is seen after treatment with Ca^{2+} antagonists. The single largest shortcoming is the absence of long-term survival studies in which the majority of the targets are examined. The existence of secondary maturational neuronal damage means that at least most histological studies employ a longer survival period, e.g., one week. The problem with most presently used histological models is the absence of major neurological deficit in the reperfusion period. Further clarification of the role of Ca^{2+} antagonists in brain ischemia can only be expected when large-scale, standardized, joint studies are performed after long survival periods in models with significant neurological deficit.

REFERENCES

1. Safar, P. 1984. Recent advances in cardiopulmonary cerebral resuscitation: a review. Ann. Emerg. Med. **13:** 856–861.
2. Siesjo, B. K. 1981. Cell damage in the brain. A speculative synthesis. J. Cereb. Blood Flow Metab. **1:** 155–185.
3. Wieloch, T. & B. K. Siesjo. 1982. Ischemic brain injury: the importance of calcium, lipolytic activities and free fatty acids. Pathol. Biol. **30:** 269–277.
4. Wauquier, A. & D. Ashton. 1985. Pharmacological approaches to the study of brain hypoxia. Mol. Physiol. **8:** 565–575.
5. Bazan, N. G., Jr. 1970. Effect of ischemia and electroconvulsive shock on free fatty acid pool in the brain. Biochim. Biophys. Acta **218:** 1–10.
6. Rehncrona, S., B. K. Siesjo & D. S. Smith. 1980. Reversible ischemia of the brain: biochemical factors influencing restitution. Acta Physiol. Scand. Suppl. **492:** 135–140.
7. Harris, R. J. 1977. The uptake and release of calcium by heart mitochondria. J. Biochem. **168:** 447–456.
8. Chan, P. H. & R. A. Fishman. 1978. Brain edema: induction in cortical slices by polyunsaturated fatty acids. Science **201:** 358–360.
9. Chan, P. H. & R. A. Fishman. 1980. Transient formation of superoxide radicals in polyunsaturated fatty acid–induced brain swelling. J. Neurochem. **35:** 1004–1007.
10. Rhoads, D. E., M. A. Kaplan, N. A. Peterson & E. Raghupathy. 1982. Effects of free fatty acids on synaptosomal amino acid uptake systems. J. Neurochem. **38:** 1255–1260.
11. van Reempts, J. & M. Borgers. 1985. Ischemic brain injury and cell calcium: morphologic and therapeutic aspects. Ann. Emerg. Med. **14:** 736–742.
12. Edmonds, H. L., Jr., A. Wauquier, W. Melis, W. A. E. van den Broeck, J. van Loon & P. A. J. Janssen. 1985. Improved short-term neurological recovery with flunarizine in a canine model of cardiac arrest. Am. J. Emerg. Med. **3:** 150–155.
13. Newberg, L. A., P. A. Steen, J. H. Milde & J. D. Michenfelder. 1984. Failure of *flunarizine* to improve cerebral blood flow or neurologic recovery in a canine model of complete cerebral ischemia. Stroke **15:** 666–671.

14. MARRANNES, R., H. L. EDMONDS, JR., A. WAUQUIER, W. MELIS & J. VAN LOON. 1986. Measurement of ischemic changes in cerebral blood flow by the hydrogen clearance technique and brain cortical temperature. Influence of flunarizine. Arch. Int. Pharmacodyn. Ther. **281:** 209–229.
15. WAUQUIER, A., G. CLINCKE, W. A. E. VAN DEN BROECK, C. HERMANS, W. MELIS & J. VAN LOON. 1984. Global incomplete ischemia in dogs assessed by quantitative EEG analysis. Effects of hypnotics and flunarizine. *In* Quantitative EEG and Imagine Techniques in Brain Ischemia. J. Pfurtscheller, E. J. Jonkman & F. H. Lopes da Silva, Eds.: 217–233. Elsevier Biomedical Press. Amsterdam, Holland.
16. DESHPANDE, J. K. & T. WIELOCH. 1986. *Flunarizine,* a calcium entry blocker, ameliorates ischemic brain damage in the rat. Anesthesiology **64:** 215–224.
17. WHITE, B. C., C. D. WINEGAR, R. F. WILSON & G. S. KRAUSE. 1983. Calcium blockers in cerebral resuscitation. J. Trauma **23:** 788–794.
18. DEAN, J. M., P. J. HOEHNER, M. C. ROGERS & R. J. TRAYSTMAN. 1984. Effect of *lidoflazine* on cerebral blood flow following twelve minutes total cerebral ischemia. Stroke **15:** 531–535.
19. MOHAMED, A. A., O. GOTOH, D. I. GRAHAM, K. A. OSBORNE, J. MCCULLOCH, A. D. MENDELOW, G. M. TEASDALE & A. M. HARPER. 1985. Effect of pretreatment with the calcium antagonist nimodipine on local cerebral blood flow and histopathology after middle cerebral artery occlusion. Ann. Neurol. **18:** 705–711.
20. GOTOH, O., A. A. MOHAMED, J. MCCULLOCH, D. I. GRAHAM, A. M. HARPER & G. M. TEASDALE. 1986. Nimodipine and the haemodynamic and histopathological consequences of middle cerebral artery occlusion in the rat. J. Cereb. Blood Flow Metab. **6:** 321–331.
21. LEBLANC, R., W. FEINDEL, L. Y. YAMAMOTO, J. G. MILTON, M. M. FROJMOVIC & C. P. HODGE. 1984. The effects of calcium antagonism on the epicerebral circulation in early vasopasm. Stroke **15:** 1017–1020.
22. LEBLANC, R., W. FEINDEL, L. YAMAMOTO, J. G. MILTON & M. M. FROJMOVIC. 1984. Reversal of acute experimental cerebral vasospasm by calcium antagonism with verapamil. Can. J. Neurol. Sci. **11:** 42–47.
23. HOFFMEISTER, F., S. KAZDA & H. P. KRAUSE. 1979. Influence of nimodipine (Bay e 9736) on the postischaemic changes of brain function. Acta Neurol. Scand. **60**(Suppl. 72): 358–359.
24. HOFFMEISTER, F., U. BENZ, A. HEISE, H. P. KRAUSE & V. NEUSER. 1982. Behavioral effects of nimodipine in animals. Arzneim. Forsch. Drug Res. **32:** 347–360.
25. WIERNSPERGER, N., P. GYGAX & A. HOFMANN. 1984. Calcium antagonist PY 108-068: demonstration of its efficacy in various types of experimental brain ischemia. Stroke **15:** 679–685.
26. HERMANS, C., R. DE REESE, J. VAN LOON, W. LOOTS & A. H. M. JAGENEAU. 1982. A cardiac arrest model in rats for evaluating the antihypoxic action of flunarizine. Eur. J. Pharmacol. **81:** 137–140.
27. FUJISAWA, A., M. MATSUMOTO, T. MATSUYAMA, H. UEDA, A. WANAKA, S. YONEDA, K. KIMURA & T. KAMADA. 1986. The effect of the calcium antagonist nimodipine on the gerbil model of experimental cerebral ischemia. Stroke **17:** 748–752.
28. STEEN, P. A., L. A. NEWBERG, J. H. MILDE & J. D. MICHENFELDER. 1984. Cerebral blood flow and neurologic outcome when nimodipine is given after complete cerebral ischemia in the dog. J. Cereb. Blood Flow Metab. **4:** 82–87.
29. STEEN, P. A., S. E. GISVOLD, J. H. MILDE, L. A. NEWBERG, B. W. SCHEITHAUER, W. L. LANIER & J. D. MICHENFELDER. 1985. Nimodipine improves outcome when given after complete cerebral ischemia in primates. Anesthesiology **62:** 406–414.
30. LANZA, R. P., D. K. C. COOPER & C. N. BARNARD. 1983. Lack of efficacy of high-dose verapamil in preventing brain damage in baboons and pigs after prolonged partial cerebral ischemia. Am. J. Emerg. Med. **2:** 481–485.
31. WAUQUIER, A., H. L. EDMONDS, JR., W. A. E. VAN DEN BROECK, W. MELIS & J. VAN LOON. 1985. Effects of flunarizine on recovery of cerebral function following cardiac arrest. Neuropsychobiology **13:** 147–151.
32. WAUQUIER, A., D. ASHTON, C. HERMANS & G. CLINCKE. 1983. Pharmacological effects in

protective and resuscitative models of brain hypoxia. *In* Brain Protection. K. Wiedeman & S. Hoyer, Eds.: 100–121. Springer-Verlag. Berlin, FRG.

33. WINEGAR, C. P., O. HENDERSON, B. C. WHITE, R. E. JACKSON, T. O'HARA, D. N. VIGOR, R. KONTRY, B. WILSON & C. SHELBY-LANE. 1983. Early amelioration of neurologic deficit by lidoflazine after fifteen minutes of cardiopulmonary arrest in dogs. Ann. Emerg. Med. **12:** 471–477.
34. HOSSMANN, K. A., W. PASCHEN & L. CSIBA. 1983. Relationship between calcium accumulation and recovery of cat brain after prolonged cerebral ischemia. J. Cereb. Blood Flow Metab. **3:** 346–353.
35. MABE, H., H. NAGAI, T. TAKAGI, S. UMEMURA & M. OHNO. 1986. Effect of nimodipine on cerebral functional and metabolic recovery following ischemia in the rat brain. Stroke **17:** 501–505.
36. SMITH, M., E. KAGSTROM, I. ROSEN & B. K. SIESJO. 1983. Effect of the calcium antagonist nimodipine on the delayed hypoperfusion following incomplete ischemia in the rat. J. Cereb. Blood Flow Metab. **3:** 543–546.
37. DATE, H. & K. A. HOSSMANN. 1984. Effect of vasodilating drugs on intracortical and extracortical vascular resistance following middle cerebral artery occlusion in cats. Ann. Neurol. **16:** 330–336.
38. BARNETT, G. H., B. BOSE, J. R. LITTLE, S. C. JONES & H. T. FRIEL. 1986. Effects of nimodipine on acute focal cerebral ischemia. Stroke **17:** 884–890.
39. STEEN, P. A., J. H. MILDE & J. D. MICHENFELDER. 1978. Cerebral metabolic and vascular effects of barbiturate therapy following complete global ischemia. J. Neurochem. **31:** 1317–1324.
40. HEFFEZ, D. S. & J. V. PASSONNEAU. 1985. Effect of nimodipine on cerebral metabolism during ischemia and recirculation in the mongolian gerbil. J. Cereb. Blood Flow Metab. **5:** 523–528.
41. DESPHANDE, J. K. & T. WIELOCH. 1985. Amelioration of ischaemic brain damage by postischaemic treatment with flunarizine. Neurol. Res. **7:** 27–29.
42. GOVONI, S., M. TRABUCCHI, M. S. MAGNONI, F. BATTAINI & R. PAOLETTI. 1985. Abnormal neurotransmitter release and calcium entry blockers. *In* Calcium Entry Blockers and Tissue protection.T. Godfraind, P. M. Vanhoutte, S. Govoni & R. Paoletti, Eds.: 151–162. Raven Press. New York, N.Y.
43. SILVERSTEIN, F. S., K. BUCHANAN, C. HUDSON & M. V. JOHNSTON. 1986. *Flunarizine* limits hypoxia-ischemia induced morphologic injury in immature rat brain. Stroke **17:** 477–482.
44. SYMON, L., R. J. HARRIS & N. M. BRANSTON. 1982. Calcium ions and calcium antagonists in ischaemia. Acta Neurochir. **63:** 267–275.
45. HARRIS, R. J., N. M. BRANSTON, L. SYMON, M. BAYHAN & A. WATSON. 1982. The effects of a calcium antagonist, nimodipine, upon physiological responses of the cerebral vasculature and its possible influence upon focal cerebral ischaemia. Stroke **13:** 759–766.
46. VAN REEMPTS, J., M. HASELDONCKX, B. VAN DEUREN, L. WOUTERS & M. BORGERS. 1986. Structural damage of the ischemic brain: involvement of calcium and effects of postischemic treatment with calcium entry blockers. Drug. Dev. Res. **8:** 387–395.
47. VAN REEMPTS, J., M. BORGERS, L. VAN DAEL, L. VAN EYNDHOVEN & M. VAN DE VEN. 1983. Protection with flunarizine against hypoxic-ischaemic damage of the rat cerebral cortex. A quantitative morphologic assessment. Arch. Int. Pharmacodyn. Ther. **262:** 76–88.
48. VAN NUETEN, J. M. 1982. Selectivity of calcium entry blockers. *In* Calcium Modulators. A. Albertini & R. Paoletti, Eds.: 199–208. Elsevier Biomedial Press. Amsterdam, Holland.
49. WAUQUIER, A., D. ASHTON, G. CLINCKE & J. FRANSEN. 1985. Calcium entry blockers as cerebral protecting agents: comparative activity in tests of hypoxia and hyperexcitability. Jpn. J. Pharmacol. **38:** 1–7.
50. KAZDA, S., B. GARTHOFF, H. P. KRAUSE & K. SCHLOSSMANN. 1982. Cerebrovascular effects of the calcium antagonistic dihydropyridine derivative nimodipine in animal experiments. Arzneim. Forsch. Drug Res. **32:** 331–338.
51. GIOIA, A. E., R. P. WHITE, B. BAKHTIAN & J. T. ROBERTSON. 1985. Evaluation of the

efficacy of intrathecal nimodipine in canine models of chronic cerebral vasospasm. J. Neurosurg. **62:** 721–728.

52. TANAKA, K., F. GOTOH, F. MURAMATSU, Y. FUKUUCHI, H. OKAYASU, N. SUZUKI & M. KOBARI. 1982. Effect of nimodipine, a calcium antagonist, on cerebral vasospasm after subarachnoid hemorrhage in cats. Arzneim. Forsch. Drug Res. **32:** 1529–1534.
53. VOLDBY, B., O. F. PETERSEN, M. BUHL, P. JAKOBSEN & R. OSTERGAARD. 1984. Reversal of cerebral arterial spasm by intrathecal administration of a calcium antagonist (nimodipine). Acta Neurochir. **70:** 243–254.
54. ESPINOSA, F., B. WEIR, T. OVERTON, W. CASTOR, M. GRACE & D. BOISVERT. 1984. A randomized placebo-controlled double-blind trial of nimodipine after SAH in monkeys. I. Clinical and radiological findings. J. Neurosurg. **60:** 1167–1175.
55. NOSKO, M., B. WEIR, C. KRUEGER, D. COOK, D. PHIL, S. NORRIS, T. OVERTON & D. BOISVERT. 1985. Nimodipine and chronic vasospasm in monkeys. I. Clinical and radiological findings. Neurosurgery **16:** 129–140.
56. BRANDT, L., B. LJUNGGREN, K. ANDERSSON, L. EDVINSSON, E. MACKENZIE, A. TAMURA & G. TEASDALE. 1983. Effects of topical application of a calcium antagonist (nifedipine) on feline cortical pial microvasculature under normal conditions and in focal ischemia. J. Cereb. Blood Flow Metab. **3:** 44–50.
57. VARSOS, V. G., T. M. LISZCZAK, D. H. HAN, J. P. KISTLER, J. VIELMA, P. MCL BLACK, R. C. HEROS & N. T. ZERVAS. 1983. Delayed cerebral vasospasm is not reversible by aminophylline, nifedipine, or papaverine in a "two-hemorrhage" canine model. J. Neurosurg. **58:** 11–17.
58. ZABRAMSKI, J., R. F. SPETZLER & C. BONSTELLE. 1986. Chronic cerebral vasospasm: effect of calcium antagonists. Neurosurgery **18:** 129–135.
59. ALLAN, G. S. & A. BAHR. 1979. Cerebral arterial spasms. X. Reversal of acute and chronic spasm in dogs with orally administered nifedipine. Neurosurgery **4:** 43–47.
60. HOLLER, M., H. DIERKING, K. DENGLER, F. TEGTMEIER & T. PETERS. 1986. Effect of flunarizine on extracellular ion concentration in the rat brain under hypoxia and ischemia. Raven Press **32:** 229–236.
61. TAKAYASU, M., Y. SUZUKI, M. SHIBUYA, T. ASANO, M. KANAMORI, T. OKADA, N. KAGEYAMA & H. HIDAKA. 1986. The effects of HA compound calcium antagonists on delayed cerebral vasospasm in dogs. J. Neurosurg. **65:** 80–85.

Pharmacological Basis and Therapeutic Efficacy of Flunarizine in Peripheral Artery Disease

T. DI PERRI, F. LAGHI PASINI, S. PECCHI, L. DOMINI, L. RALLI, M. MATERAZZI, V. DE FRANCO, A. MONACI, AND L. CECCATELLI

Institute of Medical Pathology
University of Siena
Policlinico "Le Scotte"
53100 Siena, Italy

In the last few years we have accumulated some evidence that calcium entry blockers could interfere with an endogenous purinergic mechanism, namely, with membrane adenosine receptors.[1-3] This property seemed to be shared by different groups of such drugs, independently from their chemical structure, thus opening new questions on the molecular mechanism of action.[2-4] Among these substances, first flunarizine and then dihydropyridines claimed our attention, and now we want to summarize the findings of our studies, not following the logical development of the adenosine hypothesis in our mind, but assembling our data according to the type of experimental design. In this paper the thread of the argument implies a continuous hypothetical comparison with the adenosine system. Our studies dealt with clinical pharmacological investigations on the circulatory activity of flunarizine either in control subjects or in peripheral obliterative arterial disease (POAD) patients. The design of the study included the plethysmographic investigation of the leg hemodynamics after flunarizine infusion and after treatment with drugs that either block adenosine receptors, such as theophylline, or inhibit adenosine uptake, such as dipyridamole. Finally a cellular model was approached to clarify a possible interference of calcium entry blocker with adenosine at the membrane receptor level.

CLINICAL PHARMACOLOGICAL STUDY

Twenty patients [18 males and 2 females, aged from 47 to 69, with a mean age of 60 ± 5.8 standard deviation (SD)] suffering from peripheral obliterative arterial disease (Fontaine's II stage) and 20 sex- and age-matched control subjects were selected for the study. The lower limb blood flow at the calf level in supine position was measured by means of a strain gauge plethysmograph (Periflow Janssen).

The resting flow and the peak flow after 3 minutes of ischemia were determined. Flunarizine [10 mg intravenously (IV)] was injected over 2 minutes, and hemodynamic parameters were controlled during 360 minutes. Heart rate and systemic arterial blood pressure were also registered. The effects of theophylline and dipyridamole infusion (300 μg/kg per minute and 200 μg/kg per minute IV respectively) on lower limb peak flow in 10 normal subjects were also tested, in order to evaluate the role of adenosine in the hyperemic response. Finally the acute infusion of flunarizine

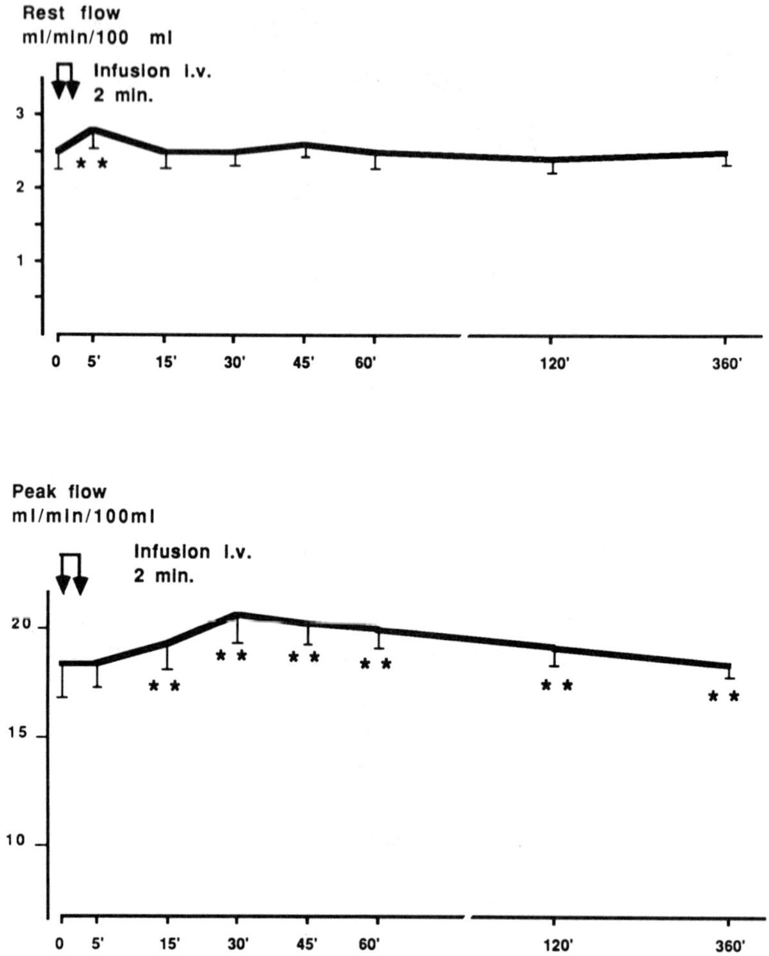

FIGURE 1. Effect of a single intravenous infusion of 10 mg flunarizine on rest flow and peak flow of lower limbs in normal subjects. Mean ± standard error (SE), n = 20, **p < 0.01. Statistical analysis was performed by means of the Student t test for paired data.

(10 mg iv in 2 minutes) was repeated in 10 normal subjects during a continuous infusion of dipyridamole (200 μg/kg per minute). In normal subjects the infusion of flunarizine induced a statistically significant but quantitatively slight increase of rest flow at the 5th minute which rapidly returned to basal values within 15 minutes (FIGURE 1). A significant increase of peak flow was observed between 15 and 30 minutes after the infusion (FIGURE 1). This effect was long lasting since a significant activity was still present at the 6th hour. Similar findings were obtained in patients with peripheral obliterative arterial disease with a more prolonged effect on resting flow (FIGURE 2). The delayed prolonged effect on peak flow was also confirmed

(FIGURE 2). Flunarizine did not induce any change in blood arterial pressure and in heart rate

The iv infusion of theophylline was followed by a relevant reduction of post-ischaemic first flow whereas dipyridamole was able to increase the peak flow significantly (FIGURE 3). These findings seem to suggest the hypothesis that adenosine may be involved in the physiological regulation of the postischemic hyperemia; in fact drugs such as methylxantines and dipyridamole are able to influence postischaemic response as theoretically expected on the basis of their pharmacological effect on adenosine function and metabolism. Theophylline, a specific receptor antagonist, is known to antagonize physiological activity of the adenosine system, whereas dipyridamole shows an opposite action since it is able to potentiate adenosine effect by blocking cellular uptake and then increasing extracellular concentration. Accordingly theophylline and dipyridamole worked in an opposite manner on peak flow in which a positive

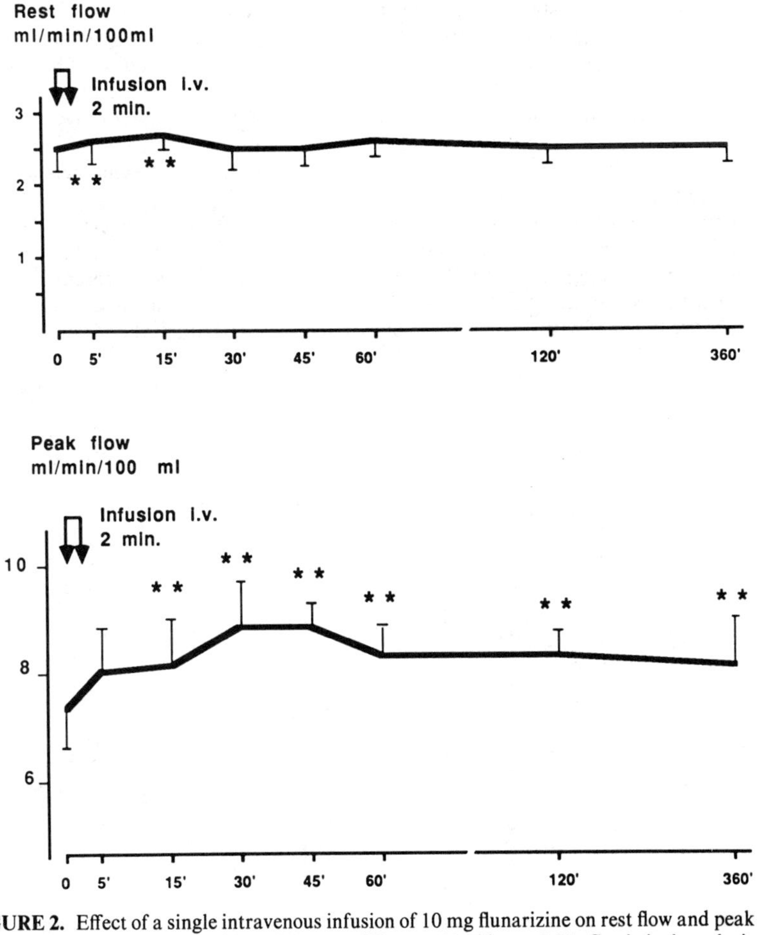

FIGURE 2. Effect of a single intravenous infusion of 10 mg flunarizine on rest flow and peak flow of lower limbs in POAD patients. Mean ± SE, $n = 20$, $^{**}p < 0.01$. Statistical analysis was performed by means of the Student t test for paired data.

role for adenosine has been suggested.[1] The iv infusion of flunarizine, while it was scarcely active on rest flow, was able to increase the peak flow significantly in normal as well as in POAD patients, and this effect was partially canceled by theophylline, thus possibly suggesting that the pharmacological effect of flunarizine may be mediated via an endogenous adenosine involvement. The observation of Snider and Murphy that nifedipine may antagonize adenosine at the membrane receptor level in smooth muscle cells[4] can be in accordance with the phenomenological results obtained in the study of the hemodynamic effects of flunarizine. Moreover evidence has recently been obtained in man that adenosine is able to block supraventricular arrhythmias, as is well known for some calcium entry blockers.[5,6] The complex interrelationships between the adenosine system and cellular calcium transport and availability are confirmed by the findings obtained with nerve terminal membrane. In fact it has been suggested that blockade of nerve terminal Ca^{2+} channels by extracellular adenosine is responsible for the inhibitory effects of adenosine and its congeners on the secretion of neurotransmitter substances.[7-11] The simplest suggestion is that a plasma membrane Ca^{2+} binding protein is structurally linked to the adenosine receptor.[7,8]

In another cellular system represented by ghost red blood cells, adenosine and inosine have been shown to be potent inhibitors of (^{3}H)-nimodipine binding in steady-state saturation experiments.[12] In particular, Glossmann and co-workers have demonstrated that the high-capacity, low-affinity sites for 1,4-dihydropyridines are linked to the nucleoside carrier (adenosine uptake system) not only in the red blood cell but in other tissues as well. They also suggest that the carrier and the channels sensitive to calcium entry blockers could be structurally related.[12,13]

In order to add some other evidence to the hypothesis of a close correlation between the adenosine system and calcium entry affecting drugs, a cellular model consisting of polymorphonuclear leucocytes (PMNs) was developed. PMNs represent a useful experimental tool to investigate definite cellular functions and the effects of different drugs. Since divalent cations have been shown to play a determinant regulatory role in

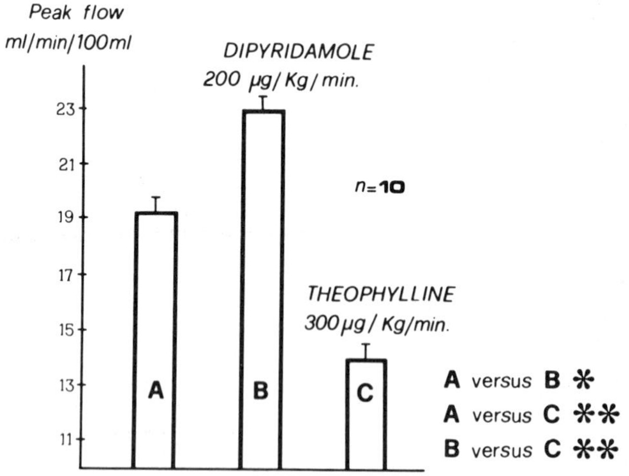

FIGURE 3. Effect of the iv infusion of dipyridamole or theophylline on peak flow in normal subjects. The postischemic hyperemia (3 minutes of ischemia) was measured at the end of 30 minutes infusion.

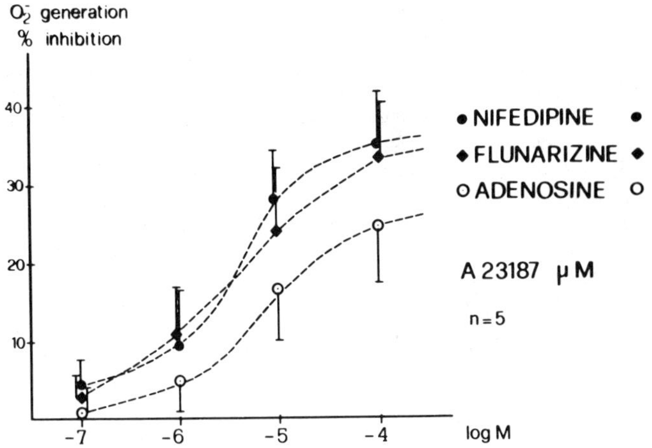

FIGURE 4. Effect of nifedipine, flunarizine, and adenosine on A 23187–induced O_2^- generation in human neutrophils (mean ± SE). O_2^- generation was quantified by the spectrophotometrical assay of the superoxide dismutase–inhibitable reduction of ferricytochrome C. The effect of drugs is expressed as percent inhibition of control sample (A 23187–stimulated and untreated neutrophils).

the expression of PMN functions, the study on the action of drugs active on membrane cation transport may be approached with such a cellular system.[14,15]

CELLULAR STUDY

Effect of Adenosine and Calcium Entry Blockers (Nifedipine and Flunarizine) on PMN Activation

A neutrophil-enriched suspension was obtained as described elsewhere.[16] The cellular activation was stimulated either by the synthetic chemoattractant oligopeptide FMLP or the divalent cation ionophore A 23187 or the phorbol myristate acetate (PMA). While the activation induced by A 23187 is completely dependent on extracellular calcium concentration and Ca^{2+} entrance, FMLP-stimulated activation is only slightly affected by extracellular Ca^{2+}, being dependent on membrane-associated Ca^{2+} availability; finally PMA-induced activation is completely independent from either extracellular or intracellular Ca^{2+} changes.[17] Accordingly the neutrophil activation by A 23187 can be considered as a specific model for the pharmacological approach to the control of intracellular calcium entrance. Adenosine only slightly affected FMLP-induced PMN activation (enzyme release and free radical formation); it did not influence PMA-dependent but it markedly inhibited A23187-induced activation.[18] The increase of Ca^{2+} concentrations in the suspension medium (from 0.5 mM to 1.5–2.0 mM) reduced the inhibitory effect of adenosine on enzyme release (lysozyme and beta-glucuronidase) and on free radical formation (superoxide anion generation and chemiluminescence), thus showing that high extracellular concentrations of Ca^{2+} are able to overwhelm adenosine activity.[18] Similar findings were observed with flunarizine and nifedipine,[19] thus confirming, in this cellular model, a phenomenological similarity between adenosine and calcium entry blockers (FIGURES 4–6).

The pretreatment of PMNs with theophylline (10^{-5} M) was able to antagonize the inhibitory effect of adenosine as previewed on the basis of its antagonistic role at the receptor level. Very interestingly theophylline, at the same final concentration, was shown to prevent calcium entry blocker effect as well (FIGURES 7–9).

Such findings could possibly be explained in terms of an endogenously released adenosine mediator of calcium entry blocker activity or in terms of a structurally linked analogy between adenosine receptor and Ca^{2+} channel binding site as previously discussed.

Such a problem has been further approached by means of a sophisticated physicochemical technique, ^{1}H-NMR spectroscopy, in order to obtain a major insight into the interrelationships between adenosine and calcium entry blocker at the membrane level.

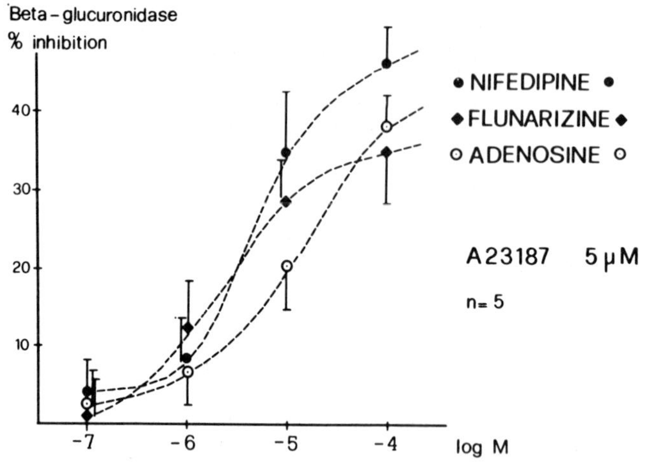

FIGURE 5. Effect of nifedipine, flunarizine, and adenosine on A 23187–induced beta-glucuronidase release in human neutrophils (mean ± SE). Beta-glucuronidase as a marker of the primary granule exocytosis was determined after 18 hours incubation with phenolphthalein glucuronic acid as substrate (beta-glucuronidase, Sigma Chemical Company). Total enzyme activities were determined in a simultaneously run duplicate reaction mixture, in which rupture of the cells was obtained with Triton X 100, 0.17%.

^{1}H-NMR Spectroscopy Study

It is known that investigations of binding interactions of a small molecule with some macromolecular receptor are suitably approached by detecting receptor-induced changes in the selective relaxation rate of any given spin system within the small molecule.[20] The NMR measurements were performed with an XL-200 NMR spectrometer (Varian Associates, Inc. Palo Alto, Calif). The methodology, the theoretical basis, and the detailed data are largely discussed elsewhere.[2,3,20] Here the findings obtained can be summarized as follows: (1) a binding interaction was detected by measuring nuclear relaxation rates of selected protons of flunarizine in the presence of neutrophils; (2) the binding, though not thoroughly delineated, involved different

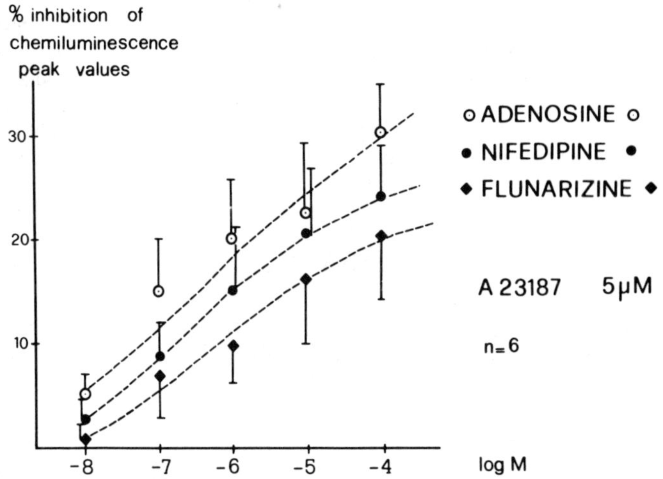

FIGURE 6. Effect of nifedipine, flunarizine, and adenosine on A 23187–induced chemiluminescence of human neutrophils (mean ± SE). Chemiluminescence enhanced by lumanol was measured by a Biocounter (Model M 2010 Luman BK).

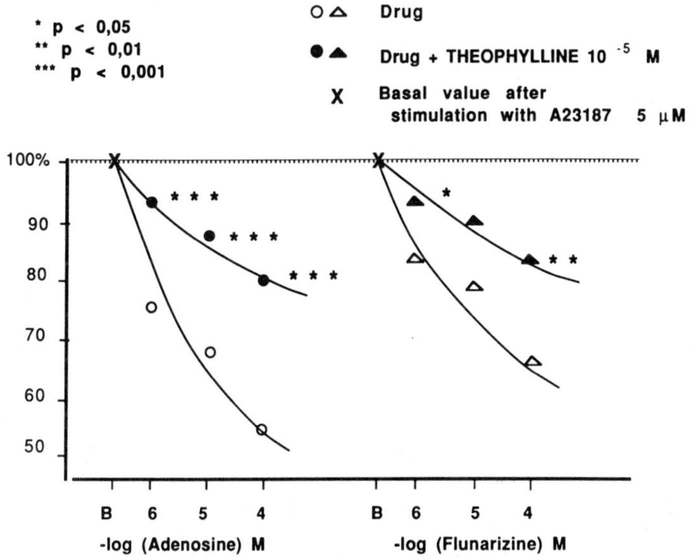

FIGURE 7. A 23187–dependent lysozyme release in human PMNs ($n = 5$). Lysozyme, as marker of the specific and primary granule exocitosis, was measured as the rate of *Micrococcus lysoideicticus* lysis at 546 nm (Testomar-Lysozyme Behringerwerke). The release of lysozyme from A 23187–stimulated and untreated neutrophils was considered as 100%. Theophylline was added to neutrophil suspension with adenosine or flunarizine 10 minutes before the addition of A 23187.

moieties of flunarizine to almost the same extent; (3) the presence of adenosine as a cosolute caused displacement of flunarizine molecules from the bound site in a concentration-dependent fashion.[2,3] Similar, unpublished data were obtained with nimodipine. From the physiological point of view it is important to underline that the endogenous mediator adenosine affects binding of flunarizine to the neutrophil surface. Such an effect could be due to a real competition at the same site as for calcium entry blockers or at a nearly site.

THERAPEUTIC EFFICACY

According to clinical pharmacological premises, a clinical trial to determine the effect of long-term treatment with flunarizine in POAD patients was planned. The

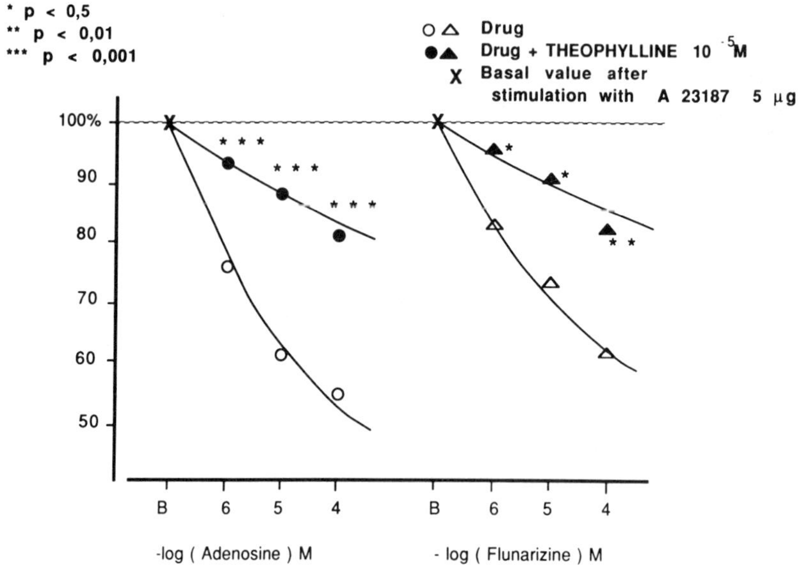

FIGURE 8. A 23187–dependent beta-glucuronidase release in human PMNs ($n = 5$). (See legends to FIGURES 5 and 7.)

study was made in 60 outpatients affected by POAD at stage II: 42 males and 18 females, aged from 44 to 70; mean age 58.0 ± 8.0 for the placebo group and 56.5 ± 7.3 for the flunarizine group (difference not statistically significant). All the patients were smokers and showed a pain-free walking distance of 50–300 m. The extent of vascular insufficiency was evaluated by means of a strain gauge plethysmography. The following patients were excluded from the study:

- Recently acute cerebral or myocardial infarction (<6 months).
- Treated diabetes or arterial hypertension.
- Heart, hepatic, or renal failure.
- Recent vascular surgery (<6 months).

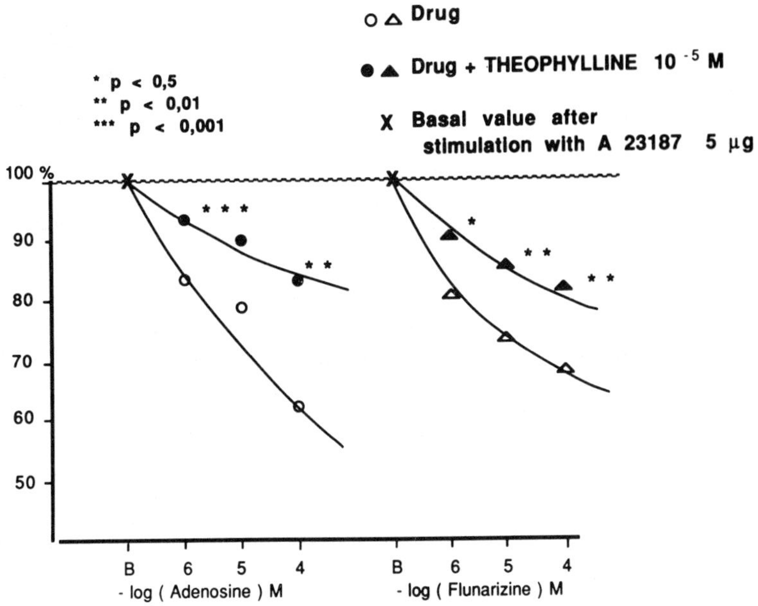

FIGURE 9. A 23187–induced O_2^- production in human PMNs ($n = 5$). (See legends to FIGURES 4 and 7.)

No concomitant drug intake was allowed during the study. Walking distance was measured by a treadmill test [at the speed of 1.5 m/second (3.5 miles/hour) at horizontal level]. The treadmill test was repeated in every patient until the walking distance measured during three sessions on different days remained unchanged. This value was considered as the starting level. After the first test, the patients were randomly allocated into two groups; after a run-in single-blind placebo period of six weeks, the double-blind study with placebo (15 mg of phenobarbital/day) or flunarizine (10 mg/day) was started.

Walking distance was measured after a single-blind run-in period and at the end of a double-blind study. Statistical analysis was performed using Student's t test for paired data. The results are summarized in TABLE 1. They show that there are no

TABLE 1. Walking Distance Values (Mean ± SD) Registered in the Flunarizine (D, E, F) and Placebo (A, B, C) Groups at Admission, after the Run-in Single-Blind Placebo Period, and at the End of the Double-Blind Study[a]

(A) −6 weeks	(B) basal	(C) +6 weeks	(D) −6 weeks	(E) basal	(F) +6 weeks
186.0 ± 68.7	188.6 ± 64.5	190.9 ± 63.3	183.1 ± 66.3	187.3 ± 56.9	278.5 ± 88.9
	t	p		t	p
A vs. B	0.06	NS	E vs. F	7.81	0.001
B vs. C	0.66	NS	B vs. E	0.147	NS
D vs. E	1.29	NS	C vs. F	4.396	0.001

[a]Statistical analysis was performed by means of Student's t test for paired data.

difference between the values registered before and after the run-in period in each group during the placebo administration. No significant difference was observed between the placebo and flunarizine groups at zero time. In flunarizine-treated patients, the pain-free distance after six weeks increased from 187.3 ± 56.9 to 278.5 ± 88.9: the difference was highly significant ($p < 0.001$). In the patients treted with placebo, the modification of walking distance was very small and not significant. The difference between placebo and flunarizine at the end of the treatment was highly significant ($p < 0.001$).

CONCLUSIONS

The final comment we can suggest is concerned with the starting hypothesis of this paper. The selective calcium entry blocker flunarizine does possess basic pharmacological activities supporting their hypothetical influence on pathophysiological mechanisms involved in the circulatory impairment. This is the basis of a clinical pharmacological study to test the possibility of the drug to modify in a theoretically useful way the hemodynamic profile of POAD patients. The finding that flunarizine acutely increases peak flow represents the rational background for extending the use of the drug to the therapeutic field. In clinical terms the pain-free walking distance is the main target to be looked for and it may be pathophysiologically correlated with the amount of the nutritive flow of muscle mass as possibly measured by reactive hyperemia after induced ischemia. In this respect a hemodynamic effect is associated with a clinical improvement and a significant correlation does exist. As regards the activity of a calcium entry blocker, namely, flunarizine, on different cellular models, our findings seem to support the hypothesis that some interrelationships exist between such drugs and the purinergic (adenosine) system. Recently much attention has been focused on interactions of humoral substances with calcium channels in membranes, especially in blood vessels.[4] There is abundant evidence that during ischemia in a variety of tissues, adenosine is released in concentrations sufficient to mediate vasodilation, particularly of coronary and cerebral blood vessels.[21] The effects of dipyridamole and theophylline on peak flow in normal subjects add more evidence, although indirect, that adenosine may be physiologically involved in the reactive hyperemia to ischemia. Alterations in calcium permeability mediate some of these effects of adenosine.[22] In our *in vitro* model, calcium entry blockers and adenosine share a calcium-dependent theophylline-sensitive inhibitory effect that could be explained in terms of a possible interference at the membrane level. This hypothesis is further suggested by the experimental evidence, by means of the ^{1}H-NMR spectroscopy study, that adenosine affects binding of flunarizine to the neutrophil surface. Such an effect could be due to a competition at the same site as for calcium entry blockers or at a nearby site allosterically linked. The hypothesis of a purine (adenosine) mediated activity of calcium entry blockers (flunarizine) does not preclude that some other mechanism may be involved as well. The role of flunarizine as a specific calmodulin inhibitor has also been determined,[23] and a possible multilevel regulatory effect of flunarizine on calcium entrance and availability and on Ca^{2+} calmodulin complex formation may be suggested.

REFERENCES

1. Di Perri, T., F. Laghi Pasini, S. Pecchi, R. Cappelli, L. Ralli & L. Domini. 1985. *In* Calcium Entry Blockers and Tissue Protection. T. Godfraind *et al.*, Eds.: 203–218. Raven Press. New York, N.Y.

2. LAGHI PASINI, F., A. ORRICO, P. L. CAPECCHI, A. L. PASQUI, L. CECCATELLI, T. DI PERRI, E. GAGGELLI & G. VALENSIN. The biological and clinical aspects of phagocyte function. Pergamon Prss. New York, N.Y. (In press.)
3. ORRICO, A., P. L. CAPECCHI, A. L. PASQUI, L. CECCATELLI, F. LAGHI PASINI & T. DI PERRI. 1986. Hematol. Rev. Commun. Abstr. (Suppl.) **1:** 58.
4. MURPHY, K. M. M. & S. H. SNIDER. 1983. *In* Ca^{++} Entry Blockers, Adenosine and Neurohormones. G. F. Merril & H. R. Weiss, Eds.: 295–306. Urban and Scharzberg.
5. GRECO, R., B. MUSTO, V. ARIENZO, A. ALBORINO, S. GAROFALO & F. MARISCO. 1982. Circ. Res. **66:** 504–508.
6. DI MARCO, J. P., T. D. SELLERS, R. M. BERNE, G. A. WEST & L. BELARDINELLI. 1983 Circ. Res. **68:** 1254–1263.
7. SILINSKY, E. M. 1986. Trends Pharmacol. Sci. **7**(5): 180–185.
8. SILINSKY, E. M. 1984. J. Physiol. London **246:** 243–256.
9. PHILLIS, J. W. & P. H. WU. 1982. *In* Trends in Autonomic Pharmacology. S. Kolsner, Ed. **2:** 237–261. Urban and Scharzenberg.
10. GINSBORG, G. L. & G. D. S. HIRST. 1972. J. Physiol. London **224:** 629–645.
11. RIBEIRO, J. A. & J. WALKER. 1975. Br. J. Pharmacol. **54:** 213–218.
12. GLOSSMANN, H., D. R. FERRY, F. LUBBECKE, R. MEWES & F. HOFMANN. 1982. Trends Pharmacol Sci. **3:** 431–437.
13. GLOSSMANN, H., D. R. FERRY, A. GOLL, J. STIESSNIG & G. ZERNIG. 1985. Arzneim. Forsch. Drug Res. **35**(II): 1917–1935.
14. WEISSMANN, G., H. M. KORCHAK, H. D. PEREZ, J. E. SMOLEN, I. M. GOLDSTEIN & S. T. HOFFSTEIN. 1979. J. Reticulo-Endothelical Soc. **26**(Suppl.): 687–692.
15. GALLIN, J. I. & A. S. ROSENTHAL. 1974. J. Cell Biol. **62:** 594–599.
16. LAGHI PASINI, F., A. L. PASQUI, L. CECCATELLI, P. L. CAPECCHI, A. ORRICO & T. DI PERRI. 1984. Tromb. Res. **35:** 527–537.
17. KORCHAK, H. M., K. VIENNE, L. E. RUTHERFORD & G. WEISSMANN. 1984. Fed. Proc. **43:** 2749–2755.
18. LAGHI PASINI, F., P. L. CAPECCHI, L. CECCATELLI, A. ORRICO, A. L. PASQUI & T. DI PERRI. 1986. Int. J. Immunother. **2**(3): 225–232.
19. DI PERRI, T., F. LAGHI PASINI, A. L. PASQUI, L. CECCATELLI, A. ORRICO & P. L. CAPECCHI. 1985. Int. J. Tissue React. **7**(4): 291–301.
20. VALENSIN, G., T. KUSHNIR & G. NAVON. 1982. J. Magn. Reson. **46:** 23–29.
21. BERNE, R. M. 1980. Circ. Res. **46:** 807–813.
22. OLSSON, R. A., E. M. KHOURI, J. L. BEDYNEK & J. MC LEAN. 1979. Circ. Res. **45:** 468–478.
23. VAN NUETEN, J. M., J. VAN BEEK & P. A. J. JANSSEN. 1978. Arzneim Forsch Drug Res. **28:** 2082–2087.

Ischemic Vasoconstriction and Parenchymal Brain pH

FREDRIC B. MEYER, THORALF M. SUNDT, JR., ROBERT E. ANDERSON, AND PHILLIP TALLY

Department of Neurosurgery
Mayo Foundation
Mayo Clinic
Rochester, Minnesota 55905

INTRODUCTION

Although it has generally been assumed that the liberation of lactic acid and other metabolites in areas of focal ischemia causes maximal vasodilatation, in actuality there is focal constriction of conducting vessels in core regions of ischemia. This ischemic vasoconstriction, sometimes termed secondary vasospasm, occurs with a temporal profile that can be related to ischemic changes of the underlying cortex.[1] The cause of this ischemic vasoconstriction is speculative, however; presented here is evidence that this phenomenon is related to the inability of ischemic smooth muscle to maintain a normal calcium gradient. It should be noted that other contributory causes of ischemic vasoconstriction include a rise in extracellular potassium, oxygen free radical injury to the endothelium, a reduction in the reuptake of norepinephrine at sympathetic synapses that terminate along penetrating arterioles, or release of vasospastic substances from ischemic tissue including serotonin.[2-6] All of these potential mechanisms reflect the rapid depletion of energy reserves in neuronal tissue under anaerobic conditions. This article however will concentrate on the potential role of calcium as the primary cause of ischemic vasoconstriction.

MICROCIRCULATORY CHANGES IN FOCAL INCOMPLETE CEREBRAL ISCHEMIA

The first microcirculatory change noted after major vessel occlusion is a darkening of the venous blood (FIGURE 1). Shortly thereafter there is a decrease in the velocity of flow of blood in both veins and venules with an aggregation of formed elements of blood.[7] This aggregation, which is often called particulate flow or sludging, results from a reduction in the shearing forces that tend to keep cells dispersed.[8] Consequently blood viscosity and resistance to flow increase. Measurements of the caliber of arteries and arterioles reveal an immediate slight increase. However at a variable time after vessel occlusion, corticol pallor develops, the earliest indication of severe ischemia. When this cortical pallor spreads to an area underlying an artery or arteriole, that vessel goes into vasoconstriction. This vasoconstriction is not simply the result of vascular collapse from lowered intraluminal pressure. In some instances this spasm becomes less severe with prolonged ischemia suggesting that there is fatigue of the constricting mechanisms of the arterial smooth muscle.

With restoration of flow to a region of ischemia, the aforementioned chain of events is reversed. The venous blood first becomes bright red, particulate flow in the venules is no longer observed, the cortex recolorizes, and finally the major vessels resume their normal caliber.[9] Often a true hyperemia develops with dilatation of conducting vessels in the cortex that were not noted in the normal state. This hyperemia is probably a function of vasomotor paralysis, partially a result of excessive lactic acidosis.[10]

THRESHOLDS OF CEREBRAL ISCHEMIA

The importance of ischemic vasoconstriction is that it may reduce potential collateral flow to jeopardized neurons during the period of major vessel occlusion. Normal tissue can accommodate to a substantial reduction in cerebral blood flow and still survive. Contrary to global ischemia, in which there is no collateral flow and irreversible neuronal damage occurs within four to eight minutes under normothermic conditions, in focal cerebral ischemia there is a potential for collateral flow.[11,12] Residual collateral flow may supply enough substrate so that neuronal basal energy requirements are satisfied.

In 1948, Kety and Schmidt first measured a normal cerebral blood flow (CBF) in humans of approximately 53 ml/100 per minute.[13] Some 25 years later two separate teams of investigators in Denmark and at the Mayo Clinic found, in patients undergoing carotid endarterectomy, that the threshold for brain electrical failure (attenuation in electroencephalograms) approximated 15 to 18 ml/100 g per minute.[14,15] Thereafter laboratory studies by Branston and associates showed that somatosensory evoked potentials were suppressed when CBF was less than 15 ml/100 g per minute.[16] Thus a threshold of electrical failure was quantitated at approximately 15 to 18 ml/100 g per minute.[17] In addition a threshold of ionic failure was substantiated at approximately 10 ml/100 g per minute.[18] At this reduced level of flow, investigators have demonstrated alterations in extracellular potassium and intracellular calcium, disturbances in brain water content, rapid depletion of adenosine triphosphate, and a profound intracellular acidosis.[19-21] This threshold of ionic failure is presumed to be a CBF at which irreversible neuronal damage rapidly occurs. Therefore between these two thresholds of electrical and ionic failure exists a small range of flow at which, despite functional loss, membrane homeostasis and structural integrity are maintained. This circumscribed range of CBF has been conceptualized in the term "ischemic penumbra" and explains why the potential for recovery exists in patients with acute focal ischemia if sufficient collateral flow is present to satisfy basal energy requirements.[22,23] Therein lies the importance of understanding the mechanism of ischemic vasoconstriction. Ischemic vasoconstriction may reduce residual CBF below this threshold for ionic failure and hasten neuronal demise.

EVIDENCE FOR THE ROLE OF CALCIUM IN ISCHEMIC VASOCONSTRICTION

We have studied the effects of the dihydropyridine calcium antagonist nimodipine when given both prior to and after middle cerebral artery occlusion in the white New Zealand rabbit.[24,25] Preliminary studies with this animal model have demonstrated that middle cerebral artery occlusion reliably produces cortical infarction similar to that observed in primates. The white New Zealand rabbit is a good model for the production of focal cerebral ischemia since the cerebral cortex is supplied solely by the internal carotid artery without contribution from the external carotid artery as found in dogs and cats.[26] The parameters that we assess during focal ischemia include measurements of cortical blood flow, intracellular brain pH, and electrocorticograms.

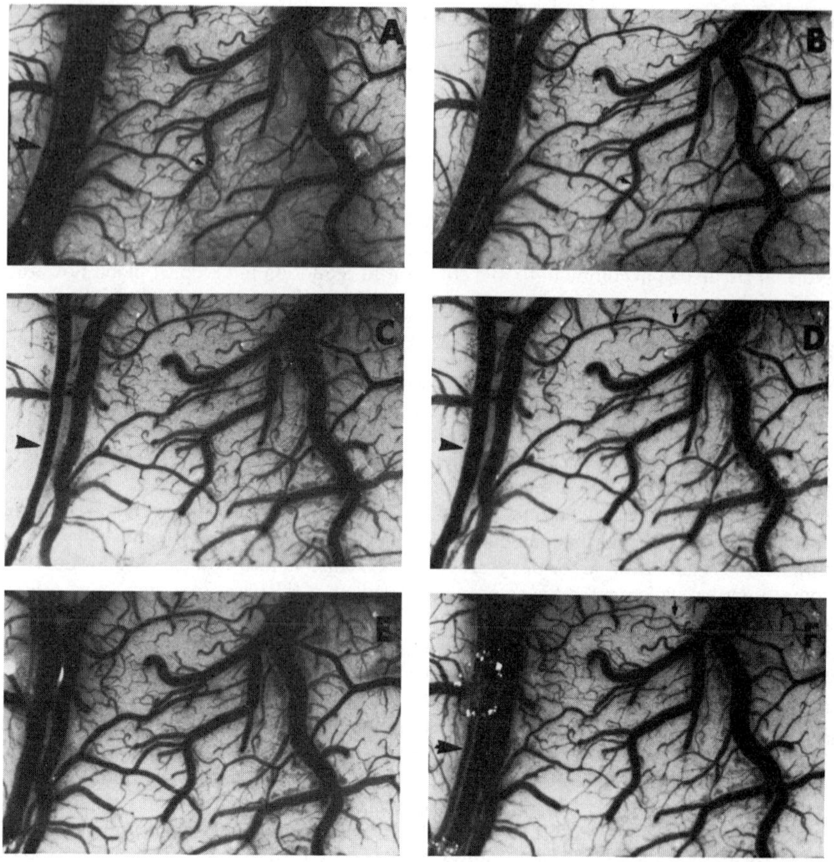

FIGURE 1. Effect of occlusion of middle cerebral artery (MCA) in the monkey. (A) Cortex before occlusion of MCA, showing normal caliber of major conducting vessel (large arrow) and location of cortical vein (small arrow). (B) Cortex shortly after occlusion of MCA. Diffuse pallor has not yet developed. (C) Cortex 1 hour after occlusion. Major artery identified in A is now constricted and cortical pallor is diffuse. Particulate flow is present in adjacent vein (arrowhead). (D) Two hours after occlusion, constricted artery has now partially dilated (arrowhead). Note anastomotic artery that was barely visible in A (small arrow). (E) Cortex 5 minutes after release of occluding clip. Artery is now more fully dilated, and particulate flow is no longer present in vein. (F) Thirty minutes after restoration of flow, brain has recolorized. Conducting vessel is fully dilated (large arrow), and anastomotic artery noted in D has decreased in size (small arrow). (Modified from Reference 7, by permission of The American Heart Association, Inc.)

Sequential *in vivo* measurements of cortical blood flow and intracellular brain pH during progressive focal ischemia are performed with the use of umbelliferone, a lipid-soluble, pH-sensitive fluorescent indicator that freely diffuses across the blood brain barrier. It is nontoxic and isolated to the intracellular compartment. Determination of parenchymal brain pH through this technique correlates closely with the calculated "equivalent pH" as determined by Siesjö and others.[27,28]

Cortical blood flow is determined by the washout curve of umbelliferone over a

60-second time period beginning after the arterial spike using the 1-minute initial slope index.[29-31] Umbelliferone clearance is a measure of perfusion through the intracellular compartment. Since this technique measures flow only in the outer 1 mm of an 80 μm region of cortex, it in effect demonstrates focal cortical blood flow. In this white New Zealand rabbit animal preparation, each is anesthetized with 4% inspired halothane and studied under 1.0%. All animals are maintained on a Harvard respirator and given 0.15 mg/kg pancuronium bromide to eliminate respiratory efforts. Catheters are inserted into the femoral artery and vein for monitoring of blood pressure and arterial blood gases and for administration of drugs. A tracheostomy is performed, and a PE-50 cannula is inserted into the ligated external carotid artery for delivery of umbelliferone into the internal carotid artery. The middle cerebral artery (MCA) is exposed through a retroorbital craniectomy similar to that used in monkeys. In the rabbit, the middle cerebral artery gives off an inferior temporal branch and then ascends over the parietal cortex, separating into two main divisions (FIGURE 2). Occlusion of one of these divisions will yield three zones of flow: (1) a zone of severe ischemia; (2) a zone of normal flow supplied by the division left intact; and (3) between these two zones a region of moderate ischemia partially supplied by the division left intact. This border zone of moderate ischemia is located approximately halfway between the occluded and

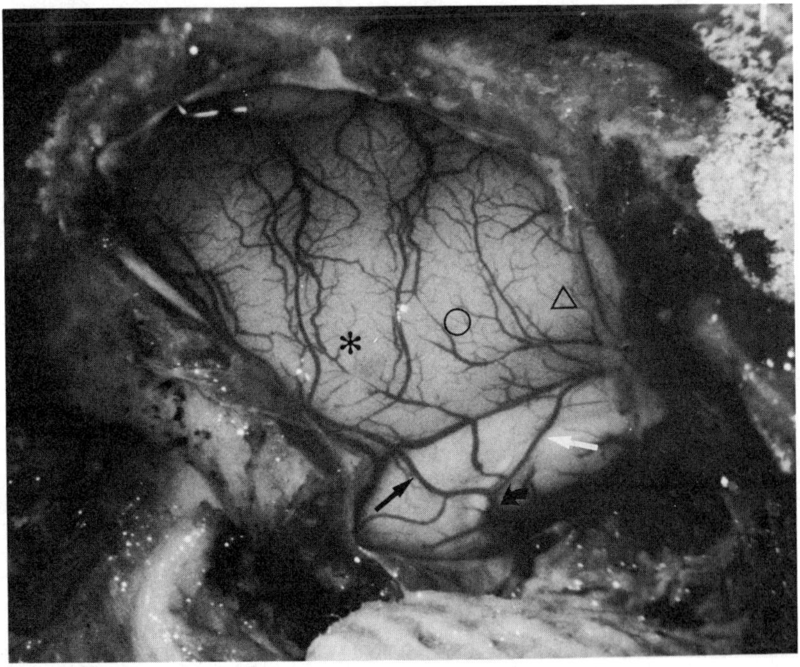

FIGURE 2. Operative exposure showing that the middle cerebral artery (curved arrow) gives off a temporal branch and then bifurcates into two parietal branches (straight black and white arrows). Occlusion of one parietal branch (straight black arrow) will give a zone of severe ischemia (asterisk). There will also be a zone of moderate ischemia (circle) and a region of normal flow (triangle), both supplied by the branch left intact (white arrow). The zone of severe ischemia represents a developing infarct while the moderate ischemia zone corresponds to a zone of ischemic penumbra.

patent branches and can be visually identified by subtle color changes of the cortex under microscopic observation. Confirmation of suspected border zones of moderate ischemia is by documentation of a 60% reduction in cortical blood flow as compared to preocclusion values with only minimal changes in intracellular brain pH. Severe ischemic regions are defined as an 80% reduction in cortical blood flow as compared to preocclusion flows with a dramatic drop in intracellular brain pH.

Effect of Calcium Antagonist When Given after Middle Cerebral Artery Occlusion

Summarized in FIGURES 3 and 4 are the results of 20 animals subjected to middle cerebral artery (MCA) occlusion, in which 10 were given nimodipine 0.5 μg/kg per

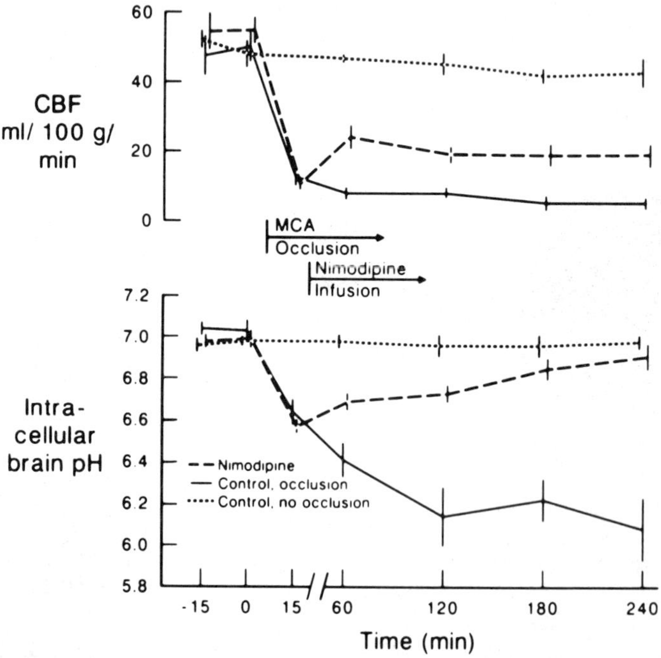

FIGURE 3. Graph of intracellular brain pH and cortical blood flow (CBF) in 10 severe ischemic sites from control rabbits (solid line) and 10 severe ischemic sites from nimodipine-treated rabbits (dashed line). In each rabbit, two measurements of flow and brain pH were performed at a $PaCO_2$ of 40 torr after a normal $PaCO_2$ response curve had been obtained and prior to middle cerebral artery (MCA) occlusion. Preocclusion cortical blood flow was 51.8 ± 4.6 ml/100 per minute and intracellular brain pH was 7.01 ± 0.04, pooling data from all 20 animals. Initial postocclusion flow was 12.7 ± 2.3 ml/100 g per minute in the control and 10.5 ± 1.3 ml/100 g per minute in the treated animals, while brain pH was 6.64 ± 0.06 and 6.57 ± 0.03 respectively. The controls demonstrated a progressive decline in both blood flow and brain pH over 4 hours. With nimodipine, blood flow increased to 24.2 ± 3.3 ml/100 g per minute in the first hour ($p < 0.001$). The improvement in blood flow in the treated vs. the control animals was significant at each hourly interval ($p < 0.001$). Intracellular brain pH improved at each interval, measuring 6.91 ± 0.06 at the fourth hour ($p < 0.001$). Three additional animals without MCA occlusion (dotted line) underwent measurements of brain pH and blood flow for 4 hours to assess the stability of the preparation. (Reproduced from Reference 25 by permission of the American Association of Neurological Surgeons, Inc.)

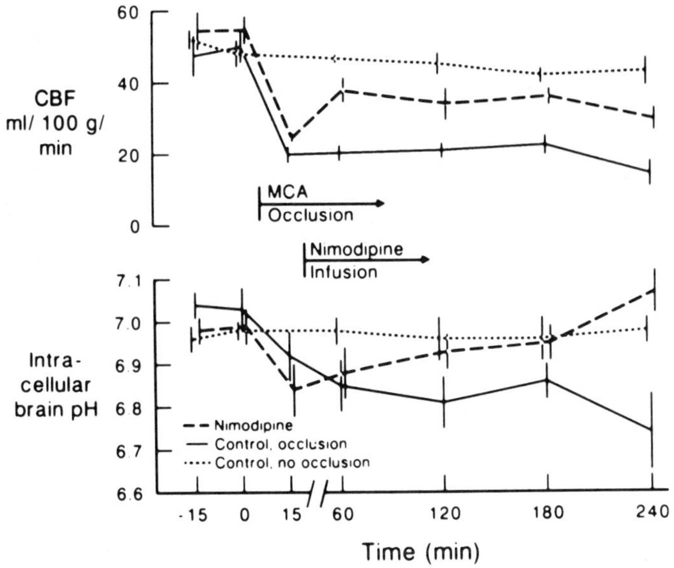

FIGURE 4. Graph of intracellular brain pH and cortical blood flow (CBF) in 10 moderate ischemic sites from control rabbits (solid line) and 10 moderate ischemic sites from nimodipine treated rabbits (dashed line). Preocclusion cortical blood flow was 51.8 ± 4.6 ml/100 g per minute and intracellular brain pH was 7.01 ± 0.04, pooling data from all 20 animals. Initial postocclusion blood flow was 20.0 ± 2.0 ml/100 g per minute in controls and 24.8 ± 1.0 ml/100 g per minute in the treated rabbits, while brain pH was 6.92 ± 0.06 and 6.84 ± 0.06 respectively. In the control group, blood flow was maintained for the first 3 hours and then dropped to 14.5 ± 3.6 ml/100 g per minute at the fourth hour. Intracellular brain pH declined in the control group and was 6.74 ± 0.09 ($p < 0.01$) at the fourth hour. The nimodipine-treated animals had an increase in blood flow to 38.0 ± 3.3 ml/100 g per minute at the first hour ($p < 0.001$). The improvement in blood flow in the treated vs. the control group was significant at each hourly interval ($p < 0.001$). Intracellular brain pH in the treated animals was stable, being 7.07 ± 0.05 at the fourth hour compared to a decline observed in the control group ($p < 0.001$). Stability of the preparation was assessed in 3 animals without middle cerebral artery occlusion (dotted line). (Reproduced from Reference 25 by permission of the American Association of Neurological Surgeons, Inc.)

minute commencing 20 minutes after middle cerebral artery occlusion. This experiment sequentially measured cortical blood flow, parenchymal brain pH, and electrocorticograms for 4 hours after middle cerebral artery occlusion. Prior to occlusion, a $PaCO_2$-CBF response curve was performed to insure that autoregulation was intact within a normal blood pressure range. Confirmation that the cortex had not been injured during the operative exposure included not only this $PaCO_2$-CBF response curve, but also measurements of brain pH. Pooling data from all 20 animals, preocclusion cortical blood flow was 51.8 ± 4.6 ml/100 g per minute and intracellular brain pH was 7.01 ± 0.04. In the 10 control animals 15 minutes after middle cerebral artery occlusion, cortical blood flow at severe ischemic sites was 12.7 ± 2.3 ml/100 g per minute with a corresponding brain pH of 6.64 ± 0.06. Observation of these sites over the ensuing 4 hours demonstrated a reduction in both intracellular brain pH and cortical blood flow. Four hours after occlusion, intracellular brain pH was 6.08 ± 0.15 and blood flow was 5.2 ± 1.5 ml/100 g per minute. Compared to the preocclusion values the reduction in both cortical blood flow and intracellular brain pH at each measured interval was statistically significant ($p < 0.001$).

In the 10 to-be-treated animals, cortical blood flow was 10.5 ± 1.3 ml/100 g per minute and intracellular brain pH was 6.57 ± 0.03 15 minutes after vessel occlusion. The difference in these values when compared to the controls was not significant. One hour after middle cerebral artery occlusion, which would correspond to 40 minutes after the commencement of the nimodipine infusion, cortical blood flow was 24.2 ± 3.3 ml/100 g per minute as compared to 8.0 ± 1.6 ml/100 g per minute in the controls and at 4 hours was 18.8 ± 3.0 ml/100 g per minute. This 90% to 130% increase in cortical blood flow was statistically significant at each hourly measurement as compared to controls ($p < 0.001$). There was also a reversal of the decline in brain pH observed in control animals with eventual normalization of intracellular brain pH at the fourth hour. Four hours after occlusion, intracellular brain pH was 6.91 ± 0.06 in the treated animals as compared to 6.08 ± 0.15 in the controls. This improvement in intracellular brain pH was statistically significant at each hourly interval ($p < 0.001$).

Similar changes in cortical blood flow and intracellular brain pH were noted at moderate ischemic sites as recorded in FIGURE 4. In the 10 control animals, initial postocclusion cortical blood flow was 20.0 ± 2.0 ml/100 g per minute or approximately a 60% reduction when compared to preocclusion values. This was associated with an intracellular brain pH of 6.92 ± 0.06. While the reduction in blood flow was significant ($p < 0.001$) the mild drop in pH was not. For the first three hours blood flow was stable but then fell significantly at the fourth hour to 14.5 ± 3.6 ml/100 g per minute ($p < 0.05$). Intracellular brain pH slowly worsened at each hourly measurement and at four hours was 6.74 ± 0.09 ($p < 0.001$).

At the moderate ischemic sites in the 10 to-be-treated animals, initial postocclusion blood flow was 24.8 ± 1.0 ml/100 g per minute, approximately a 60% reduction in preocclusion values. This was associated with an intracellular brain pH of 6.84 ± 0.06 slightly lower than the control value of 6.92 ± 0.06. However, by these two parameters the to-be-treated animals compared well with the control group. In the nimodipine infusion group, blood flow increased to 38.0 ± 3.3 ml/100 g per minute at the first hour vs. 20.4 ± 2.0 ml/100 g per minute in control animals, and was 29.7 ± 3.2 ml/100 g per minute at four hours. This 20–53% improvement in cortical blood flow in moderate ischemic regions was maintained for the duration of the experiment and was statistically significant as compared to the controls ($p < 0.001$). The nimodipine-treated animals demonstrated maintenance of a normal intracellular brain pH when compared to the data observed in the control group. For example, four-hour postocclusion intracellular brain pH was 7.07 ± 0.05 in the treated animals vs. 6.74 ± 0.09 in the control group ($p < 0.001$).

Electroencephalographic changes correlated well with the above data on cortical blood flow and brain pH. The baseline EEG of the rabbit cortex consists of a 6–10 Hz rhythm. In the 10 control animals, 8 demonstrated a loss of amplitude or a slow 1–2 Hz rhythm immediately after middle cerebral artery occlusion. In these eight rabbits the EEG continued to demonstrate progressive loss of amplitude and frequency over the ensuing four hours. None of these animals had improvement of electrical activity. In the 10 nimodipine-treated animals immediately after occlusion, 7 demonstrated initial EEG changes consisting of either a loss of amplitude or a slow 1–2 Hz delta rhythm. With the addition of nimodipine, 5 of these 7 animals had improvement in cortical electrical activity ($p < 0.05$). Two patterns of improvement were observed. Three had normalization to the 6–10 Hz baseline rhythm and 2 improved from a 1–2 Hz to a 4–6 Hz rhythm.

As demonstrated in FIGURE 5, nimodipine was visually observed to antagonize ischemic vasoconstriction. By reversal of ischemic vasoconstriction, there would be improvement in cortical blood flow which would result in improved substrate delivery promoting aerobic glycolysis. Hence, there would be a reversal of the lactic acidosis

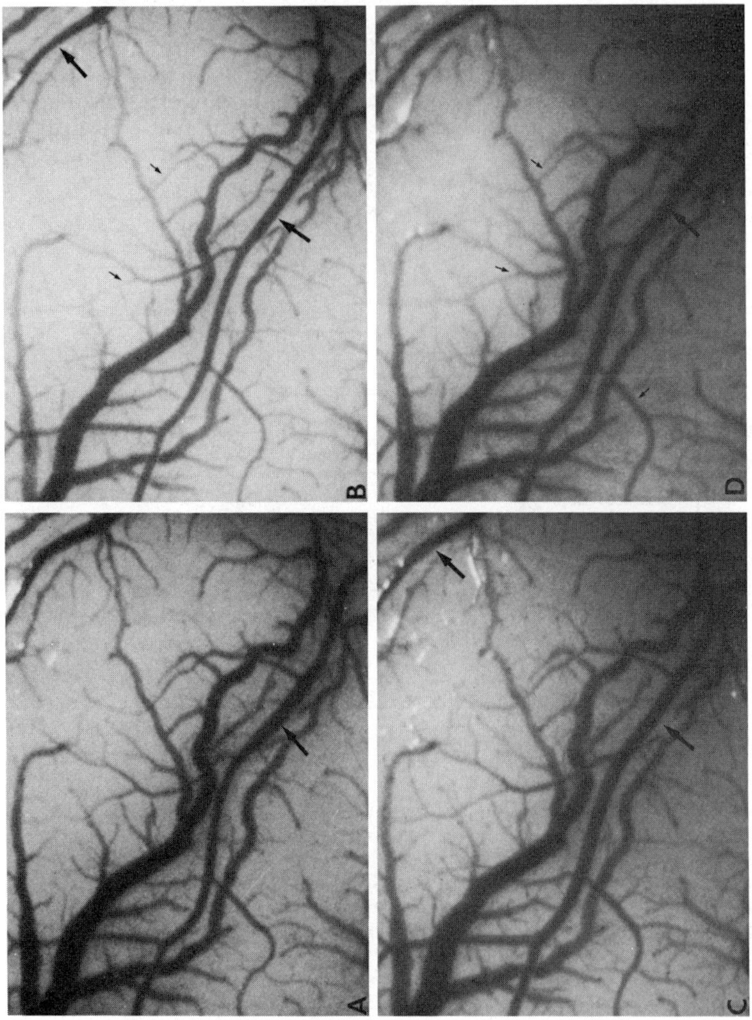

FIGURE 5. Experimental changes in the cortical vasculature of a nimodipine-treated rabbit. (A) Conducting vessels (arrows) prior to middle cerebral artery occlusion. (B) Fifteen minutes after occlusion, ischemic vasoconstriction is present evidenced by cortical pallor and by vasoconstriction of both conducting vessels (large arrows) and penetrating arterioles (small arrows). The draining veins are also constricted. (C) Fifteen minutes after nimodipine infusion there is partial reversal of this vasoconstriction. Cortical pallor is improved, and the conducting vessels (arrows) are dilated. (D) Thirty minutes after the nimodipine infusion was begun, the penetrating arterioles (small arrows), the conducting vessels (large arrows), and the draining veins are all dilated. (Reproduced from Reference 25 by permission of the American Association of Neurological Surgeons, Inc.)

observed in controls during the four hours of vessel occlusion. This improvement in brain pH indicates that there was sufficient cortical blood flow to maintain neurons above the threshold of ionic failure. The reversal in electroencephalographic patterns also suggests that blood flow was elevated above the threshold of electrical failure.

Effects of Nimodipine When Given Prior to Middle Cerebral Artery Occlusion

In a separate series of preliminary studies, the effects of nimodipine 0.5 $\mu g/kg$ per minute when given 15 minutes prior to middle cerebral artery occlusion were studied. The effects of this agent both during ischemia and during a period of reperfusion after restoration of flow through the middle cerebral artery complex were evaluated (FIGURE 6). Correlating data from all 20 animals, preocclusion cortical blood flow was

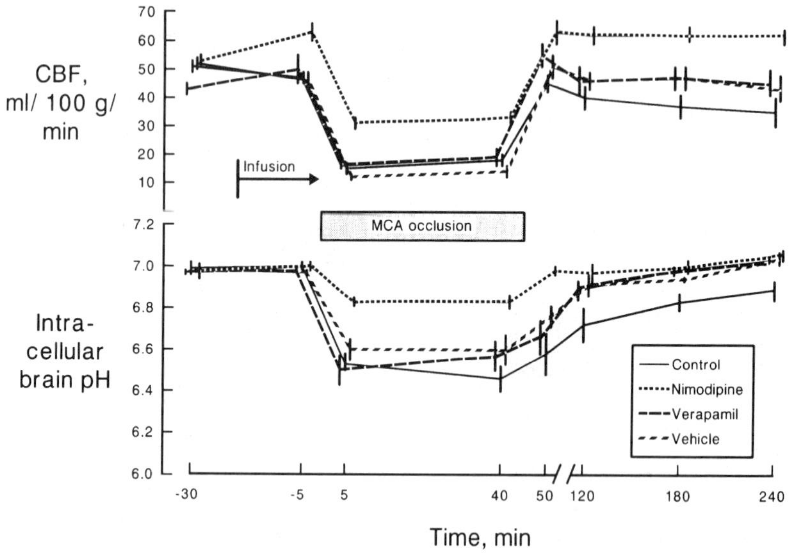

FIGURE 6. Graph of intracellular brain pH and cortical blood flow in white New Zealand rabbits subjected to 45 minutes of middle cerebral artery occlusion followed by a 3-hour period of reperfusion. In this experiment, nimodipine was infused 15 minutes prior to middle cerebral artery occlusion. Preocclusion cortical blood flow was 50.8 ± 2.1 ml/100 g per minute and intracellular brain pH was 6.99 ± 0.04 pooling data from all animals. In control animals 15 minutes after middle cerebral artery occlusion, cortical blood flow was 14.6 ± 2.3 ml/100 g per minute and brain pH was 6.53 ± 0.03. Following restoration of flow in controls, cortical blood flow rose to 45.2 ± 3.0 ml/100 g per minute but then deteriorated to 34.9 ± 3.3 ml/100 g per minute 3 hours later. Intracellular brain pH rose to 6.83 ± 0.04. In the nimodipine-treated group, 15 minutes after middle cerebral artery occlusion in regions that would have been destined to suffer from severe ischemia, focal cortical blood flow was 30.6 ± 2.2 ml/100 g per minute and brain pH was 6.83 ± 0.02. Therefore nimodipine when given prior to middle cerebral artery occlusion significantly improved both of these parameters as compared to control sites. Upon reperfusion, the nimodipine infusion prevented the deterioration in cortical blood flow as observed in controls while brain pH quickly normalized to 7.07 ± 0.03. In a similar group of experiments, the diphenylalkamine calcium antagonist verapamil was not effective in terms of stabilization of cortical blood flow during the period of ischemia.

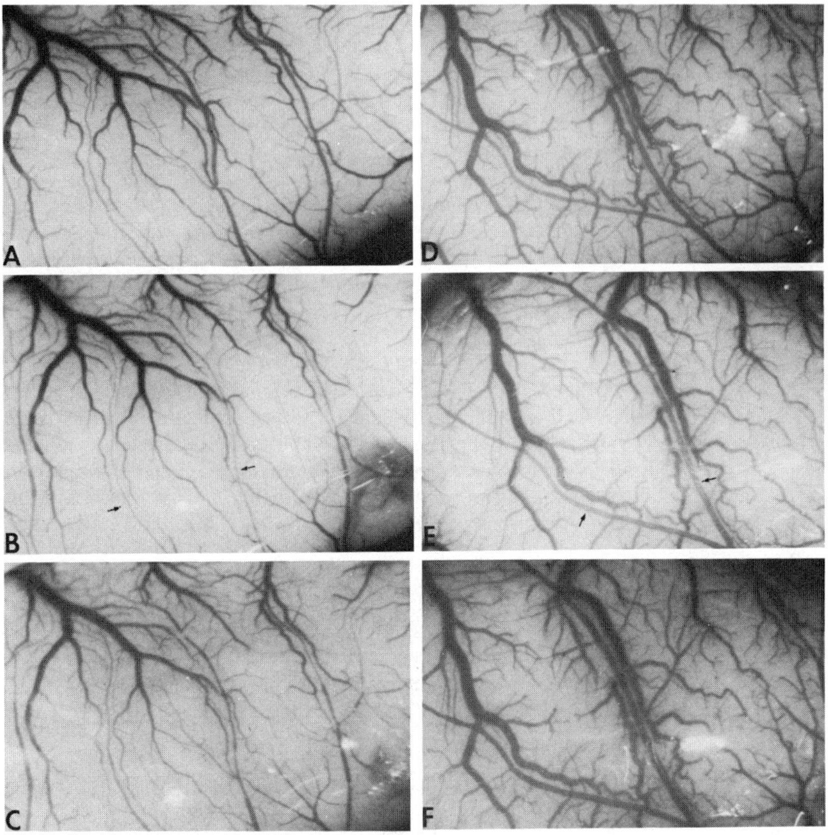

FIGURE 7. Intraoperative photographs of the cortical vasculature during temporary middle cerebral artery occlusion. The series of pictures on the left column (A, B, C) is a control animal subjected to 45 minutes of middle cerebral artery occlusion. (A) Cortical vasculature prior to middle cerebral artery occlusion. (B) Within 15 minutes of middle cerebral artery occlusion, there is cortical pallor and severe ischemic vasoconstriction (arrow). (C) Upon reperfusion, there is cortical hyperemia with both red veins and vasodilitation. Eight out of 10 animals developed severe cerebral edema along with petechial hemorrhages during the 3 hours of reperfusion. In the column on the right (D, E, F) are comparison photographs of an animal treated with nimodipine 15 minutes prior to middle cerebral artery occlusion. (D) Prior to middle cerebral artery occlusion with the addition of nimodipine, there is vasodilitation and a dense pial network as compared to the control. (E) After 15 minutes of middle cerebral artery occlusion, when compared to the control, cortical pallor is less severe and ischemic vasoconstriction is not present. (F) With reperfusion, only 3 developed mild cerebral edema and 2 of these were associated with petechial hemorrhages.

50.8 ± 2.1 ml/100 g per minute and intracellular brain pH was 6.99 ± 0.04. In the control animals, 15 minutes after middle cerebral artery occlusion with a miniature Mayfield clip, cortical blood flow was 14.6 ± 2.3 ml/100 g per minute and intracellular brain pH was 6.53 ± 0.03. Reperfusion was established by removal of the miniature Mayfield clip 45 minutes later. Immediately upon restoration of flow, cortical blood flow rose to 45.2 ± 3.0 ml/100 g per minute while intracellular brain pH was 6.58 ± 0.01. Three hours after reperfusion, cortical blood flow was 34.9 ± 3.3 ml/100 g per minute and brain pH was 6.83 ± 0.04. Therefore there was some deterioration in cortical blood flow during the period of reperfusion and intracellular brain pH never normalized after the 45 minutes of transient ischemia. In the second group of 10 animals treated with nimodipine prior to middle cerebral artery occlusion 15 minutes after middle cerebral artery occlusion in the sites that would have suffered from severe ischemia as judged by topographical analysis of the cortical vasculature, focal cortical blood flow was 30.6 ± 2.2 ml/100 g per minute and brain pH was 6.83 ± 0.02. Therefore nimodipine when given prior to vessel occlusion prevented the severe deterioration in both of these parameters as compared to the controls. Furthermore during the period of reperfusion cortical blood flow remained stable opposite that of the controls. For example, 3 hours after restoration of flow, focal cortical blood flow was 53.8 ± 3.7 ml/100 g per minute and brain pH was 7.07 ± 0.03.

Visual inspection of the cortex during this experiment yielded the following results (FIGURE 7). In 8 out of 10 animal in the control group, immediately after vessel occlusion there was darkening of the venous blood. This was followed by ischemic vasoconstriction of the cortical conducting vessels. Upon removal of the Mayfield clip, there was cortical hyperemia and red veins were clearly visible. During the second and third hours of reperfusion, hemispheric cerebral edema was visible along with cortical petechial hemorrhages.

In the nimodipine-treated rabbits it was our impression that after middle cerebral artery occlusion there was an increase in visible pial vessels with a more diffuse collateralization as compared to the control animals. Furthermore ischemic vasoconstriction was of a much less significant degree as compared to controls. During the period of reperfusion, red veins were not uniformly observed and only 3 out of the 10 animals demonstrated mild hemispheric edema. Of these, two also developed petechial hemorrhages.

RELATIONSHIP BETWEEN ISCHEMIC VASOCONSTRICTION AND INTRACELLULAR BRAIN pH

The above experiments demonstrate that the dihydropyridine calcium antagonist nimodipine when given either prior to or after vessel occlusion improved both cortical blood flow and brain pH in core regions of ischemia. Visual observation of the cortex, as demonstrated in FIGURES 5 and 7, indicated that this improvement in cortical blood flow was related to attenuation in ischemic vasoconstriction. It can be proposed that the improvement in brain pH was secondary to this improvement in cortical blood flow and not the effects of the calcium channel blocker on neuronal metabolism directly. In this regard, it is important to review briefly the metabolic derangements that occur in core regions of ischemia when cortical blood flow drops below 10–12 ml/100 g per minute.

The metabolic aberrations that occur at a reduced cortical blood flow that approaches the threshold of ionic failure are multifactorial and reflect both the rapid depletion of ATP and the accumulation of lactic acid due to the absence of oxidative phosphorylation.[32] One of the pathways that precipitates irreversible neuronal damage is thought to be an increase in intracellular calcium during ischemia.[33–36] Failure of the ATP-dependent Na^+-K^+ pump results in an increase in extracellular potassium which will depolarize the neuronal membrane. This situation will cause opening of voltage-sensitive calcium channels with an increase in intracellular free calcium. This influx of calcium is enhanced by failure of the ATP-dependent Na^+-Ca^+ antiport system, failure of the ATP-dependent sequestration of calcium by the endoplasmic reticulum, and electrophoretic accumulation of calcium by mitochondria which will uncouple oxidative phosphorylation.[37–39] This uncountered rise in intracellular free calcium is thought to activate phospholipase, which will attack membrane phospholipids with the production of free fatty acids.[40] This loss of membrane phospholipids will increase the permeability of neuronal mitochondral membranes which will further alter calcium homeostasis with additional detrimental effects on oxidative phosphorylation. It is thought that inhibition of voltage-sensitive calcium channels by calcium channel antagonists like nimodipine might attenuate the foregoing cascade of events. The potential for nimodipine to affect neuronal metabolism directly is supported by the anticonvulsant properties of this agent.[41,42] Therefore, it is possible that the improvement in brain pH observed in these experiments might have been through prevention of calcium flux into ischemic neurons as opposed to reversal of ischemic vasoconstriction.

The importance of intracellular acidosis during focal ischemia merits emphasis. As demonstrated in the experiments above, in core regions of ischemia there is a rapid drop in parenchymal brain pH as measured by umbelliferone. Currently we believe that this is a direct reflection of the fourfold increase in lactic acid that occurs during the first few minutes of severe ischemia. The decline in brain pH over the ensuing hours of ischemia presumably reflects not only the accumulation of lactic acid but also other products of deranged metabolism. This intracellular acidosis has multiple detrimental effects including the denaturing of proteins with loss of enzymatic function, increasing glial edema which will compromise potential collateral flow, suppressing regeneration of the reduced form of NADH, and possibly increasing production of free radicals.[43–48]

In summary, the improvement in neuronal metabolism as assessed by intracellular brain pH in these experiments could have been due either to prevention of ischemic vasoconstriction or to limiting calcium flux into ischemic neurons. The inhibition of ischemic vasoconstriction was visually documented. Prevention of ischemic vasoconstriction by the dihydropyridine nimodipine could be best explained by prevention of calcium flux into the sarcoplasmic reticulum. Maintenance of calcium homeostasis across the smooth muscle membrane is energy dependent.[49,50] During ischemia with the rapid depletion in ATP, there will be an increase of calcium into the smooth muscle cell and a decrease of efflux from the cytosol causing vasoconstriction through cross-linking of myosin and actin filaments. It should be emphasized that smooth muscle relaxation is also energy dependent. The muscle will remain in a contracted state until the level of intracellular free calcium in the myoplasm returns to a concentration of less than 10^{-7} M. Reuptake and sequestration of calcium into intracellular organelles and the extrusion of calcium into the extracellular space is energy dependent. Therefore during ischemia aberrant calcium metabolism will not only cause muscle contraction but prevent relaxation. The failure of these vessels to respond to dilating agents like carbon dioxide[51] but alternatively react when the animal is infused with a calcium channel antagonist like nimodipine indicates that calcium plays a central role in ischemic vasoconstriction.

REFERENCES

1. Sundt, T. J., Jr. & D. H. Davis. 1979. Reactions of cerebrovascular smooth muscle to blood and ischemia: primary versus secondary vasospasm. *In* Cerebral Arterial Spasm. R. H. Wilkins, Ed.: 244–250. Williams and Wilkins. Baltimore & London.
2. Waltz, A. G. & T. M. Sundt, Jr. 1967. The microvasculature and microcirculation of the cerebral cortex after arterial occlusion. Brain **90:** 681–696.

3. BELL, W. H., T. M. SUNDT, JR. & J. D. NOFZINGER. 1967. The response of cortical vessels to serotonin in experimental cerebral infarctin. J. Neurosurg. **26:** 203–212.
4. LITTLE, J. R., F. W. L. KERR & T. M. SUNDT, JR. 1974. Role of lysosomes in the production of ischemic nerve cell changes. Arch. Neurol. **30:** 448–455.
5. KONTOS, H. A., E. P. WEI, J. T. POVLISHOCK *et al.* 1980. Cerebral arteriolar damaged by arachidonic acid and prostaglandin G_2. Science **209:** 1242–1245.
6. CHAN, P. H., J. W. SCHMIDLEY, R. A. FISHMAN *et al.* 1984. Brain injury, edema, and vascular permeability change induced by oxygen derived free radicals. Neurology **34:** 315–320.
7. SUNDT, T. M., JR. & A. G. WALTZ. 1971. Cerebral ischemia and reactive hyperemia: studies of cortical blood flow and microcirculation before, during, and after temporary occlusion of middle cerebral artery of squirrel monkeys. Circ. Res. **28:** 426–433.
8. KNISELY, M. H., E. H. BLOCH, T. S. ELIOT *et al.* 1947. Sludged blood. Science **106:** 431–440.
9. WALTZ, A. G. 1969. Red venous blood: occurrence and significance in ischemic and nonischemic cerebral cortex. J. Neurosurg. **31:** 141–148.
10. LASSEN, N. A. 1966. The luxury-perfusion syndrome and its possible relation to acute metabolic acidosis localized within the brain. Lancet **2:** 1113–1115.
11. KABAT, H., C. DENNIS & A. B. BAKER. 1941. Recovery of function following arrest of the brain circulation. Am. J. Physiol. **132:** 737–747.
12. HOSSMANN, K. A. & Y. OLSSON. 1970. Suppression and recovery of neuronal function and transient cerebral ischemia. Brain Res. **22:** 313–325.
13. KETY, S. S. & C. F. SCHMIDT. 1948. The nitrous oxide method for the quantitative determination of cerebral blood flow in man: theory, procedure and normal values. J. Clin. Invest. **27:** 476–483.
14. TROJABORG, W. & G. BOYSEN. 1973. Relation between EEG, regional cerebral blood flow and internal carotid artery pressure during carotid endarterectomy. Electroencephalogr. Clin. Neurophysiol. **34:** 61–69.
15. SHARBROUGH, F. W., J. M. MESSICK, JR. & T. M. SUNDT, JR. 1973. Correlation of continuous electroencephalograms with cerebral blood flow measurements during carotid endarterectomy. Stroke **4:** 674–683.
16. BRANSTON, N. M., L. SIMON, H. A. CROCKARD *et al.* 1974. Relationship between the cortical evoked potential and local cortical blood flow following acute middle cerebral artery occlusion in the baboon. Exp. Neurol. **45:** 195–208.
17. MORAWETZ, R. B., R. H. CROWELL., V. DEGIROLAMI *et al.* 1979. Regional cerebral blood flow thresholds during cerebral ischemia. Fed. Proc. **38:** 2493–2494.
18. ASTRUP, J., L. SIMON, N. M. BRANSTON *et al.* 1977. Cortical evoked potential and extracellular K^+ and H^+ at critical levels of brain ischemia. Stroke **8:** 51–57.
19. SIMON, L., N. M. BRANSTON & I. O. CHIKOVANI. 1979. Ischemic brain edema following middle cerebral artery occlusion in baboons: relationship between regional cerebral water content and blood flow at one to two hours. Stroke **10:** 184–191.
20. HARRIS, R. J., L. SYMON, N. M. BRANSTON *et al.* 1981. Changes in extracellular calcium activity in cerebral ischemia. J. Cereb. Blood Flow Metab. **1:** 203–209.
21. WIELOCH, T. & B. K. SIESJÖ. 1982. Ischemic brain injury: the importance of calcium, lipolytic activities, and free fatty acids. Pathol. Biol. Paris **30:** 269–277.
22. SYMON, L., N. M. BRANSTON, A. J. STRONG *et al.* 1977. The concept of thresholds of ischemia in relation to brain structure and function. J. Clin. Pathol. **30**(Suppl. 11): 149–154.
23. ASTRUP, J., B. K. SIESJÖ & L. SYMON. 1981. Thresholds in cerebral ischemia: the ischemic penumbra. Stroke **12:** 723–725.
24. MEYER, F. B., R. E. ANDERSON, T. M. SUNDT, JR. *et al.* 1986. Intracellular brain pH, indicator tissue perfusion, electroencephalography and histology in severe and moderate focal cortical ischemia in the rabbit. J. Cereb. Blood Flow Metab. **6:** 71–78.
25. MEYER, F. B., R. E. ANDERSON, T. L. YAKSH *et al.* 1986. Effect of nimodipine on intracellular brain pH, cortical blood flow, and EEG in experimental focal cerebral ischemia. J. Neurosurg. **64:** 617–626.
26. SCREMIN, O. U., R. R. SONNENSCHEIN & E. H. RUBINSTEIN. 1982. Cerebral vascular

anatomy in blood flow measurements in the rabbit. J. Cereb. Blood Flow Metab. **2:** 55–66.
27. SIESJÖ, B. K. 1978. Brain Energy Metabolism. Wiley, New York, N.Y.
28. DAVIDIAN, N. M., T. C. BUTLER & D. T. POOLE. 1978. The effect of ketosis induced by medium chain triglycerides on intracellular brain pH of mouse brain. Epilepsia **19:** 369–378.
29. SUNDT, T. M., JR., R. E. ANDERSON & R. A. VAN DYKE. 1978. Brain pH measurements using a diffusible, lipid soluble pH sensitive fluorescent indicator. J. Neurochem. **31:** 627–635.
30. SUNDT, T. M., JR. & R. E. ANDERSON. 1980. Intracellular brain pH and the pathway of a fat soluble pH indicator across the blood-brain barrier. Brain Res. **186:** 355–364.
31. SUNDT, T. M. JR. & R. E. ANDERSON. 1980. Umbelliferone as an intracellular pH-sensitive fluorescent indicator and blood-brain barrier probe: instrumentation, calibration, and analysis. J. Neurophysiol. **44:** 60–75.
32. MICHENFELDER, J. D. & T. M. SUNDT, JR. 1971. Cerebral ATP and lactate levels in the squirrel monkey following occlusion in the middle cerebral artery. Stroke **2:** 319–326.
33. SCHANNE, F. A. X., A. B. KANE, E. E. YOUNG *et al.* 1979. Calcium dependence of toxic cell death: a final common pathway. Science **206:** 700–702.
34. FARBER, J. L., K. R. CHIEN & S. MITTNACHT, JR. 1981. The pathogenesis of irreversible cell injury in ischemia. Am. J. Pathol. **102:** 271–281.
35. SIESJÖ, B. K. 1984. Cerebral circulation and metabolism. J. Neurosurg. **60:** 883–908.
36. YANGIHARA, T. & J. T. MCCALL. 1982. Ionic shift in cerebral ischemia. Life Sci. **30:** 1921–1925.
37. GINSBERG, M. D., L. MELA, K. WROBEL-KUHL *et al.* 1977. Mitochondrial metabolism following bilateral cerebral ischemia in the gerbil. Ann. Neurol **1:** 519–527.
38. NOWICKI, J. P., E. T. MACKENZIE & A. R. YOUNG. 1982. Brain ischaemia, calcium and calcium antagonists. Pathol. Biol. Paris **30:** 282–288.
39. REHNCRONA, S., L. MELA & B. K. SIESJÖ. 1979. Recovery of brain mitochondrial function in the rat after complete and incomplete cerebral ischemia. Stroke **10:** 437–446.
40. YOSHIDA, S., S. INOH, T. ASANO *et al.* 1980. Effect of transient ischemia on free fatty acids and phospholipids in the gerbil brain. Lipid peroxidation as a possible cause of postischemic injury. J. Neurosurg. **53:** 323–331.
41. MEYER, F. B., R. E. ANDERSON, T. M. SUNDT, JR. *et al.* 1986. Selective CNS calcium channel blockers—a new class of anticonvulsant agents. Mayo Clin. Proc. **61:** 229–247.
42. MEYER, F. B., P. W. TALLY, R. E. ANDERSON *et al.* 1986. Inhibition of electrically induced seizures by a Ca^{2+} channel blocker. Brain Res. **384:** 180–183.
43. REHNCRONA, S., I. ROSEN & B. K. SIESJÖ. 1980. Excessive cellular acidosis: an important mechanism of neuronal damage in the brain? Acta Physiol. Scand. **110:** 435–437.
44. SIESJÖ, B. K., G. BENDEK, T. KOIDE *et al.* 1985. Influence of acidosis on lipid peroxidation in brain tissues in vitro. J. Cereb. Blood Flow Metab. **5:** 253–258.
45. SIESJÖ, B. K. 1982. Lactic acidosis in the brain: occurrence, triggering mechanisms and pathophysiological importance. Ciba Found. Symp. **87:** 77–100.
46. WELSH, F. A., M. J. O'CONNOR, V. R. MARCY *et al.* 1982. Factors limiting regeneration of ATP following temporary ischemia in cat brain. Stroke **13:** 234–242.
47. PLUM, F. 1983. What causes infarction in ischemic brain? The Robert Wartenberg Lecture. Neurology **33:** 222–233.
48. MYERS, R. E. 1979. Lactic acid accumulation as cause of brain edema and cerebral necrosis resulting from oxygen deprivation. *In* Advances in Perinatal Neurology. R. Korobkin & C. Guilleminault, Eds.: 85–114. Spectrum Publications. Jamaica, N.Y.
49. FITZPATRICK, D. F., E. J. LANDON, G. DEBBAS *et al.* 1972. A calcium pump in vascular smooth muscle. Science **176:** 305.
50. GODFRAIND, P., R. MILLER & M. WIBO. 1986. Calcium antagonism and calcium entry blockade. Pharmacol. Rev. **38:** 321–416.
51. KOGURE, K., M. FUJISHIMA, P. SCHEINBERG *et al.* 1969. Effects of changes in carbon dioxide pressure and arterial pressure on blood flow in ischemia regions of the brain in dogs. Circ. Res. **24:** 557.

Amlodipine

Long-Term Natriuretic and Antihypertensive Activity in Spontaneously Hypertensive Rats with Developing and Established Hypertension

R. A. BURGES, D. G. GARDINER, A. J. CARTER, AND F. F. McKAY

Pfizer Central Research
Sandwich, Kent CT13 9NJ, England

Calcium channel blockers (CCBs) differ from previous drugs used in the therapy of hypertension in that they do not generally provoke fluid retention. There are many reports suggesting that CCBs possess intrinsic natriuretic/diuretic properties; however clinical studies have generally failed to confirm that such properties are sustained on chronic administration.[1,2] We therefore set out to investigate the antihypertensive and natriuretic effects of amlodipine, a new dihydropyridine CCB with a long duration of action,[3] in a well-established animal model of hypertension, the spontaneously hypertensive rat (SHR), with the emphasis on long-term administration. We also investigated the ability of amlodipine to prevent the onset of hypertension in young animals when given during the developing phase of the disease.

The blood pressures (BP) of young (6 to 8 weeks) and mature (36 to 46 weeks) SHR were measured at weekly intervals by an automated tail-cuff method for 12 and 8 weeks, respectively. Treated animals received amlodipine in the chow at a level calculated to provide a daily dose of 8 mg/kg.

Systolic BP of untreated young SHR ($n = 25$) increased steadily over the first five weeks of the study (FIGURE 1) and thereafter remained relatively constant at approximately 40 mmHg above initial values. Amlodipine-treated animals ($n = 25$) showed a delayed rise in BP, the magnitude of which was markedly attenuated (average 18 mmHg). In mature SHR ($n = 12$), amlodipine reduced BP from 212 ± 4 to 167 ± 8 mmHg within three days and to 148 ± 7 mmHg within one week; the effect was sustained for the remaining seven weeks. Heart rate was unaffected by treatment in either group of rats.

The effect of amlodipine on water and electrolyte excretion was assessed in 20-week-old SHR, individually housed in metabolic cages, with free access to water and chow (0.05% sodium). Urine was collected in 6-hourly aliquots for 6 weeks. Treated rats ($n = 12$) received amlodipine in the chow as described above on weeks 2 through 5. Amlodipine treatment caused a marked and sustained natriuretic effect (FIGURE 2); sodium excretion was maintained at more than double that of controls ($n = 12$) for each of the 4 treatment weeks, returning to control level in the final (run-out) week. There was a parallel increase in urine volume averaging 40% above control, and potassium excretion was increased 30%.

Thus, amlodipine possesses marked antihypertensive and natriuretic properties in SHR which are well maintained during long-term treatment.

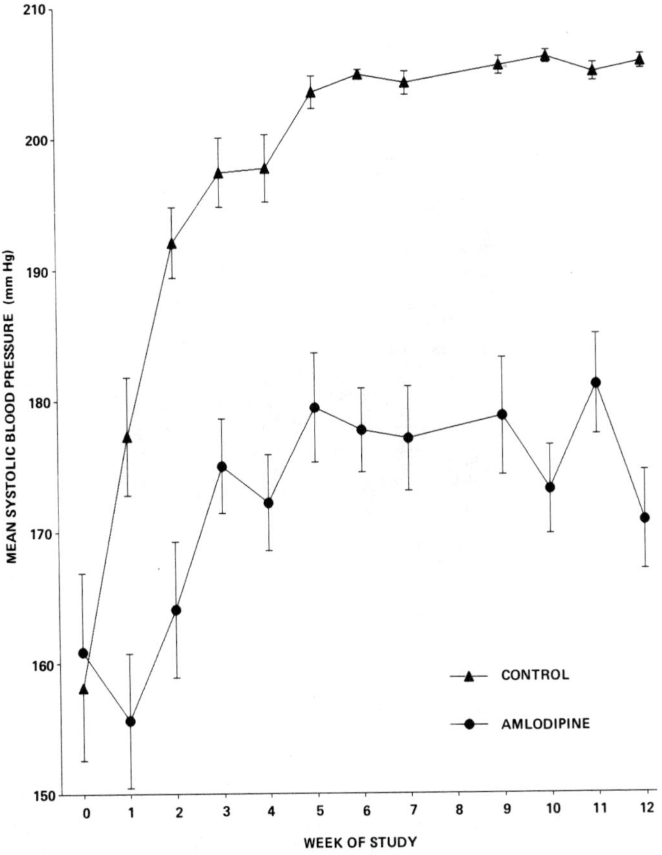

FIGURE 1. Effect of long-term amlodipine treatment on blood pressure of young SHR. Rats were 6–8 weeks old at the start of the study. Vertical bars represent standard error of the mean (SEM) for groups of 25 rats.

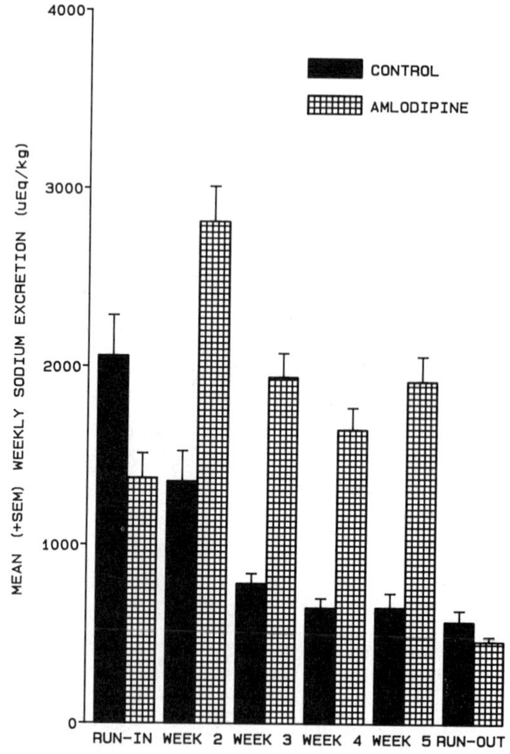

FIGURE 2. Effect of long-term amlodipine treatment on sodium excretion in SHR. Treated rats received dietary amlodipine on weeks 2 through 5. Decline in sodium excretion in control animals probably reflects continuing adaptation to 0.05% sodium diet. Vertical bars represent SEM for groups of 12 rats.

REFERENCES

1. ZANCHETTI, A. & G. LEONETTI. 1985. J. Cardiovasc. Pharmacol. **7**(Suppl. 4): S33–S37.
2. LEONETTI, G., R. GRADNIK, L. TERZOLI, M. FRUSCIO, L. RUPOLI & A. ZANCHETTI. 1984. J. Cardiovasc. Pharmacol. **6:** 392–398.
3. BURGES, R. A., D. G. GARDINER, M. GWILT, A. J. HIGGINS, K. J. BLACKBURN, S. F. CAMPBELL, P. E. CROSS & J. K. STUBBS. 1987. J. Cardiovasc. Pharmacol. **9:** 110–119.

The Antiatherosclerotic Effect of Anipamil in Cholesterol-Fed Rabbits

A. L. CATAPANO, F. M. MAGGI, AND U. CICERANO

Institute of Pharmacological Sciences
School of Pharmacy
University of Milan
Via Andrea del Sarto, 21
20129 Milan, Italy

The aim of this study was to test the antiatherosclerotic effect of anipamil (A), a calcium antagonist structurally related to verapamil, using the cholesterol-fed rabbit as a model.

METHODS

New Zealand male albino rabbits (2.5–3 kg body weight) were used for the experiments.

The animals were divided into 3 groups of 18 animals each as follows: control group (C) receiving standard pelleted chow (120 g/day); cholesterol-fed group (HC), receiving cholesterol in the diet to a total amount of 1.6 g/day; and cholesterol-fed

TABLE 1. Plasma Cholesterol and HDL Cholesterol in Control (C), Cholesterol-Fed (HC), and Cholesterol-Fed+Anipamil (HC+A) Rabbits[a]

	Plasma Cholesterol (mg/dl)	HDL Cholesterol (mg/dl)
C (17)	52 ± 28	21.2 ± 1.1
HC (18)	1373 ± 100[b]	42.3 ± 2.0[b]
HC+A (18)	1290 ± 80[b]	38.8 ± 1.7[b]

[a]Data are means ± standard error (SE); the numbers in parentheses represent the number of animals in each group.

[b]$p < 0.01$ vs. controls.

group (HC+A) receiving the drug at a dose of 10 mg/kg A per day. Plasma cholesterol, triglycerides, and high density lipoprotein (HDL) cholesterol were determined after 2 and 4 weeks of treatment using commercially available methods. In addition we determined at the end of the treatment (8 weeks) the following: (a) The uptake of ^{125}I-labeled low density lipoproteins (LDL) by the aortas of 6 animals in each group as a marker of the permeability of the arterial wall to this lipoprotein class. Human LDL were isolated from normal plasma by ultracentrifugation[1] and labeled as described by Bilheimer *et al.*[2] About 10^7 cpm were injected intravenously and the animals were sacrificed 24 hours later. The aortas were removed and counted for radioactivity. (b) To determine the area of inner surface of the aortas covered by plaques, the aortas were stained with sudan black, a dye that binds to lipids. The stainable area was then determined by planimetry by two independent observers whose determinations did not differ by more than 4%. (c) The cholesterol content of the aortas was also determined in 6 aortas from every group on the lipid extracts of the aortic tissue.[3]

RESULTS

During the experiment only one rabbit died in the control group. Feed intake was not affected by administration of the drug. Upon cholesterol feeding plasma cholesterol increased dramatically (about 25-fold), HDL cholesterol also increased but only about 2-fold (TABLE 1). These findings were also confirmed by fractionation of the lipoprotein classes by column chromatography. Anipamil at a dose of 10 mg/kg per day had no effect on plasma cholesterol levels and on HDL cholesterol (TABLE 1). The uptake of ^{125}I-labeled LDL by the aortas was significantly higher in the HC group as compared to the HC+A group. (TABLE 2). No sudan-stainable areas were detected in

TABLE 2. Aortic Surface Covered by Plaques, Relative ^{125}I-LDL Aortic Uptake, and Aortic Cholesterol in Control (C), Cholesterol-Fed (HC), and Cholesterol-Fed+Anipamil (HC+A) Rabbits[a]

	Aortic Surface Covered by Plaques	Relative ^{125}I-LDL Aortic Uptake (cpm/g aorta per 100 μl plasma)	Aortic Cholesterol (mg/g tissue)
C	0 (17)	—	0.86 ± 0.03 (6)
HC	47.8 ± 5.7 (18)[b]	11.7 ± 1.5 (6)	4.6 ± 0.2 (6)[b]
HC+A	34.8 ± 5.2 (18)[b,c]	7.2 ± 1.0 (6)[c]	3.3 ± 0.2 (6)[b,c]

[a]Data are means ± SE. Numbers in parentheses represent the number of animals in each experimental group.
[b]$p < 0.01$ vs. C.
[c]$p < 0.01$ vs. HC.

the aortas of control animals, while 48% of the aortic surface was covered by plaques in the HC group. In the HC+A animals 35% of the aortic surface was covered by plaques. ($p < 0.01$). This latter finding correlates well with the data on the aortic content of cholesterol which was also reduced in the anipamil-treated animals (TABLE 2).

From these data we conclude that:

- Anipamil at a dose of 10 mg/kg per day effectively reduces the area of the aortic surface covered by plaques and the aortic cholesterol in cholesterol-fed rabbits.
- The antiatherosclerotic effect on anipamil in this experimental model is independent of the plasma cholesterol levels.

REFERENCES

1. HAVEL, R. J., H. A. EDER & J. H. BRAGDON. 1955. The distribution and chemical composition of ultracentrifugally separated lipoproteins in human serum. J. Clin. Invest. **34:** 1345–1353.

2. BILHEIMER, D. W., S. EISENBERG & R. I. LEVY. 1972. The metabolism of very low density lipoprotein proteins. Preliminary in vitro and in vivo observations. Biochim. Biophys. Acta **260:** 212–221.
3. CHRISTIE, W. W. 1973. Lipid Analysis. Pergamon Press. Oxford, England.

Long-Lasting Protective Effect of Anipamil, a New Calcium Entry Blocker, against Myocardial Ischemia and Reperfusion Damage

R. FERRARI, C. CECONI, S. CURELLO, A. CARGNONI,
R. RADDINO, G. CIAMPALINI, AND O. VISIOLI

Department of Cardiology
University of Brescia
Brescia, Italy

It has been shown that the calcium antagonist verapamil can afford, when used prophylactically, substantial protection against the damage caused by ischemia and reperfusion.[1] However, verapamil may have several potential disadvantages when administered during the early stage of acute myocardial infarction. It can exacerbate heart failure and tachyarrhythmias[2] and, due to a relative short half-life, it has to be administered continuously. We have investigated whether the new long-acting calcium antagonist anipamil, which is a derivative of verapamil,[3] has protective effects on ischemic myocardium similar to those observed for verapamil and how long the protective effects persist after cessation of therapy.

Adult male New Zealand white rabbits were used. The control rabbits received 2 mg/kg of 0.9% sodium chloride solution subcutaneously injected for 4 or 5 days. Other rabbits (treated groups) received either 2 mg/kg of racemate of verapamil or anipamil subcutaneously, twice daily for the same period of time. The last injection was administered either 2, 6, or 12 hours before the experiment. The hearts were rapidly extracted and perfused with a Langendorff system for 120 minutes under aerobic conditions, or made ischemic for 90 minutes (by abolishing coronary flow), or made ischemic for 90 minutes and reperfused for 30 minutes as previously described.[3] Ischemic and reperfusion damage was determined in terms of mechanical function and mitochondrial ATP production.[3] FIGURE 1 shows that pretreatment with anipamil induced a reduction of developed systolic pressure. The reduction was present when anipamil injection was stopped either 2–6 or 12 hours before the isolation of the heart. The ischemic induced decline in systolic pressure was more rapid for the hearts from animals treated with anipamil. In those hearts the ischemic and reperfusion induced increase of diastolic pressure was reduced and the recovery of systolic pressure was increased. This recovery in mechanical function was concomitant with a maintenance of the ATP-producing capacities of the mitochondria (FIGURE 2). The protective effects of anipamil were still evident when the last injection was 6 or 12 hours before the isolation of the hearts. In contrast, under these conditions, verapamil was no longer protective.

In this respect anipamil provides an enormous advantage when comparing the data with verapamil because the latter drug is effective only if given to the hearts of the animals 2 hours before the isolation of the hearts. After 6 hours, its protective effect has almost completely disappeared.

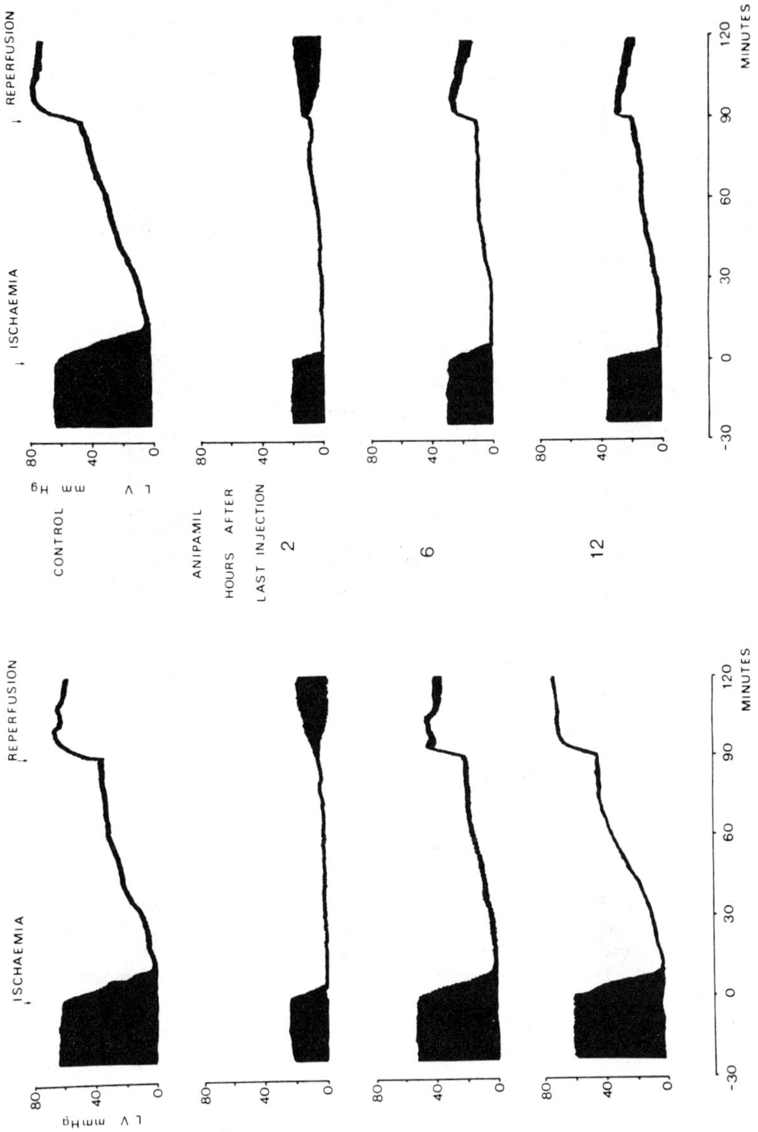

FIGURE 1. Effect of anipamil and verapamil on the mechanical function of the isolated rabbit heart.

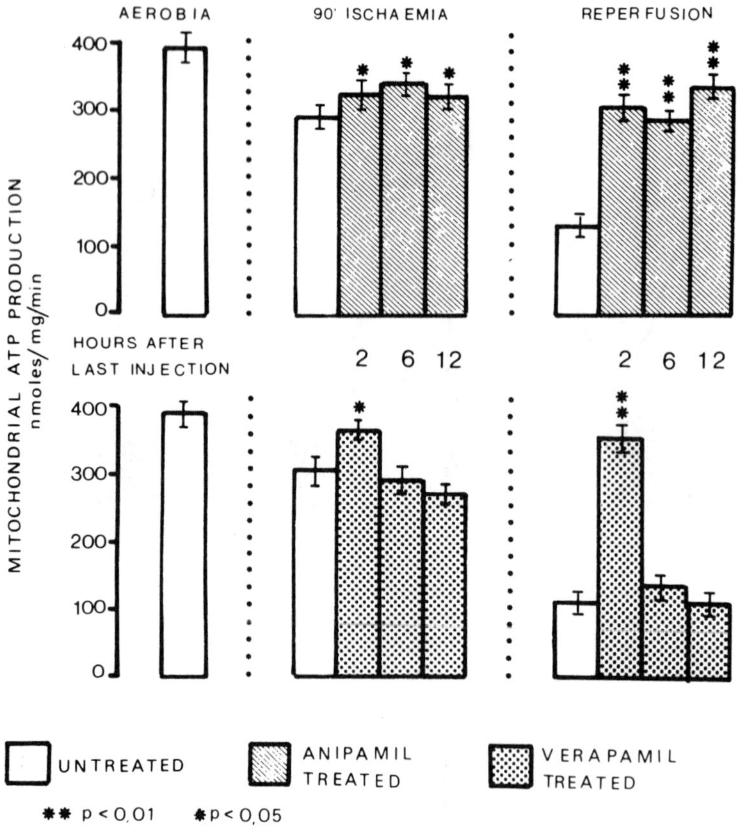

FIGURE 2. Effect of anipamil and verapamil on mitochondrial ATP production.

REFERENCES

1. Nayler, W. G., R. Ferrari & A. Williams. 1980. Protective effect of pretreatment with verapamil, nifedipine and propranolol on mitochondrial function in the ischaemic and reperfused myocardium. Am. J. Cardiol. **46:** 242–248.
2. Danish Multicenter Group on Verapamil in Myocardial Infarction. 1984. Verapamil in acute myocardial infarction. Am. J. Cardiol. **54:** 24E–28E.
3. Raschack, M. 1984. Prolonged cardioprotective effects of anipamil, a new calcium antagonist. (abstr.) Eur. Heart J. **5**(1): 14.

Effect of Nisoldipine on Diet-Induced Atherosclerosis in Rabbits

K. FRONEK

AMES-Bioengineering
University of California, San Diego
La Jolla, California 92093

The possible relationship between calcium ions and development of atherosclerosis was documented in the past. Therefore it has been hypothesized that the Ca blockers could have an antiatherosclerotic effect. In spite of numerous studies on this topic, the question remains unresolved.[3] Nisoldipine, a derivative of nifedipine, was shown to have a consistent vasodilatory effect on the peripheral circulation[2] and yet no adverse effect on the myocardial contractility.[4] Because of this characteristic of nisoldipine, we designed a set of experiments to test whether this drug possesses an inhibitory effect on diet-induced atherosclerosis.

Nineteen New Zealand White rabbits were fed (80 days) with cholesterol-supplemented rabbit chow. Nine of the rabbits were treated with 10 mg of nisoldipine every 12 hours and the rest were treated at the same intervals with placebo. The blood pressure and the plasma lipids were determined in regular intervals. By the end of this period all rabbits were sacrificed and their aortas analyzed for lipid deposits in two ways: (1) surface morphometry of lipid deposits and (2) lipid concentration in aortic tissue. Nisoldipine-treated rabbits had significantly lower systolic blood pressure than the placebo ones. There was no difference between both groups in the final cholesterol plasma concentration (TABLE 1). Considerable variations were noticeable in the size of lipid deposits, as well as in the lipid concentration. The magnitude of response to cholesterol feeding is attributed to, among others, genetic and hereditary factors.[5] Therefore the rabbits were divided into normo- and hyperresponders, using the

TABLE 1A. Systolic Blood Pressure[a]

Placebo rabbits ($n = 20$)	96.45 ± 1.15 mmHg
Nisoldipine rabbits ($n = 19$)	85.75 ± 1.48 mmHg
$p < 0.0005$	

[a]Systolic blood pressure measured on the ear artery using Grant's technique at the end of 87 days of nisoldipine treatment. Means ± standard error.

TABLE 1B. Plasma Cholesterol[a]

	Days of Cholesterol Feeding			
	0	25	48	80
Placebo ($n = 20$)	42 ± 5	2560 ± 208	3358 ± 298	2925 ± 347
Nisoldipine ($n = 19$)	44 ± 5	1952 ± 118	2568 ± 253	2906 ± 226

[a]Fluctuations of plasma cholesterol concentration in rabbits fed with cholesterol diet and treated with nisoldipine or placebo before the cholesterol feeding (0) and after 25, 48, and 80 days of cholesterol feeding. Given in cholesterol mg/dl plasma. Means from all rabbits and standard errors.

TABLE 2. Dietary Induced Lipid Deposits in Control and Nisoldipine-Treated Rabbits[a]

	Percent of Area Infiltrated	Total Lipids[b]	Total Cholesterol[b]	Cholesteryl Ester[b]
Normoresponders				
Placebo ($n = 9$)	23.0 ± 2.3	4.28 ± .32	2.04 ± .16	1.28 ± .10
p	<0.05	<0.05	<0.0025	<0.01
Nisoldipine ($n = 7$)	14.9 ± 2.6	3.43 ± .19	1.47 ± .18	.86 ± .11
	−35%	−20%	−28%	−33%
Hyperresponders				
Placebo (No. 32)	39.7	7.03	3.78	2.47
Nisoldipine (No. 41 + 42)	49.9 ± .5	6.17 ± .33	3.10 ± .34	1.96 ± .16
	+12.5%	−13%	−18%	−21%

[a]Total lipid, cholesterol, and cholesteryl ester concentration compared with the total area infiltrated by lipids. Percentage of inhibition by nisoldipine is below each column. Means ± standard error.

[b]mg/100 mg aortic tissue.

statistical methods of Dixon and Massey.[1] One rabbit from the placebo group and two nisoldipine rabbits were characterized as hyperresponders. The results are summarized in TABLE 2, and it was found that nisoldipine in normoresponders significantly decreases total lipids by 20%, cholesterol by 38%, and cholesteryl ester by 33%. The total lipid accumulation in the hyperresponder group was reduced by 13%, total cholesterol by 18%, and cholesteryl ester by 21%. The significance of these changes was not determined.

In conclusion nisoldipine significantly inhibits diet-induced atherosclerosis. Whether this beneficial effect can be primarily linked to its Ca^{2+} blocking action or to some other mechanism remains to be clarified.

REFERENCES

1. DIXON, W. J. & F. J. MASSEY, JR. 1968. Introduction to Statistical Analysis: 328–331. 3rd edit. McGraw-Hill Book Co., Inc. New York, N.Y.
2. KAZDA, S., B. GARTHOFF, K. D. RÄMSCH & G. SCLÜTER. 1983. Nisoldipine. *In* New Drugs Annual: Cardiovasc Drugs. A. Scriabine, Ed.: 243–258. Raven Press. New York, N.Y.
3. PARMLEY, W. W., S. BLUMLEIN & R. SIEVERS. 1985. Modification of experimental atherosclerosis by calcium-channel blockers. Am. J. Cardiol. **55:** 165B–171B.
4. WARLTIER, D. C., M. G. ZYVOLOSKI, G. J. GROSS & H. L. BROOKS. 1984. Comparative actions of dihydropyridine slow channel calcium blocking agents in conscious dogs: systemic and coronary hemodynamics with and without combined beta adrenergic blockade. J. Pharmacol. Exp. Ther. **230:** 367–375.
5. WEST, C. E. & D. C. K. ROBERTS. 1974. Cholesterol metabolism in two strains of rabbits differing in their cholesterolemic response to dietary cholesterol. Biochem. Soc. Trans. **2:** 1275–1277.

Cardioprotective Actions of Nisoldipine in Postreinfusion Myocardial Ischemia

RICHARD K. MENTLEY AND ALLAN M. LEFER

Department of Physiology
Jefferson Medical College
Thomas Jefferson University
Philadelphia, Pennsylvania 19107

Nisoldipine is a calcium channel blocker having a highly potent effect on vascular smooth muscle relative to cardiac muscle.[1] Previous studies in this laboratory on nisoldipine have shown it to prevent the formation and action of leukotrienes,[2] and arachidonate-induced sudden death in rabbits.[3] The aim of this study was to determine the potential protective action of nisoldipine on ischemic myocardial tissue following severe ischemia and reperfusion.

Adult male cats (2.8 to 3.8 kg) were anesthetized with sodium pentobarbital (30 mg/kg body weight) injected intravenously. Mean arterial blood pressure (MABP), heart rate (HR), and the pressure-rate index (PRI) were measured. Myocardial ischemia (MI) was produced by tightening a ligature placed around the left anterior descending (LAD) coronary artery. Infusion of nisoldipine (3 μg/kg per hour) or its vehicle (polyethylene-glycol 400, PEG + 10% ethanol) was started 30 minutes following coronary artery occlusion at a rate of 0.31 ml/hour and continued for the duration of the experiment. After two hours of ischemia, the myocardium was reperfused by opening the ligated LAD coronary artery (i.e., loosening the ligature). The animals were then monitored for 4 hours. Animals were divided into three groups: (1) Sham MI + nisoldipine (3 μg/kg per hour); (2) MI + vehicle (PEG + 10% ethanol); and (3) MI + nisoldipine (3 μg/kg per hour). At the end of the 6-hour experimental period, the ligature around the LAD coronary artery was retied. The heart was rapidly excised and transferred to a perfusion apparatus that allows perfusion of the coronary vasculature by way of the aorta with Evans blue dye. The area at risk was negatively stained while the remaining myocardium was stained dark blue by the dye. The area at risk was separated, sectioned into 1 mm thick slices and placed in nitroblue tetrazolium dye (0.1% in Sorensen's buffer) at 37°C for 10 minutes. The results were expressed as the area at risk in percent of the total left ventricular mass, and as the area of necrotic tissue in percent of the area at risk and in percent of the total left ventricular mass. The mass at risk and the mass of necrotic tissue were measured by determining the dry weight of the tissue, so as to obtain values independent of the tissue edema accompanying myocardial ischemia and reperfusion.

The MABP of the vehicle-treated group showed no significant changes during both the ischemic and reperfusion periods, although nisoldipine produced a slight decrease in MABP 2 and 4 hours following ischemia (TABLE 1). However, the PRI was not significantly reduced by nisoldipine. The total left ventricular dry weight for the three groups was not significantly different. Upon staining with nitroblue tetrazolium, no necrosis was detected in hearts of the sham-operated group and for clarity these data were excluded from FIGURE 1. The area at risk, delineated by negative staining with Evans blue dye, was 15.9 ± 0.9% in the MI + vehicle group and 16.9 ± 1.4% in the MI + nisoldipine group (not significant). The necrotic area, measured by negative staining with nitroblue tetrazolium, in the nisoldipine-treated group was 6.9 ± 3.8% of

TABLE 1. Alterations in Mean Arterial Blood Pressure (MABP), Heart Rate (HR), and Pressure-Rate Index (PRI) during Myocardial Ischemia (0 to 2 hours) and Reperfusion (2 to 6 hours)[a]

Variable	Time (hours)						
	0	1	2	3	4	5	6
MABP (mm Hg)							
Vehicle	110 ± 6	110 ± 10	108 ± 7	107 ± 9	114 ± 12	113 ± 13	111 ± 14
Nisoldipine	111 ± 9	101 ± 6	88 ± 4[b]	86 ± 6	85 ± 6[b]	88 ± 7	87 ± 5
HR (beats/minute)	147 ± 6	154 ± 9	156 ± 14	151 ± 19	151 ± 13	143 ± 14	149 ± 14
Vehicle							
Nisoldipine	156 ± 10	156 ± 8	153 ± 8	150 ± 9	154 ± 7	147 ± 9	146 ± 11
PRI (mm Hg × beats/min × 10^{-3})	16.3 ± 1.3	16.9 ± 1.9	16.8 ± 1.8	16.4 ± 1.9	16.8 ± 1.6	15.8 ± 1.7	16.0 ± 1.4
Vehicle							
Nisoldipine	17.5 ± 1.8	15.8 ± 0.9	13.6 ± 0.8	13.0 ± 1.1	13.2 ± 1.2	13.1 ± 1.6	12.9 ± 1.5

[a]Infusion of nisoldipine or its vehicle was started at 30 minutes. Six cats were studied in each group.
[b]$p < 0.05$ compared with vehicle.

the area at risk and 1.2 ± 0.7% of the total left ventricle. Respective values in the vehicle-treated group were significantly higher. The necrotic area was 29.0 ± 3.6% of the area at risk ($p < 0.001$) and 4.6 ± 0.5% of the total left ventricle ($p < 0.01$). The results shown in FIGURE 1 very clearly show a marked reduction in the amount of necrotic tissue following treatment with nisoldipine. No significant difference was observed in the area of myocardium at risk between the vehicle and nisoldipine treated MI groups. When the LAD was ligated, therefore, the animals in each group developed ischemic zones of similar size. The area at risk was a function of the position of the coronary ligation and the anatomy of the coronary vasculature, and was independent of treatment. When the area at risk was separated from the perfused tissue and incubated

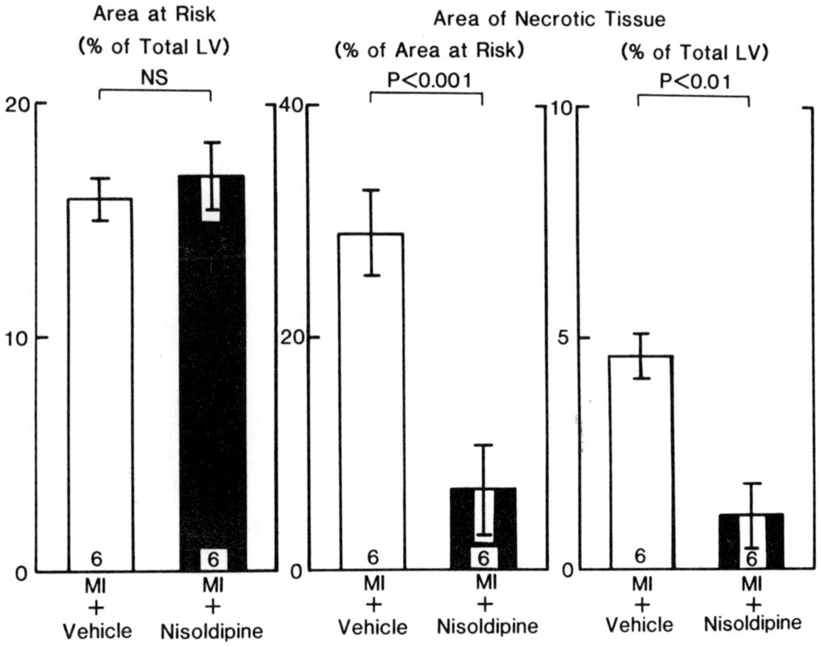

FIGURE 1. Myocardial tissue analysis following 2 hours of ischemia and 4 hours of reperfusion in nisoldipine (3 μg/kg per hour) and vehicle treated cats. Numbers inside the columns represent the number of animals in each group. LV = left ventricle.

in nitroblue tetrazolium, the necrotic area became clearly visible. Nonnecrotic tissue stained dark blue while necrotic tissue remained completely unstained and the two are very easily differentiated. The difference in the degree of necrosis between the two groups was dramatic and it was quite evident upon removing the tissue from the tetrazolium dishes.

Our results indicate that nisoldipine exerted a significant cardioprotective effect at an infusion rate that only slightly decreased arterial blood pressure and did not significantly reduce the PRI, an index of myocardial oxygen demand. This cardioprotective effect suggests that nisoldipine exerts a cytoprotective effect in the ischemic myocardium. Further work is necessary to characterize the time course and the precise mechanism of this cytoprotective effect of nisoldipine.

REFERENCES

1. Kazda, S., B. Garthoff, K. D. Ramsch & G. Schluter. 1983. New Drugs Ann. Cardiovasc. Drugs **1:** 243–258.
2. Yanagisawa, A. & A. M. Lefer. 1986. Proc. Soc. Exp. Biol. Med. **182:** 296–300.
3. Okamatsu, S., R. C. Peck & A. M. Lefer. 1981. Proc. Soc. Exp. Biol. Med. **166:** 551–555.

B 844-39, a New Dihydropyridine Derivative with Slow Onset and Long Duration of Hypotensive Action, in Comparison with Nitrendipine

K. H. SANDERS, N. KOLASSA, AND B. CETTIER

Department of Pharmacology
Byk Gulden Pharmaceuticals
P.O. Box 6500
D-7750 Konstanz, Federal Republic of Germany

Niguldipine-HCl [newly selected INN for B 844-39 = (±)-3-methyl-5-(3-(4,4-diphenyl-1-piperidinyl)-propyl)-1,4-dihydro-2,6-dimethyl-4-(3-nitrophenyl)-pyridine-3,5-dicarboxylate-hydrochloride; molecular weight, 646] is a highly lipophilic new drug (lgP Oct./H_2O at pH 7.4, 4.3). Its cardiovascular effects were studied in spontaneously hypertensive rats (SHR) and in dogs, and compared to those of nitrendipine (MW, 360) on a molar basis. Mode of action was also studied in pithed rats.

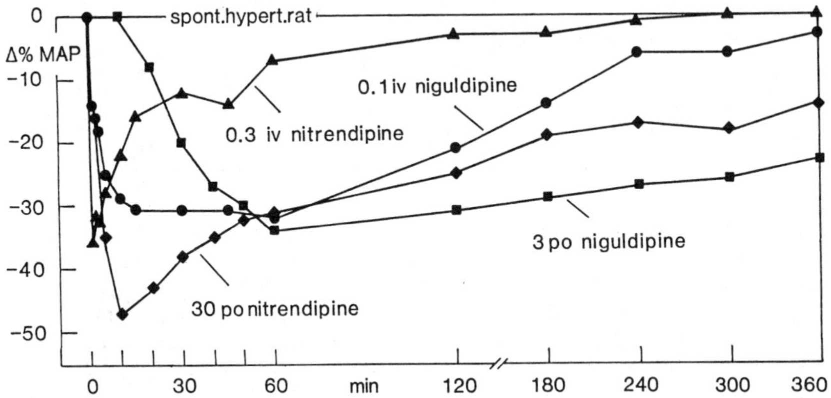

FIGURE 1. Change (%) of MAP in SHR by niguldipine and nitrendipine (doses, μmol/kg; mean, $n = 6$, global standard deviation = 10, 7, 9, 7 for iv, po niguldipine and iv, po nitrendipine).

In SHR, 0.1 μmol/kg niguldipine intravenously (iv) reduced mean arterial pressure (MAP; pretreatment value, 170–190 mmHg) by 30% as did 0.3 μmol/kg nitrendipine iv. Onset of antihypertensive action was slow and duration of action prolonged with niguldipine compared to the fast and transient effect of nitrendipine (FIGURE 1). While 0.1–0.3 μmol/kg niguldipine iv lowered blood pressure for more than 6 hours, 1 μmol/kg nitrendipine was active for 1 hour only. Three micromoles per kilogram niguldipine per orally (po) reduced MAP by 30% for more than 6 hours (FIGURE 1), and 5–25 μmol/kg for longer than 24 hours. Nitrendipine had to be dosed at 1000 μmol/kg for a 24-hour effect. Niguldipine was equieffective in solution or suspension, while initial hypotension due to nitrendipine was absent in suspension.

In the dog, niguldipine was about twice as potent as in SHR: 2.5 μmol/kg niguldipine po lowered systolic arterial pressure (SAP; pretreatment value, 160–175 mmHg) by maximal 60 mmHg after 3–5 hours and blood pressure remained reduced for 24 hours. Nitrendipine (25 μmol/kg po) caused a maximal fall of 46 mmHg after less than 1 hour. Heart rate was increased by either compound probably due to blood pressure fall, and at equieffective blood pressure lowering doses the increases in heart rate was comparable.

The area under the time-response curve (AUC) was calculated to allow a quantitative comparison despite the difference in time courses of action between niguldipine and nitrendipine. Taken the dose for a 50 mmHg reduction of MAP in SHR or 30 mmHg reduction of SAP in dog, potency of niguldipine was about 3 to 10-fold greater than that of nitrendipine (TABLE 1). In pithed rats calcium entry blocking activity was measured by antagonism to the pressor effect of the calcium entry stimulator Bay k 8644. Niguldipine (0.1 μmol/kg iv) caused a persistent blood pressure reduction (>1 hour) and inhibited the blood pressure increase after Bay k 8644, 0.1 and 1 μmol/kg iv by 77% and 34%, respectively. The pDR_2 (i.e., the antagonist dose causing a 2-fold rightward shift of the agonist dose response) was determined to 7.6 (−log mol/kg). Nitrendipine (0.3 μmol/kg) caused a short-lasting (<5 minutes) fall in blood pressure and inhibited 0.1 μmol/kg Bay k 8644 by 20%.

TABLE 1. Effect Doses (ED) for Time-Average Changes in Blood Pressure (mean, $n = 6$)

Compound	Route	ED −50 mmHg MAP (SHR) 0–10	10–60	0–60	60–360	ED −30 mmHg SAP (dog) 0-165 minutes aft. adm.
Niguldipine	iv	0.13	0.08	—	0.33	—
(μmol/kg)	po solution	—	—	11.2	3.3	—
	po suspension	—	—	9.2	4.4	2.7
Nitrendipine	iv	0.34	1.05	—	—	—
(μmol/kg)	po solution	—	—	9.3	46.0	—
	po suspension	—	—	57.0	52.0	25.8

In conscious SHR, $alpha_1$-adrenoceptor blocking activity was measured by antagonism of the pressor effect of 1-phenylephrine. Niguldipine exerted pronounced $alpha_1$-blocking activity (pDR_2, 8.4), while activity of nitrendipine was low (pDR_2, 6.0).

In conclusion, niguldipine is a potent antihypertensive with a slow onset and long duration of action in two animal species promising once daily treatment of hypertension in man. Both calcium entry blockade and $alpha_1$-adrenoceptor blockade contribute to the antihypertensive action of niguldipine.

REFERENCES

1. FISCHER, G., *et al.* 1987. J. Cardiovasc. Pharmacol. **10:** 268–273.
2. RABERGER, G., *et al.* 1986. Z. Kardiol. **75** (suppl. 1): 126.
3. SANDERS, K. H. & N. KOLASSA. 1986. 11th. Meeting of the International Society of Hypertension, Heidelberg: 31.08.–06.09.86, abstract 35.

Effect of Verapamil on Doxorubicin-Induced Cardiomyopathy[a]

F. PICCININI, E. MONTI, L. FAVALLI,[b] AND F. VILLANI[c]

Institute of Pharmacology
University of Milan
Via Celoria, 26
20133 Milan, Italy

Doxorubicin-induced cardiomyopathy has been reported to involve calcium overload: this observation suggests a possible role for Ca antagonists in preventing this adverse effect. On the other hand, Ca antagonists have been shown to reverse the resistance of some tumor cell lines to doxorubicin and other anticancer drugs, probably by inhibiting the drug's extrusion mechanism: if this effect occurs also in normal heart cells, a worsening of the cardiotoxicity should be expected. The aim of the present investigation was to evaluate the effect of verapamil on the development of doxorubicin-induced cardiomyopathy in rats and to ascertain whether a modification of doxorubicin heart pharmacokinetics might be responsible for this effect.

Doxorubicin was administered intravenously (iv) every third day at a dose of 3 mg/kg for a total of three administrations. In order to clarify whether verapamil modifies the development of doxorubicin cardiomyopathy by a modification of the drug uptake in heart, or whether the drug inhibits the Ca overload, verapamil was administered intraperitoneally (ip) at a dose of 2.5 mg/kg twice daily according to two treatment schedules: (A) from day 1 to day 21; and (B) from day 21 to day 56. These treatment schedules were suggested by the observation that in myocardial tissue isolated from rats treated with doxorubicin, the drug level and that of its metabolites—after a peak phase occurring within 2 days after doxorubicin injection—drop rapidly so that doxorubicin and its metabolites are not detectable after three weeks.[1] Doxorubicin cardiotoxicity was monitored by means of electrocardiograph (ECG); in particular we measured QaT and SaT duration since a good correlation was found between morphologic score indicating the degree of myocardial damage and QaT and SaT duration.[2] QaT and SaT duration are calculated as the interval between the Q (nS) wave and the apex of the T wave.

The influence of verapamil on myocardial cell uptake of doxorubicin was evaluated in isolated heart perfused through coronary vessels according to Langendorff with ^{14}C-doxorubicin at a concentration of 1 mcg/ml. After different perfusion periods the organs were chilled in ice-cold Tyrode solution and pump perfused with 8 ml/minute for 60 minutes in order to wash the extracellular spaces. The residual radioactivity was separately measured in left and right atria and ventricles.

As shown in FIGURE 1, doxorubicin induces a progressive and irreversible prolongation of QaT. Verapamil, when administered from day 1 to day 21, does not prevent QaT prolongation. In contrast, when administered from day 21 to day 56, it partially

[a]Supported by Grants no. 85.02561.44 and 85.02303.44. Special Project "Oncology" from the Consiglio Nazionale delle Ricerche, Rome.

[b]Institute of Pharmacology, University of Pavia, Via Taramelli 14, 27100 Pavia, Italy.

[c]To whom correspondence should be addressed at Cardiology Service, National Cancer Institute, Via Venezian 1, 20133 Milan, Italy.

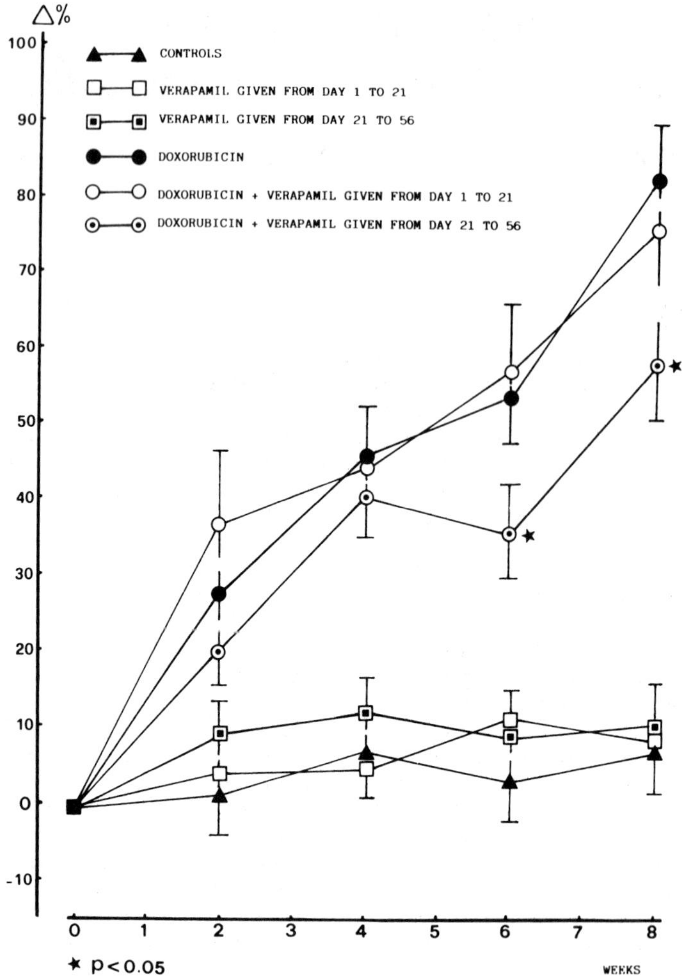

FIGURE 1. Time course of QaT duration in rats treated with doxorubicin when administered alone or in combination with verapamil. Values are expressed as percent variation from pretreatment values; means ± standard error (SE) of 7–13 animals.

TABLE 1. Effect of Verapamil on Doxorubicin Uptake in Myocardial Cells[a]

	Left Atrium	Right Atrium	Left Ventricle	Right Ventricle
Doxorubicin	21.3 ± 3.5	18.6 ± 3.4	18.7 ± 3.0	27.1 ± 2.6
Doxorubicin + verapamil 0.05 μg/ml	23.5 ± 1.3	24.4 ± 1.5	30.2 ± 0.8[b]	35.5 ± 1.3[b]
Doxorubicin + verapamil 0.1 μg/ml	24.1 ± 2.8	23.3 ± 4.9	24.4 ± 3.2	25.3 ± 4.0

[a]Values are expressed as μg/g of fresh tissue; mean ± SE of 4–7 determinations.
[b]$p < 0.05$ vs. doxorubicin.

prevents the cardiotoxic effect of doxorubicin, as shown by the significant decrease in QaT prolongation recorded 6 and 8 weeks after the first doxorubicin administration. The same results were obtained when SaT duration was considered.

Doxorubicin, as shown in TABLE 1, is taken up by both atria and ventricles, reaching slightly higher levels in the right ventricle. Preparations perfused with verapamil (0.05 μg/ml) displayed a modest increase in doxorubicin uptake which is less pronounced in the presence of the higher dose of verapamil (0.1 μg/ml). This observation is in line with the time course of development of cardiomyopathy as measured by QaT duration (FIGURE 1), showing that no significant modifications of cardiotoxicity occur when verapamil is administered from day 1 to day 21. The partially protective effect of verapamil administration from day 21 to day 56 suggests that calcium overload may play a role in the pathogenesis of doxorubicin delayed cardiotoxicity.

REFERENCES

1. MONTI E., F. PICCININI, F. VILLANI & L. FAVALLI. 1986. Myocardial contractility and heart pharmacokinetics of Doxorubicin after a single i.v. administration in the rat. Cancer Chemother. Pharmacol. **18:** 289–291.
2. VILLANI, F., E. MONTI, F. PICCININI, L. FAVALLI, E. LANZA, A. ROZZA DIONIGI & P. POGGI. 1986. Relationship between doxorubicin induced ECG changes and myocardial alterations in rats. Tumori **72:** 323–329.

Control of Cardiac Arrhythmias by Calcium Antagonism[a]

KOONLAWEE NADEMANEE AND BRAMAH N. SINGH

Department of Cardiology
Wadsworth Veterans Administration Medical Center
Wilshire and Sawtelle Boulevards
Los Angeles, California 90073

and

Department of Medicine
UCLA School of Medicine
Los Angeles, California

Since about 1970, much evidence has accumulated for the role of calcium antagonists as potent agents for the control of certain supraventricular and ventricular arrhythmias.[1] Singh and Vaughan Williams found that verapamil, the prototype of calcium antagonists, differed in its electrophysiologic properties from those of beta-blocking drugs and of local-anesthetic type of antiarrhythmic compounds such as quinidine.[2] The drug also differed from those agents (e.g., sotalol and amiodarone) that exerted their salutary effects by homogeneously prolonging the cardiac action potential and refractoriness without effect on conduction.

The antiarrhythmic action of verapamil was therefore thought to constitute a discrete mechanism for the control of cardiac arrhythmias.[2,3] Recent experimental and clinical studies have supported these earlier observations. In this paper, the role of calcium antagonists as antiarrhythmic agents is discussed in relation to their electrophysiologic properties.

ELECTROPHARMACOLOGIC CONSIDERATIONS

Most arrhythmias arise on the basis of perturbations in impulse generation (ectopic or automatic tachyarrhythmias) and in impulse conduction (reentrant arrhythmias) or from a combination of both processes.[3] An additional possibility has recently been suggested under the name of "triggered" automaticity,[4,5] but the precise role of the abnormalities of the slow channel in the genesis of such arrhythmias remains essentially inferential.

In interpreting the overall actions of a calcium blocker as antiarrhythmic agent, it is worth emphasizing that the normal atrioventricular (AV) node is slow-channel dependent. It may become the site of deranged impulse formation and impulse conduction. In the experimental setting calcium channel blockers block the slow calcium channel in a concentration- or dose-dependent fashion. Thus, in fast-channel fibers they have no significant effect on atrial, ventricular, or His-Purkinje refractory periods or on conduction velocity. In isolated preparations, they slow phase 4

[a]Supported in part by the Medical Research Service of the Veterans Administration and the American Heart Association, the Greater Los Angeles Affiliate.

depolarization in the SA and AV nodes with an associated depression of conduction. Because of their effects on the slow channel, calcium channel blockers also accelerate repolarization at the plateau phase of the action potential. However, the magnitude of this effect is such that there is little or no change in the voltage-dependent refractoriness. The major effect on the refractory period is in the AV node where both the effective and the functional refractory periods are significantly lengthened in the anterograde as well as in the retrograde directions. Some of the newer agents exert additional effects over and above their propensity to block the slow myocardial channel. For example, bepridil blocks the fast sodium channel and it prolongs the action potential duration.[6]

Clinical Electrophysiologic Effects of Calcium Antagonists

The *in vivo* and clinical effects of calcium antagonists represent a balance of their *in vitro* actions and those that result from reflex activation of the sympathetic reflexes

TABLE 1. Clinical Electrophysiologic Effects of Calcium Antagonists[a]

Effects	Verapamil[b]	Nifedipine	Diltiazem	Bepridil
R-R Interval				
QRS	0	0	0	↑
Q-Tc	0	0	0	↑
PR	↑↑	0	↑	↑
A-H	↑↑↑	0	↑↑	↑
H-V	0	0	0	↑
Atrial ERP	0	0	0	↑
AV node ERP	↑↑↑	±	↑↑	↑↑
AV node FRP	↑↑↑	±	↑↑	↑↑
Ventricular FRP	0	0	0	↑↑
His-Purkinje ERP	0	0	0	↑
Bypass tact ERP	±	0	±	↑
Sinus node recovery time	0[c]	0	0[c]	0
Ventricular automaticity	0	0	0	↓

[a]↓ = decrease; ↑ = increase; ± = variable effect; ERP = effective refractory period; FRP = functional refractory period.

[b]Effects of gallopamil and tiapamil are similar to those of verapamil.

[c]Prolonged in sick sinus syndrome.

activated by their often potent vasodilator actions. In the case of nifedipine and other dihydropyridine derivatives, such reflex actions nullify or even reverse the intrinsic actions on the sinus node. Thus, these agents do not exert measurable effects on the electrophysiologic parameters in man and appear to be devoid of antiarrhythmic actions. In the case of diltiazem, verapamil, and bepridil, the net effects are also modified by the noncompetitive sympatholytic effects of these compounds.

The major clinical electrophysiologic actions of various calcium antagonists are summarized in TABLE 1. The most significant action is on the electrophysiologic function of the AV node. This is an example of their "direct" antiarrhythmic actions. Such an action is utilized in the termination of the acute episodes and for the prevention of recurrences of paroxysmal supraventricular tachycardia (PSVT) and for the slowing of the ventricular response in atrial flutter and fibrillation. Most calcium antagonists have little or no electrophysiologic effects on ventricular muscle. Thus, they are unlikely to be potent antiarrhythmic agents in most types of ventricular tachyarrhythmias although recent experimental and clinical evidence has suggested a role of these drugs in the control of arrhythmias due to triggered automaticity (see below). There is also evidence that calcium antagonists may prevent the development of such dysrhythmias by primarily influencing the course of myocardial ischemia either by altering demand or supply or both in patients with coronary artery disease especially those prone to coronary vasospasm, an example of an "indirect" antiarrhythmic effect.

EFFECTS OF CALCIUM ANTAGONISTS IN SUPRAVENTRICULAR ARRHYTHMIAS

A somewhat simplified classification of the electrophysiologic mechanism for the clinically occurring paroxysmal supraventricular tachycardias is listed in TABLE 2. The automatic form is uncommon especially in the adult; the commonest form is the reentrant PSVT.[7] PSVTs due to sinus nodal or intraatrial reentry are uncommon and often difficult to distinguish from other types of reentrant PSVTs.

Calcium antagonists have a role in the acute termination of PSVTs when given intravenously as well as in preventing recurrences when they are administered orally. Only those calcium antagonists that depress intranodal conduction and prolong the effective refractory period of the AV node (verapamil, diltiazem, bepridil, tiapamil, and gallopamil) are effective in this regard. As might be expected, the dihydropyridines are without effect. The commonly used dosage regimens for the various agents are indicated in TABLE 3.

Acute Termination of PSVT

The major experience has been with intravenous verapamil, but tiapamil, gallopamil, diltiazem, and bepridil are also effective in terminating reentrant PSVTs in which the anterograde limb of the tachycardia circuit is the AV node, the "weakest link" of the reentrant loop. This may account for the prompt and predictable reversion

TABLE 2. Mechanisms of Paroxysmal Supraventricular Tachycardias

1. Enhanced Automaticity:
   - (a) Paroxysmal and acute
   - (b) Chronic
2. Reentry without bypass tracts:
   - (a) AV nodal reentry: slow-fast
fast-slow
   - (b) Sinoatrial nodal reentry
   - (c) Intraatrial reentry
3. Reentry in association with bypass tracts:
   - (a) Reentry with anterograde AV conduction (orthodromic)
     - (i) with evidence of preexcitation of 12-lead EDG
     - (ii) concealed WPW (bypass tract conducting only retrogradely)
   - (b) Reentry with anterograde conduction over bypass tract (antidromic) during tachycardia

TABLE 3. Dosage Regimens of Calcium Antagonists Employed in the Control of Cardiac Arrhythmias[a]

Agent	Intravenous Dose	Oral Dose	Comments
Verapamil	0.145 mg/kg (bolus)	240–480 mg/day	Oral regimen administered in 3 or 4 divided doses; formulation under investigation
	0.005 mg/kg/per min (infusion)	—	
Diltiazem	0.15 to 0.25 mg/kg (bolus)	90–360 mg/day	Oral regimen administered in 3 or 4 divided daily doses
Tiapamil	1 to 2 mg/kg (bolus)	Not established	—
Gallopamil (D_{600})	0.03 to 0.05 mg/kg (bolus)	Not established	—
Bepridil	2 to 4 mg/kg	300–400 mg/daily	Oral regimen administered in one single daily dose

[a]The dosages cited are well established for verapamil (the "reference" calcium antagonist). For the other compounds they are tentative and are given here to serve as an approximate indication.

of 80–100% of cases of PSVT given 3–5 mg (in children) to 10–15 mg (in adults) of verapamil.[8–12]

Verapamil remains the drug of choice for terminating PSVT with narrow QRS complexes due to reentry involving antegrade conduction over the AV node. Recently, it has been shown that diltiazem given intravenously (0.25 mg/kg) or orally may also terminate narrow QRS complex PSVTs,[13–16] with a potency probably comparable to that of verapamil although a direct controlled comparison has not been made. The success rate of conversion of PSVT to sinus rhythm by verapamil may be improved to nearly 100% by carotid sinus massage or the addition of 5–10 mg of edrophonium (tensilon) given in rapid succession after verapamil. The drug is equally effective in terminating slow fast as well as fast slow PSVTs. Verapamil is effective in terminating AV nodal reentrant PSVTs at all ages.

Modes of Conversion of PSVT with Calcium Antagonists

The most common mode of conversion is an abrupt termination of the tachyarrhythmia as might occur with carotid sinus massage. The cycle length of the tachycardia may prolong somewhat due to the delayed AV conduction [as evidenced by lengthening of the atrio-His (A-H) interval] followed by a short pause before conversion. The termination is usually by anterograde conduction block (FIGURE 1), rarely retrograde.[11] In some cases of PSVT, given intravenous verapamil there is frank AV dissociation followed by a junctional escape rhythm before sinus mechanism is restored. In a few patients, restoration to sinus rhythm is preceded by transient atrial fibrillation. The underlying mechanism for this is unclear. Another type of response includes the occurrence of premature ventricular contractions (rarely short runs of ventricular tachycardia) preceding conversion to sinus rhythm. This is also seen during PSVT conversion by the use of beta-adrenoceptor blocking drugs or carotid sinus massage. Neither the mechanism nor the precise clinical significance of such premature ventricular contractions is known. However, the occurrence of sustained ventricular tachycardia complicating conversion of PSVT by verapamil is not seen.

The final type of response during PSVT termination is alternating cycle length

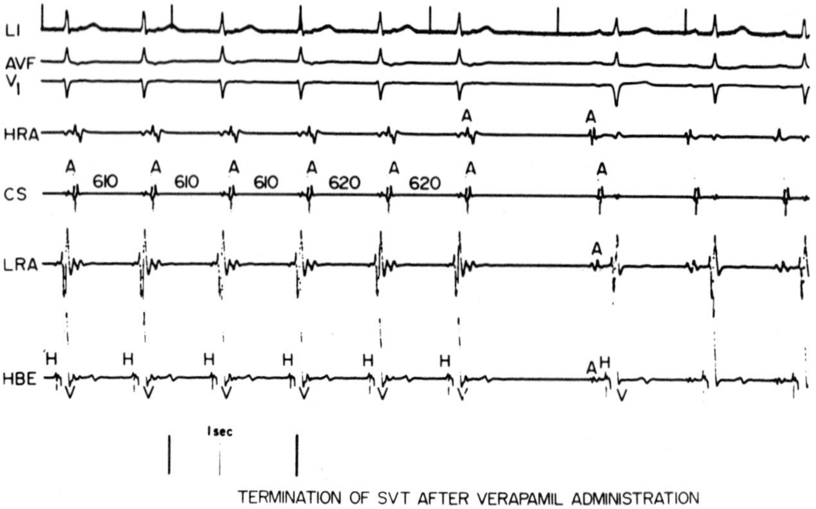

FIGURE 1. The mechanism of termination of a slow-fast form of AV nodal reentry tachycardia by iv verapamil elucidated by intracardiac recordings in the electrophysiologic laboratory. Note that the tachycardia cycle length increases to 620 mseconds before conversion to normal sinus rhythm and the site of tachycardia interruption appears to be in the anterograde slow AV nodal pathway.

preceding conversion.[9] Intracardiac recordings have shown that cycle length alternation is due to alternations in the A-H or H-A intervals,[12] but the underlying mechanism for this phenomenon is not understood. However, it is not a unique feature of the action of calcium antagonists (see Reference 9).

Acute Conversion of PSVT: Calcium Antagonists versus Other Antiarrhythmic Agents

Figures compiled from the reported experience with different agents are shown in TABLE 4. Intravenous beta-blocking drugs produce a conversion rate of 40–60% of all cases of reentrant PSVT with narrow QRS complexes. There are few systematic data on the overall efficacy of vagal maneuvers, intravenous edrophonium, alpha-agonists, or digoxin given either alone or in combination. However, verapamil is now preferred where urgent termination of PSVT is desirable since the effects of digoxin are often not apparent for 15–60 minutes or longer. In the rare event of failure of conversion with verapamil, electrical conversion maybe undertaken reasonably promptly because of the short elimination half-life of intravenous (iv) verapamil (30 minutes). In addition to the higher conversion rate, verapamil also offers significant advantages over beta-blockers in patients whose tachyarrhythmias are associated with chronic obstructive airways disease, diabetes mellitus, or peripheral vascular disease.

It is also of interest that class I agents such as quinidine,[18] disopyramide,[19] and ajamaline[20] may also convert PSVTs acutely when given either orally or intravenously (see TABLE 4). All these three compounds, which also retard conduction and prolong refractoriness over the bypass tracts in the Wolff-Parkinson-White (WPW) syndrome, prevent AV nodal reentry by the selective block of the retrograde fast intranodal pathway. The overall merit of class I agents versus that of verapamil and diltiazem is poorly defined.

Calcium Antagonists versus Adenosine and ATP in the Acute Conversion of PSVTs

Recent reports have suggested that intravenously administered adenosine or ATP may not only be as effective as verapamil but may also offer other important advantages at least in certain subsets of patients.[21] However, at present this approach is not an approved indication in the United States and many other countries. Numerous studies with intravenous ATP (3 to 15 mg in pediatric patients and 10 to 20 mg in adults) and adenosine (mean dose of 180 μg/kg) given as bolus injections have nevertheless indicated that between 90 to 95% of PSVTs are terminated within 40 seconds. The conversion may be attended by transient (lasting a few seconds) sinus arrest, AV block, bradycardia, facial flushing, bronchospasm, and even convulsions in the case of ATP. The side effects with adenosine appear to be minimal,[21] although further studies are needed especially those using blinded protocols comparing the efficacy of intravenous verapamil and adenosine.

Response in Other Forms of Reentrant or Ectopic Supraventricular Tachycardia

Verapamil and similar calcium antagonists may be of value in other forms of reentrant and automatic supraventricular tachycardia.[9] However it appears that iv verapamil is less effective in converting ectopic atrial tachycardia,[12] although paroxysmal atrial tachycardia with block due to digoxin toxicity as well as to other causes may convert to sinus rhythm following oral doses of verapamil. The mechanism mediating such a beneficial response is not known. It may be due to the drug's effect on digitalis-induced afterdepolarization.

TABLE 4. Comparative Efficacy of Verapamil and Other Antiarrhythmic Agents in the Acute Conversion of Reentrant Supraventricular Tachycardia

Agent (Reference)	Percentage Conversion	Mode of Termination
Intravenous propranolol (17)	41–44	Anterograde AV block
Intravenous ouabin (17)	44–54	Anterograde AV block
Intravenous ouabin plus intravenous propranolol (18)	58	Anterograde AV block
Intravenous procainamide	65	Retrograde AV block
Oral quinidine (18)	78	Retrograde AV block
Oral disoyramide (18)	67	Retrograde AV block
Intravenous disopyramide (19)	60	Retrograde AV block
Intravenous verapamil (9)	80–100	Anterograde AV block (see text)
Intravenous ajmaline (20)	80–100	Retrograde AV block
Intravenous bepridil	80–100	Anterograde AV block
Intravenous diltiazem (15)	over 80	Anterograde AV block
Intravenous tiapamil	over 50	Anterograde AV block
Intravenous gallopamil	over 80	Anterograde AV block
Intravenous ATP (21)	80–100	Anterograde AV block
Intravenous adenosine	90–100	Anterograde AV block
Intravenous amiodarone	?over 50	?Anterograde AV block

Calcium Antagonist and Multifocal Atrial Tachycardia

The role of calcium antagonists in multifocal atrial tachycardia (MAT) used for acute treatment or prophylactically is still uncertain. In some studies beneficial effects have been reported; in others less encouraging effects have been described. For example, Aronow *et al.* compared responses of verapamil in reentrant PSVT to those to multifocal atrial tachycardia.[22] Of the five patients with reentrant PSVT, all converted to sinus rhythm after iv verapamil, whereas only one of five with MAT responded. In contrast, a recent study by Levine *et al.* indicated a generally favorable response.[23] They found that intravenous verapamil consistently reduced the atrial and ventricular rates in a group of patients with MAT, and in one patient chronically administered drug prevented recurrences of the tachycardia. Further data are needed to deny or confirm such a beneficial response.

Chronic Prophylaxis of PSVT with Calcium Antagonists

Again, the bulk of experience has been with verapamil but even in the case of verapamil, available data[12,24–27] suggest that, in contrast to the extreme potency of the iv drug, the oral formulation (given 80 to 120 mg three or four times a day) may not have comparable efficacy in preventing recurrences of PSVT during chronic administration. However, Mauritson *et al.* found that during long-term therapy of PSVT, oral verapamil was superior to placebo.[24] Rinkenberger *et al.* found that when the drug was given orally (180–480 mg/day) to patients who had responded to iv verapamil during acute episodes of PSVT, 10 of 19 patients discontinued therapy within a month either because of side effects or lack of response.[12]

Because of the extremely variable pattern of recurrences of PSVT in different patients and in the same patient at different times, the precise efficacy of a therapeutic agent in the chronic prophylaxis of PSVT is not easily established. Nevertheless, in the case of verapamil, there are reports that indicate that this compound may be of prophylactic value in PSVT.[27]

An approach that appears to be effective in predicting the efficacy of oral calcium antagonists in the prophylaxis of PSVT is the use of electrophysiologic studies by programmed electrical stimulation.[28,29] Tonkin *et al.* made observations before and after iv verapamil, 0.15 mg/kg, in 13 patients, 12 previously resistant to other antiarrhythmic drugs.[28] The drug increased the AV nodal conduction time as well as the functional and the effective refractory periods. After the drug, reentrant PSVT could not be initiated in 5 of the 13 patients and was nonsustained in a further 3 patients. The tachycardia rate was decreased in those in whom PSVT was reinducible after iv verapamil. Over a mean follow-up period of 16 months on oral verapamil, 11 of the 13 patients had definite symptomatic improvement, with a decrease in the frequency, duration, and/or associated symptoms of their tachyarrhythmia. In only one patient were side effects severe enough to necessitate withdrawal of the drug. Very similar results have recently been reported in 8 patients by Klein *et al.*[29] Their data suggested that the response to iv verapamil could be extrapolated to predict the electrophysiologic results and outcome of long-term therapy with the oral drug; a similar predictive outcome between the acute intravenous effect and the chronic clinical response in 18 patients given diltiazem has been reported by Hung *et al.*[15] However, more extensive, controlled experiments will be needed to clearly define the role of oral verapamil, diltiazem, and other agents in the prophylaxis of PSVT.

There is a rational basis for modulating the electrophysiologic properties of the AV node by combination therapy with beta-adrenoceptor blocking drugs or digoxin; such an approach may enhance the clinical utility of verapamil in the oral prophylaxis of PSVT.

Verapamil and Paroxysmal Atrial Tachycardia with Block

Paroxysmal atrial tachycardia (PAT) with block is a relatively uncommon arrhythmia, believed in most cases to be due to digitalis intoxication. However, in the experience of Storstein and Landmark, digitalis could not be incriminated as a cause in many of their cases.[30] They found that verapamil given orally in a dose of 40 to 80 mg 3 hourly to 14 patients with PAT with block led to reversion to sinus rhythm in 10 initially, with subsequent relapse occurring in 4. The best effect was found in patients with a short duration of the arrhythmia. The mechanism of action of verapamil in this setting is uncertain, but the data suggest that the drug has a depressant effect on the ectopic pacemaker which may be mediated through the slow response.

CALCIUM ANTAGONISTS IN PREEXCITATION SYNDROMES

The major action of calcium antagonists in preexcitation syndromes is on the AV node.[9] There is a minimal effect on the bypass tracts. Thus, compounds such as verapamil, tiapamil, gallopamil, diltiazem, and bepridil are likely to be variably effective in terminating the acute paroxysms of the narrow QRS (orthodromic) PSVT. As in the case of AV nodal reentrant PSVT, the role of calcium antagonists in the oral prophylaxis of orthodromic PSVT remains to be defined, but since they prolong AV nodal refractoriness, they are likely to be of value at least in some patients. In contrast, since they have no significant effect on the refractoriness of the bypass tract, they are unlikely to terminate antidromic PSVT; nevertheless, the theoretical possibility exists that they may, in large doses, terminate the arrhythmias by inhibiting retrograde AV nodal conduction.[9]

In patients with atrial flutter and fibrillation complicating preexcitation, agents that shorten the effective refractory period of the bypass tracts (e.g., digitalis) and those that lengthen it over the AV node (digitalis and beta-adrenoceptor blocking drugs) will augment the ventricular response (FIGURE 2) and may possibly precipitate ventricular fibrillation. Calcium antagonists that increase AV nodal refractoriness (e.g., verapamil, diltiazem, tiapamil, gallopamil, and bepridil) fall into the latter category. Published data however pertain largely to verapamil (see Reference 9). They indicate that verapamil and similar calcium antagonists should not be given to patients in whom atrial fibrillation or flutter complicate the WPW syndrome with anterograde conduction over the bypass tracts. These conditions are best treated acutely by cardioversion or class I drugs (procainamide, disopyramide) and prophylactically by amiodarone or quinidine or surgery. It should be emphasized that when doubt exists regarding the nature of wide QRS tachycardia (irregular or regular), it is prudent not to use calcium antagonists for acute conversion.

TREATMENT OF OTHER ATRIAL TACHYARRHYTHMIAS BY CALCIUM ANTAGONISTS

Atrial Fibrillation

In atrial fibrillation, three types of responses to iv verapamil have been reported. The most common is the inhibition of AV conduction with subsequent slowing of the

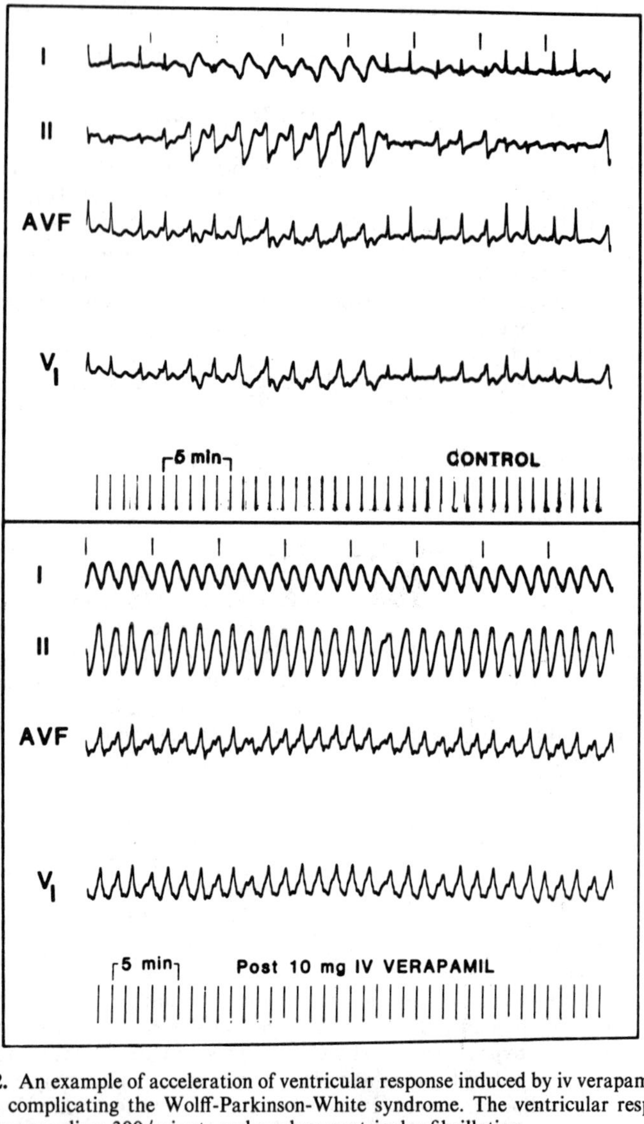

FIGURE 2. An example of acceleration of ventricular response induced by iv verapamil in atrial fibrillation complicating the Wolff-Parkinson-White syndrome. The ventricular response may reach a rate exceeding 300/minute and produce ventricular fibrillation.

ventricular response.[9] The effect is brief so that after 30 minutes the ventricular response gradually accelerates, unless a continuous infusion is instituted. The second type of response with verapamil in atrial fibrillation is what has been designated "regularization" of the ventricular response. This was noted in 25% in the series of Heng *et al.*[8] but in a higher proportion of those reported by Schamroth.[10] The precise mechanism of this phenomenon is not understood. The final type of response of atrial fibrillation to iv verapamil is reversion to sinus rhythm. This is, however, uncommon in the experience of most investigators. It usually occurs in patients with the arrhythmia of recent onset associated with normal or only mild to moderate left atrial enlargement. This observation is in line with the known findings that verapamil and similar drugs have no significant effect on atrial refractoriness.[9]

The clinical value of orally administered verapamil in controlling ventricular response in atrial fibrillation has recently been studied by a number of investigators.[9] In one study, the effects of 160–240 mg daily of verapamil on resting heart rate and that during mild exercise were studied in 23 digitalized patients with chronic atrial fibrillation of various causes. Verapamil significantly reduced the heart rate response during exercise; in a smaller number of patients, another study also confirmed the efficacy of verapamil in attenuating the ventricular response in atrial fibrillation.[31] However, in this study the higher doses were associated with significant side effects. It should be noted that verapamil tends to reduce both the resting as well as the exercise-induced increases in heart rate in the setting of atrial fibrillation whereas the major effect of digoxin is on the resting rate. In this context two recent reports are of interest.[32,33] The first deals with the effects of varying doses of verapamil in the control of the ventricular response in atrial flutter and fibrillation. Klein and Kaplinsky have clearly shown that not only does the calcium antagonist effectively control the ventricular response as well as digitalis,[32] but during exercise the attentuation of the rate increase is superior. They have raised the issue that verapamil might supplant cardiac glycosides in this setting. Roth *et al.* present similar data in the case of diltiazem.[33] It is likely that the effects of the two drugs are not due solely to calcium antagonism but may in part arise from their associated noncompetitive sympatholytic effects. It should be emphasized that the suggestion of Klein and Kaplinsky is essentially valid for most patients especially those with preserved ventricular functions.[32] In patients with impaired ventricular and atrial function, the effects of verapamil and diltiazem have not been critically evaluated and, at least for the present, cardiac glycosides may be preferred.

From the pharmacologic standpoint, it is clear that there is likely to be a subset of patients in which digoxin and verapamil (or diltiazem) might be combined in the control of the ventricular response in atrial flutter and fibrillation. However, it should be emphasized that when digoxin and verapamil are used together, their depressant effect on the AV node may summate; since a significant interaction occurs between the two compounds, the net effect may be unexpectedly exaggerated necessitating careful monitoring of serum drug concentrations. Although an interaction between diltiazem and digoxin is either minimal or absent, the electrophysiologic interaction between the two drugs on the AV node may produce a markedly depressant effect in patients with unsuspected conduction system disease.

It is clear that since verapamil and similar compounds do not exacerbate bronchospastic or vasospastic phenomena, if effective in atrial tachyarrhythmias in patients with obstructive airways or peripheral vascular disease, these drugs will have distinct advantages over beta-antagonists for the purposes of chronic prophylaxis in the above subsets of patients.

Maintenance of Sinus Rhythm

Basu *et al.* reported that patients with atrial fibrillation treated with verapamil before and after DC cardioversion, had a low rate of conversion (one out to 24) *before* electroconversion was attempted.[34] In contrast, on verapamil low energy levels were needed for conversion to sinus rhythm in the remainder, 40% of whom remained in sinus rhythm on the drug at the end of one year. The reported success rate with quinidine is 18–29%. In contrast, a recent controlled clinical trial comparing verapamil (80 mg three times a day) with quinidine (0.4 mg twice a day) demonstrated that quinidine was significantly more effective in producing conversion to sinus rhythm at 3 months postconversion.[35]

Atrial Flutter

The bulk of the clinical experience has been with verapamil.[9] The immediate effect of iv verapamil is reasonably consistent; the increased AV block slows the ventricular response, with an occasional patient converting to sinus rhythm. In some, atrial flutter alters to atrial fibrillation before sinus rhythm is restored but the rate of conversion to sinus rhythm is low, which is consistent with the known electrophysiologic effects of the drug.

A single intravenous dose of verapamil has been found to be of diagnostic value in differentiating atrial flutter with 2–1 AV conduction from paroxysmal supraventricular tachycardia when these two arrhythmias are not readily distinguished electrocardiographically. If the rhythm is atrial flutter, the AV block increases immediately after iv verapamil, thus revealing the true nature of the arrhythmias.[9] Other calcium antagonists that inhibit AV conduction may also be used in this way.

VENTRICULAR ARRHYTHMIAS

Unlike the situation with supraventricular tachyarrhythmias as outlined above, the role of calcium antagonists in ventricular dysrhythmias is poorly defined. In general, these agents are of limited value in most patients with life-threatening ventricular arrhythmias. The subject has recently been placed in perspective by Belhassen and Horowitz.[36]

Premature Ventricular Contractions

There are no controlled data to support the belief that calcium antagonists are potent agents for the suppression of premature ventricular contractions (PVCs) in the setting of chronic ischemic heart disease. Thus, if they were to prevent the incidence of sudden death in such patients, the mechanism of the salutary effect is unlikely to be mediated through the suppression of premature ventricular contractions. Similarly, while reasonably sound theoretical bases have been suggested for the role of the slow channel in the genesis of ventricular arrhythmias in obstructive cardiomyopathies[37] and for the mitral valve syndrome,[1] clinical experience with slow channel inhibitors in these conditions has not confirmed their efficacy especially in obstructive cardiomyopathies.[38] Moreover, there are few systematic data to indicate that they may be effective in reducing the frequency of symptomatic PVCs in patients without structural heart disease.

Chronic Recurrent Ventricular Tachycardia

Verapamil and other calcium antagonists have little or no effect on chronically occurring ventricular tachyarrhythmias.[36,39,40] This is consistent with the fact that the effective refractory period of the ventricle or His-Purkinje system is not lengthened by slow channel blockade.[39] Wellens *et al.* studied the effects of iv verapamil on ventricular tachycardia (VT) in patients in whom VT could be induced and terminated by programmed electrical stimulation of the heart.[39] Intravenous (10 mg) verapamil given during the tachycardia had no effect in 7 of 8 patients, and the arrhythmia could be induced readily before as well as after verapamil administration. In only one patient could the induced VT be terminated by verapamil administration.

Sung *et al.* have reported similar findings with intravenous verapamil in 10 patients with inducible ventricular tachycardia (8 with programmed stimulation and 2 with isoproterenol stimulation).[41] The drug had no effect on VT induction in any of the 10 patients. Cardioversion was required in two patients because of verapamil-induced hypotension. Mason *et al.* found verapamil to be effective in preventing VT induction in only 3 of 16 patients with chronic recurrent VT.[42] Buxton *et al.* also found that 10 mg of intravenous verapamil had no effect on nonsustained VT induced by programmed electrical stimulation of the heart in 13 patients.[43] The drug did not prevent or alter the mode of VT induction, nor did it slow the rate of the inducible tachycardia. On the other hand, in 3 of the patients the induced VT accelerated, became more prolonged and deteriorated into ventricular fibrillation in 2. The authors concluded that the mechanism of the tachyarrhythmia was unlikely to be accountable in terms of triggered activity due to afterdepolarizations.

It appears that the type of ventricular tachycardia occurring in patients with organic heart disease is probably not related to slow channel abnormality. In contrast, a recent report has suggested that there was abolition of PVCs in 7 of 8 patients who exhibited persistent frequent PVCs during the first 48 hours of acute myocardial infarction.[36] Favorable responses have also been reported in sustained arrhythmias in this setting. For example, Sclarovsky *et al.* administered 3 to 5 mg of intravenous verapamil to 8 patients with multiform accelerated idioventricular rhythm occurring during the first 12 hours of acute myocardial infarction.[44] The arrhythmia was abolished in 6, slowed in 1, and was without effect in the remaining patient. Massumi *et al.* have also reported a high success rate in the use of verapamil in controlling parasystolic ventricular tachycardia,[45] raising the possibility of triggered automaticity being due to an abnormality of the slow channel. Successful control of polymorphous ventricular tachycardia by verapamil treatment was also recently reported by Grenadier *et al.* in 3 of 4 patients during acute myocardial infarction.[46] These 3 patients had failed on lidocaine, class 1 agents, overdrive pacing, and repeated cardioversion. However, these are uncontrolled studies which raise the possibility but do not provide conclusive proof that calcium antagonism by verapamil might be effective in controlling ventricular tachyarrhythmias. It should be considered that the apparent salutary effect might result from improved ischemia and myocardial conduction rather than as a consequence of a direct antiarrhythmic effect of the drug in ventricular muscle or the Purkinje fibers. Improvement in ischemia in this situation might be effective in reversing reentry triggered as well as enhanced automaticity. Moreover, it must be emphasized that in the context of myocardial ischemia, verapamil and other calcium antagonists may exert a potent effect in reversing coronary artery spasm vasoconstriction and thus relieve ischemia and ischemia-induced ventricular tachyarrhythmia. Such an effect must be regarded as a "secondary" antiarrhythmic effect which is likely to be most readily apparent in the setting of Prinzmetal variant angina.[46]

Exercise-Triggered Ventricular Tachycardia

There have been several recent reports that have suggested that exercise-triggered ventricular tachycardia having the morphologic pattern of left bundle branch block and right axis deviation might respond predictably and promptly to intravenous verapamil. Such an arrhythmia may occur in patients without identifiable cardiac disease.[47] Wu *et al.* described three such patients;[48] in none was the tachycardia inducible by programmed electrical stimulation, but could be provoked by isoproterenol infusion. Intravenous verapamil terminated the tachycardia in all three and prevented its occurrence during exercise in two. It is of interest that propranolol and lidocaine also prevented the occurrence of the arrhythmia. Three similar cases have been reported by Sung *et al.*,[41] although in this series intravenous verapamil was not effective in preventing the ventricular tachycardia inducibility by isoproterenol; but the QRS axis in these patients during the tachycardia was not stated. Thus, it is unclear whether the nature of the arrhythmia was identical to that in those reported by Wu *et al.*[48] At present it is not clear whether the ventricular tachycardia in question is due to an automatic focus or to triggered automaticity;[49] nor is it known whether the observed response to intravenous verapamil in a small series of patients is a property unique to the drug or a common property of all type 1 calcium antagonists. In this context, it is also of interest that Coumel and Attuel recently reported a group of patients without demonstrable heart disease who experienced syncopal spells due to *torsades de pointes* in association with a normal QT and an exceptionally short coupling interval of the beat initiating the tachycardia.[49] In the authors' experience, the arrhythmia in these patients selectively responded to intravenous and oral verapamil, being resistant to other antiarrhythmic agents including amiodarone and beta-blocking drugs.

Idiopathic Ventricular Tachycardia with Right Bundle Branch Block and Left Axis Deviation Morphology

It is now increasingly appreciated that in young patients without demonstrable cardiac disease, the sustained ventricular tachycardia that occurs in a few has the morphologic pattern of right bundle branch block with left axis deviation.[50–53] This arrhythmia appears to constitute a distinct clinical entity; it is usually possible to initiate the tachycardia by both atrial and ventricular stimulation.

It is of interest that in most cases the ventricular tachycardia in these patients responds to verapamil given intravenously,[50,53] whereas beta blockers or Class 1 agents either fail or exert only a partial response.[51,53] The precise mechanism for the arrhythmia is not known; electrophysiologic studies have suggested a reentrant mechanism in the hands of some investigators[51,53] and triggered automaticity in those of others,[41] but the difficulties of such an approach in the clinical laboratory are well known.[5]

CALCIUM ANTAGONISTS AND SUDDEN DEATH

An outstanding question that needs to be dealt with is the potential of calcium antagonists to prevent sudden cardiac death in patients with coronary artery disease, especially in survivors of acute myocardial infarction. The role of coronary vasospasm in the genesis of sudden death in patients with ischemic heart disease is still unclear. In the case of beta-adrenoceptor blocking drugs, there is evidence that sudden cardiac death can be reduced significantly by prophylactic treatment in the survivors of infarction. It is however, not known whether the primary action is on electrical instability induced by myocardial ischemia. Calcium antagonists are potent antianginal drugs with the additional propensity to reverse coronary vasospasm. Calcium antagonists also have the property of minimizing myocardial ischemic damage following experimental coronary occlusion. One might therefore expect that, as a class, they should exert a salutary effect in the preservation of the ischemic myocardium during chronic prophylactic administration to patients with ischemic heart disease and to alter the incidence of ventricular arrhythmias. A controlled trials are needed to test this theoretical consideration. The results of the initial trials have been equivocal.

SUMMARY AND CONCLUSIONS

In recent years calcium channel blockers have emerged as a new class of antiarrhythmic agents for the control of certain supraventricular and ventricular arrhythmias. Electrophysiologically, they are heterogeneous but their main action is mediated through a depressant effect on the slow calcium channel in cardiac muscle. In isolated muscle, their actions are modulated by their reflex actions and by their interaction with the autonomic nervous system due to the nonocompetitive adrenergic blocking actions that some of the compounds exhibit. The major agents exerting antiarrhythmic actions are verapamil, diltiazem, gallopamil, tiapamil, and bepridil; the dihydropyridines are devoid of significant electrophysiologic actions *in vivo*. Calcium antagonists prolong intranodal conduction time, lengthen the effective and functional refractory periods in the AV node, but exert little or no effect on atrial, ventricular, His-Purkinje, or bypass tract conduction or refractoriness (except in the case of bepridil, which has additional electrophysiologic properties). These effects form the basis of the clinical antiarrhythmic effects of this class of agents. The most striking action is the predictable and prompt termination of reentrant supraventricular tachycardia by intravenous verapamil and diltiazem and the slowing of the ventricular response in atrial flutter and fibrillation. These agents may also be of value in the chronic control of ventricular response in atrial flutter and fibrillation; their role in multifocal atrial tachycardia and other ectopic tachycardias is less well defined.

Calcium antagonists reverse ischemic ventricular arrhythmias due to coronary artery spasm but exert little or no action in the usual forms of sustained ventricular tachyarrhythmias associated with severe structural heart disease. They are poor suppressants of premature ventricular contractions. Recent data have established their role in exercise-induced tachycardia occurring in the context of ischemic heart disease; they are also of value in ventricular tachycardia occurring in young subjects developing tachycardia with a right bundle branch block with left axis deviation morphology, an arrhythmia thought to be due to triggered automaticity. The role of calcium antagonists in reducing the incidence of sudden death in the survivors of acute myocardial infarction remains uncertain.

REFERENCES

1. Singh, B. N., G. Ellrodt & C. T. Peter. 1978. Verapamil: a review of its pharmacological properties and therapeutic use. Drugs **15:** 169–197.
2. Singh, B. N. & E. M. Vaughan Williams. 1972. A fourth class of antiarrhythmic action? Effects of verapamil on ouabain toxicity on atrial and ventricular intracellular potentials and on other features of cardiac function. Cardiovasc. Res. **6:** 109–119.
3. Hauswirth, O. & B. N. Singh. 1979. Ionic mechanisms in heart muscle in relation to the genesis and pharmacologic control of cardiac arrhythmias. Pharmacol. Rev. **30:** 5–63.
4. Rosen, M. R. & R. F. Redder. 1981. Does triggered activity have a role in the genesis of cardiac arrhythmias? Ann. Intern. Med. **96:** 794–801.

5. Brugada, P. & H. J. J. Wellens. 1984. The role of triggered activity in clinical ventricular arrhythmias. Pace **7:** 260–271.
6. Kato, R. & B. N. Singh. 1986. Effects of bepridil on the electrophysiologic properties of isolated canine and rabbit myocardial fibers. Am. Heart J. **111:** 271–285.
7. Josephson, M. E. & J. A. Kastor. 1977. Supraventricular tachycardia mechanism and management. Ann. Intern. Med. **87:** 869–878.
8. Heng, M. K., B. N. Singh, A. H. G. Roche, R. M. Norris & C. J. Mercer. 1975. Effects of intravenous verapamil on cardiac arrhythmias and on the electrocardiogram. Am Heart J. **90:** 487–498.
9. Singh, B. N., K. Nademanee & S. Baky. 1983. Calcium antagonists: clinical uses in treating arrhythmias. Drugs **25:** 125–153.
10. Schamroth, L., D. M. Krikler & C. Garrett. 1972. Immediate effects of intravenous verapamil in cardiac arrhythmias. Br. Heart J. **1:** 660–664.
11. Sung, R. J., B. Elser & R. G. McAllister. 1980. Intravenous verapamil for termination of reentrant supraventricular tachycardias. Intracardiac studies correlated with plasma verapamil concentrations. Ann. Intern. Med. **93:** 682–689.
12. Rinkenberger, R. L., E. N. Prystowsky, J. J. Heger, P. J. Troup, W. M. Jackman & D. P. Zipes. 1980. Effects of intravenous and chronic oral verapamil administration in patients with supraventricular tachyarrhythmias. Circulation **62:** 996–1010.
13. Rozansky, J. J., L. Zaman & A. Castellanos. 1982. Electrophysiologic effects of diltiazem hydrochloride on supraventricular tachycardia. Am. J. Cardiol. **49:** 621–628.
14. Bertin, A., B. R. Chaitman, M. G. Bourassa, G. Breuess, J. M. Scholl, P. Bruneau, P. Gague & M. Chabot. 1983. Beneficial effect of intravenous diltiazem in the acute management of supraventricular tachyarrhythmias. Circulation **67:** 88–94.
15. Hung, J. S., S. J. Yeh, F. C. Liu, M. Fu, Y. S. Lee & D. Wu. 1984. Usefulness of intravenous diltiazem in predicting subsequent electrophysiologic and clinical responses to oral diltiazem. Am. J. Cardiol. **54:** 1259–1262.
16. Yeh, S. H., F. C. Liu, Y. Y. Chan, J. S. Hung & D. Wu. 1985. Termination of paroxysmal supraventricular tachycardia with a single oral dose of diltiazem and propranolol. Circulation **71:** 104–109.
17. Bauernfeind, R. A., C. R. C. Wyndham, R. Dhingra, S. P. Swiryn, E. Palileo, B. Strasberg & K. M. Rosen. 1980. Serial electrophysiologic testing of multiple drugs in patients with atrioventricular nodal reentrant paroxysmal tachycardia. Circulation **62:** 1341–1349.
18. Wu, D., J. Hung, C. Kuo, K. Hsu & W. Shieh. 1981. Effects of quinidine on AV nodal re-entrant paroxysmal tachycardia. Circulation **64:** 169–170.
19. Swiryn, S. O., R. A. Bauernfeind, C. R. C. Wyndham, R. Dhingra, E. Palileo, B. Strasberg & K. M. Rosen. 1981. Effects of oral disopyramide phosphate on induction of paroxysmal supraventricular tachycardia. Circulation **64:** 169–178.
20. Sethi, K. K., S. Jaishankar & M. P. Gupta. 1984. Salutary effect of intravenous ajumaline in patients with paroxymal supraventricular tachycardia mediated by dual atrioventricular nodal pathways by blockade of retrograde pathways. Circulation **70**(5): 876–883.
21. Belhassen, B. & M. Pelleg. 1984. Acute management of paroxysmal supraventricular tachycardia: verapamil, adenosine triphosphate or adenosine? Am. J. Cardiol. **54:** 225–227.
22. Aronow, W. S., G. Plasencia & R. Wong. 1980. Effect of verapamil versus placebo in PAT and MAT (paroxysmal atrial tachycardia and multifocal atrial tachycardia). Curr. Ther. Res. **27:** 823–826.
23. Levine, H. J. H., J. R. Michael & T. Guarnieri. 1985. Treatment of multifocal atrial tachycardia with verapamil. N. Engl. J. Med. **312:** 21–25.
24. Mauritson, D. R., M. D. Winniford, W. S. Walker, R. E. Rude, J. R. Cary & L. D. Hills. 1982. Oral verapamil for paroxysmal supraventricular tachycardia. A longterm, double-blind randomized trial. Ann. Intern. Med. **96:** 409–412.
25. Sakurai, M., I. T. Yasuda, N. Kato, A. Nomura, M. Fujita, T. Nishino, K. Fujita, Y. Kolke & H. Saito. 1983. Acute and chronic effects of verapamil in patients with paroxysmal supraventricular tachycardia. Am. Heart J. **105:** 619–628.
26. Pritchett, E. L. C., S. C. Hammill, M. J. Reiter, K. L. Lee, E. A. McCarthy, J. M.

ZIMMERMAN & D. G. SHAND. 1983. Life-table method for evaluating antiarrhythmic drug efficacy in patients with paroxysmal atrial tachycardia. Am. J. Cardiol. **52:** 1007–1014.

27. WINNIFORD, M. D., M. D. FULTON & D. L. HILLIS. 1984. Longterm therapy of paroxysmal supraventricular tachycardia: a randomized, double-blind comparison of digoxin, propranolol and verapamil. Am. J. Cardiol. **54:** 1138–1139.
28. TONKIN, A. M., P. E. AYLWARD & S. E. JOEL. 1980. Verapamil on prophylaxis of paroxysmal atrioventricular nodal re-entrant tachycardia. J. Cardiovasc. Pharm. **2:** 473–480.
29. G. J. KLEIN, S. GULAMHUSEIN, S. G. CARRUTHERS, A. P. DONNER & P. T. KO. 1982. Comparison of the electrophysiologic effects of intravenous and oral verapamil in patients with paroxysmal supraventricular tachycardia. Am. J. Cardiol. **49:** 117–124.
30. STORSTEIN, O. & K. H. LANDMARK. 1975. Verapamil in the treatment of atrial tachycardia with block. Acta Med. Scand. **198:** 483–488.
31. KHALSA, A. & S. B. OLSSEN. 1979. Verapamil-induced ventricular regularity in atrial fibrillation. Acta Med. Scand. **205:** 509–515.
32. KLEIN, H. O. & E. KAPLINSKY. 1986. Digitalis and verapamil in atrial fibrillation and flutter. Is verapamil now the preferred agent? Drugs **31:** 185–197.
33. ROTH, A., E. HARRISON, G. MITANI, C. JORDAN, S. H. RAHIMTOOLA & U. ELKAYAM. 1986. Efficacy and safety of medium- and high-dose diltiazem alone and in combination with digoxin for the control of heart rate at rest and during exercise in patients with chronic atrial fibrillation. Circulation **73:** 316–324.
34. BASU, B., G. CHERIAN & K. A. ABRAHAM. 1977. Oral verapamil as maintenance therapy after cardioversion for atrial fibrillation. Ind. J. Chest. Dis. Allied Sci. **19:** 170–176.
35. RASMUSSEN, K., H. WANG & D. FAISA. 1981. Comparative efficacy of quinidine and verapamil in the maintenance of sinus rhythm after DC conversion of atrial fibrillation. Acta Med. Scand. (Suppl.) **645:** 23–28.
36. BELHASSEN, B. & L. N. HOROWITZ. 1984. Role of intravenous verapamil for ventricular tachycardia. Am. J. Cardiol. **54:** 1141–1133.
37. KRIKLER, D. M. & J. F. GOODWIN. 1976. Arrhythmia as a cause of sudden death in hypertrophic cardiomyopathy. Lancet **2:** 937–938.
38. MCKENNA, W. J., L. HARRIS & G. PEREZ. 1980. Hypertrophic cardiomyopathy: comparison of verapamil and amiodarone in the treatment of arrhythmia. Br. Heart J. **45:** 354–360.
39. WELLENS, H. J. J., F. W. BAR, K. I. LIE, D. R. DUREN & H. J. DOHMEN. 1977. Effects of procainamide, propranolol and verapamil on mechanism of tachycardia in patients with chronic recurrent ventricular tachycardia. Am. J. Cardiol. **40:** 579–585.
40. WELLENS, H. J. J., J. FARRE & W. B. BAR. 1980. The role of the slow inward current in the genesis of ventricular tachyarrhythmias in man. *In* The Slow Inward Current and Cardiac Arrhythmias. B. D. Zipes, J. C. Bailey & V. Elharrar, Eds.: 507–514.
41. SUNG, R. J., W. A. SHAPIRO, E. W. SHEN, F. MORADY & J. DAVIS. 1983. Effects of verapamil on ventricular tachycardias possibly caused by re-entry, automaticity, and triggered activity. J. Clin. Invest. **72:** 350–360.
42. MASON, J. W., C. D. SWERDLOW & L. B. MITCHELL. 1983. Efficacy of verapamil in chronic, recurrent ventricular tachycardia. Am. J. Cardiol. **51:** 1614–1617.
43. BUXTON, A. E., H. L. WAXMAN, F. E. MARCHLINSKI & M. E. JOSEPHSON. 1984. Electropharmacology of non-sustained ventricular tachycardia: effects of class I antiarrhythmic agents verapamil and propranolol. Am. J. Cardiol. **53:** 738–744.
44. SCLAROVSKY, S., B. STRASBERG, J. FUCHS, R. F. LEWIN, A. ARDITI, E. KLAINMAN, O. H. KRACOFF & J. AGMON. 1983. Multiform accelerated idioventricular rhythm in acute myocardial infarction: electrocardiographic characteristics and response to verapamil. Am. J. Cardiol. **52:** 43–47.
45. MASSUMI, R. A., J. MARIN & V. N. UDHOJI. 1986. Verapamil in parasystolic ventricular tachycardia and other wide QRS rhythms. Am. Heart J. **111:** 400–405.
46. GRENADIER, E., G. ALPAN, N. MAOR, S. KEIDAR, C. BINENBOIM, T. MARGUILES & A. PALANT. 1984. Polymorphous ventricular tachycardia in acute myocardial infarction. Am. J. Cardiol. **53:** 1280–1283.
47. WU, D., H. C. KOU & J. S. HUNG. 1981. Exercise-triggered paroxysmal ventricular

tachycardia. A repetitive rhythmic activity possibly related to afterdepolarization. Ann. Intern. Med. **95:** 410–414.

48. Wu, D. 1984. What is the value of calcium antagonists for ventricular tachycardia? Int. J. Cardiol. **5:** 543–547.
49. Coumel, P. & P. Attuel. 1983. Which arrhythmias are specifically susceptible to calcium antagonists. *In* Frontiers of Cardiac Electrophysiology. M. B. Rosenbaum & M. V. Elizari, Eds.: 341–348. Martines Nijhoff. Boston, Mass.
50. Belhassen, B., H. H. Rotmensch & S. Laniado. 1981. Response of recurrent sustained ventricular tachycardia to verapamil. Br. Heart J. **46:** 679–682.
51. Lin, F. C., D. Finley, S. H. Rahimtoola & D. Wu. 1983. Idiopathic paroxysmal ventricular tachycardia with a QRS pattern of right bundle branch block and left axis deviation: a unique clinical entity with specific properties. Am. J. Cardiol. **52:** 96–100.
52. German, L. D., D. L. Packer, G. H. Brady & J. J. Gallagher. 1983. Ventricular tachycardia induced by atrial stimulation in patients without symptomatic cardiac disease. Am. J. Cardiol. **52:** 1202–1207.
53. Belhassen, B., I. Shapira, A. Pelleg, I. Coperman, N. Kauli & S. Laniado. 1984. Idiopathic recurrent sustained ventricular tachycardia responsive to verapamil: an ECG-electrophysiologic entity. Am. Heart J. **108:** 1034–1036.

Calcium Antagonists in Heart Failure

SPENCER H. KUBO, MARIA TERESA OLIVARI, AND
JAY N. COHN

Cardiovascular Division
University of Minnesota
Minneapolis, Minnesota 55455

INTRODUCTION

The goals of therapy for heart failure include: (1) to improve performance of the left ventricle; (2) to improve exercise tolerance and the quality of life; (3) to prevent progression of myocardial dysfunction; and (4) to prevent suddent death which is a common terminal event in heart failure.

Ventricular performance is usually depressed in heart failure. This depression results in a decreased velocity and/or extent of muscle shortening, a decrease in ejection fraction, and an increase in end-diastolic volume and pressure. Possible mechanisms of depression in ventricular performance are listed in TABLE 1. They include a variety of specific abnormalities of the myocardium as well as the effects of the peripheral vasculature on ventricular function.

Many of the factors that depress either systolic or diastolic performance of the left ventricle may not be subject to manipulation by known therapeutic agents. Myocardial factors that certainly can be altered include ischemia related to large or small coronary artery obstruction and contractility related to alterations in excitation-contraction coupling. The effects of preload and impedance on cardiac performance can be influenced by drugs that alter the venous and arterial vasculature.[1]

The calcium antagonists as a group may exert a variety of sometimes contrasting actions on these factors influencing left ventricular performance.[2,3] By reducing myocardial cytosolic calcium concentration, a reduction of myocardial contractility from at least some of the drugs in this series would be anticipated. The reduction in cytosolic calcium could at the same time have a favorable effect on ventricular compliance which appears to be reduced in many patients with heart failure, including some who have apparently normal systolic function. If ischemia plays a role in depressed myocardial function the calcium antagonists also could have a favorable effect by relaxing the conduit coronary arteries. A small vessel coronary dilator effect also could be beneficial, but the possibility of an adverse effect on ischemia by a "steal" phenomena in individual patients with specific anatomical distribution of coronary atherosclerosis cannot be excluded.

The peripheral vascular action of the calcium antagonists should have a favorable effect on cardiac performance. Relaxation of the large and small arterial vasculature decreases the impedance to left ventricular emptying and should increase stroke volume and ejection fraction. A modest venodilator effect which results from at least some of the calcium antagonists should redistribute blood volume from the central vasculature into the venous capacitance vessels and thus reduce ventricular preload. In the presence of depressed ventricular function, the reduction in preload should have little adverse effect on stroke volume because of the relatively flat Frank-Starling curve on which most patients with heart failure function.[1]

The other therapeutic goals in the treatment of heart failure appear to depend on factors in addition to ventricular function. Changes in the peripheral vasculature, in regional vascular beds, in neurohormonal responses, and in metabolism all may contribute to exercise intolerance, progression of ventricular dysfunction, and arrhythmias. Since the mechanisms of these disorders have not been clarified, the potential role of calcium antagonists in influencing these manifestations of heart failure can only be assessed by carefully controlled prospective trials.

PHARMACODYNAMIC EFFECTS OF CALCIUM ANTAGONISTS

Although the calcium antagonists are considered as a single class of drugs, it is clear that the chemical structures, receptor affinities, and pharmacodynamic actions of these agents are quite diverse.[2,3] This diversity and heterogeneity have become even more evident as additional compounds are evaluated. It has therefore been difficult to develop a simple and coherent classification of these agents based on chemical structure or selectivity for slow calcium channels. The most useful and practical method of differentiating the various agents is to contrast their pharmocodynamic actions in the cardiovascular system, and their relative potencies.[3,4] This would include actions on coronary and peripheral vascular tone, myocardial contractility, sinoatrial nodal automaticity, atrioventricular nodal conduction, and intraventricular conduction.

TABLE 1. Factors that May Influence Left Ventricular Performance

A. Myocardial factors
1. Muscle mass
2. Muscle contractility
3. Muscle perfusion
4. Myosin species
5. Nonmuscular elements: collagen, infiltration
6. Dysynergy
7. Compliance
B. Peripheral factors
1. Capacitance (preload)
2. Impedance (afterload)

The most consistent effect of all the calcium blockers is on vascular tone. All have vasodilating properties which can be demonstrated in many different arterial beds, including the coronary, pulmonary, renal, hepatic, and mesenteric arteries. Comparative studies in the dog suggest that the increase in flow is greatest in the femoral artery, followed by the coronary, renal, and mesenteric arteries.[2] In general, on a weight basis, the dihydropyridines are more potent vasodilators than the nondihydropyridines. The arterial dilation affects both the small resistance vessels and the large muscular arteries. The calcium antagonists appear to exert at most only a modest dilating effect on the venous capacitance vessels.

Because slow inward calcium currents are also important for the normal contraction of myocardial cells, there have been concerns over negative inotropic properties of the calcium antagonists. It should be emphasized, however, that these agents are more effective in inhibiting contraction in arterial smooth muscle than in myocardial cells. Thus, while there is a definite potential for a negative inotropic effect, these drugs can generally be given in doses that exert vascular effects without significantly affecting the force of contraction of ventricular muscle. In comparative studies using equimolar doses, the relative potency of the direct negative inotropic effect is greatest for nifedipine and verapamil followed by diltiazem.[2]

Sinoatrial nodal automaticity and atrioventricular nodal conduction are both affected by diltiazem and verapamil. In contrast, nifedipine has little direct effect on these areas. One characteristic common to all three calcium channel blockers is a lack of effect on intraventricular conduction, likely related to an absence of effects on the fast sodium channel.

The hemodynamic response to the systemic administration of a calcium channel blocker represents a balance between these diverse effects on the cardiovascular system and various neurohormonal and reflex effects that may accompany their action. Moreover, the net hemodynamic response may be influenced by the underlying disease state and hemodynamic profile. For example, the administration of nifedipine in a patient with coronary artery disease might be associated with a decrease in blood pressure, but a constant cardiac output. In a patient with heart failure, the vasodilation will generally be associated with an increase in cardiac output. However, if cardiac reserve is minimal, even a slight negative inotropic effect may become clinically important.

HEMODYNAMIC AND NEUROHORMONAL RESPONSES TO CALCIUM ANTAGONISTS IN HEART FAILURE

Nifedipine

Nifedipine was the first calcium antagonist to be tested in patients with congestive heart failure and has also been the most extensively evaluated.

Several studies have shown that nifedipine, administered either orally or sublingually, can acutely improve the hemodynamic profile of patients with stable congestive heart failure.[5–9] Although the dosage (10 mg to 40 mg) and route of administration (oral versus sublingual) have been variable, most of the studies show that nifedipine will cause significant vasodilation, manifested by marked reductions in mean arterial pressure and systemic vascular resistance, accompanied by an increased cardiac output and stroke volume. In contrast to normal subjects and many patients with hypertension, reflex tachycardia usually is not observed in patients with heart failure, probably because of an acquired abnormality in reflex autonomic control in such patients.[10,11]

Although cardiac output increases considerably in response to nifedipine, this hemodynamic effect likely represents a *balance* between the effects on impedance and myocardial contractility. Similar to other forms of vasodilator therapy, the abrupt reduction in peripheral arterial tone results in better ventricular emptying and an increase in forward flow. Although a direct negative inotropic effect is difficult to demonstrate in clinical settings because of confounding effects of changes in preload, afterload, and heart rate, several studies have addressed this problem through a comparison to other vasodilators that do not have negative inotropic properties. Fifer *et al.* evaluated the hemodynamic responses to nifedipine and nitroprusside, titrating both drugs to produce equivalent degrees of vasodilatation.[12] Nifedipine decreased peak positive dp/dt from 747 ± 292 to 639 ± 238 mmHg/second ($p < 0.002$), whereas nitroprusside had no effect on this measure of left ventricular contractility. Although both drugs caused comparable increases in cardiac output and stroke volume index, left ventricular end-diastolic pressure decreased with nitroprusside, but was unchanged with nifedipine, probably because of the more prominent effect of nitroprusside on venous capacitance vessels. More recently, Rousseau and Pouleur compared the intracoronary infusions of nifedipine and nicardipine,[13] a second generation dihydropyridine calcium antagonist. In this model myocardial effects can be assessed independent of the secondary effects of afterload reduction. Nifedipine but not nicardipine caused a decrease in max dp/dt, associated with an increase in left ventricular end-diastolic pressure. Elkayam *et al.* compared nifedipine to equipotent doses of both hydralazine[14] and nitroprusside,[15] and confirmed that the magnitude of increase of cardiac output with nifedipine was less than that associated with both direct-acting vasodilators. All of these data strongly suggest that, in patients with congestive heart failure, nifedipine may exert a negative inotropic action that could attentuate the beneficial hemodynamic effects of impedance reduction. Although the acute hemodynamic responses are generally favorable, suggesting a predominant vasodilator effect, it has been speculated that the variable clinical efficacy of nifedipine in patients with chronic congestive heart failure is related to differences in the balance between these competing effects.[16] That the negative inotropic effect could predominate and be clinically relevant is supported by some adverse clinical experiences, including the precipitation of pulmonary edema and circulatory collapse.[17,18]

Several studies have shown that nifedipine will reduce preload,[5–9] but in two other studies, nifedipine administration did not cause a significant reduction in right atrial or pulmonary wedge pressures.[8,12] We further evaluated the effects of nifedipine on preload reduction by assessing the hemodynamic responses to head-up tilt.[8] This maneuver in subjects with normal cardiac function causes venous pooling in the legs, accompanied by a reduction in pulmonary wedge pressure and cardiac output. Captopril, a converting enzyme inhibitor with known effects on venous and arterial tone, can accentuate tilt-induced preload reduction.[19] However, nifedipine did not affect pulmonary wedge pressure or cardiac output during tilt testing, confirming a lack of significant effects on venous capacitance vessels. In addition, Kurnik *et al.* showed that nifedipine had no effect on venous tone measured by strain guage plethysmography.[9] This lack of preload effect would suggest that the clinical application of nifedipine in heart failure would likely require the concomitant administration of nitrates, similar to the use of hydralazine. This combination of nifedipine and nitrates has been shown to produce a beneficial and balanced arterial and venous effect.[20]

The effects of nifedipine on neurohormonal activity in patients with congestive heart failure have not been extensively evaluated. In one study a single 10 mg oral dose of nifedipine caused an increase in plasma renin activity from 10 ± 5.6 ng/ml per hour to 20 ± 9 ng/ml per hour at 30 minutes and 26 ± 12.5 ng/ml per hour at 60 minutes.[8] There was no associated change in plasma aldosterone. Plasma norepinephrine increased from 697 ± 122 to 1025 ± 264 pg/ml at 60 minutes; however, because of interpatient variability, this increase was not statistically significant. Similar findings were reported by Fifer *et al.*[12] It would be anticipated, however, that the effects of nifedipine on neurohormonal activity would be difficult to assess because of potentially competing effects. Marked vasodilatation can cause reflex stimulation of these pathways, especially if there is excessive reduction in mean arterial pressure and renal perfusion pressure. Furthermore, several studies have shown that calcium channel antagonists can directly stimulate renin secretion from the kidney[21] and that calcium channel inhibition can directly suppress aldosterone release from the adrenal gland.[22] Therefore, nifedipine may have several direct and indirect influences on neurohormonal activity.

Nicardipine

Nicardipine is a second generation calcium antagonist that is structurally and pharmacologically related to nifedipine, in that both are of the dihydropyridine class and have the ability to block slow calcium channels.[23] Nicardipine shares the same pharmacodynamic actions of nifedipine in having a predominant relaxant effect on vascular smooth muscle[24–26] with very little effect on sinus node automaticity or atrioventricular nodal conduction.[27]

Initial studies with nicardipine have suggested that it may exert less negative inotropic effects than nifedipine. In 21 patients with coronary artery disease, Rousseau and Pouleur evaluated the intracoronary infusions of nicardipine and nifedipine.[13] Nicardipine consistently increased coronary blood flow, but did not affect max dp/dt or T, the time constant of the decrease in left ventricular pressure. In contrast, nifedipine decreased max dp/dt, increased left ventricular end-diastolic pressure, and prolonged T. Other studies in patients without heart failure have shown that intravenous infusions of nicardipine will result in a marked decrease in mean aortic

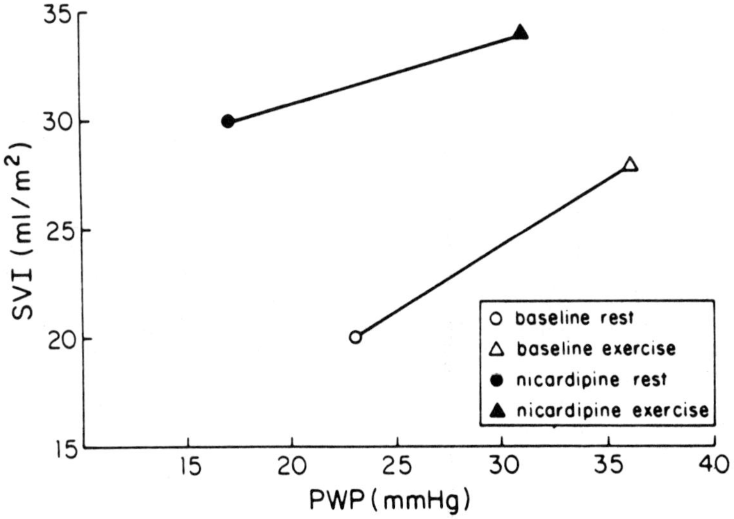

FIGURE 1. Relationship of pulmonary wedge pressure (PWP) and stroke volume index (SVI) at rest and during exercise, as an estimate of the Frank-Starling curve in heart failure patients treated with nicardipine. One week of nicardipine therapy was associated with a favoarble upward and leftward shift of the cardiac function curve, both at rest and during exercise. (Reproduced from Reference 30, with permission.)

pressure, an increase in coronary blood flow and stroke volume index, but no change in peak dp/dt or left ventricular end-diastolic pressure.[28,29] These data suggest that the peripheral vasodilating effects of nicardipine are not accompanied by a significant negative effect on myocardial contractility. Moreover, nicardipine appears to be a potent coronary vasodilator, causing increases in coronary blood flow despite a decrease in mean aortic pressure and in the absence of changes in myocardial oxygen consumption.

To evaluate further the hemodynamic actions of nicardipine in patients with heart failure, rest and exercise hemodynamics were performed before and after one week of oral nicardipine therapy.[30] At rest, nicardipine resulted in marked peripheral vasodilatation, with a decrease in mean arterial pressure from 96 ± 10 to 76 ± 10 mmHg, and in systemic vascular resistance from 2467 ± 1311 to 1424 ± 635 dynes × seconds ×

cm^{-5}. This vasodilatation was accompanied by an increase in cardiac index from 1.72 ± 0.36 to 2.56 ± 1.12 l/minute per m^2, and stroke volume index from 20 ± 5 to 30 ± 10 ml/m^2. In addition, there were reductions in mean pulmonary artery pressure from 36 ± 16 to 31 ± 13 mmHg and pulmonary wedge pressure from 23 ± 11 to 17 ± 9 mmHg. Resting heart rate, right atrial pressure, and pulmonary vascular resistance were not significantly changed with nicardipine. These data suggest that the peripheral vasodilation from nicardipine improves the resting hemodynamic profile of patients with congestive heart failure. In addition, unlike nifedipine, which has very little effect on preload reduction, nicardipine decreased both pulmonary artery and pulmonary wedge pressures.

Exercise hemodynamics were also improved on nicardipine. Peripheral vasodilatation was maintained at maximal exercise, as mean arterial pressure decreased from 110 ± 15 to 91 ± 10 mmHg, and systemic vascular resistance from 1572 ± 1326 to 1031 ± 539 dynes × seconds × cm^{-5}. There was a further increase in cardiac index from 3.42 ± 1.50 to 4.10 ± 1.91 l/minute per m^2, and stroke volume index from 28 ± 9 to 34 ± 13 ml/m^2. Finally, the salutary decreases in pulmonary artery and pulmonary wedge pressures were also maintained at maximal exercise from 55 ± 19 to 51 ± 18 and 36 ± 11 to 31 ± 12 mmHg, respectively. The relationship of pulmonary wedge pressure and stroke volume index at rest and during exercise, as an estimate of the Frank-Starling relationship, is shown in FIGURE 1. There is an upward and leftward shift with the nicardipine therapy, suggesting improved cardiac function in the setting of afterload and preload reduction.

Plasma norepinephrine was measured at rest and during exercise before and after nicardipine therapy. Plasma norepinephrine increased with exercise in the baseline state from 861 ± 486 to 1835 + 694 pg/ml and during nicardipine therapy from 843 ± 340 to 2612 ± 1325 pg/ml. Resting values of plasma norepinephrine were similar before and after nicardipine, thus suggesting the absence of significant sympathetic stimulation. Although the peak exercise norepinephrine concentration was elevated on nicardipine therapy, this increase may be related to the higher cardiac index achieved during maximal exercise while on nicardipine.

There are few data on the use of nicardipine in the long-term treatment with patients swith heart failure, as most of the chronic efficacy data are from clinical trials in patients with hypertension or coronary artery disease.[31–32] Based on these initial findings, however, long-term clinical trials assessing the efficacy of nicardipine in heart failure appear warranted.

Nitrendipine

Nitrendipine [1,4 dihydro - 2,6 dimethyl - 4 - (3 nitrophenyl) - pyridin - 3,5 - dicarbon acid - 3 - ethyl - 5 - methylester] is a dihydropyridine that has been shown to produce a prompt and sustained decrease in arterial pressure in patients with systemic hypertension by decreasing peripheral vascular resistance.[33] The hypotensive effect is comparable and longer lasting than the effect of nifedipine.[34] Nitrendipine has the advantage over nifedipine of higher vasoselectivity and has been shown to have a primary natriuretic effect[35] which may be beneficial in patients with hypertension and congestive heart failure.

The effectiveness of nitrendipine as a ventricular unloading agent for the treatment of congestive heart failure has been studied in our laboratory.[36] Eight patients with stable, chronic congestive heart failure received 10 mg of oral nitrendipine. Within one hour, there was a significant decrease in right atrial and pulmonary capillary wedge pressures, and in systemic and pulmonary vascular resistances (FIGURE 2). There was also a significant increase in cardiac index while heart rate remained unchanged. These beneficial hemodynamic changes most likely result from the direct vasodilating effect of nitrendipine on both resistance and capacitance vessels. The decrease in preload suggests that nitrendipine, in contrast to nifedipine, produces significant venodilation and confirms data obtained in animals[37] which suggest that nitrendipine has potent venous effects.

The improvement in ventricular performance with nitrendipine, as manifest by an increase in cardiac output associated with a decrease in ventricular filling pressures, was probably secondary to the reduction in systemic and pulmonary impedance and was not associated with a reflex sympathetic activation. It has been suggested that the vasodilation due to the dihydropyridine compounds is possibly associated with a reflex

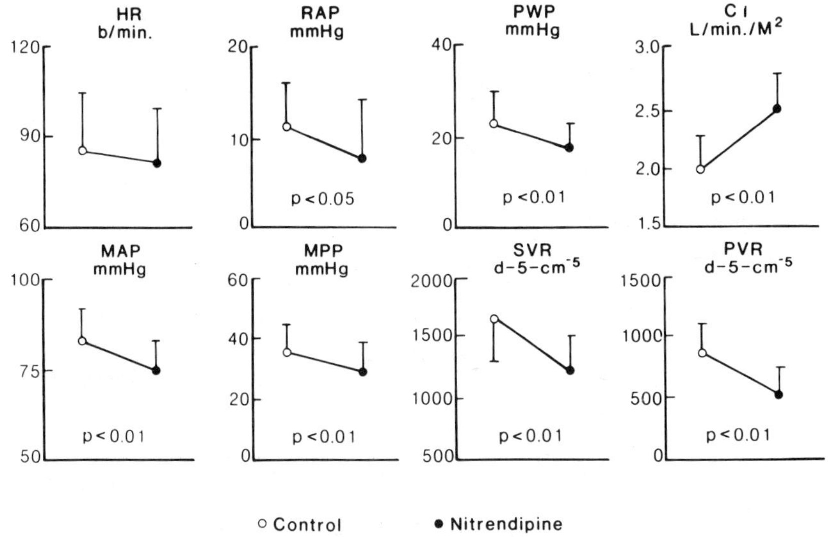

FIGURE 2. Acute hemodynamic effect of nitrendipine in congestive heart failure ($n = 8$). Peak hemodynamic response to nitrendipine, comparing control values (mean ± standard deviation; open circles) and 60 minutes after the administration of nitrendipine (filled circles). HR = heart rate, RAP = right atrial pressure, PWP = pulmonary wedge pressure, CI = cardiac index, MAP = mean arterial pressure, MPP = mean pulmonary pressure, SVR = systemic vascular resistance, PVR = pulmonary vascular resistance.

activation of the sympathetic nervous system. However, in our study heart rate was unchanged and plasma norepinephrine decreased from 830 pg/ml to 622 pg/ml after nitrendipine, thus excluding an increase in sympathetic drive as a mechanism for the improvement in ventricular function.

Verapamil

In contrast to nifedipine and nitrendipine, intravenous infusion of verapamil has been shown to exert a substantial negative inotropic effect which may overwhelm the expected improvement in ventricular performance secondary to peripheral vasodilation in patients with congestive heart failure.[38,39] Even when administered orally,[40] verapamil did not improve ventricular function despite a significant reduction in peripheral vascular resistance. Indeed, pulmonary capillary wedge pressure did not fall and left ventricular end-diastolic diameter increased, thus suggesting the predominance of the negative inotropic action. Moreover, verapamil has a significant negative chronotropic effect and may produce a substantial fall in cardiac output secondary to a decrease in heart rate.

Our experience with verapamil is limited to three patients with chronic New York Heart Association (NYHA) Class III congestive heart failure who received a five minute intravenous infusion of verapamil at 0.005 mg/kg per minute. All three patients experienced hemodynamic deterioration. One patient experienced a large

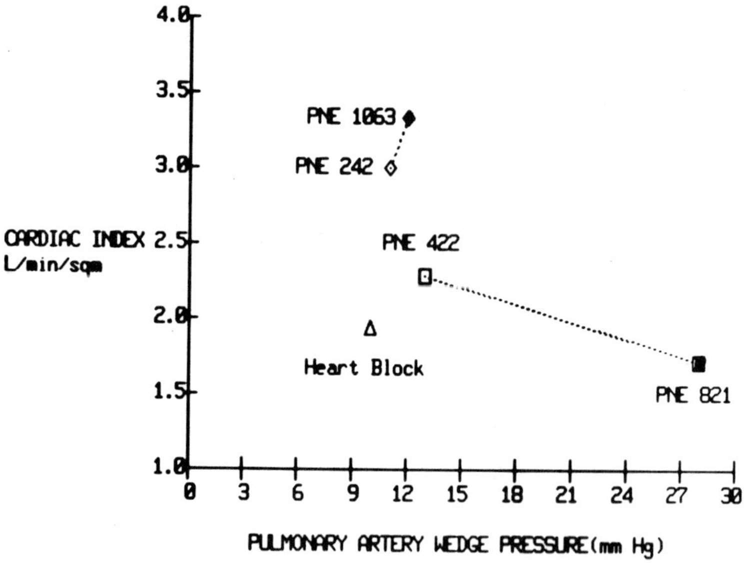

FIGURE 3. Response to verapamil in patients with congestive heart failure. Effect of intravenous verapamil on the relationship between pulmonary capillary wedge pressure (PCWP) and cardiac index (CI) and on plasma norepinephrine (PNE; pg/ml) in three patients with congestive heart failure. (Open squares = control values; filled squares = values obtained 15 minutes after intravenous verapamil.)

decrease in cardiac output secondary to third degree atrioventricular (AV) block. In the other two patients, a direct negative inotropic effect appears to be the most likely explanation for the increase in pulmonary capillary wedge pressure (FIGURE 3). Plasma norepinephrine rose abruptly in response to verapamil in two of these patients, possibly as a consequence of the deterioration of left ventricular function. However hemodynamic deterioration because of vasoconstriction induced by this sympathetic stimulation cannot be excluded.

Diltiazem

Diltiazem, a benzothiazepine derivative, has a prominent *in vitro* chronotropic effect and exerts less depression on myocardial contractility than nifedipine does. The evaluation of diltiazem has been limited to a small number of patients with congestive heart failure. Materne reported the hemodynamic effects of diltiazem (0.5 mg/kg administered intravenously) in eight patients with severe heart failure.[41] Despite a significant decrease in left ventricular positive d*p*/d*t* from 1730 ± 589 to 1404 ± 470 mmHg/second, ($p < 0.01$), stroke volume increased significantly from 60 ± 12 to 75 ± 11 ml/beat, secondary to a decrease in left ventricular impedance.

While arterial pressure and systemic vascular resistance fell significantly, right and left ventricular preload did not change. A similar effect on peripheral vascular resistance was observed by Walsh *et al.* during both intravenous and oral administration of diltiazem in eight patient with NYHA class III–IV heart failure.[42] However, in this study, the rate of left ventricular pressure development did not decrease after diltiazem and the increase in stroke volume was associated with a significant decrease in pulmonary capillary wedge pressure from 29 ± 9 to 21 ± 9 mmHg.

The explanation for these differing effects on preload and left ventricular contractility in these two studies are not clear, but may be due to different dosages of diltiazem. In addition, baseline hemodynamics were different as systemic vascular resistance was higher in the study by Walsh. It has been shown that the peripheral vasodilator effect of nifedipine is dependent on the baseline vascular tone.[43] A significant chronotropic effect was observed in both studies. Three of the four patients who were given 200 μg bolus infusion developed a transient junctional rhythm. Oxygen consumption decreased markedly in both studies as a consequence of a decrease in systemic pressure and heart rate, suggesting that diltiazem may be especially beneficial in patients with ischemic cardiomyopathy.

CONCLUSIONS

Vasodilators have now become established as effective drugs in the treatment of heart failure. Whereas their use was previously advocated only in patients who failed to improve on digitalis and diuretic therapy, the current trend is toward earlier use of these drugs.

Efficacy of these drugs has been assessed primarily by observations of improved cardiac performance and increased exercise tolerance. The drugs subjected to most intensive study have been the nitrates, hydralazine, prazosin, and the angiotensin converting enzyme inhibitors. A recently completed Veterans Administration Cooperative Study (V-HEFT) has demonstrated for the first time that a vasodilator regimen (hydralazine and isosorbide dinitrate) can prolong life in patients with heart failure already treated with digoxin and diuretics.[44] In that study prazosin did not exert a favorable effect on survival compared to placebo. Thus the favorable effect on the course of heart failure of selected vasodilator drugs is now well established.

The calcium antagonists are potent vasodilators, but their use in heart failure has been discouraged by concern regarding negative inotropic effects. Experience to date suggests that this concern may have been overstated. Favorable preliminary experience with at least some of these drugs suggests that a well-controlled trial of a calcium antagonist in heart failure is justified.

REFERENCES

1. COHN, J. N. & J. A. FRANCIOSA. 1977. Vasodilator therapy of cardiac failure. N. Engl. J. Med **297:** 27–31, 254–258.
2. STONE, P. H., E. M. ANTMAN, J. E. MULLER & E. BRAUNWALD. 1980. Calcium channel blocking agents in the treatment of cardiovascular disorders. II. Hemodynamic effects and clinical applications. Ann. Intern. Med. **93:** 886–904.

3. TAIRA, N. 1987. Differences in cardiovascular profile among calcium antagonists. Am. J. Cardiol. **59:** 24B–29B.
4. VANHOUTTE, P. M. 1987. The expert committee of the World Health Organization on classification of calcium antagonists: the viewpoint of the raporteur. Am. J. Cardiol. **59:** 3A–8A.
5. POLESE, A., C. FIORENTINI, M. T. OLIVARI & M. D. GUAZZI. 1979. Clinical use of a calcium antagonistic agent (nifedipine) in acute pulmonary edema. Am. J. Med. **66:** 825–830.
6. BELLOCI, F., G. ANSALONE, P. SANTARELLI, F. LOPERFIDO, E. SCABBIA, P. ZECCHI & U. MARJOLI. 1982. Oral nifedipine in the long term management of severe chronic heart failure. J. Cardiovasc. Pharmacol. **4:** 847–855.
7. KLUGMAN, S., A. SALVI & F. CAMERINI. 1980. Haemodynamic effects of nifedipine in heart failure. Br. Heart. J. **43:** 440–446.
8. PRIDA, X. E., S. H. KUBO, J. H. LARAGH & R. J. CODY. 1983. Evaluation of calcium mediated vasoconstriction in chronic congestive heart failure. Am. J. Med. **75:** 795–800.
9. KURNIK, P. B., A. J. TIEFENBRUNN & P. A. LUDBROOK. 1984. The dependence of the cardiac effects of nifedipine on the responses of the peripheral vascular system. Circulation **69:** 963–972.
10. OLIVARI, M. T., T. B. LEVINE & J. N. COHN. 1983. Abnormal neurohumoral response to nitroprusside infusion in congestive heart failure. J. Am. Coll. Cardiol. 2:411–417.
11. KUBO, S. H. & R. J. CODY. 1983. Circulatory autoregulation in chronic congestive heart failure: responses to head up tilt in 41 patients. Am. J. Cardiol. **52:** 512–518.
12. FIFER, M. A., W. S. COLUCCI, B. H. LORELL, B. E JASKI & W. H. BARRY. 1985. Inotropic, vascular and neuroendocrine effects of nifedipine in heart failure: comparison with nitroprusside. J. Am. Coll. Cardiol. **5:** 731–737.
13. ROUSSEAU, M. F. & H. POULEUR. 1984. Calcium antagonism free of negative inotropic effects? A comparison of intracoronary nifedipine and nicardipine. Circulation **70**(Suppl. II): II–304 (abstr.).
14. ELKAYAM, U., L. WEBER, C. R. MCKAY & S. H. RAHIMTOOLA. 1984. Differences in hemodynamic response to vasodilation due to calcium channel antagonism with nifedipine and direct acting agonism with hydralazine in chronic refractory congestive heart failure. Am. J. Cardiol. **54:** 126–131.
15. ELKAYAM, U., L. WEBER, B. TORKAN, C. R. MCKAY & S. H. RAHIMTOOLA. 1984. Comparison of hemodynamic responses to nifedipine and nitroprusside in severe chronic congestive heart failure. Am. J. Cardiol. **53:** 1321–1325.
16. ELKAYAM, U., L. WEBER, C. R. MCKAY & S. H. RAHIMTOOLA. 1985. Spectrum of acute hemodynamic effects of nifedipine in severe congestive heart failure. Am. J. Cardiol. **56:** 560–566.
17. GILLMER, D. J. & P. KARK. 1980. Pulmonary oedema precipitated by nifedipine. Br. Med. J. **280:** 1420–1421.
18. BROOKS, N., M. CATTELL, J. PIDGEON & R. BALCON. 1980. Unpredictable response to nifedipine in severe cardiac failure. Br. Med. J. **201:** 1324.
19. CODY, R. J., K. W. FRANKLIN, J. KLUGER & J. H. LARAGH. 1982. Mechanisms governing the postural response, and baroreceptor abnormalities in chronic congestive heart failure: effects of acute and long term converting enzyme inhibition. Circulation **66:** 135–142.
20. KUBO, S. H., S. C. FOX, X. E. PRIDA & R. J. CODY. 1985. Combined hemodynamic effects of nifedipine and nitroglycerine in congestive heart failure. Am. Heart J. **110:** 1032–1034.
21. NAFTILAN, A. J. & S. OPARIL. 1982. The role of calcium in the control of renin release. Hypertension **4:** 670–675.
22. FAKUNDIG, J. L. & K. J. CATT. 1980. Dependence of aldosterone stimulation in adrenal glomerulosa cells on calcium uptake: effects of lanthanum and verapamil. Endocrinology **107:** 1345–1353.
23. HOF, R. P. 1983. Calcium antagonist and peripheral circulation differences and similarities between PY-108-068, nicardipine, verapamil and diltiazem. Br. J. Pharmacol. **78:** 375–394.
24. ILIOPOULOU, S., P. TURNER & S. J. WARRINGTON. 1983. Acute haemodynamic effects of a

new calcium antagonist, nicardipine, in man. A comparison with nifedipine. Br. J. Clin. Pharmacol. **15:** 59–65.

25. HENRY, P. D. 1980. Comparative pharmacology of calcium antagonists: nifedipine, verapamil and diltiazem. Am. J. Cardiol. **46:** 1047–1058.
26. MCCREDIE, R. M., W. B. MCKENZIE & D. M. MCGILL. 1985. The acute haemodynamic effects of oral nicardipine. Br. J. Clin. Pharmacol. **20:** 1635–1685.
27. MATSUI, M., H. NISHIWAKI, J. YOSHIMO, M. ENDO, M. YOSHIKAWA, K. SUGI, H. ITO, K. NIMOMIYJA, K. EBINE, S. YABUKI & K. SEKI. 1982. Effects of nicardipine hydrochloride on the conduction system of the heart in man. Jpn. Heart J. **23:** 243–245.
28. ROUSSEAU, M. F., M. F. VINCENT, F. VAN HOOF, G. VAN DER BERGHE, A. A. CHARLIER & H. POULEUR. 1984. Effects of nicardipine and nisoldipine on myocardial metabolism, coronary blood flow and oxygen supply in angina pectoris. Am. J. Cardiol. **54:** 1189–1194.
29. LAMBERT, C. R., J. A. HILL, W. W. NICHOLS, R. L. FELDMAN & C. J. PEPINE. 1985. Coronary and systemic hemodynamic effects of nicardipine. Am. J. Cardiol. **55:** 652–656.
30. RYMAN, K. S., S. H. KUBO, J. LYSTASH, G. STONE & R. J. CODY. 1986. Effect of nicardipine on rest and exercise hemodynamics in chronic congestive heart failure. Am. J. Cardiol. **58:** 583–588.
31. JONES, R. I., R. S. HORNUNG, T. S. SONECHA & E. B. RAFTERY. 1983. The effects of a new calcium channel blocker nicardipine on 24 hour ambulatory blood pressure and the pressor response to isometric and dynamic exercise. Hypertension **1:** 85–89.
32. KHURMI, N. S., M. J. BOWLES, V. B. SUBRAMANIAN & E. B. RAFERTY. Short and long term efficacy of nicardipine, assessed by placebo controlled single and double blind crossover trials in patients with chronic stable angina. J. Am. Coll. Cardiol. **4:** 908–917.
33. HANSSON, L., L. ANDREN, L. ORO & T. RYMAN. 1983. Pharmacokinetic and pharmacodynamic parameters in patients treated with nitrendipine. Hypertension **5:**(Suppl. II): 25–28.
34. GUAZZI, M. D., N. DE CESARE, C. GALLI, G. TAMBORINI & A. SALVIONI. 1986. Nitrendipine versus long-acting nifedipine in mild, moderate and severe hypertension. Angiology 508.
35. ZANCHETTI, A., A. STELLA & R. GOLIN. 1985. Adrenergic renal sodium handling and the natriuretic action of calcium antagonists. J. Cardiovasc. Pharmacol. **7**(Suppl. 6): 194–198.
36. OLIVARI, M. T., T. B. LEVINE & J. N. COHN. 1984. Acute hemodynamic effects of nitrendipine in chronic congestive heart failure. J. Cardiovasc. Pharmacol. **6**(Suppl. 7): 1002–1105.
37. ALTURA, B. M., A. GEBREWOLD & B. T. ALTURA. 1984. Regional arteriolar and venular dilator actions of dihydropyridines versus verapamil: direct in vivo studies on the microcirculation. *In* Nitrendipine. A. Scriabine, Ed.: 219–236. Urban and Schwarzenberg. Baltimore, Md.
38. SINGH, B. & A. H. ROCHE. 1977. Effects of intravenous verapamil on hemodynamics in patients with heart disease. Am. Heart J. **94:** 593–599.
39. CHEW, C., H. HECHT, J. COLETT, R. MCCALLISTER & B. SINGH. 1981. Influence of severity of ventricular dysfunction on hemodynamic response to intravenously administered verapamil in ischemic heart disease. Am. J. Cardiol. **47:** 917–922.
40. GUAZZI, M. D., C. CIPOLLA, P. DELLA BELLA, F. FABBIOCHI, P. MONTORSI & P. SGANZERLA. 1984. Disparate unloading efficacy of the calcium channel blockers, verapamil and nifedipine, on the failing hypertensive left ventricle. Am. Heart J. **108:** 116–123.
41. MATERNE, P., V. LEGRAND, M. VANDORMOEL, P. COLLIGNON & H. E. KULBERTUS. 1984. Hemodynamic effects of intravenous diltiazem with impaired left ventricular function. Am. J. Cardiol. **54:** 733–737.
42. WALSH, R. W., C. B. PORTER, M. R. STARLING & R. O'ROURKE. 1984. Beneficial hemodynamic effects of intravenous and oral diltiazem in severe congestive heart failure. J. Am. Coll. Cardiol. **3:** 1044–1050.
43. OLIVARI, M. T., C. BARTORELLI, A. POLESE, C. FIORENTINI, P. MORUZZI & M. GUAZZI.

1979. Treatment of hypertension with nifedipine, a calcium antagonistic agent. Circulation **59:** 1056–1062.

44. Cohn, J. N., D. G. Archibald, S. Ziesche, J. A. Franciosa, W. E. Houston, F. E. Tristani, W. B. Dunkman, W. Jacobs, G. S. Francis, K. H. Flohr, S. Goldman, F. R. Cobb, P. M. Shah, R. Saunders, R. D. Fletcher, H. S. Loeb, V. S. Hughes & B. Baker. 1986. Effect of vasodilator therapy on mortality in chronic congestive heart failure. Results of a Veterans Administration cooperative study (V-HeFT). N. Engl. J. Med. **314:** 1547.

Calcium Antagonists for Angina Pectoris

P. G. HUGENHOLTZ

Thoraxcenter
University Hospital
Erasmus University
Rotterdam, the Netherlands

INTRODUCTION

Any physician intimately involved in the care of patients with coronary artery disease knows from his experience that the toughest cases, those who require the most difficult decisions in terms of management and therapy, are found in those individuals who temporarily are on the watershed between angina pectoris and myocardial infarction. This period marks the boundary between the manageable loss of tissue (by the patient) during angina and the unmanageable (by the doctor) loss of tissue that ensues once myocardial infarction has taken place.

While it is true that not every case of (un)stable angina will lead to myocardial infarction or prolonged ischemia or even sudden death, it is also not clear in how many people symptoms or signs of these unstable syndromes have actually preceded sudden death or acute myocardial infarction. In fact, we remain woefully short of a real understanding of the natural history of unstable angina in a given patient within or outside the hospital. In fact, it is the uncertainty of outcome in a specific patient that obliges us, urges us, and indeed forces us to provide maximal therapy to all.

No matter which approach one chooses, conservative,[1] intensive pharmacological,[2] or invasive,[3] such therapy should result in prompt, that is within 24 hours or less, relief of symptoms with a near absence of sequelae such as subsequent myocardial infarction or death over a one-year period. Such a goal can be achieved by a judicious choice of currently available therapies and will be much better than the 8% annual mortality and 24% myocardial infarction rate reported by Mulcahy *et al.* with a "hands off" approach.[1]

PATHOPHYSIOLOGY

It is clear that in contrast to those with stable angina where a stable atheroma causes symptoms only when O_2 demand exceeds O_2 supply during exercise, patients with unstable angina form a widely heterogeneous group in terms of the prevailing but often changing pathogenic mechanisms, the underlying state of the coronary arteriosclerosis, and the degree of associated impairment of left ventricular function. As Maseri and Foale put it: "At one end of the spectrum are patients with extremely severe reduction of coronary flow reserve in whom even a modest increase in myocardial oxygen demand is sufficient to precipitate ischaemia. At the other end are patients in whom coronary flow reserve is only marginally impaired, or even completely normal, and in whom ischaemia is caused by a transient interruption of coronary blood flow. The fixed reduction of coronary flow reserve may result from old atherosclerotic plaques, with or without an additional component (such as rupture) [References 5 and 6] or recent thrombosis. Transient impairment of flow may also result from spasm, from intravascular plugging at the site of a stenosis, from constriction of resistance vessels, or from a combination of the above factors."[4]

"The majority of patient with unstable angina appear to be between these extremes: they have a variable degree of fixed reduction of their coronary flow reserve and a variable extent of transient impairment of coronary flow, which is responsible for the spontaneous, usually unpredictable onset of anginal episodes. This proposition is supported by the angiographic observation that the severity of coronary artery stenosis in general is not dissimilar from that commonly found in patients with stable angina and by pacing studies indicating that unstable patients usually have a high threshold for tachycardia induced ischaemia. Therefore it may be reasonable to assume that most often angina becomes unstable because of the occurrence of dynamic stenosis superimposed on an old or fresh (caused by a recent thrombus) fixed stenosis of

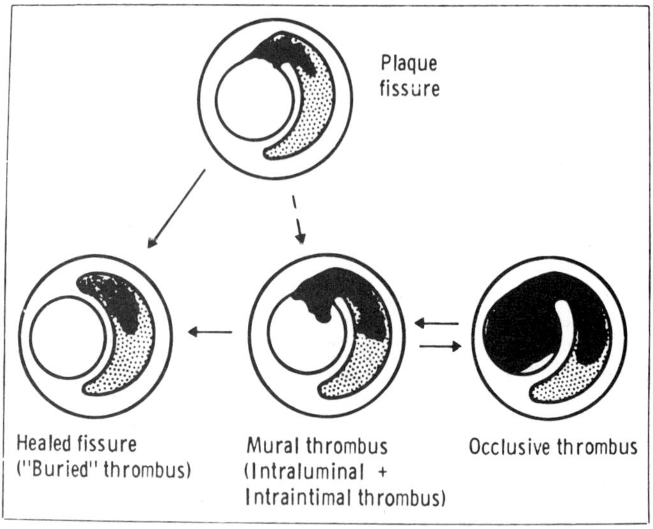

FIGURE 1. A theoretical model of the events that could lead from stable angina to ischemic myopathy, accelerated angina, unstable angina, and progression in stenosis. (Reprinted with permission from Davies.[5])

variable severity. This hypothesis seems to be gaining acceptance."[4] A schematic view of these concepts is provided in FIGURES 1 and 2.

In these "high-risk" cases, the pain is continuing or even progressive in severity and intensity despite bed rest. We are not talking here about patients who had an attack of pain which subsided spontaneously but only about those who are still considered unstable because of ongoing signs of ischemia. In such patients before "aggressive" therapy was available with persistent (>48 hours) or recurrent pain, Gazes *et al.* found a 20% one month mortality and 43% in one year.[8] Julian, combining all series since 1970 with 100 cases or more each with severe pain with coincident electrocardiogram (ECG) changes, finds a one month mortality of 4%, a one year mortality of 12%, and an early myocardial infarct rate of 8%.[9] It is therefore more the timing, the progressiveness, and the persistence rather than the character or the location of the pain that denote the unstability of this type of angina.

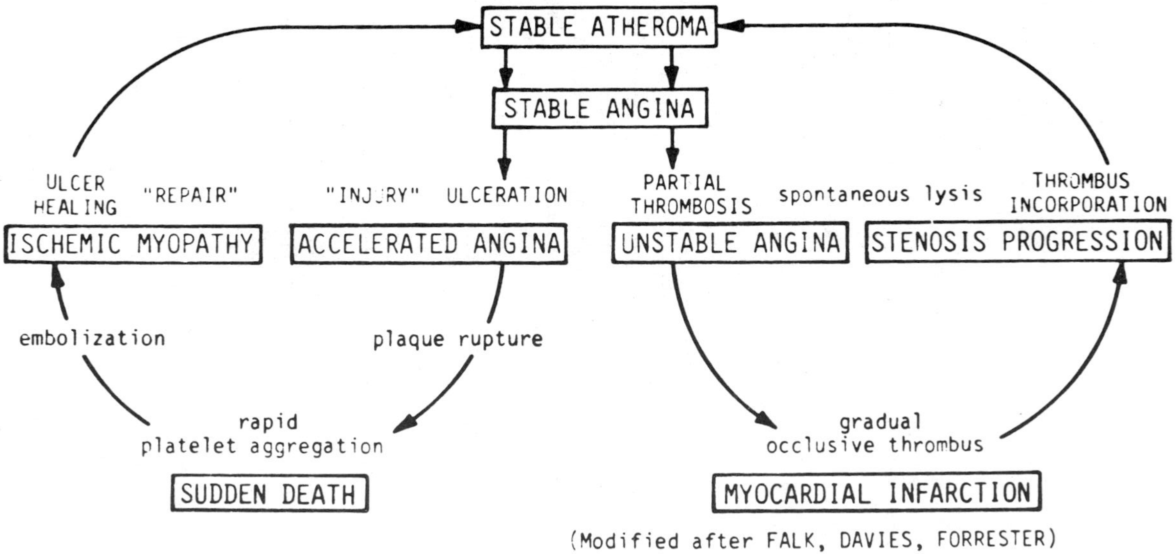

FIGURE 2. The ulceration-thrombosis cycle of coronary disease. Scheme of events after plaque rupture.

TABLE 1A[a]

Group 1: Normal or only slightly reduced coronary flow reserve
- Clinical correlates: no history of reduced effort tolerance.
- Angiographic correlates: absence of critical lesions or good collaterals.
- Objective evidence: negative maximal exercise stress test.[b]

Group 2: Moderately reduced coronary flow reserve
- Clinical correlates: history of exertional angina, but moderate efforts usually well tolerated.
- Angiographic correlates: presence of one or more severe coronary obstructions.
- Objective evidence: exercise stress test[b] produces signs or symptoms of ischemia only above 5 METS.

Group 3: Severely reduced coronary flow reserve
- Clinical correlates: severe exertional angina, even moderate efforts never tolerated.
- Angiographic correlates: one or more severe coronary obstructions.
- Objective evidence: exercise stress test[b] produces signs or symptoms of ischemia even below 5 METS.

[a]This table contains the classification in groups 1–3 depending on the extent to which coronary flow reserve is reduced. This table should be viewed in conjection with TABLE 1B.
[b]After acute administration of nitrates or calcium antagonists.

As Balakumaran *et al.* put it: "Unstable angina is doubly distressing. On the one hand the patient is confronted with the disturbing new symptomatology, namely unfamiliar pain (crescendo angina), unprovoked pain (angina at rest) or pain returning on the heels of the major blow of myocardial infarction (early postinfarct angina), on the other hand the physician knows that something potentially dangerous is afoot."[10]

Maseri feels that it is important to establish whether the ischemic episodes that characterize the instability of the syndrome are caused by an excessive increase in myocardial demand in the presence of fixed limitation of coronary blood supply or via sudden and often transient primary impairment of coronary blood supply.[4] In other words, to separate whether the ischemic episodes represent secondary or primary angina. As a second step it is necessary to assess the severity of the reduction of coronary flow reserve and the tendency to develop persistent episodes of impairment of coronary flow. TABLE 1A recognizes three groups that reflect the classification as a first step. TABLE 1B provides a guideline to classify the patient according to the assumed reduction of coronary flow reserve. (See also FIGURE 3.)

Accordingly, a patient who has reported an attack of spontaneous chest pain and who is thought to be in group 1a would be subjected to a maximal exercise test which if

TABLE 1B[a]

According to the tendency to develop persistent episodes of ischemia each group should be subdivided in:

A: Moderate tendency to develop persistent ischemic episodes
- spontaneous ischemic episodes lasting less than 5 minutes or promptly relieved by sublingual nitrates.

B: Severe tendency to develop persistent ischemic episodes
- recurring ischemic episodes lasting more than 5 minutes and responding poorly to sublingual nitrates.

[a]A subdivision is made according to the persistence of ischemia. Thus, patients with severely reduced coronary flow reserve (group 3, TABLE 1A) in whom tendency B is present would be the high-risk patients in whom therapy should be aggressive. Conversely, with group 1 and subgroup A, an expectant attitude is permitted.

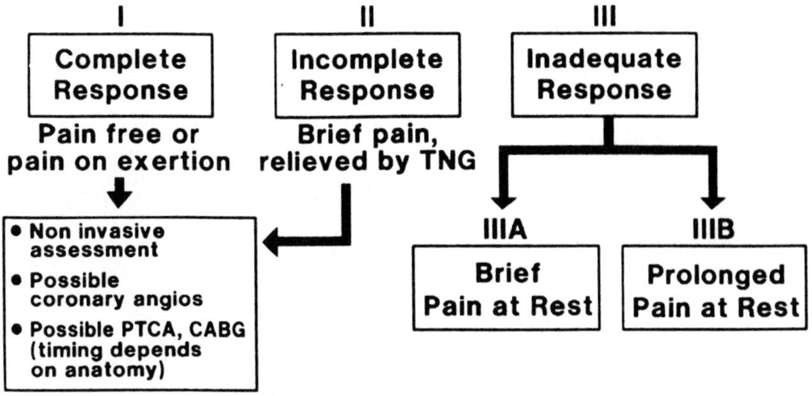

FIGURE 3A. Goldman recognizes the extent to which the patient responds to therapy. (Reproduced from Reference 24 with permission.)

negative excludes further testing. However in the long term these milder cases may still have increased mortality and late myocardial infarction. In Mulcahy's cases this was 7 resp. 15%.[1] Conversely a patient in group IIIb may have such persistent symptomatology that provocative testing such as bicycle ergometry or ergonovine provocation tests are not even indicated and semiurgent angiography must be carried out. They are the type described by de Feyter *et al.*, refractory to triple pharmacological therapy and still suffering from angina and ischemia.[3] It becomes evident therefore that when patients demonstrate anginal pain lasting longer than 15 minutes, associated with ST and T wave changes, a much more aggressive approach is warranted than in those patients classified in group I or II. In fact, the time scale of events during complete obstruction of a coronary artery is much shorter than generally realized (TABLE 2).

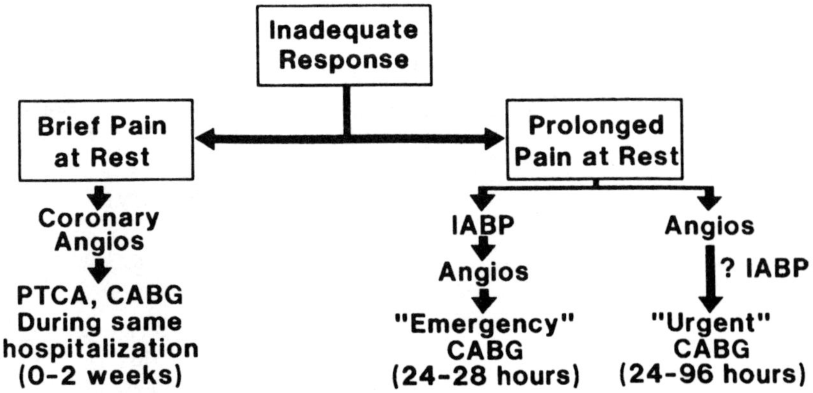

FIGURE 3B. If response is inadequate and pain is prolonged at bed rest, early angiography, with or without balloon pump support, would lead to emergency coronary artery bypass grafting or PTCA. Thus, a combination of the scheme advocated by Maseri[4] with the therapeutic responsiveness of the patient as classified by Goldman would allow for proper classification in most patients.

TABLE 2. Time Scale of Events in Myocardial Ischemia[a]

Metabolic activity (release of H^+, K^+, etc.)	0–10 seconds
Left ventricular dysfunction/E-C coupling	20 seconds
Fall of creatine phosphate	20 seconds
ECG changes, T wave, ST segment	30 seconds
Chest pain (cave "silent" episodes)	60 seconds
Release of vasoactive substances	60 seconds
Increased sympathetic activity	0–60 seconds
Fall of ATP levels	2 minutes
Irreversible damage in core	15 minutes
Ultrastructural changes	20 minutes
Malfunction of mitochondria	40 minutes
Malfunction of sarcoplasmic reticulum (Ca^{2+} transport)	40 minutes

[a]Occurrence of sequential events in myocardial ischemia induced by occlusion of a major coronary artery.

When Maseri's classification is combined with the scheme proposed by Goldman *et al.*,[12] the responsiveness to therapy as a major classification principle is recognized. As shown in FIGURE 3A, they distinguish three kinds of response from complete to inadequate. In this latter category two subsets exist (FIGURE 3B): patients with brief versus prolonged pain at rest. It is in this latter group that the most aggressive therapy should be pursued. Thus, on the basis of an initial "guestimate" of the pathogenesis in a given case, combined with the evaluation of the early (i.e., within hours) response after administration of a vasodilating, beta-blocking, or cardioprotective agent, the proper course of action can be taken (FIGURE 4). In fact, this underlies the thesis by Conti, who combines the thoughts on pathogenesis with the severity of coronary artery disease itself as reflected in the coronary arteriogram.[13] The scheme depicted in FIGURE 5 indicates quite clearly to what degree the preexistent condition of the coronary artery tree can suddenly be aggravated by six major factors. These conditions include (1) extracardiac aggravating factors (c.q. tachycardia or hypertension), (2) rapid pro-

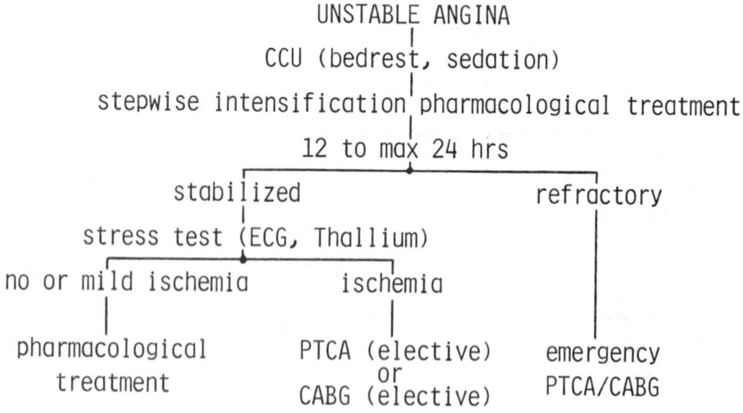

FIGURE 4. Proposed management of patients with unstable angina: presistent chest pain at rest associated with electrocardiographic changes. In this schematic flow chart, the ideal management of a patient with acute unstable angina is provided. Time intervals are obviously tentative and depend on the responsiveness of the patient.

gression of coronary atherosclerosis, (3) rapid decrease in coronary lumen size secondary to hemorrhage into an atherosclerotic plaque, (4) transient platelet aggregation in diseased vessels with intermittent distal embolization, (5) transient coronary artery thrombosis, and (6) abnormal coronary artery vasoconstriction (spasm) in normal or diseased vessels.

It may not be possible to identify the appropriate mechanism(s) responsible for unstable angina in every case but the clinician must attempt to do so, since the correct selection of therapy for the individual patient depends on the recognition of the dominant pathophysiological derangement responsible for the symptoms in that individual at that time (FIGURE 4 and TABLE 3).

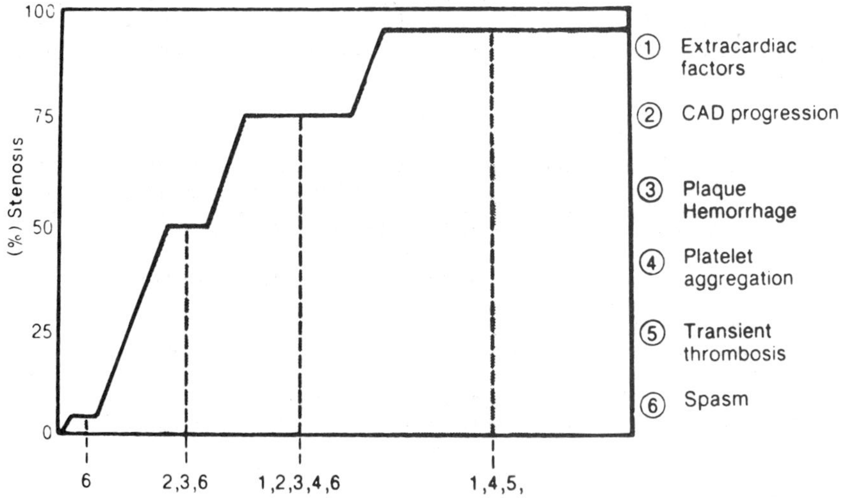

FIGURE 5. Unstable angina pathophysiology. According to Conti,[13] factors 1 to 6 at different times and to varying extent can superimpose on the existing atherosclerotic fixed stenosis (vertical axis). For example with only minimal coronary artery atherosclerosis, spasm may be a major cause of obstruction. Conversely, only minor platelet aggregation (2) can, when fixed atherosclerosis has progressed to 95% stenosis, cause occlusion.

THROMBOLYTIC THERAPY, ANTICOAGULATION

No well-designed studies are available to support the use of anticoagulants such as warfarin-derived agents in stable or unstable angina. On the other hand, heparin appears to be well accepted in the hospital environment while aspirin has been advocated for the longer term, as detailed in a later section. Since vasoactive substances, which may induce vasospasm, are released during platelet aggregation, platelet aggregation inhibitors could perhaps play a major role, although at present the usefulness of these drugs in unstable angina has not been established. In fact, no author has been able to show any clinical effect of prostaglandin derivatives and their blockers. As a consequence, short-term heparin is now advocated only in patients with prolonged bed rest or those monitored with intravascular catheters to avoid deep vein and pulmonary artery thrombosis (heparin 30,000 units/24 hours).

Recently intracoronary streptokinase has been advocated in patients with "impending infarction," a clinical situation that may follow unstable angina pectoris. Fresh data from our institute and from the Netherlands Interuniversitary Cardiological Institute have shown in 533 patients randomized either to standard therapy or to reperfusion by streptokinase (with PTCA and CABG in some) that early reperfusion halves the death rate on an intention to treat principle (16.7% in controls versus 5.9% in lysed patients).[14,15] Since 86 patients were included who from unstable angina in the hospital progressed to acute infarction and since the results in this subset did not differ from the main body, a strong argument in favor of thrombolytic therapy can be made, when the suspected mechanism is indeed proven to be thrombotic obstruction. Earlier Cowley *et al.* had shown 40 out of 69 patients with unstable angina to have intraluminal filling defects or thrombotic occlusion.[16] Similar findings have been described by Bresnahan *et al.*[17], which has led some authors to infuse streptokinase. Recently Gold *et al.* infused tissue plasminogen activator with great succes in 17 patients with unstable angina and found patent vessels in 16 with recurrent ischemia in just one case.[18]

TABLE 3. Potential Indications for Use of Ca^{2+} Antagonists as "Cardioprotective" Agents in (Pre-) or (Re-) Ischemic States on Clinical and Experimental Grounds

1. Unstable angina with signs of "tolerable" ischemia (by ECG, echo, thallium uptake or biochemical markers).
2. Within 0–3 hours after onset of symptoms and signs of myocardial ischemia without clear-cut infarction.
3. During postinfarction recurrent ischemia.
4. When "stunned" myocardium is suspected (repeated brief ischemic attacks, "crescendo angina")
5. Prophylactically after sustained infarction when residual stenoses are suspected.
6. During intentional disturbance of coronary perfusion (PTCA, aorta cross-clamping, during coronary surgery, etc.)
7. During thrombolytic therapy of coronary obstruction, provided the latter is carried out within 0–4 hours after onset of symptoms.
8. When rapid afterload reduction seems advisable with a beta blocker to avoid reflex tachycardia
9. Prophylactically when recurrent spasm as a cause of ischemia is anticipated (Prinzmetal's variant angina)

NITRATES

Nitroglycerin tablets sublingually or in an intravenous (iv) solution relieve most anginal attacks in 2/3 of the cases in the short term. Nitroglycerin's direct vasodilating effect on the venous system lowers preload and therefore wall stress and O_2 consumption of the left ventricle. An additional dilating effect on the larger arteries may decrease afterload and there may be a direct effect on coronary flow.[19] The latter has been repeatedly observed in Prinzmetal's angina where nitroglycerin, given directly into the coronary artery, was shown to relieve the obstruction caused by spasm. Recently it has been indicated that nitrates may have an antiaggregatory action, affecting blood platelets, thus augmenting its efficacy. However, unwanted side effects frequently take place and not all patients respond.[20] While hypotension and bradyarrhythmias can be managed by raising the legs to improve venous return and, if not sufficient, atropin, 0.25 to 1 mg intravenously, is usually effective, sometimes plasma infusion has to be employed. While nitroglycerin sublingually acts within minutes, its duration of action is equally short and this limits its intermediary term usefulness. Nitroglycerin ointment for topical applications has a prolonged effect as has isosorbide dinitrate. These compounds are especially effective in preventing angina attacks at night. The 5 mg tablets of isosorbide dinitrate for sublingual use begin to act within minutes and their action extends from 1 to 3 hours. The 20 mg tablets for oral administration provide an even longer lasting effect. Even so these drugs are not always effective as their blood levels and metabolism vary widely from individual to individual. Molsidomin, a completely different compound in chemical terms, has a long half-life (>6 hours) and leads to a strong reduction in preload. It is completely absorbed and is at least as effective as the nitrates. It deserves further clinical evaluation in the setting of unstable angina pectoris, given its different mode of action.

BETA-BLOCKING AGENTS

A vast literature on this subject has shown that beta-blocking agents reduce the action of catecholamines and therefore contractility and heart rate. However, when the heart is already enlarged, they may increase wall tension and thus increase O_2 consumption. Usually the net effect upon the heart not in failure is a significant reduction in oxygen consumption mainly via the induced bradycardia and this provides the major reason to use beta blockade.

Beta blockade has also been reported to redirect the limited blood supply from normally or overperfused healthy areas to ischemic areas; on the other hand, it may, by unbalancing the innervation of the coronary artery system, lead to increased receptor tone and therefore reduce coronary blood flow. It is guite understandable therefore that this drug should not be given when true spasm, such as seen in Prinzmetal's syndrome, is suspected. When spasm is not suspected and one elects to use a beta blocker, for the two reasons given above, the heart rate must be considerably slowed down for the drug to be effective. In acute ischemic conditions, propranolol (1–10 mg, at 1 mg/minute) intravenously will be most effective until a heart rate of 60 beats/minute has been reached. Oral dosage in a range of 240 to 800 mg propranolol per 24 hours is then instituted. Although much higher dosages than 800 mg of propranolol per 24 hour can be tolerated, we would rather choose acebutolol, metoprolol, or atenolol to replace propranolol when it is not effective as a first drug, although no convincing proof of their efficiency is available in randomized trials, except for metoprolol.[11]

Recently, a large-scale (5778 patients) trial in acute mocardial infarction allocated 2877 to metoprolol and 2901 to placebo.[21] A small, statistically nonsignificant difference (4.3 versus 4.9%) was found in terms of reduction in 15 day mortality, although there was quicker pain relief and less arrhythmia in the treated group. This series included some patients with unstable angina, suggesting that no major impact on death rate or infarction rate can be expected from this beta blocker. Data from Kudoch *et al.* in a coronary embolized dog model also failed to indicate a protective effect in terms of infarct size limitation.[22] Chamberlain in a recent overview of all data available on beta blockade in acute myocardial infarction states: "The influence of betablockers on acute mortality is perhaps the area of greatest controversy. Some trials have shown decreased survival, while others have shown improvement. Many of these differences may be due to variations in protocol, but as yet no firm evidence of a therapeutic effect can be claimed."[23] Even so, most clinicians, when confronted with a patient with unstable angina, obviously in sympathetic overdrive, willl choose next to the nitrate a beta blocker to reduce excessive O_2 consumption by the heart but usually in conjunction with a Ca^{2+} entry blocker.

CALCIUM ANTAGONISTS C OR Ca^{2+} ENTRY BLOCKERS

Since their introduction in the early 1970s in Japan and Europe, calcium antagonists have enjoyed great interest in the cardiological community. This is undoubtedly due to the fact that one deals with a large group of compounds with a therapeutic principle that is novel. Experience has shown that they have great clinical efficacy for hitherto difficult to treat cases of angina.[24] Inhibition of smooth muscle excitation-contraction coupling in the coronary artery wall, achieved by verapamil nifedipine and diltiazem, decreases its contractile tone resulting in vasodilation and consequently increases coronary blood flow. In the cardiac muscle cell itself, the inhibition of intracellular calcium activity reduces the contractile and mechanical function and this diminishes myocardial oxygen demand. Calcium antagonists also appear to have a protective action on ischemic cells protecting mitochondrial activity. These are highly desirable interventions when the myocardium is threatened by ischemia.[24,25] On the other hand, inhibition of the cell membrane is also important in terms of treating cardiac arrhythmias. Here major differences exist in antiarrhythmic properties between verapamil on the one hand and nifedipine on the other. It may be that the surface binding properties and the specific availabilities of receptor sites determine the extent to which a specific calcium "antagonist" antagonizes slow channel Ca transport.

In the clinical situation, the net hemodynamic and electrophysiologic effect of a given calcium antagonist remains the result of the complex interaction between its varying peripheral and central effects.[24] The degree of baroreceptor stimulation and reflex-mediated beta-adrenergic activity, which counteract and influence the intrinsic negative dromotropic, chronotropic, and inotropic effects of the calcium antagonists, are related to the degree of peripheral dilation. The search for the ideal calcium antagonist which mainly affects the coronary arteries continues therefore. Nisoldipine may turn out to be this agent.[25] Currently we share the view of Stone *et al.*: "Nifedipine is the most potent arterial vasodilator and is consequently associated with the most intense reflex adrenergic activity."[26] The net effect of nifedipine is that of relatively pure vasodilation with little electrophysiologic or negative inotropic effect, when given orally or intravenously. On the other hand, doses of verapamil and diltiazem that produce the same degree of vasodilation as nifedipine have negative dromotropic effects and the reflex-induced beta-adrenergic activity may not completely offset the direct electrophysiologic effects.

All three discussed calcium antagonists are effective in treating patients with coronary spasm or unstable angina as well as stable angina when increased vasomotor is the dominant underlying derangement. In patients with classic Prinzmetal's angina, an additional benefit might be expected (and has been demonstrated) from the combined therapy of nifedipine with verapamil and diltiazem. Nifedipine in this laboratory has become a most useful adjuvant when beta blockers and nitrates alone are not effective. It has, in fact, changed our therapeutic approach in unstable angina while in cases with proven spasm not responding to intracoronary nitroglycerin it has always relieved the spasm when given into the coronary artery. Thus for Prinzmetal's angina, short- and long-term therapies begin currently with nifedipine, and all patients with unstable angina receive nifedipine with a beta blocker when a short-term. (1–2 hours) trial with nitrates proves insufficient.[27] Often iv nifedipine is as effective as iv nitrate.

In unstable angina pectoris, the exact mechanisms of action will remain unclear in some cases, because of the uncertainties surrounding the cause(s) of unstable angina pectoris. Thus, particularly when eccentric lesions are present which leave part of the circumference of the vascular wall intact, vasoconstrictive stimuli may cause marked change in the tone of the vessel wall and therefore in the coronary blood flow. It can readily be understood why the combination of an eccentric fixed endothelial lesion and a (hyper)sensitive, but otherwise healthy, vascular wall opposite will frequently lead to intermittent ischemic episodes. In keeping with this concept, there are our early observations of the prompt and persistent relief of pain in patients with unstable angina pectoris, while still symptomatic (or perhaps worsened) after 8 hours of beta-blocker therapy.[27] The fact that 42 of the 52 patients placed on nifedipine while maintaining beta-blocker therapy experienced early and complete relief of angina, which persisted for the entire period of observation, is indeed a strong argument in favor of the overriding vasodilating effect of nifedipine in coronary arteries. Gerstenblith *et al.* in a recent study were able to duplicate our clinical observations in similar patients in a prospective randomized trial.[28] In 50% of 168 patients, nifedipine, when randomly added to conventional therapy consisting of beta blockers and nitrates, was more effective than placebo in reducing the need for urgent surgery, and also demonstrated a reduction in subsequent myocardial infarction and death rate. Since in our series, and in the study of Gerstenblith in patients who remained unresponsive to several hours of beta blockade, the subsequent response to nifedipine was so consistent (and just as effective as had been pain relief by IABP in our previous experience in the same type of patients) and since Parodi *et al.* had seen the same with verapamil,[29] there can remain little doubt that calcium antagonists in unstable angina patients were excess vasomotion is the problem are the agents that provide the extra factor tipping the balance in their favor. This is further confirmed by the nifedipine withdrawal study by Gottlieb.[30] Of 81 patients whose pain was controlled by nifedipine only 4 showed worsening after 2 years of therapy, or upon withdrawal prior to surgery. Recently Braunwald *et al.* have reviewed these arguments and stated that there now might very well be a preference for the use of calcium antagonists in patients suspected of having abnormally increased coronary vasomotor tone.[31] These experiences led to the design of a prospective randomized trial in a category of patients with moderate unstable angina, in whom an attack of 15 minutes or more had taken place within 6 hours before entry or was observed after admission with ECG changes.[11] Those in whom the severity was greater (persistent pain after nitrates or with enzyme elevation) or less (no recurrence of attacks) were excluded. Thus a group of 338 patients not treated prior to admission with a beta blocker was studied for their reaction to nifedipine, metoprolol, or their combination and all were compared to placebo. In the 177 admitted already on a beta blocker, nifedipine was added in a random fashion. Three observations that are relevant for the clinician follow from this study (HINT).[11] First, that all nonresponders to nitrates [per oral (po) and iv] were excluded, most of whom were treated by PTCA or surgery, as described hereafter. Thus this trial does not reflect on therapy in severe unstable angina. Such resistant or refractory patients in our institution reflect more than half of the patients ultimately contributed to the HINT trial. Second, when nifedipine was added to those still having unstable angina, while on beta blockade, the same effect was noted as in the earlier studies by Hugenholtz *et al.*,[27] Gerstenblith *et al.*,[28] and Moses.[32] The event rate ratio, where 1 means no effect, became 0.68 with confidence limits (0.47–0.97). Third, in the group not on beta blockade no great differences were seen between those placed on nifedipine with metoprolol vs. metoprolol alone, although a slightly more favorable effect in terms of an event rate ratio of 0.76 (confidence limits 0.49 vs. 1.16) was seen when monotherapy with metoprolol was given at the outset. The increased incidence of myocardial infarction in the nifedipine

TABLE 4A. Coronary Angioplasty for Initially Stabilized Unstable Angina

	Faxon 1983	Quigley 1986	Thoraxcenter 1986
Number of patients	442	25	71
Success rate (%)	63	81	87
Major complication rate			
• Death (%)	0.9	4	0
• MI (%)	8	12	10
• Acute surgery (%)	—	12	12
Coronary events after successful angioplasty			
• Death (%)	1.7	0	2
• MI (%)	1.5	0	2
• AP (%)	18	32	23
Mean follow-up, (months)	18	18	12

group is best explained by the chance inclusion of more high risk cases in this category. In fact the authors state that the exact onset of infarction could not be established in the study. Coupled with the small numbers and the known inefficacy of nifedipine after infarction has occurred,[33] the conclusion must follow that when infarction rather than ischemia is suspected nifedipine alone as a first-line therapy in this subset of patients had little to offer, a finding consistent with that reported in the literature.[34]

It is of interest to note that while the HINT trial[11] in the Netherlands was proceeding between 1981 and 1984, a paper by De Feyter appeared covering experiences in one of the participating hospitals for the more severe type of unstable angina,[3] the one corresponding to the definition by Conti. These patients, all of whom had not responded to triple pharmacological therapy observed for at least 24 hours, arrived in the cardiac catheterization laboratory usually with pain and underwent in the majority the PTCA procedure as an emergency procedure. It is striking to note that despite the severe form of obstruction and attendant ischemia, excellent results were obtained as soon as the vessel was desobstructed with no procedure related mortality, one delayed sudden death (at 6 months), and a 1 year myocardial infarction rate of only 6%. Similar findings are reported by others (TABLE 4).

It now becomes clear that the real issue in the management of patients with varying forms of unstable angina does not lie in the availability of appropriate treatment but in the nonavailability of adequate diagnostic procedures. As the authors of the HINT

TABLE 4B. Coronary Angioplasty for Refractory Unstable Angina

	Williams 1981	Meyer 1983	de Feyter 1985
Number of patients	17	50	60
Success rate (%)	76	74	93
Major complication rate			
• Death	0	0	0
• MI (%)	0	4	7
• Acute Surgery (%)	6	2	7
Coronary events after successful angioplasty			
• Death (%)	0	0	2
• MI (%)	0	0	0
• AP (%)	8	36	13
Mean follow-up (months)	10.5	6	9

trial observe, "these results show that it is impossible to delineate reversible ischemia (i.e. myocardial infarction) early on clinical grounds."[11] In fact, the myocardial infarction rate for the placebo group study was at best 15%, and if Q-waves are not required, 11%. It is appropriate therefore once more to review the time sequence of events that may occur immediately after the onset of angina pectoris (TABLE 2).

TIMING OF INTERVENTION

Recent studies from our laboratory have demonstrated that during balloon dilatation of a human coronary artery, up to 5 minutes of complete occlusion can be tolerated without permanent metabolic defect or severe angina, although within 10–20 seconds potassium and lactate levels in the coronary sinus efflux already increase dramatically indicating altered O_2-dependent metabolism. Shortly thereafter breakdown products of the high-energy phosphate metabolism such as inosine and hypoxanthine appear in the efflux of the coronary circulation. Such biochemical markers of ischemia denote initially a temporary metabolic disruption, but presage the onset of ECG changes and of cellular destruction which begins from the 15th minute onward. These metabolic and electric abnormalities precede other signs of ischemia as changed mechanical performance of the heart, e.g., loss of diastolic tone, impaired relaxation, as well as enzyme release, arrhythmias, and eventually anginal pain (TABLE 2).

Other clinical observations from our laboratory have shown that even when successful thrombolysis is achieved within 30 minutes after the onset of symptoms, some degree of irreversible myocardial damage has already occurred in the core of the ischemic area. Thus, in the setting of the syndrome of unstable angina, time intervals gain major importance. In this regard, the concept of a significant border zone, marginally perfused but susceptible to manipulation by interventions, must be discussed. Hearse and associates have indicated that three distinct states of reduced flow and ischemic injury may coexist and that they would determine the practicability of tissue salvage.[33] These researchers distinguish among "tolerable," "critical," and "lethal" ischemia.

In "tolerable" ischemia, flow reduction up to 50% can exist and tissue energy stores are hardly depleted. It would appear that many of the "low risk" patients in the HINT study[11] were in fact in this category. Here the vasodilator characteristic of calcium antagonist therapy and the blockade of excessive adrenergic substances by beta blockers would appear the best therapy, preferably in combination.

In "critical" ischemia, flow is reduced by as much as 80%, intracellular energy levels become rapidly reduced, and tissue is jeopardized within minutes. Only timely (30 minutes to 4 hours) reperfusion efforts can lead to recovery of part of the tissue. In this category ultimately a combination of thrombolytic therapy with PTCA and/or bypass grafting would seem mandatory, with pharmacological therapy being relegated to a secondary place.

In "lethal" ischemia, in which flow reduction exceeds 80% and tissue energy stores are very rapidly depleted, tissue is certain to die even earlier. These would be the patients with a severe plaque rupture, rapidly expanding in volume and occluding the vessel within a matter of minutes rather than hours with or without superimposed thrombus.[5] (FIGURES 1 and 2). From the recently published Netherlands Interuniversity Cardiology Trial on Streptokinase,[14,15] in which 533 patients with acute myocardial infarction were randomized either to conventional therapy in the coronary care unit or to early thrombolytic therapy with streptokinase, the results in the subset treated with intravenous streptokinase within 90 minutes of onset of symptoms and followed by desobstruction by means of intracoronary streptokinase and/or PTCA, substantiated the possibility that complete reperfusion provides major benefit. A 1 year mortality of only 2% was seen in this subset versus mortality of 16% in the randomized controls. Furthermore it was shown that in the larger group of patients who received lytic therapy before 4 hours had elapsed since onset of symptoms, infarct size was limited by up to 40%, and ventricular function preserved (average ejection fraction 53%). Furthermore in that group a 50% reduction of mortality relative to the conventionally treated patients was obtained, all analyzed according to the "intention to treat" principle.

THERAPY BY INSTRUMENTAL MEANS

From earlier sections it is now clear that while beta blockers will reduce O_2 consumption and vasodilators, in particular the nitrates and the calcium antagonists nifedipine and diltiazem, have a major effect on symptoms as well as an impact on ischemia within the first few hours after their administration, therapy-resistant cases can be identified after 8 to 12 hours. In these "refractory" instances the decision to proceed with further diagnostic procedures must be made early (FIGURE 4). Usually, significant atherosclerotic narrowing is found with or without spasm and with or without intravascular thrombus. The latter can, according to the timing of the arteriography, be seen in up to 50% of cases.

Since this form of obstruction is then most likely the major explanation for the persistence of the unstable state, mechanical recanalization must be undertaken either by means of percutaneous transluminal coronary angioplasty (PTCA) in the catheterization laboratory or by coronary artery bypass grafting (CABG) in the operating room. One can argue as de Feyter, Serruys *et al.* have done recently that PTCA always has a place when optimal pharmacological intervention has failed.[3] In fact, a period of maximally 24 hours would seem nearly too long to wait for any drug to exert its optimal effect in the face of the ongoing loss of myocardial function and cell death. Thus PTCA should not, like CABG in the past, be seen as an emergency "last ditch" treatment but rather as a semiurgent elective procedure to be initiated early in the "hot" stage of the disease when the patient proves unresponsive to a triple pharmacologic therapy approach. This would seem to be an essential and important step to be propagated in the modern concept of management of unstable angina pectoris. Furthermore the combination of aspirin, calcium antagonists, and perhaps heparin would now seem to be most advisable for the period after such mechanical dilatation of the coronary artery has taken place. Many authors have argued that residual or returning spasm can occur during the healing phase of the distended atheromatous lesion, while it is also likely that recurrent thrombosis can take place on the denuded endothelium induced by the compressing balloon.[5,7,19,20] Here calcium antagonists would be indicated.[34] The data of Cairns[35,36] and Lewis[37] indicate that aspirin has a major role to play in preventing the acute recurrence of thrombocyte aggregation on top of the fissures and cracks, which have appeared in the plaque. This is also in keeping with the findings by Born[7] and Becker.[38] The experience in Rotterdam with 139 patients with unstable angina pectoris serves as a good example of the efficacy of PTCA.[3] Other data have been recently published by Meyer *et al.*[39] in a series of 108 unstable angina pectoris patients treated with PTCA in two separate hospitals.[39] Both experiences indicate that with modern equipment, such as steerable catheters the complication rate is around 5% while the mortality rate ranged between 1 and 2%. Yet, the majority of these vessels remained patent one year after the original procedure. Our group reports an initial success rate of 84% (89% with the new steerable systems) in 117 out of 139 patients. In the 22 patients in whom the procedure was unsuccessful, coronary bypass grafting was carried out, as an emergency in 19. In the entire series there was not a single death related to PTCA or CABG although at 1 year follow-up the cumulative mortality and myocardial infarction rate was 11.5%. The mortality part was caused by one sudden cerebral death at 8 months (TABLE 4).

Thus, when unstable angina is refractory to triple therapy, (nitrates, calcium antagonists, and beta blockers) it is now recommended by major centers in Western Europe to proceed early on to mechanical dilatation which, in case it proves unsuccessful, can be followed by CABG. The importance of the data reported thus far is that while they do not form part of a randomized study design, there is a remarkably low complication rate and the virtual absence of death. Such results are at striking variance with the days of Gazes *et al.*[8] In fact the statement must now be made that when patients with unstable angina are properly managed, mortality should be absent. Not only should unneccessary death be a thing of the past, but from the data of de Feyter and Meyer *et al.*[3,37] it is likely that infarction rate in the subsequent year should not exceed 10%. Also Goldman *et al.* in their carefully documented series of unstable angina pectoris come to similar conclusions on properly timed CABG in patients unresponsive to pharmacological therapy.[12] By univariate risk factor analysis, in 299 patients with unstable angina coming to urgent surgery after failed pharmacological therapy, the only difference with similar analysis in 1003 patients with stable angina pectoris was the functional class III and IV of the New York Heart Association and the higher presence of left main coronary artery stenosis. It would seem therefore that in this category CABG should be preferable over PTCA. Again, early recognition by coronary angiography would appear to provide for a good outcome with an operative mortality of 5% and an incidence of perioperative myocardial infarction of 14%. Goldman also points to the significance of blood cardioplegia in patients with unstable angina pectoris,[12] and current research at various clinics would suggest a similar supportive role for cardioplegia with nifedipine or diltiazem added as a cardioprotective agent during cardiopulmonary bypass. Cohn reports for the period 1981–1983 an operative mortality of 3% in 222 patients considered resistant to pharmacological therapy with a perioperative myocardial infarction rate of less than 1%.[40] Yet, in that time period there has been a higher trend towards complete revascularization with multiple grafts being placed, a lower incidence of one and two vessel coronary diseases requiring operation (undoubtedly reflecting the fact that the PTCA procedure was more often carried out in this subset of patients), and increased overall patient age. Thus an increasing rather than decreasing mortality trend would have been expected. The improved results also apply to the patients with postinfarction unstable angina. Cohn furthermore underlines the need for temporary intraaortic balloon pump support in patients who appear to be at excessive risk either because of main stem disease or severe ventricular dysfunction, a point earlier argued from our laboratory. The overall outcome of early bypass surgery when PTCA has failed was underlined byHaalebos *et al.*[41] They indicate that in 53 patients who required CABG within 24 hours after a failed PTCA (out of 500 procedures in which PTCA was attempted) there were signs of myocardial damage following these procedures in roughly half of the cases while an actual myocardial infarction could be demonstrated in a quarter. Apparently, very early reperfusion after a first failed PTCA cannot avoid loss of cardiac tissue, but early complete reperfusion by CABG does prevent death.

ASPIRIN

Ever since the Veterans Administration studies reported by Lewis et al.,[37] aspirin has been in the limelight as the new therapy for unstable angina. Despite the additional evidence found by Cairns[35] and ably condensed in his "Comment to Current Medical Literature,"[36] this author must point out that aspirin as a general cyclooxygenase blocker, undoubtedly to be followed by more specific blockers for the synthesis of thromboxane A2 or by stimulators of prostacyclin,[42] has as yet failed to be of help in the acute situation. As Cairns states: "Concern over the prognosis for unstable angina, the increasing evidence that platelets might play a major role in the complications of atherosclerotic coronary artery disease and encouraging laboratory and clinical evidence of the possible efficacy of aspirin prompted the performance of two large clinical trials of antiplatelet therapy in patients with unstable angina. Both trials enrolled hospitalized patients with a clinical (non-angiographic) diagnosis of unstable angina; patients were randomly allocated to aspirin or placebo and then followed at intervals in a double blind fashion. The principal end-point of each trial was the occurrence of cardiac death or non-fatal acute myocardial infarction. In each trial a dramatic benefit with aspirin was observed. However, there were significant differences in trial design and analysis so that it is important to review these before determining what patient management decisions may be made based upon the results."[36]

In the study by Lewis *et al.* on 1338 men, treatment did not begin until 51 hours after hospitalization,[37] while Cairns *et al.* entered 555 patients who began therapy within 8 days of hospitalization.[38] Thus of the striking reductions of 41% at 3 months, respectively 30% at 18 months, for cardiac death or nonfatal acute myocardial infarction (and even higher figures for 3 month mortality, 51% respectively 56%) none apply to the acute situation. In contrast they provide the best data to recommend aspirin as secondary prevention after recovery from the leading attack of unstable angina. Thus we can mostly agree with Cairns when he states: "The present management of unstable angina includes bed rest and sedation, preferably in a coronary care unit, vigorous employment of nitrates, beta blockers and calcium antagonists. Urgent cardiac catheterisation should be performed only in those patients who fail to respond to medical management. It is clear from two recent studies that aspirin should be added to the conventional therapy for unstable angina, with the anticipation of sharp reductions in cardiac death and non-fatal acute myocardial infarction. An initial dose of 1300 mg appears a reasonable choice for most patients, and for women it is the only dose of proven efficacy. In an attempt to minimise gastro-intestinal side-effects and enhance patient compliance, the administration of 650 mg of the enteric coated form twice daily is sound. The occurrence of side-effects or poor compliance should prompt dose reductions—in men 325 mg of aspirin daily may be equally efficacious. Therapy should be continued for at least 2 years, and it should be maintained in patients undergoing aortocoronary bypass surgery."[36] Although it is clear that aspirin has no proven influence in the initial course of action and is truly a secondary prevention agent, the halving of the one year late mortality with aspirin on top of a low initial death rate with triple pharmacotherapy and/or early PTCA, indicates that unstable angina should now be truly under control (FIGURE 4 and TABLES 3 and 4).

CONCLUSION

Calcium antagonists do and will continue to play a major role in the management of all forms of angina pectoris. However rather than being recommended for increased vasomotor tone alone, the indications contained in TABLE 3 appear best to reflect current thinking.[43]

SUMMARY

Angina presents itself to us as a continuous spectrum of ischemic syndromes. The disease is multifactorial, and within the same patient different pathophysiological mechanisms may occur at different times and in succession. Several factors may be causative at a particular moment of the disease process and the very next moment a different mechanism may prevail or spontaneous improvement may occur. Among these are stable atheroma with episodic increased vasomotor tone, fissured plaques with intraluminal and/or intraintimal thrombus, thrombocyte aggregation in >70% intraluminal narrowing from ulcerated plaques, as well as frank spasm of vessels without major atherosclerosis.

Consequently, there will never be *one* therapy for *every* case of (un)stable angina nor will there ever be a best therapy for all. Rather, a stepped approach appears the most likely to be successful. This begins with bed rest and requires vasodilator therapy with nitrates and/or Ca^{2+} antagonists *and* beta blockade. If this triple therapy does not "cool" the symptoms within 6–12 hours, semiurgent arteriography is indicated. Depending on the pathophysiology found, thrombolytic therapy with streptokinase or tissue plasminogen activator, percutaneous transluminal coronary angioplasty (PTCA), or coronary artery bypass grafting (CABG) must be carried out early. Heparin in the short term and aspirin in the long term protect best against late complications. The moment is now here when infarction or death after an attack of angina pectoris should be rare.

REFERENCES

1. MULCAHY, R., A. H. AL AWADHI & M. DE BUITLEON. 1985. Natural history and prognosis of unstable angina. Am. Heart J. **109:** 753–758.
2. HUGENHOLTZ, P. G. & B. S. GOLDMAN. 1985. Unstable Angina, Current Concepts and Management: 1–10. Schattauer. Stuttgart & New York.
3. DE FEYTER, P. J., P. W. SERRUYS, M. VAN DEN BRAND *et al.* 1985. Emergency coronary angioplasty in refractory unstable angina. N. Engl. J. Med. **313:** 342–346.
4. MASERI, A. & R. FOALE. 1985. A pathophysiological classification of unstable angina. *In* Unstable Angina, Current Concepts and Management. P. G. Hugenholtz & B. S. Goldman, Eds: 71–78. Schattauer Verlag. Stuttgart & New York.
5. DAVIES, M. J. & A. THOMAS. 1984. Thrombosis and acute coronary artery lesions in sudden cardiac ischemic death. N. Engl. J. Med. **310:** 1137–1140.
6. FALK, E. 1985. Unstable angina with fatal outcome: dynamic coronary thrombosis leading to infarction and/or sudden death. Circulation **71:** 699–708.
7. BORN, G. V. R. 1985. Pathogenetic possibilities *In* Unstable Angina, Current Concepts and Management. P. G. Hugenholtz & B. S. Goldman, Eds.: 13–18. Schattauer Verlag. Stuttgart & New York.
8. GAZES P. C., E. M. MOBLEY, H. M. FARRIS *et al.* 1973. Preinfarction (unstable) angina—a prospective study—ten year follow up. Circulation **48:** 331–337.
9. JULIAN, D. G. 1985. The natural history of unstable angina. *In* Unstable Angina, Current Concepts and Management. P. G. Hugenholtz & B. S. Goldman, Eds.: 65–70. Schattauer Verlag. Stuttgart & New York.
10. BALAKUMARAN, K., P. FIORETTI, R. W. BROWER *et al.* 1985. Unstable angina and myocardial revascularisation. *In* Unstable Angina, Current Concepts and Management. P. G. Hugenholtz & B. S. Goldman, Eds.: 309–317. Schattauer Verlag. Stuttgart & New York.
11. LUBSEN, J., J. G. P. TIJSSEN, H. J. J. KERKKAMP *et al.* 1986. Report of the Holland Interuniversity Nifedipine-metoprolol Trial (HINT research group). Early treatment of unstable angina at the coronary care unit: a randomised, double blind, placebo controlled

comparison of recurrent ischaemia in patients with nifedipine and/or metoprolol. Br. Heart J. **56:** 400–413.

12. Goldman, B. S., R. D. Weisel, G. Christakis *et al.* 1985. Predictors of outcome after coronary artery bypass graft surgery for stable and unstable angina pectoris. *In* Unstable Angina, Current Concepts and Management. P. G. Hugenholtz, & B. S. Goldman, Eds.: 319–330. Schattauer Verlag. Stuttgart & New York.
13. Conti, C. R. 1985. Unstable angina: thoughts on pathogenesis. *In* Unstable Angina, Current Concepts and Management. P. G. Hugenholtz & B. S. Goldman, Eds.: 55–64. Schattauer Verlag. Stuttgart & New York.
14. Simoons, M. L., P. W. Serruys, M. van den Brand *et al.* 1985. Improved survival after early thrombolysis in acute myocardial infarction. A randomized trial conducted by the Interuniversity Cardiology Institute in the Netherlands. Lancet **2:** 578–582.
15. Serruys, P. W., M. L. Simoons, H. Suryapranata *et al.* 1986. Preservation of global and regional left ventricular function after early thrombolysis in acute myocardial infarction. J. Am. Coll. Cardiol. **7:** 729–742.
16. Cowley, M. J., G. Disciascio & G. W. Vetrovec. 1985. Coronary thrombus in unstable angina: angiographic observation and clinical relevance. *In* Unstable Angina, Current Concepts and Management. P. G. Hugenholtz & B. S. Goldman, Eds.: 95–102. Schattauer Verlag. Stuttgart & New York.
17. Bresnahan, D. R., J. L. Davis, D. R. Holmes, Jr. *et al.* 1985. Angiographic occurrence and clinical correlates of intraluminal coronary artery thrombus: role of unstable angina. J. Am. Coll. Cardiol. **6:** 285–289.
18. Zack, P. M., T. Ischinger, U. T. Aker *et al.* 1984. The occurrence of angiographically detected intracoronary thrombus in patients with unstable angina pectoris. Am. Heart J. **108:** 1408–1411.
19. Parratt, J. R. 1985. Coronary vascular endothelium, spasm and reperfusion arrhythmias; experimental approaches. *In* Unstable Angina, Current Concepts and Management. P. G. Hugenholtz & B. S. Goldman, Eds.: 19–28. Schattauer Verlag. Stuttgart & New York.
20. Furchgott, R. F. 1983. Role of endothelium in responses of vascular smooth muscle. Circ. Res. **53:** 557–573.
21. The MIAMI Trial Research Group. 1985. Metoprolol in acute myocardial infarction (MIAMI). Eur. Heart J. **6:** 199–226.
22. Kudoch, Y., M. P. Maxwell, D. J. Hearse *et al.* 1984. Inability of metoprolol to achieve a sustained limitation of infarct size in 24 hours after coronary artery embolization in the closed chest dog. J. Cardiovasc. Pharmacol. **6:** 1201–1209.
23. Chamberlain, D. A. 1985. Proceedings of the MIAMI trial, section 1. *In* The Current Status of Beta Blockers in Acute Myocardial Infarction: 4–14. Adis Pres. City, New Zealand.
24. Hugenholtz, P. G. 1985. The calcium antagonists. *In* Handbook of Experimental Pharmacology **76:** 459–538. Springer Verlag. Berlin, Heidelberg, New York & Tokyo.
25. Duncker, D. J., J. M. Hartog, P. G. Hugenholtz *et al.* 1986. The effects of nisoldipine (Bay K 5522) on cardiovascular performance and regional blood flow in pentobarbital-anaesthetized pigs with or without beta-adrenoceptor blockade. Br. J. Pharmacol. **88:** 9–18.
26. Stone, P. H. & E. M. Antman. 1983. Use of the calcium channel blocking agents in unstable angina pectoris and acute myocardial infarction. *In* Calcium Blocking Agents in the Treatment of Cardiovascular Disorders. P. H. Stone, E. M. Antman, Eds.: 321–346. Futura Publishing Company. Mount Kisco, N.Y.
27. Hugenholtz, P. G., H. R. Michels, P. W. Serruys *et al.* 1979. Nifedipine in the treatment of unstable angina, coronary spasm and myocardial ischemia. Am. J. Cardiol. **47:** 163–175.
28. Gerstenblith, G., P. Ouyang, S. C. Aschuff *et al.* 1982. Nifedipine in unstable angina: a double blind randomized trial. N. Engl. J. Med. **306:** 885–894.
29. Parodi, O., A. Maseri & D. Simonetti. 1979. Management of unstable angina by verapamil. Br. Heart J. **41:** 167–173.
30. Gottlieb, S. O., P. Ouyang, S. C. Achuff *et al.* 1984. Acute nifedipine withdrawal:

consequences of preoperative and late cessation of therapy in patients with prior unstable angina. J. Am. Coll. Cardiol. **4:** 382–388.
31. BRAUNWALD, E. 1980. Introduction: calcium channel blockers. Am. J. Cardiol. **46:** 1045.
32. MOSES, J. W., J. H. WERTHEIMER, M. M. BODENHEIMER *et al.* 1981. Efficacy of nifedipine in rest angina, refractory to propranolol and nitrates in patients with obstructive coronary artery disease. Am. Intern. Med. **94:** 425–432.
33. HUGENHOLTZ, P. G., P. W. SERRUYS, A. FLECKENSTEIN *et al.* 1986. Why Ca^{2+} antagonists will be most useful before or during early myocardial ischemia and not after infarction has been established. Eur. Heart J. **7:** 270–278.
34. HUGENHOLTZ, P. G., P. LICHTLEN, W. VAN DER GIESSEN *et al.* 1986. On a possible role of calcium antagonists in atherosclerosis. A personal view. Eur. Heart J. **7:** 546–559.
35. CAIRNS, J. A., M. GENT, J. SINGER *et al.* 1985. Aspirin, sulfinpyrazone, or both in unstable angina. Results of a Canadian multicenter trial. N. Engl. J. Med. **313:** 1369–1375.
36. CAIRNS, J. A. 1986. Aspirin in unstable angina. Comment Curr. Med. Lit. **5:** 1–4.
37. LEWIS, H. D., J. W. DAVIS, D. G. ARCHIBALD *et al.* 1983. Protective effects of aspirin against acute myocardial infarction and death in men with unstable angina: results of a Veterans' Administration cooperative study. N. Engl. J. Med. **309:** 396–403.
38. BECKER, A. E. 1985. Unstable angina revisited, the pathologist's view. *In* Unstable Angina, Current Concepts and Management. P. G. Hugenholtz & B. S. Goldman, Eds.: 29–37. Schattauer Verlag. Stuttgart & New York.
39. MEYER, J., E. ERBEL, H. J. SCHMITZ *et al.* 1985. PTCA as emergency treatment in unstable angina. *In* Unstable Angina, Current Concepts and Management. P. G. Hugenholtz & B. S. Goldman, Eds.: 239–252. Schattauer Verlag. Stuttgart & New York.
40. COHN, L. H., A. O'NEILL & J. J. COLLINS, JR. 1985. Surgical treatment of unstable angina up to 1984. *In* Unstable Angina, Current Concepts and Management. P. G. Hugenholtz & B. S. Goldman, Eds.: 279–386. Schattauer Verlag. Stuttgart & New York.
41. HAALEBOS, M., P. W. SERRUYS, V. LUYTEN *et al.* 1985. Early coronary bypass surgery following unsuccessful percutaneous transluminal coronary angioplasty. *In* Unstable Angina, Current Concepts and Management. P. G. Hugenholtz & B. S. Goldman, Eds.: 253–264. Schattauer Verlag. Stuttgart & New York.
42. GANZ, P. & R. W. ALEXANDER. 1985. New insights into the cellular mechanisms of vasospasm. Am. J. Cardiol. **56:** 11E–15E.
43. HUGENHOLTZ, P. G. 1986. Unstable angina revisited once more. Eur. Heart J. **7:** 1010–1013.

Calcium Antagonists and Their Potential for Antihypertensive Therapy[a]

F. R. BÜHLER AND W. KIOWSKI

Department of Medicine
Division of Cardiology
University Hospital
Kantonsspital Basel
CH4031 Basel, Switzerland

INTRODUCTION

Hypertension in its established phase is hemodynamically characterized by an increase in systemic vascular resistance. This derangement is due to structural differences between normotensive and hypertensive subjects[1] but also entails functional components, e.g., an increase in the sympathetically mediated component.[2–4] Since the final common pathway of all vasoconstrictor mechanisms is the free intracellular calcium concentration,[5] it has also been proposed that a defect in smooth muscle cation homeostasis in hypertension might lead to increased free cytosolic calcium concentrations and thereby to increased tension development and systemic vascular resistance.[6] A reduction of the free intracellular calcium concentration, therefore, should result in vascular smooth muscle relaxation and, consequently, vasodilatation and lowering of blood pressure. Calcium antagonists lower intracellular calcium concentrations mainly through a reduction of the transmembraneous slow calcium influx which occurs during membrane depolarization[7] and could be expected on theoretical grounds to lower blood pressure. Antihypertensive properties of calcium antagonists were noted more than 20 years ago,[8] but only in the last few years have these properties been investigated in detail. This short review focuses on the mechanisms of action of calcium antagonists on the one hand and on their clinical usefulness in hypertension on the other.

CELLULAR CALCIUM HOMEOSTASIS

The measurement of free intracellular calcium concentrations has recently been made possible by a new technique,[9] but the difficulties in obtaining and studying vascular smooth muscle cells have so far prevented the investigation of free cellular calcium contents and the effects of drugs in human hypertension. Platelets share a number of properties with vascular smooth muscle cells, e.g., adrenergic receptors[10] and calcium-dependent contractile proteins which are activated and controlled by similar mechanisms as in smooth muscle cells.[11] Consequently, platelets have been considered as a model for the study of calcium homeostasis in hypertension. When intracellular free calcium concentration in platelets of hypertensive patients was compared with normotensive subjects,[12] it was elevated in hypertensive patients and

[a]Supported in part by Schweizerische Nationalfonds, Grant No. 3.924.083.

correlated closely both with systolic ($r = 0.883$, $p < 0.001$) and diastolic ($r = 0.931$, $p < 0.001$) blood pressure, findings confirmed by others.[13] Treatment with calcium antagonists, beta blockers, and diuretics all lowered intracellular free calcium concentrations lending further evidence to the proposed, important role of intracellular calcium for the control of vascular tone and blood pressure. However, measurements in vascular smooth muscle cells must be awaited before the hypothesis of a deranged cellular cation handling and increased free cytosolic calcium concentrations as an underlying mechanism for increased vascular resistance in hypertension can be accepted.

INCREASED CALCIUM-INFLUX-DEPENDENT VASOCONSTRICTION IN HYPERTENSION

Spontaneously hypertensive rats have increased vascular relaxation when given calcium antagonists as compared to control animals,[14,15] suggesting a greater dependency of vascular tone on calcium influx in this animal model. Similar results have been obtained in human hypertension[16,17] using regional, intraarterial calcium antagonist infusions for the study of the control of vascular resistance by calcium influx. Regional, e.g., brachial artery infusions, of calcium antagonists are preferable to systemic drug administration because drug dosages can be kept sufficiently small to avoid systemic hemodynamic effects and activation of reflexes while providing high regional, e.g., forearm, drug concentrations. Therefore, changes of blood flow in these models represent changes of vascular resistance that can be ascribed solely to a particular drug's direct vascular action. Using this approach we infused various calcium antagonists intraarterially in age-matched normotensive subjects and hypertensive patients and measured the ensuing vasodilatation[16] by venous occlusion plethysmography. To account for possible differences in vascular design between normotensive and hypertensive subjects the vasodilator response to calcium entry blockade was also compared with the effects of sodium nitroprusside, a nonspecific vasodilator which does not inhibit calcium influx,[18] and with postischemic increases of forearm blood flow induced by 10 minutes of brachial artery occlusion. The results confirmed in humans the potent arterial vasodilator properties of calcium antagonists (FIGURE 1). Furthermore, calcium antagonists resulted in greater increases of forearm blood flow in hypertensive patients as compared to normotensive subjects and this finding persisted when changes in forearm blood flow during calcium antagonist administration were corrected for the individual effects of sodium nitroprusside.[16] This observation and similar results by others[17] demonstrate the existence of a functional abnormality of calcium-influx-dependent vasoconstriction in essential human hypertension and suggest that it might be specifically counteracted by calcium antagonists.

ANTIHYPERTENSIVE MECHANISMS OF ACTION OF CALCIUM ANTAGONISTS

The main hemodynamic derangement in established essential hypertension is increased systemic vascular resistance. Therefore, vasodilators in general should—at least theoretically—be ideally suited for the correction of this abnormality. However, experience with other types of arterial vasodilators shows that this kind of treatment is often associated with marked reflex tachycardia and volume retention, effects that

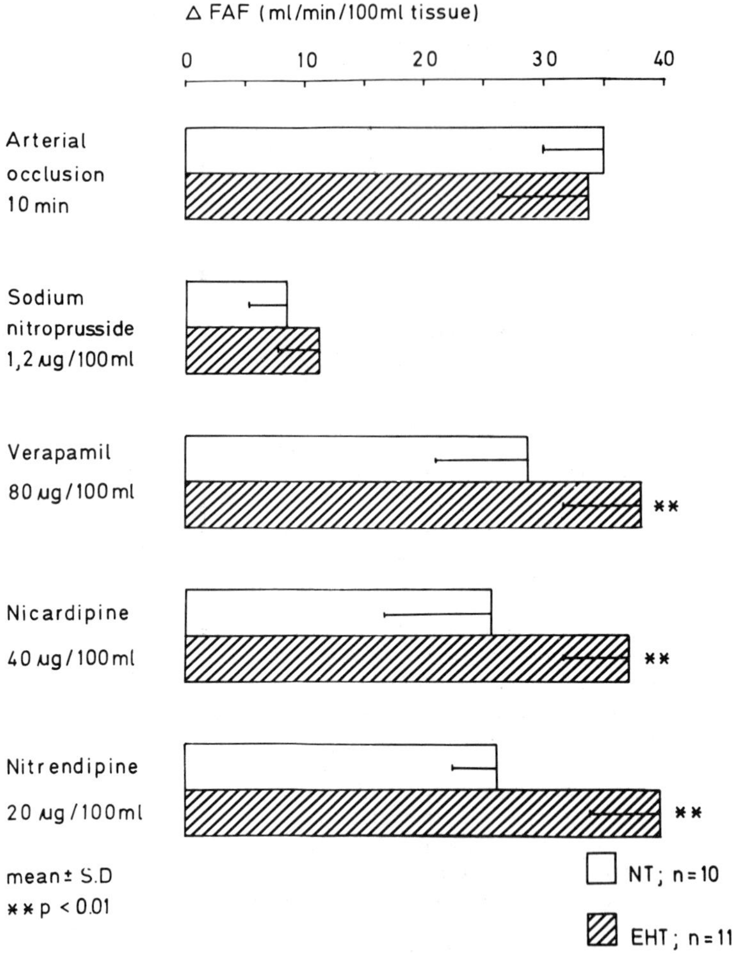

FIGURE 1. Increase in forearm blood flow (Δ FAF) during intraarterial infusion of the calcium antagonists verapamil, nicardipine, and nitrendipine as well as "nonspecific" vasodilatation by sodium nitroprusside and during reperfusion following 10 minutes of ischemia. Calcium antagonists proved to be potent arterial vasodilators increasing forearm blood to levels observed during ischemic reperfusion. In addition, each calcium antagonist caused greater increases in forearm blood flow in hypertensive patients as compared to normotensive subjects but the response to sodium nitroprusside was similar. The levels of significance refer to paired comparisons between normotensive and hypertensive subjects. NT = normotensive subjects; EHT = essential hypertensive patients.

counteract or even abolish their antihypertensive effects.[19] Accordingly, their use is limited to combination therapy with sympatholytic and diuretic agents. Calcium antagonists are also potent vasodilators but in contrast to other vasodilators several studies have demonstrated their efficacy when given as monotherapy.[20–24] There are several findings that help to explain this difference.

HEMODYNAMIC AND REFLEX RESPONSES

Acute and chronic antihypertensive effects seem to differ somewhat with respect to the underlying mechanisms, and they may also vary between the various types of calcium antagonists. Thus, when nifedipine was given sublingually to patients with hypertension there was a modest yet significant acute reduction of systolic and diastolic pressure.[25] This decrease was associated with increases of heart rate, cardiac index, and plasma norepinephrine concentrations while calculated systemic vascular resistance decreased, suggesting reflexly mediated sympathoneural activation due to arterial vasodilatation. Blood pressure was reduced further after six weeks oral therapy, but systemic vascular resistance had not decreased further as compared to the acute effect. However, heart rate, cardiac index, and plasma norepinephrine concentrations had decreased on the average and were no longer statistically different from pretreatment values, findings also noted by others.[21,26] The further decrease of blood pressure seen at six weeks, therefore, seemed to be mediated by a return towards control values of acutely increased sympathetic activity. The importance of sympathetic activity for the chronic reduction of blood pressure was further supported by the findings of an inverse correlation between chronic changes of heart rate and blood pressure (FIGURE 2). These observations would be compatible with the contention that patients with chronically elevated heart rates may still have some degree of sympathetic activation and, therefore, experience a smaller fall in blood pressure as compared to patients in whom heart rate and presumably sympathetic activity return to or even below control values. Although these findings suggest that some degree of reflexly increased sympathetic activity may persist in nonresponders, absolute increases of heart rate were small and unnoticed by the patients. The findings could be explained by a resetting of arterial baroreflexes in responders, but the assessment of the set point of the arterial baroreflexes in man is difficult. Baroreflex sensitivity on the other hand

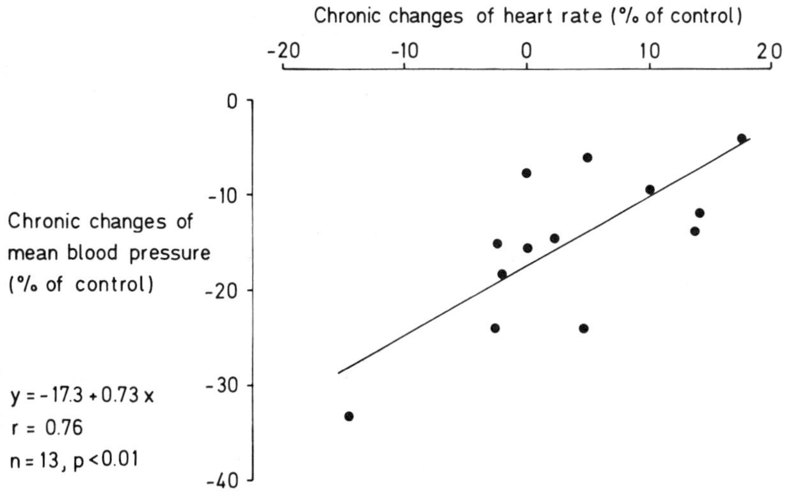

FIGURE 2. Correlation between changes of heart rate and blood pressure (as percent of control values) in 13 patients treated with nifedipine 3 × 20 mg/day for six weeks. Patients with increases of heart rate above control values had the poorest blood pressure response and vice versa.

was unchanged during therapy,[27,28] and arterial-baroreflex-mediated cardiovascular control does not seem to be impaired.

A similar pattern suggestive of mild chronic sympathetic stimulation has also been observed with another dihydropyridine, nitrendipine.[29] In contrast, verapamil and diltiazem do not seem to cause either acute or chronic reflex stimulation as judged by plasma norepinephrine measurements.[30,31] Although plasma norepinephrine concentrations may not accurately reflect sympathetic nervous system activity under all circumstances[33,34] and changes of heart rate cannot be taken as indices of sympathetic activity because of these drugs' direct negative chronotropic effects, these findings raise the possibility that counterregulatory mechanisms may differ between the dihydropyridines and verapamil and diltiazem.

Taken together, these findings suggest that calcium antagonists differ from other directly acting vasodilators with respect to the magnitude of sympathetic reflex activation, although small increases during chronic therapy may influence treatment results.

RENAL EFFECTS

Calcium antagonists differ from other vasodilators also with respect to renal effects and sodium and fluid balance. Thus, no volume retention or gain of weight was observed during therapy with nifedipine,[21,25,26] nitrendipine,[29] or verapamil.[20–24,32] The mechanisms responsible for the lack of volume retention with calcium antagonists have not been fully elucidated and may be different for the dihydropyridine calcium antagonists and verapamil. Thus, a diuretic effect has been demonstrated for nifedipine[30,35] and nitrendipine[36,37] but the situation is less clear with verapamil. Administration of verapamil did not produce a natriuresis or diuresis in some experiments,[30,38] whereas it decreased tubular sodium reabsorbtion in others.[39] In addition, an interference with aldosterone secretion has been suggested during chronic therapy with nifedipine and nitrendipine.[29,40] Although most of these findings represent acute findings the changes observed were the opposite of those found with other vasodilators such as hydralazine and minoxidil which acutely decrease sodium and water excretion.[41] Although the mechanisms responsible for the lack of volume retention are not yet completely understood, this property adds significantly to the favorable hemodynamic profile of calcium antagonists in hypertension.

INTERFERENCE WITH RECEPTOR-OPERATED VASOCONSTRICTOR MECHANISMS

Additional mechanisms may also contribute to the antihypertensive effects of calcium antagonists. Thus, vasoconstriction due to adrenergic stimulation is markedly reduced during therapy but it has been debated whether this inhibition applies to both alpha-1 and alpha-2 adrenoceptor–mediated vasoconstriction.[42–44] Recent evidence suggests that the latter system is effectively blocked by calcium antagonists.[45] However, some interference with alpha-1 adrenoceptor–mediated vasoconstriction also seems likely. Thus nifedipine reduced the blood pressure increase following the alpha-1 adrenoceptor agonist phenylephrine in patients with hypertension (FIGURE 3) both acutely and chronically. Although phenylephrine is not absolutely specific for the alpha-1-type adrenoceptor, this finding and others[46,47] suggest an interference of calcium antagonists with both alpha-1 and alpha-2 adrenoceptor–mediated vasoconstriction. However, the effect on alpha-2 adrenoceptor–mediated vasoconstriction may be more pronounced.

Calcium antagonists also interfere with angiotensin II–mediated vasoconstriction[40] and normalize blood pressure in an animal model in which hypertension was induced by continuous angiotensin II infusion.[48]

These mechanisms probably also contribute to the antihypertensive effects of calcium antagonists, but their quantitative importance remains to be defined precisely.

CLINICAL USE OF CALCIUM ANTAGONISTS

The first report of a blood-pressure-lowering effect of calcium antagonists was published more than 20 years ago.[8] However, it is only in the last 6 to 8 years after the

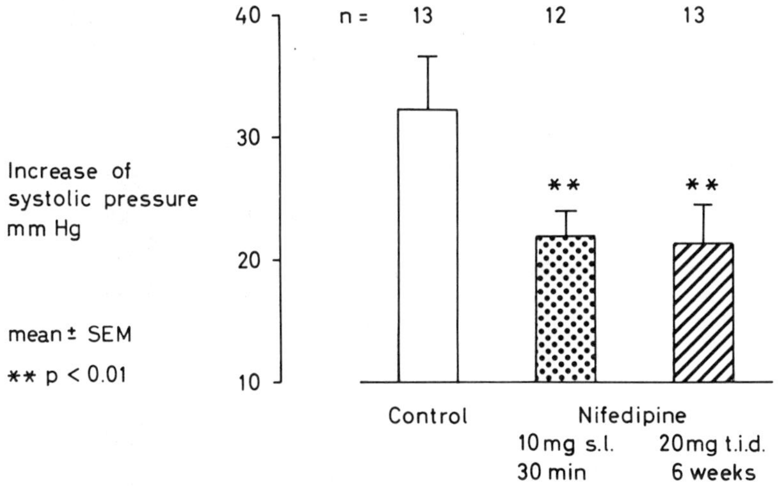

FIGURE 3. Increase of systolic blood pressure after intravenous bolus injections of the alpha-1 adrenoceptor agonist phenylephrine before and after acute (10 mg sublingually) and chronic (2 × 20 mg for six weeks) treatment with nifedipine in patients with essential hypertension. Increases were smaller during therapy despite of higher dosages.

potential usefulness of calcium antagonists for the treatment of hypertension was suggested by several trials[20–24] that this aspect has received widespread attention. Numerous trials have been performed to investigate their efficacy and tolerability alone or in combination with other drugs, and several comparative trials have assessed the relative antihypertensive potencies of the various calcium antagonists available. That literature has recently been extensively reviewed.[49]

MONOTHERAPY

All calcium antagonists lower blood pressure. Depending on the definition of "response rate" they are effective in approximately 40% to 70% of an unselected patient population, and, as shown in FIGURE 4, they all seem to lower blood pressure to a similar degree. This view is further supported by close correlations observed between the blood pressure effects of various calcium antagonists in intraindividual comparisons (FIGURE 5) and by double-blind controlled comparisons between, e.g., nifedipine and verapamil[50] or nifedipine and diltiazem.[51] The onset of the antihypertensive effect is rapid with the sublingual form of nifidipine[21,25] and occurs within hours with the tablets of all calcium antagonists. Even though most of the effect is seen within hours and days, an additional blood-pressure-lowering effect has been observed between the second and fourth week of fix dose nifedipine therapy.[52] Likewise, the response rate increased slightly during long-term monotherapy in a trial with the new dihydropyridine derivative nitrendipine and remained elevated after one year.[53] Blood pressure is reduced throughout the day and also during exercise as demonstrated by 24 hour intraarterial blood pressure monitoring.[23,54] Treatment does not lead to increases of weight, and blood pressure control is maintained during long-term therapy although a few patients have been reported to become refractory.[55] While heart rate does not change with the dihydropyridine-type calcium antagonists nifedipine[23–26,52] and nitren-

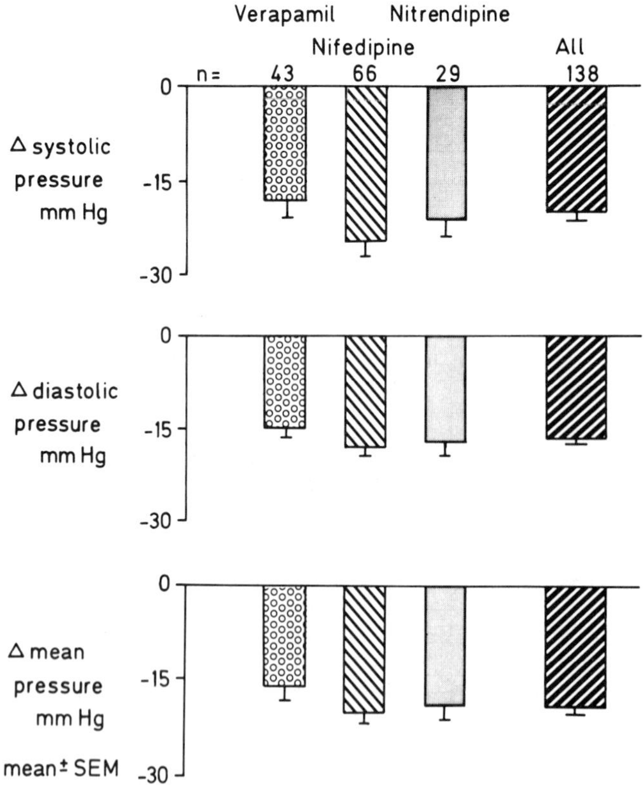

FIGURE 4. Comparison of antihypertensive effects of three calcium antagonists in three groups of patients. All drugs lowered blood pressure to a similar extent. Values are means ± standard error of the mean (SEM).

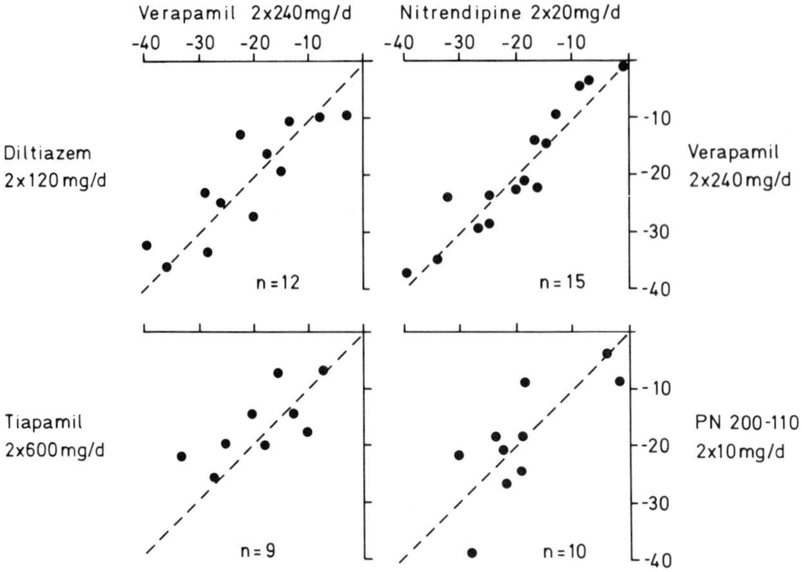

FIGURE 5. Blood pressure (mmHg) responses to various calcium antagonists in four groups of patients. Decreases of blood pressure observed with 1 compound were closely correlated with those observed after a crossover to a different drug.

dipine,[29,53,56] it is mostly reduced with verapamil[20,31,50,54] and to a lesser degree with diltiazem.[57,58] Orthostatic hypotension is uncommon.

COMPARATIVE EFFICACY

Calcium antagonists have been compared with almost all other drugs currently used in hypertension. We performed intraindividual comparisons of the efficacies of verapamil and beta blockers or diuretics (FIGURE 6) and found all three equally efficacious. Similar results or slightly better response rates in favor of calcium antagonists have been obtained in double-blind and/or crossover comparisons of nifedipine and bendroflumethiazide,[59] nifedidipine and methyldopa,[60] nitrendipine and hydrochlorothiazide,[61] verapamil and propranolol,[62] diltiazem and hydrochlorothiazide,[58] diltiazem and propranolol,[57] and verapamil and labetalol.[63]

COMBINATION WITH OTHER DRUGS

Calcium antagonists have been used in combination with most other antihypertensive drugs. They were found effective, among others, in combination with beta blockers, methyldopa,[60] prazosin,[64] and converting enzyme inhibitors[65,66] and particularly the latter combination has proved to be very efficacious in patients difficult to treat. Calcium antagonists have also been used in combination with diuretics but while some investigators found an additional, though not striking effect,[59] others failed to see any further lowering of blood pressure.[67]

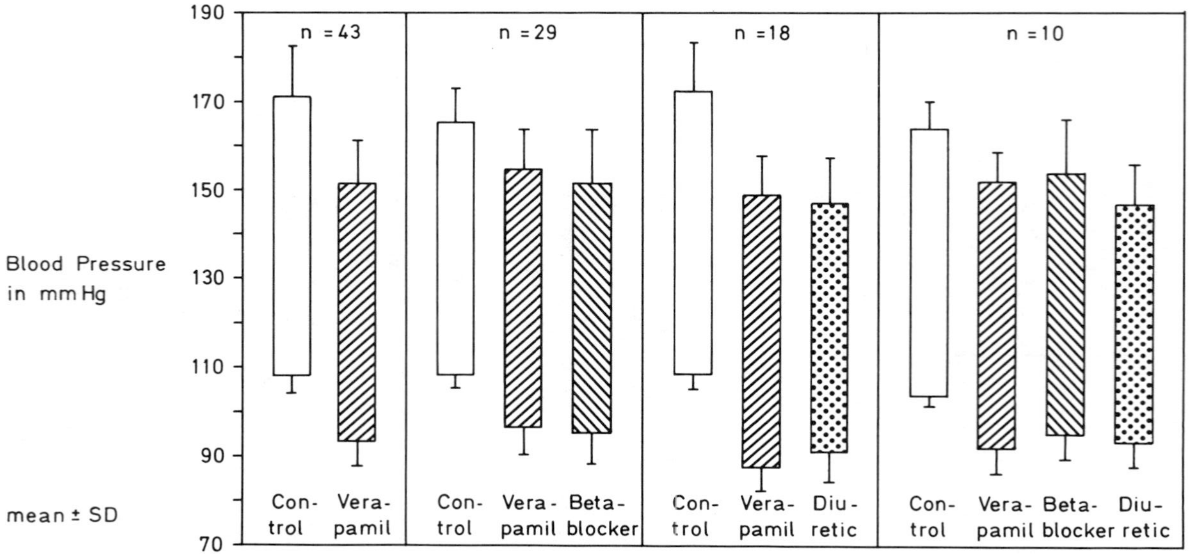

FIGURE 6. Antihypertensive response to verapamil monotherapy and intraindividual comparison of verapamil with beta blockers in a subgroup of 29 patients and diuretics in 18 patients. Comparison of all three compounds was performed in 10 of the patients. Overall antihypertensive effects were similar for all compounds.

There has been concern about the use of calcium antagonists[68,69] in combination with beta blockers. Although all calcium antagonists *in vitro* have negative inotropic effects, verapamil differs from the dihydropyridine calcium antagonists because *in vivo* it exhibits a measurable negative inotropic effect which is most pronounced in patients with already impaired myocardial function.[70] Verapamil also has a dose-dependent negative effect on atrioventricular conduction,[71,72] a property also inherent to beta blockers.[73] Although most data have come from studies in patients with coronary heart disease, this combination probably should not be sought in patients with impaired left ventricular function and when conduction disturbances are likely to occur. Since diltiazem has similar, though less pronounced, negative inotropic and dromotropic effects, its combination with a beta blocker may result in adverse effects in patients with impaired left ventricular function and/or conduction disturbances.[74] However, nifedipine has also precipitated cardiac failure.[75] Thus, more data are needed in hypertensive patients to define precisely the incidence and risk of conduction disturbances and of worsening of cardiac function for these calcium antagonists and for the newer dihydropyridines, which exhibit a greater vascular specificity and, therefore, should have fewer effects on the heart.

CALCIUM ANTAGONISTS AS THIRD-LINE DRUGS AND IN SEVERE AND ACCELERATED HYPERTENSION

Calcium antagonists have been used as vasodilators in standard triple therapy and were found at least as effective as other vasodilating agents.[76–78]

Considerable attention has been paid to the effects of calcium antagonists in severe and accelerated hypertension. Nifedipine has mostly been used for rapid control of severe hypertension, either given sublingually,[79] buccaly,[80] or orally[81] in addition to preexisting therapy. Decreases of blood pressure were correlated to pretreatment pressure,[81] and although blood pressure changes are dramatic in some patients, there seem to be few serious side effects. Nevertheless, great caution should be exercised because of the inherent risks of rapidly lowering blood pressure in patients with possibly inapparent cerebrovascular occlusive disease. Because of its efficacy and ease of administration and because no invasive monitoring is needed, nifedipine nevertheless now is often considered the treatment of choice in these situations.

PREDICTORS OF RESPONSE

The decrease of blood pressure with the use of calcium antagonists relates directly to the height of pretreatment pressure.[20,25,52] While this relationship may exist for many if not all antihypertensive drugs there is also a relationship between percent changes of blood pressure and control pressure.[52,67] Such a relationship was not observed with captopril or propranolol[67] and may indicate that calcium antagonists affect a mechanism that maintains blood pressure to a greater extent the higher the blood pressure. Furthermore, the antihypertensive response to calcium antagonists was greater in older patients who also tend to have low plasma renin activity.[20,52,56] Although the predictive value of these variables could not always be confirmed,[31,59,62] a recent analysis of a large unselected patient population showed that age, plasma renin activity, and pretreatment blood pressure had significant and independent effects on the antihypertensive response to calcium antagonists.[82] Although the relationships were not as close as previously described,[20,52] categorization of patients into age groups shows that older patients on the average have greater decreases of blood pressure and a greater likelihood to respond satisfactorily than younger and middle-aged patients (FIGURE 7). Since the opposite response pattern has been observed with beta blockers,[20,85] it has been proposed to start treatment with a beta blocker in younger and with a calcium antagonist in older patients,[83] offering a simple approach for choosing an effective antihypertensive drug. There is also evidence, though not unequivocal,[62] that black patients on the average respond well to calcium antagonists,[83,84,85] rendering them very useful in this patient group which tends to respond less well to beta blockers[86,87] or angiotensin converting enzyme inhibitors.[88]

CONCLUSION

Calcium antagonists are potent arterial vasodilators capable of correcting the underlying hemodynamic abnormality in hypertension, e.g., increased systemic vascular resistance, without concomitant reflex tachycardia or volume retention. Their excellent long-term safety record acquired in the treatment of ischemic heart disease and their well-documented efficacy and safety when given alone or in combination in hypertension make them a valuable addition to drugs already available. Monotherapy with calcium antagonists may become a first-line treatment for hypertension, particularly in older and possibly black patients.

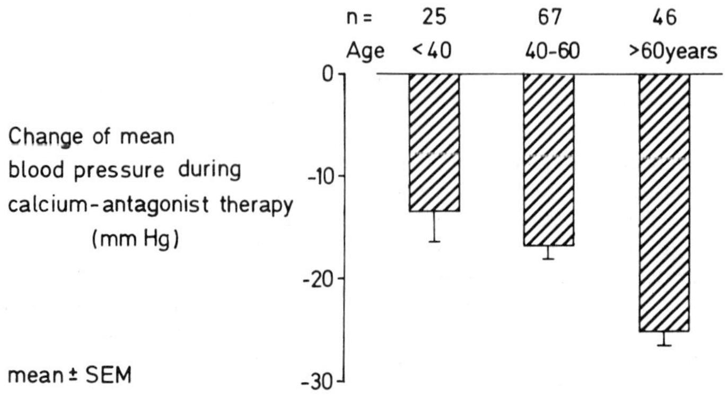

FIGURE 7. Blood pressure response to calcium antagonists in three age groups of patients after an average of three months monotherapy.

SUMMARY

Calcium antagonists are potent arterial vasodilators devoid of relevant chronic sympathetic reflex activation and sodium and volume retention. This favorable hemodynamic profile of action renders them suitable for monotherapy of hypertension where they act to reduce an enhanced, calcium-influx-dependent vasoconstrictor mechanism which may be brought about by altered smooth muscle cation handling and increased intracellular free calcium concentrations. Clinical studies have proved their efficacy, safety, and good tolerability alone or in combination with other drugs in uncomplicated hypertension where they are particularly effective in older and low-renin and possibly black patients. These properties and their efficacy in the treatment of severe and accelerated hypertension or hypertensive emergencies make them a valuable addition to already available drug therapy.

REFERENCES

1. FOLKOW, B. 1971. The hemodynamic consequences of adaptative structural changes of the resistance vessels in hypertension. Clin. Sci. **41:** 1–12.
2. KIOWSKI, W., F. R. BÜHLER, P. VAN BRUMMELEN & F. W. AMANN. 1981. Plasma noradrenaline concentrations and alpha-adrenoceptor mediated vasoconstriction in normotensive and hypertensive man. Clin. Sci. **60:** 483–489.
3. AMANN, F. W., P. BOLLI, W. KIOWSKI & F. R. BÜHLER. 1981. Enhanced alpha-adrenoceptor-mediated vasoconstriction in essential hypertension. Hypertension **3:** I-119–I-123.
4. BOLLI, P., P. ERNE, B. H. JI, L. H. BLOCK, W. KIOWSKI & F. R. BÜHLER. 1984. Adrenaline includes vasoconstriction through post-junctional alpha-2 adrenoceptors and this response is enhanced in patients with essential hypertension. J. Hypertension **2:** s115–s118.
5. BOLTON, T. B. 1979. Mechanisms of action of transmitters and other substances on smooth muscle. Physiol. Rev. **59:** 606–618.
6. BLAUSTEIN, M. P. 1977. Sodium ions, calcium ions, blood pressure regulation, and hypertension. A reassessment and a hypothesis. Am. J. Physiol. **232:** C165–173.
7. FLECKENSTEIN, A. 1977. Specific pharmacology of calcium in myocardium, cardiac pacemakers and vascular smooth muscle. Annu. Rev. Pharmacol. Toxicol. **17:** 149–166.
8. HEIDLAND, A., K. KLÜTSCH & A. OBECK. 1962. Myogen bedingte Vasodilatation bei Nierenischämie. Münch. Med. Wschr. **25:** 1636.
9. RINK, T. J., S. W. SMITH & R. Y. TSIEN. 1982. Cytoplasmic free Ca^{2+} in human platelets; Ca^{2+} thresholds and Ca-independent activation for shape-change and secretion. FEBS Lett. **148:** 21–26.
10. OWEN, N. E., H. FEINBERG & G. C. LEBRETON. 1980. Epinephrine induces Ca^{2+} uptake in human blood platelets. Am. J. Physiol. **239:** H483–488.
11. HINSSEN, H., J. D'HAESE, J. V. SMALL & A. SOBIESZEK. 1978. Mode of filament assembly of myosins from muscle and nonmuscle cells. J. Ultrastruct. Res. **64:** 282–302.
12. ERNE, P., P. BOLLI, E. BÜRGISSER & F. R. BÜHLER. 1984. Correlation of platelet calcium with blood pressure. Effects of treatment. N. Engl. J. Med. **310:** 1084–1088.
13. BRUSCHI, G., M. E. BRUSCHI, M. CAROPPO, G. ORLANDINI, M. SPAGGIARI & A. CAVATORTA. 1985. Cytoplasmic free calcium is increased in the platelets of spontaneously hypertensive rats and essential hypertensive patients. Clin. Sci. **68:** 179–184.
14. LEDERBALLE PEDERSON, O. L., E. MIKKELSEN & K. E. ANDERSSON. 1978. Effects of extracellular calcium on potassium and noradrenaline induced contractions in the aorta of spontaneously hypertensive rats. Increased sensitivity to nifedipine. Acta Pharmacol. Toxicol. **43:** 137–144.
15. MULVANY, M. J. & A. NYBORG. 1980. Increased calcium sensitivity of mesenteric resistance vessels from young and adult spontaneously hypertensive rats. Br. J. Clin. Pharmacol. **71:** 585–596.
16. HULTHEN, U. L., P. BOLLI, F. W. AMANN, W. KIOWSKI & F. R. BÜHLER. 1982. Enhanced vasodilatation in essential hypertension by calcium channel blockade with verapamil. Hypertension **4:** II-26–II-31.
17. ROBINSON, B. F., R. G. DOBBS & S. BAYLEY. 1982. Effects of forearm resistance vessels to verapamil and sodium nitroprusside in normotensive and hypertensive man. Clin. Sci. **63:** 33–42.
18. SCHULTZ, K. D., K. SCHULTZ & G. SCHULTZ. 1977. Sodium nitroprusside and other smooth muscle relaxants increase cyclic GMP levels in rat ductus deferens. Nature **265:** 750–751.

19. KOCH-WESER, J. 1974. Vasodilating drugs in the treatment of hypertension. Arch. Intern. Med. **133:** 1017–1027.
20. BÜHLER, F. R., U. L. HULTHÉN, W. KIOWSKI & P. BOLLI. 1982. Greater antihypertensive efficacy of the calcium channel inhibitor verapamil in older and low renin patient. Clin. Sci. **63:** s439–s442.
21. OLIVARI, M. T., C. BARTORELLI, A. POLESE, C. FIORENTINI, P. MORUZZI & M. GUAZZI. 1979. Treatment of hypertension with nifedipine, a calcium antagonistic agent. Circulation **59:** 1056–1062.
22. BAYLEY, S., R. J. DOBBS & B. F. ROBINSON. 1982. Nifedipine in the treatment of hypertension: report of a double blind controlled trial. Br. J. Clin. Pharmacol. **14:** 509–514.
23. HORNUNG, R. S., B. A. GOULD, R. I. JONES, T. N. SONECHA & E. B. RAFTERY. 1983. Nifedipine tablets for systemic hypertension: a study using intraarterial recording. Am. J. Cardiol. **51:** 1323–1329.
24. GUAZZI, M. D., A. POLESE & C. FIORENTINI. 1983. Treatment of hypertension with calcium antagonists. Review. Hypertension **5:** II-85–II-92.
25. KIOWSKI, W., P. ERNE, O. BERTEL, P. BOLLI & F. R. BÜHLER. 1986. Acute and chronic sympathetic reflex activation and antihypertensive response to nifedipine. J. Am. Coll. Cardiol. **7:** 344–348.
26. LUND-JOHANSSON, P. & P. OMVIK. 1983. Haemodynamic effects of nifedipine in essential hypertension at rest and during exercise. J. Hypertension **1:** 159–163.
27. KIOWSKI, W., P. ERNE, O. BERTEL, U. L. HULTHÉN, R. RITZ & F. R. BÜHLER. 1983. Unchanged baroreflex sensitivity during acute and chronic antihypertensive therapy with nifedipine. J. Hypertension **1**(Suppl. 2): 365–367.
28. MCLEAY, R. A. B., T. J. STALLARD, R. D. S. WATSON & W. A. LITTLER. 1983. The effect of nifedipine on arterial pressure and reflex cardiac control. Circulation **67:** 1084–1090.
29. FOUAD, F. M., R. PEDRINELLI, E. L. BRAVO, F. ABI-SAMRA, S. C. TEXTOR & R. C. TARAZI. 1984. Clinical and systemic hemodynamic effects of nitrendipine. Clin. Pharmacol. Ther. **35:** 768–775.
30. LEONETTI, G., C. CUSPIDI, L. SAMPIERI, L. TERZOLI & A. ZANCHETTI. 1982. Comparison of cardiovascular, renal, and humoral effects of acute administration of two calcium channel blockers in normotensive and hypertensive subjects. J. Cardiovasc. Pharmacol. **4**(Suppl. 3): 319–324.
31. MUIESAN, G., E. AGABITI-ROSEI, M. CASTELLANO, C. L. ALICANDRI, L. COREA, R. FARIELLO, M. BESCHI & G. ROMANELLI. 1982. Antihypertensive and humoral effects of verapamil and nifedipine in essential hypertension. J. Cardiovasc. Pharmacol. **4**(Suppl. 3): 325–329.
32. BRUNN, N. E., H. IBSEN, F. NIELSEN, M. D. NIELSEN, A. G. MOELBAK, & O. J. HARTLING. 1986. Lack of effect of nifedipine on counterregulatory mechanisms in essential hypertension. Hypertension **8:** 655–661.
33. FLORAS, J., J. VANN JONES, O. HASSAN, B. A. OSIKOWSKA, P. S. SEVER & P. SLEIGHT. 1986. Failure of plasma norepinephrine to consistently reflect sympathetic activity in humans. Hypertension **8:** 641–649.
34. FOLKOW, B., G. F. DI BONA, P. HJEMDAHL, P. THORN & P. E. WOLLNI. 1983. Measurements of plasma norepinephrine concentrations in human primary hypertension. A word of caution on their applicability for assessing neurogenic contributions. Hypertension **5:** 399–404.
35. KLUETSCH, K., P. SCHMIDT & J. GROSSWENDT. 1972. Der Einfluss von Bay a 1040 auf die Nierenfunktion des Hypertonikers. Arzneim Forsch **22:** 377–380.
36. THANANOPARVAN, C., M. S. GOLUB, P. EGGENA, J. D. BARRETT & M. P. SAMBHI. 1985. Renal effects of nitrendipine monotherapy in essential hypertension. J. Cardiovasc. Pharmacol. **6**(Suppl. 7): 1040–1044.
37. GARTHOFF, B., S. KAZDA, A. KNORR & G. THOMAS. 1982. Factors involved in the antihypertensive action of calcium antagonists. Hypertension **225:** 263–270.
38. LEONETTI, G., C. SALA, C. BIANCHINI, L. TERZOLI & A. ZANCHETTI. 1980. Antihypertensive and renal effects of orally administered verapamil. Eur. J. Clin. Pharmacol. **18:** 375–382.
39. DIETZ, J. R., J. O. DAVIES, R. H. FREEMAN, D. VILLAREAL & S. F. ECHTLENCAMP. 1983.

Effects of intrarenal infusions of calcium entry blockers in anaesthetized dogs. Hypertension **5:** 482–488.

40. MILLAR, J. A., K. A. MCLEAN & J. L. REID. 1983. The effects of the calcium antagonist nifedipine on pressor and aldosterone responses to angiotensin II in normal man. Eur. J. Clin. Pharmacol. **24:** 315–321.
41. O'MALLEY, K., M. VELASEO, J. WELLS & J. L. MCNAY. 1977. Control plasma renin activity and changes in sympathetic tone as determinants of minoxidil-induced increase in plasma renin activity. J. Clin. Invest. **55:** 230–237.
42. DE MEY, J. & P. VANHOUTTE. 1981. Uneven distribution of postjunctional alpha-1 and alpha-2-like adrenoceptors in canine arterial and venous smooth muscle. Circ. Res. **48:** 875–884.
43. VAN MEEL, K. A., A. DEJONGE, H. O. KALKMANN, B. WILFFERT, P. B. M. W. M. TIMMERMANS & P. A. VAN ZWIETEN. 1981. Vascular smooth muscle contraction initiated by postsynaptic-adrenoceptor activation is induced by an influx of extracellular calcium. Eur. J. Pharmacol. **69:** 205–208.
44. CAVERO, I., N. B. SHEPPERSON, F. LEFÉVRE-BORG & S. Z. LANGER. 1983. Differential inhibition of vascular smooth muscle responses to alpha-1 and alpha-2-adrenoceptor agonists by diltiazem and verapamil. Circ. Res. **52:** 169–176.
45. TIMMERMANS, P. B. M. W. M., M. J. MATHY, M. J. M. C. THOOLEN, A. DE JONGE, B. WILFFERT & P. A. VAN ZWIETEN. 1984. Invariable susceptibility to blockade by nifedipine of vasoconstriction to various alpha-2 adrenoceptor agonists in pithed rats. J. Pharm. Pharmacol. **36:** 772–775.
46. TIMMERMANS, P. B. M. W. M., M. J. MATHY, B. WILFFERT, H. O. KALKMAN, M. J. M. C. THOOLEN, A. DE JONGE & P. A. ZWIETEN. 1983. Differential effect of calcium entry blockers on alpha-1-adrenoceptor-mediated vasoconstriction in vivo. Naunyn Schmiedebergs Arch. Pharmacol. **324:** 239–245.
47. PEDRINELLI, R. & R. C. TARAZI. 1984. Interference of calcium entry blockade in vivo with pressor responses to alpha-adrenergic stimulation: effects of two unrelated blockers on responses to both exogenous and endogenously released norepinephrine. Circulation **69:** 1171–1176.
48. STERZEL, R. B., J. L. HUELSEMANN, D. E. MCKENZIE & C. S. WILCOX. 1984. Nitrendipine reverses vasoconstriction and renal hemodynamic changes in experimental hypertension. J. Cardiovasc. Pharmacol. **6**(Suppl. 7): 1032–1035.
49. HALPERIN, A. K. & L. X. CUBEDDU. 1986. The role of calcium channel blockers in the treatment of hypertension. Am. Heart J. **111:** 363–382.
50. MIDTBO, K., O. HEDS & J. VON DER MEER. 1982. Verapamil compared with nifedipine in the treatment of essential hypertension. J. Cardiovasc. Pharmacol. **4**(Suppl. 3): 363–368.
51. KLEIN, W., D. BRAND, K. VRECKO & M. HARRINGER. 1983. Role of calcium antagonists in the treatment of essential hypertension. Circ. Res. **52**(Suppl. 1): 174–181.
52. ERNE, P., P. BOLLI, O. BERTEL, U. L. HULTHÉN, W. KIOWSKI, F. B. MÜLLER & F. R. BÜHLER. 1983. Factors influencing the hypotensive effects of calcium antagonists. Hypertension **5**(Suppl. 2): II-97–II-102.
53. WEBER, M. A. A one-year experience with the calcium-channel blocking agent nitrendipine in patients with essential hypertension. J. Cardiovasc. Pharmacol. (In press.)
54. GOULD, G. A., S. MANN, H. KIESO, V. BALASUBRAMANIAN & E. B. RAFTERY. 1982. Slow channel inhibitors verapamil and nifedipine in the management of hypertension. J. Cardiovasc. Pharmacol. **4**(Suppl. 3): 369–373.
55. HUSTED, S. E., H. K. NIELSEN, C. K. CHRISTENSEN & O. L. PEDERSEN. 1982. Long-term therapy of arterial hypertension with nifedipine given alone or in combination with a beta-blocking agent. Eur. J. Clin. Pharmacol. **22:** 101–103.
56. PEDRINELLI, R., F. M. FOUD, R. C. TARAZI, E. L. BRAVO & S. C. TEXTOR. 1986. Nitrendipine, a calcium blocker: renal and humoral effects in human arterial hypertension. Arch. Intern. Med. **146:** 62–65.
57. YAMAKADO, T., N. OONISHI, S. KONDO, A. NOZIRI, T. NAKANO & H. TAKEZAWA. 1983. Effects of diltiazem on cardiovascular responses during exercise in systemic hypertension and comparison with propranolol. Am. J. Cardiol. **52:** 1023–1027.
58. INOUYE, I. K., B. M. MASSIE, N. BENOWITZ, P. SIMPSON & D. LOGE. 1984. Antihyperten-

sive therapy with diltiazem and comparison with hydrochlorothiazide. Am. J. Cardiol. **53:** 1588–1592.

59. HALLIN, L., L. ANDREN & L. HANSSON. 1983. Controlled trial of nifedipine and bendroflumethazide in hypertension. J. Cardiovasc. Pharmacol. **5:** 1083–1085.
60. GUAZZI, M. D., C. FIORENTINI, M. T. OLIVARI, A. BARTORELLI, G. NECCHI & A. POLESE. 1980. Short and long-term efficacy of a calcium-antagonistic agent (nifedipine) combined with methyldopa in the treatment of severe hypertension. Circulation **61:** 913–919.
61. MORLEDGE, J. H. Comparative study of the effects of nitrendipine and hydrochlorothiazide in hypertensive patients. J. Cardiovasc. Pharmacol. (In press.)
62. HALPERIN, A. K., K. M. GROSS, J. F. ROGERS & L. X. CUBEDDU. 1984. Verapamil and propranolol in essential hypertension. Clin. Pharmacol. Ther. **36:** 750–758.
63. ANAVEKAR, S. N., C. BARTER, W. R. ADAM, A. E. DOYLE. 1982. A double-blind comparison of verapamil and labetalol in hypertensive patients with coexisting chronic obstructive airways disease. J. Cardiovasc. Pharmacol. **4**(Suppl. 3): 374–377.
64. PASANISI, F., H. L. ELLIOTT, P. A. MEREDITH, D. R. MCSHARRY & J. L. REID. 1984. Combined alpha adrenoceptor antagonism and calcium channel blockade in normal subjects. Clin. Pharmacol. Ther. **36:** 716–723.
65. BROUWER, R. M. L., P. BOLLI, P. ERNE, D. CONEN, W. KIOWSKI & F. R. BÜHLER. 1985. Antihypertensive treatment using calcium antagonists in combination with captopril rather than diuretics. J. Cardiovasc. Pharmacol. **7**(Suppl. 4): 88–91.
66. GUAZZI, M. D., N. DE CESARE, C. GALLI, A. SALVIONI, C. TRAMONTANA, G. TAMBORINI & A. BARTORELLI. 1984. Calcium-channel blockade with nifedipine and angiotensin converting enzyme inhibition with captopril in the therapy of patients with severe primary hypertension. Circulation **70:** 279–284.
67. MACGREGOR, G. A., N. D. MARKANDU, S. J. SMITH & G. A. SAGNELLA. 1985. Does nifedipine reveal a functional abnormality of arteriolar smooth muscle cell in essential hypertension—the effect of altering sodium balance. J. Cardiovasc. Pharmacol. **7**(Suppl. 6): 178–181.
68. OPIE, L. H., & D. A. WHITE. 1980. Adverse reaction between nifedipine and beta-blockade. Br. Med. J. **281:** 1462.
69. WAYNE, V. S., R. W. HARPER, E. LAUFER, J. FEDERMANN, S. T. ANDERSON & A. PITT. 1982. Adverse interaction between beta-adrenergic blocking drugs and verapamil-report of three cases. Aust. NZ J. Med. **12:** 285–289.
70. LOW, R. I., P. TAKEDA, D. T. MASON & A. N. DE MARIA. 1982. The effects of calcium channel blocking agents on cardiovascular function. Am. J. Cardiol. **49:** 547–553.
71. MITCHELL, L. B., J. S. SCHROEDER & J. W. MASON. 1982. Comparative clinical electrophysiological effects of diltiazem, verapamil and nifedipine: a review. Am. J. Cardiol. **49:** 629–635.
72. WU, D., P. DENES, R. DHINGRA, A. KHAN & K. M. ROSEN. 1974. The effects of propranolol on induction of AV nodal reentrant paroxysmal tachycardia. Circulation **50:** 665–671.
73. WELLENS, H. J. J. 1980. Electro-physiological effects of beta-blocking agents as studied by programmed stimulation of the heart. *In* Beta-blockade and anesthesia. P. J. Poppers, B. Van Dijk & A. H. M. Van Elzakker, Eds.: 65–70. Astra Pharmaceutica. Stockholm, Sweden.
74. OESTERLE, S. N., E. L. ALDERMAN, L. BEIER-SCOTT, D. S. BAIM, M. T. ROTHMAN & J. S. SCHROEDER. 1986. Diltiazem and propranolol in combination: hemodynamic effects following acute intravenous administration. Am. Heart J. **111:** 489–497.
75. ROBSON, R. H. & M. C. VISWANATH. 1982. Nifedipine and betablockade as a cause of cardiac failure. Br. Med. J. **284:** 104.
76. EVANS, M. G., L. S. OLANOFF, G. HURWITZ, T. D. COWART & E. C. CONRADI. 1984. Use of nifedipine as an adjunct to current antihypertensive therapy. Arch. Intern. Med. **144:** 985–987.
77. SLOAN, P. J. M. & D. G. BEEVERS. 1983. Nifedipine in combination therapy for resistant hypertension. Pharmacotherapeutica **3:** 349–353.
78. KENDALL, M. J. & S. DEAN. 1983. The use of nifedipine as third line therapy in the treatment of severe hypertension. Postgr. Med. J. **59**(Suppl. 2): 119–123.

79. BEER, N., I. GALLEGOS, A. COHEN, N. KLEIN, E. SONNENBLICK & W. FRISHMAN. 1981. Efficacy of sublingual nifedipine in the acute treatment of systemic hypertension. Chest **79:** 571–574.
80. HAFT, J. I. & W. E. LITTERER. 1984. Chewing nifedipine to rapidly treat hypertension. Arch. Intern. Med. **144:** 2357–2359.
81. BERTEL, O., D. CONEN, E. W. RADÜ, C. LANG & U. C. DUBACH. 1983. Nifedipine in hypertensive emergencies. Br. Med. J. **283:** 19–20.
82. KIOWSKI, W., F. R. BÜHLER, M. FADYOMI, P. ERNE, F. B. MÜLLER, U. L. HULTHÉN & P. BOLLI. 1986. Age, race, blood pressure and renin: predictors for antihypertensive treatment with calcium antagonists. Am. J. Cardiol. **56:** 81H–85H.
83. BÜHLER, F. R., P. BOLLI, P. ERNE, W. KIOWSKI, F. B. MÜLLER, U. L. HULTHÉN & B. H. JI. 1985. Position of calcium antagonists in antihypertensive therapy. J. Cardiovasc. Pharmacol. **7**(Suppl. 4): 21–27.
84. LEARY, W. P. & A. C. ASMAL. 1979. Treatment of hypertension with verapamil. Curr. Ther. Res. **25:** 747–752.
85. MOSER, M., J. CUNN & B. J. MATERSON. 1984. Comparative effects of diltiazem and hydrochlorothiazide in blacks with systemic hypertension. Am. J. Cardiol. **56:** 101H–104H.
86. MOSER, M. & J. CUNN. 1981. Comparative effects of pindolol and hydrochlorothiazide in black hypertensive patients. Angiology **32:** 561–566.
87. Veterans Administration Cooperative Study Group. 1982. Comparison of propranolol and hydrochlorothiazide for the initial treatment of hypertension. I. Results of short term titration with emphasis on racial differences in response. JAMA **248:** 1996–2003.
88. MOSER, M. & J. CUNN. 1982. Responses to captopril and hydrochlorothiazide in black patients with hypertension. Clin. Pharmacol. Ther. **32:** 307–312.

Myocardial Protection[a]

W. FLAMENG

Department of Cardiovascular Surgery
Catholic University Leuven
University Clinic Gasthuisberg
Herestraat 49
B-3000 Leuven, Belgium

INTRODUCTION

The concept of myocardial protection has been of interest to cardiologists and cardiac surgeons for many decades. Before the introduction of coronary thrombolysis, cardiologists were primarily dealing with persistent regional myocardial ischemia induced by interruption of flow in one of the coronary arteries. Research on myocardial protection was then focused on interventions claiming a "limitation of infarct size." Not much progress was achieved in this field until it was recognized that reperfusion is an essential aspect of myocardial protection. Indeed, as Hearse stated, a severe reduction in flow (to 25% or less) in the absence of reperfusion must inevitably lead to cell death, and no intervention has yet been described that can sustain normal contractile function in tissue deprived of flow to this extent.[1] The point is that some drugs, including calcium antagonists, are able to delay irreversible myocardial injury substantially but there is much less evidence for the ability of these drugs to achieve a sustained reduction of ischemic injury unless early reperfusion is initiated.[1,2] Preservation of the myocardium during regional ischemia, however, has his own specific aspects and pitfalls such as determination and prediction of the exact infarct size, the influence of changes in general hemodynamics during ischemia, etc. This topic is out of the scope of this report and will not be discussed further: the present paper deals only with myocardial preservation during global ischemia.

Global myocardial ischemia has been the subject of many studies in the field of cardiac surgery, and there is still an ongoing quest for ideal myocardial protective techniques.[3] During prolonged periods of global ischemia myocardial ischemic injury can be substantially delayed by hypothermia and cardioplegia,[4] but there is no doubt that without timely reperfusion these "protected" globally ischemic hearts would die. Although hypothermia and cardioplegia offer adequate protection during many routine cardiac intervention,[5,6] more extended periods of aortic cross clamping are still associated with an increased incidence of postoperative low cardiac output and lethal outcome. Another topic attracting the attention of cardiac surgeons increasingly is that of prolonged organ preservation for transplantation. Donor heart preservation, i.e., cold storage after cardioplegic arrest, is limited at present to three to four hours in order to avoid postoperative low cardiac output.

[a]This study was supported in part by a grant of the NFWO (National Fonds voor Wetenschappelijk Onderzoek).

PATHWAYS LEADING TO ISCHEMIC CELL DEATH AND POSSIBLE MODIFICATIONS BY CALCIUM ANTAGONISTS

Although changes to the myocardial tissue induced by ischemia have been intensively studied in the past, the cause of the transition from reversible to irreversible or lethal injury has never been established. Nevertheless, some potential causes of irreversibility can be recognized when studying the major features of ischemia. Within a few seconds after the onset of ischemia, mitochondrial oxidative phosphorilation stops. This results in a drop of high-energy phosphate production and in an accumulation of catabolites. Creatine phosphate is almost completely depleted within the first 3 minutes of ischemia,[7] while ATP decreases to about 35% of control by 15 minutes and to less than 10% by 40 minutes.[8] A drop in high-energy phosphates is probably the trigger for a sequence of events leading to cell death. At first, energy-dependent membrane ion-pump function decreases (see FIGURE 1) and disturbs cell volume

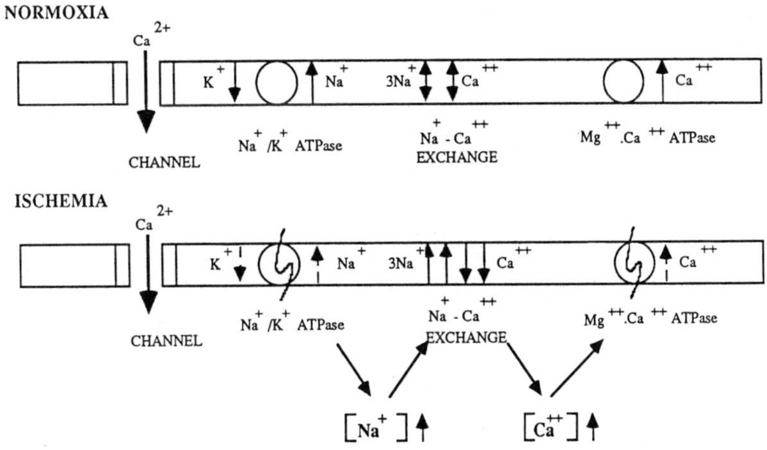

FIGURE 1. Schematic representation of the calcium shifts through the sarcolemmal membrane under normoxic (upper panel) and ischemic (lower panel) conditions.

regulation. Malfunction of the Na^+, K^+ adenosine triphosphatase enzyme induces an intracellular accumulation of Na^+ and cell swelling. An enhanced exchange between Na^+ and Ca^{2+} in turn induces an increase in cytosolic Ca^{2+}. Cytosolic Ca^{2+} is further increased by an impaired extrusion of Ca^{2+} via the energy-dependent Mg^{2+}, Ca^{2+} ATPase. Cytosolic Ca^{2+} can also be augmented by a deficiency of calcium sequestration in the sarcoplasmatic reticulum (SR) when the SR calcium pump (calcium-activated magnesium ATPase) is inhibited. Such an accumulation and redistribution of intracellular calcium has detrimental consequences for the myocyte: mitochondria start accumulating Ca^{2+} ions instead of producing ATP; calcium activates phospholipases and proteases, which in turn will destroy phospholipid bilayers and proteins. At this stage, rupture of the sarcolemma will occur and will, mainly in the presence of reperfusion, initiate a massive pathologic calcium influx. Such a *calcium overload* is the hallmark of irreversibility: massive accumulation of calcium by the mitochondria will destroy mitochondrial function completely and will induce irreversible hypercontraction of the myofibrils. Sarcolemmal rupture is also initiated by other mechanisms in the ischemic cell. Accumulation of acylcarnitine and acylCoA occurs, and these agents act as detergents on the membranes. Formation of free radicals may be induced by the increased catabolism of high-energy phosphates. Hypoxanthine, one of the final catabolites of ATP, is oxidized to xanthine and uric acid by the xanthine oxidase reaction. During ischemia, inosine and hypoxanthine rapidly accumulate and, especially when reperfusion is established, the xanthine oxidase reaction might produce an excessive load of superoxide anion. This ion is particularly toxic and produces membrane destruction. FIGURE 2 shows a schematic representation of the pathways leading to ischemic cell death.

How can calcium antagonists modify these pathways leading to ischemic cell death? As shown in FIGURE 2 calcium overload is the final and lethal feature preceding cell death. Within this concept, drugs that are able to prevent this calcium overload are potentially protective and can be called "calcium overload blockers." This by no means implies that these drugs have to prevent pathologic influx of calcium when they are administered not prior to, but together with, reperfusion. Poole-Wilson for example

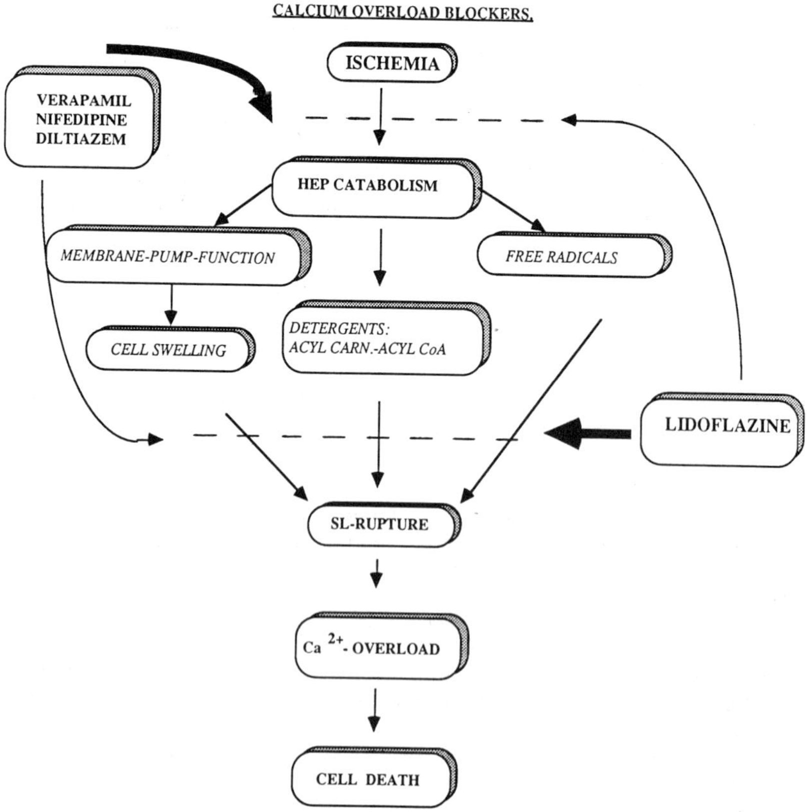

FIGURE 2. Schematic representation of the pathways leading to ischemic cell death. SL: sarcolemma. Arrows indicate the level at which calcium antagonists may interfere.

TABLE 1. Nifedipine as an Adjunct to Cardioplegia: Patient Data

	Placebo	Nifedipine
Number of patients	12	12
Age (years)	57 ± 13	56 ± 10
Sex (female—male)	4–8	5–7
Aortic stenosis, pressure gradient (mm Hg)	102 ± 26	110 ± 24
Duration of cardiopulmonary bypass (minutes)	91 ± 14	87 ± 13
Duration of aortic cross-clamping (minutes)	63 ± 20	60 ± 11

showed clearly that verapamil, administered together with reperfusion in the ischemic ventricular septum preparation, was not able to prevent massive calcium accumulation in the postischemic myocardial tissue.[9] There is however, abundant evidence that this calcium entry blocker, when given prior to ischemia, prevents calcium overload and cell death after reperfusion.[10,11] Calcium antagonistic drugs act as calcium overload blockers in the ischemic and postischemic myocardium when the heart is *pretreated* with these agents. They do so by blocking the pathways leading to calcium overload at two different levels: inhibition of ATP breakdown and stabilization of the plasma membrane. Both mechanisms, the ATP-sparing effect and membrane stabilization, are not necessarily of the same importance and the predominance of one of these interactions seems to be related to the specific type of calcium antagonist used (see FIGURE 2). For example, calcium entry blockers like verapamil, nifedipine, and diltiazem mainly act via the ATP-sparing effect[10] and also but less via a membrane stabilizing effect.[12] The calcium antagonist lidoflazine on the other hand has a predominantly protective effect on the plasma membrane and has little effect on ATP breakdown.[13,14] Both types of drugs, however, clearly prevent postischemic calcium overload and cell death when used as a pretreatment.[10,15] In this context we will assess the use of calcium antagonists as myocardial protective agents in the clinical setting.

MYOCARDIAL PROTECTIVE EFFECTS OF CALCIUM ANTAGONISTS: CLINICAL STUDIES

Clark was the first to report a well-documented clinical study on the cardioprotective effects of nifedipine during surgically induced global myocardial ischemia.[16] Ninety high-risk patients were enrolled in a randomized clinical trial. Nifedipine or placebo was added to the cardioplegic solution. The cristalloid cardioplegic solution was hyperkalemic, hypoatriemic, alkalotic, and hyperosmotic. The nifedipine concentration ranged from 100–300 μg/l such that the total dose for each patient was in the range of 1.0 to 2.0 μg per gram of estimated weight. The study showed an improved left ventricular performance (left ventricular minute work index) immediately after weaning from cardiopulmonary bypass and a lower incidence of myocardial injury as assessed by myocardial pyrophosphate scans. However, the use of nifedipine had no effect on the incidence of acute low cardiac output syndrome or death.

We studied the protective effects of nifedipine as an adjunct to St. Thomas' Hospital cardioplegia, not only in terms of functional and clinical outcome but also in relation to nucleotide metabolism.[17] This study was a double-blind placebo-controlled randomized clinical trial including 24 patients undergoing aortic valve replacement. All patients presented a significant aortic valve stenosis with a pressure gradient of at least 70 mm Hg. The patient data are given in TABLE 1. As indices of myocardial protection we used biochemical parameters (high-energy phosphates and their break-

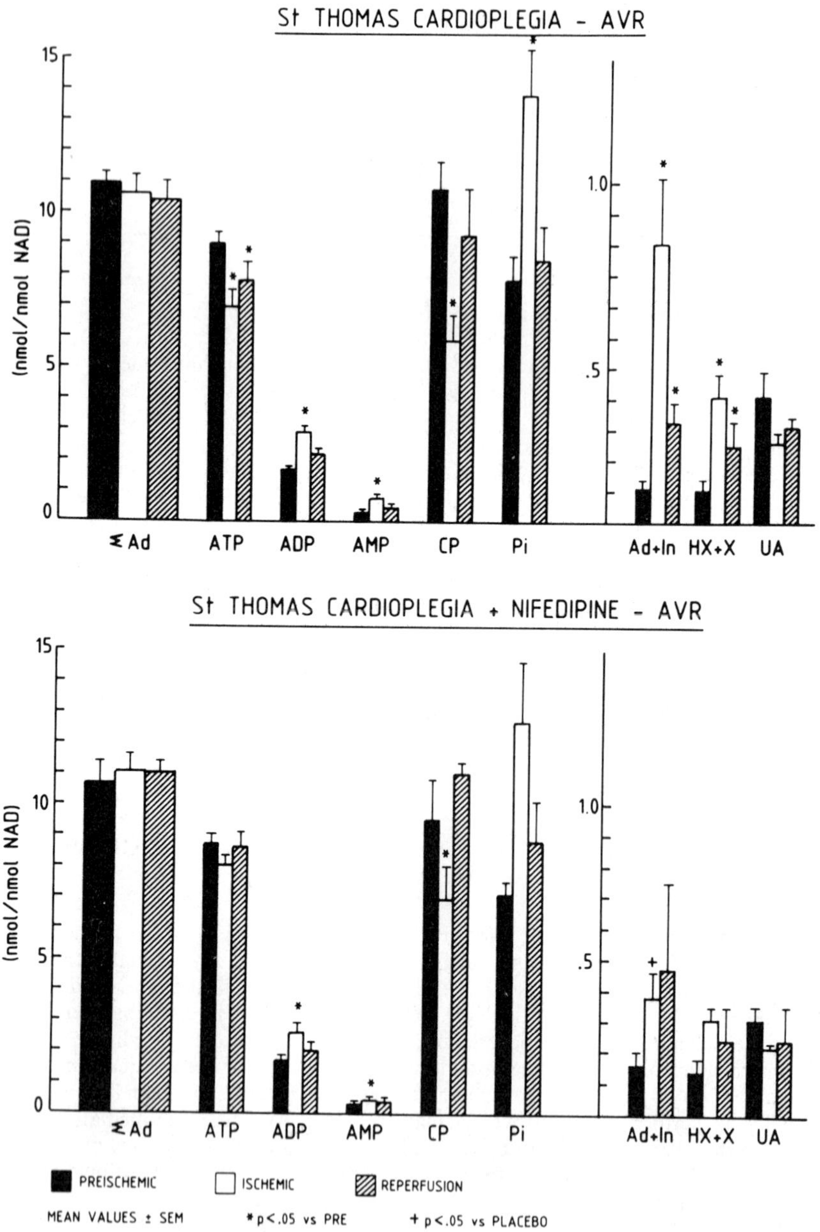

FIGURE 3. Values of high-energy phosphates and their catabolites before ischemia (black bar), during ischemia (open bars), and after reperfusion (hatched bars) in patients undergoing aortic valve replacement (AVR). ATP = adenosine triphosphate; ADP = adenosine diphosphate; AMP = adenosine monophosphate; ΣAd = sum of adenylates; CP = creatine phosphate; Pi = inorganic phosphate; Ad + In = adenosine + inosine; HX + X = hypoxanthine + xanthine; UA = uric acid.

down products), the release of CK-MB isoenzyme, recovery of hemodynamics after cardiopulmonary bypass, and clinical outcome in terms of prolongation of atrioventricular conduction, arrhythmias, low cardiac output, positive inotropic support and 15 months' follow-up. Nifedipine (200 μg/l) or placebo was added to St. Thomas' Hospital cardioplegia,[17] which is an extracellular-type cardioplegic solution. The infusion of the cardioplegic solution was stopped when septal temperature had reached 14°C and was resumed every 30 minutes. Three transmural left ventricular biopsies (each 15 mg wet weight) were taken from the anterior wall: the first before cross-clamping the aorta, the second at the end of the ischemic arrest, and the third before weaning from bypass. These biopsies were processed for analysis of ATP, ADP, AMP, adenosine, inosine, hypoxanthine, xanthine, creatine phosphate, and inorganic phosphate.

These determinations showed a preservation of ATP during ischemia in the nifedipine-treated group, associated with reduced accumulation of the catabolites adenosine, inosine, and hypoxanthine (see FIGURE 3). Obviously there was a significant ATP-sparing effect of the drug.

TABLE 2. Myocardial Protection in the Clinical Setting: Effects of Nifedipine

	Results[a]	
Effect	Study A	Study B
• ATP sparing during ischemic arrest	ND	+
• Lower incidence of myocardial injury		
• Postoperative CK-MB release	–	–
• Pyrophosphate scans	+	ND
• Better recovery of hemodynamics after weaning of CPB[b]	+	–
• Lower incidence of rhythm disturbances	–	–
• Lower incidence of postoperative LCO[c]	–	–
• Reduced mortality	–	–

[a]Study A = Reference 16. Study B = Reference 17. + = positive effect, – = no effect, ND = not done.
[b]CPB is cardiopulmonary bypass.
[c]LCO is low cardiac output.

CK-MB release, which was followed for 36 hours postoperatively, did not show a difference between groups. The time-activity curve of CK-MB showes only a slight release of the isoenzyme (the equivalent of necrosis of ±1 gram myocardial tissue), which proves that overall protection with cardioplegia is effective.

Postoperative functional recovery of the hearts was not statistically different between groups. Clinical outcome in terms of incidence of arrhythmias, conduction disturbances, need for positive inotropic support, and death was not different between groups. Actuarial survival at 15 months follow-up time was 91.5% in the whole patient population, and there was no significant difference between groups. All survivors in both groups were event free; there was no incidence of thromboembolic phenomena, endocarditis, or resurgery. Clinical status [New York Heart Association NYHA)] was 2.43 preoperatively and 1.04 postoperatively.

Both studies, Clark's study[16] as well as ours,[17] provide evidence for the protective properties of the calcium entry blocker nifedipine in the clinical setting (see TABLE 2). However, there is a definite need for more large-scale double-blind placebo-controlled randomized clinical studies in order to investigate the final goal: improvement of clinical outcome after extensive cardiac surgery. No other of the two studies presented above, although placebo controlled and randomized, contained a patient population that was large enough to allow valid conclusions on differences in clinical outcome.

In another randomized clinical study we assessed the protective properties of another calcium antagonist, lidoflazine.[13] Patient data are presented in TABLE 3. This study differed from the above-mentioned nifedipine studies in two respects. First, this study included only aortocoronary bypass operations which were performed using intermittent aortic cross-clamping at 28°C. Second, lidoflazine was administered intravenously prior to installation of cardiopulmonary bypass. Two doses of lidoflazine were tested: control group (group I, $n = 10$), 0.5 mg $\times$ kg^{-1} (group II, $n = 10$), and 1.0 mg $\times$ kg^{-1} (group III, $n = 10$). As indices of myocardial damage, biochemical, structural, and functional parameters were used as well as clinical outcome. Two pairs of transmural left ventricular biopsies were obtained, one after installation of

TABLE 3. Aortocoronary Bypass Grafting: Lidoflazine Pretreatment: Patient Data

	Group I: Hypothermia	Group II: Hypothermia + 0.5 mg $\times$ kg^{-1} Lidoflazine	Group III: Hypothermia + 1 mg $\times$ kg^{-1} Lidoflazine
Number of patients	10	10	10
Age (years)			
Mean	49	50	52
Range	54–62	48–63	34–67
Sex			
Male	8	7	8
Female	2	3	2
Number of grafts			
Mean	4.5	4.7	4.8
Range	4–5	4–6	4–7
Preoperative Ejection Fraction (%)			
Mean	56.6	62.5	55.8
Range	45–75	11–84	35–78
Angina Class			
Mean	2.8	3.0	3.1
Range	II–IV	II–IV	II–IV
Preoperative infarction (number of patients)	4	4	4

cardiopulmonary bypass but before ischemia and one shortly before weaning from bypass. Adenosine triphosphate, creatine phosphate, and glycogen were determined in the pre- and postischemic samples after immediate cooling in liquid nitrogen. Ultrastructure was assessed in a similar pair of biopsies.

The lower dose of lidoflazine (0.5 mg $\times$ kg^{-1}) did not offer substantial myocardial protection. There was only a smaller loss of ATP in the postischemic myocardium as compared to the control group ($p < 0.05$). The other parameters did not differ from those in the control group. In the group where 1.0 mg $\times$ kg^{-1} lidoflazine was given prior to ischemia, ATP, creatine phosphate, and glycogen were perfectly preserved at the end of the operation, in contrast to the control group where all these three parameters decreased significantly ($p < 0.05$). Also the electron microscopical examination of pre-and postischemic samples revealed a remarkable difference from the observations in the control group. The most striking structural abnormality in the pre-

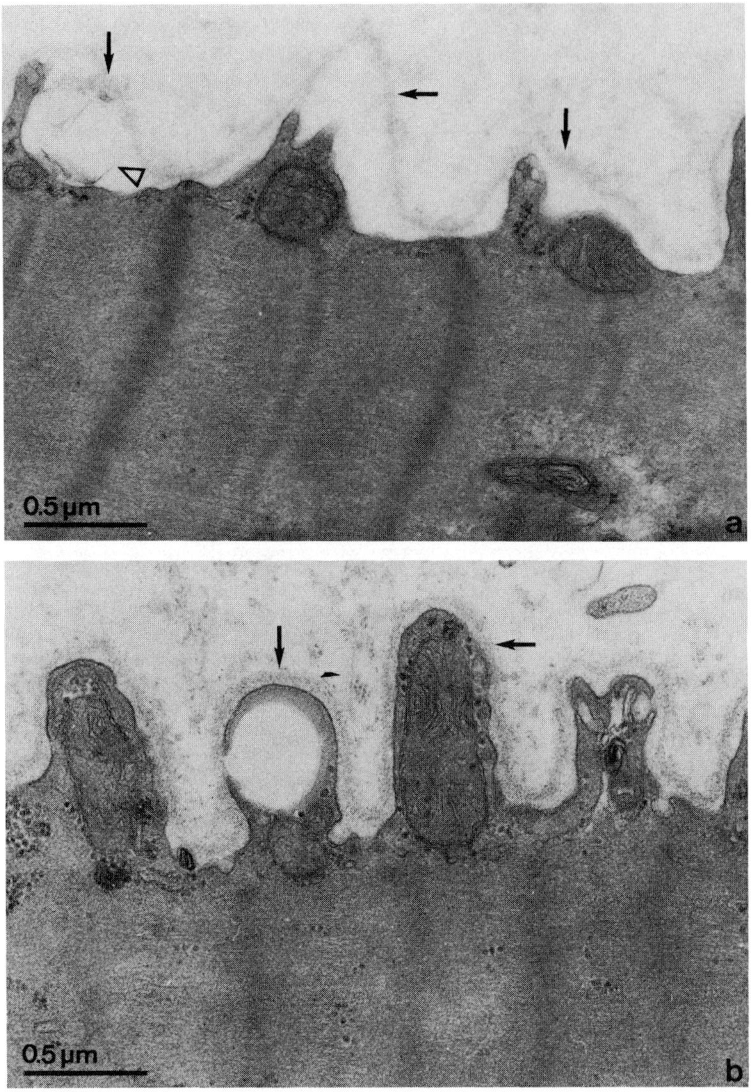

FIGURE 4. Upper panel: subendocardial postoperative biopsy specimen of a patient of group I. The close apposition of the external lamina of the glycocalyx to the sarcolemma is lost and an edematous space is seen. Lower panel: subendocardial postoperative biopsy specimen of a patient of group III, pretreated with lidoflazine 1 mg $\times$ kg^{-1}. The sarcolemma-glycocalyx complex is intact.

TABLE 4. Semiquantitative Assessment of the Ultrastructural Instability of the Sarcolemma-Glycocalyx Complex[a]

	Hypothermia				Hypothermia + Lidoflazine ($1\ mg \times kg^{-1}$)				
	Preop.		Postop.			Preop.		Postop.	
Patients	Epi	Endo	Epi	Endo	Patients	Epi	Endo	Epi	Endo
1	ND	–	–	–	1	–	–	–	–
2	–	++	+++	+++	2	–	–	+	+
3	–	++	++	++++	3	–	–	+	–
4	++	+++	++	++	4	–	–	–	–
5	+++	+++	++	++	5	+	+	–	+
6	++	++	++++	+++	6	–	–	–	–
7	++	++++	++	+++	7	+	+	+	+
8	++	++	+++	+++					

[a]Preop: preoperative biopsy specimen; Postop: postoperative biopsy specimen; these specimens were divided into subepicardial (Epi) and subendocardial (Endo) zone. Scores: ++++: frequent large blebs in all cells; +++: frequent blebs in many cells; ++: small blebs in some cells; +: occasional small blebs in few cells; –: normal close apposition of sarcolemma and glycocalyx; ND: not done.

and postischemic samples of the control group was confined to the sarcolemma-glycocalyx complex. The observed abnormality concerned the loss of close apposition of the lipid bilayer and the external coat (FIGURE 4). Fine membranous (myelinlike) blebs, derived from the lipid bilayer, protruded in the liquid-filled space between these compartments. This instability of the sarcolemma varied both in frequency and severity among the samples, ranging from occasional small interspaces in just a few cells to large edematous spaces in the large majority of cells (see TABLE 4). In the specimens obtained from patients who received $1\ mg \times kg^{-1}$ lidoflazine the sarcolemma-glycocalyx complex was remarkably preserved (see FIGURE 4 and TABLE 4). In this group recovery of hemodynamics after weaning from cardiopulmonary bypass was better than in the other two groups. Left ventricular stroke work index was 85% from the preoperative value ($p > 0.05$) in contrast to the control group (63%, $p < 0.05$ versus preoperatively) and to the low-dose lidoflazine group (62.5%, $p < 0.05$ versus

TABLE 5. Aortocoronary Bypass Surgery

Lidoflazine pretreatment ($1\ mg \times kg^{-1}$) + IXC – 28°C			
1 200 Consecutive patients			
Grafts : range 1 to 10/patient			
E.F. : range 80 to 20%			
Mortality rate			
Cardiac:	infarction	4/1 200	0.33%
	low C.D.	**2/1 200**	**0.17%**
	Causa ignota	2/1 200	0.17%
			0.67%
Noncardiac:		5/1 200	0.42%
Total			1.09%

preoperatively). Clinical outcome in terms of mortality and morbidity was excellent in all three groups: all patients survived and did well.

Encouraged by the results of this study we now use lidoflazine 1.0 mg $\times$ kg^{-1} as a pretreatment routinely in our institution. We reviewed the last 1200 consecutive cases in terms of clinical outcome and obtained excellent results. These results are presented in TABLE 5. Although we are well aware that these results are of little scientific value we feel that they are worthwhile to report. They show that the drug is safe and that an extremely low incidence of postoperative low cardiac output syndrome can be achieved with this technique.

CONCLUSIONS

In summary we conclude that calcium antagonists have the potential to delay irreversible ischemic injury to the myocardium and that they may be protective against ischemic damage provided timely reperfusion is achieved.

The protective properties of these drugs are related to an ATP-sparing effect and a membrane-stabilizing effect. The specificity of these effects will be related to the type of the drug used. Substantial evidence of an improved ischemia tolerance after pretreatment with calcium antagonists in global ischemia followed by reperfusion is provided by experimental and clinical studies. There remains, however, a definite need for well-controlled clinical trials in order to prove the final goal of myocardial protection: prevention of postischemic myocardial dysfunction and reduction of mortality.

REFERENCES

1. HEARSE, D. J. 1984. Critical distinctions in modification of myocardial cell injury. *In* Calcium Antagonists and Cardiovascular Disease. L. H. Opie, Ed.: 129–145. Raven Press. New York, N.Y.
2. YELLON, D. M., D. J. HEARSE, M. P. MAXWELL, D. E. CHAMBERS & J. M. DOWNEY. 1983. Sustained limitation of myocardial necrosis 24 hours after coronary artery occlusion: verapamil infusion in dogs with small myocardial infarcts. Am. J. Cardiol. **51:** 1409–1413.
3. McGOON, D. C. 1985. The ongoing quest for ideal myocardial protection. J. Thorac. Cardiovasc. Surg. **89:** 639–653.
4. ENGELMAN, R. M. & S. LEVITSKY, Eds. 1982. Textbook of Clinical Cardioplegia. Futura Publishing. London, England.
5. FLAMENG, W., M. BORGERS, W. DAENEN, F. THONÉ, W. A. COUMANS, G. J. VAN DER VUSSE & G. STALPAERT. 1981. St.-Thomas cardioplegia versus topical cooling: ultrastructural and biochemical studies in humans. Ann. Thorac. Surg. **31:** 339–346.
6. FLAMENG, W., G. J. VAN DER VUSSE & R. DEMEYERE. 1984. Intermittent aortic crossclamping versus St. Thomas' Hospital cardioplegia in extensive aortocoronary bypass grafting. J. Thorac. Cardiovasc. Surg. **88:** 164–173.
7. BRAASCH, W., S. GUDBJARNASON, P. S. PURI, K. G. RAVENS & R. J. BING. 1986. Early changes in energy metabolism in the myocardium following acute coronary artery occlusion in anesthetized dogs. Circ. Res. **23:** 429–438.
8. JENNINGS, R. B., H. K. HAWKINS, J. E. LOWE, M. L. HELL, S. KLOTMAN & K. A. REIMER. 1978. Relation between high energy phosphate and lethal injury in myocardial ischemia in the dog. Am. J. Pathol. **92:** 187–214.
9. BOURDELLON, P. D. & P. A. POOLE-WILSON. 1982. The effects of verapamil k, quiescence and cardioplegia on calcium exchange and mechanical function in ischemic rabbit myocardium. Circ. Res. **50:** 360–368.

10. NAYLER, W. G. 1982. Protection of the myocardium against posichemic reperfusion damage. The combined effect of hypothermia and nifedipine. J. Thorac. Cardivasc. Surg. **84:** 897–905.
11. HENRY, P. D., R. SHUCHLEIB, L. J. BORDA, R. ROBERTS, J. R. WILLIAMSON & B. E. SOBEL. 1978. Effects of nifedipine on myocardial perfusion and ischemic injury in dogs. Circ. Res. **43:** 372–380.
12. BAKER, J. E. & D. J. HEARSE. 1983. Slow calcium channel blockers and the calcium paradox: comparative studies in the rat with seven drugs. J. Mol. Cell. Cardiol. **15:** 475–485.
13. FLAMENG, W., M. BORGERS, G. J. VAN DER VUSSE, R. DEMEYERE, E. VANDERMEERSCH, F. THONÉ & R. SUY. 1983. Cardioprotective effects of lidoflazine in extensive aortocoronary bypass grafting. J. Thorac. Cardiovasc. Surg. **5:** 758–768.
14. DRAKE-HOLLAND, A. J. 1982. Biochemical features of myocardial ischemia. *In* Protection of tissues against hypoxia. A. Wauquier, Ed.: 87–94. Elsevier Biomedical Press. Amsterdam, Holland.
15. FLAMENG, W., W. DAENEN, M. BORGERS, F. THONÉ, R. XHONNEUX, A. VAN DE WATER & H. VAN BELLE. 1981. Cardio protective effects of lidoflazine during 1 hour normothermic global ischemia. Circulation **64:** 796–807.
16. CLARK, R. E., T. B. FERGUSON & J. P. MARBARGER. 1981. The first American clinical trial of nifedipine in cardioplegia. J. Thorac. Cardiovasc. Surg. **82:** 848–859.
17. FLAMENG, W., R. DEMEYERE, W. DAENEN, P. SERGEANT, V. NGALIKPIMA, J. GEBOERS, R. SUY & G. STALPAERT. 1986. Nifedipine as an adjunct to St. Thomas' Hospital Cardioplegia. A double blind placebo controlled randomized clinical trial. J. Thorac. Cardiovasc. Surg. **91:** 723–731.

Clinical Use of Calcium Antagonists in Peripheral Circulatory Disease

J. DORMANDY

Department of Vascular Surgery
St. James' and St. George's Hospitals
Sarsfeld Road, Balham
London SW12 8HW, England

THERAPY OF PERIPHERAL CIRCULATORY DISEASES

The therapy of peripheral ischemia, whether surgical or nonsurgical, is much less satisfactory than that of myocardial ischemia. So far no class of drugs has gained general acceptance as a significant and major contribution to the treatment of either the symptoms or the underlying pathology of common peripheral ischemic diseases. Yet the need for this is enormous.

FIGURE 1 is a simplified schematic representation of the possible approaches to improving blood flow along a narrowed peripheral artery. Rejecting the option of increasing the inflow pressure by raising the central arterial blood pressure, the two remaining alternatives illustrated are aimed at either increasing the caliber of the artery or improving the fluidity of the blood. The former may be achieved by preventing further atheroma or thrombus, dissolution of existing atheroma or thrombus, overcoming muscle spasm, or inducing selective dilatation. In addition, improving collateral flow and improving the efficiency of ischemic skeletal muscle metabolism are two further possibilities.

Calcium antagonists may theoretically produce a clinical improvement by acting through any of these approaches. The extent to which this class of drugs has so far been shown to be of actual benefit to patients will be considered in relation to two of the commonest manifestations of limb ischemia: intermittent claudication of the legs and Raynaud's phenomenon of the hands, diseases that have a totally different pathophysiology. Virtually all clinical evidence relating to calcium antagonists and circulation has been obtained with four drugs representing four slightly different mechanisms and specificity of action: nifedipine, flunarazine, verapamil, and diltiazem. This contribution will concentrate on an analysis of the currently available clinical evidence concerning the use of these medications in ischemia of the arms and legs.

POSSIBLE MECHANISMS OF ACTION OF CALCIUM ANTAGONISTS IN PERIPHERAL ISCHEMIA

Relaxation of Vascular Smooth Muscle

All calcium antagonists have been shown to inhibit potential-operated and receptor channels of arterial smooth muscle contraction. Calcium antagonists of the verapamil, nifedipine, and diltiazem, but not flunarazine, families have also been shown to inhibit myogenic activity in vascular smooth muscle.

It had been widely believed that general systemic vasodilators are of no benefit in patients with leg ischemia due to atherosclerosis. This view probably now needs to be slightly modified, particularly in relation to calcium antagonists. Recent experimental evidence has shown that in the presence of damaged endothelium, the increased release of serotonin and thromboxane A_2 from platelets can cause significant vasospasm. This questions the widely held belief that in ischemic tissues there is already maximal vasodilation and that a systemically acting vasodilator will only affect vessels in the normal nonischemic tissues.

Other pharmacological evidence suggests that local hypoxia may in fact alter the responsiveness of vessels preventing vasodilatation. Furthermore calcium antagonists may have a partially selective action on the vessels in ischemic areas. It has been

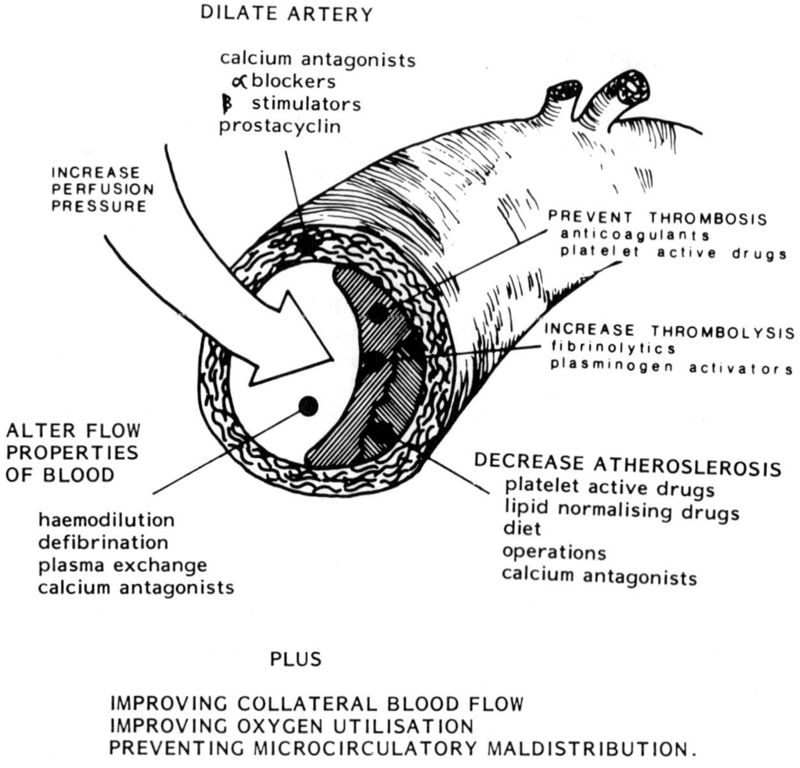

FIGURE 1. Possible therapeutic approaches to peripheral ischemia.

suggested that flunarazinelike calcium antagonists, unlike other types, have a specific vasodilator effect in ischemic regions with little generalized vasodilation of the normal vasculature. The vasodilator effect of calcium antagonists may therefore be useful in the treatment of leg ischemia due to atherosclerosis if this effect is specific to ischemic tissues, by overcoming a locally induced spasm or by dilating collaterals.

The role of arterial spasm in Raynaud's phenomenon is undisputed, although it may not be present in all cases and is not necessarily always the major pathophysiological mechanism in secondary Raynaud's. Whatever the exact trigger mechanism for such spasm, calcium antagonists should be effective in preventing or abolishing it to a large extent. The vascular smooth muscle relaxing property of calcium antagonists will therefore be particularly useful in the management of Raynaud's, where primary atherosclerosis of the arteries plays little or no part.

Antiplatelet Effect

Most platelet reactions are associated with an increase in free cytoplasmic calcium, and an increased membrane permeability to calcium. Several calcium antagonists have been shown to inhibit platelet functional changes both *in vitro* and in patients with abnormal platelet function. Both in acute ischemia, whether from thrombosis or arterial spasm, and in chronic ischemia due to atherosclerosis the possible role of activated platelets is widely accepted. Inhibition of platelet reaction by calcium antagonists may therefore be beneficial in preventing the acute ischemia of a Raynaud's attack or the progression and consequences of chronic leg ischemia.

Impaired Blood Rheology

It is becoming increasingly recognized that reduced blood flow and ischemia are not necessarily solely related to a reduction in vessel lumen, but that deterioration in the physical flow properties of the blood can also result in poor flow. Ischemia of the legs, as well as acute or chronic ischemia in other regions, is associated with decreased red cell deformability as measured by blood filtration techniques. This is partly a secondary phenomenon, with the blood passing through the ischemic region being particularly affected. The local hypoxia decreases ATP concentration, impairing the calcium pump of the blood cells and making them more rigid. The increased blood cell rigidity in turn causes further local ischemia by plugging of the microcirculation and causing maldistribution of capillary flow. Increased red cell rigidity is also an important cause of raised whole blood viscosity, which will decrease flow in the larger vessels supplying the ischemic region. This local viscous vicious cycle may be beneficially affected by the protective effect of calcium antagonists against the rigidity induced by high intracellular red cell calcium concentration. All the major types of calcium antagonists have been shown to improve red cell filterability. Calcium is thought to modify red cell rheology by an action on both the internal cytoplasmic viscosity and the viscoelastic properties of the membrane. The latter is probably by an action on spectrin phosphorylation. Conversely there is also evidence that the rheological properties of the red cell itself may influence the permeability of its membrane to calcium. A hemorheological mechanism is equally likely to be beneficial in the chronic ischemia of atherosclerotic disease affecting the legs and the acute intermittent ischemia of Raynaud's phenomenon.

In the last very few years the role of the white cells in microcirculatory ischemia is becoming recognized, particularly in situations of low perfusion pressure where in experimental models plugging of capillaries by white cells seems to play a crucial role. So far the role of calcium and calcium antagonists in white cell rheology has not been studied, but is likely to be an interesting line of new research.

Protective Effect against Damage from Calcium Overload in Vessel Wall

Part of the cytotoxic protective effect of calcium antagonists may be dampening of the atherogenic process in arterial walls. Existing evidence does not suggest that any particular type of calcium antagonist is more effective than any other in this action. Damage to the endothelial cells and the smooth muscle cells of the arterial wall is a central feature of all theories of atherogenesis and a common end point for the action of the many known risk factors for the development and progression of atherosclerosis. The general cellular protective action of calcium antagonists may therefore slow down the narrowing of the arteries that is the predominant underlying process in peripheral ischemia of the legs.

The experimental evidence in favor of and against these various possible mechanisms of action is extensively analyzed in other parts of this volume.

Most of the experimental evidence relates to protection of normal animal vessel walls against damage by risk factors like hypertension, alloxan diabetes, nicotine, or raised cholesterol diet. Calcium antagonists decrease endothelial desquamation and reduce production of growth factor, both tending to militate against atherogenesis. Calcium antagonists have rarely been looked at in the context of preventing progression of damage once it has occurred, which is the more real clinical situation. This review is primarily concerned with the clinical evidence as to whether currently available calcium antagonists do or do not significantly benefit patients with peripheral circulatory disease, in particular Raynaud's phenomenon and ischemia of the leg due to atherosclerosis. It is based on a review of all published trials that were placebo controlled and double blind.

CLINICAL USE OF CALCIUM ANTAGONISTS IN RAYNAUD'S PHENOMENON

The characteristic episodic nature of Raynaud's phenomenon in which virtually total ischemia of a finger may develop in less than a minute makes the mechanism of vascular contraction, or spasm, particularly likely and the use of a powerful vascular smooth muscle dilator particularly attractive. Indeed it is in the treatment of Raynaud's phenomenon that calcium antagonists have had their greatest successes.

To analyze critically published trials, it is important to appreciate the problems involved in the clinical assessment of a treatment of Raynaud's phenomenon:

1. The etiology is either unknown (primary Raynaud or Raynaud's disease) or it may be secondary to an almost endless list of diseases ranging from scleroderma, which is the commonest, to lupus, cervical ribs, rheumatoid disease, and myelomatosis. Moreover many cases of so-called primary Raynaud's subsequently turn out to be secondary to a connective tissue disease which was originally subclinical.
2. Between attacks most patients with Raynaud's are free of any abnormal symptoms or detectable clinical signs.
3. The frequency of attacks is extremely variable and may be provoked by a variety of changing stimuli.
4. There is no technique available for reliably reproducing an attack in the laboratory.
5. There is no generally accepted technique of measurement for quantifying the severity of the disease in the laboratory.
6. The use of daily diary cards by patients to record the frequency and severity of their attacks is inevitably difficult, although in the present circumstances it is this type of subjective record that is probably still the most reliable and relevant in the evaluation of a new therapy.

TABLE 1 summarizes 19 clinical trials of calcium antagonists used for Raynaud's phenomenon published during the past six years.[1–18] Apart from two studies using diltiazem[1,5] and one using verapamil,[3] all the rest investigated nifedipine. The vast majority were of a crossover design with a relatively short treatment period of one month. The dose of nifedipine was usually 60 mg per day (range 30 mg–80 mg). All the studies were primarily looking at subjective changes, which is not unreasonable when looking at a disease that is difficult to quantify objectively, provided always that the results were placebo controlled and double blind. However it could be argued that in view of the frequent minor side effects of a vasodilator like nifedipine, the investigators could not have been truly unaware of the treatment. Nevertheless the fact that in all but 1 of 16 placebo-controlled trials,[6] involving altogether about 300 patients, nifedipine was always significantly better than placebo in subjective terms suggests that this is a genuinely worthwhile treatment. Overall nifedipine decreased the frequency and severity of the attacks in 60% to 90% of patients treated. In 11 studies, both primary and secondary Raynaud patients were included and usually the response of the former was noted to be better. In primary Raynaud's in particular, where the natural history of the disease is benign, the aim of treatment is justifiably purely symptomatic. The fact that in only two studies[10,18] objective measurements supported the subjective findings is more a reflection on the problem of assessing Raynaud's phenomenon quantitatively than the efficacy of calcium antagonists. In two studies dasoxiben[12,19] and in one study prazosin[11] were also compared to nifedipine and shown to be no better than the placebo.

There is however no doubt that nifedipine does produce side effects, which are usually minor, such as flushing or headaches. Sometimes however patients have to abandon treatment. One of the most recent and best documented trials of Nifedipine (34 patients given 40 mg daily) reported side effects in 26 patients on active medication and 5 patients on placebo. Five of the patients receiving nifedipine had to be withdrawn.

CLINICAL USE OF CALCIUM ANTAGONISTS IN LEG ISCHEMIA

In every way ischemia of the leg is a bigger problem than Raynaud's. About 1% of all the male population below 40, rising to over 5% after the age of 50, will develop some symptoms of leg ischemia. The incidence of atherosclerotic disease in the arteries supplying the legs is even higher, but some of it is asymptomatic. The vast majority of cases will present as intermittent claudication, and it is in this group that calcium antagonists have been widely studied. Less than 10% of claudicants will progress to develop rest pain or pregangrene and at that stage long-term medication is inappropriate. Medication, that may have long-term beneficial effects on the underlying disease process may be particularly appropriate to investigate because patients presenting with claudication are at a very high risk of developing serious cardiovascular complications in other territories. Compared to the general population of comparable age the mortality of claudicators is two to three times higher after five years. Furthermore the incidence of nonfatal myocardial infarction or stroke is approximately 5% per year.

The problems of assessing a medical therapy in intermittent claudication are as severe as those involved in studying Raynaud's:

1. Intermittent claudication is the result of decades of progressive arterial disease, and it is possibly difficult to make a detectable impression on it over a period of months.

TABLE 1. Calcium Antagonists Used in the Treatment of Raynaud's Phenomenon

	Parallel (P) or Crossover (C)	Number of Patients	Primary (1°) or Secondary (2°)	Drug[a]	Dosage (mg) Daily	Duration (month)	Result of Measurements[b]	Subjective Result[b]
Vayssairat *et al.*,[1] 1981	P	26	1°2°	D	180	½	Neg.	Sig.
Kahan *et al.*,[2] 1982	C	30	1°2°	N	60	1		Sig.
Kinney *et al.*,[3] 1982	C	16	1°2°	V	160–320	3	Neg.	Sig.
Smith *et al.*,[4] 1982	C	17	1°2°	N	40	1	Neg.	Sig.
Kahan *et al.*,[5] 1983	C	16	1°2°	D		1		Neg.
Ettinger *et al.*,[6] 1984	C	22	1°2°	N	70	1	Neg.	Neg.
Rodehefer *et al.*,[7] 1983	C	15	1°	N	30–60	1	Neg.	Sig.
Winston *et al.*,[8] 1983	C	8	1°2°	N	40–80	1		Sig.
Sauza *et al.*,[9] 1984	P	18	1°2°	N	30–60	2½		Sig.
Finch *et al.*,[10] 1985	C	16	1°2°	N	60	½	Sig.	Sig.
Kahan *et al.*,[11] 1985	C	15	1°2°	N	60	½		Sig.
Malamet *et al.*,[12] 1985	C	7	1°2°	N				Sig.
Aldoori *et al.*,[13] 1986	C	13	1°2°	N	30	1	Neg.	Sig.
Corbin *et al.*,[14] 1986	C	23	1°	N	40–80	1		Sig.
					15–45	1	Neg.	Sig.
Gjorup *et al.*,[15] 1986	C	26	1°2°	N	40–80	½		Sig.
Sarkozi *et al.*,[16] 1986	P	39	1°	N	30	2½		Sig.
Waller *et al.*,[17] 1986	C	29	1°2°	N	40	2		Sig.
White *et al.*,[18] 1986	C	11	1°2°	N	60	½	Sig.	Sig.
	C	26	1°	N	40–80	1		Sig.

[a]D is diltiazem, N is nifedipine, and V is verapamil.
[b]Neg. is negative and Sig. is significant.

2. Quite exceptionally dramatic placebo effect.
3. Although there are many noninvasive technqiues for measuring leg blood flow or other variables closely related to blood flow, there is no methodology for measuring it during claudication, which is when measurements would be most relevant.

It is increasingly believed that measurement of actual claudication distance is the most relevant in assessing the efficency of a new treatment. We appear to have gone a full circle, developing increasingly subtle and ingenious techniques for trying to quantify intermittent claudication, only to have come back to simply asking the patient to say when they feel the pain while walking on the treadmill.

TABLE 2 summarizes 14 published clinical trials of calcium antagonists in the treatment of intermittent claudication. All the studies looked at flunarazine-type calcium antagonists and all but three of these showed a statistically significant benefit of active treatment compared to placebo. Only double-blind, placebo-controlled studies are quoted, and benefit was assessed in terms of pain-free walking distance. As this is the complaint of the patient, and as in the majority of cases ischemia of the legs will not progress beyong the stage of claudication, it seems the most reasonable way of assessing the efficiency of a trial medication.

There were 10 parallel groups and 5 crossover studies, the majority lasting three months and only 1 study[23] for longer than four months. The dosage of cinnarazine varied from 75 mg to 225 mg per day and of flunarazine from 10 mg to 20 mg per day. It is perhaps unfortunate that none of these studies looked at the long-term effects of treatment in a group of patients, such as claudicants, who have chronic progressive disease that is incurable. It is not possible to say at the moment whether treatment with calcium antagonists alters the amputation rate or affects the high incidence of myocardial and cerebral ischemic events in intermittent claudicants.

Altogether just over 500 patients were studied and usually the improvement in pain-free walking distance was at least twice that of the placebo group. In one study flunarazine was compared to pentoxifylline and found to be more effective.[29] By contrast to the Raynaud's studies, objective measurements of physiological variables related to ischemia of the legs usually gave significant positive results. Side effects of the active medication were not a serious problem.

CONCLUSION

The published literature on placebo-controlled double-blind trials of calcium antagonists in peripheral circulatory disease provides considerable evidence that nifedipine significantly decreases the frequency and severity of Raynaud's attacks, and that flunarazinelike drugs significantly increase the pain-free walking distance of claudicants. (There is very little evidence about the use of verapamil and diltiazemlike drugs in the periphery). There are only two serious caveats about these conclusions: firstly, that the results of negative studies may not have been published and therefore cannot be taken into account in evaluating the proper impact of positive trials; and secondly, that most of the studies involved relatively small numbers of patients treated for a short time. On the other hand, in evaluating the proper level of clinical use of calcium antagonists for either Raynaud's phenomenon or intermittent claudication, it is appropriate to take into account alternative options. By contrast to hypertension or myocardial ischemia, there is no other class of drugs that has gained universal and overwhelming acceptance for the treatment of Raynaud's or claudication. The

TABLE 2. Calcium Antagonists in the Treatment of Intermittent Claudication

	Parallel (P) or Crossover (C)	Number of Patients	Drug	Dosage (mg) Daily	Duration of Treatment (months)	Difference in Walking Distance
Adriensen,[19] 1969	C	18	C	150	2	Sig.
Schuermans,[20] 1971	P	23	C	225	3	Sig.
Verhaegen *et al.*,[21] 1974	C	12	F	25	½	Sig.
			C	75		
Staessen,[22] 1977	P	38	F	10	4	Sig.
			C	200		
Schetz *et al.*,[23] 1978	P	56	F	10	12	Sig.
Donald,[24] 1979	C	40	C	225	3	Sig.
Rudofsky,[25] 1979	P	40	F	20	1½	NS
Barber *et al.*,[26] 1980	P	46	C	225	3	Sig.
Loots *et al.*,[27] 1980	P	16	F	20	3	Sig.
Di Perri,[28] 1984	P	36	F	10	1½	Sig.
Perhoniemi,[29] 1984	C	31	F	15	3	Sig.
Balsano,[30] 1985	P	90	F	10	2	Sig.
Catalono *et al.*,[31] 1985	P	40	F	10	2	NS
Lepantalo *et al.*,[32] 1985	C	12	F	10	3	NS

evidence reviewed above may therefore suggest that the use of the two calcium antagonists considered could be advocated as reasonable general medical practice.

The mechanisms whereby nifedipine and flunarazine exert their beneficial effect are most likely to be a relaxation of vascular smooth muscle and a protective effect against the adverse hemorheological changes associated with acute or chronic ischemia. The possible protective effect against progression of atherosclerosis cannot be assessed in trials lasting one to three months. Further large-scale studies would be necessary to answer any of these questions.

REFERENCES

1. Vayssairat, M., L. Capron, J-N. Fiessinger, J-F. Mathieu & E. Housset. 1981. Calcium channel blockers and Raynaud's disease. Ann. Intern. Med. **95:** 243.
2. Kahan, A., S. Webber, B. Amor, L. Saporta, M. Hodara & M. Degeorges. 1982. Etude controlee de la nifedipine dans le traitment du phenomene de Raynaud. Rev. Rhum. Mal. Osteoarticulaires **49:** 337–343.
3. Kinney, E. L., G. G. Nicholas, J. Gallo, C. Pontoriero & R. Zelis. 1982. The treatment of severe Raynaud's phenomenon with verapamil. J. Clin. Pharmacol. **22:** 74–76.
4. Smith, C. D., R. J. R. McKendry. 1982. Controlled trial of nifedipine in the treatment of Raynaud's phenomenon. Lancet: 1299–1201.
5. Kahan, A., S. Weber, B. Amor, C. J. Menkes, L. Saporta, M. Hordara, F. Guerin & M. Degeorges. 1983. Calcium entry blocking agents in digital vasospasm (Raynaud's phenomenon). Eur. Heart J. **4:** 123–129.
6. Ettinger, W. H., R. A. Wise, D. Schaffhauser & F. M. Wigley. 1984. Controlled double-blinded trial of dazoxiben and nifedipine in the treatment of Raynaud's phenomenon. Am. J. Med. **77:** 451–456.
7. Rodeheffer, R. J., J. A. Rommer, F. Wigley & C. R. Smith. 1983. Controlled double-blind trial of nifedipine in the treatment of Raynaud's phenomenon. N. Engl. J. Med. **308:** 880–883.
8. Winston, E. L., K. M. Pariser, K. B. Miller, D. N. Salem & M. A. Creager. 1983. Nifdipine as a therapeutic modality for Raynaud's phenomenon. J. Arthritis Rheum. **26:** 1177–1180.
9. Sauza, J., A. Kraus, R. Gonzalez-Amaro & D. Alarcon-Segovia. 1984. Effect of the calcium channel blocker nifedipine on Raynaud's phenomenon. A controlled double-blind trial. J. Rheumatol. **11:**(3): 362–364.
10. Finch, M. B., G. D. Johnston & J. Dawson. 1985. The peripheral vascular effects of nifedipine in Raynaud's disease. Br. J. Clin. Pharmacol. **21**(1): 100P–101P.
11. Kahan, A., J. M. Foult, S. Weber, B. Amor, C. J. Menkes & M. Degeorges. 1985. Nifedipine and alpha$_1$-adrenergic blockade in Raynaud's phenomenon. Eur. Heart J. **6:** 702–705.
12. Malamet, R., R. A. Wise, W. H. Egginger & F. M. Wigley. 1985. Nifedipine in the treatment of Raynaud's phenomenon. Am. J. Med. **78:** 602–608.
13. Aldoori, M., W. B. Campbell & P. A. Dieppe. 1986. Nifedipine in the treatment of Raynaud's syndrome. Cardiovasc. Res. **20:** 466–470.
14. Dorbin, D. O. C., D. A. Wood, C. C. A. Macintyre & E. Housley. 1988. A randomized double blind cross-over trial of nifedipine in the treatment of primary Raynaud's phenomenon. Eur. Heart J. **7:** 165–170.
15. Gjorup, T., H. Kelbaek, O. J. Hartling & S. L. Nielsen. 1986. Controlled double-blind trial of the clinical effect of nifedipine in the treatment of idiopathic Raynaud's phenomenon. Am. Heart J. **111:** 742–745.
16. Sarkozi, J., A. A. M. Bookman, W. Mahon, C. Ramsay, A. S. Detsky & E. C. Keystone. 1986. Nifedipine in the treatment of idiopathic Raynaud's syndrome. J. Rheumatol **13**(2): 331–336.
17. Waller, D. G., V. F. Challenor, D. A. Francis & O. S. Roath. 1986. Clinical and

rheological effects of nifedipine in Raynaud's phenomenon. Br. J. Clin. Pharmacol. **22:** 449–454.
18. White C. J., W. A. Phillips, L. A. Abrahams, T. D. Watson & P. T. Singleton. 1986. Objective benefit of nifedipine in the treatment of Raynaud's phenomenon. Am. J. Med. **80:** 623–625.
19. Adriaensen, H. 1969. The treatment of intermittent claudication. Clin. Trials J. 191–193.
20. Schuermans, V., A. Boermans, H. Geivers, A. Jageneau & J. Brugmans. 1971. Cinnarizine in peripheral vascular insufficiency. Drug Res. **21:** 1541–1543.
21. Verhaegen, H., V. Roels, H. Adriaensen, J. Brugmans, W. De Cock, J. Dony, A. Jageneau & V. Schuermans. 1974. The arteriolar effects of cinnarizine and flunarizine. Angiology **25:** 261–278.
22. Staessen, A. J. 1977. Treatment of circulatory disturbances with flunarizine and cinnarizine. VASA **6:** 59–71.
23. Schetz, J., H. Bostoen, D. Clement, M. Fornhoff, A. Haerens, P. Roekaerts & A. J. Staessen. 1978. Flunerizine in chronic obstructive peripheral arterial disease: a placebo-controlled, double-blind, randomized multicentre trial. Curr. Ther. Res. **23:** 121–130.
24. Donald, J. F. 1979. A multicentre general practice study of Cinnarizine in the treatment of peripheral vascular disease. J. Int. Med. Res. **7:** 502–506.
25. Rudofsky, G., F. E. Brock, M. Ulrich & F. Noble. 1979. Clinical evaluation of flunarizine; walking distance, ergometric performance and haemodynamic and biochemical effects. Angiology **30:** 470–479.
26. Barber, J. H., C. A. Reuter, A. H. M. Jageneau & W. Loots. 1980. Intermittent claudication: a controlled study in parallel time of the short-term and long-term term effects of cinnarizine. Pharmatherapeutica **2:** 401–407.
27. Loots, W., J. Dom & C. Horig. 1980. Intermittent claudication—attempts to make this disease objective on account of the results of treatment obtainable by means of sibelium. Med. Welt **31:** 189–192.
28. Di Perri, T., F. Laghi Pasini & M. Guerrini. 1984. Calcium entry blockers in the treatment of peripheral obliterative arterial disease. *In* Calcium Entry Blockers in Cardiovascular and Cerebral Dysfunction. T. Godfraind, A. Herman & D. Wellens, Eds.: 103–110. Martinus Nighoff. The Hague, Holland.
29. Perhoniemi, V., K. Salmenkivi, S. Sundber, R. Johnsson, & A. Gordin. 1984. Effects of flunarizine and pentoxifylline on walking distance and blood rheology in claudication. Angiology **35:** 366–372.
30. Balsano, F. 1985. Chronic treatment of "claudication." *In* Calcium Entry Blockers and Tissue Protection. T. Godfraind, P. Vanhoutte, S. Giovoni & R. Paoletti, Eds.: 215–220. Raven Press. New York, N.Y.
31. Catalano M., A. Aronica, S. Belletti, E. Sacchi, M. Tommasini & A. Libretti. 1985. Flunarizine in the treatment of peripheral vascular disease. Intern. Angiol. **4:** 73–74.
32. Lepantalo, M., S. Sundberg & A. Gordin. 1985. Lack of effect of flunarizine in intermittent claudication. Intern. Angiol. **4:** 75–76.

Influence of Verapamil on the Body Sodium/Fluid Volume State and Noradrenergic-Dependent Blood Pressure Regulation in Patients with Essential Hypertension

C. BERETTA-PICCOLI, C. MARONE, P. STÄDLER, W. H. ZIEGLER, W. RIESEN, AND C. PUSTERLA

Division of Medicine
Internal Medicine and Nephrology
Italian Hospital of Lugano
CH-6962 Viganello, Switzerland

Calcium antagonists can modify the body sodium fluid volume state[1] and the cardiovascular pressor reactivity to norepinephrine without changing the endogenous adrenergic activity.[2,3] The effects of verapamil on these parameters were assessed in 15 patients with benign essential hypertension, aged 23 to 70 years; after a three week placebo phase, the calcium antagonist was administered during eight weeks at a daily dose of 240–480 mg. As compared with the placebo phase, verapamil caused a significant decrease of arterial pressure without modifying heart rate, body weight, exchangeable body sodium, and blood volume (TABLE 1). The activity of the

TABLE 1. Effects of Verapamil in Patients with Essential Hypertension

	Placebo[a]	Verapamil[a]
Blood pressure (mm Hg)	153/103 ± 19/12	140/95 ± 14/12[b]
Heart rate (bpm)	63 ± 8	62 ± 9
Body weight (kg)	79.4 ± 13.1	79.4 ± 12.4
Exchangeable sodium (mmol)	3148 ± 481	3081 ± 479
Blood volume (ml)	3871 ± 718	3942 ± 785
Plasma renin activity (ng/ml × hours)	3.3 ± 0.6	3.2 ± 0.9
Plasma aldosterone (ng/dl)	12.4 ± 4.7	12.4 ± 3.5
Plasma norepinephrine (ng/dl)	44.2 ± 12.9	37.3 ± 8.7
Norepinephrine pressor dose (ng/kg × minutes)	110 ± 65	203 ± 153

[a]Mean ± standard deviation.
[b]$p < 0.01$ versus placebo.

renin-angiotensin-aldosterone system, as judged by the plasma renin activity and plasma aldosterone concentration, as well as the sympathetic activity, as judged by the plasma norepinephrine concentration, did not change after verapamil (TABLE 1). However, the cardiovascular pressor reactivity, as assessed during an intravenous norepinephrine infusion, tended to be decreased; this was suggested by the 100% increase in mean norepinephrine pressor dose (the norepinephrine dose rate required to elevate mean arterial pressure by 20 mm Hg) (TABLE 1) and by the significant shift to the right of the dose response curve relating arterial pressure to plasma norepinephrine ($F = 5.09$; $p < 0.05$). Finally, verapamil did not modify total serum cholesterol or triglycerides as well as their lipoprotein fractions and apolipoprotein A1, A2, and B levels.

These findings suggest that verapamil given during eight weeks induces a significant fall of arterial pressure in patients with essential hypertension without causing sodium fluid volume retention or modifying the atherogenic lipid fractions. The hypotensive effect is associated with decreased cardiovascular pressor reactivity to norepinephrine without changes in endogenous sympathetic activity.

REFERENCES

1. Marone, C., S. Luisoli, F. Bomio, C. Beretta-Piccoli, M. G. Bianchetti & P. Weidmann. 1985. Body sodium–blood volume state, aldosterone, and cardiovascular responsiveness after calcium entry blockade with nifedipine. Kidney Int. **28:** 658–665.
2. Schwietzer, G., A. Distler, S. Reeck, H. M. Thiede & T. Philipp. 1983. Hypotensive action of calcium antagonists as related to plasma noradrenaline and reactivity to noradrenaline. J. Hypertension **1**(Suppl. 2): 102–104.
3. Bianchetti, M. G., C. Beretta-Piccoli, P. Weidmann, L. Link, K. Boehringen, C. Ferrier & J. J. Morton. 1983. Calcium and blood pressure regulation in normal and hypertensive subjects. Hypertension **5**(Suppl. 2): 57–65.

Acute Effects of Felodipine on Regional Blood Flow in Chronic Heart Failure

G. BINETTI, R. SPADONI, I. RUBINO, E. VARANI,
R. M. FERRETTI, S. PANCALDI, V. CERVI,
AND B. MAGNANI

Institute of Cardiology
University of Bologna
S. Orsola Polyclinic
Via Massarenti, 9
Bologna 40138, Italy

INTRODUCTION

Felodipine (F) is a new calcium antagonist agent with predominant action on vascular smooth muscle. Its efficacy in chronic heart failure has been demonstrated in previous studies.[1–3] The aim of the present work was to assess the acute hemodynamic effect of F on regional blood flow in patients with moderate to severe heart failure.

MATERIALS AND METHODS

Our study group consisted of 8 males (age 44–70, mean 55) with idiopathic (6 patients) or ischemic (2 patients) dilated cardiomyopathy in congestive heart failure (New York Heart Association III–IV). They were on chronic digitalis and diuretic therapy. All the patients underwent hemodynamic monitoring with a Swan-Ganz catheter. The following parameters were measured under basal conditions (B) and during F infusion (0.015 mg/minute bolus; 0.0075 mg/minute infusion): heart rate (HR), mean blood pressure (MBP, arm cuff), pulmonary wedge pressure (PW), cardiac index (CI, thermodilution method), muscular blood flow (MBF, strain gauge plethysmography), renal blood flow (RBF, paraaminohippuric acid clearance), and hepatic blood flow (HBF, Cardiogreen clearance). Systemic vascular resistance (SVR) and sodium clearance (C_{Na}) were also calculated.

RESULTS

The use of F induced a statistically significant increase of CI and MBF. On the other hand MBP, PW, and SVR were significantly reduced. HR and RBF were not affected. Although C_{Na} and HBF tended to increase, the changes did not reach statistical significance. The figures are presented in TABLE 1.

CONCLUSIONS

The results of this study indicate that in patients with chronic congestive heart failure (CHF), F has been able to induce an increase of cardiac output which at rest

TABLE 1. Results of Acute Intravenous Administration of Felodipine[a]

	B	F
HR (b/minute)	74.7 ± 9.07	77.8 ± 9.6[b]
MBP (mmHg)	93.8 ± 9.12	84 ± 14.12[c]
PW (mmHg)	16 ± 11.17	11.9 ± 9.73[d]
CI (1/minute × m^2)	1.98 ± 0.58	3.01 ± 0.91[d]
SVR (units)	28.5 ± 7.94	15.9 ± 4.91[d]
MBF (ml/minute × 100 g)	3.59 ± 1.63	6.23 ± 2.49[c]
HBF (mg/100 ml)	447 ± 180	512 ± 187[b]
RBF (ml/minute)	545 ± 317	566 ± 347[b]
C_{Na} (ml/minute)	1.84 ± 1.55	3.04 ± 2.83[b]

[a]For abbreviations see text. Means ± standard deviation.
[b]Not significant.
[c]$p < 0.05$.
[d]$p < 0.01$.

appears to be mainly distributed to the muscular vascular bed. Its failure to increase RBF is offset by an increased C_{Na}, probably secondary to a direct tubular mechanism[4] shared by other calcium antagonists.[5] As a consequence, the absence of sodium volume retention together with the decrease in afterload makes F a particularly beneficial agent in the treatment of CHF.

REFERENCES

1. TIMMIS, A. D., *et al.* 1984. Acute hemodynamic and metabolic effects of Felodipine in congestive heart failure. Br. Heart J. **51:** 445–451.
2. TIMMIS, A. D., *et al.* 1984. Effects of vasodilator treatment with Felodipine on hemodynamic responses to treadmill exercise in congestive heart failure. Br. Heart J. **52:** 314–320.
3. BINETTI, G., *et al.* 1987. Hemodynamic effects of Felodipine in congestive heart failure. Cardiovasc. Drug Ther. **1:** 161–167.
4. LEONETTI, G., *et al.* 1985. Antihypertensive and water and sodium balance effects of Felodipine, a new vasodilating calcium antagonist in hypertensive patients. Drugs (Suppl. 2): 185–191.
5. ENE, M. B., *et al.* 1984. Natriuretic effects of nifedipine and nitrendipine. Br. J. Clin. Pharmacol. **17:** 193.

Predictive Factors of the Acute and Chronic Blood Pressure Fall Induced by the Calcium Antagonist Nicardipine

GILLES CHATELLIER, PASCAL CLUZEL, MARC BELLET,
JOSEPH RIVALAN, PIERRE CORVOL,
AND JOËL MENARD

Arterial Hypertension Service
Broussais Hospital
Rue Didot, 96
75674 Paris Cédex 14, France

The blood pressure effect of nicardipine (N), a water-soluble dihydropyridine derivative, was studied in 87 patients (63 males) with mild to moderate uncomplicated hypertension, aged from 25 to 77 years (mean 48). Eight patients were black. A total cumulative dose of 8.75 mg of N was administered in 30 minutes by a continuous intravenous infusion. The dose administered was doubled every 10 minutes from 1.25 mg to 5 mg. Mean blood pressure (MBP) and heart rate (HR) were recorded every 2 minutes with a semiautomatic oscillometric recorder. Active renin was measured by a direct immunoradiometric assay.[1] The MBP decrease and the HR increase were both

TABLE 1. Effects of Intravenous Nicardipine on Blood Pressure, Heart Rate, and Renin Secretion[a]

		Nicardipine Infusion			
	Control	10 Minutes	20 Minutes	30 Minutes	ANOVA
Mean blood pressure (mmHg)	110.4 (12)	103.5 (11)	95.6 (10)	89.1 (9)	$p < 0.001$
Mean blood pressure changes (% of control values)	—	−6.1 (5)	−13.2 (6)	−21.3 (10)	
Heart rate (b/minute)	67.6 (10)	72.0 (11)	80.8 (13)	86.4 (14)	$p < 0.001$
Heart rate changes (% of control values)	—	+5.2 (4)	+13.2 (6)	+18.8 (8)	
Active renin (pg/ml)	20.6 (15)	22.2 (16)	27.9 (25)	41.4 (42)	$p < 0.001$
Active renin changes (% of control values)	—	+5.2 (4)	+13.2 (6)	+18.8 (8)	

[a]Data are expressed as means (one standard deviation).

dose related (TABLE 1). At the 30th minute, we observed an 18.9% MBP fall and a 28.0% HR increase by comparison to baseline values ($p < 0.001$). A significant 20.7% active renin increase was observed only at the 30th minute. The MBP fall was positively correlated with age (FIGURE 1) whereas it was negatively correlated with the HR increase ($r = -0.308$, $p < 0.01$) and the pretreatment level of renin ($r = -0.205$, $p = 0.05$).

After removing the linear effects of age by the partial correlation method, there was no link between the MBP fall and the renin level ($r = -0.046$, not significant). The positive correlation between age and the MBP fall was persistently observed after removing the renin effect ($r = 0.464$, $p < 0.001$). The baroreflex sensitivity was appreciated by the slope of the regression line HR/MBP fall, which could be calculated at the 5% statistical level in 51 among the 87 patients, and was negatively correlated to age ($r = -0.515$, $n = 51$, $p < 0.001$).

Sixteen of the 87 patients were then included in the active group of a three week, placebo controlled, double blind trial of long acting nicardipine (50 mg twice a day). The blood pressure fall observed during a 12-hour recording with the Remler device was positively correlated with the fall induced by the acute intravenous test ($r = 0.65$, $n = 17$, $p < 0.01$).

There is a complex relationship between blood pressure, age, and renin. The present work suggests that, in a group of patients with wide age ranges, age is a potent

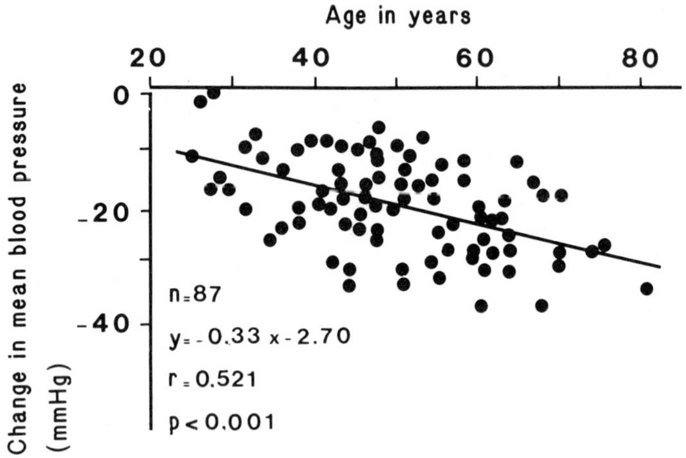

FIGURE 1. Correlation between age and the antihypertensive response to intravenous nicardipine.

predictive factor of blood response to the calcium antagonist nicardipine, whereas renin is not. It also suggests that the baroreflex triggering is a limiting factor of the acute blood pressure fall induced by calcium antagonists. Since the acute test accurately predicted the results of the chronic therapy, it is conceivable that the degree of sympathetic activation determines in part the acute and chronic response to calcium antagonists, as suggested by Kiowski *et al.*[2] Age-related alteration of these counter-regulation mechanisms could explain why these drugs are more efficient in older patients.[3]

REFERENCES

1. Ménard, J., T. T. Guyenne, P. Corvol, B. Pau, D. Simon & R. Roncucci. 1985. Direct immunometric assay of active renin in human plasma. J. Hypertension **3**(Suppl. 3): S275–S278.

2. KIOWSKI, W., P. ERNE, O. BERTEL, P. BOLLI & F. BÜHLER. 1986. Acute and chronic sympathetic reflex activation and antihypertensive response to nifedipine. J. Am. Coll. Cardiol. **7:** 344–348.
3. SHIMADA, K., T. KITAZUMI, N. SADAKANE, H. OGURA & T. OZAWA. 1985. Age-related changes of baroreflex function, plasma norepinephrine, and blood pressure. Hypertension **7:** 113–117.

Cardiovascular Effects of Dihydropyridine Calcium Channel Antagonists and Their Relation to Drug Levels in Plasma

K.-H. GRAEFE, R. ZIEGLER, W. WINGENDER,
K.-D. RÄMSCH, AND G. AHR

Department of Clinical Pharmacology
Bayer AG
Aprather Weg
D-5600 Wuppertal, Federal Republic of Germany

In a randomized, single-blind crossover study involving nine healthy male subjects, nifedipine (24 μg/kg), nitrendipine (40 μg/kg), and nisoldipine (10 μg/kg) were given intravenously on three separate occasions at intervals of 2 to 3 weeks. Before (30 minutes), during (4 minutes), and after (60 minutes) drug administration, heart rate, blood pressure, forearm blood flow, and drug levels in plasma were monitored, with the volunteers resting supine throughout. All three dihydropyridines evoked transient increases in heart rate and forearm blood flow and small decreases in blood pressure. While the oberved peak changes in heart rate were virtually identical for the three drugs (45% above baseline), the peak changes in forearm blood flow were more pronounced after administration of nitrendipine and nisoldipine (about 240% above baseline) than after administration of nifedipine (75% above baseline). Plots of the pharmacodynamic effects against the drug concentrations in plasma showed that the heart rate and forearm blood flow response to the dihydropyridines were directly dependent on the drug levels in plasma. In fact, the drug-level–response curves for both the heart rate and the forearm blood flow responses did not show any distortion by hysteresis effects and clearly obeyed Hill's equation. The analysis of these curves showed that the three drugs (although exhibiting certain differences in calculated maximum effects) differ predominantly with respect to their potencies in dilating the resistance vessels of the forearm: the relative vasodilator potencies of nifedipine, nitrendipine, and nisoldipine were 1, 2, and 13, respectively. Moreover, the values of EC_{50} (drug concentration sufficient to produce half of the maximum effect) obtained for the vasodilator responses were similar to those for the heart rate responses.

In another double-blind crossover study, which involved nine healthy male subjects, the cardiovascular effects of oral doses of 20 mg nifedipine and 20 mg nisoldipine were compared with those of placebo. In this study the volunteers rested supine for 120 minutes after dosing, during which time heart rate, forearm blood flow, and forearm venous capacity were monitored. In addition, blood was sampled from a forearm vein to determine drug levels in plasma. As in the previous study, both drugs elicited about the same increase in heart rate, but produced distinctly different increases in forearm blood flow. As far as the peak responses of the forearm blood flow are concerned, nisoldipine was about 3 times as effective as nifedipine. Neither drug produced any change in the forearm venous capacity. The drug-induced changes in forearm blood flow were again directly dependent on the plasma levels. Equieffective drug concentrations in plasma differed by about a factor of 50, with nisoldipine being more potent than nifedipine.

In conclusion, the cardiovascular effects of the dihydropyridine calcium channel antagonists observed in single-dose studies are directly dependent on the plasma levels of these drugs. There was no distortion of the effect kinetics by hysteresis effects, indicating that the compartment in which these drugs elicit their vascular effects equilibrates with the central compartment without any appreciable delay. The dihydropyridines tested here differ predominantly in their potencies as dilators of the resistance vessels. Similar heart rate responses to these drugs may well go hand in hand with dissimilar vasodilator responses. Though being quite potent arteriolar vasodilators, the dihydropyridine calcium channel blockers fail to have nitratelike effects on the venous capacitance vessels.

Comparative Evaluation of Two Calcium Antagonists, Nicardipine and Nifedipine, in Patients with Mild to Moderate Chronic Heart Failure

A Noninvasive Study

C. MAZZOLA,[a] E. E. GUFFANTI,[a] A. VACCARELLA,[a]
D. TURRI,[b] M. NAZZARI,[b] AND G. FIORELLA[b]

[a]*Department of Cardiology*
INRCA Casatenovo (Co.)
Via Monteregio 13
22064 Casatenovo, Italy

[b]*Medical Department*
Sandoz Italy S.p.A.
20135 Milan, Italy

INTRODUCTION

Several vasodilators have been extensively used in patients with congestive heart failure (CHF), and recent data suggest that some calcium channel blocker drugs might be particularly useful for the management of CHF. Nicardipine (NIC) is a new dihydropyridine derivative with strong vasodilatory properties and negligible effects on the myocardium and pacemaker cardiac cells.[1,2] The aim of the present single-blind controlled study was to compare the effectiveness and safety of orally administered NIC and nifedipine (NIF) in 20 outpatients with CHF (3/20 II and 17/20 III New York Heart Association class).

Following a two-week run-in period during which digoxin and diuretic dosages were titrated until a satisfactory hemodynamic steady state was reached, the patients (mean age 60 ± 7.6, range 45–75 years, 12/20 men) were randomly allocated to NIC ($n = 10$) or NIF ($n = 10$) for a two-week period in addition to their previous therapy. The evaluation included clinical examination (heart failure score), ergometric test, cardiothoracic ratio and echo-M-mode indexes in baseline, end-run-in, as well as end-trial conditions. The statistical significance of the results was assessed by ANOVA and Student's t-test. The results are reported in FIGURE 1.

At the end of the run-in period, a significant hemodynamic improvement was observed in both groups, and a further improvement was induced by Ca antagonist administration (FIGURE 1). The LV echocardiographic function indexes (Vcf, LVET, PEP, CI) and physical fitness (HFS) results were more favorably influenced by NIC than by NIF ($p < 0.05$).

CONCLUSION

NIC and NIF were powerful and effective unloading agents, and did not cause any detectable cardiac depressive effects in patients with mild to moderate heart failure, with a more prominent hemodynamic improvement after NIC.

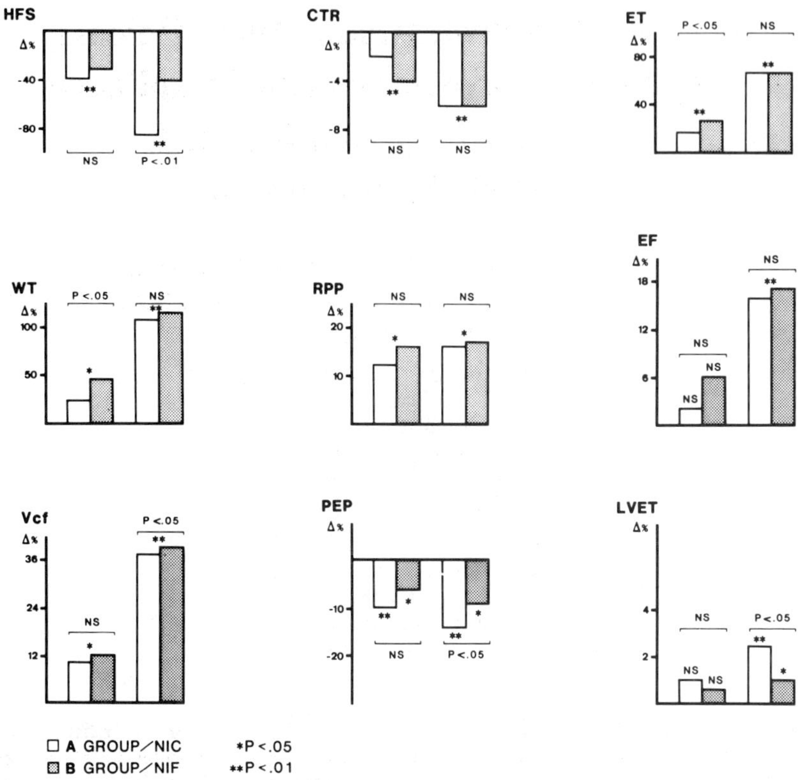

FIGURE 1. Comparative percent change from baseline values (abscissa) at the end of run-in (left) and after Ca antagonist treatment (right) ($\overline{x}$). Statistical significance is expressed in respect to the baseline conditions within the groups (*) and between the groups (horizontal line). HFS = heart failure score; CTR = cardiothoracic ratio; ET = exercise time; WT = total work performed; RPP = rate pressure product; EF = left ventricle ejection fraction; Vcf = circumferential shortening velocity of fibers; PEP = preejection time; LVET = left ventricular ejection time.

No relevant adverse reactions were induced by either drug, but NIC was overall better tolerated from a subjective standpoint.

REFERENCES

1. Lambert, C. R., J. A. Hill, W. W. Nichols, R. L. Feldman & C. J. Pepine. 1985. Coronary and systemic hemodynamic effects of nicardipine. Am. J. Cardiol. **55:** 652–656.
2. Ryman, K. S., S. H. Kubo, J. Lystash, G. Stone & R. J. Cody. 1986. Effect of nicardipine on rest and exercise hemodynamics in chronic congestive heart failure. Am. J. Cardiol. **58:** 583–588.

Chronic Administration of Slow-Release Nifedipine Improves Arterial Compliance in Elderly Hypertensives with Systolic Hypertension

S. NOVO,[a,d] G. DAVÌ,[a] E. NARDI,[a] F. ZINGONE,[a]
M. FLORIDIA,[a] G. CENTINEO,[a] G. NOTO,[a] G. LICATA,[b]
AND A. STRANO[c]

[a]*Institute of Clinical Medicine*
and
[b]*Medical Therapy*
University of Palermo
Piazza delle Cliniche, 2
90127 Palermo, Italy

[c]*Department of Internal Medicine*
Second University of Rome
Tor Vergata
Via Orazio di Raimondo, 7
00100 Rome, Italy

The concept that systolic hypertension (SH) plays an important role in the determination of cerebrovascular accident and heart failure especially in older people is well documented as far as it is clear that a decrease of arterial compliance is involved in the genesis of isolated SH in elderly patients.[1,2] The diminution of blood pressure (BP) in these patients must be regarded mainly as the systolic BP, because an inappropriate reduction of BP can induce serious disturbances of vital organ perfusion.[3] Nifedipine is a calcium channel blocker that reduces BP significantly after acute and chronic administration,[4] especially when used in a slow-release preparation (srN). The aim of our study was to evaluate the effects of srN on BP, arterial compliance, and hemodynamics in elderly patients with isolated SH.

MATERIALS AND METHODS

Ten patients (pts) (6 males and 4 females, mean age 73.7 ± 5.6 years) suffering from isolated SH (SBP > 175 mmHg) were studied after one week of pharmacological washout and after acute (20 mg) and chronic (40 mg/day for 6 months) administration of srN. Systolic (SBP), diastolic (DBP), and mean blood pressure (MBP), heart rate (HR), pulse pressure (PP), and pressure rate product (PRP) were evaluated in supine and upright positions. Pts performed also an M-Mode and a two-dimensional echocardiographic examination. The following parameters were evaluated in supine

[d]Address correspondence to Salvatore Novo, Viale Alpi no. 86, 90144 Palermo, Italy.

TABLE 1

	Acute		Chronic				
	1 Baseline Values	2 3 Hours after srN	3 Baseline Values 24 Hours after srN	4 3 Hours after srN	1 → 2 p<	1 → 3 p<	3 → 4 p<
SBP supine (mmHg)	193.75 ± 20.43	152.5 ± 22.7	178.57 ± 10.2	147.14 ± 18.4	0.005	0.025	0.0005
SBP upright (mmHg)	179.8 ± 23.5	146.25 ± 20.37	167.14 ± 5.6	142.14 ± 14.9	0.0125	0.05	0.005
DBP supine (mmHg)	81.25 ± 14.36	71.25 ± 8.69	85.7 ± 5.3	77.85 ± 6.3	0.05	NS	0.01
DBP upright (mmHg)	85.0 ± 19.14	68.75 ± 8.53	87.85 ± 2.6	78.57 ± 6.9	0.01	NS	0.01
MBP supine (mmHg)	118.75 ± 19.5	98.25 ± 9.36	116.65 ± 5.6	100.9 ± 8.6	0.01	NS	0.01
MBP upright (mmHg)	116.6 ± 20.51	94.58 ± 12.47	113.28 ± 2.5	99.74 ± 5.3	0.01	NS	0.005
HR supine (beats/minute)	59.0 ± 2.44	64.5 ± 3.0	62.7 ± 2.8	64.1 ± 3.1	0.01	NS	NS
HR upright (beats/minute)	68.75 ± 6.5	74.5 ± 4.4	72.1 ± 4.3	73.8 ± 4.2	NS	NS	NS
PRP supine	11431 ± 2935	9836 ± 1930	10479 ± 1910	9431 ± 1986	0.01	NS	0.005
PRP upright	12361 ± 3710	10895 ± 2520	12050 ± 1872	10489 ± 1672	0.025	NS	0.005
PP supine (mmHg)	112.5 ± 22.9	81.25 ± 13.5	92.85 ± 9.9	69.28 ± 17.1	0.01	0.0125	0.001
PP upright (mmHg)	94.8 ± 18.7	77.5 ± 15.0	79.28 ± 5.3	63.57 ± 18.6	0.01	0.01	0.01
EDD (cm)	5.9 ± 0.48	5.7 ± 0.43	5.4 ± 0.6	5.2 ± 0.6	0.01	0.025	0.05
ESD (cm)	3.8 ± 0.33	3.5 ± 0.25	3.7 ± 0.24	3.4 ± 0.5	0.0005	NS	0.05
SV (ml)	107.9 ± 16.0	112.4 ± 19.4	105.6 ± 15.5	114.7 ± 16.3	0.0025	NS	0.0025
CO (1/minute)	63 ± 1.17	7.2 ± 1.31	6.6 ± 1.12	7.3 ± 1.2	0.0025	NS	0.01
EF (%)	62.3 ± 2.20	68.2 ± 1.70	64.3 ± 2.1	69.5 ± 1.9	0.0025	0.025	0.005
AI	1.04 ± 0.25	0.73 ± 0.18	0.87 ± 0.21	0.60 ± 0.17	0.01	0.05	0.01
SVR (dine × sec × cm^{-5})	1504 ± 429	1094 ± 275	1412 ± 325	1097 ± 243	0.025	NS	0.01
PEP/LVET	0.19 ± 0.027	0.16 ± 0.049	0.21 ± 0.02	0.17 ± 0.03	0.0025	0.05	0.0025
SF (%)	34.2 ± 1.4	38.6 ± 1.3	31.4 ± 4.5	34.6 ± 5.4	0.005	0.05	0.01
VCF (circ/second)	1.02 ± 0.17	1.35 ± 0.05	1.14 ± 0.13	1.39 ± 0.9	0.0125	0.05	0.01

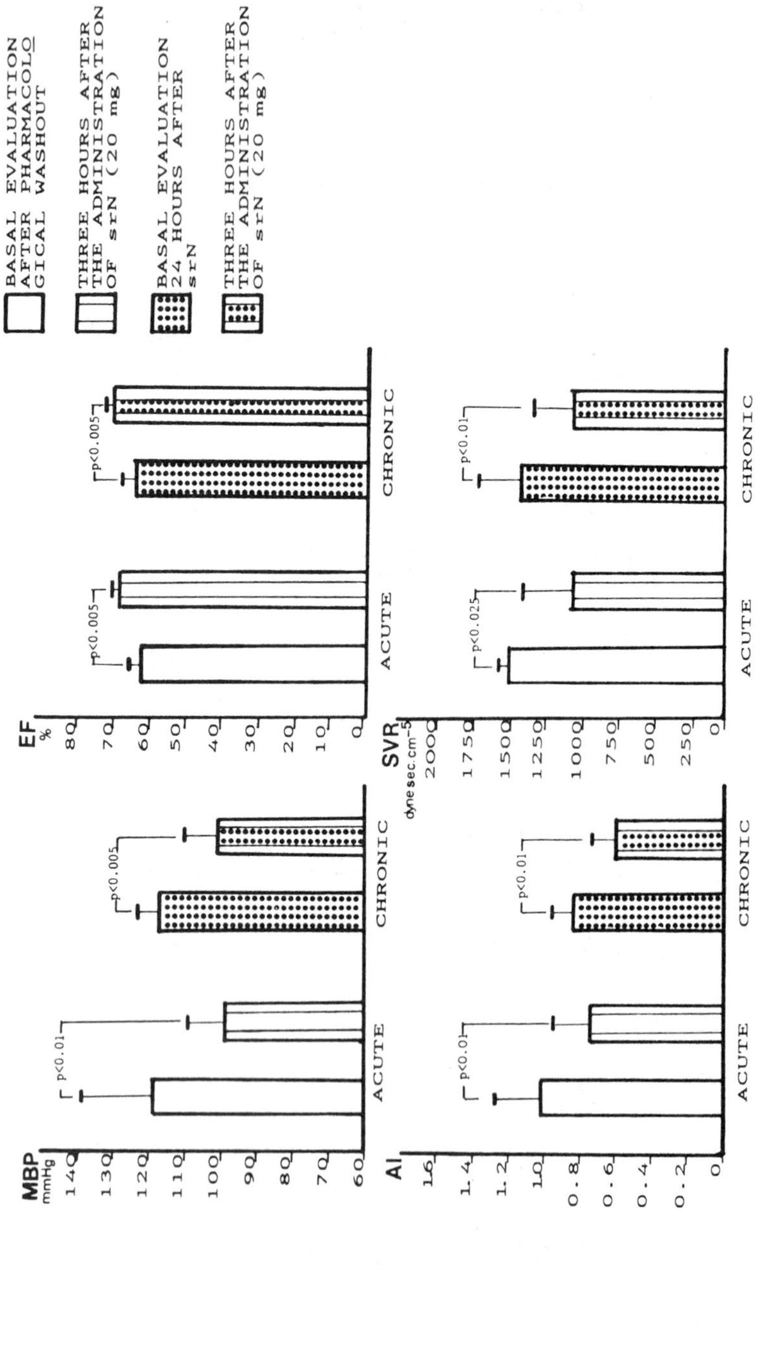
BASAL EVALUATION AFTER PHARMACOLOGICAL WASHOUT
THREE HOURS AFTER THE ADMINISTRATION OF srN (20 mg)
BASAL EVALUATION 24 HOURS AFTER srN
THREE HOURS AFTER THE ADMINISTRATION OF srN (20 mg)
MBP mmHg
p<0.01
p<0.005
EF %
p<0.005
p<0.005
AI
p<0.01
p<0.01
SVR dyne sec.cm^{-5}
p<0.025
p<0.01
ACUTE
CHRONIC

FIGURE 1

position: end-diastolic (EDD) and end-systolic diameters (ESD) of the left ventricle, shortening fraction (SF), mean rate of circumferential shortening (VCF), and PEP/LVET ratio as previously described.[5] Stroke volume (SV), cardiac output (CO), and ejection fraction (EF) were evaluated by two-dimensional images;[6] aortic index (AI) was calculated by the PP/SV ratio, and systemic vascular resistances (SVR) by the following formula: MBP $\times$ 60 $\times$ 1332/CO (ml/minute).[7] Student's t test for paired data was used to calculate statistical significance.

RESULTS AND DISCUSSION

Results are reported in TABLE 1 and FIGURE 1. The acute administration of srN determined a significant decrease of BP, especially SBP, through a significant reduction of SVR with a slight reflex increase of CO and HR, a significant diminution of PRP, index of a less MVO_2, an improvement of the indexes of myocardial function as SF, VCF, PEP/LVET ratio, and EF and an important reduction of PP and AI, expression of an increase of the compliance of the large arteries. After chronic treatment with srN for 6 months, the same modifications were evident 3 hours after the last administration of the drug, except the baroceptorial reflex increase of HR. Twenty-four hours after the last but one administration of srN, SBP, PP, and AI were significantly improved as far as the parameters exploring the myocardial function such as PEP/LVET, SF, VCF, and EF. These results confirm the usefulness of srN in the treatment of isolated SH in elderly patients because the decrease of BP goes together with an improvement of the arterial compliance, responsible in part for the isolated increase of BP[2,3] and a persistent improvement of myocardial function.

REFERENCES

1. SIMON, A. C., M. E. SAFAR, J. A. LEVENSON, G. M. LONDON, B. I. LEVY & N. P. CHAU. 1979. An evaluation of large arteries compliance in man. Am. J. Physiol. **237:** 550.
2. MESSERLY, F. H., E. D. FROHLICH & H. O. VENTURA. 1985. Arterial compliance in essential hypertension. J. Cardiovasc. Pharmacol. **7:** 33.
3. KOCH-WESER, J. 1973. The therapeutic challenge of systolic hypertension. N. Engl. J. Med. **289:** 481.
4. BOLLI, P., W. KIOWSKI, P. ERNE, L. U. HULTHÉN & F. R. BUHLER. 1985. Hemodynamic and antihypertensive treatment responses with calcium antagonists. J. Cardiovasc. Pharmacol. **7:** 126.
5. STRANO, A., S. NOVO, R. MODICA, E. NARDI & G. DONIA. 1986. Hemodynamic effects of acute administration of slow-release nifedipine in elderly patients with systolic hypertension. Am. J. Nephrol. **S1:** 453.
6. BOMMER, W. 1980. Biplane apex echocardiography versus biplane cineangiography in the assessment of left ventricular volume and function: validation by direct measurements. Am. J. Cardiol. **45:** 471.
7. NOVO, S., G. LICATA, A. PINTO, G. DAVÌ & A. STRANO. 1983. Haemodynamic effects of an antihypertensive combination between labetalol and chlorthalidone (RG 136) administered for six months. J. Hypertension **1**(Suppl. 2): 353.

Effects of Middle-Term Treatment with Nifedipine on Hemodynamic Parameters and on Left Ventricular Function in Hypertensive Patients

R. SCAGLIONE,[a] G. PARRINELLO, G. CAPUANA,
M. A. DICHIARA, G. MAZZOLA, N. ASTA,
S. NOVO, AND G. LICATA

Institute of Clinical Medicine
Chair of Medical Therapy
University of Palermo
Piazza delle Cliniche 2
90100 Palermo, Italy

Several studies have demonstrated the effect of acute and long-term oral nifedipine therapy in essential hypertension.[1–5] Moreover some papers reported a hemodynamic response observed after treatment with nifedipine in hypertensive patients.[6,7] The middle-term and the long-term effects of oral nifedipine administration on left ventricular fraction are rather less documented. The present study was carried out to verify the antihypertensive effects of middle-term treatment with nifedipine (N) and to evaluate whether N antihypertensive action is able to promote improvements on left ventricular function.

MATERIALS AND METHODS

Twenty patients (12 males and 8 females aged from 30 to 62 years with mean age of 44.96 ± 12.06 years) 12 of whom with mild and 8 with moderate hypertension (I and II World Health Organization) were consecutively studied. Subjects with severe concomitant diseases (cardiac, renal, or hepatic) as well as patients with water and electrolyte imbalances were excluded. All the patients underwent a washout period for 10 days in which no antihypertensive drugs were administered but placebo and diet with free daily water intake and a constant Na content (150 mEq/24 hours). After the washout period all the patients received an oral dose of 40 mg of N (10 mg every 6 hours) for 30 days. During the washout period and during treatment with N, systolic, diastolic, and mean blood pressure (SBP, DBP, MBP) and heart rate (HR) were recorded in a supine position 3 hours after the last administration of N. Moreover the last day of the washout period and of the treatment period computerized first-pass radionuclide angiography was performed[8] and the following hemodynamic parameters were evaluated: cardiac output (CO), stroke volume (SV), left ventricular ejection fraction (EF), and systemic vascular resistance (SVR) by the formula: MBP × 60 × 1332/CO. Student's test for paired data was used for the statistical analysis; p values below 0.05 were considered significant.

[a]Address correspondence to Rosario Scaglione, Via Lombardia 9, 90100 Palermo, Italy.

TABLE 1. Hemodynamic Parameter Behavior in 20 Hypertensive Patients before and after Treatment with Nifedipine (40 mg for 30 days)

	Before N	After N	p<
SBP (mmHg)	176.6 ± 12.5	156.7 ± 10.2	0.001
DBP (mmHg)	107.5 ± 8.21	91.1 ± 10.5	0.001
MBP (mmHg)	127.3 ± 11.07	109.3 ± 9.3	0.001
HR (beats/minute)	72.87 ± 7.12	71.77 ± 6.84	NS
CO (ml/minute)	5523 ± 358	6196 ± 384	0.02
SV (ml)	75.38 ± 4.84	83.17 ± 5.30	0.02
EF (%)	63.07 ± 4.54	65.72 ± 3.88	0.02
SVR (dyn × sec × cm^{-5})	2086 ± 211	1681 ± 161	0.005

RESULTS AND DISCUSSION

After treatment with N no relevant changes in HR, a highly significant reduction of SBP, DBP, and MBP ($p < 0.001$), a moderately significant increase of CO and SV ($p < 0.02$), a significant decrease of SVR ($p < 0.005$), and an evident but moderately significant ($p < 0.02$) increase of EF were observed (TABLE 1).

Our study demonstrates a peculiar and known hemodynamic response to therapy with N in essential hypertension[6,7] and a mild but significant increase of EF that indicates the improvement of global left ventricular function. We think that this interesting phenomenon is not due to the increase of myocardic contractility but consequent to the reduction of SVR.

So we conclude that nifedipine determines changes of hemodynamic parameters that are able to improve left ventricular function in patients with mild or moderate essential hypertension.

REFERENCES

1. GUAZZI M., M. T. OLIVARI, A. POLESE, C. FIORENTINI, F. MAGRINI & P. MORUZZI. 1977. Nifedipine, a new antihypertensive with rapid action. Clin. Pharmacol. Ther. **22:** 528.
2. LEDERBALLE PEDERSON, O. & E. MICHELSEN. 1978. Acute and chronic effects of nifedipine in arterial hypertension. Eur. J. Clin. Pharmacol. **14:** 375.
3. UEDA, K., J. KUWAIMA, H. ITO, K. KURAMOTO & M. MURAKAMI. 1979. Nifedipine in the management of hypertension. *In* International Adalat Panel Discussion: New Experimental and Clinical Results. P. R. Lichtelen, E. Kimura & N. Taira, Eds. Excerpta Medica. Amsterdam, Holland.
4. GOULD, B. A., R. S. HORNUNG & S. MANN. 1983. Nifedipine or verapamil as sole treatment of hypertension. Hypertension **5**(Suppl. 2): 91.
5. MURPHY, M. B., A. J. I. SCRIVEN & C. T. DOLLERY. 1983. Role of nifedipine in treatment of hypertension. Br. Med. J. **287:** 257.
6. GUAZZI, M. 1978. Effetti emodinamici della nifedipina nell'ipertensione. Atti della tavola rotonda "nifedipina, esperienze farmacologiche e cliniche". A. Strano, Ed., CEPI 47. Rome, Italy.
7. WATHEN, C. G., W. J. HANNAN, L. W. TURNBULL & A. L. MUIR. 1985. Afterload reduction by nifedipine—the acute hemodynamic response to exercise in hypertensive subjects. Eur. Heart J. **6:** 358.
8. LICATA, G., A. INDOVINA, S. NOVO, R. SCAGLIONE, G. PARRINELLO & G. CAPUANA. 1984. Studio della funzione ventricolare sinistra eseguito con la ventricolografia radioisotopica al primo passaggio. Cardiologia **24**(12): 615.

Historical Overview

Calcium, Ischemia, and Death of Brain Cells[a]

BO K. SIESJÖ

Laboratory for Experimental Brain Research
University of Lund
Lund Hospital, Floor EA-5
S-221 85 Lund, Sweden

and

Biochemistry Center of the CNRS
University of Nice
Parc Valrose
06034 Nice Cédex, France

Evidence derived from a variety of tissues suggests that loss of calcium homeostasis in ischemia and related disorders ("calcium overload") is a major cause of cell death. The hypothesis of calcium-related tissue injury was originally proposed to explain damage to the ischemic heart,[1-3] to ischemic or dystrophic muscle,[4,5] to ischemic liver tissue,[6] and to the traumatized spinal cord.[7,8] Some authors subsequently proposed that adverse, calcium-related reactions, elicited when the plasma membrane becomes unduly permeable to calcium, constitute more general mechanisms of cell necrosis.[9-11] At least in part, the evidence quoted in support was that removal of calcium from a suspension increases the viability of cells exposed to adverse conditions, cell viability being estimated by dye exclusion tests. It was then either assumed that calcium injured cells by causing overload and high-amplitude swelling of mitochondria, or caused structural and functional damage to plasma membranes and other targets by activating proteases and lipases.[5,12,13] One hypothesis proposed that the plasma membrane damage in muscle cells was more localized, being secondary to excessive agonist-receptor interactions.[5,14]

The hypothesis of calcium-related cell damage, as applied to brain disease, has some special features.[15-20] First, it proposes a common mechanism in the pathogenesis of ischemic, hypoglycemic, and epileptic brain damage.[16,19,20] Second, it attempts to explain selective neuronal vulnerability in terms of the special characteristics of some burst-firing neurons which, by mechanisms related to calcium influx, have a strong proclivity to epileptic firing.[16,17,21] Third, it provides a likely mediator of the postsynaptic damage which has been ascribed to the presynaptic release of the excitatory amino acids glutamate and aspartate.[22-25] Fourth, some evidence suggests that delayed neuronal death could be caused by a lingering derangement of membrane calcium transport, providing a speculative explanation for why calcium antagonists, when given after the ischemic transient, may ameliorate the final ischemic damage.[26]

Recently, the hypothesis that ischemic injury is secondary to a flooding of cells with calcium has been challenged.[27-29] The main arguments raised against the hypothesis are the following. First, it has never been shown whether calcium accumulation in

[a]Studies from the author's own laboratory were supported by grants from the Swedish Medical Research Council and the U.S. Public Health Service via the National Institutes of Health.

damaged cells precedes loss of cell viability, or if it merely occurs as a result of cell death. In fact, Cheung *et al.* quote experimental results demonstrating that cells *in vitro,* exposed to hypoxia or metabolic poisons, often fail to show an increase in the cytosolic concentration of calcium ($[Ca^{2+}]_i$)[27] (see also Reference 29). The authors also emphasize the lack of correlation between $[Ca^{2+}]_i$ and total cell calcium content—$[Ca^{2+}]_t$. Second, results demonstrating preservation of isolated cells in the absence of added calcium can be criticized on grounds that the dye exclusion tests usually used are insensitive criteria for cell viability; besides, it is emphasized that removal of calcium from cell suspensions is by itself deleterious. Third, recent results suggest that amelioration of ischemic heart damage by calcium antagonists is either due to improvement of collateral circulation or to a lowering of the work load of the ischemic tissue. Such antagonists, therefore, should be efficacious only when they are administered *before* the insult, and they do not work by preventing cellular calcium overload.

The purpose of the present article is to examine critically the hypothesis that loss of calcium homeostasis is responsible for, or contributes to, ischemic brain damage. I will begin by briefly summarizing available information on such damage, emphasizing the selectivity in neuronal response to transient ischemia, and the fact that neuronal necrosis may be of a conspicuously delayed nature. I will continue by recalling the special physiological features that may render some neurons especially vulnerable to loss of calcium homeostasis. I will then summarize data bearing on the effects of calcium antagonists in ameliorating brain damage in experimental ischemia, and speculate about the mechanisms involved. On reviewing this development, I will attempt to discuss the critical points raised by Cheung *et al.,*[27] and try to decide whether they apply, fully or in part, to the brain data. By necessity, the review must be brief, and the number of references restricted. The articles quoted, many of which are of recent origin, will hopefully provide an adequate access to the literature.

ISCHEMIC BRAIN DAMAGE

Permanent ischemia, such as that occurring following middle cerebral artery occlusion, leads to destruction of all tissue elements in the area supplied by the artery.[30,31] In the absence of reperfusion, the size of this pan-necrosis ("infarct") is mainly determined by the type of vessel affected and by the collateral circulation to the "penumbra zone" of potentially viable tissue.[32] This type of ischemia is, therefore, similar to that occurring in the heart as a result of coronary occlusion.

In many clinical conditions, brain ischemia affects larger areas, or is global. If the ischemia is transient and brief, damage may be confined to the nerve cell population, yielding a pattern of selective neuronal vulnerability.[33] With a more severe insult, neuronal destruction takes the form of laminar necrosis and, when glial cells and vascular tissue are destroyed as well, of infarction. Infarcts become more common when the ischemia is prolonged, and when tissue acidosis during ischemia is pronounced.[16,34,35]

Experiments on gerbils and rats have shown that, following brief ischemic periods, neuronal necrosis in limbic and neocortical areas occurs after a delay of many hours or a few days,[36,37] with transient resumption of cellular energy metabolism[38] and function.[39] The results, which raise the question about the mechanisms responsible for this delayed neuronal death, emphasize the importance of long-term recovery for assessment of the final ischemic damage.

With the advent of long-term recovery models, and of the routine use of histopathological techniques for subserial sectioning of the perfusion-fixed brains, it became possible to determine the rank order of neuronal vulnerability to ischemic

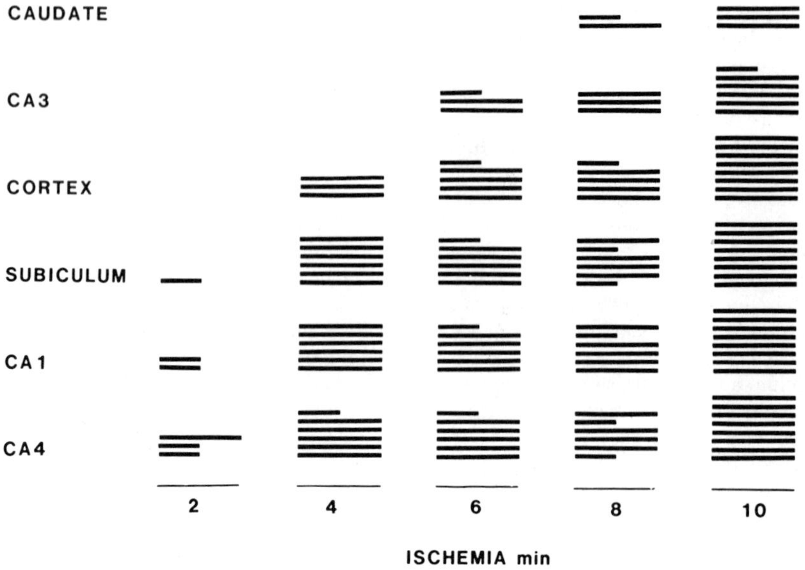

FIGURE 1. Recruitment of neuronal damage in six brain regions with increasing duration of forebrain ischemia in the rat (2–10 minutes). Long bars denote bilateral damage with more than five necrotic neurons per hemisphere. Short bars denote unilateral damage; $n = 8$ (10 minute group) or 6 (all other groups). (Reproduced with permission from Smith *et al.*)[40]

insults.[37,40] As shown in FIGURE 1, short periods of ischemia cause damage confined to the subiculum, CA 1, and CA 4 sectors of the hippocampus, while somewhat longer periods recruite hippocampal CA 3 and neocortical pyramidal neurons, as well as neurons in the caudoputamen. Notably, granule cells in the dentate gyrus are strikingly resistent. Other sensitive neurons are found in the lateral septal nucleus of the thalamus, the entorhinal cortex, and the lateral reticular nucleus of the thalamus. Models of global ischemia reveal that cerebellar Purkinje cells are equally vulnerable.[41] Such studies have also clearly demonstrated that the selective neuronal vulnerability is due to inherent functional/metabolic characteristics of affected cells rather than to vascular factors.

REGULATION OF CELL CALCIUM

Cellular calcium metabolism has been comprehensibly reviewed,[42–46] as have calcium-related mitochondrial events.[47–51] Many of the features of calcium metabolism described are similar in a variety of cells, neurons included. It seems justified to recall some of these features (FIGURE 2).[52] *First,* calcium can only fulfill its important roles as a messenger and a metabolic regulator if the cytosolic Ca^{2+} concentration—$[Ca^{2+}]_i$—is maintained around 10^{-7} M. *Second,* calcium enters the otherwise poorly permeable cell membrane via voltage- and agonist-dependent Ca^{2+} channels. Since the extracellular concentration—$[Ca^{2+}]_e$—is close to 10^{-3} M, such entry occurs along the very steep electrochemical gradient created by a 10000-fold concentration difference, and the negative membrane potential. It follows that the opening of calcium pores must inevitably cause influx of calcium, leading to an increase in $[Ca^{2+}]_i$ which is maximal at the "hot spots" where the pores are localized.[53] *Third,* reexport of the calcium gained as a result of depolarization or agonist-receptor interaction can only occur at the expense of metabolic energy. The energy source is either ATP which fuels a calcium-activated ATPase, or the sodium gradient which allows calcium extrusion by electrogenic (3:1) Na^+/Ca^{2+} exchange. Although Na^+/Ca^{2+} exchange provides a high-capacity system for Ca^{2+} extrusion, the antiporter is reversible and, especially if the external Na^+ concentration falls, it may translocate calcium into the cell.[46,54–56] *Fourth,* although long-term regulation of $[Ca^{2+}]_i$ requires energy-dependent extrusion from the cell, important short-term regulation occurs by binding and sequestration. The extent of this regulation can be appreciated if it is recalled that the total cell content of calcium (10^{-3} M) is about 10,000 times the free intracellular concentration (10^{-7} M). Thus, virtually all of the cellular calcium is bound or sequestered. It has been suggested that a large fraction of this is bound to sialic acid residues of the outer glycoprotein coat ("glycocalix") of the plasma membrane, another fraction being associated with the acidic phospholipids of the inner leaflet of the membrane.[42] Of the truly intracellular calcium some is bound to sites on calmodulin, troponin, and other effector proteins[57,58] or to special calcium-binding proteins.[59] However, many high- and

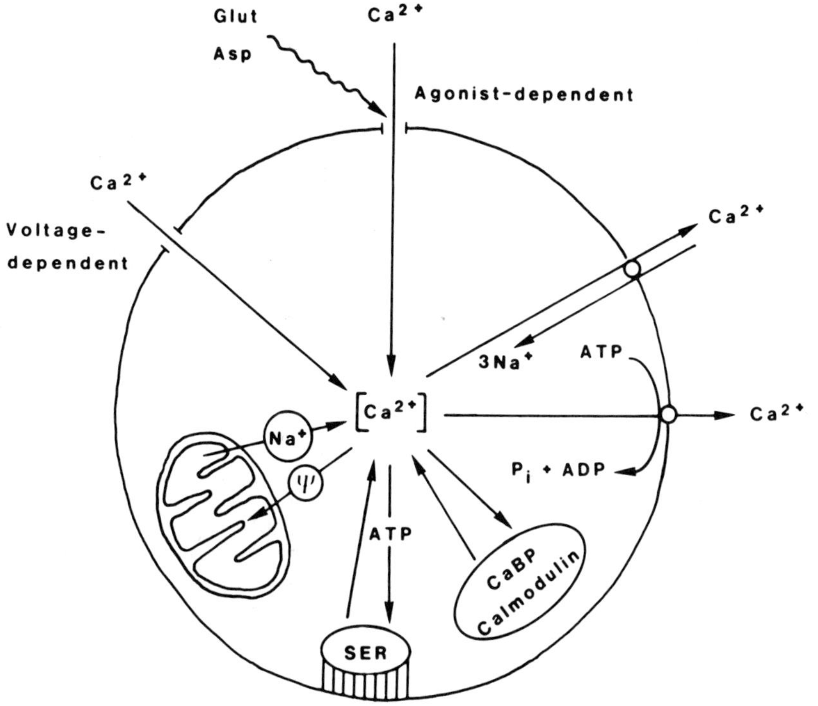

FIGURE 2. Schematic diagram illustrating transport, binding, and sequestration of calcium in an idealized cell. Calcium entry is shown to occur via voltage- and agonist-dependent gates, the latter being activated by glutamate or aspartate, and exit by Na^+/Ca^{2+} exchange and ATP-driven transport. Binding to calmodulin and calcium-binding protein (CaBP) and sequestration by mitochondria and endoplasmic reticulum (SER) are indicated. (Modified after Reference 52.)

low-molecular-weight compounds have an affinity for calcium, which can be chelated to such simple compounds as citrate. The situation is analogous to that prevailing for H^+ which can be buffered by a large number of compounds, and which is also subject to regulation by active transport.[60]

Sequestration, i.e., energy-dependent transport of calcium from cytoplasm to membrane-confined spaces, is though to occur into endoplasmic reticulum and mitochondria. In nerve cells, synaptic vesicles appear to form additional sequestration sites.[61,62] In muscle tissue, the sarcoplasmic reticulum serves as a dynamic store of calcium which is released or taken up in a sequence that is governed by electrical and chemical signals. A corresponding function in release/sequestration of calcium in nerve cells is probably fulfilled by the endoplasmic reticulum.[63,64] Inositol triphosphate, which is formed during the agonist-dependent breakdown of polyphosphoinositides, is an important modulator of calcium release from that store.[65,66]

The role of the mitochondria in calcium sequestration is more controversial.[43,47–51] It is agreed that mitochondria possess a high-capacity mechanism for calcium accumulation, a uniporter that utilizes the potential across the inner mitochondrial membrane to drag calcium electrophoretically into the matric space. Efflux of calcium from the mitochondria occurs by a separate mechanism, one in which two external Na^+ are exchanged for one internal Ca^{2+}. The maximal capacity of the efflux pathway is less than 10% of that of the uptake pathway. In the presence of physiological concentrations of Na^+ and Mg^{2+}, the "set point," i.e., the cytosolic calcium concentration at which efflux matches uptake, is reached at a $[Ca^{2+}]_i$ of about 1 μM. Therefore, if $[Ca^{2+}]_i$ increases above 10^{-6} M, the mitochondria would continuously accumulate calcium.

Opinions differ on the role played by mitochondria in regulating $[Ca^{2+}]_i$. It has often been assumed that mitochondria help regulate Ca_i^{2+} during physiological transients. If this is so, one would expect mitochondrial Ca^{2+} concentrations to vary appreciably with the physiological state. The view is compatible with a certain degree of calcium sequestration in normal mitochondria. However, two findings suggest that mitochondria do not normally regulate $Ca^{2+}{}_i$ concentrations.[49–51] First, most cells seem to have $Ca^{2+}{}_i$ concentrations far below the set point and, thereby, below those that would cause mitochondrial sequestration. Second, such sequestration is not compatible with a regulatory influence of calcium on mitochondrial dehydrogenases. In other words, mitochondria cannot both regulate cytosolic calcium concentration and have their own metabolic machinery regulated by calcium. It has been suggested, therefore, that the cycling of calcium across the inner mitochondrial membranes serves to regulate the intramitochondrial calcium concentration, rather than $[Ca^{2+}]_i$. It follows from this that any true sequestration of calcium in mitochondria is pathological. The conclusion is supported by results obtained with electron probe x-ray microanalysis, which show that accumulation of calcium in mitochondria only occurs in damaged cells.[64,67] Circumstantial evidence exists, though, that $Ca^{2+}{}_i$ concentrations can reach very high values at loci where calcium channels abound.[53] Conceivably, two populations of mitochondria exist, subserving different functions with respect to calcium metabolism.

BRAIN CALCIUM METABOLISM IN ISCHEMIA

In 1977, Nicholson *et al.* reported that anoxia is accompanied by a dramatic decrease in the extracellular calcium concentration of cerebellar cortex.[68] As shown in FIGURE 3, $[Ca^{2+}]_e$ decreased abruptly after cellular release of K^+ had begun, subsequently reaching a concentration of 10% of control, or lower. These results have been repeatedly confirmed, and extended to other species, and to different types of ischemia.[69–71] It has also been shown that a corresponding reduction in $[Ca^{2+}]_e$ occurs in hypoglycemic coma.[72] Similar, but transient, ionic changes are observed in spreading depression,[68,69] while $Ca^{2+}{}_e$ concentrations decrease much less during repetitive electrical stimulation[68] or induced epileptic seizures.[73]

Provided that calcium does not become membrane bound during ischemia or hypoglycemia, the results demonstrate rapid influx of Ca^{2+} into cells. Since such influx occurs at $K^+{}_e$ concentrations of 10–15 mM, it is tempting to assume that it is triggered by depolarization-induced opening of calcium gates.[70] However, the channels that translocate the ions have not been identified, nor can it be excluded that entry of calcium occurs by Na^+/Ca^{2+} exchange. In fact, even glial cells have been found to

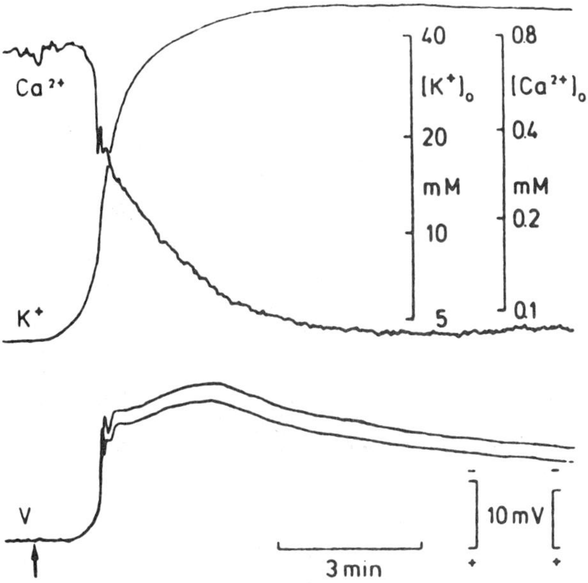

FIGURE 3. Changes in extracellular concentrations for Ca^{2+} and K^+, and slow potential changes (V), in the rat cerebellum during terminal anoxia induced by overdose of pentobarbital. The potential signals from the two reference barrels are superimposed. (Reproduced with permission from Nicholson *et al.*)[68]

possess voltage-dependent calcium channels,[74,75] and calcium precipitates can be found in astrocytes under adverse conditions (see below). The question, therefore, remains, What cells accumulate the extracellular calcium lost, and by what channels/exchangers does it enter the cells? We must also ask, To what extent is the calcium entering cells bound or sequestered, and which are the levels of $[Ca^{2+}]_i$ attained?

The common belief that $[Ca^{2+}]_i$ rises in ischemia is based on the following circumstantial evidence. *First,* the pronounced release of some neurotransmitters into extracellular fluid during hypoxia/ischemia indicates influx of calcium into presynaptic terminals.[76,77] *Second,* the increase in tissue free fatty acid concentrations[78–81] seems too rapid to be explained by cessation of ATP-dependent resynthesis, assuming a normal turnover rate of phospholipids, but suggests that calcium-dependent stimulation of phospholipase A_2 occurs. Incidentally evidence exists that phospholipase C is activated in both hypoglycemia[81] and ischemia.[82] We recognize that such activation should cause release of calcium from intracellular stores (see above). However, since the release is also dependent on other factors, such as pH_i,[83] the effect of phospholipase C stimulation is hard to predict. *Third,* histochemical and chemical results demonstrate that, at least under some circumstances, calcium is sequestered in mitochondria. Using the oxaloacetate-pyriantimonate technique of Borgers,[84] two groups of workers demonstrated calcium precipitates in mitochondria.[85,86] These were occasionally seen *during* incomplete ischemia, but more regularly during recirculation. It seems likely that such calcium sequestration, which appeared readily reversible in ischemia-resistent neurons,[21,86] reflects an increased $Ca^{2+}{}_i$ concentration. However, mitochondrial calcium sequestration is probably not extensive since it is difficult to demonstrate

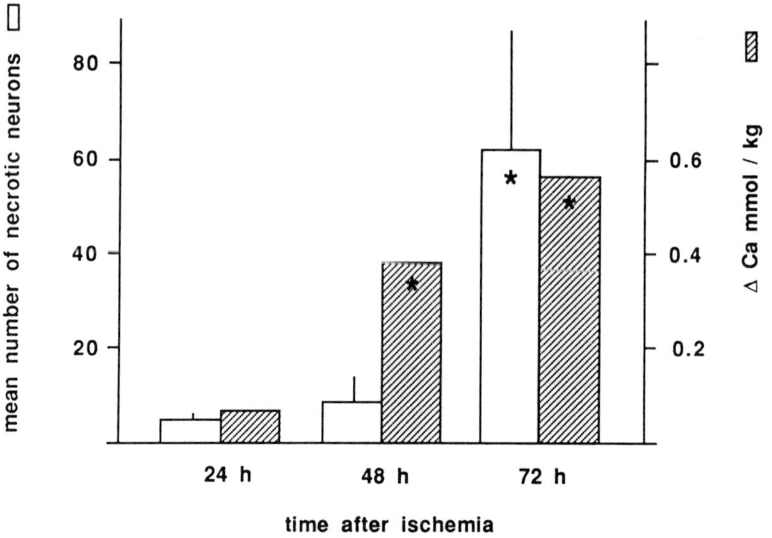

FIGURE 4. Comparison of the time-course of calcium accumulation in the CA 1 sector of the hippocampus (expressed as the change from control) and the mean number of necrotic neurons in animals subjected to ischemia and allowed recovery periods of 24, 48, and 72 hours. (Reproduced with permission from Deshpande *et al.*)[26]

in isolated mitochondria[87,88] and since it does not prevent rapid and extensive recovery of cerebral metabolism and function.[88,89]

It has usually been assumed that ischemia of a density and duration that give rise to cell damage also causes calcium to accumulate in the tissue, such accumulation then occurring during recirculation. Previous results obtained in gerbils and cats support this view.[90,91] However, subsequent data showed that 30 minutes of forebrain ischemia in rats[92] and 60 minutes of global ischemia in monkeys[89] do not necessarily cause calcium to accumulate in the tissue. Thus, calcium accumulation only occurred in selectively vulnerable regions showing dense neuronal necrosis.[92,93]

The question remains as to how calcium accumulation and cell death are related. In locust muscle, glutamate-induced morphological damage seemed to be preceded by calcium accumulation.[94] Although Dienel could clearly show that calcium accumulates in vulnerable regions of the brain after variable postischemic delays,[92] the data did not allow him to conclude whether calcium accumulation preceded cell death, or was a result of it. In a recent study, though, it was possible to demonstrate that net postischemic calcium accumulation in the CA 1 region of the hippocampus occurred *before* light microscopical criteria of necrosis developed[26] (FIGURE 4). With this model, it had previously been shown that the cell damage was ameliorated by postischemic administration of a calcium antagonist.[95] These results suggest that the ischemia could leave the membranes of injured cells with an increased permeability, causing an enhanced rate of calcium cycling and, thereby, a small increase in $[Ca^{2+}]_i$. As discussed by Rasmussen and Waisman,[44] such an increase could cause calcium overload of mitochondria after a delay which may be hours, or even days. However, this is a speculative deduction, and many other possibilities exist. For example, by inhibiting calcium-related depolarization in postsynaptic membranes, calcium antagonists could decrease the "workload" of cells that have suffered metabolic damage during the preceding insult.

In summary, therefore, evidence exists that calcium is translocated from extra- to intracellular fluids during ischemia. Other results suggest that this translocation leads to a rise in intracellular Ca^{2+} concentration of sufficient magnitude to cause transient sequestration of calcium by mitochondria. We recall that cells *in vitro* subjected to "chemical anoxia" do not usually show a rise in Ca^{2}_{i} concentration.[27] Two facts may contribute to cause such a rise in brain ischemia. First, as will be discussed below, neurons contain both voltage- and agonist-dependent Ca^{2+} gates and a high-capacity Na^{+}/Ca^{2+} exchanger which should allow calcium to enter during depolarization. Second, ischemia is accompanied by a dramatic fall in intracellular pH[96–98]. Acidosis is known to release calcium from intracellular binding/sequestration sites[99] and would certainly be expected to reduce the capacity of the cell to buffer a calcium load.

In spite of this, we lack definitive proof that the calcium transient induced by ischemia has anything to do with the subsequent ischemic damage. Thus, the transient influx/release of calcium may be too small or too short lasting to trigger adverse, calcium-related reactions. Furthermore, although the secondary accumulation of calcium appears to precede morphological damage one cannot exclude the possibility that the membrane damage that leads to cell necrosis is of a less specific nature. In order to examine this problem somewhat more closely, it is necessary to consider calcium metabolism at the cellular and regional level. Three questions arise: First, can selective vulnerability be explained in terms of differences in calcium metabolism between cell types? Second, what type of channels mediate a potentially deleterious calcium influx? Third, how is any damage caused by such calcium influx influenced by calcium antagonists?

CALCIUM CHANNELS AND CALCIUM FLUXES IN THE BRAIN

For discussing calcium metabolism in ischemia it seems warranted to recall briefly how calcium channels are distributed in the brain and to consider their responses to agonists and antagonists. According to classical neurophysiological and neurochemical concepts, one can distinguish between two main classes of calcium channels. One is the presynaptic channel which, by allowing depolarization-induced calcium entry, causes transmitter release.[100,101] The other is a postsynaptic calcium channel, mainly localized to dendrites, which is opened in response to agonist-receptor interaction.[102–105].

It has long been recognized that certain neurons fire Ca^{2+} spikes, i.e., that there is an excitatory drive on their dendrites mediated by calcium influx. However calcium has also been implicated in burst firing, i.e., a state in which a prolonged depolarizing shift (PDS) allows a series of action potentials to be fired until repolarization stops the burst.[106–108] One interpretation of such events is that the slow depolarization is due to calcium influx, and each action potential to activation of fast Na^+ and K^+ conductances, while repolarization is caused by a Ca^{2+}-activated, more long lasting increase in K^+ permeability. At synapses with this type of excitatory drive, inhibitory mechanisms must play a very important role; at least in part, these encompass pre- and postsynaptic enhancement of Cl^- conductance mediated by gamma-aminobutyric acid (GABA), serving to reduce presynaptic depolarization and to prevent postsynaptic depolarization from spreading to the perikaryon.

Pyramidal cells in the CA 3 and CA 1 sectors of the hippocampus and in the middle neocortical layers are typical examples of such calcium-excited neurons. Due to their tendency to burst firing they are considered to have a proclivity to epileptogenic behavior, obviously correlating to the high calcium conductances in their apical dendritic fields.[103,106] Normally, some of these neurons may subserve such important functions as long-term potentiation, learning and memory formation, functions that are presumably linked to calcium-triggered intracellular events.[104,109] Under adverse conditions, though, such cells may become the pacemakers of seizure discharge. In view of the importance of calcium influx for sustained depolarization it seems natural that calcium antagonists have been proposed, and used, as anticonvulsants.[110]

The localization of calcium-spiking, burst-firing neurons in the brain seemed similar to that of selectively vulnerable neurons, suggesting that the vulnerability correlates to a high density of calcium entry sites.[16,17] At first sight, some support for a correlation of that kind was obtained by the subsequent mapping of dihydropyridine-binding sites in the brain, which demonstrates high densities in, among other brain regions, the cerebral cortex, the hippocampus, and the substantia nigra.[111–113] However, the correlation is not tight since calcium channels abound in the dendritic fields of CA 3 and dentate granule cells. We recall that CA 3 pyramidal cells are less sensitive to ischemic insults than are CA 1 pyramids, and that dentate granule cells are rather resistant. What adds to the uncertainty of the relationship is that the functional correlate of dihydropyridine-binding sites is far from clear, and that calcium also enters cells by channels that are dihydropyridine resistant. It seems justified, therefore, that current information on such channels is briefly discussed.

There has been a recent surge of interest in voltage-sensitive calcium channels (VSCC) in central and peripheral neurons, and in their sensitivity to dihydrophyridines and other calcium antagonists.[114–120] It was initially difficult to explain why highly specific calcium antagonists had so few functional effects, yet displayed an abundance of binding sites in the tissue. It now seems that this discrepancy arose, at least in part, because the widely studied synaptosomal fractions contain dihydropyridine-insensitive VSCC while neurons in culture, now under intense exploration,[120] have a higher density of dihydropyridine-sensitive VSCC. Patch-clamp studies of neurons from dorsal root ganglia in culture have shown that at least three types of calcium conductances exist, differing in terms of voltage dependence of activation, slope conductances, and inactivation properties.[121] These channels have been designated L (long lasting), T (transient), and N (neither L nor T). Evidence was presented that L channels, but not T or N channels, are sensitive to agonists and antagonists of the dihydropyridine type.

On the basis of current information,[120] it is possible to construct a schematic diagram that, tentatively, assigns functions to the L, T, and N types of channels, and makes predictions about their sensitivity to calcium antagonists of the dihydropyridine type (FIGURE 5). In the presynaptic ending we envisage that calcium influx leads to the release of an undefined transmitter. This calcium influx occurs through VSCC, but these are believed to be of two types. One of them, possibly of the N type, allows

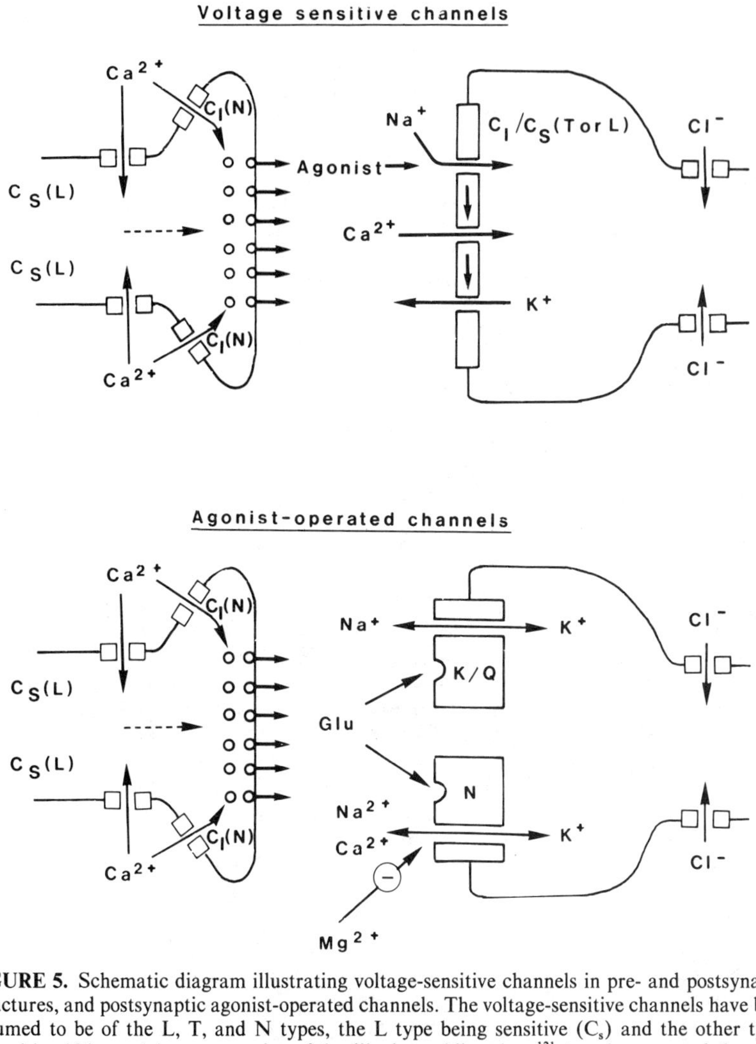

FIGURE 5. Schematic diagram illustrating voltage-sensitive channels in pre- and postsynaptic structures, and postsynaptic agonist-operated channels. The voltage-sensitive channels have been assumed to be of the L, T, and N types, the L type being sensitive (C_s) and the other types insensitive (C_i) to calcium antagonists of the dihydropyridine class.[121] Agonist-operated channels, which are activated by either glutamate or a related amino acid, have been assumed to be gated by kainate/quisqualate (K/A) or by NMDA (N) receptors. Normally, only the latter is supposed to open a conductance for Ca^{2+}.

calcium entry at the microscopic sites where vesicles abound. Since these channels are dihydropyridine insensitive (C_I), transmitter release in general is not affected by calcium antagonists. The other channel, of the L type, will allow calcium influx but, since this may occur at some distance from the vesicular apparatus, it will normally not influence transmitter release. However strong and/or long-lasting depolarizations, or calcium agonists of Bay K8644 type, can cause such pronounced calcium influx that transmitter release will be affected by a "spillover" effect. If this is the correct scenario one may envision that calcium antagonists reduce transmitter release when presynaptic depolarization is pathologically enhanced.

At postsynaptic sites (dendrites and soma) one must assume that two main types of VSCC exist which are either sensitive or insensitive to specific calcium antagonists. Some evidence exists that the relative proportions of these types vary between neuronal populations.[129,130] In FIGURE 5, one type of VSCC is shown that is activated by depolarization secondary to Na^+ influx. The agonists involved are not well known, and the sequence of ionic events is speculative. The important feature is the presence in postsynaptic membranes of VSCC that are either sensitive or insensitive to specific calcium antagonists.

Strong evidence exists that the amino acids glutamate and aspartate are ubiquitous excitatory transmitters in the brain and elsewhere.[122–127] Glutamate in particular has been identified as the major excitatory transmitter, eliciting fast excitatory responses at postsynaptic receptor sites, mainly of dendritic origin. Three major receptor types have been identified for the excitatory amino acids (EAA), selectively activated by kainate, quisqualate (Q), and *N*-methyl-D-aspartate (NMDA). These receptor types differ in their distribution within the brain, they seem to mediate different functional responses, and they are at least in part blocked by different antagonists.[125–131] I will briefly recall the main features of these differences.

Binding studies showed that the caudoputamen has the highest density of kainate-binding sites and the hippocampus of NMDA receptors, while there was less interregional variation in quisqualate receptors. With the advent of autoradiographic techniques for mapping of agonist binding, more precise information on regional distribution became available.[128–130] For example, in the hippocampus, kainate receptors could be specifically localized to the mossy fiber terminations on CA 3 pyramidal neurons, and NMDA receptors to the corresponding Schaffer collateral terminations on CA 1 pyramids, and to the terminals on CA 4 neurons. Such differences in distribution suggest corresponding differences in function. In general, whereas quisqualate/kainate receptors are thought to mediate "fast" excitation, the NMDA receptors are the ones that have been directly linked to such phenomena as long-term potentiation, and indirectly to learning and memory. In the present context, it is of particular interest that none of these amino acid receptors are blocked by the calcium antagonist types of drugs. At present, there are no specific blockers for kainate/quisqualate receptors but several dipeptides and other compounds exist that will block EAA receptors unspecifically (e.g., γ-D-glutamylglycine = γ-DGG). However, NMDA receptors are specifically blocked by the ω-phosphonic acid derivatives D-2-amino-5-phosphonovalarate (AP5) and D-2-amino-phosphonoheptanoate (AP7). It is also of interest that NMDA receptors are blocked by dissociative anesthetics such as ketamine and phencyclidine, and by sigma opiates.[126,132]

The question now arises about the relationship between activation of EAA receptors and calcium fluxes. While it has been known for long that activation of "glutamate" receptors opens a conductance for cations, the involvement of calcium has been clarified only recently.[133–137] FIGURE 5 (lower panel) summarizes current information as follows. First, when glutamate (or aspartate) acts at kainate and quisqualate receptors it causes excitation by opening a conductance to Na^+. Since this channel is unspecific for monovalent cations, it also allows efflux of K^+. Second, when acting at NMDA receptors, glutamate gates a channel that permits Ca^{2+} to pass as well. Third, the NMDA-receptor channel, and, thereby, the Ca^{2+} conductance, is strongly antagonized by Mg^{2+} which blocks the channel in a voltage-dependent manner.[126,127,137,138] Since this block is relieved at much more positive membrane potentials than the resting ones, it takes relatively strong depolarizations to open channels at NMDA receptors.

This would evidently explain the involvement of NMDA receptors in such phenomena as long-term potentiation which are only elicited by strong, repetitive stimulation.

In FIGURE 5, the channels activated by kainate/quisqualate and by NMDA have been assumed to be separate entities. Quite recently, it has been questioned if this is the case.[131,137,139] Thus, results obtained with single channel recording from hippocampal and cerebellar neurons in cell culture have suggested that the distinct conductance mechanisms discussed (kainate/quisqualate versus NMDA) could in reality represent different functional states of one and the same channel. This is an interesting and intriguing possibility since it could mean that, given sufficient time for sustained and/or repeated depolarization, receptors normally activated in the kainate/quisqualate mode would allow calcium to enter the postsynaptic elements.

AGONIST-RECEPTOR INTERACTIONS AND NEURONAL NECROSIS

It is now clear that the same synaptic events that normally provide excitation in pathways utilizing glutamate (or aspartate) as transmitter also can cause neuronal injury. The "excitotoxic" hypothesis, originally formulated to account for the toxicity of glutamate to cells unprotected by an intact blood-brain barrier, was subsequently advanced to explain neuronal necrosis in epilepsy,[140,141] as well as in Huntington's chorea and olivopontocerebellar atrophy.[142,143] Subsequent results, which demonstrated an antiepileptogenic effect of NMDA-receptor antagonists,[144,145] suggested that this subtype of glutamate receptor is involved in the generation of epileptogenic discharge.

It has recently been suggested that an excitotoxic mechanism is responsible for at least some of the features of brain damage in ischemia and hypoglycemia.[24,25,77,146–151] The hypothesis is supported by the following findings. *First,* ischemic and hypoglycemic patterns of damage have some of the dendrosomatic, axon-sparing features of excitotoxic lesions. *Second,* ischemia and hypoglycemia are accompanied by a marked cellular release of glutamate and aspartate which accumulate in extracellular fluids. *Third,* prior lesions of the excitatory innervation partly protect vulnerable neurons against ischemic and hypoglycemic insults. *Fourth,* glutamate antagonists protect against the toxic effects of EAA *in vitro* and, at least in hypoglycemia, against the presumably deleterious effects of glutamate release *in vivo. Fifth,* results obtained on primary culture *in vitro* strongly suggest that excitatory amino acids are responsible for anoxic neuronal necrosis, and amply illustrate the toxicity of added glutamate, or of glutamate analogues.

There is thus strong evidence that release of glutamate and/or aspartate, primarily acting on the NMDA receptor subtype, is at least in part responsible for ischemic and hypoglycemic neuronal necrosis. The question arises, Is the neurotoxicity of glutamate related to calcium influx? In order to respond to this question we must briefly recall a series of important *in vitro* experiments.

In 1983, Rothman exposed fetal rat hippocampal neurons maintained in dispersed tissue culture to NaCN (1 mM) or to anoxia (95% N_2, 5% CO_2).[152] He found that cells in newly plated cultures survived while those in old cultures (>2 weeks) succumbed to the anoxia. The suspicion arose that older cultures were vulnerable because the cells had developed synaptic contacts. This proved to be the case since both $MgCl_2$ (10 mM) and tetrodotoxin (TTX, 3 μM) protected against the anoxia. In a subsequent article, the author could demonstrate that a glutamate antagonist (γ-DGG) dramatically improved survival in anoxia.[147] He further showed that added glutamate or aspartate (10^{-4} M) destroyed all neurons (but not glia) after 1 hour. DGG offered marked protection against this toxicity but neither TTX nor $MgCl_2$ was efficacious. In yet another article, the author reported that the neurotoxicity of glutamate and related amino acids was not abolished by removal of calcium from the medium, but was markedly attenuated if Na^+ and Cl^- were replaced by impermeant ions.[153] On the basis of these results, the author proposed that the ionic basis of the neurotoxicity of EAA was enhanced influx of Na^+ and Cl^-, with osmotically obligated water, yielding osmolytic damage of dendrites.[25]

The subsequent work of Choi, who worked on fetal neocortical neurons in culture,[151] clarified the role of calcium in the pathogenesis of EAA-induced neuronal necrosis. When cultures were exposed to glutamate (0.5 mM) for 5 minutes, two types of cell injury were observed—an immediate one, reflected in increased darkness and granularity of cell bodies, and a delayed one, manifested as necrosis and dissolution of neurons. When NaCl in the medium was replaced by Tris-Cl or choline-Cl the immediate type of damage was abolished but delayed death still occurred. In contrast, removal of Ca^{2+} from the medium enhanced signs of immediate damage but markedly reduced cell loss at 24 hours. On the basis of these results the author concluded that the toxicity of excitatory amino acids is mediated by calcium influx. The conclusion was corroborated by Rothman *et al.*[154] It should also be emphasized that Goldberg *et al.*, inducing ischemialike conditions in neuronal cultures, obtained evidence that calcium was a mediator of cell death.[155]

Recent results reported from these two groups have yielded further information on EEA-related damage.[154,156] For example, glutamate-induced damage can be reproduced by NMDA (0.5 mM). Furthermore, glutamate antagonists that block NMDA receptors (AP5, AP7, ketamine) or act on all three subtypes (kynurenate) provided protection, while drugs that block the non-NMDA subclass of receptors produced little reduction in excitotoxic damage. Finally, addition of blockers of NMDA receptors *after* the amino acid exposure offered partial protection, suggesting the presence of a late, evoked release of NMDA agonists.

In view of these results it seems natural that excitatory amino acids have been incriminated in the pathogenesis of ischemic brain damage. Recently, Rothman and Olney suggested that released glutamate will give rise to rapid and delayed cell death, the rapid death being due to influx of Na^+, Cl^-, and H_2O with an ensuing osmolysis, and the delayed death to calcium influx, triggering changes in receptor function, proteolytic degradation of neurofilaments, mitochondrial damage, and lipolytic generation of free fatty acids.[25] We recognize that the delayed type of damage has characteristics very similar to those previously suggested to account for calcium toxicity.[16–20,34]

In summary, therefore, it seems likely that ischemic neuronal damage in general and selective neuronal vulnerability in particular are related to the innervation of vulnerable cells with fibers releasing excitatory amino acids, and that the vulnerability correlates to the density of glutamate receptors, particularly those of the NMDA type. It is highly likely that the "excitotoxic" damage is mediated by calcium influx through agonist-dependent channels in dendritic domains of these cells. However the mechanisms whereby calcium could exert its purported, adverse effects are unknown, and it has not been explained why neuronal damage can be delayed by hours or days. Although it has been suggested that altered receptor characteristics cause prolonged and harmful overactivity at excitatory synapses, it cannot be excluded that the primary damage affects inhibitory mechanisms or systems that leave normal excitatory drive unbalanced. For example, lesions of the noradrenergic innervation to the hippocampus have been found to aggravate pyramidal cell damage.[24,157] A link to calcium metabolism is suggested by findings showing that noradrenaline counteracts calcium influx at some neuronal membranes.[158] It is also of some interest that calcium has recently been reported to suppress Cl^- conductance in isolated sensory neurons by decreasing the affinity of the GABA receptor.[159]

CALCIUM ANTAGONISTS AND BRAIN DAMAGE

Since the subject is covered by others in this volume, I will confine myself to a few points relevant to the question of whether calcium influx is detrimented to cell survival, and whether this influx can be lessened by calcium antagonists. The major problem is that the channel that seems to translocate calcium into the cell, thereby causing damage, is an agonist-operated one which is not antagonized by dihydropyridines and related compounds. It would seem, therefore, that the ideal antagonist is one that would block glutamate antagonists working in the NMDA mode. So far the specific NMDA antagonists, which have been shown to block the neurotoxicity of EAAs *in vitro*,[147,151,154,156] to act as antiepileptics,[144] or to ameliorate experimentally induced hypoglycemic brain damage *in vivo*,[149] have not proved unequivocally successful in ameliorating ischemic brain damage. The situation may change quickly when new NMDA-receptor antagontists become available. Until then, it appears justified to put scrutiny on the conventional calcium antagonists, and their efficacy in preventing or ameliorating ischemic brain damage.

Calcium antagonists, notably those of the dihydropyridine type, reduce vascular resistance in the brain of normal animals, thereby increasing cerebral blood flow (CBF).[160–164] It has also been shown that pretreatment of animals with nimodipine, subjected to permanent occlusion of a middle cerebral artery (MCA), increases CBF in the perifocal areas, and significantly reduces infarct size.[164] When administered 5 minutes *after* vessel occlusion the drug neither increased CBF nor affected infarct size.[165] Clearly, these results are akin to those reported for cardiac ischemia.[27] They suggest, therefore, that with this type of focal ischemia, calcium antagonists are efficacious only when given before the insult, and that the beneficial effect seems to be exerted on vessels, rather than on neurons or glial cells. However, it may be premature to draw such firm conclusions. Thus, Germano *et al.*, inducing permanent MCA occlusion in chloral hydrate–anesthetized rats, found that nimodipine improved neurological outcome and decreased the size of the infarct when administered up to 6 hours after vessel occlusion.[166] It will remain for future studies to clarify the differences in results reported.

It may be argued that permanent MCA occlusion is bound to cause necrosis of all cells in the distribution territory of the artery, and that a therapeutic effect can only be expected if damaged cells are slowly recruited from any existing penumbra zones. Vascular occlusion in man is perhaps more amenable to postinsult therapy because clinical stroke is sometimes associated with reperfusion of ischemic areas and often progresses with time ("stroke in evolution"). Clinical trials offer some promise in this respect.[167] Definitive results are not yet available, though.

Transient ischemia, as typically occurs following cardiac arrest, is a different entity since the ultimate damage is influenced by a host of postischemic factors.[168] For example, even when an adequate reperfusion pressure is instituted, a delayed hypoperfusion develops which could possibly contribute to the final brain damage. It is of interest that dihydropyridines (nimodipine, nicardipine) ameliorate or prevent the postischemic decrease in CBF,[161,169,170] a clear effect being observed even if the treatment is postponed for up to 60 minutes after circulation has been initiated.[171]

It is currently debated whether pre- and posttreatment with calcium antagonists ameliorate ischemic brain damage and, if so, what mechanisms are involved. As discussed in two recent communications, data on large animals demonstrate that *pretreatment* with calcium antagonists somewhat improves subsequent recovery of neurological function.[170,171] It is more debatable whether posttreatment is beneficial. Three studies have demonstrated significant amelioration. In one, lidoflazine was given after asphyxial cardiac arrest in dogs[172]; in the other, nimodipine was infused following 17 minutes of complete, global ischemia in monkeys[173]; and in the third, flunnarizine was administered following forebrain ischemia in rats.[95] In the latter study the amelioration by the calcium antagonist was documented with quantitative histopathology.

These results raise two important questions. First, are different classes of calcium antagonists equipotent ? Second, if amelioration of ischemic damage is observed, what could be the mechanisms involved ? Three recent studies from the Mayo Clinic provide valuable leads. They were all carried out with complete, global ischemia of a duration that necessitated intensive care measures, and caused extensive neurological deficits, or even death. In one study on dogs subjected to 10 minutes of ischemia, flunarizine was given 10 minutes after release of vascular occlusion as a single infusion.[174] The drug did not ameliorate the postischemic, secondary hypoperfusion, nor did it improve neurological recovery. In fact, pulmonary edema developed in 5 of the 6 dogs studied and 4 died. In another study, lidoflazine was shown not to ameliorate postischemic hypoperfusion following 10 minutes of ischemia in dogs, but to possibly improve neurological outcome.[175] In order to establish whether this improvement was real the effect of lidoflazine was evaluated in monkeys subjected to 17 minutes of complete, global ischemia followed by 48 hours of intensive care.[176] This is the model previously used by the group to evaluate the effects of nimodipine. In contrast to nimodipine, lidoflazine failed to improve the outcome.

These results raise the question of whether nimodipine was efficacious because it improves postischemic blood flow. The following results seem incompatible with such a possibility. First, although nicardipine was shown to prevent secondary hypoperfusion following 10 minutes of complete ischemia in dogs, neurological outcome was not improved.[170] Second, amelioration of brain damage in rats by flunarizine occurred in spite of a similar reduction in postischemic CBF.[95] Clearly, amelioration of ischemic brain damage by postinsult administration of calcium antagonists remains a controversial subject.

CONCLUDING REMARKS

Two antagonist hypotheses exist on the pathophysiology of ischemic cell death. One proposes that influx or release of calcium, with an ensuing rise of $[Ca^{2+}]_i$, triggers adverse reactions which cause irreversible damage to mitochondrial or plasma membranes, or to cytoskeletal components. According to this hypothesis plasma membrane damage can be quite localized, and affect primarily receptor areas. Some of the purported calcium-related events, like covalent modification of receptor proteins and lipolytic/proteolytic alteration of membrane and cytoskeletal components, could conceivably be compatible with short-term but not with long-term recovery, explaining the phenomenon of delayed neuronal death. The hypothesis of calcium-related cell death in ischemia and several other adverse conditions has received considerable attention and widespread support but, admittedly, it is backed up by evidence that is largely circumstantial. Most importantly, it has been shown that cells can succumb to anoxia, or to conditions resembling anoxia, without any preceding increase in $Ca^{2+}{}_i$ concentrations. Furthermore, the amelioration of ischemic heart damage by pretreatment with calcium antagonists does not seem related to calcium "overload" of cells.

The antagonistic hypothesis, which is exclusively based on *in vitro* results, assigns no special role to calcium in triggering irreversible damage, but assumes that the crucial event is ATP depletion and a reduction in phosphorylation potential. Irreversible damage is then assumed to occur by disruption of the cytoskeleton, resulting in surface blebbing and subsequent plasma membrane breaks.

The question is whether the data supporting the second hypothesis invalidate the first. I tentatively conclude that they do not, for the following reasons. Cells studied *in vitro* may differ considerably from those existing *in vivo,* in part because they are mechanically unsupported, but also because the conditions usually employed for inducing "chemical anoxia" do not reproduce the intracellular acidosis of *in vivo* ischemia. Acidosis could conceivably induce a rise in $[Ca^{2+}]_i$ which is not observed in its absence. In fact, it cannot be excluded that acidosis enhances ischemic brain damage by provoking excessive increases in $Ca^{2+}{}_i$ concentration.

As a second point, we need an explanation for why only 5–10 minutes of transient ischemia causes extensive damage to a large population of neurons in the brain. It seems difficult to explain this in terms of a more rapid depletion of cellular ATP stores in these cells, especially since the simple procedure of inducing hyperglycemia significantly delays membrane depolarization, yet markedly enhances ischemic damage. It would seem more likely that vulnerable neurons succumb to short ischemic periods because excessive presynaptic release of excitatory transmitters triggers harmful events at the postsynaptic receptor sites, some of which are secondary to calcium influx. We recognize that recent *in vitro* results support a role for calcium in causing "excitotoxic" neuronal damage.

Conceivably, cells die by calcium-independent and by calcium-dependent mechanisms. Cell death that occurs first after long periods of ischemia could then preferentially be due to the first type of the mechanism. In the brain, cells succumbing to these could be of the "resistant" type, their resistance correlating to a low density of EAA-activated calcium channels. In contrast, when cell death occurs after only short periods of ischemia it seems justified to invoke calcium and calcium-related reactions. One characteristic of such damage is that it leads to membrane dysfunction of a type that causes delayed nerve cell death, possibly provoking a lingering calcium leak which can be lessened by calcium antagonists. If this hypothesis is correct, one can predict that calcium antagonists would normally ameliorate damage to only a portion of the neuronal population, one subserving special functions. However, it seems likely that the presently available antagonists, which act on voltage-sensitive calcium channels, will soon be replaced by drugs acting on agonist-operated channels.

ACKNOWLEDGMENTS

The author wishes to acknowledge constructive and helpful discussions with Dr. Michel Fosset and Professor Michel Lazdunski, Thanks are due to C. Roulinat-Bettelheim for expert secretarial assistance.

REFERENCES

1. FLECKENSTEIN, A., J. JANKE, H. J. DORING & O. LEDER. 1974. Myocardial fiber necrosis due to intracellular Ca overload—a new principle in cardiac hypertrophy. Recent Adv. Stud. Cardiac Struct. Metab. **4:** 563–568.
2. HEARSE, D. & P. B. GARLICK. 1977. Ischemic contraction of the myocardium: mechanisms and prevention. Am. J. Cardiol. **39:** 986–993.
3. KATZ, A. M. & H. R. REUTER. 1979. Cellular calcium and cardiac cell death. Am. J. Cardiol. **44:** 188–190.

4. WROGEMANN, K. & S. D. J. PENA. 1976. Mitochondrial calcium overload: a general mechanism for cell necrosis in muscle diseases. Lancet **1**(7961): 672–674.
5. LEONARD, J. P. & M. M. SALPETER. 1979. Agonist-induced myopathy at the neuromuscular junction is mediated by calcium. J. Cell Biol. **82:** 811–819.
6. CHIEN, K. R., J. ABRAMS, A. SERRONI, J. T. MARTIN & J. L. FARBER. 1978. Accelerated phospholipid degradation and associated membrane dysfunction in irreversible, ischemic liver cell injury. J. Biol. Chem. **253:** 4809–4817.
7. BALENTINE, J. D. & M. SPECTOR. 1977. Calcification of axons in experimental spinal cord trauma. Ann. Neurol. 2: 520–523.
8. HAPPEL, R. D., K. P. SMITH, N. L. BANIK, J. M. POWERS, E. L. HOGAN & J. D. BALENTINE. 1981. Ca^{2+}-accumulation in experimental spinal cord trauma. Brain Res. **211:** 476–479.
9. SCHANNE, F. A. X., A. B. KANE, E. E. YOUNG & J. L. FABER. 1979. Calcium dependence of toxic cell death: a final common pathway. Science **206:** 700–702.
10. FARBER, J. L. 1981. The role of calcium in cell death. Life Sci. **29:** 1289–1295.
11. TRUMP, B. F., I. K. BEREZESKY & A. R. OSORNIO-VARGAS. 1981. Cell death and the disease process. The role of calcium. *In* Cell Death in Biology and Pathology, J. D. Bower & R. A. Lockshin, Eds.: 209–242. Chapman and Hall. London & New York.
12. BEATRICE, M. C., J. W. PALMER & D. R. PFEIFFER. 1980. The relationship between mitochondrial membrane potential, and the retention of Ca^{2+} by mitochondria. J. Biol. Chem. **255:** 8663–8671.
13. KATZ, A. M. & F. C. MESSINEO. 1981. Lipid-membrane interactions and the pathogenesis of ischemic damage in the myocardium. Circ. Res. **48:** 1–16.
14. LEONARD, J. P. & M. M. SALPETER. 1982. Calcium-mediated myopathy at neuromuscular junction of normal and dystrophic muscle. Exp. Neurol. **76:** 121–138.
15. HASS, W. K. 1981. Beyond cerebral blood flow, metabolism and ischemic threshold: examination of the role of calcium in the initiation of cerebral infarction. *In* Cerebral Vascular Disease. J. S. Meyer, H. Lechner, M. Reivich, E. O. Ott & A. Arabinar, Eds. **3:** 3–17. Excerpta Medica. Amsterdam, Holland.
16. SIESJO, B. K. 1981. Cell damage in the brain: a speculative synthesis. J. Cereb. Blood Flow Metab. **1:** 155–185.
17. MELDRUM, B. S. 1983. Metabolic factors during prolonged seizures and their relation to nerve cell death. Adv. Neurol. **34:** 261–275.
18. RAICHLE, M. 1983. The pathophysiology of brain ischemia. Ann. Neurol. **13:** 2–10.
19. SIESJO, B. K. & T. WIELOCH. 1985. Cerebral metabolism in ischemia: neurochemical basis for therapy. Br. J. Anaesth. **57:** 47–62.
20. SIESJO, B. K. & T. WIELOCH. 1986. Epileptic brain damage: pathophysiology and neurochemical pathology. Adv. Neurol. **44:** 813–847.
21. GRIFFITHS, T., M. C. EVANS & B. S. MELDRUM. 1984. Status epilepticus: the reversibility of calcium loading and acute neuronal pathological changes in the rat hippocampus. Neuroscience **12:** 557–567.
22. OLNEY, J. 1978. Neurotoxicity of excitatory amino acids. *In* Kainic Acid as a Tool in Neurobiology. E. G. McGeer, J. W. Olney & P. L. McGeer, Eds.: 95–121. Raven Press. New York, N.Y.
23. COYLE, J. T., S. J. BIRD, R. H. EVANS, R. L. GULLEY, J. V. NADLER, W. J. NICKLAS & J. W. OLNEY. 1982. Excitatory amino acid neurotoxins; selectivity, specificity, and mechanism of action. Neurosci. Res. Progr. **19:** 330–427.
24. WIELOCH, T. 1985. Neurochemical correlates to regional selective neuronal vulnerability. Prog. Brain Res. **63:** 69–85.
25. ROTHMAN, S. M. & J. W. OLNEY. 1986. Glutamate and the pathophysiology of hypoxic-ischemic brain damage. Ann. Neurol. **19:** 105–111.
26. DESHPANDE, J. K., B. K. SIESJO & T. WIELOCH. 1987. Calcium accumulation and neuronal damage in the rat hippocampus following cerebral ischemia. J. Cereb. Blood Flow Metab. **7:** 89–95.
27. CHEUNG, J. Y., J. V. BONVENTRE, C. D. MALIS & A. LEAF. 1986. Calcium and ischemic injury. N. Engl. J. Med. **314:** 1670–1676.
28. SMITH, M. T., H. THOR & S. ORRENIUS. 1981. Toxic injury to isolated hepatocytes is not dependent on extracellular calcium. Science **213:** 1257–1259.

29. LEMASTERS, J. J., J. DIGUISEPPI, A. L. NIEMINEN & B. HERMAN. 1987. Blebbling, free Ca^{2+} and mitochondrial membrane potential preceding cell death in hepatocytes. Nature **325:** 78–81.
30. WALTZ, A. G. 1979. Comparative pathophysiology of ischemic stroke models: an evaluation. *In* Cerebrovascular Disease. T. R. Price & E. Nelson, Eds.: 11–17. Raven Press. New York, N.Y.
31. GARCIA, J. H. 1984. Experimental ischemic stroke: a review. Stroke **15:** 5–14.
32. ASTRUP, J., B. K. SIESJO & L. SYMON. 1981. Thresholds in cerebral ischemia. The ischemic penumbra. Stroke **12:** 723–725.
33. BRIERLEY, J. B. 1976. Cerebral hypoxia. *In* Greenfield's Neuropathology. W. Blackwood & J. Corselli, Eds. 3rd. edit.: 43–85. Arnold. London, England.
34. SIESJO, B. K. 1984. Cerebral circulation and metabolism J. Neurosurg. **60:** 883–908.
35. PLUM, F. 1983. What causes infarction in ischemic brain? The Robert Wartenberg Lecture. Neurology **33:** 222–233.
36. KIRINO, T. 1982. Delayed neuronal death in the gerbil hippocampus following ischemia. Brain Res. **239:** 57–69.
37. PULSINELLI, W. A., J. B. BRIERLEY & F. PLUM. 1982. Temporal profile of neuronal damage in a model of transient forebrain ischemia. Ann. Neurol. **11:** 491–498.
38. PULSINELLI, W. A. & T. E. DUFFY. 1983. Regional energy balance in rat brain after transient forebrain ischemia. J. Neurochem. **40:** 1500–1503.
39. SUZUKI, R., T. YAMAGUCHI, L. CHOH-LUH & I. KLATZO. 1983. The effects of 5-minute ischemia in Mongolian gerbils. II. Changes of spontaneous neuronal activity in cerebral cortex and CA1 sector of hippocampus. Acta Neuropathol. Berlin **60:** 217–222.
40. SMITH, M.-L., R. N. AUER & B. K. SIESJO. 1984. The density and distribution of ischemic brain injury in the rat following two to ten minutes of forebrain ischemia. Acta Neuropathol. Berlin **64:** 319–322.
41. DIEMER, N. H. & E. SIEMKOWICZ. 1981. Regional neuron damage after cerebral ischemia in the normo- and hypoglycemic rat. Neuropathol. Appl. Neurobiol. **7:** 217–227.
42. BORLE, A. B. 1981. Control, modulation and regulation of cell calcium. Rev. Physiol. Biochem. Pharmacol. **90:** 13–164.
43. CARAFOLI, E. 1982. The regulation of intracellular calcium. Adv. Exp. Med. Biol. **151:** 461–472.
44. RASMUSSEN, H. & D. M. WAISMAN. 1983. Modulation of cell function in the calcium messenger system. Rev. Physiol. Biochem. Pharmacol. **95:** 111–148.
45. BAKER, P. F. & R. DIPOLO. 1984. Axonal calcium and magnesium homeostatis. Curr. Top. Membr. Transp. **22:** 195–247.
46. RASSMUSSEN, H. 1986. The calcium messenger system. N. Engl. J. Med. **314:** 1094–1101, 1164–1170.
47. FISKUM, G. & A. L. LEHNINGER. 1982. Mitochondrial regulation of intracellular calcium. *In* Calcium and Cell Function. W. Y. Cheung, Ed. **2:** 39–80. Academic Press. New York, N.Y.
48. AKERMAN, K. E. O. & D. G. NICHOLLS. 1983. Physiological and bioenergic aspects of mitochondrial calcium transport. Rev. Physiol. Biochem. Pharmacol. **95:** 149–201.
49. HANSFORD, R. G. 1985. Relation between mitochondrial calcium transport and control of energy metabolism. Rev. Physiol. Biochem. Pharmacol. **102:** 1–72.
50. DENTON, R. M. & J. G. MCCORMACK. 1985. Ca^{2+} transport by mammalian mitochondria and its role in hormone action. Am. J. Physiol. **249:** E543–E554.
51. MCCORMACK, J. G. & R. M. DENTON. 1986. Ca^{2+} as a second messenger within mitochondria. Trends Biochem. Sci. **11:** 258–262.
52. BERRIDGE, M. J. 1979. Modulation of nervous activity of cyclic nucleotides and calcium. *In* The Neurosciences: Fourth Study Program. F. O. Schmitt & F. G. Worden, Eds.: 873–889. MIT Press. Cambridge, Mass.
53. SIMON, S. M. & R. R. LLINAS. 1985. Compartmentalization of the submembrane calcium activity during calcium influx and its significance in transmitter release. Biophys. J. **48:** 485–498.
54. BLAUSTEIN, M. P. 1984. The energetics and kinetics of sodium-calcium exchange in barnacle muscles, squid axons, and mammalian heart: the role of ATP. *In* Electrogenic

Transport: Fundamental Principles and Physiological Implications. M. P. Blaustein & M. Lieberman, Eds.: 129–147. Raven Press. New York, N.Y.
55. LAZDUNSKI, M., C. FRELIN &P. VIGNE. 1985. The sodium/hydrogen exchange system in cardiac cells: its biochemical and pharmacological properties and its role in regulating internal concentrations of sodium and internal pH. J. Mol. Cell. Cardiol. **17:** 1029–1042.
56. NACHSHEN, D. A., S. SANCHEZ-ARMASS & A. M. WEINSTEIN. 1986. The regulation of cystolic calcium in rat brain synaptosomes by sodium-dependent calcium efflux. J. Physiol. **381:** 17–28.
57. CHEUNG, W. Y. 1980. Calmodulin plays a pivotal role in cellular regulation. Science **207:** 19–27.
58. RHOADS, A. R., M. LULLA, P. B. MOORE & C. E. JACKSON. 1985. Characterization of calcium-dependent membrane binding proteins of brain cortex. Biochem. J. **229:** 587–593.
59. BAIMBRIDGE, K. G. & J. J. MILLER. 1982. Immunochemical localization of calcium-binding protein in the cerebellum, hippocampal formation and olfactory bulb of the rat. Brain Res. **245:** 223–229.
60. ROOS, A. & W. F. BORON. 1981. Intracellular pH. Physiol. Rev. **61**(2): 296–434.
61. FIFKOVA, E., J. A. MARKHAM & R. J. DELAY. 1983. Calcium in the spine apparatus of dendritic spines in the dentate molecular layer. Brain Res. **266:** 163–168.
62. GRIFFITHS, T., M. C. EVANS & B. S. MELDRUM. 1983. Intracellular calcium accumulation in rat hippocampus during seizures induced by bicuculline or L-allylglycine. Neuroscience **10:** 385–395.
63. BLAUSTEIN, M. P., R. W. RATZLAFF & N. K. KENDRICK. 1978. The regulation of intracellular calcium in presynaptic nerve terminals. Ann. N.Y. Acad. Sci. **307:** 195–211.
64. SOMLYO, A. P. 1984. Cellular site of calcium regulation. Cell Physiol. **309:** 516–571.
65. BERRIDGE, M. J. 1984. Inositol triphosphate and diacylglycerol as second messengers. Biochem. J. **221:** 345–360.
66. IRVINE, R. F. 1986. Calcium transients: mobilization of intracellular Ca^{2+}. Br. Med. Bull. **42**(4): 369–374.
67. SOMLYO, A. P., R. URBANICS, G. VADASZ, A. G. B. KOVACH & A. V. SOMLYO. 1985. Mitochondrial calcium and cellular electrolytes in brain cortex frozen *in situ*: electron probe analysis. Biochem. Biophys. Res. Commun. **132**(3): 1071–1078.
68. NICHOLSON, C., G. T. BRUGGENCATE, R. STEINBERG & H. STOCKLE. 1977. Calcium modulation in brain extracellular microenvironment demonstrated with ion-selective micropipette. Proc. Nat. Acad. Sci. USA **74:** 1287–1290.
69. HANSEN, A. J. & T. ZEUTHEN. 1981. Extracellular ion concentrations during spreading depression and ischemia in the rat brain cortex. Acta Physiol. Scand. **113:** 437–445.
70. HARRIS, R. J., L. SYMON, N. M. BRANSTON & M. BAYHAN. 1981. Changes in extracellular calcium activity in cerebral ischemia. J. Cereb. Blood Flow Metab. **1:** 203–209.
71. HANSEN, A. J. 1985. Effects of anoxia on ion distribution in the brain. Physiol. Rev. **65**(1): 101–148.
72. HARRIS, R. J., T. WIELOCH, L. SYMON & B. K. SIESJO. 1984. Cerebral extracellar calcium activity in severe hypoglycemia: relation to extracellular potassium and energy charge. J. Cereb. Blood Flow Metab. **4:** 187–193.
73. HEINEMANN, U., H. D. LUX & M. J. GUTNICK. 1977. Extracellular free calcium and potassium during paroxysmal activity in the cerebral cortex of the cat. Exp. Brain Res. **27:** 237–243.
74. MCVICAR, B. A. 1984. Voltage-dependent calcium channels in glial cells. Science **226:** 1345–1347.
75. NEWMAN, E. A. 1985. Voltage-dependent calcium and potassium channels in retinal glial cells. Nature **317:** 809–811.
76. BOSLEY, T. M., P. L. WOODHAMS, R. D. GORDON & R. BALAZS. 1983. Effects of anoxia on the stimulated release of amino acid neutrotransmitters in the cerebellum *in vitro.* J. Neurochem. **40:** 189–201.
77. BENVENISTE, H., J. DREJER, A. SCHOUSBOE & N. H. DIEMER. 1984. Elevation of the

extracellular concentrations of glutamate and aspartate in rat hippocampus during transient cerebral ischemia monitored by intracerebral microdialysis. J Neurochem. **43:** 1369–1374.
78. BAZAN, N. G. 1976. Free arachidonic acid and other lipids in the nervous system during early ischemia and after electroshock. Adv Exp. Med. Biol. **72:** 317–335.
79. YOSHIDA, S., S. INOH, T. ASANO, K. SANO, M. KUBOTA, H. SHIMAZAKI & N. UETA. 1980. Effect of transient ischemia on free fatty acids and phospholipids in the gerbil brain: lipid peroxidation as possible cause of postischemic injury. J. Neurosurg. **53:** 323–331.
80. REHNCRONA, S., E. WESTEREBERG, B. ÅKESSON & B. K. SIESJO. 1982. Brain cortical fatty acids and phospholipids during and following complete and severe incomplete ischemia. J. Neurochem. **38:** 84–93.
81. WEILOCH, T., R. J. HARRIS, L. SYMON & B. K. SIESJO. 1984. Influence of severe hypoglycemia on brain extracellular calcium and potassium activities, energy and phospholipid metabolism. J. Neurochem. **43:** 160–168.
82. YOSHIDA, S., M. IKEDA, R. BUSTO, M. SANTISO, E. MARTINEZ & M. D. GINSBERG. 1986. Cerebral phosphoinositide, triacylglycerol, and energy metabolism in reversible ischemia: origin and fate of free fatty acids. J. Neurochem. **47:** 744–757.
83. SIFFERT, W. & J. W. N. AKKERMAN. 1987. Activation of sodium-proton exchange is a prerequisite for Ca^{2+} mobilization in human platelets. Nature **325:** 456–458.
84. BORGERS, M. 1981. The role of calcium in the toxicity of the myocardium. Histochem. J. **13:** 839–848.
85. SIMON, R. P., T. GRIFFITHS, M. C. EVANS, J. H. SWAN & B. S. MELDRUM. 1984. Calcium overload in selectively vulnerable neurons of the hippocampus during and after ischemia: an electron microscopy study in the rat. J. Cereb. Blood Flow Metab. **4:** 350–361.
86. VAN REEMPTS, J. & M. BORGERS. 1985. Ischemic brain injury and cell calcium: morphologic and therapeutic aspects. Ann. Emerg. Med. **14:** 736–742.
87. HILLERED, L., B. K. SIESJO & K.-E. ARFORS. 1984. Mitochondrial response to transient forebrain ischemia and recirculation in the rat. J. Cereb. Blood Flow Metab. **4:** 438–446.
88. HILLERED, L., M.-L. SMITH & B. K. SIESJO. 1985. Lactic acidosis and recovery of mitochondrial function following forebrain ischemia in the rat. J. Cereb. Blood Flow Metab. **5:** 259–266.
89. HOSSMAN, K.-A. & B. GROSSE OPHOFF. 1986. Recovery of monkey brain after prolonged ischemia. I. Electrophysiological and brain electrolytes. J. Cereb. Blood Flow Metab. **6:** 15–21.
90. YANAGIHARA, T. & J. T. MCCALL. 1982. Ionic shift in cerebral ischemia. Life Sci. **30:** 1921–1925.
91. HOSSMAN, K.-A., A. PASCHEN & L. CSIBA. 1983. Relationship between calcium accumulation and recovery of cat brain after prolonged cerebral ischemia. J. Cereb. Blood Flow Metab. **3:** 346–353.
92. DIENEL, G. A. 1984. Regional accumulation of calcium in postischemic rat brain. J. Neurochem. **43:** 913–925.
93. HOSSMANN, K.-A., B. GROSSE OPHOFF, R. SCHMIDT-KASTNER & U. OSCHLIES. 1985. Mitochondrial calcium sequestration in cortical and hippocampal neurons after prolonged ischemia of the cat brain. Acta Neuropathol. Berlin **68:** 230–238.
94. DONALDSON, P. L., I. R. DUCE & P. N. R. USHERWOOD. 1983. Calcium accumulation precedes the degenerative efforts of L-glutamate on locust muscle fibres. Brain Res. **274:** 261–265.
95. DESHPANDE, J. K. & T. WIELOCH. 1986. Flunarizine, a calcium entry blocker, ameliorates ischemic brain damage in the rat. Anesthesiology **64:** 215–224.
96. KRAIG, R. P., W. A. PULSINELLI & F. PLUM. 1986. Carbonic acid buffer changes during complete brain ischemia. Am. J. Physiol. **250** (Regulatory Integrative Comp. Physiol. **19**): R348–R357.
97. VON HANWEHR, R., M.-L. SMITH & B. K. SIESJO. 1986. Extra- and intracellular pH during near-complete forebrain ischemia in the rat. J. Neurochem. **46:** 331-339.
98. SMITH, J.-L., R. VON. HANWEHR & B. K. SIESJO. 1986. Changes in extra- and intracellular pH in the brain during and following ischemia in hyperglycemic and in moderately hypoglycemic rats. J. Cereb. Blood Flow Metab. **6:** 574–583.

99. Abercrombie, R. F. & C. E. Hart. 1986. Calcium and proton buffering and diffusion in isolated cytoplasm from Myxicola axons. Am. J. Physiol. **250** (Cell Physiol. **19**): C391–C405.
100. Katz, B. 1969. The Release of Neuronal Transmitter Substances. Charles C. Thomas. Springfield, Ill.
101. Llinas, R. R. & J. E. Heuser. 1977. Depolarisation-release coupling systems in neurons. Neurosci. Res. Progr. Bull **15:** 557–687.
102. Llinas, R. R. & M. Sugimori. 1980. Electrophysiological properties *in vitro* Purkinje cell dendrites in mammalian cerebellar slices. J. Physiol. London **305:** 197–213.
103. Schwartzkroin, P. A. & A. R. Wyler. 1980. Mechanisms underlying epileptiform burst discharge. Ann. Neurol. **7:** 95–107.
104. Collingridge, G. C., S. J. Kehl & H. McLennan. 1983. Excitatory amino acids in synaptic transmission in the Schaffer collateral-commisural pathway of the rat hippocampus. J. Physiol. London **334:** 33–46.
105. Dingledine, R. 1983. *N*-Methyl aspartate activates voltage-dependent calcium conductance in rat hippocampal pyramidal cells. J. Physiol. London **343:** 385–405.
106. Wong, R. K. S. & D. A. Prince. 1978. Participation of calcium spikes during intrinsic burst firing in hippocampal neurons. Brain Res. **159:** 385–390.
107. Gorman, A. L. F., A. Hermann & M. V. Thomas. 1981. Intracellular calcium and the control of neuronal pacemaker activity. Fed. Proc. **40:** 2233–2239.
108. Johnston, D. & T. H. Brown. 1984. The synaptic nature of the paroxysmal depolarizing shift in hippocampal neurons. Ann. Neurol. **16** (Suppl.): S65–S71.
109. Lynch, G. & M. Baudry. 1984. The biochemistry of memory: a new and specific hypothesis. Science **224:** 1057–1063.
110. Meyer, F. B., R. E. Anderson, T. M. Sundt & F. W. Sharbrough. 1986. Selective central nervous system calcium channel blockers—a new class of anticonvulsant agents. Mayo Clin. Proc. **61:** 239–247.
111. Cortes, R., P. Supavilai, M. Karobath & J. M. Palacios. 1984. Calcium antagonist binding sites in the rat brain: quantitative autoradiographic mapping using the 1,4-dihydropyridines [^{3}H]PN 200-110 and [^{3}H]PY 108-068. Neural Transm. **60:** 169–197.
112. Gould, R. J., K. M. M. Murphy & S. H. Snyder. 1985. Autoradiographic localization of calcium channel antagonist receptors in rat brain with [^{3}H]nitrendipine. Brain Res. **330:** 217–223.
113. Mourre, C., P. Cervera & M. Lazdunski. 1987. Autoradiographic analysis in rat brain in the postnatal ontogeny of voltage-dependent Na^+ channels, Ca^{2+}-dependent K^+ channels and slow Ca^{2+} channels identified as receptors for tetrodotoxin, apamin and (−)desmethoxyverapamil. Brain Res. **417**(1): 21–32.
114. Hagiwara, W. & L. Syerly. 1981. Calcium channel. Annu. Rev. Neurosci. **4:** 69–125.
115. Miller, R. J. & S. B. Friedman. 1984. Are dihydropyridine binding sites voltage-sensitive channels? Life Sci. **34:** 1205–1221.
116. Godfraind, R., R. Miller & M. Wibo. 1986. Calcium antagonism and calcium entry blockade. Pharmacol. Rev. **38:** 321–414.
117. Perney, T. M., L. D. Hirning, S. E. Leeman & R. J. Miller. 1986. Multiple calcium channels mediate neurotransmitter release from peripheral neurons. Proc. Nat. Acad. Sci. USA **83:** 6656–6659.
118. Suszkiw, J. B., M. E. O'Leary, M. M. Murawsky & T. Wang. 1986. Presynaptic calcium channels in rat cortical synaptosomes: fast-kinetics of phasic calcium influx, channel inactivation, and relationship to nitrendipine receptors. J. Neurosci. **6**(5): 1349–1357.
119. Thayer, S. A., S. N. Murphy & R. J. Miller. 1986. Widespread distribution of dihydropyridine-sensitive calcium channels in the central nervous system. Mol. Pharmacol. **30:** 505–509.
120. Miller, R. J. 1987. Multiple calcium channels and neuronal function. Science **235:** 46–52.
121. Nowycky, M. C., A. P. Fox & R. W. Tsien. 1985. Three types of neuronal calcium channel with different calcium agonist sensitivity. Nature **316:** 440–443.

122. WATKINS, J. C. & R. H. EVANS. 1981. Excitatory amino acid transmitters. Annu. Rev. Pharmacol. Toxicol. **21:** 165–204.
123. FONNUM, R. 1984. Glutamate: a neurotransmitter in mammalian brain. J. Neurochem. **42:** 1–11.
124. FOSTER, A. C. & G. E. FAGG. 1984. Acidic amino acid binding sites in mammalian neuronal membranes: their characteristics in relationship to synaptic receptors. Brain Res. Rev. **7:** 103–164.
125. WATKINS, J. C. 1984. Excitory amino acids and central synaptic transmission. Trends Pharmacol. Sci. **5:** 373–376.
126. COLLINGRIDGE, G. J. 1985. Long term potentiation in the hippocampus: mechanisms of initiation and modulation by neurotransmitters. Trends Pharmacol. Sci. **6:** 407–411.
127. FAGG, G. E. 1985. L-Glutamate, excitatory amino acid receptors and brain function. Trends Neurosci. **8:** 207–210.
128. MONAGHAN, D. T., V. R. HOLETS, D. W. TOY & C. W. COTMAN. 1983. Anatomical distributions of four pharmacologically distinct ^{3}H-L-glutamate binding sites. Nature **306:** 176–179.
129. GREENAMYRE, J. T., A. B. YOUNG & J. B. PENNEY. 1984. Quantitative autoradiographic distribution of L-[^{3}H]glutamate-binding sites in rat central nervous system. J. Neurosci. **4:**(8): 2133–2144.
130. GREENAMYRE, J. T., J. M. M. OLSON, J. B. PENNEY, JR. & A. B. YOUNG. 1985. Autoradiographic characterization of *N*-methyl-D-aspartate-quisqualate- and kainate-sensitive glutamate binding sites. J. Pharmacol. Exp. Ther. **233**(1): 254–263.
131. JAHR, C. E. & C. F. STEVENS. 1987. Glutamate activities multiple single channel conductances in hippocampal neurons. Nature **325:** 522–525.
132. THOMSON, A. M., D. C. WEST & D. LODGE. 1985. An *N*-methylaspartate receptor-mediated synapse in rat cerebral cortex: a site of action of ketamine? Nature **313:** 479–481.
133. BÜHRLE, C. & U. SONNHOF. 1983. The ionic mechanism of the excitatory action of glutamate upon the membranes of motoneurones of the frog. Pfluegers Arch. **396:** 154–162.
134. HEINEMANN, U. & R. PUMAIN. 1980. Extracellular calcium activity changes in cat sensorimotor cortex induced by iontophoretic application of amino acids. Exp. Brain Res. **40:** 247–250.
135. PUMAIN, R. & U. HEINEMANN. 1985. Stimulus- and amino acid–induced calcium and potassium changes in rat neocortex. J. Neurophysiol. **53**(1): 1–16.
136. MACDERMOTT, A. B., M. L. MAYER, G. L. WESTBROOK, S. J. SMITH & J. L. BARKER. 1986. NMDA-receptor activation increases cytoplasmic calcium concentration in cultured spinal cord neurons. Nature London **321:** 519–522.
137. MAYER, M. 1987. Two channels reduced to one. Nature **325:** 480–481.
138. NOWAK, L., P. BREGESTOVSKI, P. ASCHER, A. HERBERT & A. PROCHIANTZ. 1984. Magnesium gates glutamate-activated channels in mouse central neurones. Nature **307:** 462–465.
139. CULL-CANDY, S. G. & M. M. USOWICZ. 1987. Multiple-conductance channels activated by excitatory amino acids in cerebellar neurons. Nature **325:** 525–528.
140. COLLINS, R. C. & J. W. OLNEY. 1982. Focal cortical seizures cause distant thalamic lesions. Science **218:** 177–179.
141. SLOVITER, R. S. 1983. "Epileptic" brain damage in rats induced by sustained electrical stimulation of the perforant path. I. Acute electrophysiological and light microscopic studies. Brain Res. Bull. **10:** 675–697.
142. PLAITAKIS, A., S. BERL & M. D. YAHR. 1982. Abnormal glutamate metabolism in an adult-onset degenerative neurological disorder. Science **216:** 193–196.
143. SCHWARCZ, R., A. C. FOSTER, E. D. FRENCH, W. O. WNET-SELL & C. KOHLER. 1984. Excitotoxic models for neurodegenerative disorders. Life Sci. **35:** 19–32.
144. CROUCHER, M. J., J. F. COLLINS & B. S. MELDRUM. 1982. Anticonvulsant action of excitatory amino acid antagonists. Science **216:** 899–901.
145. MELDRUM, B. 1985. Possible therapeutic applications of antagonists of excitatory amino acid neurotransmitters. Clin. Sci. **68:** 113–122.

146. JOHANSEN, F. F., M. B. JØRGENSEN, D. K. J. E. VON LUBITZ & N. H. DIEMER. 1984. Selective dendrite damage in the hippocampal CA1 stratum radiatum with unchanged axon ultra-structure and glutamate uptake after transient cerebral ischaemia in the rat. Brain Res. **291:** 373–377.
147. ROTHMAN, S. 1984. Synaptic release of excitatory amino acid neurotransmitter mediates anoxic neuronal death. J. Neurosci. **4**(7)**:** 1884–1891.
148. SIMON, R. P., J. H. SWAN, T. GRIFFITH & B. S. MELDRUM. 1984. Blockade of *N*-methyl-D-aspartate receptors may protect against ischemic damage in the brain. Science **226:** 850–852.
149. WIELOCH, T. 1985. Hypoglycemia-induced neuronal damage is prevented by a *N*-methyl-D-aspartate receptor antagonist. Science **230:** 681–683.
150. AUER, R. N. 1986. Progressive review: hypoglycemic brain damage. Stroke **17**(4)**:** 699–708.
151. CHOI, D. W. 1985. Glutamate neurotoxicity in cortical cell culture is calcium dependent. Neurosci. Lett. **58:** 293–297.
152. ROTHMAN, S. M. 1983. Synaptic activity mediates death of hypoxic neurons. Science **220:** 536–537.
153. ROTHMAN, S. M. 1985. The neurotoxicity of excitatory amino acids is produced by passive chloride influx. J. Neurosci. **5:** 1483–1489.
154. ROTHMAN, S. M., J. H. THURSTON & R. E. HAUHART. 1986. Delayed neurotoxicity of excitatory amino acids depends upon synaptic activity. Soc. Neurosci. Abstr.: 380.
155. GOLDBERG, W. J., R. M. KADINGO & J. N. BARRETT. 1986. Effects of ischemia-like conditions on cultured neurons: protection by low Na^+, low Ca^{2+} solutions. J. Neurosci. **6**(11)**:** 3144–3151.
156. CHOI, D. W., S. PETERS & M. YOKOHAMA. 1986. Glutamate neurotoxicity in cortical cell culture is attenuated by *N*-methyl-D-aspartate receptor antagonists. Soc. Neurosci. Abstr.: 381.
157. WIELOCH, T., T. KOIDE & E. WESTERBERG. 1986. Inhibitory neurotransmitters and neuromodulators as protective agents against ischemic brain damage. *In* Pharmacology of Cerebral Ischemia. J. Krieglstein, Ed.: 191–197. Elsevier Science Publishing. Amsterdam, Holland.
158. REUTER, H. 1983. Calcium channel modulation by neurotransmitters, enzymes and drugs. Nature **301:** 569–574.
159. INOUE, M., Y. OOMURA, T. YAKUSHIJI & N. AKAIKE. 1986. Intracellular calcium ions decrease the affinity of the GABA receptor. Nature **324:** 156–158.
160. HARPER, A. M., L. CRAIGEN & S. KAZDA. 1981. Effect of the calcium antagonist, nimodipine, on cerebral blood flow and metabolism in the primate. J. Cereb. Blood Flow Metab. **1:** 349–356.
161. KAZDA, S., B. GARTHOFF, H. P. KRAUSE & K. SCHLOBMANN. 1982. Cerebrovascular effects of the calcium antagonistic dihydropyridine derivative nimodipine in animal experiments. Arzneimittelforsch **32:** 331–338.
162. HAWS, C. W., J. K. GOURLEY & D. D. HEISTAD. 1983. Effects of nimodipine on cerebral blood flow. J. Pharmacol. Exp. Ther. **225:** 24–28.
163. MOHAMED, A. A., J. MCCULLOCH, A. D. MENDELOW, G. M. TEASDALE & A. M. HARPER. 1984. Effect of the calcium antagonist, nimodipine, on local cerebral blood flow: relationship to arterial blood pressure. J. Cereb. Blood Flow Metab. **4:** 206–211.
164. MOHAMED, A. A., O. GOTOH, D. I. GRAHAM, K. A. OSBORNE, J. M. MCCULLOCH, A. D. MENDELOW, G. M. TEASDALE & A. M. HARPER. 1985. Effect of pretreatment with the calcium antagonist nimodipine on local cerebral blood flow and histopathology after middle cerebral artery occlusion. Ann. Neurol. **18:** 705–711.
165. GOTOH, O., A. A. MOHAMED, J. MCCULLOCH, D. I. GRAHAM, A. M. HARPER & G. M. TEASDALE. 1986. Nimodipine and the haemodynamic and histopathological consequences of middle cerebral artery occlusion in the rat. J. Cereb. Blood Flow Metab. **6:** 321–331.
166. GERMANO, I. M., H. M. BARTKOWSKI, M. E. CASSEL & L. H. PITTS. 1987. The therapeutic value of nimodipine in experimental focal cerebral ischemia: neurologic outcome and histopathologic findings. J. Neurosurg. **67**(1): 81–87.

167. GELMERS, H. J. 1984. The effects of nimodipine on the clinical course of patients with acute ischemic stroke. Acta Neurol. Scand. **69:** 232–239.

168. HOSSMAN, K.-A. 1982. Treatment of experimental cerebral ischemia. J. Cereb. Blood Flow Metab. **2:** 275–297.

169. STEEN, P. A., L. A. NEWBERG, J. H. MILDE & J. D. MICHENFELDER. 1983. Nimodipine improves cerebral blood flow and neurologic recovery after complete cerebral ischemia in the dog. J. Cereb. Blood Flow Metab. **3:** 38–43.

170. SAKABE, T., I. NAGAI, T. ISHIKAWA, H. TAKESHITA, T. MASUDA, M. MATSUMOTO & A. TATEISHI. 1986. Nicardipine increases cerebral blood flow but does not improve neurologic recovery in a canine model of complete cerebral ischemia. J. Cereb. Blood Flow Metab. **6:** 684–690.

171. NEWBERG-MILDE, L., J. H. MILDE & J. D. MICHENFELDER. 1986. Delayed treatment with nimodipine improves cerebral blood flow after complete cerebral ischemia in the dog. J. Cereb. Blood Flow Metab. **6:** 332–337.

172. VAAGENES, P., R. CANTADORE, P. SAFAR, J. MOOSSY, G. RAO, W. DIVEN, H. ALEXANDER & W. STEZOSKI. 1984. Amelioration of brain damage by lidoflazine after prolonged ventricular fibrillation cardiac arrest in dogs. Crit. Care Med. **12**(10)**:** 846–855.

173. STEEN, P. A., S. E. GISVOLD, J. H. MILDE, L. A. NEWBERG, B. W. SCHEITHAUSER, W. L. LANIER & J. D. MICHENFELDER. 1985. Nimodipine improves outcome when given after complete cerebral ischemia in primates. Anesthesiology **62:** 406–414.

174. NEWBERG, L. A., P. A. STEEN, J. H. MILDE & J. D. MICHENFELDER. 1984. Failure of flunarizine to improve cerebral blood flow or neurologic recovery in a canine model of complete cerebral ischemia. Stroke **15:** 666–671.

175. FLEISCHER, J. E., W. L. LANIER, J. H. MILDE & J. D. MICHENFELDER. 1987. Effect of lidoflazine on cerebral blood flow and neurologic outcome when administered after complete cerebral ischemia in dogs. Anesthesiology **66**(3): 304–311.

176. FLEISCHER, J. E., W. L. LANIER, J. H. MILDE & J. D. MICHENFELDER. 1987. Lidoflazine does not improve neurologic outcome when administered after complete cerebral ischemia in primates. J. Cereb. Blood Flow Metab. **7:** 366–371.

Therapeutic Window for Pharmacological Treatment in Acute Focal Cerebral Ischemia[a]

C. FIESCHI,[b] C. ARGENTINO,[b] G. L. LENZI,[c]
L. FANTOZZI,[d] M. L. SACCHETTI,[b] A. PACE,[b]
M. RASURA,[b] S. BASTIANELLO,[d]
L. BOZZAO,[d] E. ZANETTE,[b] C. BUTTINELLI,[b]
F. GIUBILEI,[b] AND P. PANTANO[b]

[b]3rd Neurology
[c]Neuropathology
[d]Neuroradiology
Department of Neurological Sciences
University "La Sapienza" of Rome
Viale dell'Università 30
00185 Rome, Italy

Before discussing the possible guidelines for therapy of cerebral ischemia and before designing therapeutic trials, we have to figure out if there is any place for a therapy. But if a role for therapy exists, it is clear that this therapy must be applied both as soon as possible and before irreversible infarction happens. That means that we have to identify a "therapeutical window" within which active treatment may have a role, beyond which the tissue is irreversibly damaged. The concept of therapeutical window derives from experimental models.[1-2] However its clinical counterpart is not defined. For instance, the sharp limits of tissue damage in recent brain infarcts[3] cast doubt on the consistency of a border zone of penumbra where there would be a better chance of limiting the extention of damage. On the other hand the mere existence of transient ischemic attacks (TIAs), the clinical observations of a late reversibility of symptoms,[4] and the not infrequent progression of neurological signs in severe strokes[5] indicate that the first few hours, not just the first few minutes, of ischemic strokes might be a critical period, open to treatment. Unfortunately, this is still hypothetical, since our present knowledge is limited by the very few pathophysiological studies of the early hours of stroke.[6]

The present work represents a study of acute stroke patients, with a thorough assessment of their clinical, tomodensitometric, angiographic, and perfusional conditions. It has been undertaken with the working hypothesis that therapeutic trials, in order to increase the likelihood of being successful, should stratify patients with acute ischemic strokes according to the grade, severity, and duration of arterial occlusion and ischemia. Such stratification must be made as soon as possible after the onset of the stroke.

MATERIAL AND METHODS

A stroke registry has been instituted at the University Hospital in Rome. During the periods May 2 to June 15, 1986 and October 1 to January 10, 1987, all emergency

[a]Supported by Consiglio Nazionale Ricerche. Grant No. 86.01655.56.

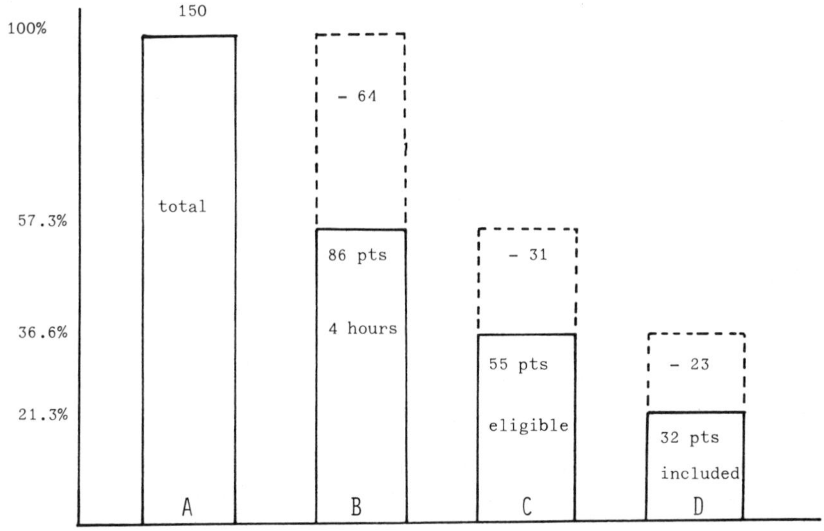

FIGURE 1. Stroke registry, May 2nd, 1986–June 15th, 1986/October 1st, 1986–January 10th, 1987. A = all patients observed; B = percent of A observed within 4 hours from the onset of symptoms; C = percent of B, excluding comatose patients, subtentorial lesions, previous strokes, TIAS, others; D = percent of C, excluding CT diagnosed hemorrages and tumors.

neurological patients were examined by a neurologist of our unit, and those with hemispheric ischemic strokes (clinical diagnosis) who were first seen within 240 minutes (4 hours) of the proven onset of acute symptoms and who were noncomatose at the time of examination were admitted to the neurological intensive care unit.

A computerized tomography (CT) scan immediately identified nonischemic strokes (hemorrhages, S.O.L.). A total of 32 patients with hemispheric ischemic stroke examined within 4 hours of onset were entered into the protocol, out of 150 (21.3%) consecutive strokes (FIGURE 1). These 32 patients were then submitted to cerebral angiography, performed within 6 hours of onset and, wherever possible, to noninvasive exams of cerebral perfusion[7] and ultrasound including transcranial doppler.[8] Criteria of exclusion, detailed elsewhere (N. Engl. J. Med. submitted), included lack of informed consent by the patient or a next-of-kin. TABLE 1 indicates sex and age of patients and side of the lesion.

TABLE 1. Details of Sex, Side of the Lesion and Age

	Side			
	Left	Right	Total	Age[a]
Males	9	8	17	68.3 ± 21.5
Females	7	8	15	63.7 ± 17.8
Totals	16	16	32	66.1 ± 20

[a]Mean ± 2 standard deviations.

TABLE 2. CT Scan Studies: Time Intervals from the Onset of Stroke and Findings

Interval between onset of symptoms and CT SCAN		Maximum	270 minutes
		Minimum	10 minutes
		Mean	187 minutes
Normal	27 cases (84.4%)		
Abnormal	5 cases (15.6%)		

RESULTS AND DISCUSSION

CT scan in the early phase (mean interval 187 minutes) was normal in the majority of patients; however, in nearly 1 out of 6 patients (15.6%) it showed indirect signs of lesion, suggesting for them limited chances of "reversible" damage (TABLE 2).

Angiography within 6 hours (mean interval 255 minutes) demonstrated a clear-cut arterial occlusion in 81.3% of cases, 26 of 32, with a very high frequency of intracranial arterial occlusions (IAOs) (TABLE 3). In 6 of these 21 IAOs, the IAO was associated—and possibly secondary—to a thrombosis at the origin of the intracranial artery (ICA). In 5 patients with ICA occlusion, only the extracranial circulation was visualized, and therefore we cannot exclude a tandem intracranial occlusion, at least in some of them.

That 81% of acute brain infarcts presented with arterial occlusion (largely intracranial) when studied at 4 hours from stroke supports the working hypothesis that intracranial arterial occlusion is the main precipitating cause of ischemic stroke, even when the original lesion is seen in the neck. The nature of intracranial occlusions seems to be largely embolic.[9] Accordingly, these occlusions may not be stable.[6,10–12] It follows that the most important single prognostic factors in ischemic strokes are the size, the site, and the duration of embolic intracranial occlusions, in conjunction with the effectiveness of collateral circulation. The relative weights of these factors realize the range of cerebral ischemia, leading from TIAs to devastating brain infarcts.

Later on, many of these emboli migrate and disappear, due to fragmentation and lysis. The dynamics of this process can perhaps be monitored noninvasively, with transcranial Doppler (TCD): 57% of our verified cases with trunk occlusion showed reperfusion of the middle cerebral artery (MCA). This technique however seems not yet sufficiently refined and fully reliable (TABLE 4).

We have evaluated the cerebral perfusion in this series, both with angiography and with SPECT (TABLE 5). With this latter technique, a severe cerebral blood flow (CBF) reduction was shown, which may persist in patients wity patent or revascularized

TABLE 3. Angiographic Findings—32 Patients[a]

	Angio ≤ 4 hours			Angio 4 hours–6 hours			
	Isol. L.		Assoc. L.	Isol. L.		Assoc. L.	Total
No occlusion	2			1			3
Carotid plaque	1	+	4	2	+	3	10
Occlusion of ICA in the neck	2	+	1	3	+	3	9
Occlusion of ICA in the siphon	1			3			4
Occlusion of the MCA	0	+	2	1	+	3	6
MCA branch occlusion	3	+	3	2	+	3	11

[a]Angiographic findings, subdivided as follows: (A) time interval from the onset of stroke; (B) presence (Assoc. L.) or absence (Isol. L.) of lesion(s) in the same arterial tree.

TABLE 4. Relationship between Angiography and TCD in 25[a] Acute Hemispheric Infarcts at 4–6 Hours

	Intracranial Angiography		
	No Trunk Occlusion	Trunk Occlusion	Total
Unrevealing	4	1	5
Normal	13	0	13
No flow in MCA	0	7	7[b]

[a]In 7 patients TCD was not performed.
[b]In 4, follow-up TCD showed recanalization.

cerebral territories, a finding perhaps related to the severity of tissue damage. It is interesting that about half of the patients show what seems to be a sufficient perfusion in spite of IAOs. The relationship between prognosis and early findings will be analyzed in a subsequent report. At this stage of analysis, we propose to separate acute ischemic patients into three groups.[13] At the two extremes are (a) early reversible ischemias with TIAs; and (b) complete persistent ischemia with early irreversible damage. An intermediate group is that of patients whose tissue is reperfused before extensive completed damage. These patients are potentially suitable for treatments aimed at brain protection. Moreover, the weight of this group, with potential recovery, might be increased in embolic strokes by very prompt fibrinolysis, with streptokinase and r-TPa.

Finally, the "therapeutic window" thus opened in strokes, might be wider the earlier the patients are studied—and treated. However suggestive and only partly supported by our preliminary data, this hypothesis is definitely worth further testing.

CONCLUSIONS

Ischemic strokes are generally precipitated by intracranial embolic arterial occlusions. Hemodynamic strokes are a minority.

Emboli tend to fragment and lyse, thus migrating to more peripheral branches or disappearing. However, trunk or branch occlusions are still present at an average time interval of 4.15 hours from stoke in over 80% of cases, but with collateral flow in 60% of them.

These findings induce us to consider prompt institution of fibrinolytic therapies. The need for a randomized clinical trial in the first 4 hours is strongly stressed if correlation is to be proven by our data between early revascularization and prognosis.

TABLE 5. Regional Perfusion in Acute Hemispheric Infarcts[a] at 4–6 Hours

	Angiography		SPECT with 99Tc—HMPAO	
	Good Revascularization	Poor Revascularization	Asymmetry ≤15%	Asymmetry ≥25%
No intracranial occlusion	—	—	60%	40%
With intracranial occlusion	62%	38%	55%	45%

[a]CBF has been studied in 16 of 32 cases; 4 cases show luxury perfusion at follow-up.

Let us consider our findings also in a different way: revascularization (spontaneous clot lysis, good collateral filling, hopefully drug-induced fibrinolysis) may be present in the majority of strokes at a time when the tissue may not be irreparably damaged, while complete persistent ischemia is rare. Therefore, pharmacological treatments directed at tissue protection and at recovery of neuronal function might have a definite role.

The validity of these assumptions leading to "very early" active treatment of strokes may however apply only to a subset of patients with clinical characteristics such as those considered here: hemispheric, sudden embolic ischemic strokes, not comatose, and without early CT hypodensity at the time of the entry. In fact, this group includes few elderly patients with severe atherosclerotic disease.

REFERENCES

1. PLUM, F. 1986. Conference closing remarks. *In* Acute Brain Ischemia Medical and Surgical Therapy. N. Battistini, P. Fiorani, R. Courbier, F. Plum & C. Fieschi, Eds. Serono Symposium Publications **32:** 356–363. Raven Press. New York, N.Y.
2. WEINSTEIN, P. R., G. G. ANDERSON & D. A. TELLES. 1986. Neurological deficit and cerebral infarction after temporary middle cerebral artery occlusion in unanesthetized cats. Stroke **17:** 318–324.
3. TORVIK, A. & A. SVINDLAND. 1986. Is there a transitional zone between brain infarcts and the surrounding brain? A Histological study. Acta Neurol. Scand. **74:** 365–370.
4. LOEB, C. 1980. Protracted transient ischemic attacks. Eur. Neurol. **19:** 1–11.
5. GAUTIER, J. C. 1985. Stroke in progression. Stroke **16**(4): 729–733.
6. SKYHOJ OLSEN, T. 1986. Regional cerebral blood flow after occlusion of the middle cerebral artery. Acta Neurol. Scand. **73:** 321–337.
7. SHARP, P. F., F. W. SMITH & H. G. GEMMEL. 1986. Technetium-99m HM-PAO stereoisomers as potential agents for imaging regional cerebral blood flow: human volunteer studies. J. Nucl. Med. **27:** 171–177.
8. AASLID, R., T. M. MARKWALDER & H. NORNES. 1982. Noninvasive transcranial doppler ultrasound recording of flow velocity in basal cerebral arteries. J Neurosurg. **57:** 769–774.
9. LHERMITTE, F., J. C. GAUTIER, C. DEROUSNÈ & B. GUIRAND. 1968. Ischemic accidents in the middle cerebral artery territory. A study of the causes in 122 cases. Arch. Neurol. **19:** 248–256.
10. DALAL, P. M., P. M. SHAF & R. R. AIYAR. 1965. Artheriographic study of cerebral embolism. Lancet **2:** 358–361.
11. FIESCHI, C. 1965. Considerazioni sulla patogenesi dei rammollimenti cerebrali derivate dallo studio di casi acuti. Arch. Psicol. Neurol. Psichiatr. **26:** 143–173.
12. FIESCHI, C. & L. BOZZAO. 1969. Transient embolic occlusion of the middle cerebral and internal carotid arteries in cerebral apoplexy. J. Neurol. Neurosurg. Phychiatry **32:** 236–240.
13. FIESCHI, C., C. ARGENTINO, M. SILVESTRINI, F. GIUBILEI, M. L. SACCHETTI, M. RASURA, P. FIORANI, L. BOZZAO & G. L. LENZI. 1986. Clinical management of acute cerebral ischemia. *In* Pharmacology of Cerebral Ischemia. S. Krieglstein, Ed.: 231–248. Elsevier Science Publishers B.V. Amsterdam, Holland.

Use of a Calcium Antagonist in Aneurysmal Subarachnoid Hemorrhage

LENNART BRANDT,[a] BENGT LJUNGGREN,[a] HANS SÄVELAND,[a] AND KARL-ERIK ANDERSSON[b]

[a]*Department of Neurosurgery*
[b]*Department of Clinical Pharmacology*
University Hospital
S-221 85 Lund, Sweden

Intracranial aneurysms are treacherous lesions which rarely give rise to any signs or symptoms until they suddenly rupture. Such rupture ensues like a bolt from the blue and turns out to be an effective tormentor, which untreated leaves less than one out of five victims alive and in good condition 10 years later.[1] The incidence of ruptured intracranial aneurysm is 6–8/100,000 per year in a western population.[2]

DIRECT EFFECTS OF ANEURYSMAL SUBARACHNOID HEMORRHAGE

The *immediate mortality* from aneurysmal subarachnoid hemorrhage (SAH) is approximately *17%* of the total population of victims. In *8%* the aneurysm rupture besides the SAH results in an associated intraparenchymal hemorrhage, which almost without exception leaves the patient in a poor condition. Another *25%* of the total population appear *severely devastated by the first bleed.*[2] Thus, only every second patient suffering from rupture of an intracranial aneurysm will pass the initial stage in a good or fairly good condition.

SECONDARY EFFECTS OF ANEURYSMAL SAH

Aside from the direct effect of the initial bleed, most of the long-term death and disability can be traced to either *recurrent bleeding* or *cerebral vasospasm.* The only way to prevent rebleeding is to occlude the ruptured aneurysm from the circulation.

EARLY ADMITTED INDIVIDUALS IN A FAVORABLE CONDITION

There remains approximately *42%* of the *total population* of victims who are admitted early and who show a *primary "recovery"* in the first days after the bleed and who are at great risk to rebleed and/or develop secondary SAH-induced cerebral vasospasm (FIGURE 1). This group of patients provides the *target group* for an immediate management program aiming to *prevent rebleeds and secondary ischemic deterioration* (symptomatic vasospasm).

PREVIOUS ATTITUDE TO TIMING OF SURGICAL INTERVENTION

Recurrences occur frequently within the first weeks. In a report (1962) 55% of patients who were alive upon admission to hospital eventually rebled with a 75% mortality rate.[3] In another series (1967) subjected to conservative treatment during the first 6–8 weeks, there was a 60% mortality from the second bleed; ¾ of the recurrences occurred within the first 8 weeks.[4] In conclusion, the second bleed occurs early and implies a more grave prognosis than the first.

The first deliberate intracranial surgical attack on a ruptured aneurysm was carried out in 1931, and the first reported series of operated aneurysms was published

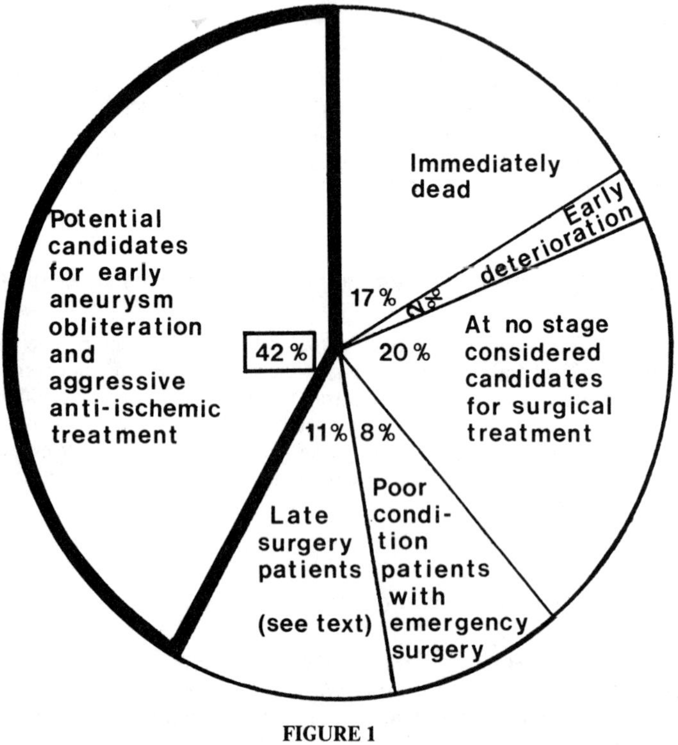

FIGURE 1

in 1944.[5] During the following decades, however, little evidence arose favoring surgical treatment as compared to the natural history of the disease.[6] In this early period of surgical treatment of ruptured intracranial aneurysms, patients operated upon in the acute stage had an unacceptably high mortality and morbidity.[7]

During the 1950s it gradually became clear that many patients did not die from rebleeding but from ischemic complications related to the hemorrhage, and the frequent occurrence of coexisting intracranial arterial spasm became recognized. Even if the pathophysiological significance of cerebral arterial spasm has been questioned as late as in 1975,[8] most investigators agree with the concept that the presence of spasm to such an extent that cerebral perfusion is affected is important in determining the clinical outcome. When the occurrence of intracranial arterial spasm was recognized, it seemed logical to assume that additional peroperative brain retraction, and sometimes induced systemic hypotension, could cause further cerebral hypoperfusion resulting in infarction. With this background, most neurosurgeons preferred *delayed operation* for ruptured intracranial aneurysms.

While awaiting surgery, many patients die or become disabled from recurrent hemorrhage(s) or from vasospasm or both. Thus, even if delayed surgery is safer as an operative procedure, the complications during the waiting period contribute to the prevailing unacceptably high management morbidity and mortality. Thus, Ropper and Zervas in 1984 reported that also in selected cases subjected to conventional late surgery, i.e., after 12–14 days, the ultimate outcome was unsatisfactory in almost half of their initially good-risk patients when viewed from a wider perspective.[9]

CEREBRAL VASOSPASM

The cause of cerebral vasospasm remains obscure. Already in 1839, John Hunter considered constriction of arteries to be one of the physiological mechanisms responsible for the control of hemorrhage. From later work it is well known that mechanical, chemical, and electrical stimulation may induce arterial constriction.

During the last two decades an immense number of studies have been undertaken to elucidate the pathophysiology of cerebral vasospasm and delayed ischemic dysfunction after aneurysmal SAH, but they "have produced more questions than answers."[10]

The significance of the various mechanisms possibly involved in this phenomenon remains controversial. A large number of different substances have been suggested to account for the pathogenesis of delayed cerebral hypoperfusion, and the list has grown as new vasoactive agents have been discovered.[11] Several studies have confirmed the presence of a variety of vasoconstrictive substances in the posthemorrhagic cerebrospinal fluid (CSF). So far, however, no complete information about the identities of these substances is available. Because of the numerous substances incriminated in delayed vasoconstriction, a variety of drugs have been tried in an effort to prevent or treat cerebral vasospasm, but despite many promising preliminary reports the results of clinical trials have been disappointing. Among other mechanisms suggested to be involved in the pathogenesis of cerebral ischemic dysfunction are lesions in the arterial wall including endothelial damage and enhanced platelet aggregability leading to thrombus formation.

CEREBRAL VASOSPASM AND SUBARACHNOID BLOOD

Not until the mid-1960s was it generally recognized that reduction of the arterial caliber after aneurysmal SAH is a time-dependent phenomenon which rarely occurs immediately after the rupture, but appears gradually following a delay of at least 3 to 4 days. Already in 1957 it was suggested that subarachnoid blood clot may cause and maintain narrowing of cerebral vessels and elicit serious ischemia.[12] With the introduction of computerized tomography (CT) scan, it was established that there is a relationship between the amount of extravasated blood in the subarachnoid space and the subsequent development of vasospasm and delayed ischemic cerebral dysfunction.[13,14] Though many surgeons still favor delayed operation as being a safer operative procedure, early surgical intervention is increasingly proposed not only with a view to improve the overall outcome by preventing rebleeding but also in an attempt to prevent ischemic complications by removal of subarachnoid blood.

The belief that the outcome from late surgical intervention is superior to that of early operation has been contradicted by several studies focused on results of a substantial amount of individuals subjected to early operation.[15–17] There is, however, so far no randomized study to document the outcome of patients undergoing early aneurysm surgery versus the outcome with delayed treatment. In a study published in 1981 comprising 81 grades I–III (Hunt and Hess)[18] patients subjected to early operation (within 3 days after SAH), a comparison was made with the outcome in a group of 55 similar patients undergoing delayed operation.[16] The comparison showed that early operation resulting in 74% good neurological recoveries, 10% morbidity, and 16% mortality was superior to delayed management, which resulted in 56% good neurological recoveries, 18% morbidity, and 26% mortality.[16] The latter outcome corresponded well with that reported the same year from North America for similar patients undergoing late operation, which had resulted in 51% good neurological recoveries, 22% morbidity, and 27% mortality.[19] We studied the incidence of symptomatic vasospasm or delayed ischemic deterioration (DID) leading to permanent neurological deficit or death and found a 13% rate of such DID in 137 grades I–III patients subjected to early operation without specific antiischemic treatment[20] (TABLE 1). In conclusion, DID is not abolished by early operation although it may be reduced by early washout of blood-contaminated CSF and clots.

Subsequent studies in the 1980s have made the timing of surgical intervention less controversial. Recently, Milhorat and Krautheim compared two series of 100 consecutive patients, each subjected to delayed and early operation, respectively.[17] The overall survival rate was 35% in the first series (delayed surgery) as compared to 80% in the other (early surgery). At an international workshop on intracranial aneurysms (IWA) in Tokyo in April 1986, it was evident that most aneurysm surgeons now favor operation in the acute stage in patients in a favorable (Hunt and Hess neurological grades I–II) clinical condition.[21]

CEREBRAL VASOSPASM AND CALCIUM CHANNEL BLOCKADE

Variations of vascular smooth muscle tone are mediated through a complex interaction between neurotransmitters, circulating as well as local hormones, and different physiochemical factors.[22] Even if important differences exist between the activation mechanisms of arterial smooth muscle in various vascular regions, many basic mechanisms seem to be common. In most types of vascular smooth muscle an influx of calcium through the cell membrane seems to be a necessary step in the activation of the muscle cell.[23] Concerning smooth muscle which exhibits spike activity triggering the mechanical events, there are reasons to believe that the action potentials are calcium mediated. The increase of free intracellular calcium, which activates the smooth muscle cell, may either occur as the result of a direct transmembrane influx or by a release of intracellularly stored calcium. The calcium influx occurs through at least two separate calcium channels, one membrane-potential dependent (potential-operated channel, POC) and one not depending on membrane potentials.[24] The latter is controlled by the interaction between an agonist and its receptor (receptor-operated channel, ROC). These channels may be involved in electromechanical and pharmacomechanical coupling, respectively.

Agents interfering with calcium at different steps in the excitation-contraction coupling process, calcium antagonists or calcium channel blockers, such as verapamil, diltiazem, nifedipine, and nimodipine, have been shown to be useful tools to elucidate the mechanisms behind potassium- and agonist-induced contractions in vascular smooth muscle, including cerebrovascular smooth muscle.[25–27] Potassium-induced contractions usually show a high sensitivity to calcium channel blockers, while contractions evoked by agonists vary considerably in their sensitivity to calcium blockers in different vascular smooth muscle preparations. Several studies have revealed a pronounced cerebrovascular dilatatory effect of calcium channel blockers of the dihydropyridine group, including experiments on human cerebral arteries *in vitro*,[28–29] as well as *in vivo*.[30–32] It has also been shown that the dilatatory effects of these drugs *in vivo* are inversely proportional to the resting vessel caliber,[30,31] and subsequent experimental studies on the dihydropyridine derivative nimodipine have revealed a relatively predominant cerebrovascular dilatatory effect.[31,33] The mechanisms behind this selectivity have not been established, but may be related to a greater dependency in cerebral than in peripheral vessels on extracellular calcium for smooth muscle activation (for a review, see Reference 34).

Since all contractile substances incriminated in cerebral vasospasm are more or less dependent on calcium for their contractile effect, a reasonable approach to the problem

TABLE 1. Incidence of Delayed Ischemic Deterioration (DID) with Permanent Neurological Deficit (PND) in Patients Subjected to Acute Stage Aneurysm Clipping (left) and the Same Combined with Intravenous Nimodipine (right)

			With Nimodipine	
Preoperative Grade[a]	Number of Patients	With DID	Number of Patients	With DID
I	43	1	20	0
II	61	10	70	3
III	33	7	28	1
Total	137	18	118	4
		13%		3%

[a]Hunt and Hess neurological grading system.

of cerebral vasospasm would be to interfere with the final step in the vascular smooth muscle contraction mechanism. Consequently, it has been proposed that calcium antagonists might be useful to counteract *any* late cerebral vasoconstriction following subarachnoid extravasation of blood.[28–32]

It has been shown that cerebral vasospasm associated with neurological deterioration observed several days following aneurysmal SAH is unaltered by pharmacological agents directed against the proposed increase in vascular smooth muscle tone.[35] Almost every drug that might have a vasodilatatory effect has been tried, and animal experiments have also demonstrated that the chronic phase of vasospasm is unaltered by vasodilators such as aminophylline, nifedipine, or papaverine.[36] This evidence of irreversibility by pharmacological agents is consistant with findings of structural alterations in the vascular wall in patients with chronic vasospasm.[37–42] It is therefore reasonable to believe that it is only the early phase of increased smooth muscle tone that can be affected by vasodilators. For this reason, it has been suggested that any treatment of delayed ischemic deterioration associated with cerebral vasospasm should

TABLE 2. Nimodipine

Continuous intravenous infusion with	2 mg/hour	at approximately 0.5 μg nimodipine/kg body weight per minute:

Steady state plasma concentration (C_{SS}):

26.6 ng/ml ± 1.8 ng/ml (SEM)

Nimodipine assay: high pressure liquid chromatography with UV detection at 254 nm.[a]

[a]Reference 47.

be prophylactic. Apart from the vasodilatatory properties of the dihydropyridines, inhibitory effects on platelet aggregation might be involved.[43]

CLINICAL RESULTS

In 1983, Allen and coauthors presented data indicating that oral nimodipine treatment of patients with a ruptured intracranial aneurysm reduces the occurrence of severe delayed ischemic dysfunction.[44] During 1984 two substantial series of patients subjected to early aneurysm surgery combined with intravenous administration of nimodipine during the critical period for cerebral vasospasm and subsequent DID revealed a very low incidence of this feared complication.[45,46] The definite answer based on incontestable scientific data to the question whether nimodipine therapy affords an additional antiischemic effect has, however, so far not been given.

In our department nimodipine is administered as follows: topical intraoperative application on exposed arterial segments immediately after clipping of the aneurysm in the acute stage followed by continuous intravenous administration of approximately 0.5 μg/kg body weight per minute (2 mg/hour) (TABLE 2) for at least 10 days. During the intravenous infusion, the mean plasma concentration was 26.6 + 1.8 ng/ml (range: <3–38.8 ng/ml)[47] (TABLE 2).

In 118 patients in Hunt and Hess neurological grades I to III who were subjected to operation of a ruptured supratentorial aneurysm in the acute stage (within 72 hours

TABLE 3. Outcome for Grades I–III[a] Patients Subjected to Acute Stage Aneurysm Clipping (left; previous series)[b] and the Same Combined with Intravenous Nimodipine (right; present series)

Outcome	Early Surgery[b]	Early Surgery + Nimodipine
Good recovery	60 (74%)	98 (83%)
Morbidity	8 (10%)	15 (13%)
Mortality	13 (16%)	5 (4)%
Total	81 (100%)	118 (100%)

[a]Hunt and Hess neurological grading system.
[b]Reference 16.

after rupture) with subsequent nimodipine treatment, the incidence of DID with permanent neurological deficit was 3% (TABLE 1).

It has been argued that the lowered mortality and very modest incidence of DID in recent series of early operated patients may be ascribed to increased surgical skill only. However, surgical expertise eventually approaches an asymptote and it is not very likely that this should be the prime reason for the reduction of DID and of mortality from 16% to 4% (TABLE 3). In the absence of any other variable it is suggested that intravenous nimodipine provides an additional antiischemic protective effect following aneurysmal SAH and early operation.

CURRENT MANAGEMENT AND OVERALL OUTCOME FOLLOWING ANEURYSMAL SAH

Following the natural course of aneurysmal SAH only 18% of all victims may be expected to be alive and well after 10 years.[1]

The overall outcome following early surgical intervention combined with additional nimodipine treatment results in 42% good neurological recoveries, 19% morbidity, and 39% mortality.[2] The outcome remains hampered by all those individuals who are permanently devastated as a result of the initial bleed. When incapacitating cognitive and psychosocial dysfunction is included in the final outcome assessment, not more than one out of every three individuals who has suffered from rupture of an intracranial aneurysm can be considered to show a good functional (neurological *and* cognitive) outcome[48] despite *recent improvements* with a near-to *elimination of rebleeds* and a *pronounced reduction of DID* in the patients who initially are in a favorable condition following rupture of an intracranial aneurysm.

REFERENCES

1. JENNETT, G. & S. GALBRAITH, Eds. 1983. An introduction to neurosurgery. 4th edit.: 187. William Heinmann Medical Books Limited. London, England.
2. LJUNGGREN, B., H. SÄVELAND, L. BRANDT & S. ZYGMUNT. 1985. Early operation and overall outcome in aneurysmal subarachnoid hemorrhage. J. Neurosurg. **62:** 547–551.
3. TAPPURA, M. 1962. Prognosis of subarachnoid haemorrhage. A study of 120 patients with unoperated intracranial arterial aneurysms and 267 patients without vascular lesions demonstrable in bilateral carotid angiograms. Acta Med. Scand. **1**(Suppl. 392): 1–75.
4. PAKARINEN, S. 1967. Incidence, aetiology, and prognosis of primary subarachnoid hemorrhage. Acta Neurol. Scand. **43**(Suppl. 29): 1–128.
5. DANDY, W. E. 1944. Intracranial arterial aneurysms. Comstock Publ. Co. New York, London, Hafner & Ithaka.
6. MCKISSOCK, W., K. W. E. PAINE & L. S. WALSH. 1960. An analysis of the results of treatment of ruptured intracranial aneurysms. Report of 772 consecutive cases. J. Neurosurg. **17:** 762–776.
7. NORLÉN, G. & H. OLIVECRONA. 1953. The treatment of aneurysms of the circle of Willis. J. Neurosurg. **10:** 404–415.
8. MILLIKAN, C. H. 1975. Cerebral vasospasm and ruptured intracranial aneurysm. Arch. Neurol. **32:** 433–449.
9. ROPPER, A. H. & N. T. ZERVAS. 1984. Outcome 1 year after SAH from cerebral aneurysm. Management morbidity, mortality, and functional status in 112 consecutive good-risk patients. J. Neurosurg. **60:** 909–915.
10. SUNDT, T. M. & D. H. DAVIS. 1980. Reactions of cerebrovascular smooth muscle to blood and ischemia: primary versus secondary vasospasm. *In* Cerebral Arterial Spasm. R. H. Wilkins, Ed. **1:** 244–250. Williams & Wilkins. Baltimore, Md.

11. WILKINS, R. H. 1986. Attempts at prevention or treatment of intracranial arterial spasm: an update. Neurosurgery **18:** 808–825.
12. JOHNSON, R. J., J. M. POTTER & R. G. REID. 1958. Arterial spasm in subarachnoid haemorrhage. Mechanical considerations. J. Neurol. Neurosurg. Psychiatry **21:** 68.
13. FISHER, C. M., J. P. KISTLER & J. M. DAVIS. 1980. Relation of cerebral vasospasm to subarachnoid hemorrhage visualized by computerized tomographic scanning. Neurosurgery **6:** 1–9.
14. PASQUALIN, A., L. ROSTA, R. DA PIAN, P. CAVAZZANI & R. SCIENZA. 1984. Role of computed tomography in the management of vasospasm after subarachnoid hemorrhage. Neurosurgery **15:** 344–353.
15. SUZUKI, J., T. ONUMA & T. YOSHIMOTO. 1979. Results of early operations on cerebral aneurysms. Surg. Neurol. **11:** 407–412.
16. LJUNGGREN, B., L. BRANDT, E. KÅGSTRÖM & G. SUNDBÄRG. 1981. Results of early operations for ruptured aneurysms. J. Neurosurg. **54:** 473–479.
17. MILHORAT, T. H. & M. KRAUTHEIM. 1986. Results of early and delayed operations for ruptured intracranial aneurysms in two series of 100 consecutive patients. Surg. Neurol. **26:** 123–128.
18. HUNT, W. E. & R. M. HESS. 1968. Surgical risk as related to time of intervention in the repair of intracranial aneurysms. J. Neurosurg. **28:** 14–19.
19. KASSELL, N. F., H. P. ADAMS, JR., J. C. TORNER & A. L. SAHS. 1981. Influence of timing of admission after aneurysmal subarachnoid hemorrhage on overall outcome. Report of the Cooperative Aneurysm Study. Stroke **12:** 620–623.
20. LJUNGGREN, B., H. SÄVELAND & L. BRANDT. 1983. Causes of unfavorable outcome after early aneurysm operation. Neurosurgery **13:** 629–633.
21. KIKUCHI, H., T. FUKUSHIMA & K. WATANABE. 1986. Intracranial Aneurysms. Surgical Timing and Techniques. Nishimura. City, Japan.
22. JOHANSSON, B. 1978. Processes involved in vascular smooth muscle contraction and relaxation. Circ. Res. **43**(Suppl. I): T14–T19.
23. ANDERSSON, K. E. 1978. Effects of calcium and calcium antagonists on the excitation-contraction coupling in striated and smooth muscle. Acta Pharmacol. Toxicol. (Suppl.) **43:** 5–14.
24. BOLTON, T. B. 1979. Mechanisms of action of transmittors and other substances on smooth muscle. Pharmacol. Rev. **59:** 606–718.
25. FLECKENSTEIN, A. 1977. Specific pharmacology of calcium in myocardium, cardiac pacemakers, and vascular smooth muscle. Annu. Rev. Pharmacol. Toxicol. **17:** 149–166.
26. ANDERSSON, K. E. 1984. Calcium entry blockers. A heterogenous family of compounds. Acta Med. Scand. Suppl. **694:** 142–152.
27. ANDERSSON, K. E. & E. HÖGESTÄTT. 1984. On the mechanism of action of calcium antagonists. Acta Med. Scand. **681:** 11–24.
28. ALLEN, G. S. & S. B. BANGHART. 1979. Cerebral arterial spasm. IX. In vitro effects of nifedipine on serotonin-, phenylephrine-, and potassium-induced contractions of canine basilar and femoral arteries. Neurosurgery **4:** 37–42.
29. EDVINSSON, L., L. BRANDT, K. E. ANDERSSON & B. BENGTSSON. 1979. Effect of a calcium antagonist on experimental constriction of human brain vessels: possible efficacy in cerebrovascular spasm. Surg. Neurol. **11:** 327–330.
30. BRANDT, L., B. LJUNGGREN, K. E. ANDERSSON, E. MACKENZIE, E. T. TAMURA & G. TEASDALE. 1982. Effects on feline cortical pial microvasculature of topical application of a calcium antagonist (nifedipine) under normal conditions and in focal ischemia. J. Cereb. Blood Flow Metab. **3:** 44–50.
31. AUER, L. M., R. W. OBERBAUER & H. V. SCHALK. 1983. Human pial vascular reactions to intravenous nimodipine-infusion during EC-IC bypass surgery. Stroke **14:** 210–213.
32. BRANDT, L., K. E. ANDERSSON, B. BENGTSSON, L. EDVINSSON, B. LJUNGGREN & E. T. MCKENZIE. 1979. Effects of nifedipine on pial arteriolar calibre: an in vivo study. Surg. Neurol. **12:** 349–352.
33. KAZDA, S. & R. TOWART. 1982. Nimodipine: a new calcium antagonistic drug with a preferential cerebrovascular action. Acta Neurochir. Wien **63:** 259–265.
34. ANDERSSON, K. E. 1986. Role of calcium ions in the excitation-contraction coupling

mechanisms of brain vessels. *In* Neural Regulation of Brain Circulation. C. Owman & J. E. Hardebo, Eds.: 67–79. Publisher, City, State, Country.

35. WILKINS, R. H. 1980. Attempted prevention or treatment of intracranial arterial spasm: a survey. Neurosurgery **6:** 198–210.
36. VARSOS, V. G., T. M. LISZCZAK, D. H. HAN, J. P. KISTLER, J. VIELMA, P. M. BLACK, R. C. HEROS & N. T. ZERVAS. 1983. Delayed cerebral vasospasm is not reversible by aminophylline, nifedipine, or papaverine in a "two-hemorrhage" canine model. J. Neurosurg. **58:** 11–17.
37. HUGHES, J. T. & P. M. SCHIANCHI. 1978. Cerebral artery spasm. A histological study at necropsy of the blood vessels in cases of subarachnoid hemorrhage. J. Neurosurg. **48:** 515–525.
38. ALKSNE, J. F. & P. J. BRANSON. 1979. Prevention of experimental subarachnoid hemorrhage–induced intracranial arterial vasonecrosis with phosphodiesterase inhibitor Phthalazinol (EG-626). Stroke **120:** 638–644.
39. ALKSNE, J. F. & P. J. BRANSON. 1982. Timing of periarterial blood removal for the prevention of vasonecrosis. Angiology **33:** 259–267.
40. ESPINOZA, F., B. WEIR, T. SHNITKA, T. OVERTON & D. BOISVERT. 1984. A randomized placebo-controlled double-blind trial of nimodipine after SAH in monkeys. J. Neurosurg. **60:** 1176–1185.
41. SMITH, R. R., B. R. CLOVER, G. M. GROTENDORST, N. YABUNO & J. M. CRUSE. 1985. Arterial wall changes in early human vasospasm. Neurosurgery **16:** 171–176.
42. GROTENHUIS, J. A., W. BETTAG, B. J. O. FIEBACH & K. DABIR. 1984. Intracarotid slow bolus injection of nimodipine during angiography for treatment of cerebral vasospasm after SAH. J. Neurosurg. **61:** 231–240.
43. TAKAHARA, K., A. KUROIWA, T. MATSUSHIMA, Y. NAKASHIMA & M. TAKASUGI. 1985. Effects of nifedipine on platelet function. Am. Heart J. **109:** 4–8.
44. ALLEN, G. S., H. S. AHN, T. J. PREZIOSI, R. BATTYE, S. C. BOONE, S. N. CHOU, D. L. KELLY, B. K. WEIR, R. A. CRABBE, P. J. LAVIK, S. B. ROSENBLOOM, F. C. DORSEY, C. R. INGRAM, D. E. MELLITS, L. A. BERTSCH, D. P. J. BOISVERT, M. B. HUNDLEY, R. K. JOHNSON, J. A. STROM & C. R. TRANSOU. 1983. Cerebral arterial spasm—a controlled trial of nimodipine in patients with subarachnoid hemorrhage. N. Engl. J. Med. **308:** 619–624.
45. AUER, L. M. 1984. Acute operation and preventive nimodipine improve outcome in patients with ruptured cerebral aneurysms. Neurosurgery **15:** 57–66.
46. LJUNGGREN, B., L. BRANDT, H. SÄVELAND, P. E. NILSSON, S. CRONQVIST, K. E. ANDERSSON & E. VINGE. 1984. Outcome in 60 consecutive patients treated with early aneurysm operation and intravenous nimodipine. J. Neurosurg. **61:** 864–873.
47. VINGE, E., K. E. ANDERSSON, L. BRANDT, B. LJUNGGREN, L. G. NILSSON & S. ROSENDAL-HELGESEN. 1986. Pharmacokinetics of nimodipine in patients with aneurysmal subarachnoid haemorrhage. Eur. J. Clin. Pharmacol. **30:** 421–425.
48. SÄVELAND, H., B. SONESSON, B. LJUNGGREN, L. BRANDT, T. USKI, S. ZYGMUNT & B. HINDFELT. 1986. Outcome evaluation following subarachnoid hemorrhage. J. Neurosurg. **64:** 191–196.

Clinical and Experimental Evidence for a Role of Calcium Entry Blockers in the Treatment of Migraine

EGILIUS L. H. SPIERINGS[a]

The Headache Research Foundation
The Faulkner Hospital
Allandale at Centre Street
Boston, Massachusetts 02130

INTRODUCTION

Migraine is a ubiquitous disorder with an estimated prevalence in modern western societies of 9% in men, 16% in women, and 3 to 4% in children.[1] It is a disorder characterized by the occurrence of attacks of which headache is the most constant feature. The attacks generally last from a couple of hours to a few days and can occur at a greatly varying frequency, up to as often as several times per week. The headache is usually severe in intensity and throbbing in nature with a preference for location in the temple, frequently one-sided but not necessarily so. It is often associated with symptoms like nausea, vomiting, photo- and phonophobia; in so-called *classical migraine* it is, in addition, preceded by transient focal neurological symptoms like the scintillating scotoma or digitolingual paresthesias (FIGURE 1) or variants thereof, generally known as aura symptoms.

The pathogenesis of migraine is basically unknown although over the last decades considerable knowledge has been acquired regarding the pathophysiology of the disorder.

The most widely accepted concept of the pathogenesis of migraine is that of Wolff,[2] which is schematically shown in FIGURE 2. It regards the mechanism underlying the headache as that of excessive dilation of blood vessels in the cranial noncerebral vascular bed. This vasodilation, in turn, occurs as an accompanying event of cerebral vasodilation which follows, as a reactive hyperemia, a phase of vasoconstriction-induced cerebral hypoxia. The cerebral hypoxia manifests itself in classical migraine in the transient focal neurological symptoms described above, and in common migraine, in which the headache is *not* preceded by such symptoms, it presumably takes place in a so-called clinically silent area of the cerebral cortex.

It is on the basis of Wolff's concept that the calcium entry blockers have been introduced into the treatment of migraine. The modes of action of the drugs considered relevant are their antivasoconstrictive effect and the protection they offer cerebral tissue against the deleterious effects of hypoxia.

In the following the clinical and experimental pharmacology of the calcium entry blockers will be reviewed and discussed, relevant to their efficacy in the treatment of migraine. The experimental pharmacology will be discussed against the background of the most recent advances in our knowledge of the pathophysiology of migraine, advances that have made an adaptation of Wolff's concept necessary.

[a]Also affiliated with the Department of Neurology, Tufts University School of Medicine.

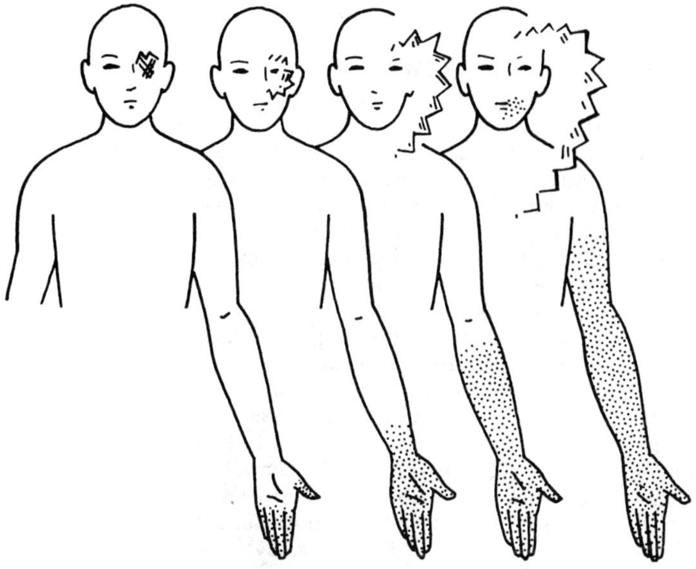

FIGURE 1. The two aura symptoms most characteristic of migraine, the scintillating scotoma and the digitolingual paresthesias, shown from left to right in their successive stages of development.

CLINICAL STUDIES

The calcium entry blockers that have been subjected to clinical studies in migraine are, in alphabetical order, diltiazem, flunarizine, nifedipine, nimodipine, and verapamil. Flunarizine has been investigated most extensively in both placebo-controlled and comparative studies. Of the other drugs only placebo-controlled studies are available, with the exception of *diltiazem* which has been examined in an open study only. This study concerned 9 patients with nadolol-resistant migraine who were treated with diltiazem 60 to 90 mg four times a day.[3] In the second month of treatment a significant decrease in mean headache score was observed but, although promising, this needs to be confirmed in double-blind placebo-controlled studies before any definite statement can be made regarding the drug's efficacy.

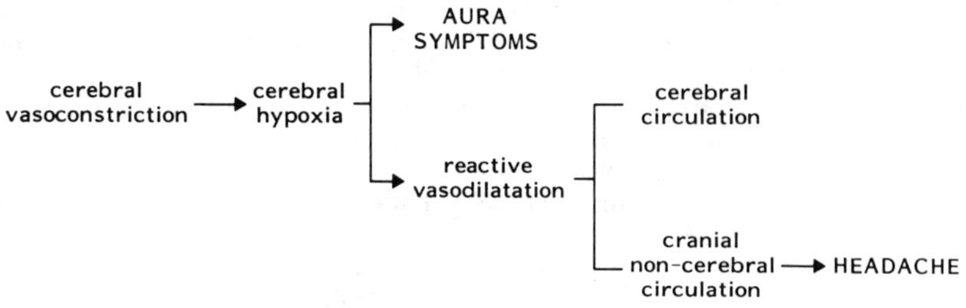

FIGURE 2. Wolff's vasoconstriction–cerebral hypoxia–vasodilation concept of the pathogenesis of the migraine attack.

FLUNARIZINE

The double-blind placebo-controlled studies of flunarizine that have been published to date are summarized in TABLE 1. Except for the one by Soelberg Sørensen *et al.*,[8] all made use of a so-called parallel or noncrossover design in which the participating patients received either flunarizine or placebo. In Soelberg Sørensen's study, which applied a crossover design, the patients received both flunarizine and placebo but successively and in randomized order. Such a study design has in general more power to detect differences as statistically significant, and also needs fewer patients. However, the duration of the study is longer resulting in a higher risk for dropouts, and the possibility of occurrence of carry-over and time-order effects complicates the analysis of the results.

A vital point of studies that make use of a parallel design is the comparability of the two groups. This is not necessarily guaranteed by the application of a randomization procedure in the assignment of the patients. A baseline observation period to collect prestudy data is therefore desirable to substantiate the claim for comparability. However, as is evident from the table, only one of the four parallel placebo-controlled studies of flunarizine in migraine included a baseline observation period!

The number of participating patients in the studies is relatively small, and this is also the case for the studies involving the other calcium entry blockers. Unfortunately in none of them except for Soelberg Sørensen's study[8] is mention made of the statistical power of the study which is closely related to the number of patients participating.

Most of the studies involved both classical and common migraine patients on the assumption that the two forms of migraine share a common pathogenesis, as inherent to Wolff's concept. However, Mendenopoulos *et al.* studied classical migraine only,[6] and Soelberg Sørensen *et al.* had only common migraine patients participate in the study.[8] The results obtained in these studies are basically similar and compare well with those of the studies with mixed patient groups.

With regard to the dose of flunarizine all studies except for the one performed in children[7] prescribed 10 mg per day, which is the standard dose for the drug. The children were given 5 mg per day which is also standard for that group. The duration of treatment was 3 to 4 months in all studies, and improvement in headache variables was generally not significant until the second month of treatment. This slow onset of the effect of flunarizine is possibly related to the long plasma half-life of the drug which is in the order of several weeks.

The improvement observed with flunarizine was in general most pronounced where it concerned the headache frequency. Reported percentages of improvement ranged from 39 to 66% and were significant in all studies. The highest rate of improvement was observed in the study of children with migraine. In contrast, significant improvement in headache duration was observed in two studies only and in intensity in one.

As mentioned earlier, the efficacy of flunarizine in the prophylactic treatment of migraine has also been studied in double-blind comparative studies. These studies are summarized in TABLE 2. In 4 out of the 5 studies the comparison was made with pizotifen which is a well-established prophylactic antimigraine drug.[14] It is an antiserotoninergic drug which also possesses antihistaminergic and anticholinergic properties. It was introduced into the treatment of migraine in 1967 as successor to methysergide, which at that time had been shown to have potentially serious side effects on prolonged use.

Pizotifen is widely used in Europe and Canada in the treatment of migraine, generally in doses of 1 to 3 mg per day; it is not available in the United States.

All comparative studies with pizotifen involved both patients with classical and common migraine. The dose of flunarizine varied from 9 to 15 mg and that of pizotifen

TABLE 1. Double-Blind Placebo-Controlled Studies of Flunarizine in the Prophylactic Treatment of Migraine[a]

Author(s)	Year	Study Design	Number of Patients: Flunarizine Group	Number of Patients: Placebo Group	Type of Migraine	Dose per Day	Baseline Observation Period	Treatment Periods	Results: Headache Frequency	Results: Headache Duration	Results: Headache Intensity
Louis[4]	1981	Parallel	29	29	Classical and common	10 mg	—	3 months	57%↓	NS	NS
Frenken and Nuyten[5]	1984	Parallel	17	18	Classical and common	10 mg	—	3 months	59% overall efficacy		
Mendenopoulos *et al.*[6]	1985	Parallel	9	11	Classical	10 mg	1 month	3 months	(50%)↓	↓	↓
Sorge and Marano[7]	1985	Parallel	24	24	Classical and common	5 mg (children)	—	3 months	66%↓	51%↓	—
Soelberg Sørensen *et al.*[8]	1986	Crossover	29		Common	10 mg	1 month	4 months	39%↓	NS	NS

[a] ↓ = significant decrease (percentage given in parentheses when applicable to last month of treatment only); NS = no significant change.

TABLE 2. Double-Blind Comparative Studies of Flunarizine in the Prophylactic Treatment of Migraine[a]

Author(s)	Year	Study Design	Drug of Comparison	Dose per Day	Number of Patients: Flunarizine Group	Number of Patients: Comparison Group	Type of Migraine	Baseline Observation Period	Treatment Periods	Headache Frequency: Flunarizine Group	Headache Frequency: Comparison Group
Drillisch and Girke[9]	1980	Parallel	Cinnarizine	9 mg vs. 225 mg	14	13	Classical	1½ months	3 months	36%↓	NS 44%↓
Louis and Spier-ings[10]	1982	Parallel	Pizotifen	10 mg vs. 2–3 mg	17	15	Classical and com-mon	—	4 months	54%↓	NS 45%↓
Wörz and Drillisch[11]	1983	Parallel	Pizotifen	10 mg vs. 2.2 mg	21	21	Classical and com-mon	?	3 months	—	NS —
Rascol *et al.*[12]	1986	Parallel	Pizotifen	10 mg vs. 2.2 mg	21	14	Classical and com-mon	—	4 months	(65%)↓	NS (45%)↓
Cerbo *et al.*[13]	1986	Crossover	Pizotifen	15 mg vs. 1.5 mg	18		Classical and com-mon	1 month	2 months	—	NS —

[a]↓ = significant decrease (percentage given in parentheses when applicable to last month of treatment only); NS = no significant difference between groups.

from 1.5 to 3. The duration of treatment was 2 to 3 months, and only one study included a baseline observation period.[13] This was also the only study that applied a crossover design, while the others made use of the parallel design.

In all studies the overall conclusion was that the drugs are comparably efficacious in the treatment of migraine. Some results for the effects on headache frequency are presented in the table, and in none of the studies were significant differences observed between the drugs. This was also the case when flunarizine was compared with its parent substance, cinnarizine.[9] Cinnarizine is an antihistamine drug with widespread use in Europe for the treatment of vertigo. It was examined in this initial study of flunarizine because of the antivasoconstrictive action it had been shown to share with that drug. Flunarizine was further developed for the treatment of migraine instead of cinnarizine especially because of its much longer plasma half-life allowing an easier dosage schedule and thereby assuring higher patient compliance.

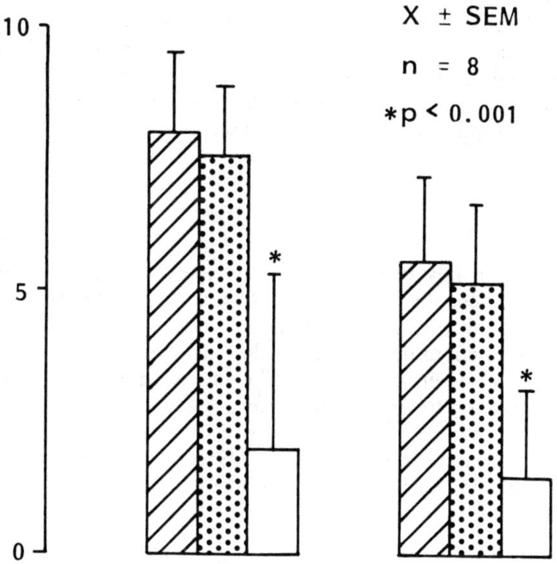

FIGURE 3. The effects of nifedipine on headache frequency (left-hand diagram) and headache intensity (right-hand diagram) as observed by Kahan *et al.*[15] in a double-blind crossover study in migraine (hatched column = baseline; dotted column = placebo; blank column = nifedipine 10 mg three times a day).

NIFEDIPINE

Nifedipine has been the subject of one double-blind placebo-controlled study in 8 patients with migraine associated with idiopathic Raynaud's phenomenon.[15] It concerns a crossover study with treatment periods of the duration of 1 month, preceded by a baseline observation period of 1 month. The dose of the drug was 30 mg per day. The results with regard to headache frequency and intensity are shown in FIGURE 3. In comparison both to baseline and placebo, a significant decrease in these variables was observed. However, the significance of these observations is compromised by the small number of patients involved and the short duration of treatment. The potential application of nifedipine in migraine is further hampered by the potent vasodilatory properties of the drug, causing considerable headaches as a side effect.

NIMODIPINE

Two double-blind placebo-controlled studies have been performed with nimodipine in the prophylactic treatment of migraine. They are summarized in TABLE 3. One is a parallel and one is a crossover study, both involving about the same number of patients with classical and common migraine. The dose prescribed was 120 mg per day and the duration of treatment amounted to 3 and 2 months, respectively. In the parallel study the treatment period was preceded by a baseline observation period of 2 weeks. In both studies a significant decrease in headache frequency and intensity was observed but not in headache duration. In the parallel study with a treatment duration of 3 months, an overall reduction in headache frequency was observed of 82%.

VERAPAMIL

Also of verapamil only two double-blind placebo-controlled studies have been performed to date. These studies are summarized in TABLE 4. They both applied the crossover design and involved only 12 and 14 patients, respectively. Patients with both classical and common migraine were included in the study. The dose of verapamil was 320 and 240 mg, respectively, and the duration of treatment 3 and 2 months. Only in the second study was the treatment preceded by a baseline observation period which lasted 1 month. In both studies a significant decrease in headache frequency was observed, in the first study in the amount of 49%. Only in the second study was a significant reduction in headache duration reported as well, while the headache intensity was unchanged in both.

WOLFF'S CONCEPT

As mentioned above, the modes of action of the calcium entry blockers considered relevant in their introduction into the treatment of migraine were their antivasoconstrictive effect and the protection they offer cerebral tissue against the deleterious effects of hypoxia. Both modes of action of the drugs have been demonstrated to occur on the basis of an interference with the influx of calcium into vascular smooth muscle cells and brain cells, respectively. Their potential efficacy in migraine was derived from Wolff's concept of the pathogenesis of the migraine attack in which vasoconstriction-induced cerebral hypoxia occupies a pivotal position (see FIGURE 2). However, this part of Wolff's concept, although central, stands on the feeble grounds of indirect evidence, predominantly pharmacological in nature. It concerns the results of experiments with the cerebral vasodilators carbon dioxide and amylnitrite on the development of the migraine aura. The experiments with carbon dioxide were conducted by Marcussen and Wolff and revealed a transient clearing of the symptoms, with return of the symptoms to their former intensity within 5 minutes after the inhalation of the gas was discontinued.[20] Cahan (in Schumacher and Wolff)[21] and Hare studied the effects

TABLE 3. Double-Blind Placebo-Controlled Studies of Nimodipine in the Prophylactic Treatment of Migraine[a]

			Number of Patients						Results		
Author(s)	Year	Study Design	Nimodipine Group	Placebo Group	Type of Migraine	Dose per Day	Baseline Observation Period	Treatment Periods	Headache Frequency	Headache Duration	Headache Intensity
Gelmers[16]	1983	Parallel	28	22	Classical and common	120 mg	2 weeks	3 months	82%↓	NS	↓
Havanka-Kanniainen *et al.*[17]	1985	Crossover	29		Classical and common	120 mg	—	2 months	↓	NS	↓

[a]↓ = significant decrease; NS = no significant change.

TABLE 4. Double-Blind Placebo-Controlled Studies of Verapamil in the Prophylactic Treatment of Migraine[a]

Author(s)	Year	Study Design	Number of Patients: Verapamil Group	Number of Patients: Placebo Group	Type of Migraine	Dose per Day	Baseline Observation Period	Treatment Periods	Results: Headache Frequency	Results: Headache Duration	Results: Headache Intensity
Solomon *et al.*[18]	1983	Crossover	12		Classical and common	320 mg	—	3 months	49%↓	—	—
Markley *et al.*[19]	1984	Crossover	14		Classical and common	240 mg	1 month	2 months	↓	↓	NS

[a] ↓ = significant decrease; NS = no significant change.

of amylnitrite on the development of their own migraine aura symptoms and also observed a transient clearing of the symptoms after inhalation of the drug.[22]

SPREADING DEPRESSION

Relatively accurate measurement of the cerebral blood flow to provide more direct evidence for Wolff's concept was not possible until the development of the Xenon clearance technique in the 1970s. The initial studies performed with this technique revealed the aura symptoms to be accompanied by a decrease in cerebral blood flow, but this decrease was generalized and bilateral despite the focal and lateralized nature of the symptoms, and also outlasted the duration of these symptoms (TABLE 5).

It took more than a decade and significant sophistication of the technique to show that the generalized decrease in cerebral blood flow was but the final step in a series of changes. These changes consisted of an initial increase in cerebral blood flow in the parietooccipital area, followed by a decrease and a gradual spreading of the decrease toward the frontal pole (FIGURE 4).[26,27] The decrease amounted to approximately 25%[27] and was considered not to be enough to cause brain cell dysfunction by ischemia, and therefore was referred to as oligemia. The rate of forward spreading of the oligemia was calculated to be in the order of and probably somewhat above 2.2 mm/minute.[27]

TABLE 5. Cerebral Blood Flow Changes of the Migraine Aura: Initial Observations

Author(s)	Observations	Comments
O'Brien[23]	18.5% ↓; $n = 6$	Changes generalized rather than focal, outlasted the duration of the symptoms and did not correlate with their laterality
O'Brien[24]	23% ↓; $n = 7$	Changes bilateral and diffuse over both hemispheres
Mathew *et al.*[25]	3/3 ↓	Changes diffuse over most of the hemispheres

The particular nature of the cerebral blood flow changes of the migraine aura and the rate of propagation of the oligemia, instead of supporting Wolff's concept, brought back a hypothesis formulated by Milner in 1958.[28] This hypothesis suggested the aura symptoms of migraine not to be caused by a primary vascular event, as Wolff suggested, but by a primary dysfunction of brain cells, described by Leão in 1944 as "spreading depression."[29] Spreading depression is, as the name implies, a wave of inhibition of the "spontaneous" cortical neuronal activity[29] which travels over the cerebral cortex at a rate of 2 to 5 mm/minute.[30] It is preceded by a short-lasting phase of intense neuronal activity,[30] and the vascular changes accompanying it are likewise an increase in cerebral blood flow of short duration followed by a long-lasting decrease.[31] The decrease in cerebral blood flow amounts to the order of 20 to 25%,[31] which is very similar to that of the spreading oligemia described above.

Thus, a similarity has been established on three levels between the vascular changes of the migraine aura and those of the spreading depression, i.e., (1) the nature of the vascular changes, (2) the depth of the decrease in cerebral blood flow, and (3) the rate of spreading of this decrease over the cerebral cortex. In addition, Gardner-Medwin has demonstrated that inhalation of carbon dioxide has the capacity of calling to a halt the development of a spreading depression after its initiation,[32] taking away the necessity to assume a vascular pathogenesis on the basis of Marcussen and Wolff's carbon dioxide experiments.

WOLFF'S CONCEPT ADAPTED

Simple incorporation into Wolff's concept of the spreading depression as the underlying mechanism of the migraine aura is not possible for two reasons: (1) there is no evidence that a spreading depression can be induced by ischemia,[33] and (2) as described above, the spreading depression is not followed by vasodilation but by prolonged vasoconstriction and decreased cerebral blood flow.[31] An adaptation of Wolff's concept to include the spreading depression is therefore necessary and a suggestion for this is presented in FIGURE 5. To be able to include the spreading depression, however, the pathogenesis of the aura symptoms has to be disconnected from that of the headache. The result is a concept in which these pathogenetic mechanisms take place as parallel rather than as sequential processes. Such a parallel

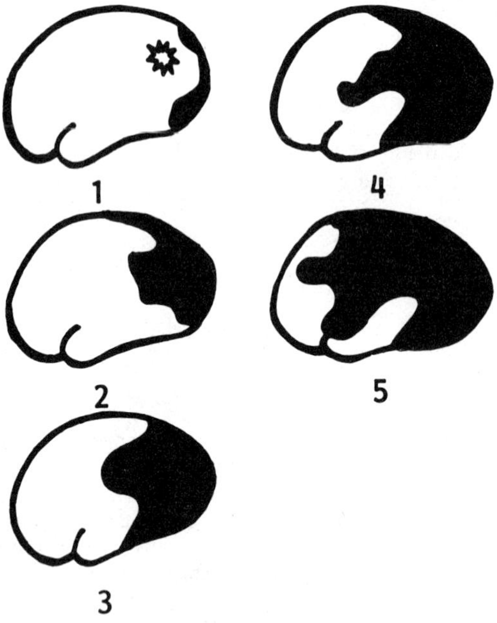

FIGURE 4. Schematic representation of the cerebral blood flow changes of the migraine aura which have recently been shown to consist of a short-lasting increase in the parietooccipital area (*), followed by a decrease and a gradual spreading of the decrease toward the frontal pole.[26,27]

occurrence also better explains the emergence of headache without aura symptoms, as in common migraine, as well as the isolated occurrence of the aura symptoms. The latter has been referred to by Fisher as transient migrainous accompaniments[34] (TMAs) and was termed by me isolated neurological migraine accompaniments[35] (INMAs), in the older age group an important differential diagnostic consideration against transient ischemic attacks (TIAs).

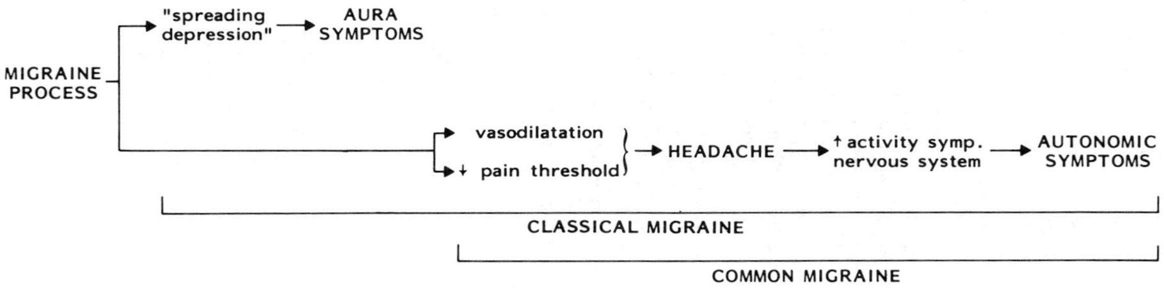

FIGURE 5. Adaptation of Wolff's concept of the pathogenesis of the migraine attack with inclusion of the spreading depression as the underlying mechanism of the migraine aura. Note that in this concept the pathogenetic processes underlying the migraine aura and headache are viewed as parallel rather than as sequential, and that the concept also includes an explanation of the autonomic symptoms of migraine.

The adapted concept also includes a possible pathogenetic mechanism for the autonomic symptoms that are usually present in abundance both in classical and common migraine. They are viewed as caused by an increase in sympathetic nervous system activity secondary to the headache. That the sympathetic nervous system is in a state of heightened activity during the migraine attack is supported by ample biochemical evidence.[36]

EPILOGUE

Of the calcium entry blockers, flunarizine has recently been shown to interfere with the initiation and propagation of spreading depression.[37] In view of the above-presented adaptation of Wolff's concept, this might be a more relevant mode of action of the drug than its antivasoconstrictive and cerebral hypoxia protective effects.[38] However, because of the parallel sequence of the pathogenetic processes of the migraine aura and headache, it would explain neither the drug's efficacy in classical migraine beyond the aura, nor that in common migraine. Of course, it is possible that the above-suggested adaptation of Wolff's concept is incorrect, but it is equally possible that the relevant mode of action of the calcium entry blockers in migraine still has to emerge from the wealth of pharmacological properties of these drugs.

REFERENCES

1. GOLDSTEIN, M. & T. C. CHEN. 1982. The epidemiology of disabling headache. Adv. Neurol. **33:** 377–390.
2. WOLFF, H. G. 1980. Headache and Other Head Pain. D. J. Dalessio, Ed. 4th edit. Oxford University Press. New York, N.Y.
3. SMITH, R. & A. SCHWARTZ. 1984. Diltiazem prophylaxis in refractory migraine. N. Engl. J. Med. **310:** 1327–1328.
4. LOUIS, P. 1981. A double-blind placebo-controlled prophylactic study of flunarizine (Sibelium®) in migraine. Headache **21:** 235–239.
5. FRENKEN, C. W. G. M. & S. T. M. NUIJTEN. 1984. Flunarizine, a new preventive approach to migraine. A double-blind comparison with placebo. Clin. Neurol. Neurosurg. **86:** 17–20.
6. MENDENOPOULOS, G., T. MANAFI, I. LOGOTHETIS & S. BOSTANTJOPOULOU. 1985. Flunarizine in the prevention of classical migraine: a placebo-controlled evaluation. Cephalalgia **5:** 31–37.
7. SORGE, F. & E. MARANO. 1985. Flunarizine v. placebo in childhood migraine. A double-blind study. Cephalalgia **5**(Suppl. 2): 145–148.
8. SOELBERG SØRENSEN, P., K. HANSEN & J. OLESEN. 1986. A placebo-controlled, double-blind, cross-over trial of flunarizine in common migraine. Cephalalgia **6:** 7–14.
9. DRILLISCH, C. & W. GIRKE. 1980. Ergebnisse der Behandlung von Migräne-Patienten mit Cinnarizin und Flunarizin. Med. Welt **31:** 1870–1872.
10. LOUIS, P. & E. L. H. SPIERINGS. 1982. Comparison of flunarizine (Sibelium®), and pizotifen (Sandomigran®), in migraine treatment: a double-blind study. Cephalalgia **2:** 197–203.
11. WÖRZ, R. & C. DRILLISCH. 1983. Migräne-Prophylaxe durch einen Kalziumeintrittsblocker. Münch. Med. Wschr. **125:** 3–9.
12. RASCOL, A., J. L. MONTASTRUC & O. RASCOL. 1986. Flunarizine versus pizotifen: a double-blind study in the prophylaxis of migraine. Headache **2:** 83–85.
13. CERBO, R., M. CASACCHIA, R. FORMISANO, M. FELICIANI, G. CUSIMANO, M. G. BUZZI & A. AGNOLI. 1986. Flunarizine-pizotifen single-dose double-blind cross-over trial in migraine prophylaxis. Cephalalgia **6:** 15–18.
14. SPIERINGS, E. L. H. 1984. Drugs for the prevention of migraine. W. H. O. Drug Bull. Rev. (6): 1–6.

15. KAHAN, A., S. WEBER, B. AMOR, F. GUERIN & M. DEGEORGES. 1983. Nifedipine in the treatment of migraine in patients with Raynaud's phenomenon. N. Engl. J. Med. **308:** 1102–1103.
16. GELMERS, H. J. 1983. Nimodipine, a new calcium antagonist, in the prophylactic treatment of migraine. Headache **23:** 106–109.
17. HAVANKA-KANNIAINEN, H., E. HOKKANEN & V. V. MYLLYLÄ. 1985. Efficacy of nimodipine in the prophylaxis of migraine. Cephalalgia **5:** 39–43.
18. SOLOMON, G. D., J. G. STEEL & L. J. SPACCAVENTO. 1983. Verapamil prophylaxis of migraine. A double-blind, placebo-controlled study. J. Am. Med. Assoc. **250:** 2500–2502.
19. MARKLEY, H. G., J. C. D. CHERONIS & R. W. PIEPHO. 1984. Verapamil in prophylactic therapy of migraine. Neurology **34:** 973–976.
20. MARCUSSEN, R. M. & H. G. WOLFF. 1950. Studies on headache. 1. Effects of carbon-dioxide mixture given during preheadache phase of the migraine attack. 2. Further analysis of pain mechanisms in headache. Arch. Neurol. Psychiatr. **63:** 42–51.
21. SCHUMACHER, G. A. & H. G. WOLFF. 1941. Experimental studies on headache. A. Contrast of histamine headache with the headache of migraine and that associated with hypertension. B. Contrast of vascular mechanisms in preheadache and in headache phenomena of migraine. Arch. Neurol. Psychiatr. **45:** 199–214.
22. HARE, E. H. 1966. Personal observations on the spectral march of migraine. J. Neurol. Sci. **3:** 259–264.
23. O'BRIEN, M. D. 1971. The relationship between aura symptoms and cerebral blood flow changes in the prodrome of migraine. *In* Proceedings of the International Headache Symposium. D. J. Dalessio *et al.*, Eds.: 141–143. Sandoz. Basel, Switzerland.
24. O'BRIEN, M. D. 1971. Cerebral blood changes in migraine. Headache **10:** 139–143.
25. MATHEW, N. T., F. HRASTNIK & J. S. MEYER. 1976. Regional cerebral blood flow in the diagnosis of vascular headache. Headache **15:** 252–260.
26. OLESEN, J., B. LARSEN & M. LAURITZEN. 1980. Focal hyperemia followed by spreading oligemia and impaired activation of rCBF in classic migraine. Ann. Neurol. **9:** 344–352.
27. LAURITZEN, M., T. S. OLSEN, N. A. LASSEN & A. B. PAULSON. 1983. Changes in regional cerebral blood flow during the course of classic migraine attacks. Ann. Neurol. **13:** 633–641.
28. MILNER, P. M. 1958. Note on a possible correspondence between the scotomas of migraine and spreading depression of Leão. EEG Clin. Neurophysiol. **10:** 705.
29. LEÃO, A. A. P. 1944. Spreading depression of activity in the cerebral cortex. J. Neurophysiol. **7:** 359–390.
30. GRAFSTEIN, B. 1956. Mechanism of spreading cortical depression. J. Neurophysiol. **19:** 154–171.
31. LAURITZEN, M., M. B. JØRGENSEN, N. H. DIEMER, A. GJEDDE & A. J. HANSEN. 1982. Persistent oligemia of rat cerebral cortex in the wake of spreading depression. Ann. Neurol. **12:** 469–474.
32. GARDNER-MEDWIN, A. R. 1981. The effect of carbon dioxide and oxygen on Leão's spreading depression: evidence supporting a relationship to migraine. J. Physiol. **316:** 23P–24P.
33. LEÃO, A. P. P. 1947. Further observations on the spreading depression of activity in the cerebral cortex. J. Neurophysiol. **10:** 409–419.
34. FISHER, C. M. 1980. Late-life migraine accompaniments as a cause of unexplained transient ischemic attacks. Can. J. Neurol. Sci. **7:** 9–17.
35. SPIERINGS, E. L. H. 1986. Migraine. Sandoz. Uden, the Netherlands.
36. SPIERINGS, E. L. H. 1980. The Pathophysiology of the Migraine Attack. Stafleu's Scientific Publishing Co. Alphen aan den Ryn, the Netherlands.
37. WAUQUIER, A., D. ASHTON & R. MARRANES. 1985. The effects of flunarizine in experimental models related to the pathogenesis of migraine. Cephalalgia **5**(Suppl. 2): 119–120.
38. AMERY, W. K., A. WAUQUIER, J. M. VAN NUETEN, F. DECLERCK, J. V. VAN TREEMPTS & P. A. J. JANSSEN. 1981. The anti-migrainous pharmacology of flunarizine (R 14950), a calcium antagonist. Drugs Exp. Clin. Res. **7:** 1–10.

Calcium Entry Blockers in the Treatment of Vertigo

J. OLESEN

Department of Neurology
Gentofte Hospital
University of Copenhagen
DK-2900 Hellerup, Denmark

INTRODUCTION

Vertigo is a symptom, not a disease. Whenever possible, a more precise diagnosis should always be used. The essence of vertigo is a feeling of illusionary movement. Either the subject feels that the surroundings move or that he moves in relation to the surroundings. The illusionary movement is either rotatory or nautic. Dizziness is a much more imprecise word which is used for uncharacteristic sensations of imbalance, lightheadedness, incipient fainting, or ataxia. Very frequently it is observed in nervous individuals, mostly as a manifestation of anxiety and sometimes associated with hyperventilation.

Vertigo can arise from lesions in the central nervous system, particularly in the nuclei of the vestibular nerve, the cerebellum, and the connections between cerebellar and vestibular nuclei. More frequently, vertigo is labyrinthine, i.e., caused by disturbance of the vestibular end organ in the inner ear. Menière's disease and vertigo cephalostatica are the main forms, but many patients with suspected labyrinthine vertigo cannot be classified. Neuritis nervi verstibularis has a typical clinical picture and is caused by a mononeuritis of the vestibular nerve.

In view of the difficulties with the classification of patients with vertigo, it is fortunate that a number of experimental procedures can be used to study labyrinthine function in normal man. From such studies much can be learned about the effect of drugs used against vertigo. Flunarizine,[1] its congener cinnarizine,[2] and nimodipine[3] are calcium entry blockers (CEBs) that, unlike most other CEBs, act preferentially at the cerebral level. These are the only CEBs that have been studied in patients with vertigo. The present paper surveys published animal work and clinical experience with flunarizine and nimodipine. Cinnarizine is not included since it has presumably the same mechanism of action as flunarizine although it is less potent in terms of vestibular depression.[4]

VESTIBULAR STUDIES IN ANIMALS

Effects of CEBs on Labyrinthine Function

Rabbits are usual laboratory animals for studying vestibular effects of drugs. After a single intraperitoneal injection of 1.25 to 40 mg/kg of flunarizine, the duration of rotation-induced nystagmus was reduced from 10 mg/kg on by 20 to 25%. Higher doses did not induce a further reduction. The effect lasted at least 2 hours after dosing.[4] In a similar rabbit model, no important effects were observed in the electronystagmograms (ENGs) some (unspecified) time after a single intravenous injection of 10 mg of flunarizine. Chronic oral dosing at 5 mg three times a day, however, reduced the nystagmus frequency by a mean of 12% and increased the amplitude by 7%.[5] The caloric-induced nystagmus was significantly reduced both in beat frequency (−26%) and duration of nystagmus (−24%) after the intravenous (iv) administration of 5 mg/kg.[6] Nimodipine, dosed at 1 and 10 mg iv, did not essentially change ENGs after rotatory stimulus.[5] Studies after chronic dosing or after higher single doses have not been reported.

Effects on Vestibular Compensation

A unilateral lesion of labyrinthine receptors results in a vestibular compensatory process. The effect of repeated oral flunarizine administrations on this process was studied in pharmacologically hemilabyrinthectomized guinea pigs, showing typical vigorous vestibular symptoms (nystagmus, head oscillations).[7] Flunarizine significantly accelerated vestibular compensation; 6, 18, and 24 hours after the labyrinthectomy, the frequency of nystagmus was reduced (versus hour 1) by >70%, >95%, and 100% after oral dosing with either 5 or 10 mg/kg of flunarizine versus 28%, 58%, and 75% in the control group. The drug effects on vestibular compensations were irreversible.

Effects after Vertebral Occlusion

Occlusion of a vertebral artery in dogs simulates the condition in patients with vertebrobasilar insufficiency. The rotation-induced nystagmus increases in frequency whereas the amplitude decreases corresponding to the ENG "petite écritine" of patients with vertebrobasilar insufficiency. The effects of 5 mg fluarizine iv and 10 mg nimodipine iv were evaluated in this model.[5] After total occlusion of the artery, the frequency of rotatory nystagmus was almost doubled, whereas the amplitude was reduced by >70%. Both drugs virtually normalized (≤15% difference with normal value) these parameters.

CLINICAL STUDIES

In Normal Subjects

The vestibular depressant effect of flunarizine has been confirmed in 4 double-blind, crossover comparisons with placebo or other vestibular drugs.[4,8–10] A single oral dose of 10 mg reduced the duration of nystagmus maximally 2.5 hours after intake (25%). A dose of 30 mg gave a similar reduction, both being significantly more effective than 45 mg cinnarizine. The reduction of the peak velocity of the nystagmus phase duration correlated well with the effect on nystagmus duration.[4] Comparable results were found by Lee *et al.*[9] Flunarizine, 10 or 30 mg, suppressed nystagmus more effectively than 5 mg prochlorperazine maleate or placebo, and caused no central depressive side effects. The effect of flunarizine lasted up to 10 hours after drug application. A high oral dose of 50 mg flunarizine significantly reduced the angular velocity of the slow phase of a caloric-induced nystagmus as compared with placebo. The peak reduction was comparable to that of naftidrofuryl but superior to that of bencyclane.[8] At this high dose of flunarizine, most volunteers reported sedation. After 1 week of dosing at 5 mg twice a day, flunarizine reduced the amplitude of the fast phase of rotational-induced nystagmus in a double-blind crossover study vs. placebo.[10]

In Vertigo Patients

Labyrinthine Vertigo

Two open and 6 double-blind studies[11–18] have been published on the response of the vestibular function and/or labyrinthine vertigo to oral treatment with flunarizine (TABLE 1). More than 250 patients with peripheral vestibular disorders and vertigo as essential symptom were treated. Controlled studies mainly included placebo as reference substance. Except in one vestibular study,[12] all patients were treated for 4 to 8 weeks mostly with a dose of 10 mg daily. In some studies, patients were started on a loading dose. In a pilot study, 4 patients with Menière's disease were treated with 30 mg nimodipine three times a day for 12 weeks.[19]

Response of Vertigo. Of the 258 patients treated with flunarizine, 230 or 81% responded favorably. Usually, associated symptoms such as tinnitus, neurovegetative symptoms, and equilibrium disorders significantly improved as well.[11,13,14,16] As a rule, a clear-cut treatment effect was observed within one month.

In three studies, the initial open run in period was followed by a double-blind placebo-controlled study phase.[15–17] The flunarizine-treated patients further improved whereas placebo-treated patients relapsed. Both the number and duration of attacks[15,16] as well as the severity of the vertigo[16] responded significantly better under flunarizine as compared to placebo. Tinnitus also improved but failed to reach statistical significance.[16] In a parallel designed placebo-controlled trial in 107 patients, however, accompanying neurovegetative symptoms, tinnitus, and hearing deficits improved significantly more on flunarizine than on placebo.[11] Flunarizine was significantly superior to nicergoline in a double-blind crossover study.[14] Vertigo, tinnitus, and hearing symptoms normalized in 3 of 4 patients with Menière's disease, treated in an open study with nimodipine for 12 weeks.[19]

Vestibular Function. Vestibular testing, often complemented by neurootological examinations, was performed in 6 studies, included recording of spontaneous, rotation- or caloric-induced nystagmus.[11–14,17,18] Some investigators specified the response of discrete ENG parameters such as the velocity of the slow nystagmus phase[12] or the asymmetry in the velocity step response to rotation, the latter in vertigo patients with a proven hyperventilation syndrome.[18] Others combined different parameters (frequency, amplitude, duration) into a single index.[11,13,14,17] All workers showed that flunarizine displayed significant vestibular depressant activity; both spontaneous and induced nystagmus were reduced. One author found that flunarizine tended to normalize both vestibular hyper- and hypoexcitability.[17]

Vertigo of "Central" Origin

A number of studies with CEBs have been performed in patients with vertigo of central nervous system etiology.[5,20–25] Most of these patients were apparently elderly persons with early dementia, previous cerebrovascular accidents, or so-called vertebro-

TABLE 1. Clinical Studies with CEBs in Labyrinthine Vertigo

Source	Trial Design[a]	CEB[b]	Daily Dose (mg)	Duration (weeks)	Results[d]	
					Vestibular Testing[e]	Vertigo
Elbaz[11]	DB vs. placebo	FNZ	10	8	Spontaneous N: improvement in 65% ($p = 0.01$) Caloric N: improvement in 69% ($p < 0.001$)	In 90% improved ($p = 0.003$) In 47% disappeared ($p = 0.05$)
Mangabeira[12]	DBCO vs. placebo	FNZ	60	0.5	Caloric N: velocity: −55% ($p < 0.05$)	—
Materna[13]	O	FNZ	10[c]	8	N index: −35%	Symptom score: −60%
Materna[14]	DBCO vs. nicergolin	FNZ	10[c]	4	N index: −41% to 53% ($p < 0.05$)	Symptom score: −84% ($p < 0.001$)
Oosterveld[15]	O + DB vs. placebo	FNZ	20[c]	12	—	Number of attacks, duration of attacks decreased in 10/13 ($p < 0.01$)
Oosterveld[16]	O + DBCO vs. placebo	FNZ	10	10	—	Severity, frequency and duration improved ($p < 0.05$)
Schwerdtfeger[17]	O + DB vs. placebo	FNZ	10[c]	6	In 79%: normalization of hyper- or hypoexcitability	—
Theunissen[18]	O	FNZ	10	4–6	Rotation N: decrease in asymmetry in velocity-step response	Improved in 11/14
Theopold[19]	O	NIM	90	12	—	3/4 patients: improved

[a] DB = double-blind; O = open; CO = crossover.
[b] FNZ = flunarizine; NIM = nimodipine.
[c] Starting dose was higher.
[d] Results of open runin not given; p values: only p values vs. control group are given.
[e] N = nystagmus.

basilar insufficiency (TABLE 2). In these studies, nearly 1000 patients were treated with flunarizine at a daily dose of 10 mg during maintenance treatment in most patients. A single dose of 40 mg or a maintenance dose of 3 × 40 mg was given in two electronystagmographic nimodipine studies in 10 and 9 patients respectively.[5]

Response of Vertigo. Of 60 patients with vertebrobasilar insufficiency, 54 patients or 90% responded favorably to flunarizine,[21,22] being significantly superior to sulpiride in a double-blind crossover study.[22] Despite a pronounced placebo effect in elderly patients with dizziness, significantly better results were obtained with flunarizine in several studies.[20,23,24] The interim data of a placebo-controlled trial revealed a marked improvement under nimodipine as compared to placebo, whereas based on similar parameters, flunarizine proved to be markedly better than pentoxifylline.[5]

ENG results. In patients with vertebrobasilar insufficiency, the ENG characteristics with a low amplitude and a high frequency improved in parallel with the clinical effects of flunarizine.[21] Similar findings have been reported for nimodipine, although the number of documented patients is low. Both the duration and the speed of the slow nystagmus phase were significantly reduced in 9 flunarizine patients as compared to 9 elderly vertigo patients treated with placebo.[20]

DISCUSSION

Flunarizine proved to be effective in both experimental vertigo of labyrinthine genesis and in double-blind trials in patients with labyrinthine vertigo. No direct vestibulodepressant effect has been described for nimodipine whereas the clinical experience is limited to a few patients, not allowing valid conclusions on the latter drug at the moment.

A number of studies in patients with vertigo of central nervous system etiology suggest that flunarizine is effective in those patients too. Comparative studies in this area reveal that the level of proof for flunarizine is at least as good as that for other substances. According to one author, nimodipine seems to give similar results, but here too, a lack of controlled data prevents final conclusions.

The calcium entry blocker flunarizine has some antihistamine activity.[1] It is therefore uncertain whether flunarizine exerts its action on the vestibular system through a calcium entry blockade. A number of antihistamines without effects on calcium entry have been shown to be effective in vertigo.[26] They have an anticholinergic and sedative effect too, however, the former not being the case for flunarizine. Moreover, flunarizine revealed a clear vestibulodepressant effect at doses that did not induce any sedative effects[4] and was more effective than prochlorperazine at sedating doses. Besides, if a histamine-1 antagonism were the primary determinant of antivertigo efficacy, affinity for H_1 receptors would be well correlated with clinical effect. As far as we know, no such correlation has been demonstrated. A vestibulodepressant effect is not limited to drugs with an H_1-antagonistic activity.[8,27,28] Apart from flunarizine, the effect of calcium entry blockers on the vestibular system has hardly been studied. Nimodipine was ineffective in a model in which flunarizine showed no significant effect either,[5] not excluding therefore an effect of nimodipine at higher doses or in other models. Moreover, flunarizine and nimodipine belong to a different class of calcium entry blockers[29] so that importantly different effects on certain organs or cells may be expected. Ca ions play an essential role in the vestibular function. Cerebellar calcium-binding protein found in cochlear and vestibular hair cells of the

TABLE 2. Clinical Studies with CEBs in Vertigo of Central Nervous System Etiology

Source	Trial Design[a]	CEB[b]	Daily Dose (mg)	Duration (weeks)	Results[d]: Vestibular Testing[e]	Results[d]: Vertigo
Boniver[20]	DB vs. placebo	FNZ	10[c]	12	Rotation (caloric) N: duration −15% (−20%); $p < 0.01$ velocity −20% (−19%); $p < 0.01$	Disappeared in 9/9 patients ($p = 0.02$ after 2 months)
Hofferberth[21]	O	FNZ	20	8	Rotation and caloric N: reduced in 17/20	Improved in 85%
Hofferberth[22]	DBCO vs. sulpiride 150 mg	FNZ	21	8	Rotation N: frequency, −30%; sulpiride, no effect	In 88% good or excellent result ($p < 0.001$)
Hofferberth[5]	O	NIM	40	Single dose	Rotation N: frequency, −41%	—
	DB vs. placebo	NIM	120	4	Rotation N: frequency, −32%	Symptom score: −62%
Nelson[23]	DB vs. placebo	FNZ	10[c]	12	—	Improved in 83% ($p < 0.001$)
Staessen[24]	O	FNZ	20	8	—	Improved
	DB vs. placebo	FNZ	10[c]	16	—	Improved in 93% ($p_c < 0.05$)
Zissis[25]	DB vs. placebo	FNZ	10	12	—	Symptom score: −57%

[a] DB = double-blind; O = open; CO = crossover.
[b] FNZ = flunarizine; NIM = nimodipine.
[c] Starting dose was higher.
[d] Results of open runin not given; p values: only p values vs. control group are given.
[e] N = nystagmus.

rat was suggested to prevent excessive concentrations of intracellular calcium.[30] Calcium entry blockers may correct such a system if insufficient. Experimentally induced endolymphatic hydrops in guinea pigs was accompanied by an increased Ca^{2+} level in light cells and melanocytes of the vestibular organ.[31]

A normalization of ENG deviations in vertebrobasilar insufficiency models does not prove a direct effect on the vestibular system. In those models, the circulatory effects of calcium entry blockers may be responsible. On balance, it is not unlikely that the calcium entry blocking properties of flunarizine explain its antivertigo effect, but further studies of its mechanism of action are needed. Also in the etiology of Menière's disease, a labyrinthine type of vertigo, microvascular mechanisms have been suggested to be responsible.[32] Flunarizine-induced increase of blood flow in the radiating arterioles of cochlea of the guinea pig may be relevant in this regard.[6]

SUMMARY

Few calcium entry blockers have been studied in the treatment of vertigo. Flunarizine and cinnarizine are the most extensively studied substances. They have been shown to be valuable drugs in the therapeutic approach to vertigo. A few pilot studies have been performed with nimodipine but controlled data are lacking.

Flunarizine has a direct long-lasting vestibulodepressant effect in both animals and humans. In patients with labyrinthine vertigo, it produced a marked symptomatic relief of symptoms significantly exceeding the effects of placebo or nicergoline. A number of studies dealing with vertigo of central etiology were also positive. Patient selection in such trials, however, is doomed to be less precise so that cautiousness must be exerted in interpreting such studies. The level of proof for flunarizine is still as good as for other substances or better.

It is discussed whether the effects are due to calcium entry blocking properties.

REFERENCES

1. HOLMES, B., R. N. BROGDEN, R. C. HEEL, T. M. SPEIGHT & G. S. AVERY. 1984. Flunarizine: a review of its pharmacodynamic and pharmacokinetic properties and therapeutic use. Drugs **27:** 6–44.
2. TOWSE, G. 1980. Cinnarizine—a labyrinthine sedative. J. Laryngol. Otol. **94:** 1009–1015.
3. BETZ, E., K. DECK & F. HOFFMEISTER, Eds. 1985. Nimodipine. Pharmacological and clinical properties. F.K Schattauer Verlag. Stuttgart, FRG.
4. OOSTERVELD, W. J. 1974. Vestibular pharmacology of flunarizine compared to that of cinnarizine. ORL **36:** 157–164.
5. HOFFERBERTH, B. 1986. Calcium entry blockers in the treatment of vertebrobasilar insufficiency. Eur. Neurol. **25**(S1): 80–85.
6. SHIOZAKI, S., K. KUBO, K. SHUTO & N. NAKAMIZO. 1982. Effects of flunarizine on nystagmus and cochlear blood flow. Folia Pharmacol. Jpn **80:** 429–439.
7. TOLU, E. & O. MAMELI. 1984. Pharmacological improvement of vestibular plasticity. Effects of a Ca^{2+}-antagonist agent. Pharmacol. Res. Commun. **16:** 1161–1173.
8. SCHERER, H., E. SCHMIDTMAYER & H. HIRCHE. 1978. Die Wirkung von Bencyclan, Flunarizin und Naftidrofuryl auf den Nystagmus eines kalorischen Dauerreizes. Laryngol. Rhinol. Otol. **57:** 773–778.
9. LEE, J. A., L. A. WATSON & G. BOOTHBY. 1986. Calcium antagonists in the prevention of motion sickness. Aviat. Space Environ. Med. **57:** 45–48.
10. ELL, J. & M. GRESTY. 1983. The effects of the "vestiblar sedative" drug, flunarizine upon the vestibular and oculomotor systems. J. Neurol. Neurosurg. Psychiatry **46:** 716–724.

11. ELBAZ, P., J.-P. HAGUENAUER, H. MULER & M. PORTMANN. 1986. Activité thérapeutique d'un inhibiteur de la surcharge calcique, la flunarizine, dans les troubles vestibulaires: etude a double-insu contre placebo. ORL **35:** 301–308.
12. MANGABEIRA-ALBERNAZ, P. L., M. M. GANANCA, N. F. NOVO & E. R. DE PAIVA. 1978. Flunarizine and cinnarizine as vestibular depressants. A statistical study. ORL **40:** 92–100.
13. MATERNA, F. 1981. Erfahrungen mit Flunarizin. Med. Welt **32:** 1157–1160.
14. MATERNA, F. 1985. Leitsymptom Schwindel: Vergleichsstudie mit Flunarizin und Nicergolin. Med. Klin. **80:** 292–295.
15. OOSTERVELD, W. J. 1974. Pilot evaluation of fluarizine (R 14950) in vertigo—a double-blind trial. J. Otolaryngol. **3:** 284–290.
16. OOSTERVELD, W. J. 1982. Flunarizine in vertigo. A double-blind placebo-controlled cross-over evaluation of a constant-dose schedule. ORL **44:** 72–80.
17. SCHWERDTFEGER, J. F. 1978. Disturbed vestibular function. Arztl. Prax. **30:** 451–452.
18. THEUNISSEN, E. J. J. M., P. L. M. HUYGEN & M. G. M. NICOLASEN. 1986. Flunarizine treatment in dizzy patients with vestibular hyperreactivity and hyperventilation. ORL **48:** 203–208.
19. THEOPOLD, H. M. 1985. Nimodipin (Bay e 9736) ein neues Therapiekonzept bei Innenohrerkrankungen? Laryngol. Rhinol. Otol. **64:** 609–613.
20. BONIVER, R. 1978. Vertigo, particularly of vascular origin, treated with flunarizine (R 14950). Arzneim. Forsch./Drug Res. **28:** 1800–1804.
21. HOFFERBERTH, B. 1980. Die Anwendung von Flunarizin bei Patienten mit vertebrobasilärer Insuffizienz. Erfahrungen aus einer Pilotstudie. Arzneim. Forsch./Drug Res. **30:** 1817–1819.
22. HOFFERBERTH, B. & K. H. GROTEMEYER. 1985. Flunarizin und Sulpiridein Vergleich zweier gebräuchlicher Antivertiginosa bei vertebrobasilärbedingtem Schwindel. Nervenarzt **56:** 553–559.
23. NELSON, M., G. DEWITZ, J. DOM & C. HORIG. 1978. Prüfung der Wirksamkeit von Sibelium (Flunarizin) bei Durchblutungsstörungen. Med. Welt **29:** 1175–1181.
24. STAESSEN, A. J. 1977. Treatment of circulatory disturbances with fluarizine and cinnarizine. VASA **6:** 59–71.
25. ZISSIS, N. P., V. ALEVIZOS & A. S. DONTAS. 1981. Flunarizine, an inhibitor of Ca^{+2}-induced vascular constriction of geriatric patients. Curr. Ther. Res. **29:** 395–400.
26. TURNER, J. S. 1977. The dizzy patient: diagnosis and treatments. Drugs **13:** 382–387.
27. OOSTERVELD, W. J. 1981. Vestibular pharmacology of domperidone in rabbits and man. ORL **43:** 175–180.
28. KOHL, R. L., S. CALKINS & A. J. MANDELL. 1986. Arousal and stability: the effects of five new sympathomimetic drugs suggest a new principle for the prevention of space motion sickness. Aviat. Space Environ. Med. **57:** 137–143.
29. VAN ZWIETEN, P. A. 1986. Differentiation of calcium entry blockers into calcium channel blockers and calcium overload blockers. Eur. Neurol. **25:** 57–67.
30. RABIE, A., M. THOMASSET & M. LEGRAND. 1983. Immuno cytochemical detection of calcium-binding protein in the cochlear and vestibular hair cells of the rat. Cell Tissue Res. **232:** 691–696.
31. MEYER, A. M. & R. KAUFMANN. 1986. Is an imbalanced calcium-homeostasis responsible for the experimentally induced endolymphatic hydrops? Acta Otolaryngol. **102:** 93–98.
32. GUSSEN, R. 1982. Vascular mechanism in Menière's disease. Arch. Otolaryngol. **108:** 544–549.

Pharmacology of Nimodipine

A Review

A. SCRIABINE[a] AND W. VAN DEN KERCKHOFF[b]

[a]*Institute for Preclinical Pharmacology*
Miles, Inc.
Post Office Box 1956
New Haven, Connecticut 06509

[b]*Pharmacological Institute*
Bayer AG
D-5600 Wuppertal, Federal Republic of Germany

This review summarizes pharmacological studies with nimodipine performed at various laboratories during the last few years. It updates and complements the earlier review on the same subject.[1]

Nimodipine, a 1,4-dihydropyridine derivative (FIGURE 1), was synthesized by Meyer *et al.*[2] Initial pharmacological studies characterized nimodipine as a potent cerebral vasodilator drug.[3–5] Nimodipine binds to cell membranes from various tissues of many different species.[6,7] Its K_D value for binding to human cell membranes is 0.27 nM.[8] Nimodipine is more lipophilic than nifedipine and its distribution volume in the brain of rats was found to be three times higher than that of nifedipine.[9]

Recent studies (reviewed below) confirmed the cerebral vasodilator activity of nimodipine and suggested that in addition to its calcium antagonistic action on smooth muscle of cerebral blood vessels, nimodipine may have direct neuronal effects.

CEREBROVASCULAR EFFECTS

On rabbit aortic strips, nimodipine is a potent antagonist of K^+-induced contractions; its IC_{50} is 5.8×10^{-9} M.[10] Contractions of rat aorta, induced by $PGF_{2\alpha}$ or by K^+ depolarization, were antagonized by nimodipine at 1×10^{-11} to 1×10^{-7} M.[11] The $^{45}Ca^+$ influx is reduced by nimodipine at the same concentrations as required for inhibition of K^+-induced contractions (FIGURE 2). 5-Hydroxytryptamine (5HT) induced contractions of basilar artery from rabbits are antagonized by nimodipine at 2×10^{-9} M (IC_{50}), while contractions of saphenous artery were not reduced by nimodipine even at 2.9×10^{-7} M.[12] Contractile responses of isolated canine basilar artery to $PGF_{2\alpha}$, thrombin, and whole blood were antagonized by nimodipine at concentrations ranging from 10^{-4} to 10^{-7} M.[13]

In anesthetized animals, nimodipine consistently increased cerebral blood flow. In dogs, nimodipine increased cerebral blood flow at single doses of 1 to 100 μg/kg intravenously (iv), 1–10 μg/kg intraarterially (ia), or 0.5 to 2 mg/kg orally (po).[4] In cats, the cerebral vasodilator effect of nimodipine was seen at 0.1–1 μg/kg ia or 10 μg/kg iv.[14]

By intravenous administration to cats, nimodipine at single doses of 1 to 100 μg/kg,[15] or by infusion at 0.5 to 1 μg/kg per minute for 5 to 20 minutes,[16] produced dose-dependent dilatation of pial vessels. An increase in cerebral blood flow after nimodipine was also seen in anesthetized and in conscious rabbits.[17] In anesthetized rabbits, nimodipine increased cerebral blood flow at 0.1 to 1.0 μg/kg per minute iv or

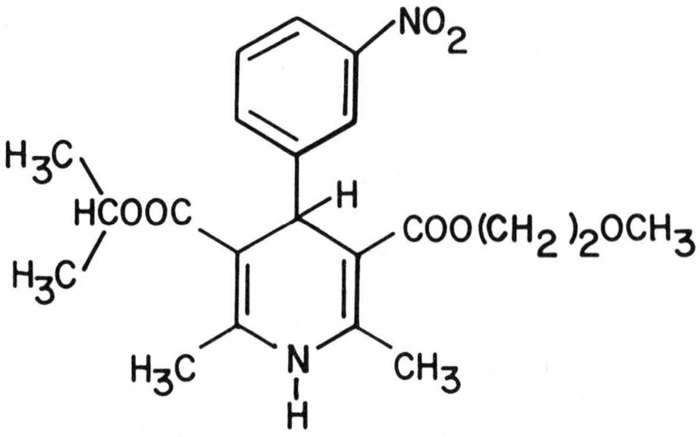

FIGURE 1. Chemical structure of nimodipine.

by intracarotid administration at 0.01 or 0.1 μg/kg per minute. In unanesthetized rabbits, nimodipine at 1.0 μg/kg per minute produced a twofold increase in cerebral blood flow.

In unanesthetized goats, nimodipine at either single intraarterial dose of 100 μg or by infusion at 10 μg/minute increased cerebral blood flow.[18] In baboons, nimodipine significantly increased cerebral blood flow at 1 μg/kg per minute iv but not at higher doses, which lowered arterial pressure.[19] In anesthetized monkeys nimodipine at 2 μg/kg/min (for one hour) increased cerebral blood flow by ca. 27%.[20]

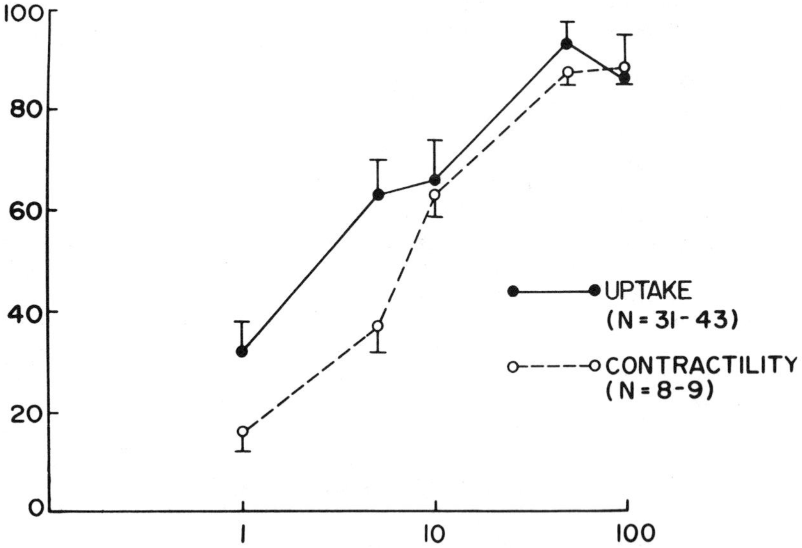

FIGURE 2. Effect of nimodipine on K^+-induced ^{45}Ca influx and contractions of isolated rabbit aortic rings. Percent inhibition is plotted against nimodipine concentration in nM. Nearly identical dose-response curves were obtained for the inhibition of ^{45}Ca uptake and of the contractile response to high K^+ (80 mM).

Hypocapnia-induced cerebral vasoconstriction was antagonized by nimodipine at 1.0 μg/kg per minute in either rabbits or primates.[21,22] Hypercapnia-induced vasodilation was slightly enhanced by nimodipine.[23]

ANTIISCHEMIC EFFECTS

Global Ischemia

Of considerable potential therapeutic importance was the observation by Kazda *et al.* that in cats, nimodipine prevents secondary postischemic impairment of cerebral blood flow after transient interruption of cerebral circulation.[4] Neurological deficits following global cerebral ischemia in dogs were reduced or prevented by nimodipine, given iv at 20 μg/kg before and at 1 μg/kg per minute for 2 hours during and after ischemia.[25] When nimodipine was given after ischemia, the neurological recovery of treated dogs was questionable.[26] Cerebral blood flow was, however, improved when nimodipine was administered as late as 15, 30, or even 60 minutes after interruption of cerebral circulation.[27] In pig-tailed monkeys subjected to transient global ischemia,[28] nimodipine at 10 μg/kg iv, given at 5 minutes after ischemia and followed by infusion at 1 μg/kg per minute for 10 hours, was effective in preventing neurological deficits.

FOCAL ISCHEMIA

In rats with middle cerebral artery (MCA) occlusion, nimodipine at 1 or 2 μg/kg per minute iv given before and during occlusion improved cerebral circulation and reduced infarct size.[29,30] Beneficial effect of nimodipine on the infarct size was detectable even in experiments in which arterial pressure of rats was reduced to 60 mmHg.[31]

In rabbits subjected to MCA occlusion, nimodipine given iv at 0.5 μg/kg per minute for the duration of the experiment (4 hours) improved cerebral blood flow in the ischemic area and normalized intracellular brain pH, which was reduced as a consequence of arterial occlusion.[32] Favorable effects of nimodipine on functional consequences of transient cerebral oligemia in rats with bilateral carotid artery occlusion were reported.[33] Also, in the "four vessel occlusion" model in rats, nimodipine, 10 μg/kg iv, followed by infusion at 1 μg/kg per minute, tended to restore brain ATP content.[34] A delay in ATP loss by nimodipine was also seen in Mongolian gerbils subjected to transient occlusion of both carotid arteries.[35]

The potential benefits of nimodipine in reduction of mortality due to stroke was dramatically demonstrated by Kazda *et al.*[36] Nimodipine added to food at 300 ppm greatly prolonged life of stroke-prone spontaneously hypertensive rats on a high-salt diet (FIGURE 3) without any significant effect on arterial pressure.

SUBARACHNOID HEMORRHAGE

As discussed above, nimodipine is an effective antagonist of contractions of isolated cerebral blood vessels.[12,13] Since vasospasm, associated with subarachnoid hemorrhage (SAH), is attributed to blood or its components, it was logical to expect that nimodipine would also antagonize cerebral vasospasm following SAH *in vivo*. This effect of nimodipine was demonstrated in dogs[37,38] and cats.[39,40] The findings suggest that nimodipine can prevent cerebral vasospasm induced by intrathecal administration of blood. The effect of nimodipine appears to be more pronounced on pial vessels than on larger cerebral arteries.

EFFECT ON CEREBRAL METABOLISM, BRAIN EDEMA, AND INTRACRANIAL PRESSURE

In vitro studies on the isolated brain slices indicated that at concentrations up to 10^{-6} M nimodipine had no effect on oxygen consumption.[4] In primates, *in vivo,* nimodipine at 1 or 2 μg/kg per minute had also no effect on oxygen consumption in spite of a significant increase in cerebral blood flow.[19,20] Under conditions of global cerebral ischemia, nimodipine had also no effect on brain oxygen consumption.[25,26]

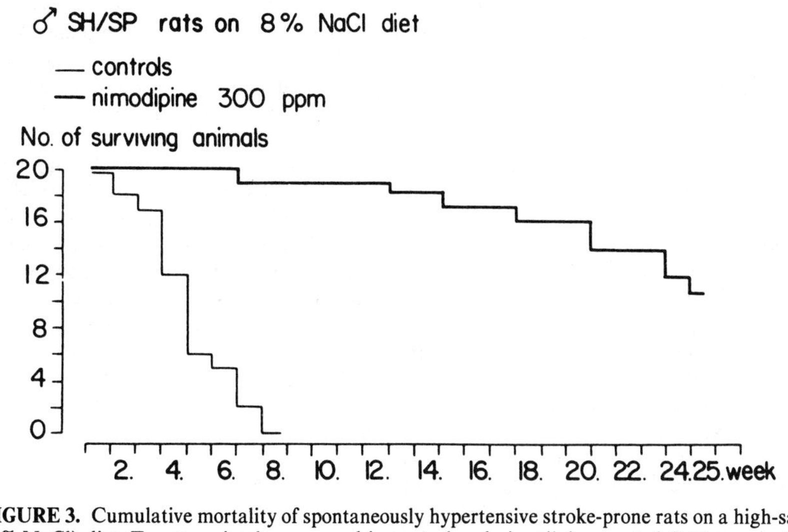

FIGURE 3. Cumulative mortality of spontaneously hypertensive stroke-prone rats on a high-salt (8% NaCl) diet. Twenty animals were used in control and nimodipine-treated (300 ppm in the diet) groups. (Reproduced from Reference 36 with permission.)

After permanent occlusion of MCA in rats, nimodipine, given either before or after occlusion, significantly reduced brain edema (water content).[41,42] In baboons with MCA occlusion, nimodipine did not further increase intracranial pressure.[43]

GENERAL HEMODYNAMIC EFFECTS

Although, as described above, nimodipine affects cerebral circulation at doses lower than required for systemic effects, at doses higher than 3 μg/kg iv nimodipine lowered systemic arterial pressure in dogs. Coronary blood flow was increased by nimodipine at 0.3 μg/kg and higher doses. The atrioventricular (AV) conduction time was slightly prolonged by nimodipine, but only at 10 μg/kg iv and higher doses.[44]

EFFECT ON CENTRAL NERVOUS SYSTEM

The above-discussed ability of nimodipine to prevent neurological deficits in various models of global or focal ischemia may represent the consequence of cerebrovascular action of this drug. It may, however, also suggest an additional neuronal site of action. During the last few years, numerous reports indicated that nimodipine could affect neuronal transmission and/or release of neurotransmitters. Nimodipine was reported to block slow inward current in hippocampal neurones and to depress transmission from the Schaffer collateral axons of CA_3 neurones onto CA_1 neurones.[45] The drug prevented naloxone-induced withdrawal signs in morphine-tolerant rats and antagonized biochemical changes in the brain caused by naloxone in morphine-treated rats.[46] Morphine-induced hyperthermia and the inhibitory effect of morphine on Ca^{2+}/Mg^{2+} ATPase activity in rat hypothalamus were found to be antagonized by nimodipine.[47] In rat cortical synaptosomes, nimodipine at 0.5 to 25 μM inhibited release of endogenous glutamate; this inhibition was correlated with the inhibition of ^{45}Ca uptake (TABLE 1).[48] *In vivo,* nimodipine has no obvious central nervous system (CNS) stimulant or depressant properties, but has demonstrable anticonvulsant activity in various animal models.[49,50]

Although no correlation was found, yet, between distribution of binding sites for dihydropyridines (DHPs) with that for any known single neurotransmitter in the brain of rats,[51] possible association of DHP binding sites with multiple neurotransmitters was not excluded. Nordström *et al.* reported that nimodipine at 10^{-7} to 10^{-5} M enhances potassium- or electrical-stimulation-evoked release of [^{3}H]dopamine while suppressing acetylcholine release from rat striatal slices.[52] DeBelleroche *et al.* found that nimodipine at 20 μM and higher concentrations had an inhibitory effect on the release of gamma-aminobutyric acid (GABA) from rat cerebral cortex.[53] At 10^{-6} M and lower concentrations, nimodipine was shown to reduce the secretion of substance P from dorsal root ganglia cells, but was without any effect on the release of norepinephrine from sympathetic neurones.[54] *In vitro* nimodipine depressed the K^+ and corticotropin-releasing factor (CRF) evoked release of ACTH from a mouse pituitary tumor cell strain (AtT 20/D16a). The drug was considerably more potent in inhibiting K^+- than CRF-evoked release of ACTH.[55] Since in most of these *in vitro* studies the effective concentrations of nimodipine were considerably higher than required for its cerebrovascular effects, nimodipine at therapeutic doses is not likely to affect release of neurotransmitters in a healthy tissue.

However, as recently demonstrated in clonal rat anterior pituitary cells (GH_4C_1),[56] nimodipine can block "slowly inactivating" Ca^{2+} channels in these endocrine cells in a time- and voltage-dependent manner. In these cells, the drug had very high affinity for its receptors, but only during maintained depolarization. This finding suggests that hypoxic or otherwise damaged cells with depolarized membranes can be expected to be much more susceptible to nimodipine than are normal, healthy endocrine or possibly

TABLE 1. Effect of Nimodipine on Inhibition of ^{45}Ca Uptake and on the Release of Endogenous Glutamate from Rat Cortical Synaptosomes[a]

Concentration of Nimodipine (μM)	Percent of Control ^{45}Ca Uptake	Percent of Control Glutamate Release
0.5	90	75
1.0	47	63
10.0	30	37
25.0	10	0
50.0	12	0

[a] Adapted from Reference 48.

TABLE 2. Inhibition of ^{45}Ca Uptake by NCB-20 (Neuroblastoma) Cells by Ca^{2+} Antagonists[a]

Ca^{2+} Antagonists	IC_{50}(nM)
Nimodipine	5.6
Nifedipine	9.2
Flunarizine	750.0
Verapamil	1800.0

[a] Adapted from Reference 58.

also neuronal cells. The release of neurotransmitters under conditions of sustained depolarization of cell membrane could, therefore, conceivably be affected by nimodipine even at therapeutic concentrations.

A correlation between affinity of 1,4-dihydropyridines for their binding sites and their activity in blocking Ca^{2+} uptake was described for the NCB-20 clonal cell line (neuroblastoma × Chinese hamster brain hybrid).[57] Comparison of abilities of various Ca^{2+} channel antagonists to block ^{45}Ca uptake into NCB-20 cells and their affinities for binding to cell fragments of rat cerebral cortex revealed that nimodipine was more potent than nifedipine as an inhibitor of Ca^{2+} uptake and had also higher affinity for 1,4-dihydropyridine binding sites in the rat cerebral cortex.[58] Non-dihydropyridine-type Ca^{2+} channel antagonists were considerably less potent than nimodipine (TABLE 2). Depolarization-induced Ca^{2+} uptake into rat cerebellar granule cells was also shown to be antagonized by nitrendipine at 100 nM.[59]

The importance of dihydropyridine-controlled Ca^{2+} channels for at least some functions of the central nervous system was confirmed with the help of the Ca^{2+} channel agonist BAY K 8644,[60] which can produce behavioral changes in mice, including ataxia, Straub tail, limb clonus and tonus, and increased sensitivity to auditory stimulation. All these effects were antagonized by nifedipine, but not verapamil.[61,62] BAY K 8644 was also shown to have hypothermic activity in rats and to stimulate hypothalamic Ca^{2+}/Mg^{2+} ATPase. These effects of BAY K 8644 were antagonized by nimodipine, but not by verapamil or diltiazem.[63]

Although the existence of calcium channels in neurones was first described 28 years ago,[64] only recently have we begun to appreciate their physiological and pharmacological significance.[65] The sensitivity of some voltage-sensitive calcium channels to nimodipine and other dihydropyridines suggests new therapeutic applications for these drugs, not only in the treatment of global or focal ischemia, but also in the therapy of other diseases of the central nervous system, which may or may not involve elevation of brain levels of neurotransmitters.

SUMMARY AND CONCLUSIONS

The major pharmacological findings with nimodipine reviewed in this chapter are summarized in TABLE 3. On the basis of these findings, the following conclusions appear to be justified:

1. Nimodipine is a 1,4-dihydropyridine with Ca^{2+} channel antagonist properties. It is more lipophilic than nifedipine and its distribution volume in the brain of rats is higher than that of nifedipine.
2. Nimodipine dilates cerebral vessels at considerably lower concentrations than required for dilatation of peripheral blood vessels. It can, therefore, improve cerebral blood flow at doses that do not reduce systemic arterial pressure.

TABLE 3. Selected Pharmacological Findings with Nimodipine

Observations	References
Postischemic secondary decrease in cerebral blood flow in cats can be prevented by nimodipine.	4
Nimodipine antagonizes hypoxia-induced amnesia in rats and pentylenetetrazole-induced convulsions in mice.	49
Survival rate of stroke-prone SH rats is increased by nimodipine.	36
Nimodipine reduces neurological deficits in dogs or pig-tailed monkeys subjected to transient global cerebral ischemia.	25, 28
Nimodipine reduces the area of focal cerebral ischemia in rat brains.	24, 30
Nimodipine normalizes brain pH and reduces focal brain ischemia in rabbits.	32
Nimodipine antagonizes experimental seizures in rabbits.	50
Distribution volume of nimodipine in the brain of rats is considerably higher than that of nifedipine.	9
Nimodipine inhibits release of GABA from rat cerebral cortex.	53
Nimodipine reduces secretion of substance P from dorsal root ganglia cells.	54
Morphine-induced hyperthermia is antagonized by nimodipine in rats.	47
Naloxone-induced withdrawal symptoms in morphine-tolerant rats are prevented by nimodipine.	46

3. Nimodipine inhibits ^{45}Ca uptake into vascular smooth muscle and neuronal cells.
4. Nimodipine antagonized postischemic cerebral hypoperfusion in cats and prolonged life of stroke-prone spontaneously hypertensive (SH) rats at doses that have little if any effect on arterial blood pressure.
5. Nimodipine reduced neurological deficits in dogs and monkeys with global cerebral ischemia. In focal ischemia (MCA occlusion) nimodipine reduced infarct size and neurological deficits and normalized intracellular brain pH.
6. In addition to its cerebral vasodilator effect, nimodipine appears to have a direct neuronal action. The suggested evidence for the neuronal site of action of nimodipine includes:

   a. Presence of nimodipine binding sites in brain.
   b. Blockade by nimodipine of Ca^{2+} channels in single nerve cells and in endocrine cells under conditions of sustained depolarization.
   c. Interactions with centrally acting drugs.
   d. Effects on release of various neurotransmitters from neuronal tissue or endocrine cells.
   e. Demonstration of anticonvulsant action of nimodipine.
   f. Blockade of behavioral effects of Ca^{2+} channel agonists by calcium channel antagonists.

REFERENCES

1. Scriabine, A., *et al.* 1985. New Cardiovasc. Drugs **3:** 197–218.
2. Meyer, H., *et al.* 1983. Arzneim. Forsch. **33:** 106–112.
3. Kazda, S. & F. Hoffmeister. 1979. Arch. Pharmacol. **307**(Suppl.): R43.
4. Kazda, S., *et al.* 1982. Arzneim. Forsch. **32:** 331–338.
5. Kazda, S. & R. Towart. 1982. Acta Neurochirurg. **63:** 259–265.
6. Bellemann, P., *et al.* 1983. Proc. Nat. Acad. Sci. USA **80:** 2356–2360.

7. GLOSSMANN, H., *et al.* 1983. Naunyn-Schmiedeberg's Arch. Pharmacol. **323:** 1–11.
8. PEROUTKA, S. J. & G. S. ALLEN. 1983. J. Neurosurg. **59:** 933–937.
9. VAN DEN KERCKHOFF, W. & L. R. DREWES. 1985. J. Cereb. Blood Flow Metab. **5:** 459–460.
10. TOWART, R. & S. KAZDA. 1985. *In* Nimodipine, Pharmacological and Clinical Properties. Schattauer-Verlag. Stuttgart & New York.
11. GODFRAIND, T., *et al.* 1985. *In* Nimodipine, Pharmacological and Clinical Properties. Schattauer-Verlag. Stuttgart & Munich.
12. TOWART, R. 1981. Circ. Res. **48:** 650–657.
13. WHITE, R. P., *et al.* 1982. Neurosurgery **10:** 344–348.
14. MOHAMMED, A. A., *et al.* 1983. J. Cereb. Blood Flow Metab. **1:** 578–579.
15. TANAKA, K., *et al.* 1980. Arzneim. Forsch. **30:** 1494–1497.
16. AUER, L. M. 1981. Arzneim. Forsch. **31:** 1423–1425.
17. HAWS, C. W., *et al.* 1986. J. Pharmacol. Exp. Ther. **225:** 24–28.
18. ALBORCH, E., *et al.* 1985. Rev. Espan. Cardiol. **38:** 163–169.
19. MCCALDEN, T. A. 1984. Bibl. Cardiol. **38:** 244–249.
20. HARPER, A. M., *et al.* 1981. J. Cereb. Blood Flow Metab. **1:** 349–350.
21. HAWS, C. W. & D. D. HEISTAD. 1983. J. Cereb. Blood Flow Metab. **3**(Suppl. 1): 524–525.
22. HARPER, A. M., *et al.* 1981. J. Cereb. Blood Flow Metab. **1:** 349–356.
23. MCCALDEN, T. A., *et al.* 1984. Stroke **15:** 527–530.
24. BARTKOWSKI, H. M., *et al.* 1985. Paper presented at the Annual Meeting of the American Society of Neurological Surgeons, Atlanta, April 21–25.
25. STEEN, P. A., *et al.* 1983. J. Cereb. Blood Flow Metab. **3:** 38–43.
26. STEEN, P. A., *et al.* 1984. J. Cereb. Blood Flow Metab. **4:** 82–87.
27. NEWBERG-MILDE, L., *et al.* 1986. J. Cereb. Blood Flow Metab. **6:** 332–337.
28. STEEN, P. A., *et al.* 1985. Anesthesiology **62:** 406–414.
29. MOHAMMED, A. S., *et al.* 1985. Ann. Neurol. **18:** 705–711.
30. GERMANO, I. M., *et al.* 1986. Stroke **17**(1): 144.
31. GRAHAM, D. I., *et al.* 1984. *In* Circulation Metabolism and Infarction—An Integrated Approach. Bes *et al.*, Eds.: 91–102. Elsevier. Amsterdam, Holland.
32. MEYER, F. B., *et al.* 1986. J. Neurosurg. **64:** 617–626.
33. BORZEIX, M. G. & J. CAHN. 1983. Naunyn-Schmiedeberg's Arch. Pharmacol. **324**(Suppl.): R46.
34. MABE, H., *et al.* 1986. Stroke **17:** 501–505.
35. HEFFEZ, D. S. & J. V. PASSONNEAU. 1985. J. Cereb. Blood Flow Metab. **5:** 523–528.
36. KAZDA, S., *et al.* 1982. *In* Calcium Modulators. T. Godfraind, A. Albertini & R. Paoletti, Eds.: 155–167. Elsevier. Amsterdam, New York & Oxford.
37. COHEN, R. J. & G. S. ALLEN. 1980. *In* Proceedings of the 2nd International Workshop on Vasospasm. R. H. Wilkins, Ed.: 527–553. William and Wilkins. Baltimore, Md.
38. GIOIA, A. E., *et al.* 1985. J. Neurosurg. **62:** 721–728.
39. TANAKA, K., *et al.* 1982. Arzneim. Forsch. **32:** 1529–1534.
40. ULRICH, F., *et al.* 1985. *In* Cerebral Vascular Spasm. D. Voth & P. Glees, Eds.: 179–189. de Gruyter. Berlin & New York.
41. GERMANO, I. M., *et al.* 1987. Stroke **18:** 288.
42. OBANA, W. G., *et al.* 1985. Clin. Res. **33:** 286.
43. HADLEY, M. N., *et al.* 1987. J. Neurosurg. **66:** 387–393.
44. SATOH, K., *et al.* 1984. Arzneim. Forsch. **34:** 563–568.
45. BROWN, D. A., *et al.* 1985. *In* Cardiovascular Effects of Dihydropyridine-Type Calcium Antagonists and Agonists. A. Fleckenstein, C. van Breemen, R. Gross & F. Hoffmeister, Eds.: 74–87. Springer. Berlin, Heidelberg, New York & Tokyo.
46. BONGIANNI, R., *et al.* 1986. Br. J. Pharmacol. **88:** 561–567.
47. PILLAI, N. P. & D. H. ROSS. 1986. Pharmacol. Biochem. Behav. **25**(3): 555–560.
48. WHITE, E. J. & H. G. BRANFORD. 1985. Trans. Biochem. Soc. London **13:** 985–987.
49. HOFFMEISTER, F., *et al.* 1982. Arzneim. Forsch. **32:** 347–360.
50. MEYER, F., *et al.* 1986. Mayo Clin. Proc. **61:** 239–247.
51. CORTÉS, R., *et al.* 1984. J. Neurol. Transm. **60:** 169–197.
52. NORDSTRÖM, Ö., *et al.* 1986. Acta Physiol. Scand. **126:** 115–119.
53. DEBELLEROCHE, J. S., *et al.* 1986. Br. J. Pharmacol. **88:** 446P.

54. PERNEY, T. M., *et al.* 1986. Biophys. J. **49:** 200a.
55. RICHARDSON, U. I. 1986. Life Sci. **38:** 41–50.
56. COHEN, C. J. & R. T. MCCARTHY. 1987. J. Physiol. **387:** 195–225.
57. FREEDMAN, S. B., *et al.* 1984. J. Neurosci. **4:** 1453–1467.
58. FREEDMAN, S. B. & R. J. MILLER. 1984. *In* Nitrendipine. A. Scriabine, S. Vanov & K. Deck, Eds.: 79–90. Urban and Schwarzenberg. Baltimore & Munich.
59. CARBONI, E., *et al.* 1985. Neuropharmacology **24:** 1123–1126.
60. SCHRAMM, M., *et al.* 1983. Nature **303:** 535–537.
61. BOLGER, G. T., *et al.* 1985. Naunyn-Schmiedeberg's Arch. Pharmacol. **328:** 373–377.
62. BOURSON, A., *et al.* 1986. Br. J. Pharmacol. **89:** 624.
63. PILLAI, N. P. & D. H. ROSS. 1986. Pharmacol. Biochem. Behav. **25:** 549–554.
64. HAGIWARA, S. & S. SAITO. 1959. J. Physiol. **148:** 161–177.
65. MILLER, R. J. 1987. *In* Structure and Physiology of the Slow Inward Calcium Channel. J. C. Venter & D. Triggle, Eds.: 161–246. A. R. Liss. New York, N.Y.

Improvement of Parkinsonism after Withdrawing Long-Term Flunarizine Treatment

F. BENVENUTI,[a] A. BARONI,[a] S. BANDINELLI,[a]
R. CORRADETTI,[b] N. MARCHIONNI,[c]
F. M. ANTONINI,[c] AND T. PANTALEO[d]

[a]*Geriatric Department*
I.N.R.C.A.
Via dei Massoni 21
50139 Florence, Italy

[b]*Department of Clinical and Preclinical Pharmacology*
[c]*Department of Geriatrics*
[d]*Department of Physiological Sciences*
University of Florence
50134 Florence, Italy

Recently it has been reported that some patients presenting parkinsonism during flunarizine treatment showed partial or complete recovery after drug withdrawal.[1] Parkinsonism in general can be assessed clinically and investigated further by studying kinematic and electromyographic (EMG) variables of ballistic movements. Patients with Parkinson's disease have been proved to be unable to perform ballistic actions within a single cyle of alternating EMG agonist and antagonist activity as normal subjects do,[2,3] thus providing a physiological explanation for bradykinesia.[2] The aim of this study was to ascertain whether parkinsonism, and bardykinesia in particular, observed in patients during flunarizine treatment shared common features with Parkinson's disease, by analyzing clinical features and kinematic and EMG variables of ballistic arm abduction movements performed in a step-tracking task.[3]

Twenty-two patients (15 women, 7 men; aged 66–88 years, mean 74) with parkinsonism noticed during long-term flunarizine therapy (10 mg daily; 2–48 months) were studied. Clinical assessment, scored with the Webster rating scale, and the analysis of ballistic movements were carried out before and one month after drug withdrawal. Ten healthy subjects of similar age were studied for comparison.

Before withdrawing flunarizine treatment, all patients showed mild to moderate parkinsonism: mild to severe bradykinesia and rigidity were present in all the patients, whereas tremor, posture, and gait disturbances were not constantly observed. All the patients displayed abnormal ballistic movements characterized by a lower mean velocity and altered EMG patterns (see B, FIGURE 1).

One month after flunarizine discontinuation, all patients clinically improved mainly in rigidity and bradykinesia (TABLE 1). In general, when present, tremor and gait disturbances were not affected by drug withdrawal. Ballistic movements were performed with higher mean velocity, and underlying EMG patterns became more similar to those recorded in normal subjects (see C, FIGURE 1).

After a 60-day washout, seven patients were diagnosed as affected by Parkinson's disease and successfully treated with L-dopa whereas the others completely recovered.

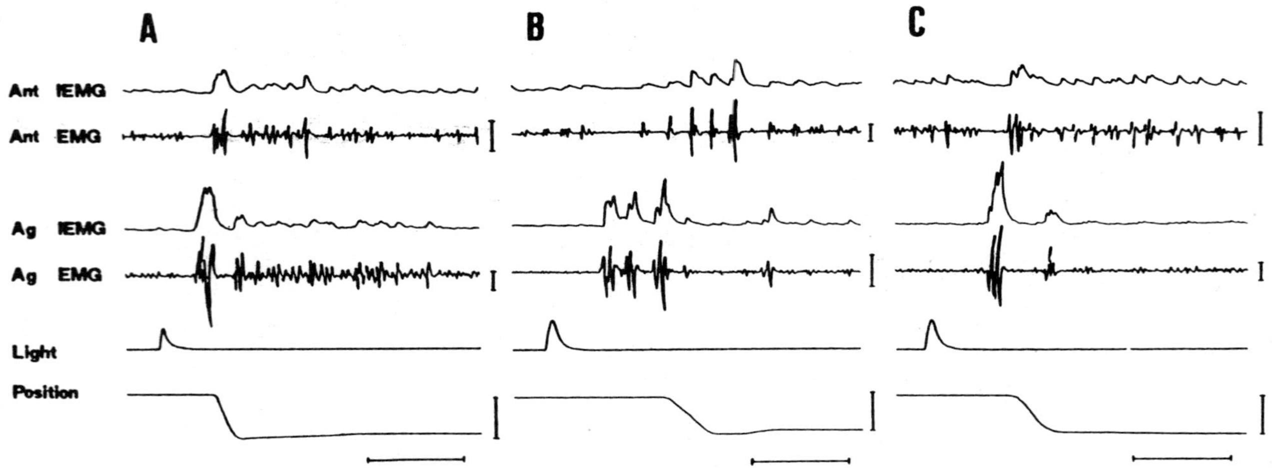

FIGURE 1. An example of the effects of flunarizine treatment withdrawal on fast arm abduction movements. From left to right: (A) healthy subject; (B) a patient during flunarizine treatment; (C) the same patient one month after treatment discontinuation. From top to bottom: Ant IEMG, "integrated" electromyogram of the antagonist muscle; Ant EMG, electromyogram of the antagonist muscle; Ag IEMG, "integrated" electromyogram of the agonist muscle; Ag EMG, electromyogram of the agonist muscle; Light, signal of switching on of the target light; Position, signal of hand movement. In A, the recordings show the characteristic EMG triphasic pattern of ballistic movement in normal subjects. In B, unlike normal subjects, the initial EMG agonist activity (i.e., before and at the onset of movement) does not consist of a single burst, but of multiple bursts with a trend of increasing intensity. Note, in correspondence to the activation of the agonist muscle, a prolonged duration of the antagonist inhibition which seems to be a characteristic feature in patients with Parkinson's disease.[3] In C, the EMG pattern assumes a ballistic aspect. Calibration bars: 1 mV, 500 ms, 10 cm in A; 0.5 mV, 500 ms, 10 cm in B and C.

TABLE 1. Comparisons of Clinical Data (Webster Rating Scale) Recorded before and after Flunarizine Withdrawal

	During Treatment[a]		After Drug Withdrawal[a]	
Bradykinesia of hands (including handwriting)	1.6	0.7	0.8[b]	0.6
Rigidity	1.6	0.7	0.9[b]	0.6
Posture	1.0	0.6	0.7[c]	0.6
Upper extremity swing	1.0	1.0	0.5[b]	0.8
Gait	0.8	0.7	0.7	0.7
Tremor	0.5	0.6	0.4	0.5
Facies	1.0	0.4	0.8	0.5
Seborrhea	0.3	0.4	0.2	0.4
Speech	0.8	0.4	0.3[b]	0.5
Self-care	0.9	0.7	0.5[b]	0.6
Total scores	9.3	3.4	5.9[b]	4.2

[a]Mean ± standard deviation.
[b]$p < 0.01$, signed rank test.
[c]$p < 0.05$, signed rank test.

With present methods we are unable to assess whether the observed syndrome was an iatrogenic parkinsonism or initial idiopathic Parkinson's disease unmasked by the drug. Nevertheless the fact that all patients improved after drug withdrawal leads to the suggestion that this drug acts on some central neural mechanisms that are involved in the pathophysiology of Parkinson's disease. Furthermore, since tremor and gait disturbances were not constantly present and, when present, not consistently ameliorated by flunarizine withdrawal, it is conceivable that the drug affects mainly those mechanisms responsible for motor planning and muscle tone.

From our study and previous ones,[1] the appearance of these side effects seems related to ages over 60. The age-related decline in control of calcium entry associated with a decline in the efficiency of dopaminergic systems could give an explanation of the sensitivity of the elderly to this drug.

REFERENCES

1. Chouza, C., A. Scaramelli, J. L. Caamano, O. De Medina, R. Aljianati & S. Romero. 1986. Parkinsonism, tardive dyskinesia, akhatisia, and depression induced by flunarizine. Lancet **i:** 1303–1304.
2. Hallett, M. & S. Khoshbin. 1980. A physiological mechanism of bradykinesia. Brain **103:** 301–314.
3. Baroni, A., F. Benvenuti, L. Fantini, T. Pantaleo & F. Urbani. 1984. Human ballistic arm abduction movements: effects of L-dopa treatment in Parkinson's disease. Neurology Cleveland **34:** 868–876.

Flunarizine in Epilepsy

C. D. BINNIE

Department of Clinical Neurophysiology
The Maudsley Hospital
Denmark Hill
London SE5 8AZ, England

All completed trials of flunarizine in epilepsy have been add-on studies in therapy-resistant patients, predominantly with partial seizures and a diagnosis of partial or secondary generalized epilepsy (see TABLES 1 and 2). All studies have produced some evidence of therapeutic response; where a 50% seizure reduction was used as an outcome criterion, this was attained by 25% to 40% of patients.

There is no evidence of interactions affecting blood levels of comedication, but the metabolism of flunarizine is accelerated by enzyme-inducing drugs. The therapeutic level is of the order of 50 ng/ml, and the daily dose required to achieve this in patients on enzyme-inducing drugs is in the range of 10 to 25 mg.

The chief side effects have been sedation and weight gain, and the former was not generally a significant problem at therapeutic blood levels.

TABLE 1. Open Trials[a]

Investigator	Patients	Flunarizine (mg/day)	Seizure Reduction	Results
Binnie *et al.*[1]	Adults	10–25	>50%	16/47
Curatolo *et al.*[3]	Children	10 (>10 kg) 5 (<10 kg)	>50%	8/21
Declerck *et al.*[4]	Adults + children	10	>25% >50%	10/14 1/14
Overweg *et al.*[7]	Adults	15	>50%	18/77
Sorel[8]	Adults	20	>50%	10/20
Treiman *et al.*[9]	Adults	30–60–120 ng/ml	>50%	8/12

[a]All dated 1986.

TABLE 2. Double-Blind Trials

Investigator	Design	Patients	Flunarizine (mg/day)	Seizure Reduction	Results: Placebo	Results: Flunarizine
Declerck & Wauquier (1983)[5]	Parallel	Children	10	>50%	0/5	3/7
Overweg *et al.* (1984)[7]	Crossover	Adults	10	>50%	0	7 (*n* = 30)
Froscher *et al.* (unpublished)	Crossover	Adults	15	>50%	2	4 (*n* = 22)
Cavazutti *et al.* (1986)[2]	Crossover	Children	5 (<12 yrs) 10 (>12 yrs)	>50%	0	4 (*n* = 14)
Starreveld *et al.* (unpublished)	Crossover	Adults	15	>50% minor major	3 1	5 (*n* = 22) 5 (*n* = 13)
Mancia *et al.* (1986)[6]	Crossover	Adults	10–25	20% reduction mean Sz. frequency on flunarizine		(*n* = 72)

Interesting incidental findings in some trials include an abolition of the initial events of secondarily generalized partial seizures, relief of postictal headache, and a mild euphoria even where there was no seizure reduction.

Flunarizine clearly shows promise as an antiepileptic drug, although its value can be assessed only after completion of further trials including monotherapy in less resistant patients.

REFERENCES

1. BINNIE, C. D., F. DE BEUKELAAR, J. W. A. MEIJER, H. MEINARDI, J. OVERWEG, A. WAUQUIER & A. VAN WIERINGEN. 1985. Open dose-ranging trial of flunarizine as add-on therapy in epilepsy. Epilepsia **26**(5): 424–428.
2. CAVAZZUTTI, G. B., V. GALLI & A. BENATTI. 1986. Use of flunarizine in pediatric epilepsy. Suppl. Giornale Neuropsicofarmacol. **8**(2): 19–20.
3. CURATOLO, P., O. BRUNI, I. BRINDESI, D. PRUNA & R. CUSMAI. 1986. La flunarizina nelle epilessie farmaco-resistenti dell'infanzia e dell'adolescenza. Estratto Rivi. Neurol. **61:** 1.
4. DECLERCK, A., L. T. OEI & A. WAUQUIER. 1985. Flunarizine in mentally retarded children with therapy-resistant epilepsy. *In* Health Science Review International Workshop on Flunarizine in Epilepsy: 68–73. Publisher, City, State.
5. DECLERCK, A. C. & A. WAUQUIER. 1983. Flunarizine, a double-blind study in therapy resistant mentally retarded epileptic children. Suppl. Boll. Chimi. Farma. **122:** 9CL–16CL.
6. MANCIA, D., B. BERGAMASCO, A. MOGLIA & R. DI PERRI. 1985. Double-blind placebo-controlled cross-over study of the efficacy of flunarizine as add-on therapy in epilepsy. *In* Health Science Review International Workshop on Flunarizine in Epilepsy: 89–92.
7. OVERWEG, J., C. D. BINNIE, J. W. A. MEIJER, H. MEINARDI, S. T. M. NUIJTEN, S. SCHMALTZ & A. WAUQUIER. 1984. Double-blind placebo-controlled trial of flunarizine as add-on therapy in epilepsy. Epilepsia **25:** 217–222.
8. SOREL, L. 1987. La flunarizine dans L'épilepsie: evaluation d'un traitment "additif" de quatre mois chez des patients resistants an traitment antiépileptique existant. Acta Neurol. Belg. **87:** 140–147.
9. TREIMAN, D. M., C. M. DEGIORGIO, J. W. CORNISH & J. J. CEREGHINO. 1986. Efficacy and toxicity of flunarizine in partial onset seizures at serum concentrations of 30, 60, and 120 ng/ml. Epilepsia **27**(5): 649–650.

Safety Profile of Flunarizine

A Retrospective Study in Migraine and Cerebrovascular Disorders

G. BONO,[a] N. MARTUCCI,[b] P. MERLO,[a] R. CERBO,[c]
G. NAPPI,[a] AND A. AGNOLI[c]

[a]*Department of Neurology*
C. Mondino Foundation
University of Pavia
Pavia, Italy

[b]*Italian Institute of Neurotraumatology*
Grottaferrata
Rome, Italy

[c]*Department of Neurosciences*
University of Rome "La Sapienza"
Rome, Italy

INTRODUCTION

Pharmacodynamic and pharmacokinetic investigations have produced during the last 10 years a wide series of experimental data about flunarizine, thus contributing to the development of several clinical indications. These have included, so far, various pathological conditions, some with different pathophysiology (vestibular disorders; venous insufficiency; epilepsia), some others linked by similarities in the pharmacological postulates (rationale) for treatment (migraine syndromes; ischemic cerebrovascular disorders).[5]

The ubiquity of calcium-dependent biological processes and events can account for the wide spectrum of clinical indications that characterize, in general, all the calcium entry blockers (CEBs); these substances, however, represent an etherogenous group of compounds, each one with different effects on the cardiovascular system as well as on the central nervous system (CNS).[4,8] In the neurological literature, as a consequence, besides reports on new therapeutic strategies (CEBs as prophylactic agents in migraine, cluster headache, vasospasm following subarachnoid hemorrhage), information has also been growing (sometimes controversial) about the safety patterns of these drugs.

Particularly during the last two years, flunarizine has been claimed to be responsible for the onset of CNS disturbances related to mood and motor activity.[1,3,6] The aim of the present report is therefore a retrospective and prospective analysis of the safety pattern of flunarizine administered in over 1200 cases for treatment of migraine or cerebrovascular disorders (CVDs) of ischemic origin (monotherapy; 10 mg/day, at bedtime; treatment duration, range 3–24 months). Only patients with a sufficient definition of the disease and other baseline clinical characteristics were admitted to the survey protocol.

TABLE 1. Flunarizine Side Effects Requiring Withdrawal: Incidence among 1270 Consecutive Cases[a]

Nature of Complaints	Migraine Patients (total 840 cases)				CVD Patients (tot. 430 cases)			
	n	M/F	Mean Age (years)	Mean Time of Onset (months)	*n*	M/F	Mean Age (years)	Mean Time of Onset (months)
Drowsiness	23	14/9	41 ± 7	1st–2nd	56	34/22	65 ± 11	1st–2nd
Weight gain	9	2/7	34 ± 5	5 ± 2	8	2/6	60 ± 15	9 ± 7
Depression	11	2/9	43 ± 8	9 ± 15	6	4/2	64 ± 7	6 ± 4
Motor disturbances	—	—	—	—	14	6/8	69 ± 11	2 ± 4
Combinations (one or more of the above)	6	—/6	39 ± 4	7 ± 12	9	8/1	66 ± 9	4 ± 7
Total	49 (5%)				93 (22%)			

[a]Migraine patients: M = 228; F = 612; mean age = 39 ± 12 years. CVD patients: M = 286; F = 144; mean age 62 ± 14 years. Depression: scored by the Hamilton rating scale (26 to 35) and requiring treatment in all cases (recovery within the 4th–7th week). Motor disturbances: akinesia and rigidity clinically scored (rated neurological examination). Weight gain: mean 5.5 kg.

RESULTS

TABLE 1 shows the list of the complaints requiring treatment withdrawal: their different incidence between the two groups of patients may indicate that the phenomena occurring under treatment are correlated with the pathology and the respective characteristics. This holds particularly true for weight gain and motor disturbances. Drowsiness, even if more remarkable among CVD patients, certainly is the earliest and most frequent side effect, having been complained about, even if not severely, by over 65% of the general population.

The different distribution of some patients' characteristics has then been analyzed with the aim of defining cases prone to develop certain side effects. Among migraine patients depressive symptoms (slight to severe) occur in 8.5% of the cases. The incidence of depressive symptoms among patients with family and/or personal history of affective disorders and/or baseline elevated (14 to 22) depression scores and/or abnormal personality profiles (Minnesota Multiphasic Personality Inventory) is striking. Weight increase has a high frequency of occurrence (30.6%), but no significant correlation with patients' characteristics (pretreatment body weight included).

Among CVD patients depressive symptoms occur in 9.5%, while motor disturbances reach 31% and include mostly akinetic/rigid symptoms. Their incidence, independently by the severity, seems to be correlated with the duration of the disease and both severity and extent of the ischemic damage: a particular risk belongs to cases with subcortical involvement (lacunar syndromes and Binswanger's type encephalopathy).

COMMENT

The present results confirm previous data[1] and indicate that, despite the pharmacological rationale, the drug has sustained and frequent side effects among chronic CVD patients, in particular when signs and symptoms of diffuse brain damage are present (basal ganglia involvement).

Most of the adverse affects, however, are reversible. This stresses the importance of a more accurate selection and definition of patients that are entered into long-term treatment with flunarizine, considering that, in our experience, the nature (mood/motricity) of the side effects is often predictable. About pathophysiology of adverse effects, there is enough evidence[2] to exclude a direct interference with a single neurotransmitter (dopamine receptor blockade in particular). The CNS effects that we observed, in fact, depend on different pathophysiological mechanisms and involve different neurotransmitters (DA, 5HT, CA) in different areas of the CNS (basal ganglia, limbic system, etc.). The most probable hypothesis is therefore that flunarizine can cause a general (nonspecific) inhibition of neural transmission, directly correlated to its calcium-antagonistic properties.[7] The different features of CNS side effects might therefore be the expression of a preexisting risk correlated with age and the different diseases treated (migraine or CVD).

REFERENCES

1. BONO, G., G. C. MANZONI, N. MARTUCCI *et al.* 1985. Cephalalgia **5**(Suppl. 2): 155–158.
2. CAERS, I., W. K. AMERY, F. DE BEUKELAAR *et al.* 1983. Janssen Research Products Information Service N36608.

3. CHOUZA, C., J. L. CAAMANO, ALJANATI, *et al.* 1986. Lancet **i:** 1303–1304.
4. GOVONI, S., F. BATTAINI, M. S. MAGNONI, *et al.* 1985. Cephalalgia **5**(Suppl. 2): 115–118.
5. HOLMES, B., R. N. BROGDEN, R. C. HEEL *et al.* Drugs **27:** 6–44.
6. MEYBOOM, R. H. B., M. D. FERRARI & B. P. DIELEMAN. 1986. Lancet **ii:** 292.
7. SIESJÖ, B. K. 1986. Mayo Clin. Proc. **61:** 299–302.
8. SNYDER, S. H. & I. REYNOLDS. 1985. N. Engl. J. Med. **16:** 995–1002.

Specific Effects of Nimodipine on the Auditory System[a]

P. J. JASTREBOFF[b] AND J. F. BRENNAN[c]

[b]*Department of Surgery*
Yale University School of Medicine
333 Cedar Street
New Haven, Connecticut 06510

[c]*Department of Psychology*
University of Massachusetts
Harbor Campus
Boston, Massachusetts 02125

Since calcium ions are crucial in determining cochlear micromechanics and for the transduction properties of hair cells,[1,2] we hypothesize that calcium channel antagonists and agonists may interact directly with cochlear functions without the intermediary of changing cochlear blood supply. In a pilot study, we evaluated the interaction of nimodipine (Bay e 9736) on the auditory system using 9 albino guinea pigs and 60 pigmented rats. In the first series of experiments, we sampled perilymph, cerebrospinal fluid (CSF), and blood from anesthetized rats at different time intervals after intraperitoneal (ip) injection of 1 mg/kg nimodipine dissolved in alcohol. The serum concentration of nimodipine peaked at 20 μg/l 30 minutes after injection, gradually declining to lower levels (FIGURE 1A, open circles). Interestingly, the levels in perilymph (FIGURE 1A, filled circles) were higher than in CSF (FIGURE 1A, squares) for times below 1 hour and above 3 hours. This finding not only indicates possible direct action of nimodipine on cochlear structure due to its presence in the perilymph, but suggests that nimodipine enters the perilymph directly from the blood, without the dominant participation of passive transport from CSF.

Amplitude and latency characteristics of cochlear microphonics and auditory nerve potentials before and after nimodipine (1–2 mg/kg) indicate the presence of recruitment-type properties induced for low levels of stimuli. More interestingly, nimodipine (2 mg/kg) seemed to partially reverse the effect of 30 minutes 125 dB sound pressure level (SPL) noise on cochlear microphonics and latencies of auditory nerve potentials (FIGURE 1B). Spontaneous activity of single cells recorded from the inferior colliculus and cerebellar vermis of 9 guinea pigs before and after nimodipine injection revealed that, while the activity of inferior colliculus cells significantly increased from 29.5 ± 1.5 Hz [mean ± standard error of the mean (SEM), $n = 177$] to 63.3 ± 8.3 Hz ($n = 35$, $p < 0.01$), the activity of cerebellar cells remained stable: 52.2 ± 6.1 ($n = 27$) before and 57.8 ± 8.5 Hz ($n = 25$) after (FIGURE 1C). Since nimodipine influenced cell activity recorded from a nucleus belonging to auditory pathways, without affecting cerebellar cell activity, its action can be related more to a specific effect on the auditory system than to general nonspecific influences on the nervous system.

We tested the action of nimodipine on tinnitus using a behavioral model we have developed[3] consisting of a Pavlovian conditioning paradigm of licking response

[a]This project was supported by a grant from Miles Laboratories, Inc. and partially by a Deafness Research Foundation Grant 1987.

suppression. Our results have measured apparent phantom auditory sensation evoked by salicylate injection when compared to control subjects (FIGURE 2A). Control groups showed that solvent alone (alcohol), had no significant influence on salicylate-evoked behavior in our procedure (FIGURE 2B). Nimodipine injected simultaneously with salicylate (2 mg/kg) completely abolished the action of salicylate (FIGURE 2C)),

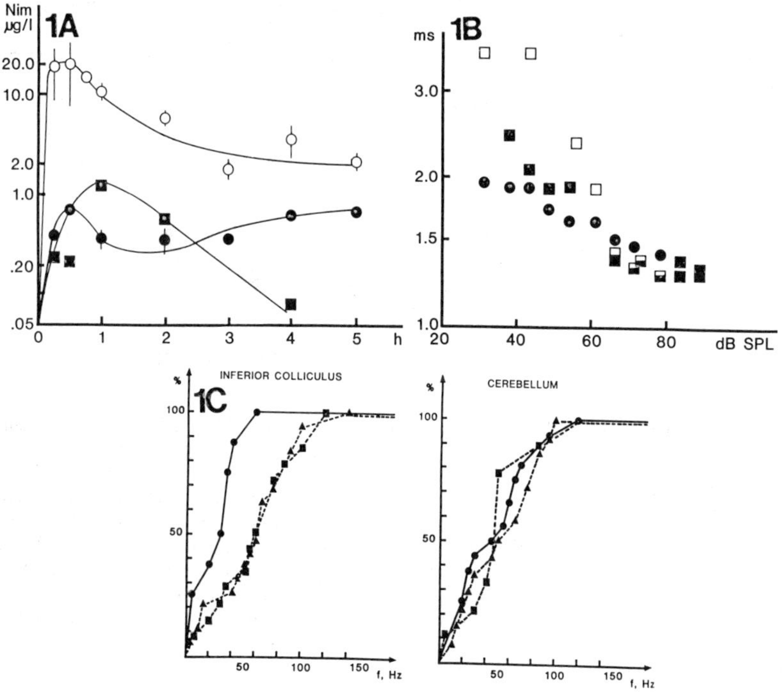

FIGURE 1. Concentration of nimodipine in body fluids, its action on auditory nerve potential characteristics, and on spontaneous activity of single cells recorded from inferior colliculus and cerebellum. (A) Concentration of nimodipine in serum (open circles), cerebrospinal fluid (squares), and perilymph (filled circles) as a function of time after nimodipine injection (1 mg/kg, ip). Bars, SEM. (B) Latency characteristics of auditory nerve potentials before (open circles), after (open squares) 125 dB SPL noise expoisition, and after nimodipine (2 mg/kg, ip). Note shortening of latencies after nimodipine for low levels of stimuli as compared to the after-noise situation. (C) Cumulative distribution of spontaneous cell activity recorded from inferior colliculus and lobulus V of cerebellar vermis before (continuous line) and after (dashed line) ip injections of nimodipine: squares, 1 mg/kg; triangles, 2.5 mg/kg. Note shift of distributions after nimodipine for inferior colliculus ($p < 0.01$) and overlapping of curves for cerebellum.

indicating that nimodipine may be alleviating tinnitus in animals. Thus, our preliminary data indicate that nimodipine may directly influence the auditory system and may have clinical application in elevation of noise-induced threshold shift, as well as in the treatment of tinnitus. Recently published clinical data support the possibility of alleviation of tinnitus and other auditory and vestibular disorders after nimodipine administration.[4]

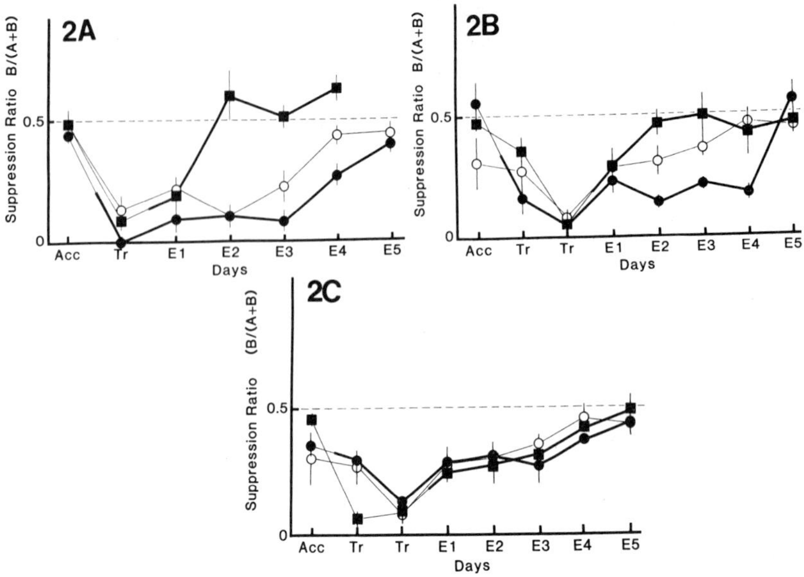

FIGURE 2. Behavioral assessment of nimodipine action in abolishing salicylate-induced tinnitus. (A) Suppression ratios of control and salicylate groups during the experiment. Acc, acclimation; Tr, training; E, extinction; Bars, SEM; the thick lines show time period when animals are subject to salicylate. Control group, open circles; salicylate introduced before training, filled circles; salicylate introduced after training, filled squares. Note rapid extinction in the group with salicylate introduced *after* training, contrasting significantly ($p < 0.001$) with strong suppression and prolonged extinction in the group where salicylate was introduced *before* training. (B) Animals' suppression ratios when alcohol was injected simultaneously with salicylate. Note persistence of the salicylate effects. (C) Animals' suppression ratios when nimodipine (2 mg/kg, subcutaneously) was injected simultaneously with salicylate. Note absence of salicylate effects indicating the disappearance of salicylate-evoked tinnitus.

REFERENCES

1. KRONESTER-FREI, A. 1979. Hearing Res. **1:** 81–94.
2. HUDSPETH, A. J. 1983. Annu. Rev. Neurosci. **6:** 187–215.
3. JASTREBOFF, P. J., *et al.* 1988. Behav. Neurosci. (In press.)
4. THEOPOLD, H. M. 1985. Laryngol. Rhinol. Otol. **64:** 609–613.

Pharmacokinetics and Metabolism of Radiolabeled Nimodipine

J. LETTIERI,[a] G. KROL,[a] K.-D. RÄMSCH,[c] S. YEH,[a]
F. G. McMAHON,[b] J. RYAN,[b] A. JAIN,[b] AND B. KAMATH[b]

[a]*Miles Pharmaceuticals*
400 Morgan Lane
West Haven, Connecticut 06516

[b]*Clinical Research Center*
147 South Liberty Street
New Orleans, Louisiana 70112

[c]*Bayer AG*
Aprather Weg
Postfach 101709
5600 Wuppertal 1, Federal Republic of Germany

Six healthy male volunteers were each given single 20 mg oral doses of ^{14}C-nimodipine in the form of a liquid suspension. Plasma, urine, and fecal samples were collected and analyzed for total radioactivity. Plasma and urine samples were also assayed by capillary gas chromatography for unchanged nimodipine and several metabolites. The average recovery of radioactivity in the urine over 96 hours was 52.9% ± 4.4% of the dose. In the same period, 32.4 ± 4.4% of the dose was recovered in the feces. Plasma concentrations of radioactivity were considerably higher than those of unchanged drug. Whereas peak plasma concentrations of nimodipine averaged 4.1 ng/ml, radioactivity data indicated a mean peak level of 255 ng/ml as nimodipine equivalents. The discrepancy demonstrates that most of the radioactivity in plasma was due to labeled metabolites. The elimination half-life of unchanged nimodipine was 5.7 hours, compared to a value of 14 hours derived from total radioactivity data.

The areas under the plasma-time curves (AUC) for total radioactivity and unchanged nimodipine were 3270 ng-hr/ml and 19 ng-hr/ml, respectively. Three metabolites (M1, M2, M3) had AUCs of 9, 81, and 33 ng-hr/ml respectively. Upon glucuronidase treatment, plasma concentrations of metabolites M2 and M3 increased approximately threefold.

The urinary excretion of conjugated M2 and M3 metabolites was 200 to 400 times higher than that of the corresponding free forms. Cumulative urinary excretion of nine free and conjugated metabolites accounted for about 20% of the dose. Since 53% of the dose was excreted in the urine, about 40% of radioactivity measured in urine was excreted in the form of known metabolites. Urinary excretion of nimodipine and metabolite M1 accounted for less than 0.1% of the dose. The above results indicate that nimodipine is well absorbed and eliminated primarily in the form of urinary metabolites.

Calcium Entry Blockers in the Prophylaxis of Migraine

JES OLESEN

Department of Neurology
Gentofte Hospital
University of Copenhagen
2900 Hellerup, Denmark

Migraine prophylaxis is indicated when patients have two or more attacks a month. Existing prophylactic treatments are not universally effective, and all have considerable side effects. The need for novel treatment principles is therefore obvious.

Recently our understanding of migraine pathophysiology has been greatly increased by measurements of regional cerebral blood flow during attacks.[1] Marked depression of regional cerebral blood flow occurs in classic migraine, but not in common migraine, where neuronal mechanisms are more likely. Calcium entry blockers exert effects both on arteries and on neurons, and are therefore interesting as potential migraine drugs. This paper reviews trials of calcium entry blockers in migraine prophylaxis.

CRITICAL EVALUATION OF PUBLISHED DOUBLE-BLIND TRIALS

The effect of flunarizine has been examined in seven double-blind trials including a total of 277 patients (TABLE 1). Results from one of the trials are given in FIGURE 1. In four of the trials, flunarizine was significantly better than placebo, and in the three other studies it was equal to pizotiphen, a drug with known prophylactic effect against migraine. Also two large, long-term, open studies have demonstrated efficacy of flunarizine. Side effects were few and mild in the double-blind studies.

Nimodipine was significantly better than placebo in two fairly large and well-planned double-blind trials including a total of 79 patients.

Verapamil has been evaluated in two double-blind trials, each including 12 patients. This sample size is clearly too small to justify any conclusions, and furthermore the studies were afflicated by other methodological problems.[2]

DISCUSSION

It is clear from existing studies that flunarizine is an effective prophylactic agent in migraine. There have been few and mild side effects, but it should be noted that the onset of effect is slow, being maximal only after two months. The evidence in favor of nimodipine is quite good, but not sufficient for general recommendation, whereas the evidence for verapamil is clearly insufficient.

Since the activity profiles of calcium entry blockers vary widely, as discussed in this volume, effectiveness of one calcium entry blocker in the prophylaxis of migraine cannot justify the use of other calcium entry blockers that have not themselves been sufficiently tested in controlled double-blind trials.

TABLE 1. Double-Blind Studies of Calcium Entry Blockers in Migraine Prophylaxis

	Number of Patients	Type of Patients		Type of Design		Duration of Periods (weeks)	Dose (mg/kg)	Drug Compared to	Results			
									Attack Frequency			Headache Index
		Common	Classical	Group	Crossover				Reduction	Duration	Severity	
Flunarizine												
Louis	58	+	+	+		13	10	Placebo	57% $p < 0.01$	NS[a]	NS	?
Frenken & Nuijten	35	+	+	+		12	10	Placebo	53% $p < 0.05$	?	?	?
Mendenopoulos *et al.*	20		+?	+		13	10	Placebo	?	?	NS	$p < 0.05$
Sørensen *et al.*	27	+			+	16	10	Placebo	38% $p < 0.01$	$p < 0.05$	NS	$p < 0.01$
Louis & Spierings	75	+	+	+		18	10	Pizotiphen 2–3 mg	NS	NS	NS	NS
Rascol *et al.*	35	+	+	+		13	10	Pizotiphen 2,19 mg	NS	NS	NS	?
Cerbo *et al.*	27	+	+		+	9	15	Pizotiphen 1,5 mg	NS	NS	?	?
Nimodipine												
Gelmers	50	+	+	+		13	120	Placebo	$p < 0.05$	NS	?	$p < 0.01$
Havanka-Kanniainen	29	+	+		+	8	120	Placebo	28% $p < 0.01$	NS	?	$p < 0.01$
Verapamil												
Solomon *et al.*	12	+	+		+	13	320	Placebo	42% $p < 0.05$	?	?	$p < 0.05$
Markley *et al.*	12	+	+		+	8	240	Placebo	17% $p < 0.05$	$p < 0.05$	NS	$p < 0.05$

[a]NS means not significant.

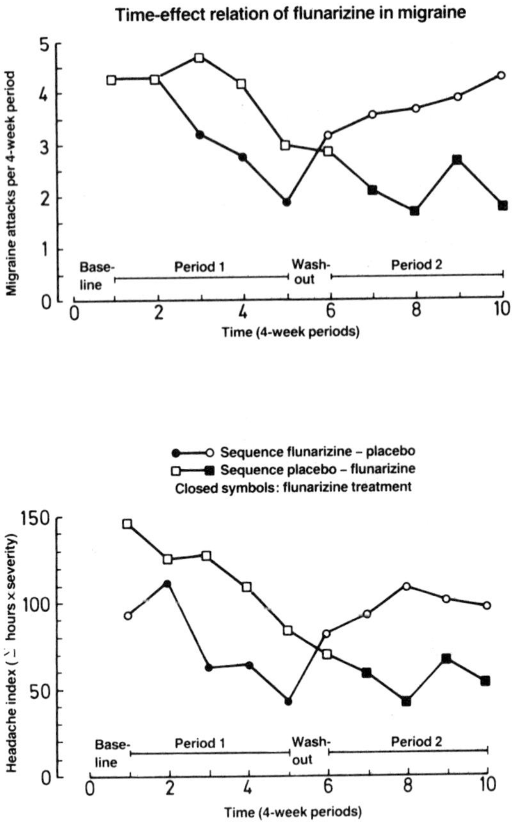

FIGURE 1. The effect of flunarizine in migraine prophylaxis. (Reproduced from Reference 3 with permission from the publisher.)

Further studies of the mechanism of action of calcium entry blockers in migraine prophylaxis may help to improve our understanding of migraine pathophysiology.

REFERENCES

1. OLESEN, J. 1986. The pathophysiology of migraine. *In* Handbook of Clinical Neurology. Headache. F. C. Rose, Ed. **4**(48): 59–83. Elsevier. Amsterdam, Holland.
2. OLESEN, J. 1986. Role of calcium entry blockers in the prophylaxis of migraine. Eur. Neurol. **25**(Suppl. 1): 72–79.
3. SOELBERG SØRENSEN, P., K. HANSEN & J. OLESEN. 1986. A placebo controlled, double-blind, cross-over trial of flunarizine in common migraine. Cephalalgia **6:** 7–14.

Lumbar and Cisternal Cerebrospinal Fluid Level of Arachidonate Metabolites in Nimodipine-Treated Patients after Subarachnoid Hemorrhage[a]

RICCARDO RODRIGUEZ Y BAENA,[b] PAOLO GAETANI,[b] VITTORIO SILVANI,[b] GUIDO GRIGNANI,[c] GIANCARLO FOLCO,[d] AND PIETRO PAOLETTI[b]

[b]*Department of Surgery*
Section of Neurosurgery
[c]*Department of Internal Medicine*
University of Pavia
27100 Pavia, Italy

[d]*Institute of Pharmacology and Pharmacognosy*
University of Milan
20133 Milan, Italy

INTRODUCTION

Several naturally occurring compounds have been proposed as possible vasoactive agents.[1] Recently, the role of arachidonic acid (AA) metabolites in the biological response of arterial wall to subarachnoid blood is investigated as one of the most important factors in vasospasm (VSP) onset. Samuelsson stated that despite a common precursor, two different pathways of AA metabolism differently act on physiopathological responses of the brain after subarachnoid hemorrhage (SAH).[2] Metabolites of cyclooxygenase primarily act as vasoactive agents, while AA metabolites of lipoxygenase are mostly involved in modifications of cell membrane permeability, inflammatory processes, and edema formation.[3] Calcium channel entry blockers, mainly nimodipine (Bay e 9736), were proposed in order to reduce or reverse ischemic complications following VSP.[4] Nimodipine improves clinical results in long-term follow-up of SAH patients, without a significant reduction of VSP incidence.

MATERIAL AND METHODS

Thirty-five selected SAH patients entered the study: 18 of them were treated with nimodipine [24–36 mg intravenously (iv)/24 hours for 10–14 days, then 240 mg orally until operation]. Lumbar cerebrospinal fluid (CSF) samples were obtained between day 4 and day 10 after the hemorrhage. Cisternal CSF samples were obtained by intraoperative cisternal puncture. CSF was immediately centrifuged (5700 × *g* for 5 minutes at 4°C), then frozen in liquid nitrogen and stored at −80°C until analysis.

[a]This Research was supported in part by a Grant of Regione Lombardia (Milano, 1984) and by Bayer Italia S.p.A.

Control CSF samples were obtained from 10 patients undergoing myelography for disc lesion.

Prostaglandin (PG) D_2, 6-Keto-PG F_{1alpha}, leucotriene (LT) C_4, and thromboxane (Tx) B_2 were measured with a radioimmunological assay (RIA) technique as described in previous experiments.[3]

RESULTS AND DISCUSSION

The overall incidence of angiographic symptomatic VSP was not significantly reduced by nimodipine, while cognitive impairment after a mean follow-up period of six months was significantly reduced in the nimodipine group.[5] After SAH there was a significant increase of the CSF level of AA metabolites in both groups. TABLE 1 reports mean cisternal level for each metabolite in comparison to lumbar CSF level: in perianeurismatic cisterns the level of TxB_2, LTC_4 and PGD_2 was significantly higher than lumbar CSF level in both groups of patients. Cisternal CSF level was significantly higher in patients with symptomatic VSP suggesting the importance of the "clotting phenomenon" around the ruptured aneurysmal wall as an important source of vasoactive agents. Nimodipine did not significantly modify CSF level of AA metabolites in both groups of patients and did not influence AA metabolism and CSF level of eicosanoids, mainly in perianeurismatic cisterns, the site most exposed to biochemical reactions promoting VSP (TABLE 2). This could be related to the hypothetical activity of calcium channel blockers in antagonizing the passage of Ca^{2+} from the extracellular to the intracellular compartment, without a significant antagonism of the passage of intracellular Ca^{2+} to the intracytoplasmatic free fraction.[6] There is experimental evidence on the role of AA metabolites in the modulation of contractile proteins enhancing the passage of extracellular and intracellular stored calcium to the intracytoplasmatic free fraction: calcium channel entry blockers could partially antagonize this reaction, causing an incomplete prevention of the AA-metabolite-mediated smooth muscle contraction mechanism. Moreover, release of AA metabolites is cell specific and depends on a receptor activation which enhances calcium-dependent reactions: nimodipine probably fails to interfere with the specific receptor. On the

TABLE 1. Arachidonate Metabolite Levels (pg/ml) in Lumbar and Cisternal CSF of SAH Patients[a]

	Control Cases	Standard Treatment	Nimodipine Treatment
Lumbar			
PGD_2	79.10 ± 17.3	411.11 ± 81.04	365.88 ± 76.82
6-K-$PGF_{1\,alpha}$	21.90 ± 6.6	195.13 ± 25.93	154.36 ± 32.45
LTC_4	107.50 ± 42.73	437.50 ± 73.57	286.67 ± 83.67
TxB_2	187.60 ± 47.50	760.00 ± 204.13	1072.00 ± 437.68
Cisternal			
PGD_2		759.05 ± 131.24	712.63 ± 123.16
6-K-$PGF_{1\,alpha}$		193.70 ± 52.09	328.67 ± 129.16
LTC_4		800.38 ± 356.10	1300.00 ± 349.02
TxB_2		4972.31 ± 1162.04	4611.87 ± 952.99

[a]Control patients, $n = 10$; nimodipine treatment, $n = 18$; standard treatment, $n = 17$. Nimodipine = standard treatment (Student's t-test).

TABLE 2. Arachidonate Metabolite Cisternal CSF Levels (pg/ml) in SAH Patients (n = 35) with and without Vasospasm and Who Have Undergone Nimodipine or Standard Treatment

	Group "Spasm"		Group "No Spasm"	
Cisternal CSF	Nimodipine (n = 6)	Standard (n = 8)	Nimodipine (n = 11)	Standard (n = 10)
PGD_2	1246.67 ± 231.90[a]	1017.78 ± 236.67	466.15 ± 83.37[a]	481.67 ± 76.64
6-K-PGF_{1alpha}	201.25 ± 37.66[a]	134.00 ± 45.78	203.82 ± 33.67[a]	225.85 ± 76.16
LTC_4	1858.00 ± 714.43[a]	1607.00 ± 837.16	1021.00 ± 172.07[b]	296.25 ± 92.52
TxB_2	5022.00 ± 2289.36[a]	5723.33 ± 1641.48	4425.45 ± 1008.67[a]	4328.57 ± 1715.40

[a] Difference not significant.
[b] $p < 0.005$ in nimodipine vs. standard treatment (Student's t-test).

other hand, nimodipine is effective in preventing the liberation of AA metabolites from membrane phospholipids, reducing the neuronal toxic effect. Nimodipine, in our opinion, does not interfere with pathogenetical mechanisms of VSP following aneurysm rupture, but it improves neuronal resistance to hypoperfusion and modified metabolic patterns after SAH.

ACKNOWLEDGMENT

The help and the advice of P. Salvini, M.D., L. Caresia, M.D., and G. Fenu, Ph.D. are gratefully recognized.

REFERENCES

1. KASSELL, N. F., T. SASAKI, A. R. T. COLOHAN & G. NAZAR. 1985. Cerebral vasospasm following aneurysmal subarachnoid hemorrhage. Stroke **16:** 562–572.
2. SAMUELSSON, B. 1981. Prostaglandins, thromboxanes and leukotrienes. Formation and biological roles. The Harvey Lectures 1979–1980, Series 75: 1–41. Academic Press. New York, N.Y.
3. RODRIGUEZ Y BAENA, R., P. GAETANI, G. FOLCO, T. VIGANÒ & P. PAOLETTI. 1986. Arachidonate metabolites and vasospasm after subarachnoid hemorrhage. Neurol. Res. **8:** 25–32.
4. WHITE, R. P. 1983. Vasospasm. I. Experimental Findings. *In* Intracranial Aneurysms. J. L. Fox, Ed.: 218–249. Springer Verlag. Heidelberg, New York & Tokyo.
5. LJUNGGREN, B., L. BRANDT & H. SAEVELAND. 1984. Outcome in 60 consecutive patients treated with early aneurysm operation and intravenous nimodipine. J. Neurosurg. **61:** 864–873.
6. HUBSCHMANN, O. R. & D. C. NATHANSON. 1985. The role of calcium and cellular membrane dysfunction in experimental trauma and subarachnoid hemorrhage. J. Neurosurg. **62:** 698–703.

New Opportunities with a Calcium Overload Blocker in Brain Protection?

T. PETERS AND K. U. SEILER

Departments of Experimental and Clinical Pharmacology
Janssen Research Laboratoria
D-4040 Neuss 21, Federal Republic of Germany

In a variety of animal models the sequence of events occurring under conditions of oxygen shortage in brain tissue could be defined more accurately during recent years. This has become possible because simultaneous determination of interstitial concentration of different ions by means of double- and triple-barreled electrodes can be done in parallel to biochemical determination of intermediary metabolism.[4,7]

Immediately upon cessation of oxygen supply the pH value in the interstitial space decreases. Coincidingly the electrical activity superimposed in the DC potential stops, and a slight hyperpolarization is observed. The K^+ activity slowly rises to a threshold of about 12 mM and thereafter abruptly increases to more than 70 mM. Coincidingly, the DC potential negativates. The calcium ion activity increases slightly and, when the K^+ activity attains the threshold value, falls drastically. All the events described so far proceed in spite of a diminished but still sufficient ATP reserve. Nevertheless, with the exception of K^+ and DC potential, a reversal of the situation proceeds but slowly, even if reperfusion starts immediately upon the steep deflection of the K^+ curve.[5,8]

Sound pharmacological evidence has accumulated that flunarizine, a calcium overload blocker, favorably influences the pathophysiological sequence involved in brain ischemia, hypoxia, or anoxia and in intracerebroventricular bleeding. Flunarizine acted protectively under these conditions either used as a pre- or a posttreatment.[2,3,5,6,10]

Flunarizine pronouncedly prolonged the period of anoxia tolerance by elevating the threshold at which extracellular potassium induces calcium overload of both neuronal tissue[5] (Höller et al., 1986) and vascular smooth muscle.[1,9] The effects in animals were obtained at plasma and brain concentrations of flunarizine identical to or even lower than those obtained in man after intravenous application of well-tolerated doses. In volunteers cardiohemodynamic parameters remained almost unchanged, the main side effect being dizziness during the period of intravenous application.

The major advantage of the drug was prolonged pharmacodynamic activity on the brain over a period of at least 24 hours after once-daily application. Phase I and phase II trials were extended to a seven-day treatment by daily infusions of 50 mg. Also under these conditions the drug appeared to be reasonably safe. This led to the conclusion to design and conduct phase II and phase III trials in the following fields of indication: stroke, cardiac arrest, and subarachnoidal bleeding.

REFERENCES

1. Borgers, M., F. De Clerck, J. Van Reempts, R. Xhonneux & J. Van Nueten. 1984. Intern. Angiol. **3:** 25–31.
2. Deshpande, J. K. & T. Wieloch. 1985. Neurol. Res. **7:** 27–29.
3. Edmonds, H. L., Jr., A. Wauquier, W. Melis, W. A. E. Van den Broeck, J. Van Loon, & P. A. J. Janssen. 1985. Am. J. Emerg. Med. **3:**150–155.

4. HANSEN, A. J. 1985. Physiol. Rev. **65:** 101–148.
5. HÖLLER, M., H. DIERKING, K. DENGLER, F. TEGTMEIER & T. PETERS. 1986. *In* Acute Brain Ischemia Medical and Surgical Therapy. Noé Battistine, *et al.*, Eds.: 229–236. Raven Press. New York, N.Y.
6. JAGENEAU, A., W. MELIS, J. VAN LOON & A. WAUQUIER. 1986. *In* Acute Brain Ischemia Medical and Surgical Therapy. Noé Battistine, *et al.*, Eds.: 237–243. Raven Press. New York, N.Y.
7. SIESJÖ, B. K. 1986. Eur. Neurol. **25**(Suppl. 1): 45–56.
8. TEGTMEIER, F., K. DENGLER, E. ZACHARIAS, R. EICHHORN & M. HÖLLER. 1987. Brain concentrations and effect of cerebroprotective drugs—investigations with flunarizine and R 56865. Preclinical Research Report. Janssen Research Department. Neuss, FRG.
9. VAN NUETEN, J. M., P. M. VANHOUTTE. 1981. *In* Vasodilatation. P. M. Vanhoutte & I. Leusen, Eds.: 459–468. Raven Press. New York, N.Y.
10. VAN REEMPTS, J., M. BORGERS, L. VAN DAEL, J. VAN EYNDHOVEN & M. VAN DE VEN. 1983. Arch. Int. Pharmacodyn. **262:** 76–88.

Nimodipine Oral Treatment in Subarachnoid Hemorrhage

Overview of Results from Three Randomized Controlled Trials

G. TAQUOI,[a] L. PORTO,[b] AND D. TETTENBORN[c]

[a]*Medical Department*
Bayer France
F-92815 Puteaux Cedex, France

[b]*Medical Department*
Bayer U.K.
Newbury Berkshire RG13 1JA, United Kingdom

[c]*Medical Department*
Bayer AG
D5600 Wuppertal, Federal Republic of Germany

Three double-blind placebo-controlled trials of nimodipine in the prevention of ischemic complications due to cerebral vasospasm following aneurysmal subarachnoid hemorrhage (SAH) have been conducted from 1979 to 1985.[1–3] In each of the studies a reduction of mortality and severe morbidity due to cerebral vasospasm had been found. As the number of patients in these three trials was relatively small, a further analysis was conducted in which all previously excluded patients from all trials were included in the analysis (metaanalysis) of the pooled data.

METHOD

Patients (285) were enrolled [142 on nimodipine (N), 143 on placebo (P)] within 96 hrs of aneurysmal rupture and received 60 mg N or 0.35 mg N/kg every four hours. Hunt and Hess grade on entry into the study was 1 to 2, 1 to 3, or 1 to 5. Glasgow Outcome Scale (GOS) or 5 steps scale was used to assess functional clinical status after 21 days of treatment.

The metaanalysis statistical[4] test was applied to the data of *all* patients allocated to the treatment. The test was performed three times on the same criteria of efficacy, that is, number of deaths and severe neurological deficits (ND) assessed after 21 days (4th week after the bleeding). Each calculation was based on data depending on the cause of death or severe ND.

RESULTS

Results are shown in TABLES 1 and 2.

First Test—Mortality and Severe Morbidity Due to Vasospasm Alone

In the treated group (N), the relative risk of mortality and severe morbidity due to vasospasm alone is significantly decreased ($p < 0.001$), the risk of severe disablement or death being four times greater for a control patient than for a nimodipine-treated patient (14.7% and 2.8% respectively).

Second Test— Mortality and Severe Morbidity Due to Vasospasm Alone or to Vasospasm and Other Complications

The relative risk in the treated group is significantly decreased (at the 6% level of significance) ($p < 0.052$), the risk of severe disablement or death being two times greater for a control patient than for a nimodipine-treated patient (22.4% and 13.4% respectively).

Third Test—Total Mortality and Severe Morbidity

The relative risk in the treated group (N) is decreased and the difference is significant at the 12% level ($p < 0.12$), the risk of severe disablement or death being

TABLE 1. Main Characteristics of Randomized Controlled Trials of Oral Nimodipine Treatment after SAH Due to Aneurysmal Rupture

	United Kingdom[1]	United States[2]	France[3]
Double blind	Yes	Yes	Yes
Randomization of trial treatment	Yes	Yes	Yes
Number of centers	1	5	2
Nimodipine oral therapy	30 mg tab	10 mg cap	30 mg tab
Galenic form			
Dosage	60 mgm Q4H	0.35 mg/kg Q4H	60 mg Q4H
Duration of treatment	21 days	21 days	21 days
Patients	75	129	81
Number			
Hunt and Hess grade on entry into study	1 to 5	1 to 2	1 to 3
Delay between bleeding and treatment	less than 96 hours	less than 96 hours	less than 72 hours
Scale of clinical assessment	GOS	5 step scale	GOS
Time of assessment	3 months[a] (21 days)	21 days	21 days
Main results	Decreased[b]	Decreased	Decreased
Global mortality			
Mortality due to spasm alone	Decreased	Decreased	Decreased
Mortality and severe morbidity due to spasm alone	Decreased	Decreased[b]	Decreased[b]

[a]Data analysis on the 21st day was performed when randomization code had been broken for this overview.

[b]Significant statistical decrease at least at the 5% level.

TABLE 2. Statistical Analysis

		Cause of Death or Severe Neurological Deficit		
		Vasospasm Alone	Vasospasm Alone or Vasospasm Associated with Other Cause	All Causes
Mortality + severe morbidity (No. patients)	N	4	19	38
	P	21	32	51
Mortality + severe morbidity (%)	N	2.8%	13.4%	26.8%
	P	14.7%	22.4%	35.7%
Statistical significance of the meta-analysis (p value)		0.001	0.06	0.12
Pooled relative risk for N (risk of P = 1)		0.229	0.547	0.666
95% confidence interval of the pooled relative risk		0.1–0.52	0.30–1.01	0.40–1.10
Chi-square test for heterogenicity		$\chi^2 = 0.23$ homogenous	$\chi^2 = 0.28$ homogenous	$\chi^2 = 1.51$ homogenous

1.5 times greater for a control patient than for a nimodipine-treated patient (35.7% and 26.8% respectively).

CONCLUSION

For the three double-blind studies of nimodipine (285 patients) the metaanalysis test confirms that nimodipine given as preventive oral therapy after SAH due to aneurysmal rupture is effective in preventing death and/or severe neurological deficits; this applies in particular to patients suffering from delayed ischemic syndrome related to cerebral vasospasm.

REFERENCES

1. MEE, E. W., *et al.* 1986. J. Neurol. Neurosurg. Psychiatry **49:** 469.
2. ALLEN, G. S., *et al.* 1983. N. Engl. J. Med. **308:** 619–624.
3. PHILIPPON, J., *et al.* 1986. Acta Neurochir. **82:** 110–114.
4. ARMITAGE, P. 1985. Statistical methods in medical research. Blackwell Scientific Publications Ltd. Oxford, England.

The Role of Calcium Channel Blockers in Reactive Airway Disease

ROBERT G. TOWNLEY, J. CHENG, A. K. BEWTRA,
N. NAIR, R. HOPP, AND D. K. AGRAWAL

Department of Internal Medicine
Pulmonary Allergy Division
School of Medicine
Creighton University
California at 24th Street
Omaha, Nebraska 68178

Bronchial asthma is a disease characterized by episodic and reversible narrowing of the smaller bronchi and bronchioles through a combination of smooth muscle constriction, edema, mucus formation, and cellular secretions containing a high percentage of eosinophils. All asthmatic patients are exquisitely sensitive to methacholine aerosol.[1] Asthmatic individuals react excessively to pharmacologic bronconstricting agents such as histamine, cholinergic agonists, serotonin, bradykinin, leukotriene C_4 and D_4, and the prostaglandins PGF_2 and PGD_2.[2] They also react to exercise, hyperventilation of cold dry air, or inhalation of hypotonic or hypertonic solutions (such as distilled water or hypertonic saline) and adenosine.[3]

Airway smooth muscle constriction, mast cell mediator release, mucus gland secretion, and vagal cholinergic reflex activity are all calcium-related events.[4] Increased availability of free calcium ions for excitation-contraction coupling, stimulus-secretion coupling, and nerve impulse conduction might account for the augmented smooth muscle contractibility, increased mast cell mediator release, and increased mucus gland secretion. Consistent with this is the finding that stimulation of beta-adrenergic receptors results in formation of cyclic adenosine monophosphate (AMP), which mediates muscle relaxation by favoring Ca^{2+} movement out of the cell or Ca^{2+} sequestration within cell depots. Conversely, stimulation of cholinergic receptors causes elevation of cyclic guanosine monophosphate (GMP), enhancement of Ca^{2+} movement back into the cell, and subsequent muscle contraction.

The available evidence does not permit a definitive biochemical explanation of the membrane events that account for the hyperreactivity of the airways in asthma. There may be a defect in membrane receptors, in calcium influx, in phospholipid metabolism, or in some other process.

The overriding factor in the development of symptoms, irrespective of which mediators are released in the lung by immunologic or nonimmunologic means, is the hypersensitivity to these mediators in the asthmatic individual.

The hyperreactivity of the airways to the various mediators that is noted in asthma patients could have a common mechanism since they all require calcium for their smooth muscle stimulating activity. Thus, it is possible that airway hypersensitivity is due to a partial depolarization of the smooth muscle. Although the basic cause of the hypersensitivity is unknown, it may be related to an increased permeability of smooth muscle cell membrane to calcium ions, which activate the contractile mechanism.

If the critical pathogenetic pathways in asthma are ultimately related to free calcium ion availability in smooth muscle mast cells and mucous glands, it follows that effective therapy must reduce calcium availability to the essential contractile and secretory functions.[4] In this regard, there have been several recent reviews on this topic.[5–7] It is now possible to evaluate the role of calcium channel blockade in the management of asthma.

EFFECT OF MAST CELLS AND BASOPHILS

Calcium ions may play an important role in allergic reactions, mainly by relating to the release mechanism of chemical mediators from target cells. The requirement for Ca^{2+} in the anaphylactic release of chemical mediators from target cells is well established.[8–10] Nonimmunologic stimuli such as concanavalin A, compound 48/80, dextran, and ATP also require Ca^{2+} for histamine release.[11]

Recently, Ishizaka *et al.* reported that increased phospholipid methylation of cell membrane induced by bridging of immunoglobulin E (IgE) receptors, causes influx of Ca^{2+} into the cells and subsequent histamine release.[12] A close relation between the rate of histamine release and the amount of Ca^{2+} uptake has been observed in stimulated cells.[13,14] When the entry of Ca^{2+} into target cells is inhibited by certain agents, histamine release from the cells is also inhibited. Theophylline also inhibits both the increase in calcium uptake and histamine release from mast cells due to antigen.[15] Thus it seems possible that allergic reactions could be suppressed by inhibiting Ca^{2+} influx into target cells at the early stage of the release mechanism.

In our preliminary studies the inhibitory effect of nifedipine was observed on passive cutaneous anaphylaxis (PCA) reactions in rats elicited by IgE antibody, and on the ^{45}Ca uptake of rat peritoneal mast cells stimulated by reaginic antibody, concanavalin A, compound 48/80, or Ca ionophore A23187. At the same time, the effect of nifedipine was compared to that of sodium cromolyn in rat skin reactions and the *in vitro* mast cell reactions.[16]

Our results can be summarized as follows:

1. The rat PCA response induced by IgE antibody was inhibited by intravenous administration of nifedipine (100 μg per rat). Cromolyn sodium (5 mg per rat) also inhibited the rat PCA response.
2. The ^{45}Ca uptake of actively or passively sensitized mast cells with stimulation by ovalbumin antigen was suppressed by preincubation with nifedipine (FIGURE 1). The inhibitory effect of nifedipine and cromolyn sodium on the ^{45}Ca uptake of the stimulated cells was dose dependent and biphasic. Nifedipine was more potent than cromolyn sodium in inhibiting calcium uptake; however, cromolyn sodium was more potent in inhibiting histamine release.
3. The ^{45}Ca uptake of mast cells stimulated by concanavalin A or compound 48/80 was inhibited by nifedipine. The inhibitory effect was very similar to that seen in antigen-stimulated cells.

The effects of the calcium antagonists on anaphylactic histamine release from human basophils are still controversial.[17,18] Verapamil reportedly suppresses the anaphylactic human basophil degranulation at a concentration of 100 μM.[19] Our data suggest that verapamil may influence the receptor-operated calcium channels on human basophils, but nifedipine has little effect. These agents reportedly inhibit a Ca ionophore A23187 induced histamine release from human basophils.[18,20] We confirmed an effect by nifedipine and an equal or more pronounced effect by verapamil. However, the effects were observed only at 10 and 100 μM.[21]

The release of inflammatory mediators from mast cells and platelets also depends

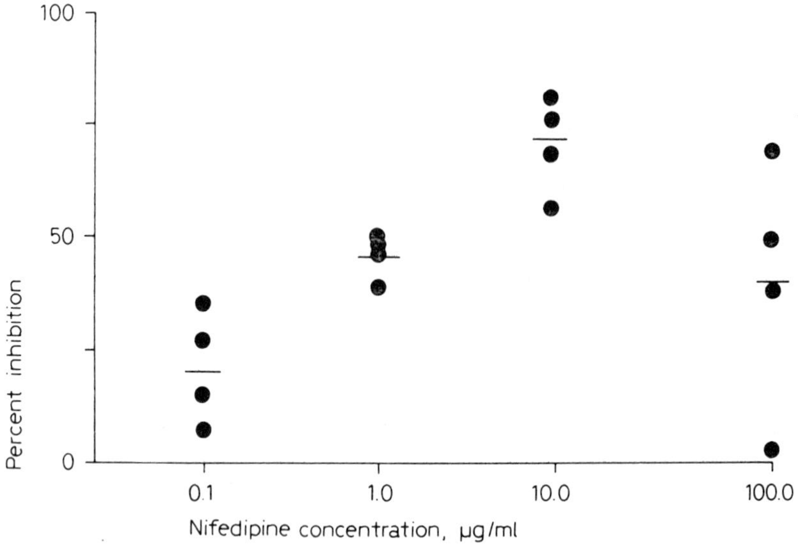

FIGURE 1. Effect of nifedipine on ^{45}Ca uptake on passively sensitized mast cells stimulated with ovalbumin. The ordinate refers to percent inhibition of ^{45}Ca uptake. The horizontal bars represent the mean for four experiments. The initial concentrations of nifedipine are shown on the abscissa; the final concentrations are one-half of three initial values.

upon extracellular Ca^{2+}. When stimulated by phagocytosis or Ca^{2+} ionophore, purified human polymorphonuclear neutrophils (PMNs) liberate performed proteases and two mediators involved in inflammatory processes, platelet-activating factor (PAF) and slow-reacting substance (SRS), i.e., leukotrienes.[22]

The Ca^{2+} antagonist nifedipine used at physiological concentrations decreases the release of PAF, SRS, and to a lesser degree the lysosomal enzyme β-glucuronidase. In addition it also diminished the uptake of $^{45}Ca^{2+}$ by these cells. These results confirm that the secretion of the PAF is Ca^{2+} dependent[23,24] and indicate that organic Ca^{2+} antagonists can inhibit the release of inflammatory mediators.

Blood levels of nifedipine after oral administration of 20 mg are 3 and 0.1 μM at 30 minutes and 4 hours, respectively.[25] These concentrations are within the range of those used in these experiments. These investigators have found an inhibitory effect on the PAF release from PMNs in five patients taking nifedipine. Further studies are necessary to clarify the physiological and pathological consequences of the use of Ca^{2+} blockers in human inflammatory processes.

The directly mediated contractile activity of leukotriene LTD_4 on isolated guinea pig trachea and lung parenchyma was dependent upon the presence of calcium in the bathing buffer.[26] Whereas 8-(*N*,/*N*-diethylamino)-octyl-3,4,5-trimethoxybenzoate (TMB-8), a calcium antagonist believed to act intracellularly, completely antagonized the LTD_4-induced contraction, the calcium channel entry blockers nifedipine and verapamil only partially inhibited LTD_4 contractile activity; diltiazem was inactive. TMB-8, nifedipine, and verapamil were more effective in blocking the contraction of the trachea elicited by KCl-induced membrane depolarization than the contraction induced by LTD_4. Of the channel entry blockers only nifedipine appeared capable of partially relaxing an established LTD_4 contraction.[26] The strict stereochemical requirement for the LTD_4-induced contraction of the trachea supported the hypothesis that LTD_4 may indeed operate via a receptor mechanism.[27,28]

To explore the biochemical aspects of the airway leukotriene receptor, we set out to use $[^3H]LTD_4$ to quantitate its binding to guinea pig lung homogenates and to assess directly interactions of leukotrienes and many other compounds with the binding sites.[29]

None of the calcium entry blockers at 10^{-5} or 10^{-4} M, including verapamil, nifedipine, diltiazem as well as TMB-8, or cromolyn sodium, had an effect on the IC_{50} value in competition experiments for leukotriene receptors. Thus calcium entry blockers have no direct action on the leukotriene receptors.

AIRWAY CHALLENGES *IN VIVO* IN ANIMALS

Calcium channel blockers, such as nifedipine, verapamil, and diltiazem, exert their effect on only one of these pathways, the voltage-operated channels,[7] which can be opened by depolarization of cellular membrane. Increased intracellular calcium ion concentration may also be due to influx of calcium via receptor-operated channels, and by release of calcium from intracellular calcium stores such as sarcoplasmic reticulum and mitochondria. Potassium-induced contractions and to a lesser extent leukotriene-induced contractions are mainly dependent on voltage-operated channels, and are therefore blocked by calcium-channel blockers such as nifedipine,[30] whereas histamine is less dependent on extracellular calcium and also appears to release internal calcium.[31,32]

The effects of calcium channel blockers nifedipine and verapamil [intravenous (iv) and aerosol] were investigated in beagle dogs natively allergic to *Ascaris suum* antigen.[33] Control exposures to an aerosol of ascaris antigen provoked significant

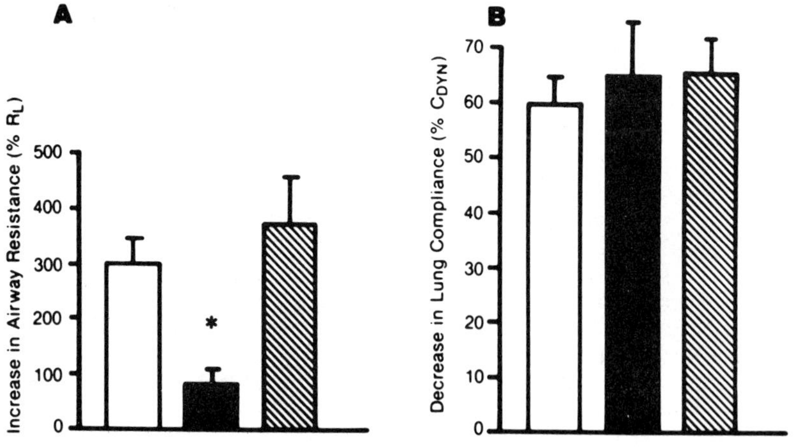

FIGURE 2. Effect of nifedipine (iv and aerosol) pretreatment versus ascaris-antigen-induced bronchospasm in anesthetized dogs. Each bar represents the mean percent change ± standard error of the mean (SEM) in airway resistance (R_L) or dynamic lung compliance (C_{dyn}) for five animals; $p < 0.005$ when value compared to ascaris response alone. Ascaris antigen alone; nifedipine (200 μg/kg, iv) + ascaris antigen 15 minutes later; nifedipine aerosol (1.0%; 10 breaths) + ascaris antigen 15 minutes later. (Reproduced from Reference 33 with permission.)

bronchopulmonary changes, i.e., increases in pulmonary resistance (R_L) and decreases in dynamic lung compliance (C_{dyn}) (FIGURE 2). Pretreatment with either nifedipine or verapamil (200 μg/kg iv) provided significant inhibition in R_L and responses to ascaris antigen ($p < 0.015$), while neither agent significantly affected C_{dyn} changes. When administered by aerosol, verapamil (1.0%, 10 breaths) significantly inhibited both the R_L and C_{dyn} responses to ascaris antigen ($p < 0.05$), whereas a similar concentration of nifedipine was without effect. Resting basal levels of R_L and C_{dyn} were unaffected by either nifedipine or verapamil by the iv route or by aerosols. The results suggest that calcium channel blockers may have beneficial effects against allergen-provoked bronchoconstriction. However, differences appear to exist in the choice of agent, route of administration, and site of action.

Brugman *et al.* investigated the ability of a calcium channel blocker, nifedipine, given as an aerosol to attenuate bronchoconstriction induced by citric acid, ascaris antigen, and methacholine in Basenji greyhound dogs.[34] They conclude that nifedipine effectively attenuates bronchoconstriction induced by citric acid, ascaris antigen, and methacholine in dogs with hyperreactive airways.

Russi *et al.* treated sheep allergic to *Ascaris suum* antigen with the calcium antagonist verapamil prior to airway challenge with an aerosol of *Ascaris suum* antigen and also investigated the response without pretreatment.[35] Aerosolized *Ascaris suum* antigen increased mean pulmonary resistance (R_L) to 530% of baseline ($n = 6$). Pretreatment with intravenously administered verapamil (150 μg/kg) increased the mean R_L to 225% of baseline but bronchoconstriction produced by subsequent antigen challenge was completely prevented. Verapamil did not modify bronchoconstriction produced by aerosols of histamine and carbachol, agents that act upon airway smooth muscle. Furthermore it did not reverse the increase in R_L induced by intravenous infusion of carbachol. These results suggest that verapamil, at the dosage used, did not prevent allergic bronchoconstriction by direct action on smooth muscle and therefore was effective by inhibiting the release of mast cell mediators.

Another possible effect of calcium channel blockers in asthma has recently been suggested. Nifedipine appeared to enhance nonadrenergic inhibitory nerve effects in airway smooth muscle contraction.[36] It has also been reported that there is a synergistic effect between isoprenaline and nifedipine on the inhibition of contraction evoked by electrical field stimulation of airway smooth muscle.[37] Thus, calcium channel blockers can enhance bronchodilatory effects, either by exogenous beta-agonists or by endogenous inhibitory transmitters.

AIRWAY CHALLENGES IN HUMANS

Synergistic relaxing effect on bronchial smooth muscle of beta-adrenoceptor stimulation and calcium channel blockade has been reported.[37] Also in clinical studies pretreatment with nifedipine results in a more pronounced bronchodilation with increasing doses of intravenous terbutaline[38] and the effect of inhaled β_2-adrenoceptor agonist treatment after nifedipine is prolonged compared to placebo.[39,40] There is also a spasmolytic effect, i.e., relaxation of precontracted bronchial smooth muscle, against histamine-induced bronchoconstriction.[41] The duration of bronchoconstriction was shortened by nifedipine compared to placebo. These effects correspond to the *in vitro* finding that nifedipine is more potent in reversing contraction of airway smooth muscle than in preventing its development.[42]

These findings are consistent with those of Patel, who also observed failure of verapamil and nifedipine to inhibit methacholine and histamine-induced bronchoconstriction in humans,[43,44] whereas exercise-induced fall in forced expiratory volume in one second was prevented by both verapamil[45] and nifedipine.[46] The effect of calcium channel blocking agents on allergen-induced bronchoprovocation has also been investigated in humans, and the results are controversial. So and co-workers compared the protective effects of inhaled verapamil (estimated dose 2.4 mg) and sublingual nifedipine (20 mg) against allergen-induced asthma.[47] This was assessed by the administration of the above calcium antagonists 30 minutes before bronchial provocation tests using *Dermatophagoides pteronyssinus* extracts on eight young perennial asthmatics.[47] Neither drug changed the basal forced expiratory volume in one second (FEV_1) or the provocation dose of allergen required to cause a 20% fall in FEV_1 ($PD_{20}FEV_1$).

However, more recently Henderson *et al.* investigated the effects of the calcium antagonist nifedipine on antigen-induced bronchoconstriction *in vivo* and *in vitro*.[48] Eight grass-pollen-sensitive asthmatics were given either nifedipine (20 mg sublingually) or placebo 30 minutes before antigen challenge. The fall in forced expiratory volume in 1 second after pretreatment with placebo was 42.8 ± 10.1%. After nifedipine this was significantly reduced to 26.5 ± 11.7% ($p < 0.005$). The protective effect of oral administration of verapamil on allergen-induced asthma was investigated by Miadonna *et al.*[49] As a whole, in eight patients, the mean fall of FEV_1 was 27.5 ± 4.9% with no pretreatment, while the treatment with 80 mg three times a day for 3 days the decrease was only 11.1 ± 2.2% ($p < 0.01$).

Although verapamil can induce a relaxation of smooth muscle, some clinical experiments performed by Patel[43] as well as by Miadonna's group[49] have demonstrated that the drug cannot prevent the bronchoconstriction induced by inhalation of histamine and methacholine. Therefore the activity of verapamil in the prevention of the allergen-induced asthma seems to be predominantly mediated by inhibition of specific mast cell degranulation.

Recently, So and co-workers pointed out the lack of activity of verapamil in preventing allergen-induced asthma.[47] Although these results differ from those of Miadonna *et al.*,[49] it should be noted that the methods, the dosages of verapamil, and the selections of the patients were different.

POSSIBLE MECHANISMS OF ACTION

TABLE 1 summarizes and compares the effect of cromolyn sodium, nifedipine, and verapamil on the bronchoconstrictive effect of exercise, hyperventilation of cold dry air, allergen, water challenge, methacholine, and histamine. From the above studies it is clear that although calcium channel blockers consistently protect against exercise-induced asthma, their effect on allergen-induced asthma is controversial. For the most part, these agents are ineffective against histamine or methacholine challenges. The reason for these differences may be patient selection, timing of drug administration, dosage, and the end point of judging efficacy. Perhaps what is needed is to determine the efficacy of these agents on allergen, exercise, and methacholine airway responses in the same group of asthma subjects using the same drug timing and route of administration. Protection against exercise and allergen challenge but not against methacholine would suggest an effect on airway mast cells.

Although most earlier studies have reported no effect of calcium channel blockers on basal bronchial tone in humans, two recent studies do show that nifedipine does decrease bronchial tone.

In 11 patients with bronchial asthma and regular overnight falls in peak expiratory flow rate (PEFR) of 15%, Patakas *et al.* demonstrated significant bronchodilation restricted only to large airways after the administration of a single dose of 10 mg of

TABLE 1. Protective Effect on Bronchoprovocation

Bronchoprovocation	Cromolyn Na^+	Nifedipine	Verapamil	Comments
Exercise	+	+	+	All studies report protection
Hyperventilation of cold dry air	+	+	+	Fanta and McFadden (personal commun.) Henderson and Costello found protection against hyperventilation of cold dry air[48]
Allergen	+	+	+	Controversial[47–49]
H_2O inhalation	+	+	+	S. Anderson *et al., Thorax,* May 1983
Methacholine	–	–	–	
Histamine	–	–	–	Although some investigators report a twofold protection, the effect is not biologically significant
Leukotriene D_4	–	–	–	J. A. Roberts *et al., Thorax* **41:** 753, 1986.

nifedipine.[50] A statistically significant increase in PEFR, specific conductance of airways (SG_{aw}), and FEV_1 was noted at 1 hour and especially 2 hours after nifedipine administration. During 4 days of nifedipine treatment (10 mg three times a day), the overnight fall in mean of PEFR was statistically significant ($p < 0.02$) and less than the mean fall of PEFR during the 4 days of placebo treatment. Thus nifedipine does modify the basal bronchial tone of patients with asthma and diminishes the circadian swing of airway resistance.[50]

In vitro studies have demonstrated nifedipine to be a smooth muscle relaxant of guinea pig,[42,51] canine, and human trachea.[52] A few studies have reported on the effect of "prolonged treatment by calcium channel blockers" in asthma.[53,54] Asthmatics were treated with 60 mg nifedipine per day for 3 weeks compared to placebo.[53] Eleven patients with severe chronic asthma were studied, and during nifedipine treatment the duration of asthma attacks decreased and the use of inhaled beta-adrenoceptor stimulants decreased.

It is possible that drugs may be developed in the future that interact with calcium entry by receptor-operated channels, or with the release of calcium from intracellular stores.

To pursue the possibility of an *in vivo* effect a prospective study was undertaken to evaluate the effect and safety of nifedipine on a total of 60 subjects, 15 with asthma, 15 with chronic obstructive pulmonary disease (COPD), 15 with angina, and 15 normals. All subjects received nifedipine, 20 mg sublingually[54] (FIGURE 3). Except for the normal subjects, there was a significant ($p < 0.05$) improvement in FEV_1 and forced vital capacity (FVC) postnifedipine. The maximum bronchodilating effect was noted one hour after administration of the drug and maintained through the second hour. There was no tachyphlaxis at the end of two weeks. Nifedipine, because of the bronchodilating effect, is safe in patients with angina and COPD or asthma.

This is of clinical importance to patients with angina pectoris and COPD or bronchial asthma. These patients could represent a difficult problem to the physician, owing to the inability to use beta-adrenergic blocking agents to control the symptoms of angina, since these agents are reported to induce marked bronchoconstriction in patients with COPD and bronchial asthma.[55,56]

There are several characteristics that are common to both variant angina and bronchial asthma including the provocation with methacholine, serotonin agonists, cold air, histamine, and beta-adrenergic blockade.[57,58] The provocation of bronchospasm or coronary vasospasm with the neurotransmitters acetylcholine, serotonin, or histamine may activate specific receptors that open calcium channels. The cytoplasmic concentration of free calcium appears to be the primary intracellular signal controlling smooth muscle tissue tonus. However, the cyclic nucleotides play a role in modulating the intracellular availability of calcium. An increase in cAMP, whether by stimulation of adenylate cyclase with beta-adrenergic agonists or inhibition of phosphodiesterase by theophylline, has been shown to relax smooth muscle. Beta-adrenergic blocking agents alone or in combination with alpha-adrenergic stimulation would result in decreased removal of calcium and/or an increase in calcium influx, respectively. The exacerbation of asthma or variant angina by beta-adrenergic blocking agents could be explained by the above mechanism. Futhermore, the resultant adrenergic imbalance by beta-adrenergic blockade alone or in combination with alpha adrenergic stimulation has been shown in animal models of asthma,[59] as well as in patients with allergic rhinitis[60] and asthma[61] to increase the sensitivity to serotonin, histamine, and methacholine.

The hyperreactivity of the airways that occurs in asthma patients could have a common mechanism since they all require calcium for their smooth muscle stimulating activity. Thus, it is possible that airway hyperreactivity is due to a partial depolarization of the smooth muscle. Although the basic cause of the hypersensitivity is unknown, it suggests an increased permeability of smooth muscle cell membrane to calcium ions, which activate the contractile mechanism.

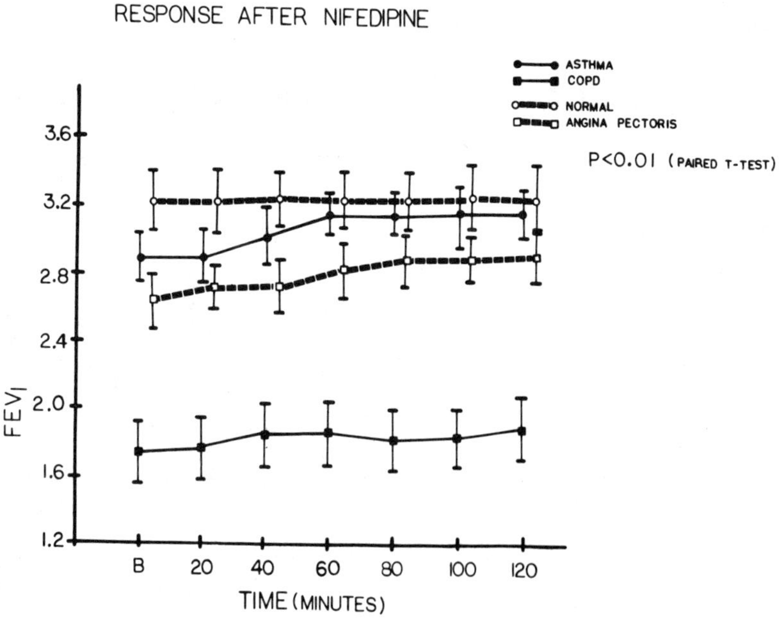

FIGURE 3. FEV_1 response after nifedipine at different time intervals in the four groups on initial visit.

Weiss and Vismanath reported on the possible role of an abnormality in calcium homeostasis in the pathogenesis of airway hyperreactivity.[62] The finding of an increased sensitivity of resting isometric tension to extracellular calcium following *in vitro* anaphylaxis in guinea pig trachealis was the basis for this hypothesis. The reactivity of airway smooth muscle to a variety of nonspecific stimuli or agonists, as occurs in asthmatic airways, could be due to an increase in free myoplasmic Ca^{2+}. Other observations provide added evidence for this model. In this regard, exogenous arachidonate metabolites cause a specific, rapid, and significant increase in the permeability of the plasma membrane to $^{45}Ca^{2+}$ of rabbit peritoneal neutrophils.[63] The facts that lipoxygenase products augment the response to histamine in human bronchi[64] and methacholine responses in man can be increased by cyclooxygenase products[65] suggest that inflammatory mediators are involved in airway smooth muscle reactivity.

Using nonimmune guinea pigs that were natively highly sensitive to histamine,

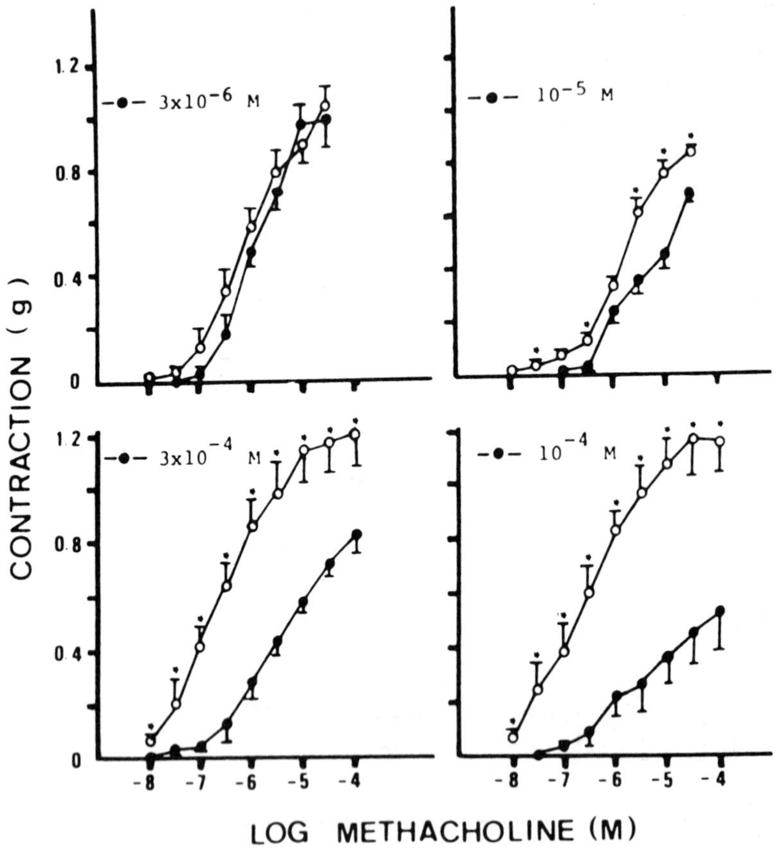

FIGURE 4. Effects of verapamil on the contractile response of rat tracheal muscle to methacholine. Each point represents the mean ± SEM of 3–6 experiments. Open circles, control; filled circles, verapamil treated. *Significantly different from the corresponding control ($p < 0.05$). (Reproduced from Reference 42 with permission.)

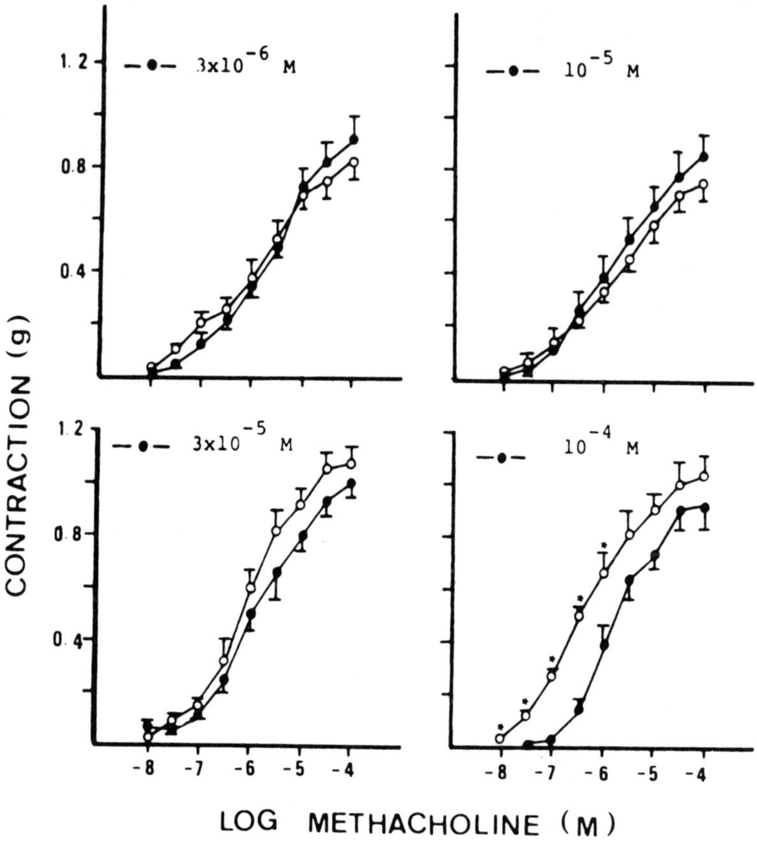

FIGURE 5. Effects of nifedipine on the constractile response of rat tracheal muscle to methacholine. Each point represents the mean ± SEM of 3–5 experiments. Open circles, control; filled circles, nifedipine treated. *Significantly different from the corresponding control ($p < 0.05$). (Reproduced from Reference 42 with permission.)

Nath and colleagues found that an increased tracheal lysophosphatidyl choline (LPC) content correlated with airway sensitivity.[66] Although LPC has many other biochemical effects, increased membrane LPC could alter membrane permeability to calcium, resulting in a higher concentration of intracellular calcium, and further contribute to airway hyperreactivity.

The success of long-term prophylactic treatment of asthma with Ca^{2+} channel blockers must await clinical verification. So little is known about the Ca^{2+} binding properties of the respiratory system (e.g., lung and airway smooth muscle) that nothing absolute can be proposed. For example, the sites of action for inhibition of Ca^{2+} influx and the affinity of the channel blockers for these sites probably vary with the tissues and species being examined. To induce their effect in respiratory muscle, the currently available Ca^{2+} channel blockers must be used at considerably greater concentrations than those used with vascular smooth muscle. These calcium channel binding sites have recently been identified using [^{3}H]nitrendipine in tracheal smooth muscle.[67]

[^{3}H]Nitrendipine binding to the bovine tracheal muscle membrane at 25°C was rapid, saturable (B_{max} = 74.8 ± 3.9 fmol/mg protein), and of high affinity (K_d = 0.14 ± 0.04 nM). The rank order of Ca^{2+} antagonists competing for airway [^{3}H]nitrendipine binding was nitrendipine = nisoldipine = nifedipine ≫ verapamil. Cromolyn, however, neither inhibited nor increased the binding. In a similar bovine tracheal muscle preparation, the number of muscarinic and beta-adrenergic receptor sites is about 190- and 13-fold, respectively,[68] greater than that of [^{3}H]nitrendipine binding sites when the numbers are expressed per milligram protein.

We found that verapamil (10^{-5}–10^{-4} M) reduced contraction of rat tracheal muscle to methacholine[42] (FIGURE 4), a finding consistent with its inhibition on binding of [^{3}H]QNB (quinuclidinyl benzilate) to bovine tracheal muscle membranes. Unlike verapamil, nifedipine (10^{-5}–3×10^{-5} M) inhibited neither methacholine response

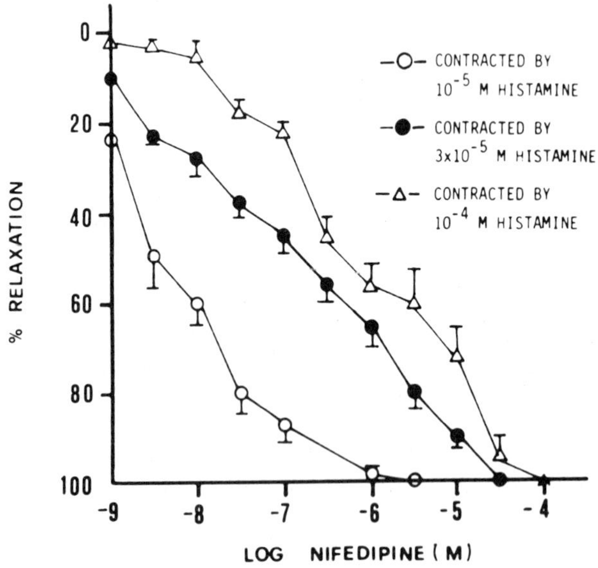

FIGURE 6. Effect of nifedipine on the relaxation of guinea pig tracheal muscle precontracted with 10^{-5} M, 3×10^{-5} M, and 10^{-4} M histamine. Each point represents the mean ± standard error of 8 to 10 experiments.

(FIGURE 5) nor [^{3}H]QNB binding.[42] Verapamil but not nifedipine decreased the affinity of binding sites. Neither of them affected the concentration of [^{3}H]QNB binding sites.

An important observation is that effects on isolated airways indicate that inhibition of mechanical responses occur at doses 1000 times greater than for vascular tissue. Although significant variations apparently depend on tissue type and agonist used, the IC_{50} values for airway smooth muscle range from 10^{-6} to 10^{-4} M. It is not known why calcium channel blockers exert their effects on airway tissue at higher concentrations than required for equivalent effects on vascular tissue. Although we observed that rat trachea responses to potassium depolarization were attenuated by nifedipine at 10^{-8} M,[42] this is one of the few instances where the potency of calcium channel inhibitors approaches that observed for nonairway smooth muscle. One possible reason is that airway smooth muscle and cardiovascular smooth muscle contain different receptors for calcium channel inhibitors, contributing to the apparent selectivity of these compounds for cardiovascular smooth and cardiac muscle. A more likely possibility is that these differences occur at the postreceptor level and the release of calcium from intracellular sites.

Although it (10^{-8}–10^{-7} M) blocked the contraction of the rat tracheal muscle to KCl and $CaCl_2$, nifedipine (10^{-7}–10^{-6} M) did not significantly inhibit histamine-, methacholine-, or serotonin-induced muscle contractions in guinea pigs and the methacholine contraction in rats. Nifedipine produced a potent relaxation on contracted tracheal muscle. The extent of the nifedipine-induced relaxation could be modified by the baseline and active contracted tension (FIGURE 6). Our results indicate that nifedipine exerts a potent dilatory effect directly on airway muscle, and suggest that this effect could be one of its pharmacological actions of relieving bronchospasm.

A final comment concerning the possible mechanism of action pertains to the fact that cromoglycate and similar antiallergics act in some way to prevent an increased flux of calcium into mast cells, which is associated with antigen challenge of mast cells and subsequent mediator release.[69] The ability to measure directly calcium channel receptors[67] as well as cromolyn sodium receptors on mast cells[70] provides an opportunity to gain further insight into the possible mechanism of action at a molecular level.

To induce their effect in respiratory muscle, the currently available Ca^{2+} channel blockers must be used at considerably greater concentrations than those used with vascular smooth muscle. This suggests that these channels are either different from or less sensitive than those previously described for the cardiovascular system. However, the relative ineffectiveness of these agents as bronchodilators is still unexplained.

REFERENCES

1. TOWNLEY, R. G., U. Y. RYO, B. M. KOLOTKIN, *et al.* 1975. Bronchial sensitivity to methacholine in current and former asthmatic and allergic rhinitis patients and control subjects. J. Allergy Clin. Immunol. **56:** 429.
2. TOWNLEY, R. G. 1987. Asthma. *In* Principles of Immunology and Allergy. Eds. R. F. Lockey & S. C. Bukanty, Eds.: Chapter 3. W. B. Saunders Co. Philadelphia, Pa.
3. HOLGATE, S. T., J. S. MAUN & M. J. CUSHLEY. 1984. Adenosine as a bronchoconstrictor in asthma and its antagonism by methylxanthine. J. Allergy Clin. Immunol. **74:** 302–306.
4. MIDDLETON, E. 1980. Antiasthmatic drug therapy and calcium ions: review of pathogenesis and role of calcium. J Pharm. Sci. **69:** 234.
5. RUSSI, E. W. & T. AHMED. 1984. Calcium and calcium antagonists in airway disease. A review. Chest **86:** 475.
6. BARNES, P. J. 1985. Clinical studies with calcium antagonists. Br. J. Clin. Pharmacol. **20:** 289S.
7. TRIGGLE, D. J. 1984. Cellular calcium metabolism: activation and antagonism. J. Asthma **21:** 375.
8. MONGAR, J. L. & H. O. SCHILD. 1958. The effect of calcium and pH on the anaphylactic histamine release. Br. J. Pharmacol. **46:** 741.
9. KALINER, M. & K. F. AUSTEN. 1973. A sequence of biochemical events in the antigen-induced release of chemical mediators from sensitized human lung tissue. J. Exp. Med. **138:** 1077.
10. DIAMANT, B., N. GROSSMAN, P. STAHLSKOV & S. THOMPLE. 1974. Effect of divalent cations and metabolic energy on the anaphylactic histamine release from rat peritoneal mast cells. Int. Arch. Allergy Appl. Immunol. **47:** 42.
11. DIAMANT, B. & S. A. PATKAR. 1975. Stimulation and inhibition of histamine release from isolated rat muscle cells. Dual effects of ionophore A23187. Int. Arch. Allergy Appl. Immunol. **49:** 183.

12. ISHIZAKA, T., P. HIRATA, K. ISHIZAKA & J. AXELROD. 1980. Stimulation of phospholipid methylation Ca^{2+} influx and histamine release by bridging IgE receptors. Proc. Nat. Acad. Sci. USA **77:** 1903.
13. ISHIZAKA, T., J. C. FOREMAN, A. R. STERK & K. ISHIZAKA. 1979. Induction of calcium flux across the rat cell membrane by bridging IgE receptors. Proc. Nat. Acad. Sci. USA **76:** 5858.
14. RYO, U. Y., B. KANG & R. G. TOWNLEY. 1976. Cromolyn therapy in patients with bronchial asthma. J. Am. Med. Assoc. **236:** 927.
15. FOREMAN, J. C., M. B. HALLETT & J. L. MONGAR. 1977. The relationship between histamine and ^{45}Ca uptake by mast cells. J. Physiol. **271:** 193.
16. TANIZAKI, Y., K. AKAGI, K. N. LEE & R. G. TOWNLEY. 1983. Inhibitory effect of nifedipine on skin reactions and ^{45}Ca uptake of mast cells induced by various stimulating agents. Int. Arch. Allergy Appl. Immunol. **72:** 102–109.
17. MIDDLETON, E., JR., G. DRZEWIECKI & D. TRIGGLE. 1981. Effects of smooth muscle antagonists on human basophil histamine release. Biochem. Pharmacol. **30:** 2867.
18. SKOV, P. S., C. JENSEN & S. NORN. 1982. *In vivo* and *in vitro* effect of calcium antagonists on basophil histamine release. (Abstr.) XII Congress Allergol. Clin. Immunol. **12:** 114.
19. NASSAR, A., F. LEYNADIER & J. DRY. 1982. Inhibition of the human basophil degranulation by verapamil. Nouv. Presse Med. **11:** 3572. (In French.)
20. BEDARD, R. M. & W. W. BUSSE. 1983. Nifedipine inhibition of human basophil histamine release (HR). (Abstr.) J. Allergy Clin. Immunol. **71:** 104.
21. AKAGI, K. & R. TOWNLEY. Unpublished.
22. JOUVIN-MARCHE, E., J. CERINA, E. COEFFIER, P. DUROUX & J. BENVENISTE. 1983. Effect of the Ca^{2+} antagonist nifedipine on the release of platelet-activating factor (PAF-acether), slow-reacting substance and β-glucuronidase from human neutrophils. Eur. J. Pharmacol. **89:** 19.
23. BENVENISTE, J., P. M. HENSON & C. G. COCHRANE. 1972. Leukocyte-dependent histamine release from rabbit platelets: the role of IgE, basophils and a platelet-activating factor. J. Exp. Med. **136:** 1377.
24. BETZ, S. J. & P. M. HENSON. 1980. Production and release of platelet-activating factor (PAF); dissociation from degranulating and superoxide production in the human neutrophil. J. Immunol. **125:** 2756.
25. PATZSCHKE, K. K., K. SCHLOSSMANN & F. HORSTER. 1975. Nifedipine—Pharmakokinetik und Biotransformation. Ther. Berlin **47:** 197.
26. WEICHMAN, B. M., R. A. MUCCITELLI, S. S. TUCKER & M. A. WASSERMAN. 1983. Effect of calcium antagonists on leukotriene D_4–induced contraction of the guinea pig trachea and lung parenchyma. J. Pharmacol. Exp. Ther. **225:** 310.
27. TSAI, B. S., P. BERSTEIN, R. A. MACIA, J. CONATY & R. D. KRELL. 1982. Comparative potency and pharmacology of isomers of leukotriene D_4 on guinea pig trachea: requirement for a 5(S)6(r) configuration. Prostaglandin **23:** 489.
28. JONES, T. R., C. DAVIS & E. E. DANIEL. 1983. Pharmacological study of the contracile activity of leukotriene C_4 and D_4 on isolated human airway smooth muscle. Can. J. Physiol. Pharmacol. **60:** 638.
29. CHENG, J. B. & R. G. TOWNLEY. 1984. Identification of leukotriene D_4 receptor binding sites in guinea pig lung homogenates using (^3H)leukotriene D_4. Biochem. Biophys. Res. Commun. **118:** 20.
30. AHMED, F., R. W. FOSTER & R. C. SMALL. 1985. Some effects of nifedipine in guinea-pig isolated trachealis. Br. J. Pharmacol. **84:** 861.
31. CREESE, B. R. & M. A. DENBOROUGH. 1981. Sources of calcium for contraction of guinea pig isolated tracheal smooth muscle. Clin. Exp. Pharmacol. Physiol. **8:** 175.
32. SASAKI, T., K. TAKAGI, T. SATAKE, S. SUGIYAMA & T. OZAWA. 1984. Mechanism of leukotriene-induced contraction isolated guinea pig tracheal smooth muscle. Lung **162:** 369.
33. MALO, P. E., M. A. WASSERMAN & R. L. GRIFFIN. 1983. The effects of nifedipine and verapamil on antigen-induced bronchoconstriction in dogs. Eur. J. Pharmacol. **92:** 69.
34. BRUGMAN, T. M., M. L. DARNELL & C. A. HIRSHMAN. 1983. Nifedipine aerosol attenuates airway constriction in dogs with hyperreactive airways. Am. Rev. Respir. Dis. **127:** 14.
35. RUSSI, E. W., B. MARCHETTE, L. YEAGER, W. M. ABRAHAM & T. AHMED. 1983.

Modification of allergic bronchoconstriction by a calcium antagonist: mode of action. Am. Rev. Respir. Dis. **127:** 675.

36. Cuss, F. M., J. M. Palmer & P. J. Barnes. 1985. Effect of nifedipine on autonomic control of airway smooth muscle in vitro. Am. Rev. Respir. Dis. **131**(4)Suppl: A283.
37. Lofdahl, C. G., L. G. Carlsson, N. Svedmyr & B. E. Skoogh. 1985. Calcium channel blockade and beta-adrenoceptor stimulation have synergistic effects on relaxation of ferret tracheal smooth muscle. Am. Rev. Respir. Dis. **131**(4)Suppl: A283.
38. Svedmyr, K., C. G. Lofdahl & N. Svedmyr. 1984. Nifedipine—a calcium channel blocker—in asthmatic patients. Allergy **39:** 17.
39. Lever, A. M. L., P. A. Corris & G. J. Gibson. 1984. Nifedipine enhances the bronchodilator effect of salbutamol. Thorax **39:** 576.
40. Cuss, F. M., S. E. Mannix & P. J. Barnes. 1984. Nifedipine prolongs isoprenaline induced bronchodilation in normal subjects. Clin. Sci. **67:** 62P.
41. Cuss, F. M. & P. J. Barnes. 1985. Inhaled nifedipine and histamine-induced bronchoconstriction. Am. Rev. Respir. Dis. **131**(4): A50.
42. Cheng, J. B. & R. G. Townley. 1983. Pharmacological characterization of effects of nefedipine of isolated guinea-pig and rat tracheal smooth muscle. Arch. Int. Pharmacodyn. **263:** 228.
43. Patel, K. R. 1981. The effect of verapamil on histamine and methacholine induced brochoconstriction. Clin. Allergy **11:** 441.
44. Patel, K. R. 1981. Effect of nifedipine on bronchomotor tone and histamine reactivity in asthma. Br. Med. J. **283:** 348.
45. Patel, K. R. 1981. Calcium antagonists in exercise-induced asthma. Br. Med. J. **282:** 932.
46. Patel, K. R. 1981. The effect of calcium antagonist, nifedipine in exercise-induced asthma. Clin. Allergy **11:** 429.
47. So, S. Y., W. K. Lam & D. Y. C. Yu. 1982. Effect of calcium antagonists on allergen-induced asthma. Clin. Allergy **12:** 595.
48. Henderson, A. F., R. W. Heaton, L. S. Dunlop & J. F. Costello. 1983. Effects of nifedipine on antigen-induced bronchoconstriction. Am. Rev. Respir. Dis. **127:** 549.
49. Miadonna, A., A. Tedeschi, E. Leggieri, M. Conttini, M. Restuccia & C. Bianchini. 1983. Effect of verapamil on allergen-induced asthma in patients with respiratory allergy. Ann. Allergy **51:** 201.
50. Patakas, D., E. Vlachoianni, V. Tsara, G. Louridas & P. Argiropoulou. 1983. Nifedipine in bronchial asthma. J. Allergy Clin. Immunol. **72:** 269.
51. Williams, D. O., P. J. Barnes, H. P. Vickers & M. Rudolph. 1981. Effect of nifedipine on bronchomotor tone and histamine reactivity in asthma. Br. Med. J. **283:** 348.
52. Tran, K., K. Lee, M. Hoff, A. Bewtra & R. Townley. 1982. Effect of temperature and nifedipine on tracheal muscle responses to methacholine. (Abstr.) J. Allergy Clin. Immunol. **69:** 131.
53. Ozenne, G., N. D. Moore, A. Leprevost, G. Tardif, F. Boismare, P. Pasquis & J. P. Lemercier. 1985. Nifedipine in chronic bronchial asthma. A randomized double-blind crossover trial against placebo. Eur. J. Respir. Dis. **67:** 233.
54. Nair, N., R. G. Townley, A. Bewtra & C. K. Nair. 1984. Safety of nifedipine in subjects with bronchial asthma and COPD. Chest **86:** 515.
55. Anderson, E. G., B. Calcrall, A. G. Jariwaiia & M. Ai-Zaibak. 1979. Persistent asthma after treatment with beta blocking drugs. Br. J. Dis. Chest **73:** 407.
56. Raine, J. M., M. G. Palazzo, J. H. Kerr & R. Slight. 1981. Near-fatal bronchospasm after oral nadolol in a young asthmatic and response to ventilation with halothane. Br. Med. J. **282:** 548.
57. Townley, R. G. 1982. Calcium channel antagonists in coronary artery spasm and bronchial spasm. Chest **82:** 401.
58. Ginsburg, R., M. R. Bristow, D. C. Harrison & E. B. Stinson. 1980. Studies with isolated human coronary arteries. Some general observations, potential mediators of spasm, role of calcium antagonists. Chest **78:** 180.
59. Townley, R. G., I. L. Trapani & A. Szentivanyi. 1967. Sensitization of anaphylaxis and some of its pharmacological mediators by blockade of the beta-adrenergic receptors. J. Allergy **39:** 3.
60. Townley, R. G., S. McGeady & A. Bewtra. 1976. The effect of beta-adrenergic

blockade on bronchial sensitivity to acetyl-beta-methacholine in normal and allergic rhinitis subjects. J. Allergy **57:** 358.

61. RYO, U. Y. & R. G. TOWNLEY. 1976. Comparison of respiratory and cardiovascular effect of isoproterenol, propranolol and practolol in asthmatic and normal subjects. J. Allergy Clin. Immunol. **57:** 12.

62. WEISS, E. B., & S. G. WISWANATH. 1983. Calcium hypersensitivity in airways smooth muscle: calcium dependency and verapamil inhibition. Prostaglandins Leukotrienes Med. **12:** 53.

63. VOLPI, M., P. H. NACCARCHE & R. I. SHA'AFI. 1980. Arachidonate metabolite(s) increase the permeability of the plasma membrane of neutrophils to calcium. Biochem. Biophys. Res. Commun. **92:** 1231.

64. COPAS, J. L., P. BORGEAT & P. J. GARDINER. 1982. The actions of 5-, 12- and 15-HETE on tracheobronchial smooth muscle. Prostaglandins Leukotrienes Med. **8:** 105.

65. WALTERS, E. H., *et al.* 1982. Time-dependent effect of prostaglandin E_2 inhalation on airway responses to bronchoconstrictor agents in normal subjects. Thorax **37:** 438.

66. NATH, P., A. P. JOSHI & K. P. AGRAWAL. 1983. Biochemical correlates of airway reactivity in guinea pigs: role of lysophosphatidylcholine. J. Allergy Clin. Immunol. **72:** 351.

67. CHENG, J. B., A. BEWTRA & R. G. TOWNLEY. 1984. Identification of calcium channel receptor binding sites using (^{3}H)nitrendipine in bovine tracheal smooth muscle membranes. Experientia **40:** 267.

68. CHENG, J. B. & R. G. TOWNLEY. 1982. Comparison of muscarinic and beta adrenergic receptors between bovine peripheral lung and tracheal smooth muscle: a striking difference in the receptor concentration. Life Sci. **30:** 2079.

69. CHAKRAVARTY, N. 1978. The role of plasma membrane Ca^{+2}-MG^{+2} activated adenosine triphosphastase of rate mast cells on histamine release. Acta Pharmacol. Toxicol. **47:** 281.

70. MAXUREK, N., G. BERGER & I. PECKT. 1980. A binding site on mast cells and basophils for the anti-allergic drug cromolyn. Nature London **286:** 722.

Calcium Antagonists and Dysmenorrhea

K.-E. ANDERSSON

Department of Clinical Pharmacology
University of Lund
S-221 85 Lund, Sweden

UTERINE ACTIVITY IN PRIMARY DYSMENORRHEA

Even if the cause of pain in primary dysmenorrhea may be attributable to several factors, there is general agreement that an increased uterine activity is of main importance.[1–4] High intensity "well-coordinated" contractions producing extremely high intrauterine pressures as well as "dysrhythmic" contractions with high or low pressures may be found.[1] Filler and Hall suggested, however, that an elevated basal tonus was more important than the intensity of the contractions for pain production.[2] This suggestion was supported by the observation of Csapo *et al.* that the magnitude of intrauterine pressure changes was not influenced, but resting pressure and frequency decreased in a patient who became pain free after administration of a prostaglandin synthetase inhibitor.[5] The increased contractile activity of the myometrium may compromise uterine blood flow, and thereby induce ischemia and pain. Whether or nor primary vasoconstriction may contribute to this has not been established.[6,7]

Several workers have produced evidence that increased endometrial prostaglandin production and release are involved in the production of uterine hyperactivity and dysmenorrhea.[8] Prostaglandins may also sensitize afferent nerve terminals mediating pain, thus lowering their threshold to physical and chemical stimuli. In addition, prostaglandins (PG) $F_{2\alpha}$ and E_2 were found to contract vascular preparations of the ascending branches of the uterine artery, suggesting that a vasoconstrictor effect of these agents may contribute to ischemic pain in primary dysmenorrhea.[9] However, Maigaard *et al.* found that the vascular responses to prostaglandins differed markedly between human extra- and intramyometrial arteries. In extramyometrial arteries $PGF_{2\alpha}$ and PGE_2 produced relaxation at low, and contraction at high, concentrations. In small intramyometrial arteries, on the other hand, $PGF_{2\alpha}$ had negligible contractile effects, and PGE_2 produced relaxation only. It is reasonable to expect that effects on intramyometrial arteries are more important for uterine blood flow than effects on extramyometrial vessels. Thus, these data do not support the view that a direct vasoconstrictor effect of $PGF_{2\alpha}$ and PGE_2 contributes significantly to the development of dysmenorrheic uterine ischemia.

Vasopressin has been suggested to be a factor of etiological importance in primary dysmenorrhea.[10,11] During menstruation the uterus is highly sensitive to this hormone,[12] and inhibition of release of neurohypophyseal hormones by water diuresis or ethanol produces a marked inhibition of uterine activity.[13–15] Forsling *et al.* found that plasma vasopressin concentrations varied throughout the menstrual cycle with the highest levels found during menstruation.[16] In dysmenorrhea patients, plasma vasopressin levels were four times higher than in controls on the first day of menstruation, and it was suggested that this could be of importance for the symptoms of the patients.[17,18] It could not be excluded that vasopressin activated the uterus via a final step of prostaglandin synthesis and release.[18] However, Strömberg *et al.*[11] and Laudanski *et al.*[19] found that the contractant effects of vasopressin on the myometrium and uterine arteries could be obtained without an obligatory last step of prostaglandin synthesis and release. In addition, vasopressin antagonists were found to inhibit vasopressin-induced effects on myometrial activity both *in vitro*[10] and *in vivo*.[20]

The postulated central role of prostaglandins in the genesis of dysmenorrhoic pain makes it attractive to use agents that inhibit prostaglandin synthesis to treat the condition. About 70% of patients treated with prostaglandin synthetase inhibitors respond with significant pain relief.[21] However, as uterine hyperactivity obviously is a main characteristic in primary dysmenorrhea, it would be expected that drugs inhibiting myometrial activity are effective irrespective of how the activity is initiated,[22] spontaneously, by a myogenic mechanism, or directly by local or circulating hormones. As prostaglandins and vasopressin are of suggested importance for the production of this activity, the mechanisms by which they stimulate the myometrium are of particular interest.

EXCITATION-CONTRACTION COUPLING IN THE MYOMETRIUM

As in other types of smooth muscle, spontaneous and drug-induced contractions of the myometrium are related to the concentration of intracellular calcium ions. Conceptually the increase in intracellular free calcium associated with contraction may be produced by (1) an increased influx from the extracellular medium, (2) translocation of calcium ions in or near the cell membrane, or (3) the release of calcium from intracellular stores.[23] In experiments *in vitro*, the importance of extracellular calcium in the activation of the myometrium has been demonstrated. Calcium seems to play dual roles in the electrical activity of uterine smooth muscle. It has an excitatory role in the spike potential,[24–26] and an inhibitory role by means of membrane stabilization.[24,27]

Several investigators have shown that the electrical spike activity triggering contraction in, e.g., the rat myometrium is associated with an influx of calcium.[25,28–30] This was found to be the case also in the human pregnant myometrium.[31,32] In this tissue three types of action potential could be distinguished, the spike, plateau, and intermediate types.[31] The amplitude of the contraction depended on the frequency of the spikes in the spike-type action potential. In case of the plateau-type potential, the plateau was associated with the amplitude and particularly the duration of the contraction, which was proportional to the plateau duration.

An increase in extracellular calcium from 2.5 mM up to 7.0 mM caused a gradual suppression of both spike- and plateau-type potentials and of contraction. When the external calcium concentration was lowered from 2.5 to 2.0 and 1.25 mM, the amplitude and duration of both types of action potential were gradually reduced, and so were the accompanying contractions.[32] Removing the extracellular calcium abolished spontaneous contractions in human myometrium within 10 minutes.[33] It thus seems obvious that extracellular calcium is of main importance for uterine contraction.

Mironneau, working with voltage-clamped uterine strips of the pregnant rat, suggested that tension elicited by depolaration consisted of two components.[28] The first component depended on a slow inward current and the contraction was related to the extracellular calcium concentration and to calcium influx (it could be inhibited by Mn, La, and D-600). It was suggested that the slow inward current may directly activate the myofibrils, or release a part of calcium bound inside the cell. The second contraction component could be observed in an Mn-containing solution and was therefore suggested to be due to release of calcium from intracellular stores presumed to be located in the sarcoplasmic reticulum. This would mean that inhibition of the slow inward current also can have consequences for the calcium release from intracellular stores.

Mechanism of Prostaglandin-Induced Contraction

$PGF_{2\alpha}$[26] and PGE_2[34] increase spike activity in the rat myometrial cells. Grosset and Mironneau analyzed the effects of PGE_1 on pregnant rat myometrium and found that the prostaglandin did not affect the phasic contraction or the inward current obtained with depolarization.[35] However, when the inward current was blocked with D-600, the tonic contraction was increased. It was therefore suggested that PGE_1 acts essentially by increasing the intracellular calcium concentration by translocation of membrane-bound calcium from surface microvesicles or sarcoplasmic reticulum. The view that intracellular structures are important sources of calcium for contractile activation of the myometrium by prostaglandins lends support from studies on isolated subcellular fractions. Thus PGE_2 stimulated net calcium release from microsomes isolated from human term myometrium.[36] Also uterine smooth muscle mitochondria can effectively store and release calcium.[37]

In the isolated human pregnant myometrium, $PGF_{2\alpha}$ was found to increase the amplitude and duration of contractions associated with both spike-type and plateau-type action potentials, but affected the frequency to a lesser degree.[38] $PFG_{2\alpha}$ enhanced the plateau potentials and changed spike-type action potentials into plateau-type. It was suggested that $PGF_{2\alpha}$ increased contractions by affecting the plateau part of the action potential.[38]

It is well known that in isolated human nonpregnant as well as pregnant myometrium, $PGF_{2\alpha}$ stimulates spontaneous contractions.[39] $PGF_{2\alpha}$-evoked responses have been found to be sensitive to removal of calcium from the extracellular medium and to calcium antagonists. In calcium-free medium and in the presence of 4 mM [ethylene-bis(oxyethylenenitrile)] tetraacetic acid (EGTA), $PGF_{2\alpha}$ induced no contractile response.[33] These results suggested that intracellular calcium stores are not the primary target for $PGF_{2\alpha}$ in the human myometrium, but rather that transmembrane calcium influx sensitive to calcium antagonists is an important step in the activation.[33] Rubanyi and Csapo arrived at a similar conclusion, studying the effects of $PGF_{2\alpha}$ on the rabbit uterus.[40]

Mechanism of Vasopressin/Oxytocin-Induced Contractions

The membrane response of pregnant rat myometrium to oxytocin consists of increased spike activity.[34,41] In the pregnant human myometrium, Kawarabayashi and Sugimori[38] and Kawarabayashi *et al.*[42] found oxytocin to have effects on the electrical activity similar to those of prostaglandin $F_{2\alpha}$. Thus, spontaneous contractions were increased by enhancement of the plateau-type potentials. The effects were highly dependent on the extracellular calcium concentration. Even in the absence of calcium in the extracellular medium causing disappearance of spontaneous electrical activity, oxytocin evoked electrical and mechanical activity, although of greatly reduced amplitude. When spontaneous electrical activity was abolished by an increase of extracellular calcium to 5 mM, oxytocin induced reappearance of plateau type potentials and markedly increased contractions.[42] Corresponding electrophysiological studies on the effects of vasopressin on human myometrium seem to be lacking.

In potassium-depolarized myometrium, oxytocin produced a slowly developing contractile response.[42,43] Kawarabayashi *et al.* suggested this to mean that oxytocin could mobilize calcium from intracellular storage sites.[42] This cannot be excluded and is in line with the finding that oxytocin can displace calcium from an isolated myometrial microsomal fraction.[44] However, as this contractile response could be completely blocked by calcium antagonists,[43] it seems (if direct intracellular effects of the calcium antagonist can be excluded) that a step involving calcium influx is necessary for the mobilization. Calcium flux studies on rat myometrium also support the view that oxytocin-induced contractions are largely dependent on an influx of extracellular calcium.[45]

Maigaard *et al.* verified the well-known contractant effect of vasopressin on nonpregnant myometrium and myometrial vessels.[46] They also found that at a time of exposure to calcium-"free" medium when vasopressin-induced contractions in the myometrium were abolished, 25% of the vascular response remained. The threshold concentration for contractile activation of the intramyometrial arteries was similar to that needed for stimulation of the myometrium, which is in contrast to findings with $PGF_{2\alpha}$.[7] These results suggest that vasopressin may play a role as a vasoconstrictor in the nonpregnant uterus[47] and that such an effect can contribute to dysmenorrhoic pain.

Effects of Calcium Antagonists on Isolated Human Myometrium

Although the influx of calcium ions may not be the only source of calcium used for activation of the contractile proteins, inhibition of this inflow could be expected to significantly reduce myometrial contraction.[48] Fleckenstein *et al.*[49] and Grün and Fleckenstein[50] demonstrated in animal as well as in human uterine smooth muscle that calcium antagonists (verapamil, D-600, prenylamine) were capable of blocking spontaneous as well as induced (K^+, oxytocin) contractile activity. Ulmsten *et al.*[51] and Forman *et al.*[43] found that nifedipine concentration-dependently inhibited spontaneous contractions in both nonpregnant and pregnant human myometrium. The drug reduced amplitude more than frequency of contraction, and also inhibited K^+-induced contraction in a concentration-dependent manner. This effect seemed to be more pronounced in pregnant than in nonpregnant tissue. Nifedipine also depressed the contraction induced by vasopressin in isolated nonpregnant myometrium as well as contraction induced by oxytocin in pregnant myometrium. The frequency of contractions induced by oxytocin and vasopressin was sometimes increased in the presence of the drug.[43]

Maigaard *et al.* compared the effects of nicardipine and nifedipine on isolated human myometrium.[52] It was found that nicardipine as well as nifedipine relaxed pregnant as well as nonpregnant myometrial preparations contracted by K^+ and also reduced or abolished contractions occurring spontaneously or induced by $PGF_{2\alpha}$, oxytocin, and vasopressin. However, the effect of nicardipine had a slower onset of action than that of nifedipine, and the drug was significantly more potent than nifedipine in pregnant, but not in nonpregnant, myometrium.

Kawarabayashi *et al.* investigated the effects of diltiazem on isolated human pregnant myometrium.[32,42] They found that the drug concentration-dependently inhibited amplitude and duration of spontaneously occurring contractions, but increased the frequency. The drug also concentration-dependently inhibited spike- and plateau-type action potentials in myometrial tissue. Also contractions induced by oxytocin were inhibited by diltiazem. However, even at a diltiazem concentration of 10^{-4} g/ml, which completely suppressed the electrical activity, a small increase in basal tension was induced by oxytocin.

As in other types of smooth muscle, the inhibitory effects of calcium antagonists on myometrial and uterine vascular contractions have been attributed to their ability to block calcium channels (preferentially voltage operated) in the cell membrane.[33,53,54] On the other hand, it is well known that calcium antagonists enter the cell and may have intracellular effects.[55] The importance of these effects for their ability to inhibit smooth muscle contraction has not been definitely established. However, Sakamoto and Huszar found that the concentrations of nitrendipine needed to inhibit myosin light chain phosphorylation by 50% were at least 10,000 times higher than the concentrations needed to produce myometrical relaxation *in vivo* and *in vitro*.[56] This would mean that the direct intracellular actions of dihydropyridine calcium antagonists could not be expected to contribute significantly to their *in vivo* effects on myometrium and uterine vasculature.

EFFECTS OF CALCIUM ANTAGONISTS ON UTERINE ACTIVITY IN WOMEN

It has been convincingly demonstrated that the spontaneous contractile activity of the nonpregnant human uterus occurring during the menstrual cycle is most pronounced around the onset of menstruation.[47,57–59] Nifedipine 20–30 mg given orally as capsules to 10 healthy females on their first menstrual days effectively and rapidly reduced uterine activity recorded as changes in intrauterine pressure by means of a recording catheter.[51] The effect was observed after approximately 15 minutes in women who were asked to chew the capsules. There was a dose-dependent decrease in amplitude, frequency, and basal tone. After a dose of 30 mg the myometrial activity was more or less completely inhibited in all investigated women. The duration of the effect varied, but in no case was the initial uterine activity resumed during the first 3–4 hours after drug intake. When myometrial activity returned frequent contractions of low amplitude were seen. No rebound phenomenon was observed. At the time of maximum effects of the drug on myometrial activity, most patients felt warm and experienced facial flushing. There was a moderate increase in heart rate by 20 beats/minute, but the effects on blood pressure were insignificant.

Andersson and Ulmsten investigated the effects of nifedipine on myometrial activity and lower abdominal pain in women with primary dysmenorrhea.[4] Ten women were investigated on their first menstrual day, and intrauterine pressure was recorded. When given orally, nifedipine (capsules) 20–40 mg within 20–40 minutes effectively reduced the myometrial activity and pain (FIGURE 1). The amplitude, frequency, and duration of the contractions were all reduced and there was a marked decrease in basal tone. This effect was most marked in recordings from the uterine fundus. Recordings continued for up to 3 hours after drug administration. During this time there was a gradual increase in myometrial activity. All women reported pain relief within 10–40 minutes of drug taking. When myometrial activity was abolished patients were completely pain free. Rapid low-amplitude contractions appearing about 40 minutes after drug administration were not associated with pain. The duration of pain relief was up to 5 hours. At the maximum effect on the myometrium there was a feeling of facial warmth and transient flushing. Some of the patients receiving 30 or 40 mg nifedipine and chewing the capsules before swallowing had a slight transient headache, but no other side effects were noted.

The effectiveness of prostaglandin synthetase inhibitors in dysmenorrhea is well documented.[21] This may occur without complete inhibition of uterine activity.[60] In dysmenorrhoic patients becoming pain free after treatment with diflunisal but retaining some uterine activity, this activity was completely blocked by nifedipine. It was therefore suggested that in cases with persistent pain after treatment with prostaglandin synthetase inhibitors, nifedipine may be added to evaluate the significance of residual uterine activity in the genesis of pain.[22,61] If the combination may also have a therapeutic potential remains to be studied.

In line with the *in vitro* findings that calcium antagonists were even more effective on pregnant than on nonpregnant myometrium and vessels,[43,52,62] uterine activity in the pregnant uterus can be effectively counteracted by these drugs. This has been shown not only in patients with preterm labor,[63,64] but also when uterine activity was induced by $PGF_{2\alpha}$ and PGE_2 for midtrimester abortion,[65] and postpartum on $PGF_{2\alpha}$, oxytocin, and methylergometrine-induced activity.[66,67]

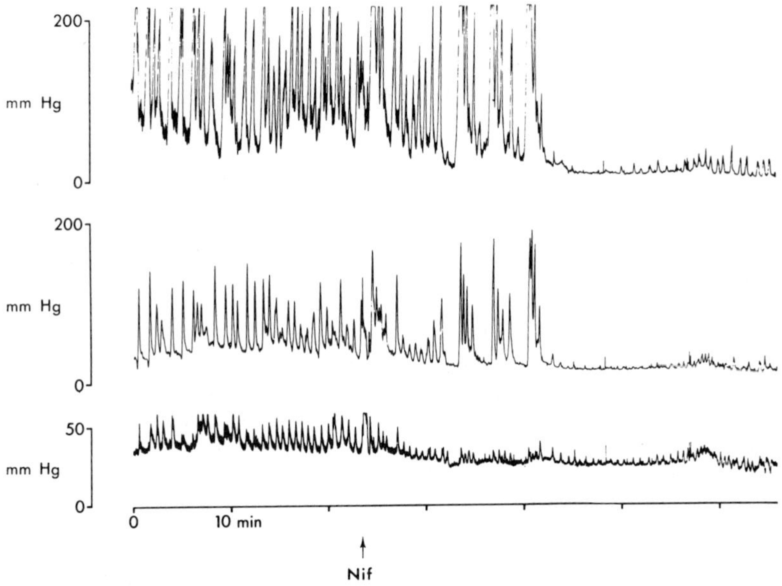

FIGURE 1. Effects of nifedipine 30 mg given orally (arrow) to a 35-year-old woman with severe primary dysmenorrhea. Intrauterine pressure was recorded by means of a three-channel microtransducer catheter. The microtransducers were placed in uterine fundus (upper tracing), uterine isthmus (middle tracing), and cervix (lower tracing). Complete pain relief was reported 20 minutes after drug intake. (Reproduced from Reference 4 with permission from the publisher).

CLINICAL TRIALS OF CALCIUM ANTAGONISTS IN DYSMENORRHEA

The promising acute effects of nifedipine in women with severe primary dysmenorrhea[4] prompted clinical trial of the effectiveness of the drug. In an open study comprising 40 women with severe primary dysmenorrhea, 36 could be observed over 3 consecutive menstrual cycles.[68] They received an initial dose of 20 mg nifedipine and the maximum daily intake was restricted to 90 mg/day. Twenty-six patients experienced good pain relief, 10 moderate relief, and 4 reported no benefit. The frequency of symptoms associated with menstrual pain (e.g., headache, gastrointestinal disturbances, and malaise) was not reduced. Side effects were encountered in almost half of the patients (19/40). The most common were headache (in 15 patients) and palpitations (in 5 patients). There was a transient facial flushing in all patients and a moderate increase in pulse rate. Nevertheless, 25 of the 36 women who completed the three-month trial wanted to continue nifedipine therapy regularly.

In another open study, Vaquez Camacho reported excellent effects of nifedipine 10 mg sublingually in 57 patients with idiopathic dysmenorrhea.[69] In 29 of the patients dysmenorrhea was abolished, and in the remaining 28 different degrees of improvement were obtained. Side effects were, however, frequently encountered including headache (14 patients), nausea (12 patients), palpitations (7 patients), and hypotension (5 patients).

Mondero studied the effects of nifedipine in 24 women with primary dysmenorrhea.[70] The patients were randomized to receive 10 mg nifedipine capsules or placebo at the onset of menstrual cramping. Of 19 nifedipine-treated patients, 3 obtained no pain relief, 2 had some relief, whereas 14 reported good or excellent pain relief. None of the 5 patients taking placebo noted any marked improvement. Side effects were found in 15 of the 19 nifedipine-treated patients including headache (8 patients), but this was also found in 3 of the 5 on placebo. The side effects were overall not considered bothersome, and 12 out of 19 patients were willing to use the drug as their monthly analgesic.

Audebert *et al.* reported in a short communication on a placebo-controlled trial with diltiazem 240 mg/day given to 14 patients who completed 4 treatment cycles, 2 on diltiazem and 2 on placebo.[71] They found that 78% of the patients were improved when on diltiazem compared with 42% when on placebo. The symptoms associated with the dysmenorrheic pain were not improved. The tolerance to diltiazem was considered to be good with only one patient stopping the trial because of nausea when treated with the drug.

The lack of adequately designed and controlled trials of calcium antagonists in dysmenorrhea makes it impossible to assess their overall efficacy and side effects. Furthermore, no comparisons with prostaglandin synthetase inhibitors seem to have been performed. Before such information is available the value of calcium antagonists as therapeutic alternatives in dysmenorrhea cannot be established. However, the potent inhibitory effects of these drugs on the activity of the pregnant as well as nonpregnant uterus deserve further clinical evaluation.

REFERENCES

1. Woodbury, A., R. Torpin, G. P. Child, H. Watson & M. Jarboe. 1947. Myometrial physiology and its relation to pelvic pain. J. Am. Med. Assoc. **134:** 1081–1085.
2. Filler, W. W., Jr. & W. C. Hall. 1970. Dysmenorrhea and its therapy: a uterine contractility study. Am. J. Obstet. Gynecol. **106:** 104–109.
3. Åkerlund, M., K. E. Andersson & I. Ingemarsson. 1976. Effects of terbutaline on myometrial activity, uterine blood flow, and lower abdominal pain in women with primary dysmenorrhea. Br. J. Obstet. Gynecol. **83:** 673–678.
4. Andersson, K.-E. & U. Ulmsten. 1978. Effects of nifedipine on myometrial activity and lower abdominal pain in women with primary dysmenorrhea. Br. J. Obstet. Gynaecol. **85**(2): 142–148.
5. Csapo, A. J., M. D. Pulkkinen & M. R. Henzl. The effect of naproxen-sodium on the intrauterine pressure and menstrual pain of dysmenorrhoic patients. Prostaglandins **13**(1): 193–199.
6. Wiqvist, N., B. Lindblom, M. Wikland & L. Wilhelmsson. 1983. Prostaglandins and uterine contractility. Acta Obstet. Gynecol. Scand. Suppl. **113:** 2329.
7. Maigaard, S., A. Forman & K.-E. Andersson. 1985. Different responses to prostaglandin $F_{2\alpha}$ and E_2 in human extra- and intramyometrial arteries. Prostaglandins **30**(4): 599–607.

8. YLIKORKALA, O. & M. YUSOFF. 1978. New concepts in dysmenorrhea. Am. J. Obstet. Gynecol. **130:** 833–847.
9. WILHELMSSON, L., B. LINDBLOM, M. WIKLAND & N. WIQVIST. 1981. Effects of prostaglandins on the isolated uterine artery of non-pregnant women. Prostaglandins **22:** 223–233.
10. ÅKERLUND, M., A. KOSTRZEWSKA, T. LAUDANSKI, P. MELIN & H. VILHARDT. 1983. Vasopressin effects on isolated non-pregnant myometrium and uterine arteries and their inhibition by deamino-ethyl-lysine-vasopressin and deamino-ethyl-oxytocin. Br. J. Obstet. Gyn. **90:** 732–738.
11. STRÖMBERG, P., ÅKERLUND, M. L. FORSLING & H. KINDAHL. 1983. Involvement of prostaglandins in vasopressin stimulation of the human uterus. Br. J. Obstet. Gyn. **90:** 332–337.
12. COUTINHO, E. M. & H. C. V. LOPES. 1968. Response of the non-pregnant uterus to vasopressin as an index of ovarian function. Am. J. Obstet. Gynecol. **102:** 479–489.
13. FUCHS, A. R., E. M. COUTINHO, R. XAVIER, P. E. BATES & F. FUCHS. 1968. Effect of ethanol on the activity of the nonpregnant uterus and its reactivity to neurohypophyseal hormones. Am. J. Obstet. Gynecol. **101:** 997–1003.
14. FUCHS, A.-R. & E. M. COUTINHO. 1971. Suppression of uterine activity during menstruation by expansion of the plasma volume. Acta Endocrinol. **66:** 183–192.
15. COBO, E., R. CIFUENTES & M. DE VILLAMIZAR. 1978. Inhibition of menstrual motility during water diuresis. Am. J. Obstet. Gynecol. **132:** 313–320.
16. FORSLING, M. L., M. ÅKERLUND & P. STRÖMBERG, 1981. Variations in plasma concentrations of vasopressin during the menstrual cycle. J. Endocrinol. **89:** 263–266.
17. ÅKERLUND, M., P. STRÖMBERG & M. L. FORSLING. 1979. Primary dysmenorrhea and vasopressin. Br. J. Obstet. Gynaecol. **86:** 484–487.
18. STRÖMBERG, P., M. L. FORSLING & M. ÅKERLUND. 1981. Effects of prostaglandin inhibition on vasopressin levels in women with primary dysmenorrhea. Obstet. Gynecol. **58:** 206–208.
19. LAUDANSKI, T., A. KOSTRZEWSKA & M. ÅKERLUND. 1984. Interaction of vasopressin and prostaglandins in the non-pregnant human uterus. Prostaglandins **27**(3): 441–452.
20. ÅKERLUND, M., A. HAUKSSON, S. LUNDIN, P. MELIN & J. TROJNAR. 1986. Vasotocin analogues which competitively inhibit vasopressin in stimulated uterine activity in healthy women. Br. J. Obstet. Gynaecol. **93:** 22–27.
21. OWEN, P. R. 1984. Prostaglandin synthetase inhibitors in the treatment of primary dysmenorrhea. Outcome trials reviewed. Am. J. Obstet. Gynecol. **148:** 96–103.
22. FORMAN, A., K. E. ANDERSSON & U. ULMSTEN. 1983. Aspects of inhibition of myometrial hyperactivity in primary dysmenorrhea. Acta Obstet. Gynecol. Scand. Suppl. **113:** 71–76.
23. KURIYAMA, H., T. OSA, Y. ITO & H. SUZUKI. 1975. Excitation-concentration coupling mechanism in visceral smooth muscle. Adv. Biophys. **8:** 115–190.
24. ABE, Y. 1970. The hormonal control and the effects of drugs and ions on the electrical and mechanical activity of the uterus. *In* Smooth Muscle. E. Bulbring, A. F. Brading, A. W. Jones & T. Tomita, Eds.: 396–417. Edward Arnold. London, England.
25. ABE, Y. 1971. Effects of changing the ion environment on passive and active properties of pregnant rat uterus. J. Physiol. **214:** 173–190.
26. REINER, O. & J. M. MARSHALL. 1975. Action of D-600 on spontaneous and electrically stimulated activity of the parturitent rat uterus. Naunyn-Schmiedeberg's Arch. Pharmacol. **290:** 21–28.
27. OSA, T. 1973. The effects of sodium, calcium and manganese on the electrical and mechanical activities of the myometrial smooth muscle of pregnant mice. J. Physiol. **23:** 113–133.
28. MIRONNEAU, J. 1973. Excitation-contraction coupling in voltage clamped uterine smooth muscle. J. Physiol. **233:** 127–141.
29. VASSORT, G. 1975. Voltage-clamp analysis of transmembrane ionic currents in guinea-pig myometrium: evidence for an initial potassium activation triggered by calcium influx. J. Physiol. **252:** 713–734.
30. OSA, T. & T. KAWARABAYASHI. 1977. Effects of ions and drugs on the plateau potential in the circular muscle of pregnant rat myometrium. Jpn. J. Physiol. **27:** 111–121.

31. KAWARABAYASHI, T., M. IKEDA, H. SUGIMORI & H. NAKANO. 1986. Spontaneous electrical activity and effects of noradrenaline on pregnant human myometrium recorded by the single sucrose-gap method. Acta Physiol. Hung. **67**(1): 7172.
32. KAWARABAYASHI, T., T. KISHIKAWA & H. SUGIMORI. 1986. Effects of external calcium and calcium antagonist, diltiazem, on isolated segments of human myometrium. Asia-Oceania J. Obstet. Gynaecol. **12**(3): 409–417.
33. FORMAN, A. 1984. Calcium entry blockade as a therapeutic principle in the female urogenital tract. Acta Obstet. Gynecol. Scand. Suppl. **121:** 1–26.
34. KURIYAMA, H. & H. SUZUKI. 1976. Effects of prostaglandin E_2 and oxytocin on the electrical activity of hormone-treated and pregnant rat myometria. J. Physiol. **260:** 335–349.
35. GROSSET, A. & J. MIRONNEAU. 1977. An analysis of the actions of prostaglandin E_1 on membrane currents and concentration in uterine smooth muscle. J. Physiol. **270:** 765–784.
36. CARSTEN, M. E. 1973. Prostaglandins and cellular calcium transport in the pregnant human uterus. Am. J. Obstet. Gynecol. **117:** 824–832.
37. BATRA, S. 1977. The importance of calcium binding by subcellular components of smooth muscle in excitation-contraction coupling. *In* Excitation-contraction coupling in smooth muscle. R. Casteels, T. Godfraind & J. C. Rügg, Eds.: 225–231 Elsevier/North Holland. Amsterdam, Holland.
38. KAWARABAYASHI, T. & H. SUGIMORI, 1985. Effects of oxytocin and prostaglandin $F_{2\alpha}$ on pregnant human myometrium recorded by the single sucrose-gap method—comparison of an *in vitro* experiment and an *in vivo* trial. Asia-Oceania J. Obstet. Gynaecol. **11**(2): 247–253.
39. BYGDEMAN, M. 1964. The effect of different prostaglandins on human myometrium in vitro. Acta Physiol. Scand. **63**(Suppl. 242): 1–78.
40. RUBANYI, G. & A. J. CSAPO. 1977. The effect of prostaglandin $F_{2\alpha}$ on the activator calcium of the uterus. Life Sci. **20:** 2061–2074.
41. MIRONNEAU, J. 1976. Effects of oxytocin on ionic currents underlying rhythmic activity and contraction in uterine smooth muscle. Pflügers Arch. **363:** 113–118.
42. KAWARABAYASHI, T., T. KISHIKAWA & H. SUGIMORI. 1986. Effect of oxytocin on spontaneous electrical and mechanical activities in pregnant human myometrium. Am. J. Obstet. Gynecol. **155**(3): 671–676.
43. FORMAN, A., K.-E. ANDERSSON, C. G. A. PERSSON & U. ULMSTEN. 1979. Relaxant effects of nifedipine on isolated human myometrium. Acta Pharmacol. Toxicol. **45:** 81–86.
44. CARSTEN, M. E. 1979. Calcium accumulation by human uterine microsomal preparations: effects of progesterone and oxytocin. Am. J. Obstet. Gynecol. **113:** 598–601.
45. BATRA, S. 1986. Effect of oxytocin on calcium influx and efflux in the rat myocardium. Eur. J. Pharmacol. **120:** 57–61.
46. MAIGAARD, S., A. FORMAN & K.-E. ANDERSSON. 1985. Differences in contractile activation between human myometrium and intramyometrial vessels. Acta Physiol. Scand. **124:** 371–379.
47. ÅKERLUND, M. & K.-E. ANDERSSON. 1976. Vasopressin response and terbutaline inhibition of the uterus. Obstet. Gynecol. **48**(5): 528–536.
48. ANDERSSON, K.-E. 1977. Inhibition of uterine activity by the calcium antagonist nifedipine. *In* Premature Labour: 101–114. Royal College of Obstetricians and Gynaecologists. London, England.
49. FLECKENSTEIN, A., G. GRÜN, H. TRITTHART & K. BYON. 1971. Uterus-Relaxation durch hochaktive Ca^{++}-antagonistische Hemmstoffe der elektro-mechanischen Koppelung wie Isoptin (Verapamil, Iproveratril), Substanz D600 und Segontin (Prenylamin) (Versuchen am isolierten Uterus virginellen Ratten). Klin. Wschr. **49:** 32–41.
50. GRÜN, G., A. FLECKENSTEIN & K. BYON. 1971. Hemmung der Motilität isolierter Uterus—Streifen aus graviden und nicht-graviden meschlichen Myometrium durch Ca^{++}-Antagonisten und Sympathomimetica. Arzneimittelforsch. (Drug. Res.) **21:** 1585–1590.
51. ULMSTEN, U., K.-E. ANDERSSON & A. FORMAN. 1978. Relaxing effects of nifedipine on the non-pregnant human uterus *in vitro* and *in vivo*. Obstet. Gynecol **52:** 436–441.
52. MAIGAARD, S., A. FORMAN, K.-E. ANDERSSON & U. ULMSTEN. 1983. Comparison of the

effects of nicardipine and nifedipine on isolated human myometrium. Gynecol. Obstet. Invest. **16:** 354–366.

53. FORMAN, A., K.-E. ANDERSSON & U. ULMSTEN. 1981. Inhibition of myometrial activity by calcium antagonists. Semin. Perinatol. **5**(3): 288–294.
54. FORMAN, A., K.-E. ANDERSSON & S. MAIGAARD. 1986. Effects of calcium channel blockers on the female genital tract. Acta Pharmacol. Toxicol. **58**(Suppl. II): 183–192.
55. ANDERSSON, K.-E. 1986. Pharmacodynamic profiles of different calcium channel blockers. Acta Pharmacol. Toxicol. **58**(Suppl. II): 31–42.
56. SAKAMOTO, H. & G. HUSZAR. 1986. Pharmacologic levels of nitrendipine do not affect actin-myosin interaction in the human uterus and placenta. Am. J. Obstet. Gynecol. **154:** 402–407.
57. HENDRICKS, C. H. 1966. Inherent motility patterns and response characteristics of the non-pregnant human uterus. Am. J. Obstet. Gynecol. **96:** 1152–1158.
58. MOAWAD, A. H. & L. P. BENGTSSON. 1967. In vivo studies of the motility patterns of the non-pregnant human uterus. Am. J. Obstet. Gynecol. **98**(8): 1057–1064.
59. BAUMGARTEN, K. 1970. Die Uterusmotilitet beim weiblichen Zyklus. Geburtsh. Frauenheilk. **30:** 921–933.
60. FORMAN, A., K.-E. ANDERSSON & U. ULMSTEN. 1982. Combined effects of diflunisal and nifedipine on uterine contractility in dysmenorrhoic patients. Prostaglandins **23:** 237–246.
61. ULMSTEN, U. 1985. Calcium-blockade as a rapid pharmacological test to evaluate primary dysmenorrhea. Gynecol. Obstet. Invest. **20:** 78–83.
62. SURESH, M. S., S. H. NELSON, T. E. NELSON & O. S. STEINSLAND. 1985. Pregnancy: increased effect of verapamil in human uterine arteries. Eur. J. Pharmacol. **112:** 387–391.
63. ULMSTEN, U., K.-E. ANDERSSON & L. WINGERUP. 1980. Treatment of premature labor with the calcium antagonist nifedipine. Arch. Gynecol. **229:** 1–5.
64. READ, M. D. & D. E. WELLBY. 1986. The use of a calcium antagonist (nifedipine) to suppress preterm labor. Br. J. Obstet. Gynaecol. **93:** 933–937.
65. ANDERSSON, K.-E., I. INGEMARSSON, U. ULMSTEN & L. WINGERUP. 1979. Inhibition of prostaglandin induced uterine activity by nifedipine. Br. J. Obstet. Gynaecol. **86:** 175–179.
66. FORMAN, A., P. GANDRUP, K.-E. ANDERSSON & U. ULMSTEN. 1982. Effects of nifedipine on oxytocin and prostaglandin $F_{2\alpha}$–induced activity in the postpartum uterus. Am. J. Obstet. Gynecol. **144:** 665–670.
67. FORMAN, A., P. GANDRUP, K.-E. ANDERSSON & U. ULMSTEN. 1982. Effects of nifedipine on spontaneous and methylergometrine-induced activity post partum. Am. J. Obstet. Gynecol. **144:** 442–448.
68. SANDAHL, B., U. ULMSTEN & K.-E. ANDERSSON. 1979. Trial of the calcium antagonist nifedipine in the treatment of primary dysmenorrhea. Arch. Gynecol. **227:** 147–151.
69. VAQUEZ-CAMACHO, L. 1983. Tratamiento de la dismenorrea esencial con un vasodilatador coronario. Ginecol. Obstet. Mexico **51:** 187–190.
70. MONDERO, N. A. 1983. Nifedipine in the treatment of dysmenorrhea. J. Am. Osteopath. Assoc. **89:** 704–708.
71. AUDEBERT, A. J. M., M. COLLE, J. P. COQUELIN & J. C. EMPERAIRE. 1985. Essai d'un inhibiteur calcique dans la dysmenorrhee. Press Med. **14:** 163.

Protection of Liver by Calcium Entry Blockers[a]

RONALD G. THURMAN,[b] ELIZABETH APEL,[b]
MOSTAFA BADR,[b] AND JOHN L. LEMASTERS[c]

[b]*Department of Pharmacology*
[c]*Department of Anatomy*
University of North Carolina at Chapel Hill
Chapel Hill, North Carolina 27514

The first suggestion that drugs that reduce cell calcium could play a role in protection against toxic injury by chemicals and hypoxia was made by Rees and Spector.[1] They observed that phenergan, an antihistaminic drug, protected the liver against toxic chemical injury, an effect that was thought to be due to calcium. While pathlogists have long recognized that massive increases in intracellular calcium are associated with the death of cells, the exact role of calcium in the initiation of events that lead to cell death remains controversial. A review of the data in support of or against the idea that calcium must enter the liver cell to initiate toxicity is beyond the scope of this review. Briefly, groups working with freshly prepared hepatocytes observe toxicity of chemicals predominantly in the absence of extracellular calcium[2] whereas others working with cultured hepatocytes report an absolute requirement for extracellular calcium for cell death due to chemicals and hypoxia.[3] Others, however, report no change in cytosolic free calcium preceding hepatocellular death in cultured cells.[4] Furthermore, Israel and his colleagues found that removal of Ca^{2+} from the media reduced cell damage induced by anoxia in the perfused liver but not in freshly prepared hepatocytes. They suggest that the mechanism of cell death may be different in isolated hepatocytes from models in which the structure of the liver is preserved.[5]

The purpose of this article is to review a small but growing literature that has accumulated over the past few years on calcium entry blockers in the liver. We will address the following questions: (1) Do calcium entry blockers protect liver against chemical and hypoxic damage? (2) Does evidence for more than one class of Ca^{2+} entry blocker in liver exist? and (3) Would Ca^{2+} entry blockers be beneficial in treating alcoholic liver disease?

CALCIUM ENTRY BLOCKERS AND INJURY TO LIVER BY TOXIC CHEMICALS

One of the more convincing studies on the hepatoprotective effect of calcium entry blockers comes from Erwin Landon and his colleagues at Vanderbilt.[6] Twenty-four hours after administration of hepatotoxic doses of several chemicals *in vivo,* calcium was measured in liver homogenates and tissues were scored for centrilobular necrosis. As expected, carbon tetrachloride, chloroform, dimethylnitrosamine, thioacetamide,

[a]Supported, in part, by AA-03629, ES-02759, and AM 37034 from the National Institutes of Health and Miles Pharmaceuticals. J.J.L. is an Established Investigator of the American Heart Association.

and acetaminophen all caused massive increases in hepatocellular calcium content and produced pericentral necrosis (e.g., see FIGURE 1). However, if the calcium entry blockers nifedipine, verapamil, or chlorpromazine were administered 1 hour before and 7 hours after the hepatotoxins, the increase in cellular calcium content and necrosis were diminished markedly (FIGURE 1). These studies *in vivo* clearly demonstrate a protective effect of calcium channel blockers against chemical injury in the liver. However, little is known about their mechanism of action since information about the

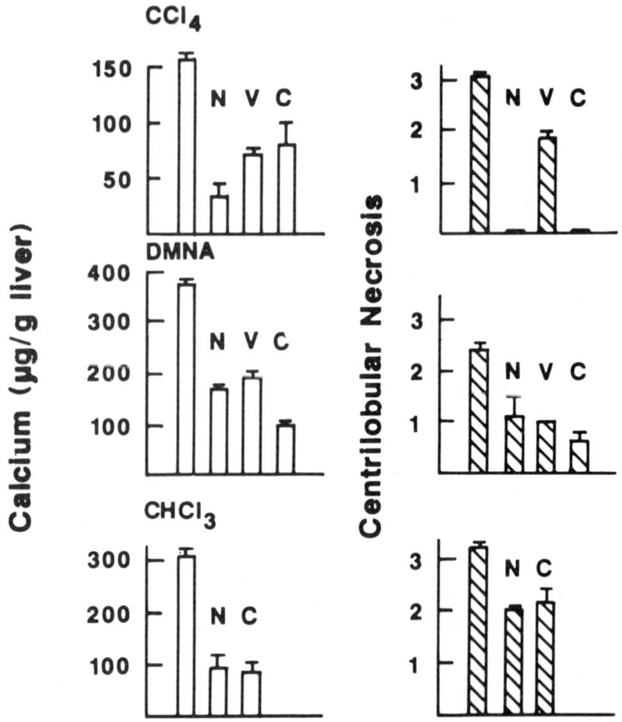

FIGURE 1. Protective effect of calcium channel blocking agents on the liver. Calcium content and the mean histological score of centrilobular necrosis were assessed 24 hours after the administration of hepatotoxic agents. Calcium channel blocking agents were administered 1 hour before and 7 hours after the hepatotoxic agent. N is nifedipine, V is verapamil, and C is chlorpromazine. Because necrosis extends in three dimensions, the percent protection is determined from the cubic function of the histological score. Partial protection was greater than it appears in the figure. (From Reference 6. Reproduced by permission of publisher and authors.)

nature of Ca^{2+} channels in the liver is scarce. Carbon tetrachloride and related compounds decrease the ability of the endoplasmic reticulum to sequester calcium,[7] so presumably calcium entry blockers can blunt the increase in calcium due to toxins by blocking Ca^{2+} channels in the plasma membrane. Dihydropyridine-type calcium channel blockers bind to liver tissue weakly,[8] but voltage-dependent, agonist-dependent, or calcium-dependent Ca^{2+} channels have yet to be characterized in the liver. More work is needed before it can be determined whether Ca^{2+} channel blockers protect the liver against chemical injury via the direct action of calcium on channels.

A useful model which is nearly physiological and easier to manipulate than the liver *in vivo* is the perfused liver. The perfused rat liver makes bile, maintains normal architecture of the liver lobule, and metabolizes many toxins. We have used this model to study mechanisms of zone-specific hepatotoxicity of allyl alcohol, a periportal toxin. Allyl alcohol is actually an O_2-dependent toxin in the liver.[9,10] Its action on the liver is depicted in FIGURE 2. Infusion of allyl alcohol (350 μM) for 60 minutes into livers from fed rats perfused in the anterograde direction damaged virtually all cells in periportal areas of the liver lobule as indexed by trypan blue uptake. Half-maximal dye uptake occurred at 38 minutes. Under these conditions, oxygen uptake was inhibited only in periportal regions of the liver lobule. Increasing the time of infusion of allyl alcohol to 90 minutes, however, caused dye uptake in virtually all cells across the liver lobule, with half-maximal staining in pericentral regions occurring at 70 minutes. This finding indicates that hepatocytes in pericentral areas are not immune to damage by allyl alcohol. Perfusion in the retrograde direction reverses the oxygen gradient in the liver. When allyl alcohol was infused in the retrograde direction for 60 minutes, cells in pericentral regions took up trypan blue while those in periportal areas were not damaged. Concomitantly, oxygen uptake was decreased only in pericentral regions. Infusion of allyl alcohol in oxygen-saturated buffer perfused in either direction caused release of lactate dehydrogenase and malondialdehyde. However, if oxygen tension was decreased by lowering the flow rate or perfusing with air-saturated buffer, malondialdehyde release and dye uptake due to allyl alcohol was reduced markedly. Desferrioxmine, an iron trapping agent, (+)-cyanidanol-3, an oxygen radical scavenger, and allopurinol, an inhibitor of xanthine oxidase, each prevented allyl alcohol–induced damage.[9,10] These data indicate that local O_2 tension is an important determinant of zone-specific hepatotoxicity due to allyl alcohol.

These studies led to the hypothesis that acrolein, the toxin produced from allyl alcohol metabolism, reacts with critical -SH groups on Ca^{2+} pumps thereby increasing cytosolic Ca^{2+}. In support of this idea, we observed that the calcium entry blocker nitrendipine decreased hepatotoxicity due to acrolein in the perfused liver (FIGURE 3). Most importantly, nitrendipine was hepatoprotective at very low doses (e.g., 10 μM). Based on these studies *in vitro,* it would be interesting to compare liver disease in workers in the chemical industry who are taking dihydropyridine-type Ca^{2+} channel blockers with appropriate controls. These studies *in vitro* predict that liver disease due to certain toxic chemicals might be diminished in humans by Ca^{2+} entry blockers.

PROTECTION AGAINST HYPOXIC DAMAGE IN THE LIVER BY CALCIUM ENTRY BLOCKERS

Pericentral regions of the liver lobule have lower O_2 tension than periportal areas due to the natural O_2 gradient in the liver.[11] Therefore, one would predict that pericentral areas would be more susceptible to hypoxic damage. Indeed, in a study of over 1000 autopsy cases with congestive heart failure, damage to pericentral regions of the liver lobule occurred with a frequency of about 10%.[12] Evidence has also been presented in support of the hypothesis that hypoxia plays a role in alcohol-induced liver damage.[11,12] This idea is based on the fact that alcohol damages pericentral regions that are furthest from input O_2 and on the observation that alcohol increases oxygen requirements in the liver.[14,15] In addition, hypoxia may play an important role in damage to human livers during storage prior to transplantation.

The first study to demonstrate a protective effect of a calcium entry blocker in

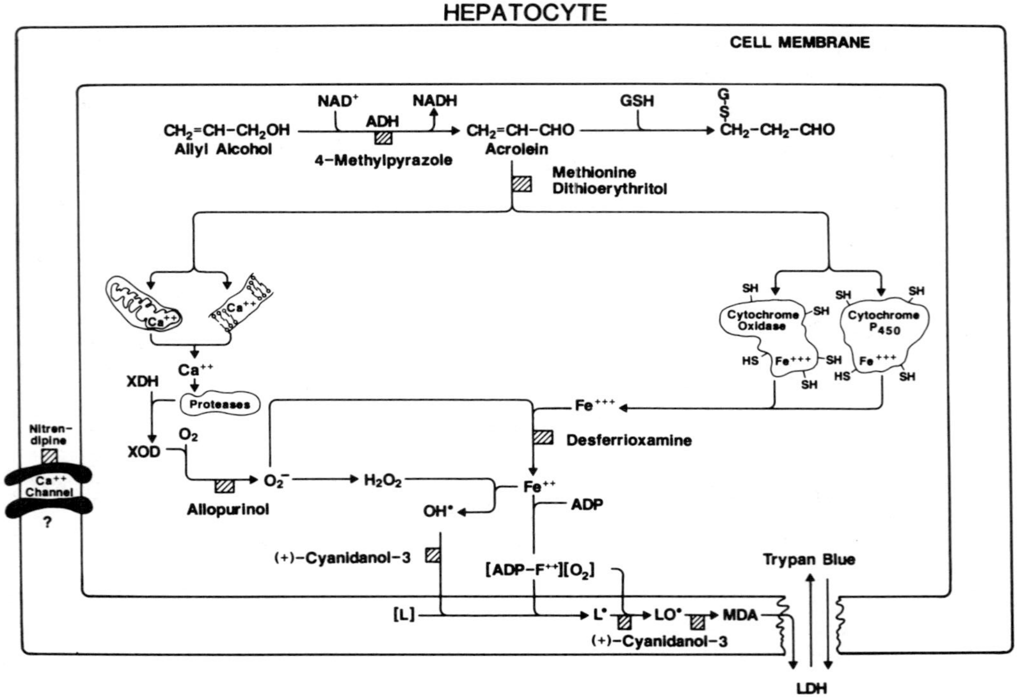

FIGURE 2. Schematic representation of suggested mechanism of allyl alcohol–induced cell damage. ADH, alcohol dehydrogenase; ALDH, aldehyde dehydrogenase; LDH, lactate dehydrogenase; MDA, malondialdehyde; L, lipid; $L^{\cdot}$ and $LO^{\cdot}$, lipid radicals; SH, free sulfhydryl group; XDH, xanthine dehydrogenase; XOD, xanthine oxidase; $O_2^{\overline{\cdot}}$, superoxide anion; $OH^{\cdot}$, hydroxyl radical.

hypoxia injury was performed by Peck and Lefer in 1981.[16] They demonstrated that the release of lactate dehydrogenase (LDH) during hypoxia could be prevented nearly completely by nifedipine in perfused cat liver (FIGURE 4). Similar studies have been performed with nitrendipine,[17] anipamil,[18] and ronipamil[18] with similar results.

Recently, models were developed in our laboratory to study hypoxic damage in the liver following ischemia, perfusion with hypoxic buffer, or periods of low-flow perfusion followed by reflow.[19,20] We observed that nutritional status was an important

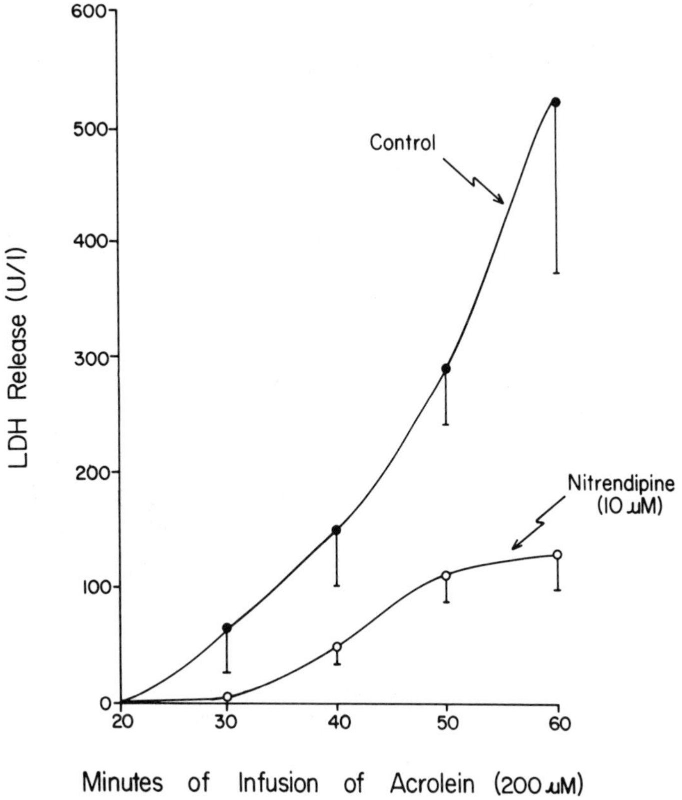

FIGURE 3. Effect of nitrendipine on release of lactate dehydrogenase by perfused rat liver. Livers were perfused with N_2-saturated buffer as described by Bradford *et al.*[17] Nitrendipine (10 μM) and acrolein (200 μM) were infused during normoxic perfusion 8 minutes prior to anoxia. Samples of effluent perfusate were collected at 10-minute intervals and analyzed for LDH enzymatically. Mean ± standard error of the mean (SEM) ($n = 4$).

determinant of hypoxic damage in the liver. Perfusion with N_2-saturated buffer damaged nearly all cells in livers from 24-hour-fasted rats yet failed to damage livers from fed rats during perfusion periods of up to 2 hours.[19] We demonstrated that 30 minutes of perfusion of livers from fasted rats with N_2-saturated buffer caused massive cell damage reflected by release of lactate dehydrogenase (>2000 U/l) and staining of nuclei by trypan blue.[19] This damage was observed both in the presence and absence of extracellular calcium, suggesting that release of Ca^{2+} from intracellular stores might be involved in the mechanism of hypoxia-induced damage.

Using our hypoxic perfusion model, we have recently evaluated the effect of a dihydropyridine-type calcium channel blocker, nitrendipine, on hypoxia-induced hepatocellular damage in the isolated, perfused rat liver.[21] In these studies, an experimental design depicted by FIGURE 5 was employed. Livers were preperfused for 10 minutes prior to the infusion of nitrendipine (0.1 to 60 μM). O_2 uptake during the early phase of the experiment was monitored with a Clark-type O_2 electrode placed in the effluent perfusate line. The subsequent infusion of nitrendipine (0.5 μM) in ethanol vehicle or vehicle alone had no effect on O_2 uptake. At 20 minutes, the perfusate was switched from one saturated with 95% O_2:5% CO_2 to one saturated with 95% N_2:5% CO_2. Concomitantly, O_2 tension in the effluent perfusate declined rapidly and anoxia was

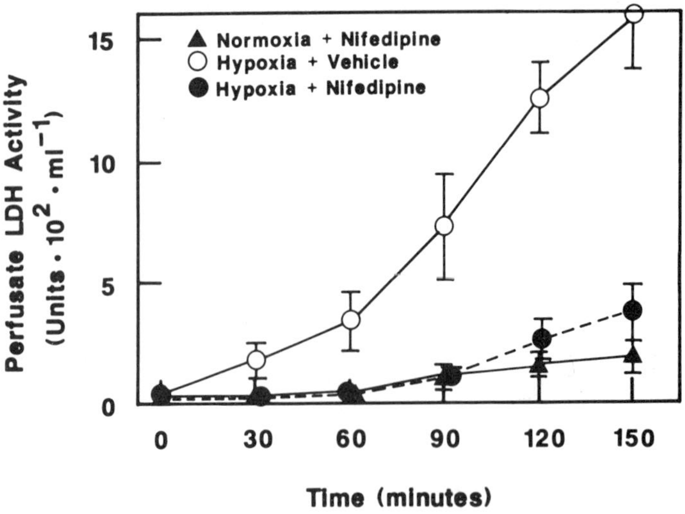

FIGURE 4. Effect of nifedipine on LDH activity in perfusate of normoxic cat livers. All points are means and brackets indicate SEM. Significant differences occurred between hypoxia + vehicle and the other two groups at 60 minutes ($p < 0.05$), 90 minutes ($p < 0.01$), and 120 and 150 minutes ($p < 0.001$). (From Reference 16. Reproduced by permission of publisher and authors.)

established (<10 μM oxygen) in less than 5 minutes (FIGURE 5). Infusion of nitrogen-saturated buffer was continued for 40 minutes. During the final 10 minutes of perfusion, trypan blue was infused to stain the nuclei of damaged cells. The effect of nitrendipine on irreversible cell damage in this model is depicted in TABLE 1. As can be seen from the data, nitrendipine was hepatoprotective in the micromolar range. Interestingly, it also prevented damage in the absence of extracellular calcium. Nitrendipine also protected the liver from ultrastructural alterations during anoxic injury. After 10 minutes of anoxic perfusion (FIGURE 6A), hepatocytes that received vehicle only were covered with surface blebs similar to those observed previously during the early stages of hypoxic injury.[20] With nitrendipine, however, bleb formation was prevented totally (FIGURE 6B) and cellular architecture was similar to that of normoxic livers. After 30 minutes of anoxic perfusion with vehicle (FIGURE 6C),

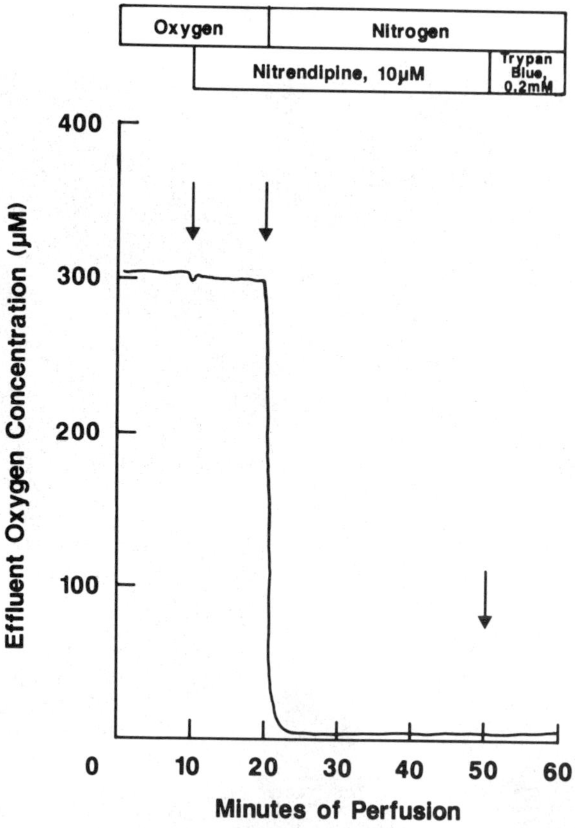

FIGURE 5. Experimental design for studies of effect of nitrendipine on hypoxic damage in perfused liver. Livers from fasted normal rats were perfused with oxygenated Krebs-Henseleit bicarbonate buffer for 10 minutes. Nitrendipine (1 to 60 μM) was infused subsequently as indicated by the horizontal bars and arrows. After 8 minutes of perfusion, the buffer was changed from O_2 to N_2 saturation as depicted by the horizontal bars. O_2 concentration in the effluent perfusate was monitored continuously with a Clark-type platinum electrode. At 50 minutes, trypan blue was infused for 10 minutes. The liver was then fixed with paraformaldehyde and prepared for light microscopy. Typical experiment.

TABLE 1. Effect of Nitrendipine on Hypoxia-Induced Cell Damage[a]

Nitrendipine (μM)	Percent Cells Stained with Trypan Blue: Calcium 1.2 mM		No Calcium	
	Periportal	Pericentral	Periportal	Pericentral
0	66 ± 4	51 ± 5	89 ± 3	71 ± 10
0.5	46 ± 9	48 ± 9	58 ± 9	37 ± 8
1.0	13 ± 6	6 ± 3	63 ± 4	54 ± 3
5.0	28 ± 5	19 ± 5	53 ± 7	36 ± 9
10.0	12 ± 2	5 ± 2	44 ± 8	29 ± 9

[a]Livers were perfused with the experimental design depicted in FIGURE 5. Livers were exposed to N_2 for 50 minutes (30 minutes N_2-saturated buffer, 10 minutes of trypan blue followed by a 10-minute washout period). Tissue was stained with eosin only and examined by light microscopy. Regions were defined as cells radiating 5 layers from the central or portal vein. Mean ± SEM. Four to five livers per group.

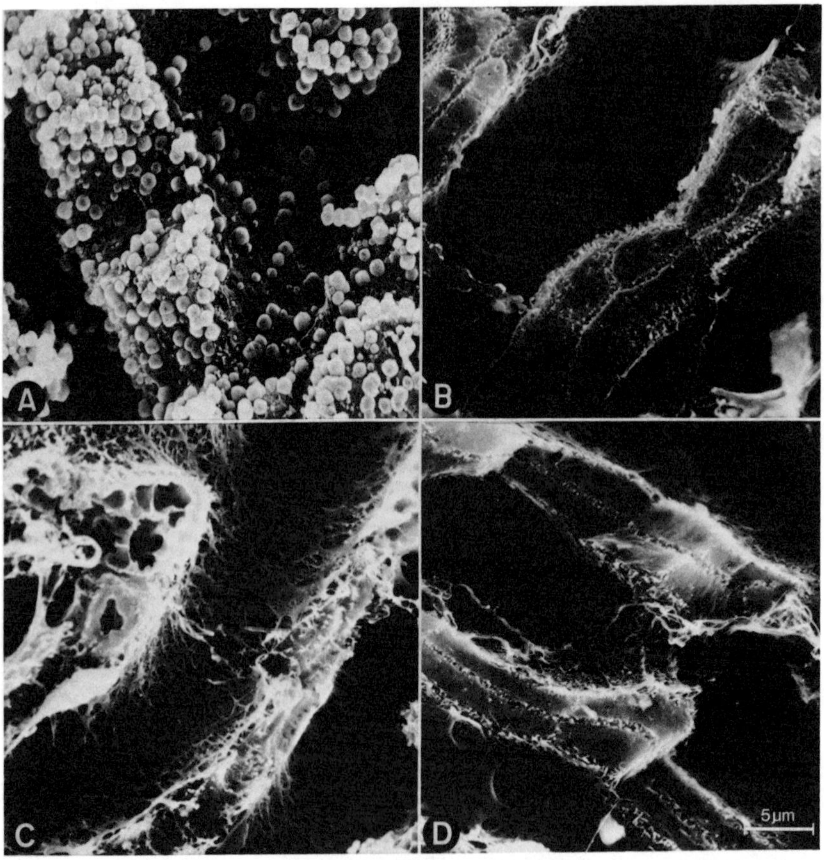

FIGURE 6. Effect of nitrendipine on scanning electron micrographs of anoxic perfused rat liver. **A,** 10 minutes of anoxic perfusion; **B,** 10 minutes of anoxic perfusion with 1 µM nitrendipine; **C,** 30 minutes of anoxic perfusion; **D,** 30 minutes of anoxic perfusion with 1 µM nitrendipine. Bar is 5 µm.

hepatocytes were fragmented and shrunken indicative of irreversible injury. In the presence of nitrendipine, hepatocytes looked nearly normal (FIGURE 6D).

The mechanism of hypoxic damage remains unknown; however, evidence from the study described above suggests a complex interaction with calcium. As mentioned above, the role of calcium in hepatotoxicity remains controversial. In freshly prepared hepatocytes, blebbing due to toxic chemicals was greater in the absence than in the presence of calcium,[2] whereas damage was dependent on extracellular calcium in cultured hepatocytes.[3] Since nitrendipine provided protection in both the presence and absence of extracellular calcium (TABLE 1; FIGURE 6), an obligatory role for extracellular calcium in hypoxic hepatocellular injury in the intact liver seems unlikely.

The sequence of events occurring during hypoxia may be as follows (see FIGURE 7). After removal of oxygen, ATP levels decline rapidly in the fasted state. Ca^{2+} pumps in the plasma membrane, endoplasmic reticulum, and mitochondria are inhibited, and there is a redistribution of Ca^{2+} between subcellular compartments. As a result of the decline in ATP and/or redistribution of Ca^{2+}, blebs develop due to an alteration in the cytoskeleton. Finally, the plasma membrane ruptures, LDH is released, and trypan blue is taken up reflecting irreversible cell death.

Since nitrendipine protects in the absence of extracellular Ca^{2+} (TABLE 1), its action may not be on a calcium channel in the plasma membrane. Furthermore, cytosolic free Ca^{2+} did not increase during bleb formation preceding cell death in cultured hepatocytes exposed to the metabolic inhibitors cyanide and iodoacetic acid.[4] How, then, is nitrendipine acting as a hepatoprotective drug? One possibility is that nitrendipine prevents the release of Ca^{2+} from intracellular stores. Alternatively, it could stabilize the plasma membrane and prevent cell contents from leaking. Nitrendipine could also block a voltage-dependent Ca^{2+} channel that has not yet been discovered in the plasma membrane, the endoplasmic reticulum, or the mitochondrial membrane. Nitrendipine[22] and nifedipine[23] have been shown to increase hepatic blood flow *in vivo;* this could be involved in their mechanism of action. More work will be needed in the future to evaluate these interesting hypotheses.

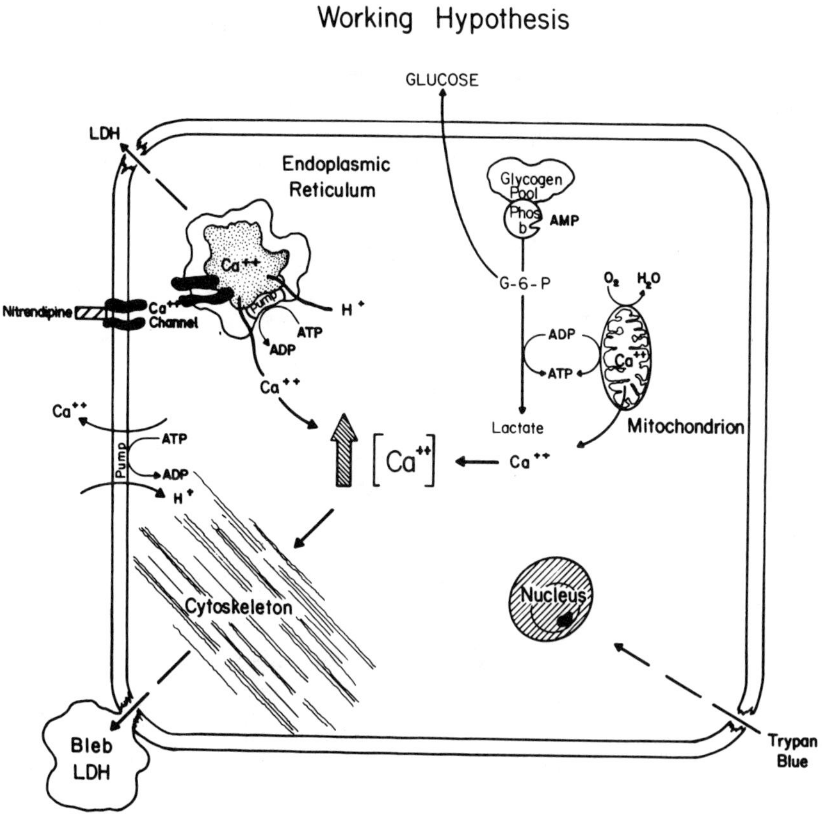

FIGURE 7. Schematic representation of the suggested mechanism of hypoxic cell damage. LDH, lactate dehydrogenase; ATP, adenosine triphosphate; ADP, adenosine diphosphate; G-6-P, glucose-6-phosphate; Phos b, glycogen phosphorylase b; AMP, adenosine monophosphate.

TABLE 2. Effect of Nitrendipine on Ischemic Damage in the Rat Liver *In Vivo*[a]

Treatment	Hours of Ischemia	Index of Ischemic Damage
None (8)	4	8.1 ± 0.6
Nitrendipine (8)	4	4.6 ± 1.2[b]

[a]The hepatic artery and left branch of the portal vein were ligated under light ether anesthesia. Rats were pretreated with nitrendipine (10 mg/kg) or vehicle 1 hour prior to surgery. Index of ischemic damage is from a rating score of 0 to 2 based on five structural parameters: cellular swelling, acidophilic nuclear inclusions, nuclear pyknosis, cellular deposition, and cytoplasmic vacuolization. Mean ± SEM for number of rats in parentheses.

[b]$p < 0.05$.

Since we demonstrated that nitrendipine (5 to 30 μM) prevented enzyme release and trypan blue uptake during hypoxia in the isolated, perfused rat liver,[21] we evaluated the effect of nitrendipine on ischemic liver damage in the rat *in vivo*. Following light ether anesthesia, the hepatic artery and the left branch of the portal vein, which supplies blood to about 50% of the liver, were ligated. Livers were removed 4 hours following surgery, and the tissue was cut into 1 cm pieces, placed in 4% paraformaldehyde in phosphate buffer, and prepared for histology. Plastic sections were viewed after staining with methylene blue–acid fuchsin and a rating score from 0 to 2 (0, normal; 1, moderate alterations; 2, massive changes) was used to evaluate five structural parameters: cellular swelling as indexed by sinusoidal patency, appearance of acidophilic nuclear inclusions, nuclear pyknosis, loss of cellular definition, and cytoplasmic vacuolization. Four hours following surgery, ischemia produced a score of

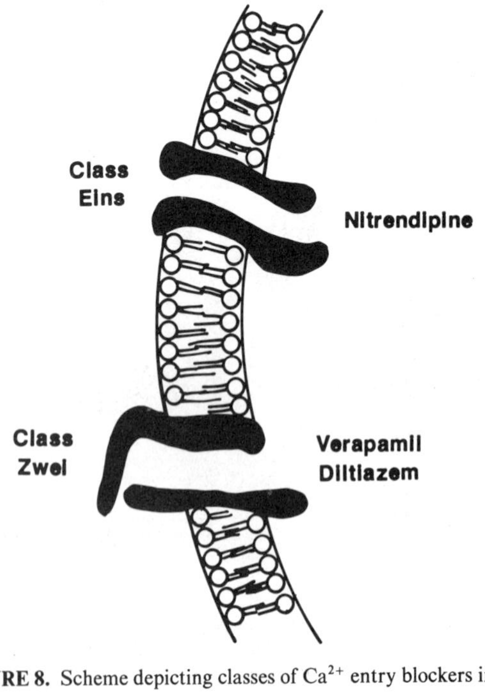

FIGURE 8. Scheme depicting classes of Ca^{2+} entry blockers in liver.

8.1 ± 0.6 out of a possible score of 10 (TABLE 2). Pretreatment of rats 1 hour prior to surgery with nitrendipine (10 mg/kg) reduced the total score significantly to 4.6 ± 1.2. In these experiments, significant reductions in scores for sinusoidal patency, nuclear inclusions, pyknosis, and loss of cellular definition were observed without changes in vacuolization. These data indicate that nitrendipine and possibly other dihydropyridine-type calcium channel blockers protect against ischemic damage in the liver *in vivo*.

EVIDENCE FOR TWO CLASSES OF Ca^{2+} ENTRY BLOCKERS IN LIVER

As mentioned above, direct evidence for the existence of Ca^{2+} channels in the liver is lacking. Liver is not an excitable tissue and therefore may not have voltage-sensitive

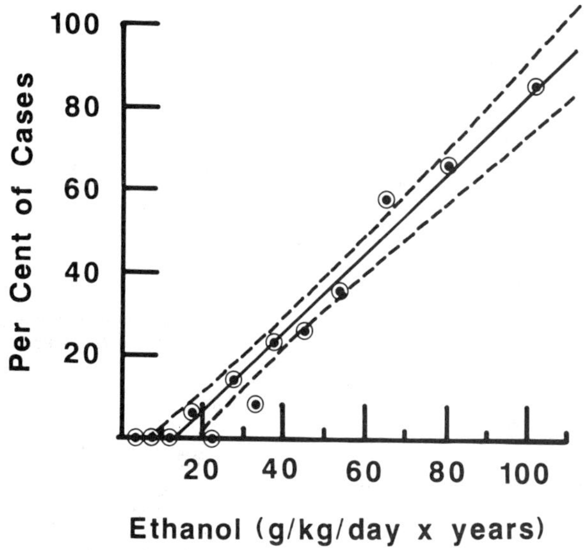

FIGURE 9. Correlation between total amount of ethanol consumed during drinking life and incidence of cirrhosis of the liver in alcoholics. Data from 265 alcoholics. (From reference 24. Reproduced by permission of the publisher.)

Ca^{2+} channels; however, the evidence reviewed above argues strongly for the existence of Ca^{2+} channels in the liver. If one assumes that many forms of cell death involve an initial increase in cytosolic Ca^{2+}, an argument that has many proponents, then Ca^{2+} entry blockers should be hepatoprotective by decreasing cytosolic Ca^{2+}. Nitrendipine, but not verapamil or diltiazem (unpublished), protects against hypoxic injury in the liver. However, all three classes of Ca^{2+} entry blockers protect against chemical injury. Therefore, we propose that at least two classes of Ca^{2+} channels exist in the liver, one sensitive only to dihydropyridines and the other sensitive to all three classes of entry blockers. In honor of Professor Fleckenstein and the scientists at Bayer, we have used German and named these classes "eins" (dihydropyridine-sensitive) and "zwei" (sensitive to all three classes) (see FIGURE 8).

WOULD Ca^{2+} CHANNEL BLOCKERS BE USEFUL IN ALCOHOLIC LIVER DISEASE?

Lelbach demonstrated a direct dose-response relationship between the amount of alcohol consumed and the incidence of cirrhosis of the liver[24] (FIGURE 9). Thus, drugs that prevent liver disease should be beneficial.

Ethanol-induced liver damage is often confined to the O_2-poor pericentral region of the liver lobule. Israel *et al.* postulated that ethanol-induced pericentral necrosis results from an accentuated gradient of decreasing oxygen tension from the portal to the central venous end of the sinusoid leading to pericentral hypoxia.[13] This hypothesis is based on the observations that ethanol treatment increases the rate of oxygen uptake in liver slices[15] and perfused liver.[25] In support of this postulate it was demonstrated that pericentral necrosis was greater in ethanol-treated rats than in controls after brief

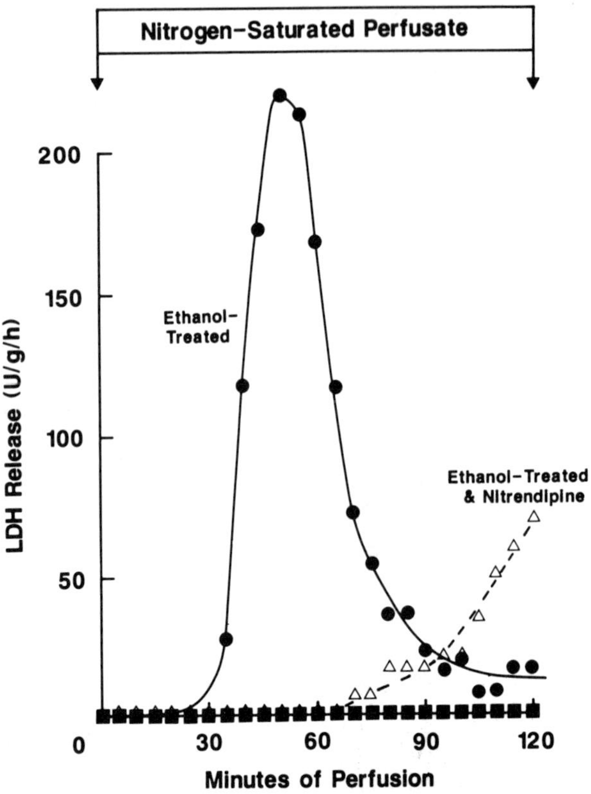

FIGURE 10. Effect of nitrendipine on release of lactate dehydrogenase by perfused rat liver. Rats were treated with ethanol (4 g/kg) via gastric intubation 4 hours before surgery. Experimental conditions as in FIGURE 5, except that total time of anoxic perfusion was 2 hours. Samples of effluent perfusate were collected at 5-minute intervals and analyzed for LDH enzymatically.

exposure to hypoxia.[26] More recently, French and his colleagues have developed an *in vivo* model of alcohol-induced liver damage[27] and suggest that hypoxia is an important determinant of hepatocellular damage due to alcohol.[28]

We have measured the effect of ethanol on the O_2 gradient in the liver directly. In livers from rats administered ethanol, the lobular oxygen gradient increased from less than 300 to over 400 torr in the perfused liver.[11] This increase in the oxygen gradient was accompanied by a similar increase in hepatic oxygen uptake and was confined primarily to pericentral regions of the lobule. This finding is of interest because ethanol causes pericentral injury in experimental animals and man. These experiments show that increased hepatic oxygen uptake caused by chronic treatment with ethanol indeed increases the oxygen gradient along the sinusoid. The mechanism by which alcohol increases energy demands in the liver is not totally clear, but involves a swift increase in alcohol metabolism (SIAM). SIAM is an activation of hepatic O_2 and ethanol uptake after only a few hours of exposure to ethanol. The metabolic sequences most likely responsible for SIAM are as follows. First, hormone-stimulated glycogenolysis leads to a depletion of glycogen which in turn causes rates of glycolysis to decline. Since glycolysis converts ADP to ATP, the ADP that is not phosphorylated by glycolysis enters the mitochondria and is phosphorylated by the electron transport chain. This causes NADH to be reoxidized at a faster rate to NAD^+, the cofactor for alcohol dehydrogenase (ADH). The increased availability of NAD^+ leads to an increased rate of oxidation of ethanol via ADH resulting in a faster rate of ethanol elimination, the SIAM response.

Extensive studies evaluating protection against alcoholic liver injury by Ca^{2+} channel blockers have yet to be carried out. In preliminary experiments depicted in FIGURE 10, however, we observed that nitrendipine prevented hypoxic damage in livers from ethanol-treated rats. Livers from fed rats did not release LDH for up to 2 hours of perfusion; however, in livers from fed, ethanol-treated rats, LDH release was detected beginning at 30 minutes of anoxic perfusion and was maximal in about 50 minutes (FIGURE 10). Infusion of nitrendipine (35 μM) prevented this damage nearly completely. Clearly, more basic and clinical research needs to be done in this important area.

CONCLUSION

Studies with rats *in vivo* and with the perfused liver have demonstrated that verapamil, diltiazem, and dihydropyridine-type calcium entry blockers prevent hepatotoxicity due to a variety of chemicals. In contrast, damage due to hypoxia appears to be sensitive only to dihydropyridine-type calcium entry blockers. Based on these differences, we propose that at least two distinct classes of calcium entry blockers exist in the liver. We have named these two classes of calcium channels in livers "eins" and "zwei." Of possible clinical importance, we observed that nitrendipine protects against alcohol-induced hepatocellular injury in the perfused rat liver.

REFERENCES

1. REES, K. R. & W. G. SPECTOR. 1961. Nature London **90:** 821–822.
2. JEWEL, S. A., G. BELLOMO, H. THOR, S. ORRENIUS & M. T. SMITH. 1982. Science **207:** 125–1259.
3. SCHANNE, F., A. B. KANE, E. E. YOUNG & J. L. FARBER. 1979. J. Biol. Chem. **206:** 700–702.

4. LEMASTERS, J. J., J. D. DIGUISEPPI, A. L. NIEMINEN & B. HERMAN. 1987. Nature London **325:** 78–81.
5. OKUNO, F., H. ORREGO & Y. ISRAEL. 1983. Res. Commun. Chem. Pathol. Pharmacol. **39**(3): 437–444.
6. LANDON, E. J., R. J. NAUKAM & B. V. R. SASTRY. 1986. Biochem. Pharmacol. **30:** 697–705.
7. LOWREY, K., E. A. GLENDE & R. O. RECKNEGAL. 1981. Biochem. Pharmacol. **30:** 135.
8. TRIGGLE, D. J. & R. A. JANIS. 1984. *In* Nitrendipine. A. Scriabine, S. Vanov & K. Deck, Eds.: 33–52. Urban & Schwarzenberg. Baltimore, Md.
9. BELINSKY, S. A., M. Z. BADR, F. C. KAUFFMAN & R. G. THURMAN. 1986. J. Pharmacol. Exp. Ther. **238:** 1132–1137.
10. BADR, M. Z., S. A. BELINSKY, F. C. KAUFFMAN & R. G. THURMAN. 1986. J. Pharmacol. Exp. Ther. **238:** 1138–1142.
11. JI, S., J. J. LEMASTERS, V. CHRISTENSON & R. G. THURMAN. 1982. Proc. Nat. Acad. Sci. USA **79:** 5415–5419.
12. DE LA MONTE, S., J. M. ARCIDI, G. W. MOORE & G. M. HUTCHINS. 1984. Gastroenterology **86:** 627–631.
13. ISRAEL, Y., H. KALANT, H. ORREGO, J. M. KHANNA, L. VIDELA & J. M. PHILLIPS. 1975. Proc. Natl. Acad. Sci. USA. **72:** 1137–1141.
14. YUKI, T. & R. G. THURMAN. 1980. Biochem. J. **186:** 119–126.
15. BERNSTEIN, J., L. VIDELA & Y. ISRAEL. 1973. Biochem. J. **134:** 515–522.
16. PECK, R. G. & A. M. LEFER. 1981. Agents Actions **11:** 421–424.
17. LEFER, A. M. & G. L. STAHL. J. Cardiovasc. Pharmacol. Suppl. **2.** (In press.)
18. LEFER, A. M. & G. PAPARICOLAOU. 1985. Methods Findings Exp. Clin. Pharmacol. **7**(2): 59–63.
19. BRADFORD, B. U., M. MAROTTO, J. J. LEMASTERS & R. G. THURMAN. 1986. J. Pharmacol. Exp. Ther. **236:** 263–268.
20. LEMASTERS, J. J., C. J. STEMKOWSKI, S. JI & R. G. THURMAN. 1983. J. Cell Biol. **97:** 777–786.
21. THURMAN, R. G., J. N. KING & J. J. LEMASTERS. 1986. J. Cardiovasc: Pharmacol. Suppl. **2:** (In press.)
22. MOLS, P., R. NAEIJE, R. MALLEMANS, C. MELOT, P. LEJEUNE & M. ENGLERT. 1986. J. Cardiovasc. Pharmacol. **8:** 77–81.
23. LEIER, C. V., T. J. PATRICK, J. MERMILLER, K. D. PACHT, P. HUSS, R. D. MAGORIENM & D. V. UNVERFERTH. 1984. Am. Heart J. **108**(6): 1461–1468.
24. LELBACH, W. K. 1975. *In* Alcohol Liver Pathology. J. M. Khanna, Y. Israel & H. Kalant, Eds.: 1–18. Addiction Research Foundation. Ontario, Canada.
25. THURMAN, R. G., W. R. MCKENNA & T. B. MCCAFFREY. 1975. Mol. Pharmacol. **12:** 156–166.
26. ISRAEL, Y., H. KALANT, H. ORREGO, J. M. KHANNA, M. J. PHILLIPS & D. J. STEWART. 1979. *In* Biochemistry and Pharmacology of Ethanol. E. Majchrowice & E. P. Noble, Eds.: 433–444. Addiction Research Foundation. Ontario, Canada.
27. TSUKAMOTO, H., R. REIDELBERGER, S. W. FRENCH & C. LARGMAN, 1984. Am. J. Physiol. **247:** R595–R599.
28. FRENCH, S. W., N. C. BENSON & P. S. SUN. 1984. Hepatology. **4:** 912–917.

Calcium Antagonists and the Renal Hemodynamic Response to Vasoconstrictors[a]

RODGER LOUTZENHISER AND MURRAY EPSTEIN

Nephrology Section
Veterans Administration Medical Center
1201 N.W. 16th Street
Miami, Florida 33125

Department of Medicine
University of Miami School of Medicine
Miami, Florida 33101

INTRODUCTION

Since the pioneering work of Fleckenstein in the early 1960s,[1,2] considerable progress has been made in elucidating the mechanisms of action and physiological effects of calcium channel blocking agents, or calcium antagonists. The ability of these agents to disrupt excitation-contraction coupling of vascular smooth muscle, improve perfusion of the ischemic heart, and reduce systemic vascular resistance have been major areas of investigation. Only recently has attention been focused on the renal effects of calcium antagonists. It is increasingly apparent that calcium antagonists also possess unique renal effects, which have important clinical applications.[3–9] In order to understand the renal hemodynamic effects of calcium antagonists, however, one must consider the cellular mechanisms by which these agents inhibit vasoconstriction, and the unique characteristics of the renal microcirculation.

Calcium antagonists represent a unique class of vasodilators. These agents bind to and modulate the function of specific types of proteinic calcium channels of vascular smooth muscle cells.[10,11] By preventing depolarization-mediated[12–15] or receptor-mediated[13] activation of these calcium channels, calcium antagonists disrupt smooth muscle excitation-contraction coupling. Unlike agents that block receptor occupation (i.e., phentolamine, saralasin), calcium antagonists can inhibit a broad range of vasoconstrictor agents. Thus, the responses to diverse agonists that activate the same class of potential-dependent calcium channels are inhibited by the blockade of this channel. On the other hand, agonists may vary with respect to activating mechanisms and sensitivity to calcium antagonists.

The renal hemodynamic response to calcium antagonists, thus, depends upon the setting in which the calcium antagonists are administered. As anticipated, the magnitude of underlying renal vasoconstriction greatly influences the renal hemodynamic effects of calcium antagonists (for review see Reference 3). Thus, the greater the basal renal vascular resistance, the greater the response to calcium antagonists. Furthermore, the renal vasodilatory response to calcium antagonists also depends upon which vasoactive hormones, neurotransmitters, and autacoids are exerting the predom-

[a]These studies were supported in part by a grant from the Veterans Administration (No. 2456).

inant influence on basal renal vascular resistance. Thus, in evaluating the renal actions of calcium antagonists, the basal renal vascular state must be defined.

Finally, smooth muscle heterogeneity influences the renal hemodynamic response to calcium antagonists. Within the circulation, different vessel types may exhibit different sensitivities to calcium antagonists.[13,14] The resistance vessels of the kidney are of two types, the afferent and efferent arteriole, separated by the glomerular capillary bed. This unique anatomic organization, combined with the physiologic requirement for independent control of pre- and postglomerular resistances, constitutes a setting in which regional heterogeneity plays an important role in determining the pharmacologic effects of calcium antagonists.

The above considerations illustrate the need to examine the renal hemodynamic response to calcium antagonists in a setting in which the factors establishing basal renal vascular tone are carefully controlled and defined. The isolated kidney perfused at constant pressure represents one approach to this problem. In the present communication, we review our observations using this model to elucidate the nature of the renal hemodynamic response to calcium antagonists in the presence of diverse renal vasoconstrictors.

METHODS

Isolated Kidney Studies

Adult male Sprague-Dawlcy rats were used as kidney donors. Following anesthesia with 5-sec-butyl-5-ethyl-ethiobarbituric acid (Inactin, 100 mg/kg body weight), the right kidney was cannulated and initially perfused *in situ* by introducing the cannula through the superior mesenteric artery. The perfused kidney was excised and placed in a recirculating perfusion apparatus, designed to provide warmed (37°C), oxygenated medium at a constant pressure.[16–18] Perfusion pressure was derived from the inflow of 95% O_2 and 5% CO_2 into a sealed reservoir, and was set by means of a back-pressure-type regulator placed in the gas escape line. Renal arterial pressure was maintained at 100 mmHg as described previously.[16] Perfusate flow was measured with an electromagnetic flow meter (model 501, Carolina Medical Electronics).

Kidneys were perfused with a Kreb-Ringer bicarbonate buffer containing 5 mM D-glucose, 10 mM sodium acetate, 8 g/dl albumin (fraction V, Reheiss Chemical), and a complement of amino acids. Urine was collected from a stretched PE-50 catheter inserted into the right ureter. Urine volume was gravimetrically determined. Glomerular filtration rate (GFR) was estimated from the clearance of [^{14}C]carboxyinulin (New England Nuclear, Boston, Mass).

In the experimental procedures, vasoconstrictors [i.e., noradrenaline (Sigma), angiotensin II (Sigma), or KCl] were added to the medium at concentrations that elicited a 50% decrease in perfusate flow (e.g. 3×10^{-7} M, 3×10^{-10} M, and 30 mM, for norepinephrine, angiotensin II, and KCl, respectively). Since norepinephrine and angiotensin II are metabolized by the isolated kidney, sustaining infusions of these agents (10^{-9} mol/minute and 10^{-11} mol/minute for norepinephrine and angiotensin II, respectively) were required to elicit a sustained level of renal vasoconstriction. In order to avoid the beta-adrenergic effects of norepinephrine, this agent was added after the kidneys were pretreated with 3×10^{-6} M propranolol.

Following the administration of a vasoconstrictor agent, calcium antagonists were added directly to the perfusion medium and the renal hemodynamic response was ascertained. Administration of the vehicle (PEG 400) alone had no effect on renal hemodynamics (data not shown). All studies with dihydropyridines were performed in sodium lighting, to avoid photoinduced degradation.

Hydronephrotic Kidney Studies

In order to facilitate direct examination of the afferent arteriole, studies were conducted with the isolated perfused hydronephrotic kidney. As described by Steinhausen *et al.*,[19] studies in the hydronephrotic kidney facilitate direct visualization of the renal microvessels. We have modified this model by combining it with the isolated perfusion technique to facilitate direct visualization of the afferent arteriole under specific modes of activation.[20] In brief, chronic unilateral hydronephrosis is established by ligation of the right ureter. Following 8–10 weeks, the kidney was removed and perfused on the stage of an inverted microscope equipped with a video camera. The images were recorded (Panasonic model NV-8950) for subsequent quantitative analysis on an IBM-AT equipped with a video acquisition board (Datacube Inc. IVG-128, Peabody, Mass). The afferent arteriole was visualized and vasoconstrictor stimuli were applied (i.e., increased perfusion pressure or the thromboxane A_2 mimetic (U44069). Nifedipine was then added to the perfusate to reverse the afferent arteriolar response.

All data are expressed as a mean followed by the standard error, as an index of dispersion. Student's t-test was used to determine the statistical significance of differences between means.

RESULTS AND DISCUSSION

Isolated Kidney Studies

Renal Perfusate Flow

The isolated perfused rat kidney has little intrinsic vascular tone. In the absence of exogenous vasoconstrictor agents, calcium antagonists do not alter renal hemodynamics in the preparation.[17,18,21] In contrast, when the isolated kidney is pretreated with vasoconstrictors, calcium antagonists exert dramatic effects on renal hemodynamics. The response to calcium antagonists in this setting varies, however, with the type of underlying renal vasoconstriction.

FIGURE 1 summarizes the differing responses to nitrendipine, a prototypic dihydropyridine, obtained following renal ischemia induced by either norepinephrine (NE), angiotensin II (AII), or potassium (KCl). Each vasoconstrictor was administered at a concentration sufficient to produce a 50% decrease in renal perfusate flow (RPF) (i.e., 3×10^{-7} M NE, 3×10^{-10} g/ml AII, and 30 mM KCl). Nitrendipine was then administered in the continued presence of each agent.

As illustrated in FIGURE 1, nitrendipine was most potent and efficacious in reversing the renal vasoconstriction elicited by KCl-induced depolarization. At 0.1 micromolar, nitrendipine completely reversed the vasoconstriction induced by KCl. The contractile response to KCl is exclusively dependent on calcium entry through potential-dependent calcium channels. Since this channel type is the primary molecular target for calcium antagonists, it is not surprising that KCl-induced vasoconstriction is completely inhibited by calcium antagonists.

In contrast to KCl, the renal vasoconstrictions elicited by norepinephrine and angiotensin II were markedly less sensitive to nitrendipine. As illustrated in FIGURE 1, nitrendipine only modestly reversed the renal vasoconstriction elicited by NE. Similar results have been obtained using other dihydropyridines (e.g., nifedipine and nisoldipine,[22] and the benzothiazepine diltiazem).[18]

The renal vasoconstriction elicited by AII is more effectively reversed by nitrendipine than that elicited by norepinephrine (FIGURE 1), suggesting that the renal

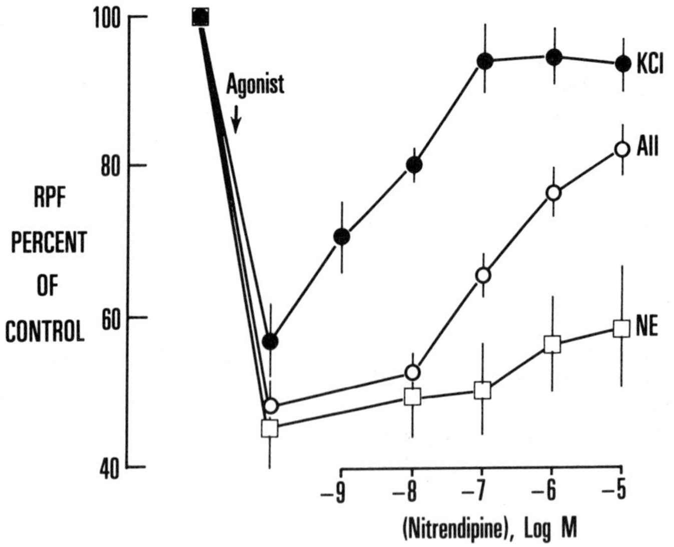

FIGURE 1. Dose-dependent effects of nitrendipine on the vasoconstrictor response of the isolated perfused rat kidney. Norepinephrine (NE), angiotensin II (AII), and KCl were utilized to elicit equivalent vasoconstrictor responses. Nitrendipine completely reversed KCl-induced vasoconstriction, but was less effective in reversing the response to norepinephrine. A component of the response to angiotensin II was also refractory to nitrendipine. (Reproduced from Reference 22 with permission.)

vascular effects of these two agonists involve differing mechanisms. However, the AII-induced vasoconstriction was also much less sensitive to reversal by nitrendipine than was the vasoconstriction elicited by KCl. Furthermore, as was observed with NE, a component of the AII-induced vasoconstriction was resistant to inhibition even at the highest concentration of nitrendipine employed (i.e., 10 μM). Thus, in contrast to KCl, the renal vasoconstriction elicited by both NE and AII appear to involve complex mechanisms. A fraction of the renal vasoconstriction elicited by NE and AII is blocked by calcium antagonists, while another component is refractory.

The Renal Microcirculation

The renal microcirculation is unique. Renal vascular resistance is determined by the summation of segmental resistances of two types of vessels, the afferent and efferent arterioles. These arterioles are arranged in series and are separated by the glomerular capillary bed (FIGURE 2). The afferent arteriole is proximal and regulates the pressure drop between the interlobular artery and the glomerular capillaries. Under conditions of constant perfusion pressure, a vasoconstriction of this vessel results in a decrease in glomerular capillary hydrostatic pressure, a primary determinant of the glomerular filtration rate (GFR). The efferent arteriole is the distal vessel, arising from the glomerular capillary bed and terminating either at the peritubular capillaries or vasa recta. Vasoconstriction of this vessel would reduce renal perfusion, but may result in an increase rather than decrease in glomerular capillary hydrostatic pressure. Thus, these two resistance vessels act in concert to regulate renal perfusate flow, but have opposing effects on the hydraulic driving force for GFR. This unique vascular architecture is the major determinant of the actions of calcium antagonists on GFR.

Glomerular Filtration Rate

Many investigators have suggested that calcium antagonists are unique among vasodilators in their ability to augment GFR. Certainly, in *in vivo* settings with underlying renal vasoconstriction, the administration of calcium antagonists often results in an increase in GFR.[3] In the absence of enhanced basal renal vascular tone, such effects are not always observed.[7–9] Similarly, in the isolated perfused rat kidney, calcium antagonists increase GFR only in the presence of underlying vasoconstriction.[16–18,20–22,24]

As depicted in FIGURE 3, the response of GFR differs from that of RPF. First, although the three vasoconstrictors elicited identical reductions in RPF, they produced

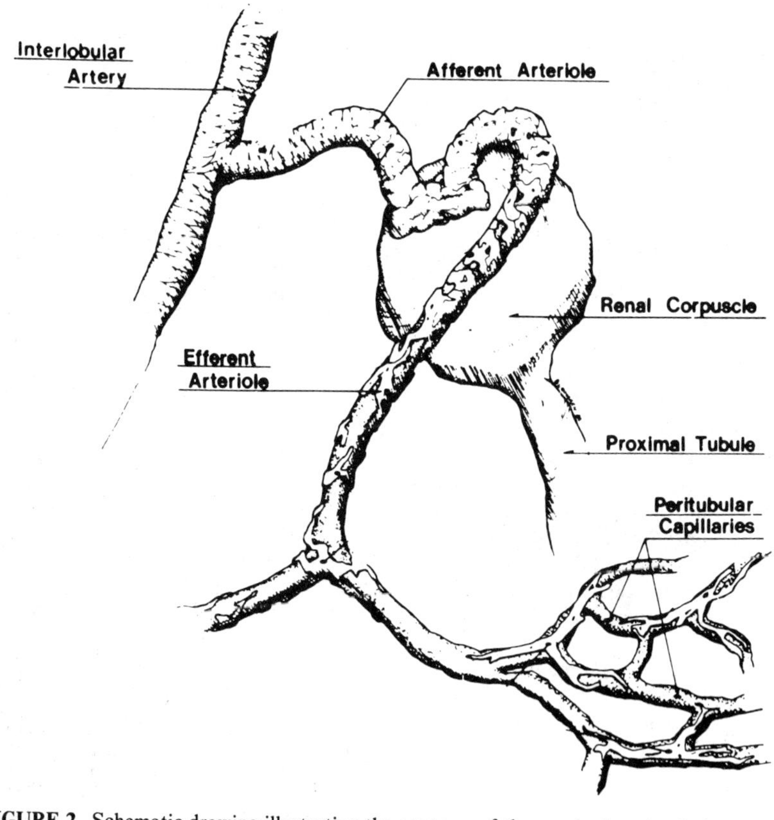

FIGURE 2. Schematic drawing illustrating the anatomy of the renal microcirculation. (Reproduced from Reference 23 with permission.)

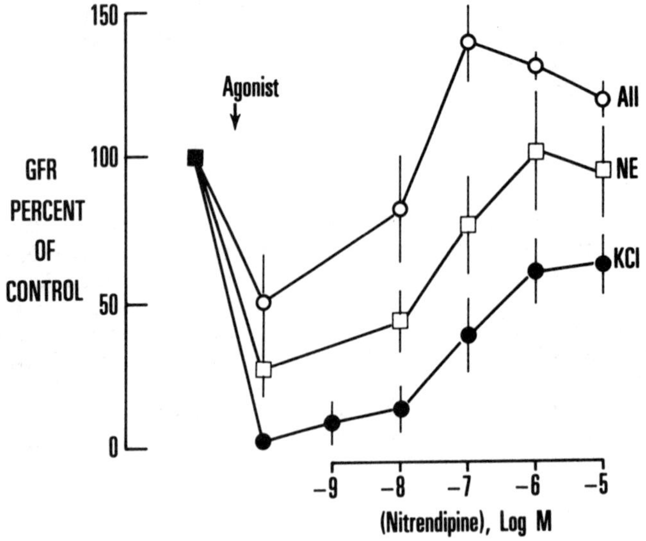

FIGURE 3. Dose-dependent effects of nitrendipine on the GFR response of the isolated perfused rat kidney. Equivalent vasoconstrictor doses of norepinephrine (NE), angiotensin II (AII), and KCl elicited divergent effects on GFR. Nitrendipine exerted a preferential augmentation of GFR during AII- and NE-induced vasoconstriction (refer to FIGURE 6) but not during KCl-induced vasoconstriction. (Reproduced from Reference 22 with permission.)

dissimilar effects on GFR. Thus, 30 mM KCl reduced GFR to 3 ± 2% of control; whereas, 3×10^{-7} M NE and 3×10^{-10} g/ml AII reduced GFR to 24 ± 10% and 51 ± 15% of control, respectively. Such observations reflect different relative effects of these vasoconstrictors on afferent and efferent tone in addition to possible differences in the effects of these agents on the nonvascular determinants of GFR.

Secondly, nitrendipine exerted effects on GFR that were quantitatively dissociated from its effects on RPF. Thus, as depicted in FIGURE 3, in the presence of AII and NE, nitrendipine elicited an augmentation of GFR that greatly exceeded its effects on RPF (FIGURE 1). During NE-induced vasoconstriction, nitrendipine caused GFR to return to pre-NE levels, but was less effective in reversing the NE-induced reduction in RPF. Similarly, in the presence of AII, nitrendipine caused GFR to return to control levels at concentrations that had only modest effects on RPF. At higher concentrations, nitrendipine increased GFR of AII-treated kidneys to values greatly exceeding pre-AII levels. In contrast, this preferential augmentation of GFR was not observed with KCl. Rather, in the presence of KCl, nitrendipine caused parallel increases in both GFR and RPF.

The preferential augmentation of GFR in the presence of agonist-induced (e.g., NE, AII) renal vasoconstriction is observed with calcium antagonists,[17,18,21] but not with the inorganic calcium entry blocker manganese.[3,18] FIGURE 4 summarizes the relative effects of a number of calcium antagonists and manganese on GFR and RPF of kidneys pretreated with norepinephrine. In contrast to the organic calcium antagonists, manganese exerted equal effects on RPF and GFR. This difference in selectivity reflects the differing actions of these two types of calcium entry blockers. Organic calcium antagonists appear to act on specific channels, whereas inorganic divalent cations block a wider variety of calcium translocating processes.[25,26] Since the preferential augmentation of GFR occurs only with organic calcium antagonists, this indicates that their preferential effects on GFR reflect their selectivity of action rather than calcium entry blockade per se.

Regional Heterogeneity

Since calcium antagonists act on specific calcium channels, they possess an unusual type of selectivity. Their effects exhibit regional heterogeneity. This follows from the observation that the activating mechanisms utilized by a single agonist vary within different regions of the circulation.[13] Accordingly, calcium antagonists block the actions of a vasoconstrictor in one region of the vasculature, while leaving the response intact at another site. Within the kidney, calcium antagonists appear to act preferentially on the preglomerular or afferent arteriolar resistance. A preferential dilation of the afferent arteriole could, thus, account for the observed augmentation of GFR.

To test this hypothesis, we determined stop-flow (ureteral) pressure in isolated kidneys during norepinephrine and nisoldipine administration.[17] Norepinephrine produced a decrement in stop-flow pressure which was markedly reversed by nisoldipine (FIGURE 5). Since RPF was affected only modestly, these data suggest a preferential action of the calcium antagonist on preglomerular vasoconstriction. This interpretation implies that norepinephrine evokes differing activating mechanisms in preglomerular and postglomerular vessels. Analogous regional heterogeneity has been suggested for norepinephrine in other vascular beds.[13,14]

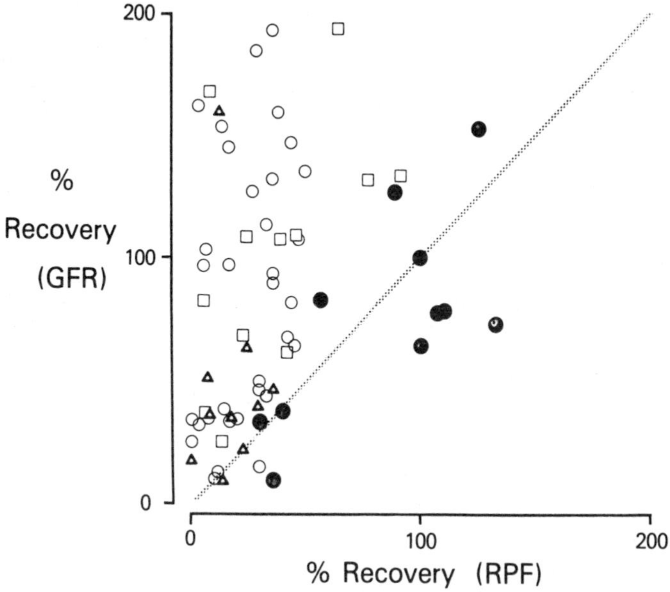

FIGURE 4. Comparison of reversal by calcium antagonists of norepinephrine-induced decrement in RPF and GFR of isolated perfused kidney. Nitrendipine, nisoldipine, and diltiazem (open circles, squares, and triangles, respectively) preferentially augment GFR; whereas manganese (closed circles) does not. (Reproduced from Reference 3 with permission.)

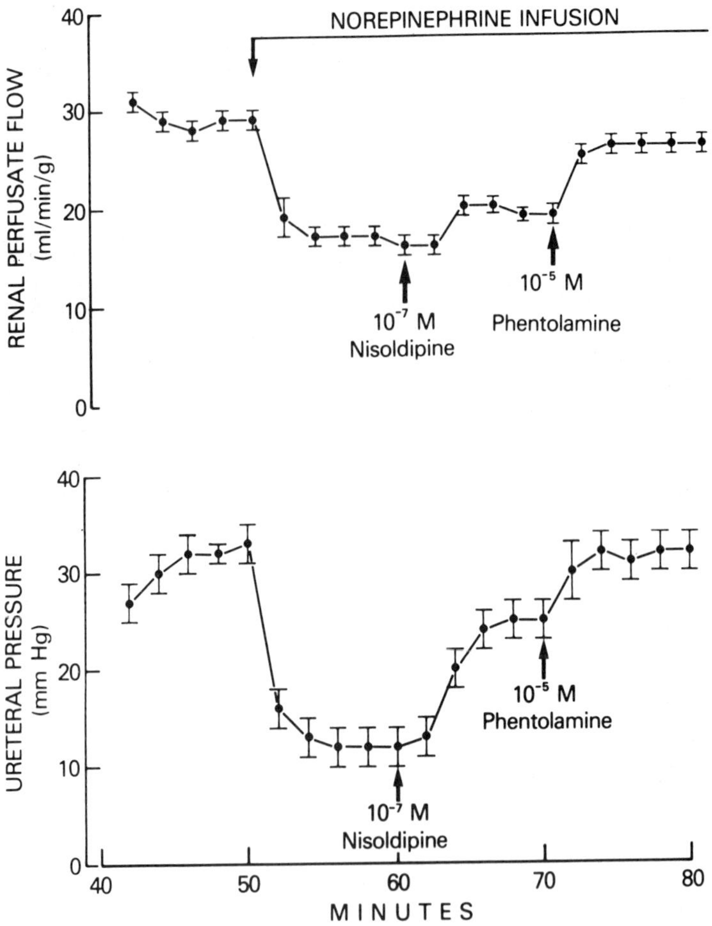

FIGURE 5. Effects of norepinephrine, nisoldipine, and phentolamine on ureteral (stop-flow) pressure and RPF of isolated perfused kidneys. Norepinephrine caused a decrease in both perfusate flow and ureteral pressure. Nisoldipine reversed the decrement in ureteral pressure even though RPF was only modestly affected. This suggests a preferential action of nisoldipine on preglomerular vasoconstriction and an increase in filtration pressure. Phentolamine readily reversed that component of the norepinephrine-induced vasoconstriction that was resistant to nisoldipine. (Reproduced from Reference 17 with permission.)

In this regard, it is of interest that a selective augmentation of GFR by calcium antagonists did not occur during KCl-induced renal vasoconstriction. In contrast to the mechanisms linking receptor occupation to vasoconstriction, the mechanism of KCl-induced vasoconstriction does not exhibit regional heterogeneity.[13,14] Accordingly, vessels that demonstrate dissimilar sensitivities to calcium antagonists when activated by norepinephrine exhibit similar sensitivities when activated by KCl.[13,14]

The selective augmentation of GFR by calcium antagonists, thus, requires the presence of an agonist that acts upon afferent and efferent resistance vessels by

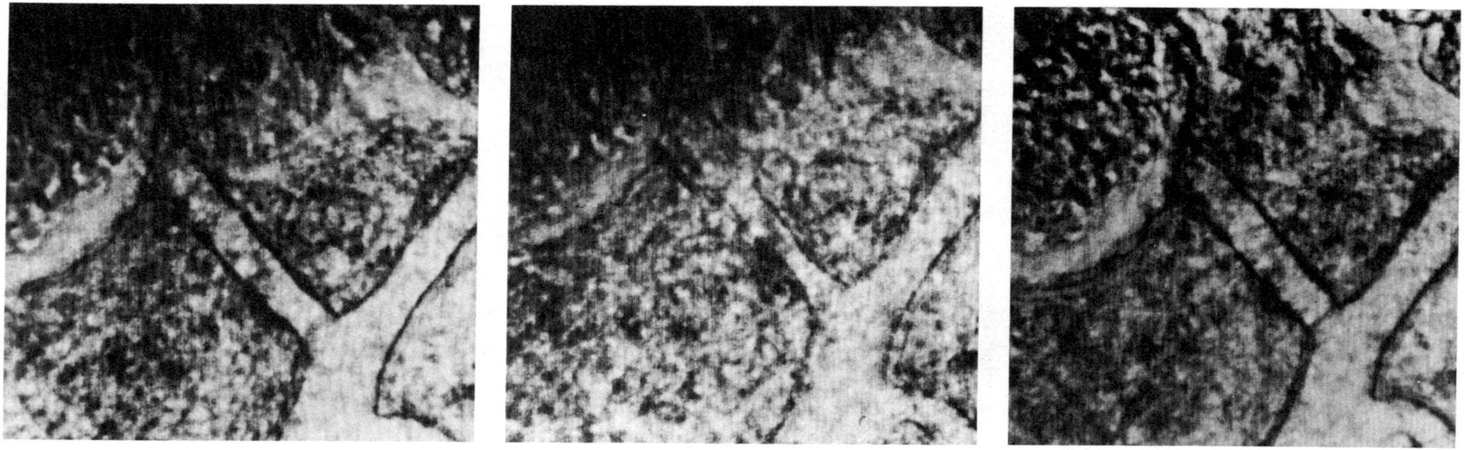

FIGURE 6. Photomicrographs of an isolated perfused hydronephrotic kidney during the control perfusion (left), and the administration of the thromboxane A_2 mimetic U44069 (1.0 μM, center), followed by the administration of 1.0 μM nifedipine (right). U44069 caused an afferent arteriolar vasoconstriction which was reversed by nifedipine. (Reproduced from Reference 28 with permission.)

differing activating mechanisms. Such agonists may elicit membrane depolarization and activate potential-dependent calcium channels in afferent but not efferent arteriolar smooth muscle. Since organic calcium antagonists selectively inhibit the function of this calcium channel type, they increase GFR by preferentially attenuating afferent arteriolar tone. In support of this formulation, Flemming *et al.* recently presented direct, *in vivo* evidence that the afferent arteriole is more sensitive to calcium antagonists than is the efferent arteriole.[27]

Direct Visualization of Afferent Arteriolar Vasodilation

In order to assess directly the effects of calcium antagonists on afferent arteriolar vasoconstriction in an *in vitro* setting, we have modified the hydronephrotic rat kidney model which was originally described by Steinhausen *et al.*[19,27] In the normal rat kidney, the renal tubular elements obscure direct visualization of the renal resistance vessels. Chronic hydronephrosis induced by unilateral ureteral ligation results in progressive atrophy of the renal tubules. The structure of the renal microcirculation remains intact in the hydronephrotic kidney and can be directly observed using videomicroscopy. We have developed a model combining the hydronephrotic kidney with isolated perfusion techniques to study the microvessels in an *in vitro* setting, in which the vasoconstrictor stimuli can be accurately controlled.

We recently assessed the effects of a renal vasoconstrictor postulated to play a role in renal dysfunction, thromboxane A_2, with this model.[28] Thromboxane A_2 is an unstable prostanoid which has been implicated in mediating the alterations in renal hemodynamics accompanying nephrotoxic serum nephritis,[29] glycerol-induced renal failure,[30] and ureteral obstruction.[31] The stable endoperoxide analogue U44069 mimics

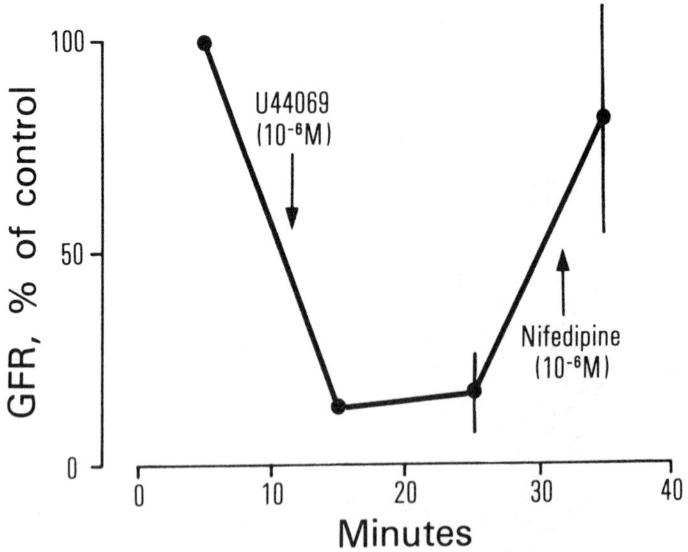

FIGURE 7. Effects of U44069 and nifedipine on GFR of isolated perfused normal rat kidneys. The U44069-induced decrement in GFR was reversed with nifedipine. (Reproduced from Reference 28 with permission.)

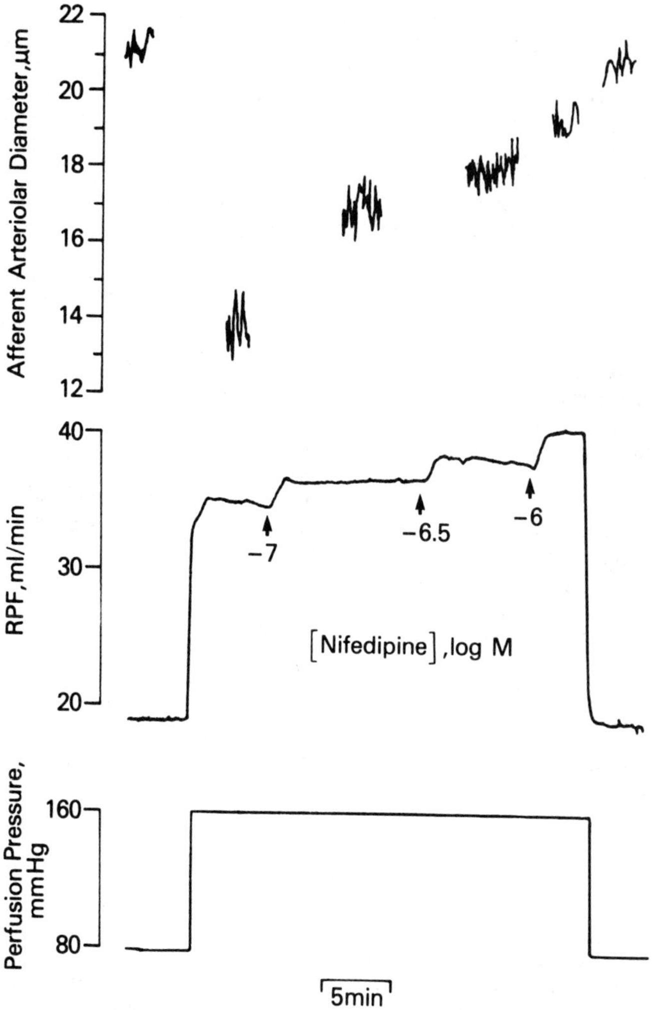

FIGURE 8. Effects of elevating perfusion pressure and nifedipine on afferent arteriolar diameter and RPF of the isolated perfused hydronephrotic kidney. Increasing renal arterial pressure (lower panel) elicited a vasoconstriction in the afferent arteriole (upper panel). Nifedipine returned afferent arteriolar diameter to control levels and increased RPF.

many biological effects of thromboxane A_2 and has been demonstrated to reduce GFR *in vivo.*[32] Similarly, we previously reported that U44069 causes an 80% decrement in GFR of the normal isolated perfused rat kidney while reducing perfusate flow by only 18% and suggested that this reflects a predominant action on afferent resistance.[24]

The photomicrographs in FIGURE 6 illustrate directly the effects of U44069 on the afferent arteriole of the isolated perfused hydronephrotic kidney. U44069 elicited a marked afferent arteriolar vasoconstriction. This afferent vasoconstriction was completely reversed by nifedipine.

The actions of U44069 and nifedipine on the afferent arteriole of the hydronephrotic kidney parallel their effects on GFR in the normal *in vitro* perfused kidney. As depicted in FIGURE 7, the reduction in GFR associated with administration of U44069 is also reversed by nifedipine. We have previously demonstrated that the dose dependency of the effects of calcium antagonists on GFR coincides precisely with their effects on isolated vascular smooth muscle.[24] Thus, in the presence of this putative mediator of renal dysfunction,[29–31] calcium antagonists augment GFR by reversing a selective afferent arteriolar vasoconstriction. Further studies are required to investigate the obvious clinical implications of these findings.

Effects on Renal Autoregulation

Finally, basal renal vascular resistance is influenced by a variety of vasoconstrictor stimuli under normal physiologic conditions. Since renal blood flow exhibits autoregulation, perfusion pressure itself exerts direct and indirect effects on the microcirculation. Though renal autoregulation is a complex phenomenon involving renal autacoids and tubuloglomerular feedback,[33,34] intraarteriolar pressure may contribute directly to the response. In the isolated perfused hydronephrotic kidney, acute alterations in perfusion pressure elicit direct changes in afferent arteriolar caliber which are also sensitive to inhibition by calcium antagonists.[20]

FIGURE 8 depicts the effects of elevating renal arterial pressure on afferent arteriolar diameter and renal perfusate flow. As illustrated, increasing perfusion pressure elicited an afferent arteriolar vasoconstriction. RPF increased, but not in proportion to the increase in pressure, indicating an increase in renal vascular resistance. The administration of nifedipine dose dependently and completely reversed these effects. Thus, afferent diameter returned to basal levels and RPF increased in proportion to renal arterial pressure. These observations are in accord with other reports[35–37] suggesting that calcium antagonists inhibit the autoregulatory response of the kidney.

Summary

These findings demonstrate that calcium antagonists reverse renal vasoconstriction in a variety of settings. The ability of calcium antagonists to augment GFR of the vasoconstricted kidney is striking and has also been demonstrated in a number of *in vivo* settings.[3] These observations and others[38,39] raise the possibility that calcium antagonists have potential utility in the treatment of a number of disorders characterized by renal ischemia and consequent renal insufficiency. Further studies to evaluate this possibility are required. The unique effects of calcium antagonists on GFR reflect a regional heterogeneity within the renal microcirculation and a preferential action of calcium antagonists on the afferent arteriole. Final resolution of the pharmacological basis for the renal hemodynamic actions of calcium antagonists will require a more complete understanding of the divergent activating mechanisms within the renal microcirculation.

ACKNOWLEDGMENT

The authors are indebted to Charles Horton for his expert technical assistance.

REFERENCES

1. FLECKENSTEIN, A. 1964. Die bedeutung der energiereichen phosphate fur kontraktilitat und tonus des myokards. Verh. Dtsch. Bes. Inn. Med. **70:** 81–99.
2. FLECKENSTEIN, A., H. KAMMERMEIER, H. J. DORING & H. J. FREUND. 1967. Zum wirjungsmechanismus neuartiger koronardilatoren mit gleichzeitig sauerstoff-einsparenden myokard-effeckten, prenylamin und iropveratril. Z. Kreislaufforsch. **56:** 716–744.
3. LOUTZENHISER, R. & M. EPSTEIN. 1985. Effects of calcium antagonists on renal hemodynamics. Am. J. Physiol. **249:** F619–F629.
4. BELL, A. J. & A. LINDNER. 1984. Effects of verapamil and nifedipine on renal function and hemodynamics in the dog. Renal. Physiol. **7:** 329–343.
5. DIETZ, J. R., J. O. DAVIS, R. H. FREEMAN, D. VILLARREAL & S. F. ECHTENKAMP. 1983. Effects of intrarenal infusion of calcium entry blockers in anesthetized dogs. Hypertension **5:** 482–488.
6. ABE, Y., T. KOMORI, K. MIURA, *et al.* 1983. Effects of the calcium antagonist nicardipine on renal function and renin release in dogs. J. Cardiovasc. Pharmacol. **5:** 254–259.
7. LEONETTI, G., C. CUSPIDI, L. SAMPIERI, L. TERZOLI & A. ZANCHETTI. 1982. Comparison of cardiovascular, renal and humoral effects of acute administration of two calcium channel blockers in normotensive and hypertensive subjects. J. Cardiovasc. Pharmacol. **4:** S319–S324.
8. WALLIA, R., A. GREENBERG & J. B. PUSCHETT. 1985. Renal hemodynamic and tubular transport effects of nitrendipine. J. Lab. Clin. Med. **105:** 498–503.
9. YOKOYAMA, S. & T. KABURAGI. 1983. Clinical effects of intravenous nifedipine on renal function. J. Cardiovasc. Pharmacol. **5:** 67–71.
10. GLOSSMANN, H. & D. R. FERRY. 1983. Molecular approach to the calcium channel. *In* New Calcium Antagonists. Recent Developments and Prospects, A. Fleckenstein, K. Hashimoto, H. Mermann, A. Schwartz & L. Siepel, Eds.: 63–98. Fischer-Verlag. Stuttgart, FRG.
11. HESS, P., J. B. LANSMAN & R. W. TSIEN. 1985. Mechanism of calcium channel modulation by dihydropyridine agonists and antagonists. *In* Cardiovascular Effects of Dihydropyridine-Type Calcium Antagonists and Agonists. A. Fleckenstein, C. van Breemen, R. Gross & F. Hoffmeister, Eds.: 34–55. Springer Verlag. Heidelberg, FRG.
12. LOUTZENHISER, R. & M. EPSTEIN. 1984. Activation mechanisms of human renal artery: effects of KCl, norepinephrine and nitrendipine upon tension development and ^{45}Ca influx. Eur. J. Pharmacol. **106:** 47–52.
13. CAUVIN, C. & C. VAN BREEMEN. 1985. Effects of Ca+2 antagonists on isolated rabbit mesenteric resistance vessels as compared to rabbit aorta. *In* Cardiovascular Effects of Dihydropyridine-Type Calcium Antagonists and Agonists. A. Fleckenstein, C. van Breemen, R. Gross & F. Hoffmeister, Eds.: 259–269. Springer Verlag. Heidelberg, FRG.
14. CAUVIN, C., R. LOUTZENHISER & C. VAN BREEMEN. 1983. Mechanisms of calcium antagonist-induced vasodilation. Annu. Rev. Pharmacol. **23:** 373–396.
15. MEISHERI, K., O. HWANG & C. VAN BREEMEN. 1981. Evidence for two separate Ca+2 pathways in smooth muscle plasmalemma. J. Membr. Biol. **59:** 19–25.
16. LOUTZENHISER, R., C. HORTON & M. EPSTEIN. 1982. Flow-induced errors in estimating perfusion pressure of the isolated rat kidney. Kidney Int. **22:** 693–696.
17. LOUTZENHISER, R., M. EPSTEIN, C. HORTON & P. SONKE. 1985. Reversal by the calcium antagonist nisoldipine of norepinephrine-induced reduction of GFR: evidence for preferential antagonism of preglomerular vasoconstriction. J. Pharmacol. Exp. Ther. **232:** 382–387.
18. LOUTZENHISER, R., C. HORTON & M. EPSTEIN. 1985. Effects of diltiazem and manganese on renal hemodynamics: studies in the isolated perfused rat kidney. Nephron **39:** 382–388.
19. STEINHAUSEN, M., H. SNOEI, N. PAREKH, R. BAKER & P. C. JOHNSON. 1983. Hydronephrosis: a new method to visualize vas afference, efferens, and glomerular network. Kidney Int. **23:** 794–806.
20. LOUTZENHISER, R., M. EPSTEIN & C. HORTON. 1987. Inhibition by diltiazem of pressure-

induced afferent vasoconstriction in the isolated perfused rat kidney. Am. J. Cardiol. **59:** 72A–75A.

21. STEELE, T. & L. CHALLONER-HUE. 1984. Renal interactions between norepinephrine and calcium antagonists. Kidney Int. **26:** 719–724.
22. LOUTZENHISER, R., M. EPSTEIN & C. HORTON. 1987. Modification by dihydropyridine-type calcium antagonists of the renal hemodynamic response to vasoconstrictors. J. Cardiovasc. Pharmacol. **9**(Suppl. 1): S70–S75.
23. GATTONE, V. H., F. C. LUFT & A. P. EVAN. 1984. Renal afferent and efferent arterioles of the rabbit. Am. J. Physiol. **247:** F219–F228.
24. LOUTZENHISER, R., M. EPSTEIN, C. HORTON & P. SONKE. 1986. Reversal of renal and vascular smooth muscle actions of the thromboxane mimetic U44069 by diltiazem. Am. J. Physiol. **250:** F619–F626.
25. DETH, D. & C. LYNCH. 1981. Inhibition of alpha-receptor induced Ca+2 release and Ca+2 influx by Mn+2 and La+3. Eur. J. Pharmacol. **71:** 1–11.
26. HAGIWARA, S. & L. BYERLY. 1981. Calcium channel. Annu. Rev. Neurosci. **4:** 69–125.
27. FLEMING, J. T., N. PAREKH & M. STEINHAUSEN. 1987. Calcium antagonists preferentially dilate preglomerular vessels of hydronephrotic kidney. Am. J. Physiol. **253** (Renal Fluid Electrolyte Physiol. 22): F1157–F1163.
28. LOUTZENHISER, R. & M. EPSTEIN. 1987. Modification of the renal hemodynamic response to vasoconstrictors by calcium antagonists. Am. J. Nephrol. **7**(Suppl. 1): 7–16.
29. LIANOS, E. A., G. A. ANDRES & M. J. DUNN. 1983. Glomerular prostaglandin and thromboxane synthesis in rat nephrotoxic serum nephritis. J. Clin. Invest. **72:** 1439–1448.
30. BENABE, J. E., S. KLAHR, M. H. HOFFMAN & A. R. MORRISON. 1980. Production of thromboxane A_2 by the kidney in glycerol-induced acute renal failure. Prostaglandins **19:** 333–347.
31. MORRISON, A. R., K. NISHIKAWA & P. NEEDLEMAN. 1978. Thromboxane A_2 biosynthesis in the ureter obstructed isolated perfused kidney of the rabbit. J. Pharmacol. Exp. Ther. **205:** 1–8.
32. GERBER, J. G., E. ELLIS, J. HOLLIFIED & A. NIES. 1979. Effect of prostaglandin endoperoxide analogue on canine renal function, hemodynamics and renin release. Eur. J. Pharmacol. **53:** 239–246.
33. NAVAR, G. L. & L. ROSIVALL. 1984. Contribution of the renin-angiotensin system to the control of intrarenal hemodynamics. Kidney Int. **25:** 857–868.
34. NAVAR, L. G. 1978. Renal autoregulation: perspectives from whole kidney and single nephron studies. Am. J. Physiol. **234:** F357–F370.
35. ONO, H., H. KOKUBUN & K. HASHIMOTO. 1974. Abolition by calcium antagonists of the autoregulation of renal blood flow. Naunyn Schmiedebergs Arch. Pharmacol. **285:** 201–207.
36. NAVAR, L. G., W. J. CHAMPION & C. E. THOMAS. 1986. Effects of calcium channel blockade on renal vascular resistance responses to changes in perfusion pressure and angiotensin-converting enzyme inhibition in dogs. Circ. Res. **58:** 874–881.
37. COHEN, A. J. & J. C. S. FRAY. 1982. Calcium ion dependence of myogenic renal plasma flow autoregulation: evidence from the isolated perfused rat kidney. J. Physiol. London **330:** 449–460.
38. LEE, S. M., B. J. HILLMAN, R. L. CLARK & U. F. MICHAEL. 1985. The effects of diltiazem and captopril on glycerol-induced acute renal failure in the rat: functional, pathologic, and microangiographic studies. Invest. Radiol. **20:** 961–970.
39. BAKRIS, G. L. & J. C. BURNETT. 1985. A role for calcium in radiocontrast-induced reductions in renal hemodynamics. Kidney Int. **27:** 465–468.

Effects of Calcium Antagonists on Renal Function

JOHN H. BAUER AND GARRY P. REAMS

Hypertension Section
Nephrology Division
University of Missouri Health Sciences Center
One Hospital Drive
Columbia, Missouri 65212

INTRODUCTION

Although calcium antagonists were initially characterized by their pharmacological ability to produce coronary vasodilation with myocardial depression, the individual members of this family of drugs differ not only in their pharmacokinetic properties, but also in their pharmacodynamic effects. They all, however, appear to alter vascular tone by selectively blockading potential-dependent calcium channels. Some may also selectively blockade receptor-operated (alpha-adrenoceptor) calcium channels, and/or inhibit calcium release from intracellular stores. Since most, if not all, vasoconstrictor hormones activate vascular smooth muscle by modifying cellular calcium handling, it is not surprising that calcium antagonists attenuate the effects of exogenously administered norepinephrine and angiotensin II on systemic resistance vessels.[1–4] Presumably, this is a primary mechanism whereby calcium antagonists diminish total peripheral vascular resistance in hypertensive diseases.

RENIN-ANGIOTENSIN-ALDOSTERONE

Since calcium may inhibit renin secretion by a direct action on juxtaglomerular cells,[5,6] the administration of a calcium antagonist might be expected to stimulate renin secretion, and thus increase the angiotensin II concentration in circulating plasma. However, only the dihydropyridine derivative calcium antagonists appear to produce this effect with some consistency[7] (see TABLE 1). When renin stimulation is present, it is not associated with aldosterone release. Although angiotensin II is a major regulator of aldosterone secretion from the adrenal glomerulosa cells, angiotensin II employs calcium as a second messenger to couple stimulus to secretion.[7,8] Calcium antagonists block this angiotensin II steroidogenic response by inhibiting the rise in cytosolic free calcium.[7,8]

RENAL FUNCTION AND HEMODYNAMICS

The renal effects of calcium antagonists are only now being characterized[7] (see TABLE 2). Among the currently studied calcium antagonists, diltiazem, nifedipine, and nicardipine have been reported to increase acutely glomerular filtration rate and/or effective renal plasma flow.[7] However, only diltiazem[9,10] and amlodipine[11] have been reported to produce sustained increases in glomerular filtration rate and/or effective renal plasma flow.

TABLE 1. Calcium Antagonists: Renin-Angiotensin-Aldosterone

	PRA[a]	A_{II}[b]	Aldo[c]
Acute			
Diltiazem	No Δ	—	No Δ
Amlodipine	—	—	—
Nifedipine	Increase	Increase	No Δ
Nitrendipine	No Δ	—	No Δ
Nicardipine	No Δ/↑	—	No Δ
Verapamil	No Δ	—	No Δ
Chronic			
Diltiazem	No Δ	—	No Δ
Amlodipine	No Δ	—	No Δ
Nifedipine	No Δ/↑	—	No Δ
Nitrendipine	No Δ/↑	—	No Δ
Nicardipine	No Δ/↑	—	No Δ
Verapamil	No Δ	—	No Δ

[a]PRA = plasma renin activity.
[b]A_{II} = plasma angiotensin II.
[c]Aldo = plasma aldosterone.

There are at least two potential mechanisms for the observed increase in glomerular filtration rate and/or effective renal plasma flow following calcium antagonism therapy: (1) reversal of angiotensin II–induced vasoconstriction (mesangium and/or efferent arteriolar tone), and (2) reversal of norepinephrine-induced vasoconstriction (afferent arteriolar tone). The effect of calcium antagonists to prevent an increase in cytosol ionized calcium would be expected to decrease the sensitivity of the renal vasculature and/or the mesangium to both angiotensin II and norepinephrine. Indeed, diltiazem, nifedipine, nitrendipine, and verapamil have all been reported to attenuate the intrarenal effects of exogenously administered angiotensin II,[12–20] and norepinephrine,[16,20–24] producing marked increases in renal perfusion and glomerular filtration.

TABLE 2. Calcium Antagonists: Renal Function and Hemodynamics

	GRF[a]	ERPF/RBF[b]	RVR[c]
Acute			
Diltiazem	No Δ/↑	No Δ/↑	—
Amlodipine	—	—	—
Nifedipine	No Δ/↑	No Δ/↑	—
Nitrendipine	No Δ	No Δ	—
Nicardipine	No Δ/↑	No Δ/↑	↓
Verapamil	No Δ	—	—
Chronic			
Diltiazem	No Δ/↑	No Δ/↑	No Δ/↑
Amlodipine	↑	↑	↓
Nifedipine	No Δ	No Δ	—
Nitrendipine	No Δ	No Δ	No Δ
Nicardipine	No Δ/↑	—	—
Verapamil	No Δ	No Δ	↓

[a]GFR = glomerular filtration rate.
[b]ERPF/RBF = effective renal plasma flow/renal blood flow.
[c]RVR = renal vascular resistance.

In general, calcium antagonists do not adversely effect renal function or hemodynamics. However, there are two reports in the literature suggesting that nifedipine[25] and/or diltiazem[26] may produce acute reversible deterioration in renal function. In these case reports, the patients were hemodynamically unstable, and they were receiving a variety of cardiovascular drugs prior to the prescription of the calcium antagonist. The causal relationship of acute renal failure to the institution of the calcium antagonist suggests that calcium antagonism prevented angiotensin II–mediated augmentation in efferent arteriolar tone, abolishing renal autoregulations. These observations, however, are not likely to be extrapolated to essential hypertensive patients.

TABLE 3. Pathophysiology of Essential Hypertensive Renal Disease

Time (age-years)	
(20–30) Phase I:	Rise in renal vascular resistance due to functional disturbance of renal vasculature: ? active vasoresponse to endogenous angiotensin II, norepinephrine.
(30–40) Phase II:	Further rise in renal vascular resistance; both functional and structural disturbances in renal vasculature; preservation glomerular filtration rate (although glomeruli may be ischemic); rise in filtration fraction; microalbuminuria.
(40–50) Phase III:	Further rise in renal vascular resistance; structural disturbances involving both renal vasculature and glomeruli (arteriolar nephrosclerosis); reduction in perfusion disproportionately greater than filtration; sustained rise in filtration fraction; proteinuria.
(50–) Phase IV:	End-stage renal disease: chronic renal failure.

RENAL PROTECTIVE EFFECTS

Renal function and hemodynamic factors have been studied intensively in hypertensive diseases for more than 50 years. From such studies, a pathophysiological sequence for the progression of essential hypertensive renal disease may be proposed[27] (see TABLE 3). Recent studies with two classes of antihypertensive drugs, calcium antagonists[9–11] and angiotensin converting enzyme inhibitors,[28,29] suggest that functional renal disturbances (phases I and II) can be reversed in essential hypertension. The ability to reverse these functional changes appears dependent not only on lowering systemic blood pressure, but also on blunting angiotensin II–mediated vasoconstriction of the renal vasculature and mesangial beds. Unique to both calcium antagonists and angiotensin converting enzyme inhibitors are their ability to attenuate the intrarenal effects of angiotensin II. If systemic blood pressure is not controlled, and/or functional disturbances are not corrected, irreversible structural change may occur (phase III), ultimately leading to end-stage renal disease (phase IV).

When structural change does occur, and there is a reduction in renal mass, the remaining nephrons undergo adaptive changes resulting in glomerular hyperperfusion and hyperfiltration.[30] Elevation of glomerular capillary plasma flow rate is due to afferent and efferent renal arteriolar vasodilation; elevation in glomerular filtration is due to elevation of glomerular capillary hydraulic pressure, resulting from the proportionately greater reduction in afferent arteriolar resistance. It is now clear from experimental studies that elevation of glomerular capillary hydraulic pressure results in glomerular destruction, and that prevention of glomerular capillarly hypertension protects against the development of glomerular structural injury.[31,32]

The transmission of systemic hypertension to the glomerular capillary network may be one of the most important mechanisms for the progression of renal disease accompanying hypertensive states. What has not been appreciated, until only recently, is that reduction in systemic blood pressure does not invariably result in reduction of glomerular capillary pressure.[32] Both diuretics and vasodilators stimulate the renin-angiotensin system. Drug-mediated elevation of intrarenal angiotensin II may vasoconstrict efferent arterioles, maintaining high glomerular capillary pressures, in spite of a reduction in systemic blood pressure. Indeed, it has been demonstrated experimentally that triple drug therapy, employing a diuretic, reserpine, and hydralazine, does not reduce glomerular capillary hydraulic pressure, in spite of a significant drop in systemic blood pressure.[32] The net clinical result is that glomerular injury is not abated.

Drug-mediated elevation of angiotensin II may also impair salt and water homeostasis, compromise glomerular perfusion and filtration, and enhance the transglomerular passage of albumin.[33] Interruption of the intrarenal renin-angiotensin system has the potential to decrease efferent arteriolar resistance, enhance renal blood flow, enhance glomerular filtration rate, decrease urinary protein excrtion, and maintain sodium and water homeostasis. Drug therapy, with angiotensin converting enzyme inhibitors, has now been described, both experimentally[31,32] and clinically,[33] that can mediate the above renal protective events. Initial observations would suggest that many of the intrarenal effects of calcium antagonists mimic the intrarenal effects of angiotensin converting enzyme inhibitors (see TABLE 4). The potential role for these two classes of drugs to modify the pathophysiology of hypertensive renal disease, and/or to attenuate the progression of chronic renal disease, has generated considerable experimental and clinical attention, prompting ongoing clinical trials.

TABLE 4. Comparative Effects: ACEI vs. Ca^{2+} Antagonist[a]

	ACEI		Ca^{2+} Antagonist	
	Acute	Chronic	Acute	Chronic
GRF	No Δ/↑	No Δ/↑	No Δ/↑	No Δ/↑
ERPF/RBF	↑	No Δ/↑	No Δ/↑	No Δ/↑
Filt. fract.	↓	No Δ	No Δ	No Δ
RVR	↓	↓	↓	↓
Uprotein	↓	↓	No Δ	No Δ
$\dot{V}$	↑	No Δ	↑	No Δ
$U_{Na}V$	↑	No Δ	↑	No Δ

ACEI = angiotensin converting enzyme inhibitor, inhibits AII. Calcium antagonist blocks calcium influx (second messenger for AII). GRF = glomerular filtration rate. ERPF/RBF = effective renal plasma flow/renal blood flow. Filt. fract. = filtration fraction (GFR/ERPF). RVR = renal vascular resistance. Uprotein = urinary protein excretion. $\dot{V}$= urine flow rate. $U_{Na}V$ = urinary sodium excretion.

TABLE 5. Calcium Antagonist: Salt and Water/Body Fluids

	$\dot{V}$	$U_{Na}V$[b]	U_KV[c]	PV/ECF[d]
Acute				
Diltiazem	Increase	Increase	No Δ	—
Amlodipine	—	—	—	—
Nifedipine	Increase	Increase	No Δ	—
Nitrendipine	Increase	Increase	No Δ	—
Nicardipine	Increase	Increase	No Δ	—
Verapamil	Increase	Increase	No Δ	—
Chronic				
Diltiazem	No Δ	No Δ	No Δ	No Δ
Amlodipine	No Δ	No Δ	No Δ	No Δ
Nifedipine	No Δ	No Δ	No Δ	No Δ
Nitrendipine	No Δ/↑	No Δ/↑	No Δ	No Δ
Nicardipine	No Δ/↑	No Δ/↑	No Δ	No Δ
Verapamil	No Δ	No Δ	No Δ	No Δ

[a] $\dot{V}$ = urine flow rate.
[b] $U_{Na}V$ = urinary sodium excretion.
[c] U_KV = urinary potassium excretion.
[d] PV/ECF = plasma volume/extracellular fluid volume.

Calcium antagonists may also protect the failing kidney by mechanisms independent of any systemic or renal hemodynamic effect, by diminishing cellular calcium accumulation.[34,35] Enhanced calcium uptake is common in chronic renal disease, and might be expected to cause cellular damage by injuring cell mitochondria secondary to calcium overload, injuring cell membranes via activation of phospholipases, or enhancing free oxygen radical formation.[35] Recent studies suggest that calcium antagonism may protect against the progression of experimental chronic renal failure by decreasing nephrocalcinosis and tubular ultrastructural abnormalities.[34,35]

Finally, calcium antagonists have been demonstrated to have a renal protective role in several experimental models of acute renal failure, including (1) norepinephrine-induced acute renal failure,[36,37] (2) warm and cold ischemia in the isolated perfused kidney,[38] (3) ischemia induced by complete renal artery occlusion,[39] and (4) radiocontrast-induced acute renal failure.[40] A recent report suggests that verapamil may prevent posttransplant acute renal failure, if given to renal donors prior to nephrectomy.[41] However, the mechanism by which calcium antagonism protects ischemic tissues is unknown. It is currently hypothesized that calcium accelerates death of viable, but jeopardized, cells during reperfusion, by potentiating the damaging effects of free oxygen radicals on the mitochondrial electron transport chain.[42] Calcium antagonism, via abolition of renal vasoconstriction responses and/or inhibition of cellular calcium influx, represents a significant new therapeutic potential for the treatment of ischemic and/or nephrotoxic acute renal failure.

SALT AND WATER EXCRETION

All of the calcium antagonists induce an acute natriuresis and diuresis[7] (see TABLE 5). The effects appear to be independent of any hemodynamic action of the drugs, most likely relating to a direct effect on both proximal segments and segments located more distally than the loop of Henle.[43,44] However, none of the calcium antagonists have been demonstrated to have a clincially important sustained effect on salt and water excretion. This conclusion is supported by the absence of an observed effect of calcium antagonists on serum electrolytes or body fluid composition. Body weight may, or may not, be decreased. Anecdotal case reports do attest to the potential for these drugs to produce edema formation. However, the mechanism and frequency of this side effect are unknown. Since calcium antagonists generally lower blood pressure, without producing salt and water retention, these drugs can be positioned as a first-step therapy for the treatment of hypertensive diseases.

CONCLUSIONS

Calcium antagonists can be expected to assume a prominent role in the treatment of hypertensive diseases because of their ability to lower blood pressure, while preserving renal perfusion, glomerular filtration, and sodium homeostasis. The potential roles for calcium antagonists to reverse or prevent the pathophysiological progression of hypertensive renal disease, to attenuate the progression of chronic renal disease, and/or to alter the course of ischemic or nephrotoxic acute renal failure are currently unknown, but represent promising new areas for research, with important therapeutic consequences.

REFERENCES

1. Ikeda, F., T. Kono, F. Oseko, H. Imura & J. Endo. 1980. Effects of diltiazem hydrochloride on pressor and steroidogenic actions of angiotensins and norepinephrine in man. Endocrinol. Jpn. **27:** 779–784.
2. Vierhapper, H. & I. Waldhausl. 1982. Reduced pressor effect of angiotensin II and noradrenaline in normal man following the oral administration of the calcium-antagonist nifedipine. Eur. J. Clin. Med. **12:** 263–267.
3. Guthrie, G. P., R. G. McAllister & T. A. Kotchen. 1983. Effect of intravenous and oral verapamil upon pressor and adrenal steroidogenic responses in normal man. J. Clin. Endocrinol. Metabl. **57:** 339–343.
4. Magometschnigg, D., H. Hortnagl & H. Ramlis. 1984. Diltiazem and verapamil: functional antagonism of exogenous noradrenalin and angiotensin II in man. Eur. J. Clin. Pharmacol. **26:** 303–307.
5. Kotchen, T. A., K. I. Maull, R. Luke, D. Rees & W. Flamenbaum. 1974. Effect of acute and chronic calcium administration on plasma renin. J. Clin. Invest. **54:** 1279–1286.
6. Watkins, B. E., J. O. Davis, T. E. Lohmeier & R. H. Freeman. 1976. Intrarenal site of action of calcium on renin secretion in dogs. Circ. Res. **39:** 847–853.
7. Bauer, J. H. & G. P. Reams. 1987. Short-term and long-term effects of calcium entry blockers on the kidney. Am. J. Cardiol. **59:** 66A–71A.
8. Millar. J. A. & A. D. Struthers. 1984. Calcium antagonists and hormone release. Clin. Sci. **66:** 249–255.
9. Sunderrajan, S., G. P. Reams & J. H. Bauer. 1986. Renal effects of diltiazem in primary hypertension. Hypertension **8:** 238–242.
10. Sunderrajan, S., G. P. Reams & J. H. Bauer. 1987. Long-term effects of diltiazem in primary hypertension. Am. Heart J. **114:** 383–388.
11. Reams, J. P., A. Lau, A. Hamory & J. H. Bauer. 1987. Amlodipine therapy corrects renal vascular abnormalities encountered in the hypertensive state. Am. J. Kidney Dis. **10:** 446–451.
12. Sakurai, T., T. Kurita, S. Nagano & T. Sonoda. 1972. Antihypertensive, vasodilating and sodium diuretic actions of D-*cis*-isomer of benzothiazepine derivative (CRD-401). Acta Urol. Japonica **18:** 695–707.

13. YAMAGUCHI, I., K. IKEZAWA, T. TAKODA & A. KIYOMOTO. 1974. Studies on a new 1,5-benzothiazepine derivative (CRD-401). IV. Effects on renal blood flow and renal function. Jpn. J. Pharmacol. **24:** 511–522.
14. HIRAKAWA, M., Y. SHIWAKU, T. AJI & F. KOSAKA. 1975. Experimental and clinical studies on diuretic action of CRD-401. Anesth. Resusc. **11:** 159–170.
15. ICHIKAWA, I, J. F. MIELE & B. M. BRENNER. 1979. Reversal of renal cortical actions of angiotensin II by verapamil and manganese. Kidney Int. **16:** 137–147.
16. JOVER, B., M. DUPONT, D. CASELLAS & A. MIMRAN. 1983. Comparative effects of nifedipine and diltiazem on vascular responses to norepinephrine and angiotensin II. Eur. Heart J. **4**(Suppl. G): 21–25.
17. SEINO, M., K. ABE, S. ITO, M. YASUJIMIA, S. CHIBA, M. HIWATARI, K. SATO, T. GOTO, K. OMATA, J. TAJIMA, M. TANNO & K. YOSHINAGO. 1984. Effects of nifedipine on renal vascular responses to vasoactive agents in rabbits. Tohoku J. Exp. Med. **142:** 67–76.
18. BELL, A. J. & A. LINDNER. 1984. Effects of verapamil and nifedipine on renal function and hemodynamics in the dog. Renal Physiol. Basel **7:** 329–343.
19. HUELSEMANN, J. L., R. B. STERZEL, D. E. MCKENZIE & C. S. WILCOX. 1985. Effects of a calcium entry blocker on blood pressure and renal function during angiotensin-induced hypertension. Hypertension **7:** 374–379.
20. IMAGAWA, J. I., M. KUSABA-SUZUKI & S. SATOH. 1986. Preferential inhibitory effect of nifedipine on angiotensin II–induced renal vasoconstriction. Hypertension **8:** 897–903.
21. STEELE, T. H. & L. CHALLONER-HUE. 1984. Renal interactions between norepinephrine and calcium antagonists. Kidney Int **26:** 719–724.
22. STEELE, T. H. & L. CHALLONER-HUE. 1985. Glomerular response to verapamil by isolated spontaneously hypertensive rat kidney. Am. J. Physiol. **248:** F668–F673.
23. LOUTZENHISER, R., C. HORTON & M. EPSTEIN. 1985. Effects of diltiazen and manganese on renal hemodynamics: studies in the isolated perfused rat kidney. Nephron **39:** 382–388.
24. LOUTZENHISER, R., M. EPSTEIN, C. HORTON & P. SONKE. 1985 Reversal by the calcium antagonist nisoldipine on norepinephrine-induced reduction of GFR: evidence for preferential antagonism of preglomerular vasoconstriction. J. Pharmacol Exp. Ther. **232:** 382–387.
25. DIAMOND, J. R., J. Y. CHEUNG & L. S. FANG. 1984. Nifedipine-induced renal dysfunction. Am. J. Med. **77:** 905–909.
26. TER WEE, P. M., J. B. ROSMAN & S. VAN DER GEEST. 1984. Acute renal failure due to diltiazen. Lancet **2:** 1337–1338.
27. BAUER, J. H., C. S. BROOKS & R. N. BURCH. 1982. Renal function and hemodynamic studies in low- and normal-renin essential hypertension. Arch. Intern. Med. **142:** 1317–1323.
28. BAUER, J. H. & P. GADDY. 1985. Effects of enalapril alone, and in combination with hydrochlorothiazide, on renin-angiotensin-aldosterone, renal function, salt and water excretion, and body fluid composition. Am. J. Kidney Dis. **6:** 222–232.
29. REAMS, G. P. & J. H. BAUER. 1986. Long-term effects of enalapril monotherapy and enalapril/hydrochlorothiazide combination therapy on blood pressure, renal function, and body fluid composition. J. Clin. Hypertension **2:** 55–63.
30. HOSTETTER, T. H. & J. L. OLSON, H. G. RENNKE, M. A. VENKATACHALAM & B. M. BRENNER. 1981. Hyperfiltration in remnant nephrons: a potentially adverse response to renal ablation. Am. J. Physiol. **241:** F85–F93.
31. ANDERSON, S., T. W. MEYER, H. G. RENNKE & B. M. BRENNER. 1985. Control of glomerular hypertension limits glomerular injury in rats with reduced renal mass. J. Clin. Invest. **76:** 612–619.
32. ANDERSON, S., H. G. RENNKE & B. M. BRENNER, 1986. Therapeutic advantage of converting enzyme inhibitors in arresting progressive renal disease associated with systemic hypertension in the rat. J. Clin. Invest. **77:** 1993–2000.
33. BAUER, J. H. & G. P. REAMS. 1986. Renal effects of angiotensin converting enzyme inhibitors in hypertension. Am. J. Med **81**(Suppl. 4C): 19–27.
34. GOLIGORSKY. M. S., C. CHAIMOVITZ, J. RAPOPORT, F. GOLDSTEIN & R. KOL. 1985. Calcium metabolism in uremic nephrocalcinosis: preventive effect of verapamil. Kidney Int **27:** 774–779.

35. HARRIS, D. C. H., W. S. HAMMOND, T. J. BURKE & R. W. SCHRIER. 1987. Verapamil protects against progression of experimental chronic renal failure. Kidney Int. **31:** 41–46.

36. MALIS, C. D., J. Y. CHEUNG, A. LEAF & J. V. BONVENTRE. 1983. Effects of verapamil in models of ischemic acute renal failure in the rat. Am. J. Physiol. **245:** F735–F742.

37. BURKE T. J., P. E. ARNOLD, J. A. GORDON, R. E. BULGER, D. C. DOBYAN & R. W. SCHRIER. 1984. Protective effect of intrarenal calcium membrane blockers before or after renal ischemia. J. Clin. Invest. **74:** 1830–1841.

38. SHAPIRO, J. I., C. CHEUNG, A. ITABASHI, L. CHAN & R. W. SCHRIER. 1985. The effect of verapamil on renal function after warm and cold ischemia in the isolated perfused rat kidney. Transplantation **40:** 596–600.

39. GINGRICH, G. A., G. R. BARKER, P. LIU & S. C. STEWART. 1985. Renal preservation following severe ischemia and prophylactic calcium channel blockade. J. Urol. **134:** 408–410.

40. BAKRIS, G. L. & J. C. BURNETT. 1985. A role for calcium in radiocontrast-induced reductions in renal hemodynamics. Kidney Int **27:** 465–468.

41. DUGGAN, K. A., G. J. MACDONALD, J. A. CHARLESWORTH & B. A. PUSSELL. 1985. Verapamil prevents post-transplant oliguric renal failure. Clin. Nephrol. **24:** 289–291.

42. CHEUNG, J. Y., J. V. BONVENTRE, C. D. MALIS & A. LEAF. 1986. Calcium and ischemic injury. N. Engl. J. Med. **314:** 1670–1676.

43. ZANCHETTI, A. & G. LEONETTI. 1985. Natriuretic effect of calcium antagonists. J. Cardiovasc. Pharmacol. **7**(Suppl. 4): S33–S37.

44. ZANCHETTI, A., A. STELLA & R. GOLIN. 1985. Adrenergic sodium handling and the natriuretic action of calcium antagonists. J. Cardiovasc. Pharmacol. **7**(Suppl. 6): S194–S198.

Dihydropyridine Calcium Channel Blocking Agents in Hepatotoxic and Ethanol-Induced Liver Cell Injury

ERWIN J. LANDON, MELANIE SURBER,
AND B. V. RAMA SASTRY

Department of Pharmacology
Vanderbilt University School of Medicine
Nashville, Tennessee 37232

The present study measures cell injury, calcium entry, ATP, and glucose-6-phosphate in the rat liver and protective effects of the dihydropyridine calcium channel blocking compounds nitrendipine and nifedipine when hepatotoxic agents are administered *in vivo.* In preceding studies carbon tetrachloride and thioacetamide 12 hours or more after administration *in vivo* to rats initiated a progressive centrilobular necrosis and a large parallel increase in the calcium content of the liver. Several compounds known to block membrane calcium channels (nifedipine, nitrendipine, verapamil, and chlorpromazine) reduced the calcium entry and the centrilobular necrosis.[1,2] Carbon tetrachloride initiated an immediate progressive rise in membrane fluidity which was maximal at 18 hours.[1] A similar but smaller fluidity change occurred with thioacetamide. In the present study 24 hours after *in vivo* administration of carbon tetrachloride or thioacetamide, ATP and glucose-6-phosphate in the rat liver were decreased. Employing several doses of carbon tetrachloride, the centrilobular necrosis and decrease in glucose-6-phosphate were dose dependent but the decrease in ATP was similar at the several doses of carbon tetrachloride tested (TABLE 1). Treatment of rats with dihydropyridine compounds (nitrendipine or nifedipine) reduced or prevented the fall in glucose-6-phosphate and the liver cell necrosis. Dihydropyridine compounds did not affect ATP levels with carbon tetrachloride and only partially increased ATP with thioacetamide. Within this experimental framework, the levels of glucose-6-phosphate appeared to be related to levels of calcium (FIGURE 1). Dihydropyridine compounds did not prevent the destruction of endoplasmic reticulum calcium pumps by carbon tetrachloride and in an earlier study had only a partial effect on the membrane fluidity change.[1] High levels of chronic ethanol ingestion resulted in biochemical evidence of liver cell injury (increased enzyme levels in the serum) wihtout any change in liver cell calcium. Nifedipine administered chronically had no effect on this ethanol-induced cell injury. Chronic ingestion of ethanol enhanced low dosc carbon tetrachloride toxicity and the dihydropyridine effccts were complex. They protected at the lowest carbon tetrachloride dose and caused significant mortality at a higher dose. Pretreatment of rats with the antithyroid compound 6-propyl-2-thiouracil reduced this mortality. The dihydropyridine compound protection in liver toxicity is both similar to and different from the protection obtained in cardiac ischemia followed by reperfusion. The cardiac ischemia greatly reduces ATP and the subsequent reperfusion leads to uncontrolled calcium entry which is prevented by dihydropyridine compounds. Calcium entry in the heart via voltage-dependent calcium channels is a major pathway of calcium entry specifically inhibited by low levels of dihydropyridine compounds. In liver, calcium influx in the basal state is extensive and metabolic regulation of this entry is critical. Voltage-dependent calcium entry is a lesser component of the total

TABLE 1. The Effect of Carbon Tetrachloride, Thioacetamide, and Dihydropyridine Calcium Channel Blocking Agents on ATP and Glucose-6-phosphate Content of the Rat Liver[a]

	ATP (μmol/g liver)	Glucose-6-phosphate (μmol/g liver)	Necrosis (0 to 4+)
Control (25)	3 ± 0.03	0.8 ± 0.07	0
Nitrendipine 20 mg/kg 24 hours (7)	2.9 ± 0.1	0.9 ± 0.08	0
CCl_4 2 mmol/kg 24 hours (6)	2.1 ± 0.17	0.9 ± 0.1	0.5 ± 0.1
CCl_4 5 mmol/kg 24 hours (10)	2.0 ± 0.05	0.6 ± 0.06	1.25 ± 0.17
CCl_4 13 mmol/kg 24 hours (18)	2.2 ± 0.07	0.4 ± 0.08	2.7 ± 0.17
CCl_4 13 mmol/kg 24 hours + nitrendipine 20 mg/kg −1 hour and 7 hours (8)	2.1 ± 0.12	1 ± 0.1	1 ± 0.17
CCl_4 13 mmol/kg 24 hours + nifedipine 5 mg/kg −1 hour, 7 hours, and 13 hours (17)	2.3 ± 0.08	0.63 ± 0.07	2.1 ± 0.1
Thioacetamide 8.6 mmol/kg 24 hours (6)	1.6 ± 0.05	0.3 ± 0.04	1.8 ± 0.16
Thioacetamide 8.6 mmol/kg 24 hours + nitrendipine 20 mg/kg −1 hour (8)	2 ± 0.06	0.76 ± 0.1	0.15 ± 0.1

[a]Values are means ± standard error; the numbers in parentheses indicate the number of experiments.

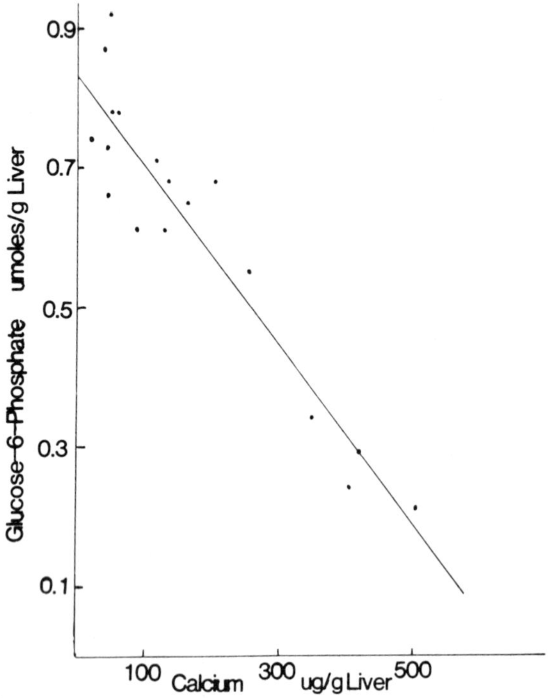

FIGURE 1. The linear regression plot of an experimental group of rat liver glucose-6-phosphate values (y-axis) versus the corresponding values for liver calcium content (x-axis) measured 24 hours after the administration of 5 and 13 mmol/kg carbon tetrachloride. The r value for these 18 points was 0.94.

possible calcium influx. In the present study relatively high levels of dihydropyridine compounds were employed in the liver so that mechanisms conceivably may be different. The dihydropyridine compounds did protect against hepatotoxic liver cell injury, prevented a fall in glucose-6-phosphate, and reduced calcium entry. These events appear to be associated. Coupling of the metabolic regulation of calcium with enzymes of glycolysis in the liver is postulated.

REFERENCES

1. LANDON, E. J., R. K. JAISWAL, R. J. NAUKAM, & B. V. R. SASTRY. 1984. Biochem. Pharmacol. **33:** 3553–3560.
2. LANDON, E. J., R. J. NAUKAM & B. V. R. SASTRY. 1986. Biochem. Pharmacol. **35:** 697–705.

Nitrendipine

An Antidote to the Lethal Toxicity of Cocaine

G. NAHAS,[a] R. TROUVÉ, C. LATOUR, M. SITBON,
AND J.-F. DEMUS

[a]Department of Anesthesiology
College of Physicians & Surgeons
Columbia University
630 West 168th Street
New York, New York 10032
and
INSERM U26
Paris, France

Cocaine, an "indirectly acting sympathomimetic amine," is a potent topical vasoconstrictor which inhibits the reuptake of noradrenaline.[1] Self-administration of cocaine is associated with dysrhythmia and myocardial infarction in healthy young adults and also with stroke and intracranial hemorrhage and with convulsions and death.[2] The selection of a Ca^{2+} modulator as an antidote to cocaine was predicated on its properties of inhibiting the vasoconstrictive effects of norepinephrine which accumulates in body fluid and tissues as a result of cocaine intoxication. Nitrendipine, a dihydropyridine, was selected because of its coronary vasodilator effect in the presence of maintained contractile force of the myocardium. It was already reported that nitrendipine prevents functional and morphological cardiac toxicity due to cocaine intravenous administration.[3]

Ten fasting Sprague Dawley rats weighing 292 ± 31 g are fitted, under ether anesthesia, with a catheter in the caudal artery. The catheter is connected to a constant microinfusion pump and to a recorder for on-line recording of arterial blood pressure which is analyzed and processed by a microcomputer. Heart rate and pulse pressure are displayed every 30 seconds. Five rats are administered 60 mg/kg of cocaine solution intraperitoneally, a lethal dose. Five other animals are given the same amount of cocaine, followed by nitrendipine 4 to 5 minutes after cocaine. Nitredipine is given intraarterially first in a loading dose of 7.4 μg, followed by a constant infusion of 1.22 μg/kg per minute lasting 85 ± 20 minutes. The end point of the perfusion was reached when the rat was active and restless. The 5 control animals had a survival time of 8′06″ ± 5′20″. Death could be attributed to convulsions and respiratory arrest. The 5 animals treated with nitrendipine survived. Total dose of nitrendipine administered was 129 ± 23 μg/kg. The animals were replaced fully conscious in their cage and 24 hours later were active and feeding themselves. Survival of the animals could be attributed not only to the cardioprotective effect of the Ca^{2+} modulator[3] but also to its stabilizing effect on the central nervous system. The animals treated with nitrendipine were quiet and did not convulse. This dihydropyridine might be considered for clinical trials in the treatment of acute toxicity of cocaine in man.

REFERENCES

1. FLECKENSTEIN, A. & J. H. BURN. 1953. Uber Neurosympathomimetica. Ver. Dtsch. Inn. Med. **59:** 17–22.

TABLE 1. Effects of Cocaine Administration (60 mg/kg intraperitoneally) on Blood Pressure and Heart Rate of the Rat[a]

		Minutes after Cocaine Administration							
	Control	2	4[b]	6[c]	8[c]	10[c]	12[a]	14[d]	15[d]
Mean pressure (mmHg)	94 ± 13	100 ± 12	89 ± 9	94 ± 6	100 ± 1	107 ± 10	96 ± 4	97	21[f]
Heart rate (per minute)	418 ± 26	392 ± 46	371 ± 23[a]	365 ± 35[e]	370 ± 40	374 ± 39	443 ± 75	372	242[f]

[a]No animals survived (mean survival time 8′06″ ± 5′20″).
[b]Measurement on 4 surviving animals.
[c]Measurement on 3 surviving animals.
[d]Measurement on 1 surviving animal.
[e]$p < 0.05$.
[f]$p < 0.005$.

TABLE 2. Effects of Nitrendipine Administered Five Minutes following a Lethal Dose of Cocaine (60 mg/kg intraperitoneally) on Blood Pressure and Heart Rate of the Rat[a]

		Minutes after Cocaine Administration						
	Control	4	30	60	90	120	150	180
Mean pressure (mmHg)	102 ± 18	94 ± 8	103 ± 13	105 ± 17	100 ± 9	110 ± 11	112 ± 6	113 ± 26
Heart rate (per minute)	416 ± 26	372 ± 23[b]	392 ± 46	371 ± 23	365 ± 35	370 ± 40	374 ± 39	443 ± 75

↑ Nitrendipine (between 4 and 30 minutes)

[a]All animals survived.
[b]$p < 0.05$.

2. PASTERNAK, P. F., S. B. COLVIN & G. F. BAUMANN. 1985. Cocaine induced angina pectoris and acute myocardial infarction in patients younger than 40 years. Am. J. Cardiol. **55:** 847.
3. NAHAS, G. G., R. TROUVÉ R. & M. MAILLET. 1985. Prevention de la cardiotoxicite de la cocaine par un bloqueur du Ca2+. Bull. Acad. Nat. Med. **169:** 1151–1155.

Index of Contributors